Manual of

Medical-Surgical Nursing Care

Nursing Interventions and Collaborative Management

Manual of
Medical-Surgical Nursing Care

Nursing Interventions and Collaborative Management

Pamela L. Swearingen, RN
Special Project Editor

Dennis G. Ross, RN, PhD, MAE
Professor of Nursing
Castleton State College
Castleton, Vermont;
Nursing Faculty
Regents College
Albany, New York

Fourth Edition

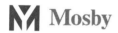 Mosby

St. Louis   Baltimore   Boston   Carlsbad
Chicago   Minneapolis   New York   Philadelphia   Portland
London   Milan   Sydney   Tokyo   Toronto

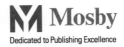
Mosby
Dedicated to Publishing Excellence

A Times Mirror Company

Publisher: Nancy L. Coon
Editor: Barry Bowlus
Developmental Editor: Cindi Anderson
Project Manager: John Rogers
Project Specialist: Betty Hazelwood
Designer: Yael Kats

Fourth Edition
Copyright© 1999 by Mosby, Inc.
Previous editions copyrighted 1986, 1990, 1994

Composition by Graphic World, Inc.
Printing/binding by R.R. Donnelley & Sons Company

Mosby, Inc.
11830 Westline Industrial Drive
St. Louis, Missouri 63146

Library of Congress Cataloging in Publication Data
Manual of medical-surgical nursing care: nursing interventions and
    collaborative management / Pamela L. Swearingen, special
project editor; Dennis G. Ross. — 4th ed.
        p.   cm.
    Includes bibliographical references and index.
    ISBN 0-8151-2744-8
    1. Nursing—Handbooks, manuals, etc.   2. Surgical nursing—
Handbooks, manuals, etc.   3. Nursing diagnosis—Handbooks, manuals,
etc.   I. Swearingen, Pamela L.   II. Ross, Dennis.
    [DNLM: 1. Nursing Assessment handbooks.   2. Nursing Care
handbooks.   WY 49 M2938 1998]
RT51.M365   1998
610.73—dc21
DNLM/DLC
for Library of Congress   98-22562
                                                                CIP

98 99 00 01 02 / 9 8 7 6 5 4 3 2 1

Contributors

Lolita M. Adrien, RN, MS, CETN
Enterostomal Therapy Clinical Nurse Specialist
Ostomy/Enterostomal Therapy Services
John Muir Medical Center
Walnut Creek, California

Linda S. Baas, RN, PhD, CCRN
Assistant Professor
Adult Health Nursing—College of Nursing and Health
University of Cincinnati
Cincinnati, Ohio

Marianne Saunorus Baird, RN, MN, CCRN
Case Manager/Clinical Nurse Specialist
Patient Care Management
St. Joseph's Hospital of Atlanta
Atlanta, Georgia

Bernice N. Beaulac, RN, MS, C
Assistant Professor of Nursing
Department of Nursing
Castleton State College
Castleton, Vermont

Linda Frank, RN, MSN, PhD, ACRN
Assistant Professor, Director, Pennsylvania AIDS Education & Training Center
Department of Infectious Disease, Graduate School of Public Health
University of Pittsburgh
Pittsburgh, Pennsylvania

Pamela Feeney Godwin, RN, MA, CS
Adult Nurse Practitioner
Internal Medicine
Rockville, Maryland

Cheri A. Goll, RN, MSN
Assistant Program Director
Nursing and Patient Care Services
Indiana University Hospital
Indianapolis, Indiana

Patricia Hall, RN, PhD
Clinical Nurse Specialist, Cardiac Services
Department of Patient Services
Promina Kennestone Hospital
Marietta, Georgia

Judith A. Headley, RN, PhD, AOCN
Assistant Professor
School of Nursing
University of Texas-Houston Health Science Center
Houston, Texas

Mima M. Horne, RN, MS, CDE
Diabetes Clinical Nurse Specialist
Coastal Diabetes Center
New Hanover Regional Medical Center
Wilmington, North Carolina

Marguerite McMillan Jackson, RN, PhD, CIC, FAAN
Administrative Director, Nursing Research and Education & Epidemiology Unit
UCSD Medical Center;
Associate Clinical Professor of Family and Preventive Medicine
UCSD School of Medicine
University of California—San Diego
San Diego, California

Patricia Jansen, RN, MSN, CS
Geriatric Clinical Nurse Specialist; Consultant
San Jose, California

Janet Hicks Keen, RN, MS(N), CCRN, CEN
Consultant in Emergency, Trauma, and Critical Care Nursing
Staff Nurse, Level II
St. Joseph's Hospital of Atlanta
Atlanta, Georgia

Cynthia M. Ladabouche, RN, BSN, OCN
Independent Consultant in Oncology Nursing
Rutland, Vermont

Maryann B. McDonough, RN, MS
Assistant Professor of Nursing
Department of Nursing
Castleton State College
Castleton, Vermont

Dennis G. Ross, RN, PhD, MAE
Professor of Nursing
Castleton State College
Castleton, Vermont;
Nursing Faculty
Regents College
Albany, New York

Nancy A. Stotts, RN, MN, EdD
Professor
Department of Physiological Nursing
University of California San Francisco
San Francisco, California

Carol Monlux Swift, RN, BSN
Clinical Nurse III
Critical Care Unit
El Camino Hospital
Mountain View, California

Diane Wind Wardell, RN, PhD, C
Associate Professor
School of Nursing
University of Texas, Houston Health Science Center
Houston, Texas

Karen S. Webber, RN, MN
Assistant Professor
Department of Nursing
Memorial University of Newfoundland
St. John's, Newfoundland
Canada

Consultants

Beverly Carlson, RN, MS, CCRN
Cardiac Research Project Director
Sharp Health Care;
Adjunct Faculty, School of Nursing
San Diego State University;
Adjunct Faculty, School of Nursing
Grossmont College
San Diego, California

Sharon Childs, RN, CRNP, MS, CS, CEN, ONC
Certified Adult Nurse Practitioner, Orthopedic Clinical Specialist
Associate Faculty, College of Notre Dame of Maryland;
Independent Practice Nurse Practitioner
Concertia Medical Center
Baltimore, Maryland

Mary E. Lough, RN, MS, CCRN, CNS
Critical Care Cardiovascular Clinical Nurse Specialist
Sequoia Hospital
Redwood City, California;
Associate Clinical Professor
University of San Francisco at California
San Francisco, California

Sally S. Russell, RN, C
Instructor/Course Coordinator
St. Elizabeth Hospital School of Nursing;
Education Director, Past President
Academy of Medical Surgical Nurses
Lafayette, Indiana

Mary Gritzmaker Schira, RN, PhD
Faculty, Acute Care Nurse Practitioner Program
School of Nursing
University of Texas at Arlington
Arlington, Texas

Kathleen M. Stacy, RN, MS, CCRN
Critical Care Clinical Nurse Specialist
Cardiopulmonary Clinical Outcomes Manager
Tri-City Medical Center
Oceanside, CA

Preface

Manual of Medical-Surgical Nursing Care: Nursing Interventions and Collaborative Management is designed to enable both staff and student nurses to plan and evaluate care of the adult medical-surgical patient. Focusing on NANDA-approved nursing diagnoses that are specific to each disorder, the manual provides a brief review of pathophysiology, physical assessment, diagnostic testing, collaborative management, and patient/family teaching and discharge planning data. The order of presentation of the information in each health alteration provides a hierarchy of data that enables the nurse to make nursing diagnoses and to plan interventions specific to each patient. More generic information can be found in the appendixes, where nursing diagnoses and interventions for preoperative and postoperative patients, patients on prolonged bedrest, patients with cancer and other life-disrupting illnesses, and older adults are discussed.

Staff and student nurses can use this reference to obtain clinical information formerly found only in medical-surgical textbooks or large manuals. It is the first reference of its size to feature the application of nursing diagnoses and interventions to more than 145 health alterations. A consistent, easy-to-use format is incorporated to enhance the quick-reference feature of this book.

This edition was thoroughly revised and updated. The outcome criteria are specific, positive statements that facilitate evaluation of care. Timeframes are incorporated into the outcome criteria, where appropriate, to facilitate nurses in setting more realistic goals for nursing outcomes. Timeframes are provided as guidelines—individual patients having their own unique response times—and to serve as reminders that Medicare and other third-party payors monitor the fine lines between quality, cost-effective care, and premature discharge. This manual advocates use of Standard Precautions as stated by the Centers for Disease Control and Prevention (CDC) to reduce the risk of transmission of infectious diseases to patients and health care workers.

New in this edition are suggested interventions from the Iowa Intervention Project's Nursing Intervention Classification (NIC). (From McCoskey JC, Bulechek GM, editors: *Iowa Intervention Project: Nursing Interventions Classification (NIC),* ed 2, St. Louis, 1996, Mosby.) This taxonomy of nursing interventions forms the beginning of a nursing classification system for interventions used by nurses in a wide variety of settings. This classification system shows promise for becoming the basis of nursing interventions for the Minimum Data Set of Nursing, a national classification system similar to those used by the medical profession, for example, International Classification of Diseases (ICD and ICD-CM) or The Diagnostic and Statistical Manual of Mental Disorders (DSM). NIC is advocated to:
- Standardize nursing nomenclature
- Expand nursing knowledge about the links between nursing diagnoses, treatments, and outcomes
- Aid in the development of nursing and health care information systems
- Facilitate teaching of decision making to nursing students
- Clearly delineate the cost of services provided by nurses
- Identify the impact of nursing care on patient outcomes
- Aid in planning for resource needs in nursing practice settings
- Articulate the unique function of nursing to other health care providers

Suggested NIC alternative interventions are listed for each nursing diagnosis.

A variety of information resources have been added wherever possible to facilitate the staff and student nurse in obtaining additional information and patient teaching services. These sources include internet addresses, when available.

Throughout this text we use the phrase "health care provider" instead of the traditional "physician" or "doctor." This reflects the current trend to use Advanced Practice Nurses and Physician Assistants to aid in providing care in the acute care setting.

In this edition we also encourage the reader to include sensory information when providing any patient teaching. This is consistent with current nursing research by Johnson, which has determined that outcomes of patient education are improved when sensory experiences associated with tasks or procedures are explained to the patient. For example, if a procedure will involve some discomfort, the nurse should describe any discomfort that the patient may encounter. Or, if an MRI is scheduled, the nurse should explain that the patient will be placed in a narrow tube within a large structure and that he or she may sense some claustrophobia, which may be minimized by doing the relaxation and deep-breathing exercises taught by the nurse.

Finally, a word about the health alterations we selected: we chose those that are either commonly seen as primary admission diagnoses or frequently seen as secondary diagnoses in hospitalized patients. To control the number of pages and ensure a portable, handbook-size reference, we did not include discussions of pediatric, critical care, mental health, or other specialized areas.

Manual of Medical-Surgical Nursing Care was designed to help students and staff nurses apply nursing diagnoses in the "real world" of the acute care hospital. Reviewers indicate that it achieves this objective. The ultimate judgment rests with those nurses who read and use the manual on a daily basis. We welcome comments on how we could enhance its usefulness in subsequent editions.

Pamela L. Swearingen
Dennis G. Ross

Acknowledgments

The contributors and the editors want to thank the many individuals whose input was of value in the development of this manuscript. In particular, we wish to acknowledge the third edition contributions of Barbara Tueller Steuble, RN, MS; Ellen L. Hellman, RN, MN, CFNP; Kathryn Schroeder, RN, BSN; Kenneth Miller, RN, MS, PhD; and Mary E. Cooley RN, CRNP, MSN, OCN.

P.L.S. and D.G.R.

Contents

5 Endocrine Disorders
Marianne Saunorus Baird

6 Gastrointestinal Disorders

Appendixes

Manual of
Medical-Surgical Nursing Care

Nursing Interventions and Collaborative Management

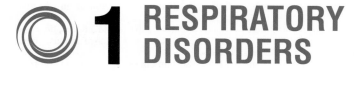

1 RESPIRATORY DISORDERS

Section One: Acute Respiratory Disorders

Acute respiratory disorders are short-term diseases or acute complications of chronic conditions. They can occur once and respond to treatment or recur to further complicate an underlying disease process.

Atelectasis

Atelectasis is a spontaneous collapse of alveolar lung tissue secondary to persistent hypoinflation. It is most commonly seen following major abdominal or thoracic surgery and results from hypoventilation of dependent portions of the lungs or inadequate clearing of secretions. Atelectasis can be an acute or a chronic condition, and it occurs most frequently in individuals with COPD. In the postoperative period atelectasis can be precipitated by the effects of anesthesia, sedation, and decreased mobility. Other precipitating factors include mucus plugs, foreign objects in the airways, pleural effusion, bronchogenic carcinoma, history of smoking, and obesity. Atelectasis can lead to pulmonary infection.

ASSESSMENT

The clinical picture is determined by the site of collapse, rate of development, and size of the affected area.

Signs and symptoms: Pleuritic chest pain, tachypnea, SOB, fever, dyspnea.

Physical assessment: Decreased chest wall movement on affected side, dullness to percussion, decreased or absent breath sounds, crackles (rales) persisting after deep inspiration or cough, restlessness, agitation, change in LOC, cyanosis.

DIAGNOSTIC TESTS

Oximetry: Bedside oximetry may demonstrate decreased O_2 saturation ($\leq$92%).

Chest x-ray: Reveals higher density in affected lung, elevation of the hemidiaphragm on affected side, and compensatory hyperinflation of adjacent lobes on the opposite side.

ABG values: May reveal acute respiratory acidosis, with pH <7.35 and $Paco_2$ >45 mm Hg. Pao_2 may be <80 mm Hg, which is consistent with hypoxemia.

COLLABORATIVE MANAGEMENT

Management is aimed at preventing this condition in all patients. If atelectasis occurs and is left untreated, the affected lung area may eventually become infected, fibrotic, and functionless.

Deep breathing and coughing exercises: To expand alveoli deep in the lungs and mobilize/clear secretions.

Chest physiotherapy: To mobilize secretions.

Hyperinflation therapy: For example, incentive spirometry to expand partially collapsed lung areas, thereby improving gas exchange.

Analgesics: To reduce pain, thereby facilitating production of an effective cough.

Bronchoscopy: Procedure in which patient is intubated and a fiberoptic scope is passed into the bronchi to visualize the area and remove mucus plugs, retained secretions, or foreign objects.

Oxygen therapy: To maintain Pao_2 >80 mm Hg or within patient's normal baseline range.

NURSING DIAGNOSES AND INTERVENTIONS

*For patients at **risk** for atelectasis*

Ineffective breathing pattern related to decreased lung expansion secondary to inactivity or omission of deep breathing

Desired outcomes: Patient demonstrates deep breathing and effective coughing at least hourly and is eupneic (RR 12-20 breaths/min with normal depth and pattern) at all other times, and auscultation of the patient's lungs reveals no adventitious sounds.

- Auscultate breath sounds at least q2-4hr (or as indicated by the patient's condition) and during hyperinflation therapy. Report any decrease in breath sounds or presence of/increase in adventitious breath sounds.
- Instruct patient in the use of hyperinflation device (e.g., an incentive spirometer). Instruct the patient that the emphasis of this therapy is on inhalation to expand the lungs maximally. Ensure that patient inhales slowly and deeply 2× normal tidal volume and holds the breath at least 5 sec at the end of inspiration. Ten breaths per hour is recommended to maintain adequate alveolar inflation. Deep breathing expands the alveoli and aids in mobilizing secretions to the airways, and coughing further mobilizes and clears the secretions. Monitor patient's progress and document in nurses' notes.
- Administer analgesics as prescribed to reduce pain, which may facilitate patient's ease with coughing and deep-breathing exercises.
- When appropriate, instruct the patient in methods of splinting wounds or painful areas to enable cough.
- Instruct patients who are unable to cough effectively in cascade cough, i.e., a succession of more short and forceful exhalations.
- Encourage activity as prescribed to help mobilize secretions and promote effective airway clearance.
- When not contraindicated, instruct patient to increase fluid intake (>2.5 L/day) to decrease viscosity of pulmonary secretions and facilitate their mobilization.
- When appropriate, coordinate deep breathing and coughing exercises with the peak effectiveness of bronchodilator therapy to maximize potential for mobilization of secretions.

You may also wish to refer to the following interventions from the Nursing Interventions Classification (NIC)

NIC: Airway Management; Analgesic Administration; Cough Enhancement; Exercise Promotion; Respiratory Monitoring; Vital Signs Monitoring

PATIENT-FAMILY TEACHING AND DISCHARGE PLANNING

When providing patient-family teaching, focus on sensory information; avoid giving excessive information; and initiate a visiting nurse referral for necessary

follow-up teaching. Consider including verbal and written information about the following:

- Use of hyperinflation device if patient is to continue this therapy at home. Conduct a predischarge check of patient's technique, and document assessment in the progress notes.
- Importance of maintaining activity level as prescribed to promote optimal lung expansion, mobilize secretions, and promote effective airway clearance.
- Importance of maintaining fluid intake (>2.5 L/day) to decrease viscosity of pulmonary secretions.
- Medications, including drug name, purpose, dosage, schedule, precautions, drug/drug and food/drug interactions, and potential side effects.
- Precipitating factors in the development of atelectasis.
- Importance of notifying health care provider if signs and symptoms recur.
- Importance of medical follow-up. Review date and time of next appointment.

Pneumonia

Pneumonia is an acute bacterial or viral infection that causes inflammation of the lung parenchyma (alveolar spaces and interstitial tissue). As a result of the inflammation the involved lung tissue becomes edematous and the air spaces fill with exudate (consolidation), gas exchange cannot occur, and nonoxygenated blood is shunted into the vascular system, causing hypoxemia. Bacterial pneumonias involve all or part of a lobe, whereas viral pneumonias appear diffusely throughout the lungs.

Pneumonias generally are classified into two groups: community acquired and hospital associated (nosocomial). A third type is pneumonia in the immunocompromised individual.

Community acquired: Individuals with community-acquired pneumonia generally do not require hospitalization unless an underlying medical condition, such as COPD, cardiac disease, or diabetes mellitus or an immunocompromised state, complicates the illness.

Hospital associated (nosocomial): Nosocomial pneumonias usually occur following aspiration of oropharyngeal flora in an individual whose resistance is altered or whose coughing mechanisms are impaired (e.g., a patient who has decreased LOC, dysphagia, diminished gag reflex, or a nasogastric tube or who has undergone thoracoabdominal surgery). Bacteria invade the lower respiratory tract via three routes: aspiration of oropharyngeal organisms (most common route), inhalation of aerosols that contain bacteria, or hematogenous spread to the lung from another site of infection (rare). Gram-negative pneumonias have a high mortality, even with appropriate antibiotic therapy. *Aspiration pneumonia* is a nonbacterial cause of hospital-associated pneumonia that occurs when gastric contents are aspirated. If the alveolar-capillary membrane is affected, adult respiratory distress syndrome (ARDS) may be seen.

Pneumonia in the immunocompromised individual: Immunosuppression and neutropenia are predisposing factors in the development of nosocomial pneumonias, from both common and unusual pathogens. Severely immunocompromised patients are affected not only by bacteria but also by fungi *(Candida, Aspergillus),* viruses (cytomegalovirus), and protozoa *(Pneumocystis carinii).* Most commonly, *P. carinii* is seen in persons with HIV disease or in persons who are immunosuppressed therapeutically following organ transplants.

ASSESSMENT

Findings are influenced by the patient's age, extent of the disease process, underlying medical condition, and pathogen involved. Generally, any factor that alters the integrity of the lower airways, thereby inhibiting ciliary activity, increases the likelihood of developing pneumonia (Table 1-1).

TABLE 1-1   Assessment Guidelines by Pneumonia Type

Type/pathogen	Risk groups	Onset	Defining characteristics	Complications/comments
Community-acquired				
Pneumococcal (*Pneumococcus pneumoniae, Streptococcus pneumoniae*)	Persons >40 yr, especially males; risk increased with alcoholism and debilitating diseases (e.g., COPD, heart failure, multiple myeloma, sickle cell disease); often preceded by viral URIs	Abrupt	Single shaking chill, fever, pleuritic chest pain, severe cough, SOB, rust-colored sputum, diaphoresis. Many patients also have herpes labialis, abdominal pain and distention, and paralytic ileus	Pleural effusions, empyema, impaired liver function, bacteremia, meningitis. Incidence of pneumococcal pneumonia peaks in winter and early spring. Mortality increases if more than one lobe is involved
Mycoplasma (*Mycoplasma pneumoniae*)	School-aged children to young adult (5-30 yr); intrafamilial spread common	Gradual	Cough, sore throat, fever, headache, chills, malaise, anorexia, nausea, vomiting, diarrhea. In children arthralgias involving large joints are common	Rare. Persistent cough and sinusitis possible. Pulse-temperature dissociation is common
Legionnaires' (*Legionella pneumophila*)	Middle-aged, elderly (males at increased risk) populations; smokers; individuals with malignancy, immunosuppression, or chronic renal failure; exposure to contaminated construction site	Abrupt	Malaise, headache within 24 hr, fever with normal HR, shaking chills, progressive dyspnea, cough that may become productive; GI symptoms, including anorexia, vomiting, diarrhea; arthralgias, myalgias	Respiratory failure, hypotension, shock, acute renal failure

Organism	Population	Onset	Symptoms	Comments
Viral influenza A	Elderly persons with chronic diseases (e.g., COPD, diabetes mellitus, heart failure); pregnancy	1 wk after onset of influenza symptoms	Severe dyspnea, cyanosis, scant sputum occasionally with blood, fever, persistent and dry cough	Rapid course leading frequently to acute respiratory failure; secondary bacterial pneumonia
Haemophilus influenzae	Adults (especially ≥50 yr of age) with chronic diseases (e.g., diabetes mellitus, COPD, chronic alcohol ingestion)	2–6 wk after URI	Fever, chills, dyspnea, cough, nausea, vomiting, pain	Fever may be minimal or absent; HR and RR may be normal
Nosocomial				
Klebsiella (*Klebsiella pneumoniae*); also may be acquired in the community	Males >40 yr, alcoholics; patients with diabetes mellitus, COPD, or heart disease; those previously treated with antibiotics or ET intubation	Abrupt	Chills, fever, productive cough (copious purulent green or "currant jelly" sputum), severe pleuritic chest pain, dyspnea, cyanosis, jaundice, vomiting, diarrhea	Lung abscess and empyema, necrotizing pneumonitis with cavitation, acute respiratory failure. High mortality (~50%). Aspiration of oropharyngeal flora is responsible for nosocomial and community-acquired cases
Pseudomonas; also may be acquired in the community	Patients neutropenic from chemotherapy or immunosuppressed secondary to cortisone therapy or other illnesses	Gradual	Fever, chills, confusion, delirium, bradycardia, purulent sputum (green, foul smelling)	Rarely occurs in previously healthy adults; high mortality

COPD, Chronic obstructive pulmonary disease; *URI,* upper respiratory infection; *SOB,* shortness of breath; *HR,* heart rate; *GI,* gastrointestinal; *RR,* respiratory rate; *ET,* endotracheal.

Continued

TABLE 1-1   Assessment Guidelines by Pneumonia Type—cont'd

Type/pathogen	Risk groups	Onset	Defining characteristics	Complications/comments
Nosocomial—cont'd				
Proteus	Older adults with debilitating underlying diseases	Abrupt	High fever, chills, pleuritic chest pain	Rare. Localizes to areas that are already damaged. Occurs as a mixed infection; has four pathogenic species with differing antibiotic susceptibilities
Staphylococcus aureus	Patients with debilitating diseases (e.g., diabetes mellitus, renal failure, liver disease, COPD); those with a prior viral or influenza infection; injecting drug users	Abrupt with community acquired; insidious with hospital associated	Cough, chills, high fever, pleuritic pain, progressive dyspnea, cyanosis, bloody sputum	Pulmonary abscesses, empyema, pleural effusions; slow response to antibiotics
Aspiration of gastric contents	Patients with impaired gag/cough reflexes; general anesthesia; presence of NG/ET tube	Gradual; latent period between aspiration and onset of symptoms	Fever, wheezes, crackles (rales), rhonchi, dyspnea, cyanosis	Physiologic response depends on pH of material aspirated; ≥2.5, little necrosis occurs; <2.5, atelectasis, pulmonary edema, hemorrhage, and necrosis can occur

NOTE: *Enterobacter* and *Serratia* are enteric organisms that cause pneumonia with the same clinical pattern as *Klebsiella* organisms.

Immunocompromised patient			
Pneumocystis (*Pneumocystis carinii*)	Patients with AIDS or organ transplants	Insidious	Several weeks of fever, nonproductive cough, night sweats, dyspnea; hypoxemia with few auscultatory signs	Bronchoscopy with transbronchial biopsy usually required for diagnosis
Aspergillosis (*Aspergillus*)	Patients with AIDS, COPD, and transplants (especially autologous bone marrow transplant); also those receiving cytotoxic agents or steroids	Abrupt with immunosuppression; insidious with COPD	High fever; fungal ball within lung cyst or cavity; nonproductive cough; pleuritic chest pain	Cavitation frequently occurs; hematogenous spread common in immunocompromised patient

COPD, Chronic obstructive pulmonary disease; *NG*, nasogastric; *ET*, endotracheal; *AIDS*, acquired immunodeficiency syndrome.

General signs and symptoms: Cough (productive and nonproductive); increased sputum (rust colored, discolored, purulent, bloody, or mucoid) production; fever; pleuritic chest pain (more common in community-acquired bacterial pneumonias); dyspnea; chills; headache; myalgia. Older adults may be confused or disoriented and run low-grade fevers but may present with few other signs and symptoms.

General physical assessment findings: Restlessness; anxiety; older adults may exhibit mental status changes, decreased skin turgor, and dry mucous membranes secondary to dehydration; presence of nasal flaring and expiratory grunt; use of accessory muscles of respiration (scalene, sternocleidomastoid, external intercostals); decreased chest expansion caused by pleuritic pain; dullness on percussion over affected (consolidated) areas; tachypnea (RR >20 breaths/min); tachycardia (HR >100 bpm); increased vocal fremitus; egophony ("e" to "a" change) over area of consolidation; decreased breath sounds; high-pitched and inspiratory crackles (rales) (increased by or heard only after coughing); low-pitched inspiratory crackles (rales) caused by airway secretions; and circumoral cyanosis (a late finding). **Note:** Findings may be normal, even with an abnormal chest x-ray.

DIAGNOSTIC TESTS

Chest x-ray: Confirms the presence of pneumonia (i.e., vague haziness to consolidation in the affected lung fields).

Sputum for Gram stain and culture and sensitivity tests: Sputum is obtained from the lower respiratory tract before initiation of antibiotic therapy in order to identify the causative organism. It can be obtained via expectoration, suctioning, transtracheal aspiration, bronchoscopy, or open-lung biopsy.

WBC count: Will be increased (>11,000/mm^3) in the presence of bacterial pneumonias. Normal or low WBC count may be seen with viral or mycoplasma pneumonias.

Blood culture and sensitivity: To determine presence of bacteremia and aid in the identification of the causative organism.

Oximetry: May reveal decreased O_2 saturation (≤92%).

ABG values: May vary, depending on the presence of underlying pulmonary or other debilitating disease. May demonstrate hypoxemia (Pao_2 <80 mm Hg) and hypocarbia ($Paco_2$ <35 mm Hg), with a resultant respiratory alkalosis (pH >7.45), in the absence of an underlying pulmonary disease.

Serologic studies: Acute and convalescent antibody titers are drawn to diagnose viral pneumonia. A relative rise in antibody titers suggests a viral infection.

Acid-fast stains and cultures: To rule out tuberculosis.

COLLABORATIVE MANAGEMENT

Oxygen therapy: Administered when oximetry or ABG results demonstrate hypoxemia. Special consideration must be given to patients with chronic CO_2 retention. (Normally, the respiratory drive is stimulated by increasing $Paco_2$ levels. In patients with CO_2 retention the respiratory drive is paradoxically stimulated by decreasing Pao_2 levels. Therefore, in the presence of high concentrations of oxygen, the respiratory drive actually may be depressed in these patients.) Initially, oxygen is delivered in low concentrations, and oximetry or ABG levels are watched closely. If O_2 saturation or Pao_2 does not rise to acceptable levels (≥92% or ≥60 mm Hg, respectively), FIo_2 is increased in small increments, with concomitant checks of ABG values.

Antibiotic agents: Prescribed empirically based on presenting signs and symptoms, clinical findings, and chest x-ray results until sputum or blood culture results are available. Erythromycin is the most commonly used antibiotic in community-acquired pneumonia. Many organisms responsible for nosocomial pneumonias are resistant to multiple antibiotics. Proper identification of the organism and determination of sensitivity to specific antibiotics are critical for appropriate therapy.

Hydration: IV fluids may be necessary to replace fluids lost from insensible sources (e.g., tachypnea, diaphoresis, fevers) and decreased oral intake.

Percussion and postural drainage: Indicated if deep breathing and coughing are ineffective in mobilizing secretions.

Hyperinflation therapy: Prescribed for patients with inadequate inspiratory effort.

Antitussives: Given in the absence of sputum production if coughing is continuous and exhausting to the patient.

Antipyretics and analgesics: Prescribed to reduce fever and provide relief from pleuritic pain or pain from coughing.

Standard precautions: See discussion in Appendix Two, p. 817.

NURSING DIAGNOSES AND INTERVENTIONS

For patients with pneumonia

Impaired gas exchange related to altered oxygen supply and alveolar-capillary membrane changes secondary to inflammatory process in the lungs

Desired outcomes: Following intervention/treatment, patient has adequate gas exchange as evidenced by RR of 12-20 breaths/min with normal depth and pattern; absence of signs and symptoms of respiratory distress; and lung sounds clear to auscultation. At least 24 hr before hospital discharge, patient's O_2 saturation is >92% or ABGs reveal Pao_2 is $\geq$80 mm Hg, $Paco_2$ is 35-45 mm Hg, and pH is 7.35-7.45 (or values consistent with patient's baseline).

- Observe for signs and symptoms of respiratory distress (e.g., restlessness, anxiety, mental status changes, SOB, tachypnea, use of accessory muscles of respiration). Remember that cyanosis of the lips and nail beds may be a late indicator of hypoxia.
- Monitor and document VS q2-4hr. Be alert to a rising temperature and other changes in VS that may indicate infection (e.g., increased HR, increased RR).
- Auscultate breath sounds at least q2-4hr or as indicated by the patient's condition. Monitor for decreased or adventitious sounds (e.g., crackles, wheezes).
- Monitor oximetry readings; report O_2 saturation $\leq$92% because this can indicate a need for O_2 therapy.
- Monitor ABG results. A decreasing Pao_2 often indicates the need for oxygen therapy.
- Position patient for comfort (usually semi-Fowler's position) to promote diaphragmatic descent, maximize inhalation, and decrease WOB. In patients with unilateral pneumonia, positioning on the unaffected side (i.e., "good side down") will promote ventilation-perfusion matching.
- Deliver oxygen with humidity as prescribed; monitor oximetry or Flo_2 to ensure that oxygen is within prescribed concentrations. Be aware that patients with COPD may not tolerate oxygen at a delivery >2 L/min, which can suppress the centrally mediated respiratory drive.
- Facilitate coordination across health care providers to provide rest periods between care activities to decrease oxygen demand. Allow 90 min for undisturbed rest.

NIC: Acid-Base Management: Respiratory Acidosis; Airway Management; Bedside Laboratory Testing; Cough Enhancement; Energy Management; Laboratory Data Interpretation; Oxygen Therapy; Respiratory Monitoring

Ineffective airway clearance related to presence of tracheobronchial secretions secondary to infection or related to pain and fatigue secondary to lung consolidation

Desired outcomes: Patient demonstrates effective cough. Following intervention, patient's airway is free of adventitious breath sounds.

- Maintain a patent airway, and ensure that secretions are removed at least q2hr. Suction as indicated/prescribed.
- Auscultate breath sounds q2-4hr (or as indicated by the patient's condition), and report changes in the patient's ability to clear pulmonary secretions.
- Inspect sputum for quantity, odor, color, and consistency; document findings. As patient's condition worsens, the sputum can change in color from clear→white→yellow→green, or it may show other discoloration characteristic of underlying bacterial infection (e.g., rust colored; "currant jelly").
- Ensure that patient performs deep breathing with coughing exercises at least q2hr. Assist patient into position of comfort, usually semi-Fowler's position, to facilitate effectiveness and ease of these exercises.
- Assess need for hyperinflation therapy (i.e., patient's inability to take deep breaths). Report complications of hyperinflation therapy to health care provider, including hyperventilation, gastric distention, headache, hypotension, and signs and symptoms of pneumothorax (SOB, sharp chest pain, unilateral diminished breath sounds, dyspnea, cough).
- Teach patient to splint chest with pillow, folded blanket, or crossed arms when coughing to reduce pain.
- Ensure that patient gets prescribed chest physiotherapy. Document patient's response to treatment.
- Assist patient with position changes q2hr to help mobilize secretions. If the patient is ambulatory, encourage ambulation to patient's tolerance.
- Suction as prescribed and indicated.
- When not otherwise indicated, encourage fluid intake (≥2.5 L/day) to decrease viscosity of the sputum.

For other interventions, see "Atelectasis" for **Ineffective breathing pattern,** p. 2.

NIC: Airway Management; Airway Suctioning; Chest Physiotherapy; Cough Enhancement; Oxygen Therapy; Positioning; Respiratory Monitoring

Fluid volume deficit related to increased insensible loss secondary to tachypnea, fever, or diaphoresis
Desired outcome: At least 24 hr before hospital discharge, patient is normovolemic as evidenced by urine output ≥30 ml/hr with specific gravity 1.010-1.030, stable weight, HR and BP within patient's normal limits, CVP >2 mm Hg (5 cm H_2O), fluid intake approximating fluid output, moist mucous membranes, and normal skin turgor.
- Monitor I&O. Consider insensible losses if patient is diaphoretic and tachypneic. Be alert to urinary output <30 ml/hr; report urinary output <30 ml/hr for 2 hr or urinary specific gravity >1.030.
- Weigh patient daily at the same time of day and on the same scale; record weight. Report weight decreases of 1-1.5 kg/day.
- Encourage fluid intake (at least 2.5 L/day in the unrestricted patient) to ensure adequate hydration.
- Maintain IV fluid therapy as prescribed.
- Promote oral hygiene, including lip and tongue care to moisten dried tissues and mucous membranes.
- Provide humidity for oxygen therapy to decrease convective losses of moisture.

NIC: Fluid/Electrolyte Management; Fluid Monitoring; Intravenous Insertion; Intravenous Therapy; Venous Access Device (VAD) Management

*For patients at **risk** for developing pneumonia*
Risk for infection (nosocomial pneumonia) with risk factors from inadequate primary defenses (e.g., decreased ciliary action), invasive procedures (e.g., intubation), and/or chronic disease

Desired outcome: Patient is free of infection as evidenced by normothermia, WBC count ≤11,000/mm^3, and sputum clear to whitish in color.

- Perform good hand-washing technique before and after contact with patient (even though gloves were worn).
- Identify presurgical candidate who is at increased risk for nosocomial pneumonia because of the following: older adult (>70 yr), obesity, COPD, other chronic pulmonary conditions (e.g., asthma), history of smoking, abnormal pulmonary function tests (especially decreased forced expiratory flow rate), intubation, and upper abdominal/thoracic surgery.
- Provide preoperative teaching, explaining and demonstrating the following pulmonary activities that will be used postoperatively to prevent respiratory infection: deep breathing, coughing, turning in bed, splinting wounds, ambulation, maintaining adequate oral fluid intake, and use of hyperinflation device. Make sure that patient verbalizes knowledge of the exercises and their rationale and returns the demonstrations appropriately.
- Encourage individuals who smoke to discontinue smoking, especially during preoperative and postoperative periods. Refer to a community-based smoking cessation program as needed. When appropriate, discuss the possibility of the health care provider's prescription of transdermal nicotine patches to facilitate smoking cessation.
- Control pain, which interferes with lung expansion, by administering analgesics ½ hr before deep-breathing exercises. Support (splint) surgical wound with hands, pillows, or folded blanket placed firmly across site of incision.
- Identify patients who are at increased risk for aspiration: individuals with a depressed LOC, dysphagia, or an NG or enteral tube in place. Maintain HOB at 30-degree elevation, and turn patient onto side rather than back. When patient receives enteral alimentation, recommend continuous rather than bolus feedings.
- Recognize risk factors for patients with tracheostomy: presence of underlying lung disease or other serious illness, increased colonization of oropharynx or trachea by aerobic gram-negative bacteria, greater access of bacteria to lower respiratory tract, and cross-contamination caused by manipulation of tracheostomy tube.
- Use "no-touch" technique or wear sterile gloves on both hands until tracheostomy wound has healed or formed granulation tissue around the tube.
- Suction prn rather than on a routine basis, because frequent suctioning increases risk of trauma and cross-contamination.
- Use sterile catheter for each suctioning procedure and sterile solutions if secretions are tenacious and catheter flushing is necessary. Consider use of closed suction system to further minimize the risk of contamination; replace closed suction system q8hr or per agency policy.
- Always wear gloves on both hands to suction.
- Recognize the following ways in which nebulizer reservoirs can contaminate patient: introduction of nonsterile fluids or air, manipulation of nebulizer cup, or back flow of condensate from delivery tubing into reservoir or into patient when tubing is manipulated.
- Use only sterile fluids, and dispense them using sterile technique.
- Replace (rather than replenish) solutions and equipment at frequent intervals. For example, empty reservoir completely and refill with sterile solution q8-24hr, according to agency protocol.
- Change breathing circuits q48hr or according to agency policy; if used for multiple patients, replace breathing circuit with sterilized or disinfected breathing circuit between patients.
- Fill fluid reservoirs immediately before use (not far in advance).
- Discard any fluid that has condensed in tubing; do not allow it to drain back into reservoir or into patient.

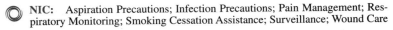

NIC: Aspiration Precautions; Infection Precautions; Pain Management; Respiratory Monitoring; Smoking Cessation Assistance; Surveillance; Wound Care

PATIENT-FAMILY TEACHING AND DISCHARGE PLANNING

When providing patient-family teaching, focus on sensory information; avoid giving excessive information; and initiate a visiting nurse referral for necessary follow-up teaching. Consider including verbal and written information about the following:

- Techniques that promote gas exchange and minimize stasis of secretions (e.g., deep breathing, coughing, use of hyperinflation device, increasing activity level as appropriate for patient's medical condition, percussion and postural drainage as necessary).
- Medications, including drug name, purpose, dosage, frequency or schedule, precautions, drug/drug and food/drug interactions, and potential side effects, particularly of antibiotics (see p. 581).
- Signs and symptoms of pneumonia and the importance of reporting them promptly to health professional should they recur. Teach patient's significant others that changes in mental status may be the only indicator of pneumonia if patient is elderly.
- Importance of preventing fatigue by pacing activities and allowing frequent rest periods.
- Importance of avoiding exposure to individuals known to have flu and colds. Recommend that patient receive a pneumococcal vaccination and annual influenza vaccination.
- Minimizing factors that can cause reinfection, including close living conditions, poor nutrition, and poorly ventilated living quarters or work environment.
- Phone numbers to call should questions or concerns arise about therapy or disease after discharge. Additional general information can be obtained by contacting:

  American Lung Association
  1740 Broadway
  New York, NY 10019-4374   (212) 315-8700
  WWW address: *http://www.lungusa.org*

- Information about the following free brochures that outline ways to help patients stop smoking:

  How to Help Your Patients Stop Using Tobacco: A National Cancer Institute Manual for the Oral Health Team, from the Smoking and Tobacco Control Program of the National Cancer Institute; call 1-800-4-CANCER.

  Clinical Practice Guideline: A Quick Reference Guide for Smoking Cessation Specialists, from the Agency for Health Care Policy and Research (AHCPR); call 1-800-358-9295.

Pleural effusion

A pleural effusion is an accumulation of fluid (blood, pus, chyle, serous fluid) in the pleural space. Generally, fluid gravitates to the most dependent area of the thorax, and the adjacent lung becomes compressed. Pleural effusion is rarely a disease in itself, but rather it is caused by a number of inflammatory, circulatory, or neoplastic diseases. *Transudate effusion* results from changes in hydrodynamic forces in the circulation and usually is caused by heart failure (increased hydrostatic pressure) or cirrhosis (decreased colloidal osmotic pressure). *Exudate effusion* results from irritation of the pleural membranes secondary to inflammatory, infective, or malignant processes. More exact nomenclature can be used once the nature of the fluid in the pleural effusion has been identified, that is, hydrothorax (a transudate or exudate of serous fluid), pyothorax or empyema (a collection of purulent material), hemothorax (bloody fluid), or chylothorax (effused chyle).

ASSESSMENT

Clinical indicators of pleural effusion are related to the underlying disease. With a small effusion (<300 ml) the patient may be asymptomatic. Dyspnea is present when there is a large effusion. Effusion >1000 ml may be associated with a contralateral mediastinal shift.

Signs and symptoms: Pleuritic chest or shoulder pain, diaphoresis, cough, fever.

Physical assessment: Decreased breath sounds, dullness to percussion, decreased tactile fremitus, egophony ("e" to "a" change) over the effusion site, tracheal deviation away from affected side, pleural friction rub.

DIAGNOSTIC TESTS

Chest x-ray: Will show evidence of effusion if >300 ml of fluid in the pleural space. The costophrenic angle will be obliterated, and opacification of the hemithorax, as evidenced by shadiness on the x-ray, increases as the effusion increases. With a large effusion the x-ray may show a mediastinal shift away from the affected lung.

Thoracentesis: Removal of fluid from the pleural space for examination to provide the definitive diagnosis and determine type of effusion.

Pleural biopsy: Aids in diagnosing cause of effusion. Tissue is removed (via biopsy needle or pleuroscopy) and sent to pathologist for examination.

COLLABORATIVE MANAGEMENT

Therapeutic thoracentesis: Removal of fluid, thereby allowing the lung to reexpand. The rate of recurrence and time span for return of symptoms are recorded.

Chest tube insertion: To provide continuous drainage of larger effusions through a 26-30 Fr catheter that is connected to a closed chest-drainage system.

Sclerosing pleurodesis: Instillation of sclerosing agent (tetracycline, bleomycin, or nitrogen mustard) via the chest tube to produce pleural fibrosis and symphysis (a line of fusion below the pleura and chest wall).

NURSING DIAGNOSES AND INTERVENTIONS

Ineffective breathing pattern related to decreased lung expansion secondary to fluid accumulation in the pleural space

Desired outcome: Following intervention, patient's breathing pattern moves toward eupnea.

- Auscultate breath sounds q2-4hr (or as indicated by the patient's condition), monitoring for decreasing breath sounds or the presence of a pleural friction rub.
- Monitor oximetry readings; report O_2 saturation $\leq 92\%$ because this can indicate a need for O_2 therapy.
- Ensure patency of chest drainage system (see guidelines, p. 24, in "Pneumothorax/Hemothorax")
- Position patient for maximum chest expansion, generally semi-Fowler's position.
- If hyperinflation therapy is prescribed, instruct patient in its use. Reinforce teaching, and document patient's progress.
- For patients with gross pleural effusion, provide the following instructions for apical expansion breathing exercises:
  —Sit upright.
  —Position fingers just below the clavicles.

—Inhale and attempt to push upper chest wall against the pressure of the fingers.

—Hold breath for a few seconds, and then exhale passively.

When performed at frequent intervals, this exercise will help expand the involved lung tissues, minimize flattening of the upper chest, and mobilize secretions.

NIC: Airway Management; Cough Enhancement; Pain Management; Positioning; Respiratory Management; Tube Care: Chest

---

See Also: "Pneumonia" for **Impaired gas exchange,** p. 9; "Atelectasis" for **Ineffective breathing pattern,** p. 2; "Pneumothorax/Hemothorax" for **Pain,** p. 25.

PATIENT-FAMILY TEACHING AND DISCHARGE PLANNING

When providing patient-family teaching, focus on sensory information; avoid giving excessive information; and initiate a visiting nurse referral for necessary follow-up teaching. Consider including verbal and written information about the following:

- Importance of smoking cessation. Provide patient with resources related to community smoking cessation programs. When appropriate, discuss the possibility of the health care provider's prescription of transdermal nicotine patches to facilitate smoking cessation.
- Signs of respiratory distress, such as restlessness, mental status changes, agitation, changes in behavior, and complaints of SOB or dyspnea, and the importance of rapidly notifying health care provider if these signs occur.
- Use of equipment at home (e.g., hyperinflation device, nebulizer, oxygen).
- Medications, including drug name, dosage, purpose, schedule, precautions, drug/drug and food/drug interactions, and potential side effects.

Pulmonary embolus

The most common pulmonary perfusion abnormality is a pulmonary embolus (PE); it is caused by the passage of a foreign substance (blood clot, fat, air, or amniotic fluid) into the pulmonary artery or its branches, with resulting obstruction of the blood supply to lung tissue and subsequent collapse. The most common source is a dislodged blood clot from the systemic circulation, typically the deep veins of the legs or pelvis. Thrombus formation is the result of the following factors: blood stasis, alterations in clotting factors, and injury to vessel walls. A fat embolus is the most common nonthrombotic cause of pulmonary perfusion disorders. It is the result of the release of free fatty acids, causing a toxic vasculitis, followed by thrombosis and obstruction of small pulmonary arteries by fat.

Total obstruction leading to pulmonary infarction is rare because the pulmonary circulation has multiple sources of blood supply. Early diagnosis and appropriate treatment reduce mortality to less than 10%. Although most pulmonary emboli resolve completely and leave no residual deficits, some patients may be left with chronic pulmonary hypertension.

ASSESSMENT

Signs and symptoms often are nonspecific and variable, depending on the extent of the obstruction and whether the patient has infarction as a result of the obstruction.

Pulmonary embolus: Sudden onset of dyspnea and sharp chest pain, restlessness, anxiety, nonproductive cough or hemoptysis, palpitations, nausea, and syncope. With a large embolism, oppressive substernal chest discomfort will be present.

Pulmonary infarction: Fever, pleuritic chest pain, and hemoptysis.

Physical assessment: Tachypnea, tachycardia, hypotension, crackles (rales), decreased chest wall excursion secondary to splinting, S_3 and S_4 gallop rhythms, transient pleural friction rub, jugular venous distention, diaphoresis, edema, and cyanosis. Temperature may be elevated if infarction has occurred.

History and risk factors

Prolonged immobility: Especially significant when it coexists with surgical or nonsurgical trauma, carcinoma, or cardiopulmonary disease. Risk increases as duration of immobility increases.

Cardiac disorders: Atrial fibrillation, heart failure, myocardial infarction, rheumatic heart disease.

Surgical intervention: Risk increases in postoperative period, especially for patients with pelvic, thoracic, and abdominal surgery and for those with extensive burns or musculoskeletal injuries of the hip or knee.

Pregnancy: Especially during the postpartum period.

Chronic pulmonary disease

Trauma: Especially fractures of the lower extremities and burns. The degree of risk is related to the severity, site, and extent of trauma.

Carcinoma: Particularly neoplasms involving the breast, lung, pancreas, and genitourinary and alimentary tracts.

Obesity: A 20% increase in ideal body weight is associated with an increased incidence of PE.

Varicose veins or prior thromboembolic disease

Age: Risk of thromboembolism is greatest for patients between 55 and 65 years of age.

Specific findings for fat embolus: Typically, patient is asymptomatic for 12-24 hr following embolization; this period ends with sudden cardiopulmonary and neurologic deterioration: apprehension, restlessness, mental status changes, confusion, delirium, coma, and dyspnea.

Physical assessment for fat embolus: Tachypnea, tachycardia, and hypertension; fever; petechiae, especially of the conjunctivae, neck, upper torso, axillae, and proximal arms; inspiratory crowing; pulmonary edema; profuse tracheobronchial secretions; fat globules in the sputum; and expiratory wheezes.

History and risk factors for fat embolus

Multiple long bone fractures: Especially fractures of the femur and pelvis.

Trauma to adipose tissue or liver

Burns

Osteomyelitis

Sickle cell crisis

DIAGNOSTIC TESTS

General findings for pulmonary emboli

ABG values: Hypoxemia (Pao_2 <80 mm Hg), hypocarbia ($Paco_2$ <35 mm Hg), and respiratory alkalosis (pH >7.45) usually are present. A normal Pao_2 does not rule out the presence of pulmonary emboli.

Chest x-ray: Initially, the chest x-ray is normal or an elevated hemidiaphragm may be present. After 24 hr, x-ray examination may reveal small infiltrates secondary to atelectasis that result from the decrease in surfactant. If pulmonary infarction is present, infiltrates and pleural effusions may be seen within 12-36 hr.

ECG: If PEs are extensive, signs of acute pulmonary hypertension may be present: right-shift QRS axes, tall and peaked P waves, ST-segment changes, and T-wave inversion in leads V_1-V_4.

Pulmonary ventilation-perfusion scan: Used to detect abnormalities of ventilation or perfusion in the pulmonary system. Radiopaque agents are inhaled and injected peripherally. Images of both agents' distribution through-out the lung are scanned. If the scan shows a mismatch of ventilation and perfusion (i.e., a pattern of normal ventilation with decreased perfusion), vascular obstruction is suggested.

Pulmonary angiography: The definitive study for PE. It is an invasive procedure that involves right heart catheterization and injection of dye into the pulmonary artery (PA) to visualize pulmonary vessels. An abrupt vessel "cutoff" may be seen at the site of embolization. Usually, filling defects are seen. More specific findings are abnormal blood vessel diameters (i.e., obstruction of right PA would cause dilation of left PA) and shapes (i.e., the affected blood vessel may taper to a sharp point and disappear).

Findings specific for fat emboli

ABG values: Should be drawn on patients at risk for fat embolus for the first 48 hr following injury because early hypoxemia indicative of fat embolus is apparent only with laboratory assessment. Hypoxemia (Pao_2 <80 mm Hg) and hypercarbia ($Paco_2$ >45 mm Hg) will be present with a respiratory acidosis (pH <7.35).

Chest x-ray: A pattern similar to adult respiratory distress syndrome (ARDS) is seen: diffuse, extensive bilateral interstitial and alveolar infiltrates.

CBC: May reveal decreased hemoglobin (Hgb) and hematocrit (Hct) secondary to hemorrhage into the lung. In addition, thrombocytopenia ($\leq$150,000/mm^3) is indicative of fat embolism.

Serum lipase: Will rise with fat embolism.

Urinalysis: May reveal fat globules following fat embolus.

COLLABORATIVE MANAGEMENT

The three goals of therapy are as follows: (1) prophylaxis for individuals at risk for development of PE; (2) treatment during the acute embolic event; and (3) prevention of future embolic events in the individual who has experi-enced a PE.

General management of pulmonary emboli

Oxygen therapy: Delivered at appropriate concentration to maintain a Pao_2 of >60 mm Hg.

IV heparin therapy: Treatment of choice; it is started immediately in patients without bleeding or clotting disorders and in whom PEs are strongly suspected.

Initial dose: IV bolus of 5,000-10,000 U.

Maintenance dose: From 2-4 hr after initial dose, usually a continuous heparin infusion is begun with the rate of infusion based on evaluation of the PTT (1.5-2.5 × normal). Once established, daily or twice daily PTT levels are determined to ensure a therapeutic dosage is maintained. If continuous heparin infusion is not feasible, IV boluses of 5000-7500 U q4hr may be provided and monitored via serial PTT determination.

Goals of therapy: To inhibit further thrombus growth, promote resolution of the formed thrombus, and prevent further embolus formation.

Protamine sulfate: Heparin antidote, which should be readily available dur-ing heparin therapy. Fatal hemorrhage occurs in 1%-2% of patients undergoing heparin therapy. Risk of bleeding is greatest in women >60 yr of age.

Oral anticoagulants (warfarin sodium):   Started 48-72 hr after initiation of heparin therapy. The two are given simultaneously for a few days to allow time for warfarin to inhibit vitamin K-dependent clotting factors before heparin is discontinued.

Prothrombin time (PT):   Monitored daily, with the goal of 1.25-1.50 × normal. Once the patient has stabilized and the heparin is discontinued, weekly monitoring of PT is acceptable. After hospital discharge, the PT should be monitored q2wk for as long as the patient continues to take oral anticoagulants.

International Normalized Ratio (INR): Has been advocated by the World Health Organization (WHO) to compensate for variations encountered with various reagents and methods used in prothrombin tests. The INR goal for oral anticoagulant therapy is 2.0-3.0.

Maintenance: Usually 5-10 mg/day continued for 6 mo, based on the continued presence of risk factors. Certain tumors (e.g., Trousseau syndrome) necessitate lifetime therapy.

Vitamin K (vitamin K₁ [Mephyton or phytonadione] or K₃ [menadione]): Reverses the effects of warfarin in 24-36 hr. Fresh frozen plasma may be required in cases of serious bleeding.

> **Caution:** Warfarin crosses the placental barrier and can cause spontaneous abortion and birth defects.

Thrombolytic therapy (i.e., streptokinase, urokinase): May be given in the first 24-72 hr after PE to speed the process of clot lysis via conversion of plasminogen to plasma. After the first 24-72 hr of thrombolytic therapy, heparin therapy is initiated. Thrombolytic therapy may be preferred for initial treatment of PE in patients with hemodynamic compromise, >30% occlusion of pulmonary vasculature, and in whom therapy has been initiated no later than 3 days after onset of PE.

Streptokinase: Loading dose of 250,000 IU in normal saline or 5% dextrose in water (D_5W) given IV over a 30-min period. Maintenance dose is 100,000 IU/hr given IV for 24-72 hr.

Urokinase: Loading dose of 4400 IU/kg of body weight in 5 ml of solution given IV over a 10-min period. Maintenance dose is 4400 IU/kg/hr for 12 hr.

Thrombin time: Monitors therapy for both drugs. The test is repeated q4hr during therapy to ensure adequate response, which should be between 2 and 5 × normal. PTT can be used instead of thrombin time and should be 2-5 × control. Once thrombolytic therapy is stopped, thrombin time or PTT should be checked frequently until values fall below 2 × normal. When the values are below 2 × normal, heparin is started and continued as described under IV heparin therapy, above.

Contraindications: Active internal bleeding, cerebrovascular accident, or intracranial bleeding within 2 mo of PE. Other contraindications include trauma or surgery within 15 days of PE, diastolic hypertension >100 mm Hg, recent cardiopulmonary resuscitation, pregnancy, and <10 days postpartum.

> **Caution:** As many as 33% of patients receiving thrombolytic therapy have hemorrhagic complications. Discontinuing the drug and administering fresh frozen plasma are the appropriate treatments.

Surgical interventions: Used only in select cases because anticoagulant therapy is usually successful.

Vena caval interruption/ligation: To interrupt passage of venous thrombi through the inferior vena cava. These include the following FDA-approved filters: Greenfield filters, Venatech filter, Simon Nitinol filter, and Bird's Nest filter.

Pulmonary embolectomy: To remove clots from the pulmonary circulation. Generally, the use of thrombolytic agents eliminates the need for this procedure.

Management of fat emboli

Oxygen: Concentration of oxygen is based on clinical picture, ABG results, and patient's prior respiratory status. Intubation and mechanical ventilation may be required.

Steroids: Cortisone, 100 mg, or methylprednisone, 30 mg/kg, is used to decrease local injury to pulmonary tissue and pulmonary edema.
Diuretics: Approximately 30% of patients with fat emboli develop pulmonary edema, necessitating use of diuretics.

NURSING DIAGNOSES AND INTERVENTIONS

Impaired gas exchange related to altered oxygen supply secondary to ventilation-perfusion mismatch

Desired outcomes: Following intervention/treatment, patient exhibits adequate gas exchange and ventilatory function as evidenced by RR 12-20 breaths/min with normal pattern and depth (eupnea), no significant changes in mental status, and orientation to person, place, and time. At a minimum of 24 hr before hospital discharge patient has O_2 saturation >92% or Pao_2 $\geq$80 mm Hg, $Paco_2$ 35-45 mm Hg, and pH 7.35-7.45 (or values consistent with patient's acceptable baseline parameters).

- Monitor patient for signs and symptoms of increasing respiratory distress: RR increased from baseline, increasing dyspnea, anxiety, restlessness, confusion, and cyanosis.
- As indicated, monitor oximetry readings; report O_2 saturation $\leq$92% because this can indicate a need for O_2 therapy.
- Position patient for comfort and optimal gas exchange. Ensure that the area of the lung affected by the embolus is not dependent when patient is in the lateral decubitus position. Elevate HOB 30 degrees to improve ventilation.
- Avoid positioning patient with knees bent (i.e., gatching the bed) because this impedes venous return from the legs and can increase the risk of PE. Instruct the patient not to cross the legs when lying in bed or sitting in a chair.
- Decrease metabolic demands for oxygen by limiting or pacing patient's activities and procedures.
- Ensure that patient performs deep-breathing and coughing exercises 3-5 times q2hr.
- Ensure delivery of prescribed concentrations and humidity of oxygen.
- Monitor serial ABG values, assessing for the desired response to treatment. Report lack of response to treatment or worsening ABG values.

NIC: Acid-Base Monitoring; Airway Management; Bedside Laboratory Testing; Cough Enhancement; Embolus Precautions; Oxygen Therapy; Respiratory Monitoring

Altered protection related to risk of prolonged bleeding or hemorrhage secondary to anticoagulation therapy

Desired outcome: Patient is free of frank or occult bleeding; body secretions/excretions test negative for blood.

- Monitor VS for indicators of profuse bleeding or hemorrhage resulting from anticoagulant therapy: hypotension, tachycardia, and tachypnea.
- At least once each shift use a reagent stick to check stool, urine, emesis, and NG drainage for blood via agency-approved protocols.
- At least once each shift inspect wounds, oral mucous membranes, any entry site of an invasive procedure, and nares for evidence of bleeding.
- At least once each shift inspect the torso and extremities for petechiae or ecchymoses.
- To prevent hematoma formation, do not give an IM injection unless it is unavoidable. If parenteral medications are mandatory, attempt to administer SC using a small-gauge needle.
- Apply pressure to all venipuncture or arterial puncture sites until bleeding stops completely.
- Ensure easy access to antidotes for prescribed treatment:
    —*Protamine sulfate:* 1 mg counteracts 100 U of heparin. Usually initial dose is 50 mg.

—*Vitamin K (vitamin K$_1$ [Mephyton or phytonadione] or K$_3$ [menadione]):* 20 mg given SC to counteract the effects of oral anticoagulants.

—*Aminocaproic acid (e.g., Amicar):* administered via slow IV infusion of 5 g to reverse the fibrinolytic condition related to thrombolytic therapy.

- If patient is receiving heparin therapy, monitor serial PTT (desired range is 1.5-2.5 × control). If patient is receiving warfarin (Coumadin) therapy, monitor serial PT. Desired range is 1.25-1.5 × control, or an INR value of 2.0-3.0. Report values outside the desired range.
- To prevent negative interactions with anticoagulants or thrombolytic therapy, establish compatibility of all drugs before administering them.
  —*Heparin:* digitalis, tetracycline, nicotine, and antihistamines decrease the effect of heparin therapy. Consult pharmacist about compatibility before infusing other IV drugs through heparin IV line.
  —*Warfarin sodium:* numerous drugs result in a decrease or increase in response to treatment with warfarin. Consult pharmacist to obtain specific information about patient's medication profile.
  —*Thrombolytic therapy (e.g., streptokinase, urokinase):* no specific drug interactions are noted. However, consult pharmacist before infusing any other medication through the same IV line.
- Because aspirin and NSAIDs, such as ibuprofen, are platelet aggregation inhibitors and can prolong episodes of bleeding, avoid use of *any* drug that contains these medications.
- Discuss with patient and significant others the importance of reporting promptly the presence of bleeding, such as any of the following: hematuria, melena, frank bleeding from the mouth, epistaxis, hemoptysis, excessive vaginal bleeding (menometrorrhagia).
- Teach patient the necessity of using sponge-tipped applicators and mouthwash for oral care to minimize the risk of gum bleeding. Instruct patient to shave with an electric rather than a straight or safety razor.
- If patient is restless and combative, provide a safe environment: pad the side rails, restrain patient as necessary to prevent falls, and use extreme care when moving patient to avoid bumping extremities into side rails.

NIC: Bleeding Precautions; Nutritional Counseling; Risk Identification; Self-Care Assistance; Teaching: Individual

Knowledge deficit: Oral anticoagulant therapy, potential side effects, and foods and medications to avoid during therapy

Desired outcome: Within the 24-hr period before hospital discharge, patient verbalizes knowledge of the prescribed anticoagulant drug, the potential side effects, and foods and medications to avoid while receiving oral anticoagulant therapy.

- Determine patient's knowledge of oral anticoagulant therapy. As appropriate, discuss the drug name, purpose, dose, schedule, precautions, food/drug and drug/drug interactions, and side effects.
- Inform patient of the potential side effects/complications of anticoagulant therapy: easy bruising, prolonged bleeding from cuts, spontaneous nosebleeds, bleeding gums, black and tarry or bloody stools, vaginal bleeding, and blood in urine and sputum.
- Discuss with patient the importance of laboratory testing and follow-up visits with health care provider.
- Explain the importance of informing all health care providers (e.g., dentists and other health care providers) that patient is taking an anticoagulant. Suggest that patient wear a Medic-Alert tag or other method of informing health care providers about the anticoagulant therapy.
- Teach patient to avoid foods high in vitamin K (e.g., fish, bananas, dark green vegetables, tomatoes, cauliflower), which can interfere with anticoagulation.
- Caution patient that a soft-bristled, rather than hard-bristled, toothbrush and an electric, rather than a straight or safety, razor should be used during

anticoagulant therapy to minimize the risk of injury that could cause bleeding.
- Instruct patient to consult health care provider before taking over-the-counter (OTC) or prescribed drugs that were used before initiating anticoagulants. Aspirin, cimetidine, and trimethaphan are among the many drugs that enhance the response to warfarin. Drugs that decrease the response include antacids, diuretics, oral contraceptives, and barbiturates, among others.

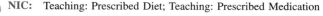 NIC: Teaching: Prescribed Diet; Teaching: Prescribed Medication

> **See Also:** If appropriate, Appendix One, "Caring for Preoperative and Postoperative Patients," p. 717; "Caring for Patients on Prolonged Bed Rest," p. 738.

PATIENT-FAMILY TEACHING AND DISCHARGE PLANNING

When providing patient-family teaching, focus on sensory information; avoid giving excessive information; and initiate a visiting nurse referral for necessary follow-up teaching. Consider including verbal and written information about the following:
- Risk factors related to the development of thrombi and embolization and preventive measures to reduce the risk.
- Signs and symptoms of *thrombophlebitis:* swelling of the calf, tenderness or warmth in the involved area, possible presence of pain in affected calf when ankle is dorsiflexed, slight fever, and distention of distal veins, coolness, edema, and pale color in the distal affected leg.
- Signs and symptoms of *pulmonary embolism:* sudden onset of dyspnea and anxiety, nonproductive cough or hemoptysis, palpitations, nausea, syncope.
- Rationale and application procedure for antiembolism hose. Explain that patient should put them on in the morning before getting out of bed.
- Importance of preventing impairment of venous return from the lower extremities by avoiding prolonged sitting, crossing legs, and constrictive clothing.

> **Note:** Rehabilitation and family teaching concepts for fat emboli are nonspecific.

Pneumothorax/Hemothorax

Pneumothorax is an accumulation of air in the pleural space, which leads to increased intrapleural pressure. Risk factors include blunt or penetrating chest injury, COPD, previous pneumothorax, and positive pressure ventilation. There are three types:

Spontaneous: Also referred to as *closed pneumothorax* because the chest wall remains intact with no leak to the atmosphere. It results from the rupture of a bleb or bulla on the visceral pleural surface, usually near the apex. Generally, the cause of the rupture is unknown, although it may result from a weakness related to a respiratory infection or from an underlying pulmonary disease (e.g., COPD, tuberculosis, malignant neoplasm). The affected individual is usually young (20-40 yr), previously healthy, and male. Generally, onset of symptoms occurs at rest, rather than with vigorous exercise or coughing. Potential for recurrence is great, with the second pneumothorax occurring an average of 2-3 yr after the first.

Traumatic: Can be open or closed. An open pneumothorax occurs when air enters the pleural space from the atmosphere through an opening in the chest wall, such as with a gunshot wound, stab wound, or invasive medical procedure (e.g., lung biopsy, thoracentesis, or placement of a central line into a subclavian vein). A sucking sound may be heard over the area of penetration during inspiration, accounting for the classic wound description as a "sucking chest wound." A closed pneumothorax occurs when the visceral pleura is penetrated but the chest wall remains intact with no atmospheric leak. This usually occurs following blunt trauma that results in a fracture and dislocation of the ribs. It also may occur from the use of PEEP or after CPR.

Tension: Generally occurs with closed pneumothorax; also can occur with open pneumothorax when a flap of tissue acts as a one-way valve. Air enters the pleural space through the pleural tear when the individual inhales, and it continues to accumulate but cannot escape during expiration because the tissue flap closes. With tension pneumothorax, as the pressure in the thorax and mediastinum increases, it produces a shift in the affected lung and mediastinum toward the unaffected side, which further impairs ventilatory efforts. The increase in pressure also compresses the vena cava, which impedes venous return, leading to a decrease in cardiac output and, ultimately, to circulatory collapse if the condition is not diagnosed and treated quickly. Tension pneumothorax is a life-threatening medical emergency.

Hemothorax is an accumulation of blood in the pleural space. Hemothorax generally results from blunt trauma to the chest wall, but it can also occur following thoracic surgery, after penetrating gunshot or stab wounds, as a result of anticoagulant therapy, after the insertion of a central venous catheter, or following various thoracoabdominal organ biopsies. Mediastinal shift, ventilatory compromise, and lung collapse can occur, depending on the amount of blood accumulated.

ASSESSMENT

Clinical presentation will vary, depending on the type and size of the pneumothorax or hemothorax (Table 1-2).

DIAGNOSTIC TESTS

Chest x-ray: Will reveal the presence of air or blood in the pleural space on the affected side, size of the pneumothorax/hemothorax, and any shift in the mediastinum.

ABG values: Hypoxemia (Pao_2 <80 mm Hg) may be accompanied by hypercarbia ($Paco_2$ >45 mm Hg) with resultant respiratory acidosis (pH <7.35). Arterial oxygen saturation may be decreased initially but usually returns to normal within 24 hr.

Oximetry: Will reveal decreased O_2 saturation (≤92%).

CBC: May reveal decreased Hgb proportionate to the amount of blood lost in a hemothorax.

COLLABORATIVE MANAGEMENT

Management is determined by the signs and symptoms. A small pneumothorax may heal itself via reabsorption of the free air, making invasive procedures unnecessary unless an underlying disease process or injury is present. Hemothorax nearly always requires intervention.

Oxygen therapy: Administered when ABG values or oximetry demonstrates the presence of hypoxemia, which usually occurs when the pneumothorax/hemothorax is large.

Thoracentesis: For hemothorax to remove blood from the pleural space. For cases of tension pneumothorax, it is performed immediately to remove air from the pleural space. A large-bore needle is inserted in the second intercostal space, midclavicular line, which correlates to the superior portion of the anterior axillary lobe. A sudden rushing out of air confirms the diagnosis of tension pneumothorax. To decrease risk of further pleural laceration as the chest reexpands, a stylet introducer needle with a plastic sheath may be used. The

TABLE 1-2   Assessment of the Patient With Pneumothorax or Hemothorax

	Spontaneous or traumatic pneumothorax		Tension pneumothorax	Hemothorax
	Closed	Open		
Signs and symptoms				
	SOB, cough, chest tightness, chest pain	SOB, sharp chest pain	Dyspnea, chest pain	Dyspnea, chest pain
Physical assessment				
	Tachypnea, decreased thoracic movement, cyanosis, subcutaneous emphysema, hyperresonance over affected area, diminished breath sounds, paradoxical movement of chest wall (may signal flail chest), change in mental status	Agitation, restlessness, tachypnea, cyanosis, presence of chest wound, hyperresonance over affected area, sucking sound on inspiration, diminished breath sounds, change in mental status	Anxiety, tachycardia, cyanosis, jugular vein distention, tracheal deviation toward the unaffected side, absent breath sounds on affected side, distant heart sounds, hypotension, change in mental status	Tachypnea, pallor, cyanosis, dullness over affected side, tachycardia, hypotension, diminished or absent breath sounds, change in mental status

SOB, Shortness of breath.

needle is removed after penetration, and the plastic catheter sheath is left in place to allow decompression of the chest cavity. Following release of entrapped air, chest tubes are inserted.

Chest tube placement (tube thoracotomy):   A chest tube (thoracic catheter) may be inserted in any patient who is symptomatic. During insertion the patient should be in an upright position so that the lung falls away from the chest wall. The position of the thoracic catheter will depend on whether the health care provider wants to drain air, fluid, or both. The thoracic catheter must be connected to an underwater-seal drainage system or a one-way flutter valve device. Usually, simple underwater-seal drainage is all that is necessary for 6-24 hr. Suction may be used, depending on size of the pneumothorax or hemothorax, patient's condition, and amount of drainage. If drainage is minimal and no suction is required, a one-way flutter valve may be used instead of an underwater-seal drainage system. After chest tube insertion and removal of air or fluid from the pleural space, the lung begins to reexpand. A chest tube may produce inflammation of the pleura, causing pleuritic pain, slight temperature elevation, and pleural friction rub.

Thoracotomy: Often indicated if patient has had two or more spontaneous pneumothoraces on one side, because of the risk of continuous recurrence, or if resolution of the pneumothorax does not occur within 7 days. With a hemothorax, a thoracotomy is performed to locate the source and control bleeding if blood loss exceeds 200 ml/hr for 2 hr. Thoracotomy may include mechanical abrasion of the pleural surfaces with a dry sterile sponge or chemical abrasion via an agent such as tetracycline solution or talc, which results in pleural adhesions (pleurodesis) that help prevent recurrence of pneumothorax. A partial pleurectomy may be performed instead of mechanical or chemical abrasion.

IV therapy: If there is significant loss of fluids or blood.

Analgesia: Because of rich innervation of the pleura, chest tube placement is painful and significant analgesia is usually required.

NURSING DIAGNOSES AND INTERVENTIONS

Impaired gas exchange related to altered oxygen supply secondary to ventilation-perfusion mismatch

Desired outcomes: Following treatment/intervention, patient exhibits adequate gas exchange and ventilatory function as evidenced by RR ≤ 20 breaths/min with normal depth and pattern (eupnea), no significant mental status changes, and orientation to person, place, and time. At a minimum of 24 hr before hospital discharge, patient's ABG values are as follows: Pao_2 ≥ 80 mm Hg and $Paco_2$ 35-45 mm Hg (or values within patient's acceptable baseline parameters); or oximetry readings demonstrate O_2 saturation >92%.

- Monitor serial ABG results to detect decreasing Pao_2 and increasing $Paco_2$, which can signal impending respiratory compromise; or monitor oximetry readings for O_2 saturation $\leq 92\%$. Report significant findings to health care provider.
- Observe for indicators of hypoxia, including increased restlessness, anxiety, tachycardia, and changes in mental status. Cyanosis may be a late sign.
- Assess patient's VS and breath sounds q2hr or as indicated by the patient's condition.
- Following tube or exploratory thoracotomy the patient will require checks q15min until stable for signs of respiratory distress: increased RR, diminished or absent movement of chest wall on affected side, paradoxical movement of the chest wall, increased WOB, use of accessory muscles of respiration, complaints of increased dyspnea, unilateral diminished breath sounds, and cyanosis. Evaluate HR and BP for indications of shock (i.e., tachycardia and hypotension).

- Position patient to allow for full expansion of the unaffected lung. Semi-Fowler's position usually provides comfort and allows adequate expansion of chest wall and descent of diaphragm.
- Change patient's position q2hr to promote drainage and lung reexpansion and facilitate alveolar perfusion.
- Encourage patient to take deep breaths, providing necessary analgesia to decrease discomfort during deep-breathing exercises. Instruct the patient in splinting the thoracotomy site with either the arms, a pillow, or a folded blanket. Deep breathing will promote full lung expansion and decrease the risk of atelectasis. Coughing will facilitate mobilization of tracheobronchial secretions, if present.
- Deliver and monitor oxygen and humidity as indicated.

NIC: Acid-Base Management; Cough Enhancement; Oxygen Therapy; Positioning; Respiratory Monitoring; Surveillance; Tube Care: Chest

Ineffective breathing pattern (or risk of same) related to decreased lung expansion secondary to malfunction of chest drainage system
Desired outcome: Following intervention, patient becomes eupneic.
- Monitor patient at frequent intervals (q2-4hr, as appropriate) to assess breathing pattern while chest-drainage system is in place. Auscultate breath sounds, reporting diminished sounds; be alert for and report signs of respiratory distress, including tachycardia, restlessness, anxiety, and changes in mental status.
- Assess and maintain the closed chest-drainage system:
  —Tape all connections, and secure chest tube to thorax with tape. Avoid all kinks in the tubing, and ensure that the bed and equipment are not compressing any component of the system.
  —Eliminate all dependent loops in tubing. These may impede removal of air and fluid from the pleural space.
  —Maintain fluid in underwater-seal chamber and suction chamber at appropriate levels.
- Be aware that the suction apparatus does not regulate the amount of suction applied to the closed chest-drainage system. The amount of suction is determined by the water level in the suction control chamber. Minimal bubbling in this chamber is acceptable and desirable. **Note:** Suction aids in the reexpansion of the lung, but removing suction for short periods of time, such as for transporting, will not be detrimental or disrupt the closed chest-drainage system.
- Follow institution's policy about chest-tube stripping. Be aware that this mechanism for maintaining chest-tube patency is controversial and has been associated with creating high negative pressures in the pleural space, which can damage fragile lung tissue. Chest-tube stripping may be indicated when bloody drainage or clots are visible in the tubing. Squeezing alternately hand-over-hand along the drainage tube may generate sufficient pressure to move fluid along the tube. Use of mechanical or hand-held tube-stripping devices should be avoided.
- Be aware that fluctuations in the underwater-seal chamber are characteristic of a patent chest tube. Fluctuations stop when either the lung has reexpanded or there is a kink or obstruction in the chest tube:
  —Bubbling in the underwater-seal chamber occurs on expiration and is a sign that air is leaving the pleural space. Continuous bubbling in the underwater-seal chamber may be a signal that air is leaking into the drainage system. Locate and seal the system's air leak, if possible.
- Keep necessary emergency supplies at the bedside:
  —Petrolatum gauze pad to apply over insertion site if the chest tube becomes dislodged; use of this dressing provides an airtight seal to prevent recurrent pneumothorax.

—A bottle of sterile water in which to submerge the chest tube if it becomes disconnected from the underwater-seal system.

- *Never* clamp a chest tube without a specific directive from the health care provider, inasmuch as clamping may lead to tension pneumothorax because air in the pleural space no longer can escape.

NIC: Analgesia Administration; Emotional Support; Pain Management; Positioning; Respiratory Monitoring; Tube Care: Chest

Pain related to impaired pleural integrity, inflammation, or presence of a chest tube

Desired outcomes: Within 1 hr of intervention, patient's subjective perception of pain decreases, as documented by a pain scale. Objective indicators, such as grimacing, are absent or diminished.

- At frequent intervals, assess patient's degree of discomfort, using patient's verbal and nonverbal cues. Devise a pain scale with patient, rating pain from 0 (no pain) to 10 (worst pain).
- Medicate with analgesics as prescribed, using the pain scale to evaluate and document the effectiveness of the medication. Encourage the patient to request analgesic before pain becomes severe.
- Premedicate patient 30 min before initiating coughing, exercising, or repositioning.
- Teach patient to splint affected side when coughing, moving, or repositioning.
- Facilitate coordination across health care providers to provide rest periods between care activities to decrease oxygen demand. Allow 90 min for undisturbed rest.
- Stabilize chest tube to reduce pull or drag on latex connector tubing. Tape chest tube securely to thorax.
- For additional interventions, see **Pain,** p. 719, in Appendix One.

NIC: Anxiety Reduction; Environmental Management: Comfort; Pain Management; Patient-Controlled Analgesia (PCA) Assistance; Progressive Muscle Relaxation; Simple Relaxation Therapy; Sleep Enhancement

---

See Also: "Abdominal Trauma" for **Fluid volume deficit,** p. 469; psychosocial nursing diagnoses and interventions in Appendix One, "Caring for Patients With Cancer and Other Life-Disrupting Illnesses," p. 791.

PATIENT-FAMILY TEACHING AND DISCHARGE PLANNING

When providing patient-family teaching, focus on sensory information; avoid giving excessive information; and initiate a visiting nurse referral for necessary follow-up teaching. Consider including verbal and written information about the following:

- Purpose for chest-tube placement and maintenance.
- Potential for recurrence of spontaneous pneumothorax. Average time between occurrences is 2-3 yr. Explain the importance of seeking medical care immediately if the symptoms recur (see Table 1-2).
- Medications, including drug name, purpose, dosage, schedule, precautions, drug/drug and food/drug interactions, and potential side effects.

Pulmonary tuberculosis

Tuberculosis (TB) was a leading cause of death in the United States until the late 1940s and early 1950s, when antituberculosis drug therapy was introduced, resulting in a decline in the disease until the 1980s. In 1990 the WHO reported that 2.9 million deaths occurred from TB, the largest pathogen-related cause of death in the world. In 1991 the WHO estimated that approximately one third of the world's population was infected with *Mycobacterium tuberculosis*. Recently rates of TB have also been increasing in the United States. Factors contributing to the rise include immigration of individuals to the United States from countries where TB is endemic and increasing prevalence of individuals who are immunocompromised (i.e., those receiving immunosuppressive therapy or with a disease that impairs the immune response, such as HIV disease).

TB is a highly infectious disease spread by contact with respiratory droplets containing mycobacteria, generally the *Mycobacterium tuberculosis* bacillus in humans. The most common mode of transmission is inhalation of bacilli in airborne mucus droplets from sputum of persons with active disease. Less frequently, transmission may result from ingestion or skin penetration. When infection with tubercle bacilli occurs, lung parenchyma become inflamed. Natural body defenses attempt to counteract the infection, and lymph nodes in the hilar region of the lung may begin to filter drainage from the infected site. The inflammatory process and cellular reaction produce a small, firm white nodule called the primary tubercle, the center of which contains tubercle bacilli. Cells gather around the center, and the outer portion becomes fibrosed. As blood vessels become compressed, nutrition to the tubercle ceases and the center begins to necrose. The area is further walled off by fibrotic tissue, and the center becomes soft and cheesy in consistency, a process known as caseation. This fluid may calcify (calcium deposits) or liquefy (liquefaction necrosis). Most individuals (90%) infected with the tubercle bacillus do not progress to active disease, because the disease usually settles into the latency phase.

ASSESSMENT

It is important to assess whether the patient was exposed to a person with active TB. Also, close contacts of the patient require identification so that they can undergo evaluation for the presence of infection.

Signs and symptoms: Cough, afternoon temperature elevation, night sweats, anorexia, weight loss, chest pain, lethargy, and dyspnea.

DIAGNOSTIC TESTS

Sputum culture: To ascertain presence of *M. tuberculosis;* will not be positive during latency period.

Acid-fast stain: Culture of sputum positive for acid-fast bacilli (AFB) in the presence of active TB. Specimens may be collected by tracheal washing, thoracentesis of pleural fluid, and lung biopsy.

Chest x-ray: Involvement is most characteristically evident in the apex and posterior segments of the upper lobes. Although not diagnostically definitive, will reveal calcification at original site, enlargement of hilar lymph nodes, parenchymal infiltrate, pleural effusion, and cavitation.

Intradermal injection of antigen: Purified protein derivative (PPD); old tuberculin (OT). Considered positive when an area of induration >10 mm is present within 48-72 hr after injection. A positive test indicates past infection and presence of antibodies; it is not definitive of active disease.

Gastric washings: May reveal presence of tubercle bacilli secondary to swallowed sputum.

COLLABORATIVE MANAGEMENT

AFB isolation: Until antimicrobial therapy is successful as indicated by AFB smears. AFB isolation (or "airborne precautions" in the nomenclature of Standard Precautions) requires a private room with special ventilation that dilutes and removes airborne contaminants and controls the direction of air flow. To allow adequate function of this negative air-flow system, the door to this room should be kept closed as much as possible. High-efficiency masks (e.g., particulate respirators) designed to provide a tight face seal and filter particles in the 1- to 5-μm range are worn by all individuals entering the patient's room and by the patient if it is necessary to leave the room.

Pharmacologic agents: A combination of antiinfective agents is recommended to prevent development of resistant strains of tubercle bacillus. The drug of choice, along with the dosage and duration of administration, depends on the stage of the infection or disease, presence of extrapulmonary disease, and sensitivity of the patient to the chemotherapeutic agent. The most common combination is isoniazid (INH) and rifampin, which is given for 6-12 mo. Other drugs, which may be added to this protocol if the organism shows resistance to the first-line drugs, include ethambutol (EMB), streptomycin (SM), and aminosalicylic acid (PAS). Second-line pharmacotherapy may include ethionamide, cycloserine, pyrazinamide (PZA), capreomycin, viomycin, and kanamycin.

Surgery: Resection for persistent cavitary lesions; surgical intervention for massive hemoptysis, spontaneous pneumothorax, abscess drainage, and other complications.

NURSING DIAGNOSES AND INTERVENTIONS

Knowledge deficit: The spread of TB and the procedure for AFB isolation

Desired outcome: Following instruction, patient and significant others verbalize how TB is spread and the measures necessary to prevent the spread.

- Teach patient about TB and the mechanism by which it is spread (respiratory droplet aerosol).
- Explain AFB isolation to patient and significant others. Post a notice of AFB isolation/airborne precautions on the patient's room door.
- Remind staff and visitors of the need to keep the door closed to allow effective function of the ventilation system.
- Explain to staff and visitors the importance of wearing high-efficiency masks, including their proper fit and use. Provide masks at doorway or other convenient place.
- Teach patient the importance of covering mouth and nose with tissue when sneezing or coughing and disposing of used tissue in container suitable for biohazardous waste disposal.
- Stress the importance of good hand-washing technique to reduce the risk of ingesting the organism.

NIC: Health Education; Infection Control; Teaching: Disease Process; Teaching: Individual; Teaching: Prescribed Medication

PATIENT-FAMILY TEACHING AND DISCHARGE PLANNING

When providing patient-family teaching, focus on sensory information; avoid giving excessive information; and initiate a visiting nurse referral for necessary follow-up teaching. Consider including verbal and written information about the following:

- Importance of good hand-washing technique.
- Antituberculosis medications, including drug name, purpose, dosage, schedule, precautions, drug/drug and food/drug interactions, and potential side effects. Remind patient that medications are to be taken without interruption for the prescribed period of time. Remind the patient of the need for continued laboratory monitoring for complications of pharmacotherapy.
- Importance of periodic reculturing of sputum.
- Phone numbers to call should questions or concerns arise about therapy or disease after discharge. Additional general information can be obtained by contacting:

American Lung Association
1740 Broadway
New York, NY 10019-4374   (212) 315-8700
WWW address: *http://www.lungusa.org*

Section Two: Acute Respiratory Failure

Acute respiratory failure (ARF) develops when the lungs are unable to exchange O_2 and CO_2 adequately. Clinically, respiratory failure exists when Pao$_2$ is <50 mm Hg with the patient at rest and breathing room air. Paco$_2$ $\geq$50 mm Hg or pH <7.35 is significant for respiratory acidosis, which is the common precursor to ARF.

Although a variety of disease processes can lead to the development of respiratory failure (Table 1-3), four basic mechanisms are involved:

Alveolar hypoventilation: Occurs secondary to reduction in alveolar minute ventilation. Because differential indicators (cyanosis, somnolence) occur late in the process, the condition may go unnoticed until tissue hypoxia is severe.

Ventilation-perfusion mismatch: Considered the most common cause of hypoxemia. Normal alveolar ventilation occurs at a rate of 4 L/min, with normal pulmonary vascular blood flow occurring at a rate of 5 L/min. Normal ventilation/perfusion ratio is 0.8:1. Any disease process that interferes with either side of the equation upsets the physiologic balance and can lead to respiratory failure as a result of the reduction in arterial O_2 levels.

Diffusion disturbances: Processes that physically impair gas exchange across the alveolar-capillary membrane. Diffusion is impaired because of the increase in anatomic distance the gas must travel from alveoli to capillary and capillary to alveoli.

Right-to-left shunt: Occurs when the above processes go untreated. Large amounts of blood pass from the right side of the heart to the left and out into the general circulation without adequate ventilation; therefore blood is poorly

---

TABLE 1-3   Disease Processes Leading to the Development of Respiratory Failure

Impaired alveolar ventilation
  Chronic obstructive pulmonary
    disease (emphysema, bronchitis,
    asthma, cystic fibrosis)
  Restrictive pulmonary disease
    (interstitial fibrosis, pleural effusion,
    pneumothorax, kyphoscoliosis,
    obesity, diaphragmatic paralysis)
  Neuromuscular defects (Guillain-
    Barré syndrome, myasthenia gravis,
    multiple sclerosis, muscular
    dystrophy)
  Depression of respiratory control
    centers (drug-induced cerebral
    infarction, inappropriate use of
    high-dose O_2 therapy)

Diffusion disturbances
  Pulmonary/interstitial fibrosis
  Pulmonary edema
  Adult respiratory distress syndrome
  Anatomic loss of functioning lung
    tissue (tumor pneumonectomy)

Ventilation or perfusion disturbances
  Pulmonary emboli
  Atelectasis
  Pneumonia
  Emphysema
  Chronic bronchitis
  Bronchiolitis
  Adult respiratory distress syndrome

Right-to-left shunting
  Atelectasis
  Pneumonia
  Pulmonary edema
  Pulmonary emboli
  O_2 toxicity

From Howard C. In Swearingen PL, Keen JH: *Manual of critical care: applying nursing diagnoses to adult critical illness,* ed 3, St Louis, 1995, Mosby.

oxygenated. This mechanism occurs when alveoli are atelectatic or fluid filled, inasmuch as these conditions interfere with gas exchange. Unlike the first three responses, hypoxemia secondary to right-to-left shunting does not improve with the administration of O_2, because the additional FIo_2 is unable to cross the alveolar-capillary membrane.

ASSESSMENT

Clinical indicators of ARF vary according to the underlying disease process and severity of the failure. ARF is one of the most common causes of impaired LOC. Often it is misdiagnosed as heart failure, pneumonia, or cerebrovascular accident.

Early indicators: Restlessness, changes in mental status, anxiety, headache, fatigue, cool and dry skin, increased BP, tachycardia, cardiac dysrhythmias.
Intermediate indicators: Confusion, lethargy, tachypnea, hypotension caused by vasodilation, cardiac dysrhythmias.
Late indicators: Cyanosis, diaphoresis, coma, respiratory arrest.

DIAGNOSTIC TESTS

ABG analysis: Assesses adequacy of oxygenation and effectiveness of ventilation and is the most important diagnostic tool. Typical results are Pao_2 ≤ 60 mm Hg, $Paco_2$ ≥ 45 mm Hg, and pH <7.35, which are consistent with severe respiratory acidosis.
Chest x-ray: Ascertains presence of underlying pathophysiology or disease process that may be contributing to the failure.

COLLABORATIVE MANAGEMENT

Treatment is aimed at correcting the acid-base disturbance while treating the underlying pathophysiology in an effort to prevent or correct ARF. Although the general rule is to bring the Pao_2 to >60 mm Hg and the $Paco_2$ to 35-45 mm Hg, patients with COPD may be clinically stable with a $Paco_2$ >45 mm Hg, so determination of pH is critical with these individuals. For example, the patient with a chronically high $Paco_2$ whose pH drops below baseline is at risk for development of respiratory failure.

O_2 therapy: As determined by ABG values. O_2 therapy at an FIo_2 of 0.50 or less and chest physiotherapy in conjunction with pharmacotherapy (e.g., bronchodilators, steroids, antibiotics) often improve ABGs sufficiently to get the patient out of danger. Persistent respiratory acidosis following medical intervention may indicate the need for intubation and mechanical ventilation.
IV aminophylline: To treat bronchospasms. Therapeutic range is 10-20 µg/ml. Daily serum levels are drawn to evaluate the patient.
Bronchodilator therapy: Delivered via nebulizer or intermittent positive-pressure breathing (IPPB) machine q2-4hr to minimize CO_2 retention.
Chest physiotherapy: To assist in mobilization of secretions.
Coughing/deep breathing exercises: To mobilize secretions and promote full lung expansion. If the cough is ineffective, suctioning may be necessary to stimulate cough reflex and clear secretions.
IV fluids: To maintain fluid balance and prevent dehydration.
Antibiotics: If infection is present.
Intubation and mechanical ventilation: To prevent further airway collapse and tissue injury. The patient may require intubation and mechanical ventilation to provide adequate respiratory function and stabilize ABGs if ARF progresses. Mechanical support is used until the underlying cause of the failure can be corrected and the patient can resume ventilatory efforts independently.

NURSING DIAGNOSES AND INTERVENTIONS

See "Pneumonia" for **Impaired gas exchange,** p. 9, and **Fluid volume deficit,** p. 10. Also see "Pleural Effusion," p. 13, "Pulmonary Embolus," p. 18, "Pneumothorax/Hemothorax," p. 23, "Asthma," p. 35, "Chronic Bronchitis,"

p. 38, "Emphysema," p. 41, "Pulmonary Fibrosis," p. 44, "Pulmonary Edema," p. 104, "Guillain-Barré Syndrome," p. 213, and "Multiple Sclerosis," p. 207, because these disorders may be precursors to ARF. For psychosocial nursing diagnoses and interventions, see Appendix One, "Caring for Patients With Cancer and Other Life-Disrupting Illnesses," p. 791.

PATIENT-FAMILY TEACHING AND DISCHARGE PLANNING

ARF is an acute condition that is symptomatically treated during the patient's hospitalization. Discharge planning and teaching should be directed at educating the patient and significant others about the underlying pathophysiology and treatment specific for that process. See sections in this chapter that relate specifically to the underlying pathophysiology contributing to the development of ARF.

Section Three: Chronic Obstructive Pulmonary Disease

COPD is the second leading cause of disability in the United States. It is a chronic respiratory condition that obstructs the flow of air to or from the bronchioles. Causative factors include smoking, allergens, and environmental and occupational pollutants. This section discusses the following types of COPD: asthma, chronic bronchitis, and emphysema.

Asthma

Asthma is a broad clinical syndrome in which there is recurrent, reversible obstruction of air flow in the bronchioles and smaller bronchi secondary to bronchospasm, mucosal edema, and excessive mucus production. It can occur in any age-group, and its symptoms are intermittent and usually alleviated with treatment. Approximately 12 million Americans have asthma, and incidence and mortality have increased in the past 2 decades (speculated to be related to air pollution). Approximately 5000 people per year die from asthma, a 46% increase from 1980-1989. Asthma-related health care costs an estimated $6.2 billion per year.

Asthma has been classified as *extrinsic* and *intrinsic.*

Extrinsic asthma is associated with a classic antigen-antibody response triggered by exposure to environmental allergens (e.g., pollens, dust, feathers, animal dander, foods). During the antigen-antibody reaction, chemical mediators (histamine, slow-releasing substance of anaphylaxis, eosinophilic chemotactic factor of anaphylaxis) are released. These mediators result in constriction of the smooth muscle of the airways, which leads to bronchospasm; increased capillary permeability leading to mucosal edema; and increased mucous gland secretion with increased mucus production.

Intrinsic asthma occurs secondary to factors that cannot fully be defined and occurs more frequently in individuals older than 35 yr. Most commonly, intrinsic asthma develops as a sequela to a severe respiratory infection with progressive symptoms that develop into asthma. It is speculated that damage to airway epithelium by mediator substances exposes sensitive nerve endings that are then directly stimulated by comparatively minor irritants. Intrinsic asthma most frequently develops in persons with a family history of hypersensitivity reactions such as eczema, rhinitis, urticaria, or hay fever. In intrinsic forms, the triggering mechanism for an attack is nonallergic, such as infection, irritant inhalants, cold air, laughing, or exercise. Whatever the triggering agent, the pathologic response is very similar to that of extrinsic asthma, that is, bronchospasm, mucosal edema, and excess mucus production. Nonallergic triggering mechanisms may also cause the patient with extrinsic asthma breathing problems.

ASSESSMENT

Signs and symptoms: Coughing (frequently paroxysmal), chest tightness, increased sputum production, SOB, dyspnea on exertion (DOE), anxiety, orthopnea, and dyspnea.

Physical assessment: Agitation, prolonged expiratory phase, nasal flaring, use of accessory muscles of respiration, tachypnea, chest retractions (supraclavicular area, intercostal and suprasternal spaces), hyperexpansion of the thorax, expiratory wheezing, coarse rhonchi, diminished or "distant" breath sounds, hyperresonance, tachycardia, pulsus paradoxus, diaphoresis, and pallor.

> **Caution:**   If symptoms are untreated, an acute asthmatic attack can progress to status asthmaticus (SA), a severe and unrelenting asthma attack. SA is an exhausting condition that results in respiratory insufficiency, dehydration (from prolonged dyspnea), and hypoxia and may result in death if untreated.

DIAGNOSTIC TESTS

Oximetry: Will reveal decreased O_2 saturation ($\leq 92\%$).

ABG values: Reveal status of oxygenation and acid-base balance. Generally, acute respiratory acidosis is present during an acute asthma attack ($Paco_2$ >45 mm Hg and pH <7.35).

Chest x-ray: X-ray examination usually shows lung hyperinflation caused by air trapping and a flat diaphragm related to increased intrathoracic volume. Because of paroxysmal cough, pneumothorax is a risk in these patients and may be identified on x-ray examination. Patients with long-standing asthma may exhibit changes associated with emphysema, that is, flattened diaphragms and increased anteroposterior (AP) diameter of the thoracic cage.

CBC: May show increased WBCs with concurrent infection. Differential may show increased eosinophils (in patients with extrinsic forms not taking corticosteroids), which indicate an allergic response.

Sputum: Gross examination may reveal increased viscosity or actual mucus plugs. Culture and sensitivity may reveal microorganisms if infection was the precipitating event. Cytologic examination of sputum will reveal esosinophils in extrinsic forms.

Serum theophylline level: Important baseline indicator for patients who are receiving this therapy. Acceptable therapeutic range is 10-20 µg/ml. The therapeutic level is close to the toxic level, and the patient must be monitored for toxic side effects (e.g., nausea, central nervous system [CNS] stimulation, seizures, dysrhythmias). Serial levels are drawn at frequent intervals. Theophylline agents until recently were used as first-line therapy for asthma prophylaxis, but because of the frequency of life-threatening side effects, their use is being curtailed.

Pulmonary function tests (PFTs):   To evaluate the degree of obstruction. Forced expiratory volume (FEV) is decreased during acute episodes because of severely narrowed airways, which prevent forceful exhalation of inspired volume (Table 1-4). Metacholine, metabisulfite, exercise, and antigen-specific challenges may be used to induce an asthmatic response, which is measured using PFTs. After determining baseline PFTs, the patient is exposed to one of the above triggers and the PFTs are repeated. Metacholine is 100% specific for asthma and is becoming a standard test for patients with nonspecific symptoms.

Peak expiratory flow rate (PEFR):   Provides objective measurement of lung function via a small hand-held gauge called a peak flowmeter. The patient is

TABLE 1-4   Pulmonary Function Tests Used in Individuals With Asthma

Test	Description	Normal values	Parameters in asthma
FVC	Total amount of gas exhaled as forcefully and as rapidly as possible after maximal inspiration	≥80% of predicted normal	Normal or slightly decreased because of air trapping
FEV_1	Volume of gas exhaled over first second of FVC (FEV_2 and FEV_3 may also be measured, at 2 and 3 sec, respectively)	≥75% of predicted normal	Decreased because of airway obstruction; may return to normal after administration of aerosolized bronchodilator
FEF, formerly called maximal midexpiratory flow	Average rate of flow during middle half of FEF. It is an accurate estimate of airway resistance	≥80% of predicted normal	Decreased because of small airways obstruction; may return to normal after administration of aerosolized bronchodilator

FVC, Forced vital capacity; *FEV₁,* forced expiratory volume in 1 sec; *FEF,* forced midexpiratory flow; *FEV₂,* forced expiratory volume in 2 sec; *FEV₃,* forced expiratory volume in 3 sec.

instructed to inhale deeply and forcibly exhale rapidly into the flowmeter, providing a reading in liters per minute (L/min). The higher the number, the better the air flow. Normal peak flow rates vary across individuals and are based on gender, height, and age. Each patient should monitor daily morning peak flow rates for 1 mo to determine normal values. A peak flowmeter costs $25-$50 and is useful to monitor therapy for asthmatics.

ECG: Sinus tachycardia is an important baseline indicator because use of some bronchodilators (e.g., metaproterenol, terbutaline) may produce cardiac stimulant effects and dysrhythmias. Prominent P waves appear in long-term asthma.

COLLABORATIVE MANAGEMENT

Primarily, management is directed toward decreasing bronchospasm and increasing pulmonary ventilation.

Acute phase

O₂ therapy: Generally, these patients experience mild to moderate hypoxemia. Low-flow (1-3 L/min) O_2 is delivered via nasal cannula with humidity.

Pharmacotherapy: Initiated to relieve bronchospasm and continued until wheezing subsides and PFTs return to baseline.

Bronchodilators: Dilate smooth muscles of the airways (Table 1-5).

Corticosteroids: To inhibit the inflammatory response.

IV STEROIDS (HYDROCORTISONE OR METHYLPREDNISOLONE):   To gain control of inflammation in severe attacks. Dosage varies according to severity of the episode and whether patient is currently taking steroids.

ORAL STEROIDS (PREDNISONE OR METHYLPREDNISOLONE):   Once stabilized in acute phases the patient begins taking oral steroids (dosage depends on severity of symptoms and patient weight, but commonly 1 mg/kg daily). Steroids are contraindicated in patients with TB, diabetes, and peptic ulcer.

> **Caution:**   Acute adrenal insufficiency can develop in patients who take steroids routinely at home if these drugs are not given to the patient during hospitalization.

Antibiotics: Initiated if there is concurrent fever, leukocytosis, changes in color and amount of sputum, or other indicators of superimposed infection.

Fluid replacement: To maintain adequate hydration. Generally, crystalloid fluids (i.e., 5% dextrose in water or 5% dextrose in normal saline) are used.

Chest physiotherapy: Generally contraindicated in acute phases because of the hyperreactive state of airways. The patient may benefit from the cautious use of percussion and postural drainage to help mobilize secretions.

Chronic phase

Nebulizer/aerosolized bronchodilators: Usually prescribed for short-term, acute exacerbations of symptoms. However, some patients require maintenance doses to prevent recurrent attacks.

Steroids

Oral steroids (prednisone or methylprednisolone):   Usually, patients are gradually weaned from the steroids over 2-3 wk. Some patients may require low-dose steroids indefinitely, that is, 5 mg qd or qod.

Inhaled steroids (beclomethasone, flunisolide, triamcinolone acetonide):   Have become the mainstay of interim therapy to prevent or reduce the incidence of acute asthmatic attacks. Dosage is commonly 2-4 inhalations 2-4 times per day. Some patients use inhalant bronchodilators simultaneously with the steroid inhalers. To maximize effectiveness of the steroid inhaler, these patients should be taught to use the bronchodilator as prescribed, wait

TABLE 1-5   Bronchodilators Used in the Treatment of Acute Asthma

Medication	Usual dosage	Action	Side effects
Epinephrine	0.2-0.5 ml of 1:1000 solution given SC q15-30min	Immediate adrenergic effects; activates adrenergic sympathomimetic receptors; acts on α-, β_1-, and β_2-receptors; relieves bronchospasm	Cardiac stimulation, palpitations, anxiety
Sympathomimetic drugs (ephedrine, isoproterenol, isoetharine, metaproterenol, albuterol, bitolterol, pirbuterol, salmeterol, terbutaline)	Varies with each agent; many are given as 2 inhalations 3 or 4 times daily	β_2-Selective adrenergic agonists, allow bronchodilation	Restlessness, anxiety, tremor, headaches, dizziness, palpitations, tachycardia, hypertension, dysrhythmias, weakness, hyperglycemia, urinary retention, muscle tremors
Anticholinergic drugs (ipratropium, glycopyrrolate)	2 inhalations 4 times daily	Anticholinergic, antimuscarinic, and parasympatholytic; depress bronchial secretions and dilate bronchi	Nervousness, dizziness, headache, blurred vision, dry mouth, nausea, urinary hesitance and retention, dysphagia
Methylxanthines (theophylline, aminephylline)	*Loading dosage:* 6 mg/kg given as IV bolus. **Note:** Loading dose may be omitted if patient is already taking oral methylxanthine and serum level is therapeutic. *Maintenance dosage:* 0.1-0.5 µg/kg/hr given via continuous IV infusion	Short-acting nonadrenergic; directly relaxes smooth muscle of bronchial airways and pulmonary vasculature	Nausea, vomiting, GI bleeding, gastric distress, HR >120 bpm, decreased BP, restlessness. **Note:** Because toxic levels are close to therapeutic loads, serum levels should be monitored to ensure correct dosage adjustment; dysrhythmias may result from toxic levels of theophylline

SC, Subcutaneous; *IV*, intravenous; *GI*, gastrointestinal; *HR*, heart rate; *BP*, blood pressure.
Note: Isoproterenol and isoetharine are two inhalants usually avoided during acute asthma because the patient's gas flow may be too minimal to provide adequate distribution of medication.

10-15 min, and then use the steroid inhalant. Steroid inhalers may result in fungal overgrowth of the mouth or pharynx; patients should rinse their mouth after each dose.

Nonsteroidal antiinflammatory inhalers (cromolyn, nedocromil sodium): To treat exacerbations in extrinsic asthma. These agents are suspected to mediate endothelial response to allergens and thus prevent bronchospasm. Cromolyn is thought to inhibit secretion of the slow-reacting substance of anaphylaxis (SRS-A) from mast cells. Not all patients benefit from cromolyn. Usual dosage is 20-mg capsules given with a spinhaler. (A spinhaler is an inhaler that uses a medication capsule, which is crushed when the inhaler is conpressed.) Nedocromil sodium is a pyranoquinoline that acts to inhibit a variety of airway inflammatory cells. Nedocromil is more potent than cromolyn and used for more severe forms of asthma.

Methylxanthines (aminophylline, theophylline): Although methylxanthines were formerly first-line therapeutic agents, their use is being curtailed because of the prominence of life-threatening side effects. When methylxanthines are used, dosage is carefully monitored by blood levels of theophylline.

NURSING DIAGNOSES AND INTERVENTIONS

Impaired gas exchange related to altered oxygen supply secondary to decreased alveolar ventilation as a result of narrowed airways

Desired outcomes: Following treatment/intervention, patient has adequate gas exchange as evidenced by RR 12-20 breaths/min (or values consistent with patient's baseline). Before hospital discharge, patient's ABG values are as follows: Pao_2 ≥80 mm Hg, $Paco_2$ 35-45 mm Hg, and pH 7.35-7.45; or oximetry readings demonstrating O_2 saturation >92%.

- Observe for signs and symptoms of hypoxia (e.g., agitation, mental status changes, anxiety, restlessness, changes in mental status or LOC). Remember that cyanosis of the lips and nail beds is a late indicator of hypoxia.
- Position patient for comfort and to promote optimal gas exchange. Usually this is accomplished using high Fowler's position, with the patient leaning forward and elbows propped on the over-the-bed table to promote maximal chest expansion. Pad the over-the-bed table with pillows or blankets to decrease patient discomfort. Record patient's response to positioning.
- Auscultate breath sounds q2-4hr or more frequently as indicated by the patient's condition. Monitor for decreased or adventitious sounds (e.g., crackles [rales], rhonchi, wheezes).
- Monitor oximetry readings; report O_2 saturation ≤92% because this can indicate a need for O_2 therapy.
- Monitor ABG results. Be alert to decreasing Pao_2 and increasing $Paco_2$, which can signal respiratory compromise.
- Deliver and monitor O_2 and humidity as prescribed. **Note:** Be aware that patients with long-standing asthma may have developed concurrent COPD and may not tolerate oxygen at a delivery of >2 L/min, which can suppress the centrally mediated respiratory drive.

NIC: Acid-Base Monitoring; Airway Management; Bedside Laboratory Testing; Oxygen Therapy; Respiratory Monitoring; Teaching: Disease Process; Teaching: Individual

See Also: "Emphysema" for **Ineffective breathing pattern,** p. 41; for anxiety, see Appendix One, p. 791. For other nursing diagnoses related to psychosocial interventions, see Appendix One, "Caring for Patients With Cancer and Other Life-Disrupting Illnesses," p. 791.

PATIENT-FAMILY TEACHING AND DISCHARGE PLANNING

When providing patient-family teaching, focus on sensory information; avoid giving excessive information; and initiate a visiting nurse referral for necessary follow-up teaching. Consider including verbal and written information about the following:

- Irritants that can precipitate an attack and the importance of removing these irritants from patient's environment.
- Signs and symptoms of pulmonary infection (e.g., increased cough, increasing sputum production, change in color of sputum from clear white to yellow-green, fever) or bronchial irritation (e.g., dry, hacking cough).
- Medications, including drug name, route, purpose, dosage, precautions, drug/drug and food/drug interactions, and potential side effects.
- Teach the patient the proper use of metered-dose inhalers, including use of a spacer (if indicated) to facilitate medication inhalation. Document adequate return demonstration by discharge. Remind the patient that OTC inhalers contain medications that can interfere with prescribed therapy. Instruct the patient to contact his or her health care provider before taking *any* OTC medications. Instruct the patient in the sequencing of inhalers, that is, bronchodilator inhalers 15 min before administration of steroidal inhalers.
- If the patient will take corticosteroids while at home, provide instructions accordingly to ensure that the patient takes the correct amount, particularly during the period in which the medication will be tapered.
- Signs and symptoms of pneumonia and the importance of reporting them promptly to a health care professional should they recur. Teach patient's significant others that changes in mental status may be the only indicator of pneumonia if patient is elderly.
- Importance of avoiding contact with infectious individuals, especially those with respiratory infections.
- Recommend that patient receive a pneumococcal vaccination and annual influenza vaccination.
- Importance of follow-up care. Confirm date and time of next appointment.
- Phone numbers to call should questions or concerns arise about therapy or disease after discharge. Additional general information can be obtained by contacting:

  American Lung Association
  1740 Broadway
  New York, NY 10019-4374   (212) 315-8700
  WWW address: *http://www.lungusa.org*

- For patients who smoke: elimination of smoking; refer patient to a "stop smoking" program, as appropriate. The following free brochures outline ways to help patients stop smoking:

  How to Help Your Patients Stop Using Tobacco: A National Cancer Institute Manual for the Oral Health Team, from the Smoking and Tobacco Control Program of the National Cancer Institute; call 1-800-4-CANCER.

  Clinical Practice Guideline: A Quick Reference Guide for Smoking Cessation Specialists, from the Agency for Health Care Policy and Research (AHCPR); call 1-800-358-9295.

Chronic bronchitis

Chronic bronchitis is the most common respiratory disease in the United States. It occurs in individuals who have smoked cigarettes for a long time or lived in areas of severe air pollution. The extent of the disease depends on the length of time the lungs have been exposed to pollutants.

Airway changes that occur with this disease result from chronic airway inflammation and irritation. Pathologic changes in the airways include loss of ciliary action, hypertrophy of mucosal glands (goblet cell hyperplasia), and edema of bronchial mucosa, all of which contribute to increased mucus production. Increased mucus, decreased mucociliary movement, and corresponding loss of moisture by convection allow the formation of mucus plugs. Mucus plugs can eventually obstruct the bronchioles. As the disease progresses, there is associated destruction of lung tissue used in gas exchange, resulting in inadequate ventilation. Recurrent upper respiratory infections (URIs) with *Streptococcus pneumoniae* and *Haemophilus influenzae* are common in this population secondary to the inability to clear the bronchial tree of mucus. As the disease progresses, acute exacerbations increase in severity and duration. Respiratory failure and cardiac problems can develop.

ASSESSMENT

Chronic indicators: Morning cough, clear and copious secretions, anorexia, cyanosis, dependent edema.

Acute indicators (exacerbation):   Fever; dyspnea, SOB, orthopnea; discolored, thick, tenacious sputum.

Physical assessment: Use of accessory muscles of respiration, prolonged expiratory phase, digital clubbing, decreased thoracic expansion, dullness over areas of consolidation, adventitious breath sounds (especially coarse rhonchi and wheezing), ankle edema, distended neck veins, bloated appearance.

DIAGNOSTIC TESTS

Chest x-ray: Will reveal normal AP diameter, nearly normal diaphragm position, and increased peripheral lung markings.

ABG values: Will reveal hypoxemia (Pao_2 <60 mm Hg) and hypercapnia ($Paco_2$ >50-60 mm Hg) in most patients. Baseline pH may be 7.35-7.38, but during acute exacerbation, as the $Paco_2$ increases, pH may fall below 7.35.

Oximetry: Will reveal decreased O_2 saturation (≤92%).

Sputum culture: May reveal presence of infective organisms. Sputum specimens are best collected when the patient first wakes in the morning.

CBC: Will reveal chronically elevated Hgb in the presence of chronic hypoxemia and elevated WBC count in the presence of acute bacterial infection.

Pulmonary function tests: Will show reduced vital capacity, increased residual volume caused by trapping of air, and increased expiratory reserve volume. For descriptions and normal values of these tests, see Table 1-4.

COLLABORATIVE MANAGEMENT

O_2 therapy: To treat hypoxemia. It is used cautiously and at a low flow rate (1-2 L/min) in patients with chronic CO_2 retention for whom hypoxemia, rather than hypercapnia, stimulates the respiratory drive.

Pharmacotherapy

Bronchodilators: To open the airways by relaxing smooth muscles. The resultant increased air flow may help loosen mucus (see Table 1-5).

Steroids (i.e., prednisone):   To decrease inflammation, thereby increasing air flow. **Note:** Acute adrenal insufficiency can develop in patients who take steroids routinely at home if these drugs are not given during hospitalization.

Antibiotics: Based on sensitivity studies from sputum cultures.

Chest physiotherapy: To help loosen and mobilize pulmonary secretions.

IV or oral fluids: To promote adequate hydration.

Diuretics or sodium (Na^+) restriction: To reduce fluid overload in the presence of cardiac complications, such as heart failure.

NURSING DIAGNOSES AND INTERVENTIONS

Ineffective airway clearance related to decreased energy, which results in ineffective cough, or related to presence of increased tracheobronchial secretions

Desired outcome: Following intervention, patient coughs appropriately and has effective airway clearance as evidenced by absence of adventitious breath sounds.

- Auscultate breath sounds q2-4hr (or as indicated by the patient's condition) and after coughing. Be alert to and report changes in adventitious breath sounds.
- Teach patient the "double cough" technique:
  —Sit upright with upper body flexed forward slightly.
  —Take two to three breaths, and exhale passively.
  —Inhale again, but only to the mid-inspiratory point.
  —Exhale by coughing quickly two to three times.
  This technique prevents small airway collapse, which can occur with forceful coughing.
- Administer chest physiotherapy as prescribed to mobilize secretions.
- When not otherwise indicated, encourage fluid intake (≥ 2.5 L/day) to decrease viscosity of the sputum.

NIC: Airway Management; Airway Suctioning; Chest Physiotherapy; Cough Enhancement; Oxygen Therapy; Positioning; Respiratory Monitoring

Altered nutrition: Less than body requirements related to decreased intake secondary to fatigue and anorexia

Desired outcome: For a minimum of 24 hr before hospital discharge, patient has adequate nutrition as evidenced by stable weight, positive nitrogen (N) state on N studies, total lymphocyte count ($1500\text{-}4500/mm^3$), and serum albumin 3.5-5.5 g/dl.

- Monitor patient's food and fluid intake. If indicated, obtain dietary consultation for calorie counts.
- Provide diet in small, frequent meals that are nutritious and easy to consume.
- Request a dietitian consultation so that patient can verbalize food likes and dislikes.
- Unless otherwise indicated, provide calories more from unsaturated fat sources (Table 1-6) than from carbohydrate sources. During the process of carbohydrate metabolism, the body uses O_2 and produces CO_2, which is then excreted by the lungs. The patient with COPD takes in less O_2 and retains CO_2. A high-fat diet minimizes this problem because fat generates the least amount of CO_2 for a given amount of O_2 used, whereas carbohydrates generate the most.
- Discuss with the patient and significant others the importance of good nutrition in the treatment of chronic bronchitis.

NIC: Fluid Monitoring; Nutrition Management; Nutrition Counseling; Teaching: Disease Process; Teaching: Prescribed Diet

See Also: "Asthma" for **Impaired gas exchange,** p. 35; "Emphysema" for **Ineffective breathing pattern,** p. 41, and **Activity intolerance,** p. 41; "Heart Failure" for **Fluid volume excess,** p. 70; Appendix One for **Anxiety,** p. 791

TABLE 1-6   Recommended Calorie Sources for Patients With COPD

Foods high in fat	Foods to avoid
Whole milk	Cakes
Cream	Cookies
Evaporated milk	Jams
Cream soups	Pastries
Custards	Sugar-concentrated snacks
Cheese	
Salad and cooking oils	
Margarine	
Mayonnaise	
Nuts	
Meat	
Poultry	
Fish	

COPD, Chronic obstructive pulmonary disease.

PATIENT-FAMILY TEACHING AND DISCHARGE PLANNING

When providing patient-family teaching, focus on sensory information; avoid giving excessive information; and initiate a visiting nurse referral for necessary follow-up teaching. Consider including verbal and written information about the following:

- Use of home O_2, including instructions for when to use it, importance of not increasing prescribed flow rate, precautions, and community resources for O_2 replacement when necessary. Request respiratory therapy consultation to assist with teaching related to O_2 therapy, if indicated.
- Medications, including drug name, route, purpose, dosage, schedule, precautions, drug/drug and food/drug interactions, and potential side effects. If the patient will take corticosteroids while at home, provide instructions accordingly to ensure that the patient takes the correct amount, particularly during the period in which the medication will be tapered.
- Signs and symptoms of heart failure that necessitate medical attention: increased dyspnea; fatigue; increased coughing; changes in the amount, color, or consistency of sputum; swelling of the ankles and legs; fever; and sudden weight gain. Patients with COPD often have right-sided heart failure secondary to cardiac effects of the disease. For more information, see "Heart Failure," p. 68.
- Importance of avoiding contact with infectious individuals, especially those with respiratory infections.
- Recommend that patient receive a pneumococcal vaccination and annual influenza vaccination.
- Review of Na^+-restricted diet (see Table 3-2, p. 133) and other dietary considerations as indicated.
- Importance of pacing activity level to conserve energy.
- Follow-up appointment with health care provider; confirm date and time of next appointment.
- Introduction to local chapter of American Lung Association activities and pulmonary rehabilitation programs. Physical training programs may improve ventilation and cardiac muscle function, which may compensate for nonreversible lung disease.

- Phone numbers to call should questions or concerns arise about therapy or disease after discharge. Additional general information can be obtained by contacting:

  American Lung Association
  1740 Broadway
  New York, NY 10019-4374   (212) 315-8700
  WWW address: *http://www.lungusa.org*

- For patients who smoke: elimination of smoking; refer patient to a "stop smoking" program as appropriate. The following free brochures outline ways to help patients stop smoking:

  How to Help Your Patients Stop Using Tobacco: A National Cancer Institute Manual for the Oral Health Team, from the Smoking and Tobacco Control Program of the National Cancer Institute; call 1-800-4-CANCER.

  Clinical Practice Guideline: A Quick Reference Guide for Smoking Cessation Specialists, from the Agency for Health Care Policy and Research (AHCPR); call 1-800-358-9295.

Emphysema

Pulmonary emphysema is a degenerative process characterized by enlargement of the air spaces distal to the terminal bronchioles accompanied by destruction of the alveolar walls (coalescence of the alveoli). Because of the destruction of the alveoli, terminal airways lose support of surrounding pulmonary parenchymal structure, allowing terminal airways to collapse. Because more pressure can be created on inhalation than on exhalation, it is possible to inspire air past these collapsed terminal airways, but there the air becomes trapped. Distal airways and coalesced alveoli become hyperinflated. Hyperinflation contributes to the loss of lung elasticity, further contributing to inability to adequately exhale inspired air. Emphysema is a progressive disease, and affected individuals can become totally disabled because they must use all available energy for breathing. In the later stages of the disease, pulmonary hypertension develops, leading to cor pulmonale, or right-sided heart failure, a condition that produces cardiac symptoms as well as complicating respiratory problems.

ASSESSMENT

Chronic indicators: Nonproductive cough (unless patient also has bronchitis), dyspnea on exertion, orthopnea, SOB.
Acute indicators (exacerbation):   Increased dyspnea, productive cough, fever, peripheral edema, fatigue.
Physical assessment: Emaciation, increased AP chest diameter, pursed-lip breathing, hypertrophy of accessory muscles of respiration, decreased fremitus over affected lung fields, decreased thoracic excursion, hyperresonance over affected lung fields, decreased breath sounds, and prolonged expiratory phase. Digital clubbing occurs late in the disease.

DIAGNOSTIC TESTS

Chest x-ray: Will show hyperinflation of the lungs, an increased AP diameter, lowered and flattened diaphragm, and a small cardiac silhouette. With cor pulmonale the pulmonary vasculature may appear engorged and the heart size enlarged.
ABG values: May reveal a slight decrease in Pao_2. As disease progresses, the Pao_2 will continue to decrease and $Paco_2$ may increase because of hypoventilation and CO_2 retention. Early in the disease process, however, the $Paco_2$ may

be normal if the patient has good ventilation-perfusion matching. The pH will be low-normal once CO_2 retention begins.

Oximetry: May reveal decreased O_2 saturation ($\leq$92%).

CBC: May reveal a chronically elevated RBC count (polycythemia) later in the disease process as a compensatory response to chronic hypoxemia. Leukocytosis may be evident with overlying respiratory tract infection.

Pulmonary function tests: Will show an increased total lung capacity, increased residual volume, and decreased forced expiratory reserve volume. The vital capacity will be normal or slightly decreased. For descriptions and normal values of these tests, see Table 1-4.

ECG: May reveal atrial and ventricular dysrhythmias. Most patients will have an atrial dysrhythmia as a result of atrial dilation and right ventricular hypertrophy caused by pulmonary hypertension.

Sputum culture: May be requested to determine presence of pulmonary infection.

COLLABORATIVE MANAGEMENT

See "Chronic Bronchitis," p. 37.

NURSING DIAGNOSES AND INTERVENTIONS

Ineffective breathing pattern related to decreased lung expansion secondary to chronic air flow limitations

Desired outcome: Following treatment/intervention, patient's breathing pattern improves as evidenced by reduction in or absence of dyspnea and movement toward a state of eupnea.

- Assess patient's respiratory status q2-4hr, being alert for indicators of respiratory distress (i.e., agitation, restlessness, changes in mental status, decreased LOC, use of accessory muscles of respiration). Auscultate breath sounds; report a decrease in breath sounds or an increase in adventitious breath sounds.
- Instruct patient in the use of pursed-lip breathing, which increases intraluminal air pressure and thus internal stability to the airways and may prevent airway collapse during expiration, as follows:
  —Sit upright with hands on thighs, or lean forward with elbows propped on the over-the-bed table.
  —Inhale slowly through the nose with the mouth closed.
  —Form lips in an *O* shape as though whistling.
  —Exhale slowly through pursed lips. Exhalation should take twice as long as inhalation (e.g., count to 5 on inhalation; count to 10 on exhalation).

Record patient's response to breathing technique.
- Administer bronchodilator therapy as prescribed. Monitor patient for side effects, including tachycardia and dysrhythmias.
- Monitor patient's response to prescribed O_2 therapy. Be aware that high concentrations of O_2 can depress the respiratory drive in individuals with chronic CO_2 retention.
- Monitor oximetry readings; report O_2 saturation $\leq$92% because this can indicate a need for O_2 therapy.
- Monitor serial ABG values. Patients with chronic CO_2 retention may have chronically compensated respiratory acidosis with a low-normal pH (7.35-7.38) and a $Paco_2$ >45 mm Hg.

NIC: Airway Management; Cough Enhancement; Oxygen Therapy; Respiratory Management; Teaching: Procedure/Treatment; Teaching: Psychomotor Skill

Activity intolerance related to imbalance between oxygen supply and demand secondary to inefficient work of breathing

Desired outcome: Patient reports decreasing dyspnea during activity or exercise and rates his or her perceived exertion at $\leq$3 on a 0-10 scale.

- Maintain prescribed activity levels, and explain rationale to patient.
- Monitor patient's respiratory response to activity. Activity intolerance is indicated by excessively increased respiratory rate (e.g., >10 breaths/min above baseline) and depth, dyspnea, and use of accessory muscles of respiration. Ask patient to rate perceived exertion (see p. 739 for a description). If activity intolerance is noted, instruct patient to stop the activity and rest.
- Facilitate coordination across health care providers to provide rest periods between care activities to decrease oxygen demand. Allow 90 min for undisturbed rest.
- Assist patient with active ROM exercises to build stamina and prevent complications of decreased mobility. For more information, see **Risk for activity intolerance** in Appendix One, "Caring for Patients on Prolonged Bed Rest," p. 738.

NIC: Activity Therapy; Body Mechanics Promotion; Energy Management; Exercise Promotion; Respiratory Monitoring; Teaching: Prescribed Activity/ Exercise

---

See Also: "Asthma" for **Impaired gas exchange,** p. 35; "Chronic Bronchitis" for **Ineffective airway clearance,** p. 38, and **Altered nutrition: less than body requirements,** p. 38; psychosocial nursing diagnoses and interventions in Appendix One, "Caring for Patients With Cancer and Other Life-Disrupting Illnesses," p. 791.

PATIENT-FAMILY TEACHING AND DISCHARGE PLANNING
See "Chronic Bronchitis," p. 36.

Section Four: Restrictive Pulmonary Disorders

Restrictive lung disease is a category of pulmonary pathologic conditions in which restricting alveolar inflation impairs lung function. Restrictive disorders are characterized by decreased vital capacity, reduced resting volumes, and normal airway resistance. Lung compliance (distensibility) decreases, and elastic recoil (deflating force) increases, resulting in an increase in the WOB. Physiologic consequences are similar for all restrictive processes and can be mildly, moderately, or severely debilitating for the patient. See Table 1-7 for some of the pathologic conditions identified as causes of restrictive lung disease. This section discusses pulmonary fibrosis.

Pulmonary fibrosis

The physiologic mechanisms in the development of pulmonary fibrosis are not clearly defined. It is theorized that pulmonary fibrosis occurs as a reaction to the inhalation of noxious materials or exposure to radiation. The fibrotic process is a continuous one and does not abate, even when the causative agent is no longer present. Fibrotic tissue forms as a natural process of tissue repair following infection, inflammation, or destruction of tissue. The fibrosis affects primarily the alveoli and causes an increase in the bronchial diameter in relation to lung volume. WOB is increased because of decreased lung compliance, and affected individuals adopt a rapid, shallow breathing pattern since it requires less energy. Cardiac complications can occur as a result of pulmonary hypertension.

T A B L E 1 - 7   Causative Factors in Development of Restrictive Lung Disease

Extrapulmonary (involves respiratory muscles, pleura, and chest wall)	Intrapulmonary (involves lung parenchyma)
Bony deformities	Alveolar fibrosis, secondary to:
Scoliosis	Infection
Ankylosing spondylitis	Chronic aspiration
Neuromuscular disorders	Inhalation of toxins
Guillain-Barré syndrome	Chemotherapy
Amyotrophic lateral sclerosis	Radiation therapy
Myasthenia gravis	Alveolar cell cancer
Muscular dystrophy	Goodpasture's syndrome
Pleural effusion	Idiopathic
Pleural thickening	Pneumoconioses
Pneumothorax	Asbestosis
Ascites	Silicosis
Obesity	Black lung
Pregnancy	Atelectasis
	Pulmonary edema
	Lung resection

ASSESSMENT

The causative factors in pulmonary fibrosis are very difficult to uncover. A meticulous history of life-style, occupation, habits, and background can provide valuable information.

Signs and symptoms: Dyspnea, cough.

Physical assessment: Tachypnea, shallow respirations, cyanosis, digital clubbing, use of accessory muscles of respiration, and crackles.

Risk factors: See Table 1-7.

DIAGNOSTIC TESTS

Chest x-ray: Reveals the extent of the fibrosis as evidenced by diffuse, mottled shadowing of the lung fields (honeycombing).

Pulmonary function tests: Will demonstrate concentric reduction in lung volumes; normal airway resistance.

ABG values: Pao_2 may be normal at rest but may decrease with exercise. $Paco_2$ may be within normal limits secondary to tachypnea but may increase in late stages of the disease.

Oximetry: May reveal decreased O_2 saturation ($\leq 92\%$), especially with exercise.

Lung biopsy: To determine cause and pathologic mechanism of the process.

COLLABORATIVE MANAGEMENT

Oxygen therapy: To correct the hypoxemia, which will relieve the dyspnea. Generally, low-flow (2-4 L/min) oxygen therapy is indicated.

Corticosteroids: To decrease inflammation. Prednisone is usually given, at 1 mg/kg daily.

Lung transplantation: Emerging as a therapy for patients who have a functional disability refractory to conventional therapies and a life expectancy <18 mo without transplantation.

NURSING DIAGNOSES AND INTERVENTIONS

Ineffective breathing pattern related to decreased lung expansion secondary to fibrotic condition in the lungs

Desired outcomes: Following treatment/intervention, patient verbalizes a subjective relief of dyspnea; patient resumes normal respiratory pattern (eupnea).

- Assess respiratory status q2-4hr. Auscultate breath sounds, and report increasing crackles (rales) or other adventitious sounds.
- Monitor patient's serial ABG values for decreasing Pao_2 or oximetry readings demonstrating O_2 saturation <92% and be alert to early signs of hypoxia (restlessness, changes in mental status, anxiety, dyspnea), especially with activity.
- Assist patient in identifying ways to conserve energy during daily activities (e.g., planning frequent rest periods before and after activities as needed, stopping the activity and resting if dyspnea increases, waiting for 1 hr after eating before engaging in activities, because digestion draws blood and hence O_2 away from the muscles). As indicated, arrange for a consultation with occupational therapist or physical therapist.
- Deliver O_2 as prescribed. Remember that the Pao_2 may be normal at rest but may decrease with exercise. The patient may require supplemental O_2 with activity.

NIC: Emotional Support; Energy Management; Exercise Promotion; Oxygen Therapy; Respiratory Management; Teaching: Procedure/Treatment

Knowledge deficit: side effects of corticosteroids

Desired outcome: Within the 24 hr before hospital discharge, patient verbalizes knowledge of the side effects of corticosteroids and the importance of reporting them promptly to the staff or health care provider should they occur.

- Corticosteroids are potent medications used to suppress the immune system that have potentially serious side effects. Alert the patient taking steroids to the potential for the following, depending on the dosage and duration of therapy: poor resistance to infection, increasing BP, mental changes (euphoria, depression, psychosis), hyperglycemia, capillary fragility, and GI bleeding.
- Stress the importance of avoiding individuals known to have infections.
- If the patient receives prolonged corticosteroid therapy, instruct the patient to monitor for sodium and water retention, hypokalemia, edema, buffalo hump, hirsutism, moon face, skin striae and thinning, weight gain, peptic ulcer, headache, muscle wasting, nervousness, insomnia, and metabolic acidosis.

See Also: "Chronic Bronchitis" for **Altered nutrition: less than body requirements,** p. 38; "Glomerulonephritis" for **Knowledge deficit:** Side effects of corticosteroids, p. 134; psychosocial nursing diagnoses in Appendix One, "Caring for Patients With Cancer and Other Life-Disrupting Illnesses," p. 791.

PATIENT-FAMILY TEACHING AND DISCHARGE PLANNING

When providing patient-family teaching, focus on sensory information; avoid giving excessive information; and initiate a visiting nurse referral for necessary follow-up teaching. Consider including verbal and written information about the following:

- Importance of pacing activities to tolerance and avoiding strenuous exercises that would increase cardiac and respiratory symptoms.
- Medications, including drug name, dosage, purpose, schedule, precautions, drug/drug and food/drug interactions, and potential side effects. It is likely

that the patient will take corticosteroids while at home. Provide instructions accordingly to ensure that the patient takes the correct amount, particularly during the period in which the medication will be tapered.

- Use of O_2 and the necessary precautions if it is to be used at home.
- Importance of avoiding contact with infectious individuals, especially those with respiratory infections.
- Recommend that patient receive a pneumococcal vaccination and annual influenza vaccination.
- Date and time of follow-up visit.
- Phone numbers to call should questions or concerns arise about therapy or disease after discharge. Additional general information can be obtained by contacting:

American Lung Association
1740 Broadway
New York, NY 10019-4374   (212) 315-8700
WWW address: *http://www.lungusa.org*

- For patients awaiting lung transplantation, provide the following information as appropriate:

The United Network for Organ Sharing
UNOS Communication Department
P.O. Box 13770
Richmond, VA 23225   (804) 330-8561 or (800) 243-6667 (voice mail)
WWW address: *http://www.unos.org*

Section Five: Lung Cancer

Lung cancer is the most common cause of cancer death in both American men and women. Each year about 150,000 new cases of lung cancer are diagnosed and about 100,000 people die of lung cancer. Of individuals diagnosed with lung cancer, 87% die in less than 5 yr. The length of survival depends on the tumor histology and stage of the disease at the time treatment begins. Statistically, 80%-90% of lung cancers occur among people who smoke tobacco. Patients at high risk for cancer began smoking before 25 yr of age, smoked ≥ one pack each day for 20 yr, and are older than 50 yr. In addition, other environmental and occupational exposures to chemicals, toxins, and pollutants contribute to the development of this disease; for example, living in an environment with asbestos significantly increases the risk of lung cancer.

Lung cancer can be categorized as small cell or non–small cell cancer. *Small cell lung cancer (SCLC)* is composed of classic or "oat" cells, intermediate cells, and mixed cells. SCLC accounts for 25%-30% of all lung cancers and has the following characteristics: (1) it arises from basal lining of bronchial mucosa; (2) it shows rapid cell growth (is highly proliferative); (3) it has a propensity for widespread dissemination; and (4) it is highly sensitive to cytotoxic drugs and radiation therapy. When first seen, approximately 60% of patients with SCLC have extensive disease and 40% have limited disease. The period of time between onset of symptoms and diagnosis is approximately 3-4 mo, and a change in the character of a chronic cough is the typical presenting symptom. Tumors generally form in larger, central bronchi, causing obstruction, wheezing, coughing, and dyspnea. Hemoptysis occurs as cancers erode blood vessels and capillaries in the airways. The tumors can compress nerves, causing radiating chest pain.

Non–small cell lung cancer (NSCLC) is composed of epidermoid (squamous cell), adenocarcinoma, and large cell cancer. NSCLC accounts for approximately 70%-75% of all lung cancers and possesses the following characteristics: (1) it arises from large bronchi (squamous) or periphery of lung (adenocarcinoma); (2) it is slower growing (less proliferative); (3) squamous cell generally is less disseminated; (4) adenocarcinoma and large cell often have distant metastases; (5) response to therapy is limited except for surgical excision (only form of treatment currently considered curative); and (6) it is generally not curable once metastasized outside the thoracic cavity.

Most patients have advanced disease at the time of diagnosis and receive multimodality therapy with minimal or partial response. Ultimately patients succumb to both local and distant disease with multiple complications. Tumors generally grow in the small peripheral bronchi and alveoli and may press against nerves in the pleural tissues. Typical presenting symptoms include shortness of breath and sharp chest pain on inspiration.

ASSESSMENT

Patients often are asymptomatic in early stages of the disease process. When symptoms do occur, they are likely to be vague and easily confused with other pulmonary conditions.

Early indicators: Cough, dyspnea, SOB, change in character of sputum, hemoptysis, fatigue, dull chest pain, wheezing, frequent respiratory infections.

Advanced disease: Weakness, anorexia, dysphagia, hoarseness, weight loss. Metastasis can occur to the liver, adrenal glands, brain, skeleton, and kidney, in decreasing order of frequency, and result in symptoms associated with pathologic conditions of these tissues.

Physical assessment: Presence of adventitious breath sounds and pleural friction rub. In advanced disease, the patient may exhibit use of accessory muscles of respiration, nasal flaring, cyanosis, pleural effusion, and severe muscle wasting.

DIAGNOSTIC TESTS

Chest x-ray: To define tumor outline. X-ray examination may reveal presence of solitary nodules and possibly pleural effusion, atelectasis, and lymph node enlargement.

Sputum for cytology: Generally, a first morning specimen is obtained for 3 consecutive days. Sputum contains cells that shed from the tumor, which aids in identifying tumor type.

Flexible fiberoptic bronchoscopy: To visualize central tumor directly and take tissue samples for biopsy, along with bronchial washings. May be done with conscious sedation or general anesthesia.

Fine-needle aspiration: Needle biopsy with fluoroscopic or computed tomographic (CT) guidance to obtain tissue samples from peripheral tumor for histologic examination.

Thoracoscopy: Uses an endoscope placed into the thoracic cavity to allow direct visualization and biopsy of suspicious growths. This may be done with the patient under general or local anesthesia.

Lung tomogram: To locate tumor and determine depth and extent.

Other tests: Once the cancer has metastasized from the primary site to nearby lymph nodes or distant organs, tests may include fluoroscopy; abdominal and chest CT scan; radionuclide studies of liver, bone, and brain; bone marrow aspiration; and mediastinoscopy to obtain a biopsy specimen from hilar nodes.

COLLABORATIVE MANAGEMENT

The most effective intervention is prevention. Treatment of disease is planned according to histology, location, and extent of the disease.

Grading and staging the disease: To formulate a prognosis and guide treatment. The degree of grading and staging is determined by the extent of metastasis and tissue involvement: the more tissue involved and the greater the metastasis, the higher the grade and stage. The TNM criteria of the American Joint Committee for Cancer Staging and End Results Reporting are commonly used. In this system, "T" is defined by the size and location of the tumor. Nodes

("N") are graded as follows: negative (N_0); involving only ipsilateral hilar nodes (N_1); involving ipsilateral mediastinal or subcarinal nodes (N_2); or involving a wider variety of nodes (N_3). The "M" indicates metastasis as either negative (M_0) or present (M_1).

Surgery: To excise a tumor confined to lung tissue and remove involved lymph nodes. This may involve lobectomy, bilobectomy on the right side, or pneumonectomy. A secondary function of surgical excision is to permit accurate staging of the disease.

Radiation therapy: Use can be curative, adjuvant to chemotherapy/surgery, or palliative. It is used if the tumor has grown to adjacent tissues or if cancer has produced clearly defined secondary tumors elsewhere in the body. Usual dose is 2500-6000 cGy delivered over a 5- to 6-wk period. This therapy generally shrinks tumors more often than eradicating them. Side effects include anorexia, esophagitis, dysphagia, radiation pneumonitis, and skin changes.

Chemotherapy: Used when primary tumor extends beyond the lungs into surrounding tissues or metastasizes outside the lungs. It is also given to patients with SCLC whose disease has not yet spread beyond the lung. Treatment agents are generally used in combination. Drugs commonly used include cyclophosphamide, doxorubicin, methotrexate, procarbazine, mitomycin C, vinblastine, vincristine, etopside, cisplatin, and bleomycin.

Brachytherapy: Used as an alterative palliative therapy or for unresectable tumors. Radioactive seeds of iodine-125 are surgically placed into the tumor mass, and iridium-192 is instilled through thoracic catheters into the mediastinum.

Antiemetics: To control nausea and vomiting associated with chemotherapy. Generally, phenothiazines, metaclopramide, or ondansetron is used.

Analgesics: To control pain.

Sedatives: Benzodiazepines are given for their amnesic effects, helping patients forget unpleasantness of the chemotherapy and thus promoting therapy continuation.

NURSING DIAGNOSES AND INTERVENTIONS

Pain related to biologic and physiologic agents secondary to compression of nerves by the tumor

Desired outcome: Within 1 hr of intervention, patient's subjective perception of pain decreases, as documented by a pain scale.

- Assess and document the following: location, description, onset, duration, and factors that precipitate and alleviate patient's pain. Devise a pain scale with the patient rating pain from 0 (no pain) to 10 (worst pain).
- Offer prescribed analgesics. Encourage patient to ask for pain medication before pain becomes severe. If patient has more than one analgesic, confer with patient regarding which would be more beneficial for pain control. Document the patient's subjective pain rating before and after receiving medication, using the pain scale.
- Position patient for comfort.
- Encourage patient to use relaxation techniques (e.g., deep breathing, imagery, meditation, biofeedback) and diversional activities (e.g., television, books, radio, crafts). For a description of an effective relaxation technique, see "Coronary Artery Disease" for **Health-seeking behaviors:** Relaxation technique effective for stress reduction, p. 59.

For other effective pain interventions, see Appendix One, "Caring for Preoperative and Postoperative Patients," **Pain,** p. 719.

NIC: Analgesic Administration; Coping Enhancement; Environment Management: Comfort; Pain Management; Patient Controlled Analgesia (PCA) Assistance; Simple Guided Imagery; Simple Relaxation Therapy; Sleep Enhancement

> **See Also:** "Pulmonary Fibrosis" for **Ineffective breathing pattern** related to decreased lung expansion, p. 44; Appendix One, "Caring for Preoperative and Postoperative Patients," p. 717, and "Caring for Patients With Cancer and Other Life-disrupting Illnesses," p. 747.

PATIENT-FAMILY TEACHING AND DISCHARGE PLANNING

When providing patient-family teaching, focus on sensory information; avoid giving excessive information; and initiate a visiting nurse referral for necessary follow-up teaching. Consider including verbal and written information about the following:

- Signs and symptoms of respiratory complications that may necessitate medical attention: increased dyspnea, cyanosis, agitation.
- If surgery was performed, the indicators of wound infection: redness and swelling at wound site, local warmth, purulent drainage, pain, fever.
- Medications, including drug name, purpose, dosage, schedule, precautions, drug/drug and food/drug interactions, and potential side effects.
- Operation of all equipment that will be used at home, including O_2.
- Need for follow-up care with health care provider; confirm date and time of next appointment.
- Phone numbers to call should questions or concerns arise about therapy or disease after discharge. Additional general information can be obtained by contacting:

  The American Cancer Society
  1599 Clifton Road NE
  Atlanta, GA 30329   (800) ACS-2345
  WWW address: *http://www.cancer.org*

  National Cancer Institute Information Service (CIS)
  Bldg. 31, Room 10A16
  9000 Rockville Pike
  Bethesda, MD 20892   (800) 422-6237

  American Lung Association
  1740 Broadway
  New York, NY 10019-4374   (212) 315-8700
  WWW address: *http://www.lungusa.org*

- Phone numbers to call should questions or concerns arise about hospice after discharge. Information for these patients can be obtained by contacting:

  National Hospice Association
  1901 North Moore St., Suite 901
  Arlington, VA 22209   (703) 243-5900; (703) 525-5762 FAX
  WWW address: *http://www.nho.org*

- For patients who continue to smoke: elimination of smoking; refer patient to a "stop smoking" program as appropriate. The following free brochures outline ways to help patients stop smoking:

  How to Help Your Patients Stop Using Tobacco: A National Cancer Institute Manual for the Oral Health Team, from the Smoking and Tobacco Control Program of the National Cancer Institute; call 1-800-4-CANCER.

  Clinical Practice Guideline: A Quick Reference Guide for Smoking Cessation Specialists, from the Agency for Health Care Policy and Research (AHCPR); call 1-800-358-9295.

Selected Bibliography

Abou-Shala N, MacIntyre N: Emergent management of acute asthma, *Med Clin North Am* 80(4):677-699, 1996.

Allen EA: Tuberculosis and other mycobacterial infections of the lung. In Thurlbeck WM, Chung AM, editors: *Pathology of the lung,* New York, 1995, Thieme Medical Publishers.

Apple S: New trends in thrombolytic therapy, *RN* 59(1):30-35, 1996.

Bartter T et al: The evolution of pleural effusion, *Chest* 106(4):1209-1214, 1994.

Baum GL, Wolinsky E: *Textbook of pulmonary disease,* Boston, 1994, Little, Brown.

Borkgren M, Gronckiwicz C: Update your asthma care from hospital to home, *Am J Nurs* 95(1):26-35, 1995.

Brooks-Brunn JA: Postoperative atelectasis and pneumonia, *Heart Lung* 24(2):94-115, 1995.

Celli B: Current thoughts regarding treatment of chronic obstructive pulmonary disease, *Med Clin North Am* 80(3):589-609, 1996.

Eisenbeis C: Full partner in care: teaching your patient how to manage her asthma, *Nursing* 26(1):48-51, 1996.

Esler R et al: Patient centered pneumonia care: a case management success story, *Am J Nurs* 94(11):34-38, 1994.

Finkelstein L: Sputum testing for TB: getting good specimens, *Am J Nurs* 96(2):14, 1996.

Goldstone J: Veins & lymphatics. In Way LW, editor: *Current surgical diagnosis and treatment,* ed 10, Norwalk, Conn, 1994, Appleton & Lange.

Greenfield LJ, Proctor MC: Endovascular methods for caval interruption, *Semin Vasc Surg* 10(4):310-314, 1997.

Held J: Caring for a patient with lung cancer, *Nursing* 25(10):34-45, 1995.

Holcroft JW, Wisner DH: Shock and acute pulmonary failure in surgical patients. In Way LW, editor, *Current surgical diagnosis and treatment,* ed 10, Norwalk, Conn, 1994, Appleton & Lange.

Howland W: Defending your patient against nosocomial pneumonia, *Nursing* 25(8):62-62, 1995.

Interqual, *The ISD-A review system with adult ISD criteria,* Northhampton, NH, and Marlboro, Mass, August 1992, Interqual.

Keep NB: Identifying pulmonary embolism, *Am J Nurs* 95(4):52, 1995.

Kim MJ, McFarland GK, McLane AM: *Pocket guide to nursing diagnoses,* ed 7, St Louis, 1997, Mosby.

Majoros K et al: Pulmonary embolism: targeting an elusive enemy, *Nursing* 26(4):27-32, 1996.

McCloskey JC, Bulechek GM, editors: *Nursing interventions classification (NIC),* ed 2, St Louis, 1996, Mosby.

Moine P et al: Severe community acquired pneumonia: etiology, epidemiology and prognosis factors, *Chest* 105(5):1487-1495, 1994.

Peloquin C: Pharmacology of antimicrobacterial drugs, *Med Clin North Am* 77(6):1253-1262, 1993.

Quigley R: Thoracentesis and chest tube drainage, *Crit Care Clin* 11(1):111-126, 1995.

Repasky TM: Tension pneumothorax, *Am J Nurs* 94(9):47, 1994.

Rutter K: Tension pneumothorax, *Nursing* 25(4):33, 1995.

Savin MA, Shlansky-Goldberg RD: Greenfield filter fixation in large venae cavae, *J Vasc Interv Radiol* 9(1 Pt1):75-80, 1998.

Schreur H et al: Abnormal lung sounds in patients with asthma during episodes with normal lung function, *Chest* 106(1):91-99, 1994.

Sperry S, Birdsall C: Outcomes of a pneumonia critical path, *Nurs Econ* 12(6):332-339, 1992.

Turley K: Thoracic wall, pleura, mediastinum & lung. In Way LW, editor: *Current surgical diagnosis and treatment,* ed 10, Norwalk, Conn, 1994, Appleton & Lange.

Wolff G, Crystal R: Biology of pulmonary fibrosis. In Crystal R, West JB, editors: *The lung: scientific foundations,* Philadelphia, 1997, Lippincott.

2 CARDIOVASCULAR DISORDERS

Section One: Degenerative Cardiovascular Disorders

Cardiomyopathy

Cardiomyopathy is a disorder of the heart muscle, usually of unknown origin. It is classified according to abnormalities in structure and function. The disorder involves the heart muscle and usually results in heart failure.

Dilated (or congestive) cardiomyopathy: Characterized by dilation of all four heart chambers, especially the ventricles. Contractile dysfunction usually is the first sign, followed by heart failure. There is progressive deterioration of cardiac muscle function caused by toxic (e.g., alcohol), metabolic (e.g., thyrotoxicosis), or infectious (e.g., bacterial, viral) agents. Pathophysiologic changes include loss of functioning myofibrils, decreased contractile strength, and dilation, followed by sympathetic nervous system stimulation, increased myocardial oxygen consumption, increased pulmonary pressures, increased venous pressures, and heart failure.

Hypertrophic cardiomyopathy: Characterized by an abnormally hypertrophied left ventricle that is not accompanied by a concomitant increase in cavity size. Therefore filling is restricted and there is the potential for outflow obstruction. This causes increased left atrial and left ventricular pressures, resulting in increased workload and increased pulmonary pressures causing dyspnea. Cardiac function can remain normal for varying periods of time before decompensation occurs. Symptoms include increased diastolic BP, decreased cardiac output, pulmonary hypertension, and right ventricular failure. Although it is theorized that hypertrophic cardiomyopathy has a strong hereditary link, the etiology is unknown. Possible causes include increased circulating catecholamine levels, subendocardial ischemia, or abnormal conduction patterns that lead to abnormal ventricular contraction.

Restrictive cardiomyopathy: Least common in Western countries, it is characterized by restrictive ventricular filling caused by fibrosis, infiltration, hypertrophy, and cardiac stiffness.

ASSESSMENT

Signs and symptoms: Dyspnea usually is the symptom that brings the patient to the health care provider. Decreased exercise tolerance, fatigue, weakness, syncope, peripheral edema, palpitations, right or left ventricular failure, and peripheral or pulmonary emboli also can occur. Chest pain may occur because of ischemia of the hypertrophied muscle.

Physical assessment: Presence of S_3 or S_4 heart sounds and valve murmurs, systolic murmur, prominent apical pulse, increased venous pressure and pulsations, crackles (rales), decreased BP, and increased heart rate (HR) and respiratory rate (RR) related to decreased cardiac output. In addition, hepatomegaly and mild to severe cardiomegaly may be present.

DIAGNOSTIC TESTS

Chest x-ray: To detect cardiac enlargement, particularly of the ventricle and left atrium. Pulmonary hypertension also may be seen.

ECG results: Determined by the extent and location of myocardial involvement. ECG changes indicative of cardiomyopathy include left ventricular hypertrophy, conduction defects, nonspecific ST-segment changes, and Q waves that resemble those found with infarction.

Echocardiography: Will identify thickened ventricular walls, septal thickening, and chamber dilation or restriction, depending on the type of cardiomyopathy. Poor contractility also may be seen if myocardial muscle deterioration has progressed.

Cardiac catheterization: Does not confirm cardiomyopathy, but it can be valuable for ruling out other disorders, such as ischemic heart disease. Findings may include decreased cardiac output, decreased ventricular movement, increased filling pressures, and valvular regurgitation. For further detail, see "Cardiac Catheterization, Angioplasty, and Atherectomy," p. 109.

Endomyocardial biopsy: Sometimes necessary to identify the type of pathologic agent; it can be done during the cardiac catheterization procedure.

Radionuclide studies: May demonstrate contractile dysfunction.

COLLABORATIVE MANAGEMENT

Medical management is aimed toward support, maintenance of normal function for as long as possible, and delaying disease progression.

Controlling symptoms of heart failure: See "Heart Failure," p. 68.

Limiting or restricting activity: To decrease O_2 demand. Activity is increased gradually.

Prohibiting alcohol intake: Alcohol can worsen myopathy.

Pharmacotherapy

Antidysrhythmic agents: To control dysrhythmias.

β-Blockers: To decrease outflow obstruction during exercise (used mainly in hypertrophic forms).

Calcium antagonists: To produce arterial vasodilation, decrease cardiac workload, and improve symptoms and exercise capacity.

Anticoagulants (warfarin sodium):   To prevent embolus formation.

Diuretics: To decrease pulmonary congestion.

Vasodilators: To decrease cardiac workload.

Inotropic agents: To increase contractile strength.

Surgical replacement of valves: See "Cardiac Surgery," p. 113.

Heart transplant (for end-stage disease):   Used for patients in New York Heart Association (NYHA) class IV heart failure (see Table 2-5).

NURSING DIAGNOSES AND INTERVENTIONS

Decreased cardiac output related to negative inotropic changes in the heart (decreased cardiac contractility) secondary to cardiac muscle changes

Desired outcomes: By at least 24 hr before hospital discharge, patient has adequate cardiac output as evidenced by systolic BP ≥90 mm Hg, HR ≤100 bpm, urinary output ≥30 ml/hr, stable weight, eupnea, normal breath sounds, and edema ≤1+ on a 0-4+ scale. By at least 48 hr before hospital discharge, patient is free of new dysrhythmias. Patient does not exhibit significant changes in mental status and remains oriented to person, place, and time.

• Assess for, document, and report evidence of decreased cardiac output, such as edema, jugular venous distention, adventitious breath sounds, shortness of breath (SOB), decreased urinary output, extra heart sound such as S_3, changes in mental status or level of consciousness (LOC), cool extremities, hypotension, tachycardia, and tachypnea.

- Keep accurate I&O records; weigh patient daily.
- Assist with ADL and facilitate coordination of health care providers to provide rest periods between care activities to decrease cardiac workload. Allow 90 min for undisturbed rest. If necessary, limit visitors to allow adequate rest.
- Administer medications as prescribed, such as β-blockers, calcium channel blockers, and antidysrhythmic agents.
- Assist patient into position of comfort, usually semi-Fowler's position (head of bed [HOB] up 30-45 degrees).

You may also wish to refer to the following interventions from the Nursing Interventions Classsification (NIC):

NIC: Cardiac Care; Hemodynamic Regulation; Medication Management; Oxygen Therapy; Respiratory Monitoring; Vital Signs Monitoring

Activity intolerance related to imbalance between oxygen supply and demand secondary to decrease in cardiac muscle contractility

Desired outcome: During activity, patient rates perceived exertion at ≤3 on a 0-10 scale and exhibits cardiac tolerance to activity as evidenced by RR ≤20 breaths/min, systolic BP within 20 mm Hg of resting range, HR within 20 bpm of resting HR, and absence of chest pain and new dysrhythmias.

- Monitor patient's physiologic response to activity. Report chest pain, new dysrhythmias, increased SOB, HR increased >20 bpm over resting HR, and systolic BP >20 mm Hg over resting systolic BP. Ask patient to rate perceived exertion (see p. 739 for a description).
- Monitor BP and other vital signs (VS) q4hr, and report changes such as irregular HR, HR >100 bpm, or decreasing BP.
- Observe for and report signs of acute decreased cardiac output, including oliguria, decreasing BP, decreased mentation, and dizziness.
- Assess integrity of peripheral perfusion by monitoring peripheral pulses, distal extremity skin color, and urinary output. Report changes such as decreased amplitude of pulses, pallor or cyanosis, and decreased urinary output.
- In the presence of acute decreased cardiac output, ensure that the patient's needs are met so that activity can be avoided (e.g., by keeping water at the bedside and urinal or commode nearby, maintaining a quiet environment, and limiting visitors as necessary to ensure adequate rest).
- Facilitate coordination of health care providers to provide rest periods between care activities to decrease cardiac workload. Allow 90 min for undisturbed rest.
- Administer medications as prescribed.
- To help prevent complications caused by immobility, assist patient with passive and some active or assistive ROM and other exercises, depending on patient's tolerance and prescribed limitations.

NIC: Activity Therapy; Cardiac Care; Energy Management; Environmental Management; Exercise Promotion; Surveillance

---

See Also: Appendix One, "Caring for Patients on Prolonged Bedrest," **Risk for activity intolerance,** p. 738; **Risk for disuse syndrome,** p. 740, for discussion of a progressive in-bed exercise program; "Pulmonary Embolus" for **Altered protection** related to risk of prolonged bleeding or hemorrhage secondary to anticoagulation therapy, p. 18; "Pulmonary Hypertension" for **Activity intolerance,** p. 75; "Coronary Artery Disease" for **Knowledge deficit:** Precautions and side effects of β-blockers, p. 60; "Heart Failure" for **Knowledge deficit:** Precautions and side effects of diuretic therapy, p. 71; **Knowledge deficit:** Precautions and side effects of vasodilators, p. 72; **Fluid volume excess,** p. 70; Appendix One, "Caring for Patients on Prolonged Bedrest," p. 738; psychosocial nursing diagnoses and interventions in "Caring for Patients With Cancer and Other Life-disrupting Illnesses," p. 791.

PATIENT-FAMILY TEACHING AND DISCHARGE PLANNING

When providing patient-family teaching, focus on sensory information; avoid giving excessive information; and initiate a visiting nurse referral for necessary follow-up teaching. Consider including verbal and written information about the following:

- Medications, including drug name, purpose, dosage, schedule, precautions, drug/drug and food/drug interactions, and potential side effects.
- Signs and symptoms that necessitate immediate medical attention: dyspnea, decreased exercise tolerance, alterations in pulse rate/rhythm, loss of consciousness (caused by dysrhythmias or decreased cardiac output), oliguria, and steady weight gain (caused by heart failure).
- Reinforcement that cardiomyopathy is a chronic disease requiring lifetime treatment.
- Importance of abstaining from alcohol, which increases cardiac muscle deterioration.
- Need for physical support from family and outside agencies as disease progresses.
- Availability of community and medical support, such as American Heart Association. Either provide the address or phone number for the local chapter or encourage the patient to write for information to the following address:

American Heart Association
7320 Greenville Avenue
Dallas, TX 75231   (800) 242-8721
WWW address: *http://occ.com/amerh*

Coronary artery disease

The coronary arteries are the vessels that supply the myocardial muscle with O_2 and the nutrients necessary for optimal function. Atherosclerotic lesions within these arteries are a major cause of obstruction and subsequent ischemia, which ultimately can lead to myocardial infarction (MI). Other mechanisms include spasm, platelet aggregation, and thrombus formation. The most common symptom of coronary artery disease (CAD) is angina (Table 2-1), a result of decreasing blood flow and decreased O_2 supply through narrowed or obstructed arteries (ischemia). This often occurs during exercise, but it may occur at rest or during a condition of decreased perfusion, such as an episode of hypotension. Often, CAD is diagnosed only after the patient is seen for angina or MI. It is important to note that symptoms do not appear until approximately 75% of the artery is occluded. CAD is the number one killer of both men and women in the United States. After 65 yr of age, death from CAD occurs slightly (11%) more frequently in women than men.

TABLE 2-1 Classification of Angina

Stable angina: pattern of frequency, duration, and severity stable over several months
Unstable angina: pattern of frequency, duration, and severity changed or increased; associated with decreased exercise or exertion. This broad category includes:
- Wellen's syndrome: unstable angina usually associated with left arterial descending (LAD) lesions
- Rest angina
- New-onset angina
- Preinfarction (also called *crescendo*): unstable angina with progression to myocardial infarction (MI) possible (this term sometimes is used interchangeably with *unstable angina*)

Prinzmetal's angina (also called **variant angina**): often occurs at rest (unrelated to exercise) or during sleep; usually caused by coronary artery spasm

ASSESSMENT
Chronic indicators: Stable or progressively worsening angina that occurs when myocardial demand for O_2 is more than the supply, such as during exercise. The pain usually is described as pressure or a crushing or burning substernal pain that radiates down one or both arms. It can be felt also in the neck, cheeks, and teeth. Usually it is relieved by discontinuation of exercise or administration of nitroglycerin (NTG).
Acute indicators: CAD is considered unstable (acute) when angina becomes more frequent and is unrelieved by NTG and rest, when it occurs during sleep or rest, or when it occurs with progressively lower levels of exercise.
Risk factors: Family history, race, increasing age, male gender, smoking, high serum lipid levels, hypertension, obesity, glucose intolerance, sedentary and stressful life-style.

DIAGNOSTIC TESTS
ECG: Usually normal unless MI has occurred or the individual is experiencing angina at the time of the test. If ECG is performed during angina, characteristic changes include ST-segment depression in leads over the area of ischemia.
Serum enzymes: To rule out acute MI.
Chest x-ray: Usually normal unless heart failure is present.
Treadmill exercise test: To determine the amount of exercise that causes angina, as well as the degree of ischemia and the ECG changes produced. Significant findings can include 1-mm or more ST-segment depression or elevation and ventricular ectopic beats.
Radionuclide studies
- Infarct imaging: use of an imaging agent, usually technetium pyrophosphate, that concentrates in the infarcted zone.
- Myocardial perfusion imaging: use of an imaging agent, usually thallium, that concentrates in "normal" tissue.
- Radionuclide ventriculography: enables visualization of the ventricular muscle during the cardiac cycle.

Ambulatory monitoring: A 24-hr ECG monitoring that can show activity-induced ST-segment changes or ischemia-induced dysrhythmias.
Coronary arteriography via cardiac catheterization: Provides the ultimate diagnosis of CAD. Arterial lesions (plaque) are located, and the amount of

occlusion is determined. At this time, feasibility for coronary artery bypass grafting (CABG) or angioplasty is determined. For details, see "Cardiac Surgery," p. 113, and "Collaborative Management," below.

Intravascular ultrasound (IVUS):   To assess the degree of atherosclerosis. A flexible catheter with a miniature transducer at the tip is threaded from an arteriotomy (commonly femoral) retrograde to the coronary arteries to provide information on the interior of the coronary arteries. Ultrasound is used to create a cross-sectional image of the three layers of the arterial wall and its lumen.

Dobutamine two-dimensional echocardiography (2D-Echo):   Aids in determining occult CAD via noninvasive testing.

COLLABORATIVE MANAGEMENT

Management of risk factors: Eliminating tobacco, reducing BP, reducing serum lipid levels, controlling weight and stress, and initiating an exercise program.

Oxygen by nasal cannula: During periods of angina.

Pharmacotherapy

Sublingual NTG: During angina to increase microcirculation, perfusion to the myocardium, and venous dilation.

β-Blockers: To decrease O_2 demand of the myocardium.

Angiotensin-converting enzyme (ACE) inhibitor (e.g., enalapril, perindopril, quinapril, ramipril):   To reduce O_2 demands by decreasing BP.

Long-acting nitrates (isosorbide preparations) or topical NTG: For anginal prophylaxis.

Calcium channel blockers (e.g., nifedipine, diltiazem):   To decrease coronary artery vasospasm and decrease O_2 demand.

Diet: Low in cholesterol (Table 2-2), saturated fat (Table 2-3), Na^+ (see Table 3-2), calories, and triglycerides, as appropriate.

Percutaneous transluminal coronary angioplasty (PTCA):   A procedure that improves coronary blood flow by using a balloon inflation catheter to compress plaque material into the vessel wall. Performed in the cardiac catheterization laboratory with the patient under local anesthesia and mild sedation, it is a common alternative to bypass surgery for individuals with discrete lesions.

Directional coronary atherectomy: A procedure for removal of atherosclerotic deposits in the coronary arteries. It involves use of a special catheter and contains a balloon (for stabilization of the catheter), a cutting device that "shaves" the lesion, and a nose cone in which the shaved lesions are placed. Usually it is performed in the catheterization laboratory. For more information, see "Cardiac Catheterization, Angioplasty, and Atherectomy," p. 109.

NURSING DIAGNOSES AND INTERVENTIONS

Pain (angina) related to decreased oxygen supply to the myocardium

Desired outcomes: Within 30 min of onset of pain, patient's subjective perception of angina decreases, as documented by a pain scale. Objective indicators, such as grimacing and diaphoresis, are absent.

- Assess the location, character, and severity of pain. Record the severity on a subjective 0 (no pain) to 10 (worst pain) scale. Also record the number of NTG tablets needed to relieve each episode, the factor or event that precipitated the pain, and alleviating factors. Document angina relief obtained, using the pain scale.
- Keep sublingual NTG within reach of patient, and explain that it is to be administered as soon as angina begins, repeating q5min × 3 if necessary.
- Stay with patient and provide reassurance during periods of angina. If indicated, request that visitors leave the room.
- Monitor HR and BP during episodes of chest pain. Be alert to and report irregularities in HR and changes in systolic BP >20 mm Hg from baseline.

TABLE 2-2   Guidelines for a Low-cholesterol Diet

Foods to avoid	Foods to choose
Egg yolks (no more than 3/wk)	Egg whites, cholesterol-free egg substitutes
Foods made with many egg yolks (e.g., sponge cakes)	Lean, well-trimmed meats (minimize servings of beef, lamb, pork)
Fatty cuts of meat, fat on meats	Fish (except shellfish), chicken and turkey (without the skin)
Skin on chicken and turkey	
Luncheon meats or cold cuts	Dried peas and beans as meat substitutes
Sausage, frankfurters	Nonfat (skim) or low-fat (2%) milk
Shellfish (e.g., lobster, shrimp, crab)	Partially skim milk cheeses
Whole milk, cream, whole milk cheese	Ice milk and sherbet
Ice cream	Polyunsaturated oils for cooking and food
Commercially prepared foods with hydrogenated shortening (saturated fat)	preparation: corn, safflower, cottonseed, sesame, sunflower
Coconut and palm oils and products made with them (e.g., cream substitutes)	Margarines that list one of the above oils as their first ingredient
Butter, lard, hydrogenated shortening	Foods prepared "from scratch" with the above suggested oils
Fried meats and vegetables	Meats (in acceptable quantity) and vegetables prepared by broiling,
Seasonings containing large amounts of sugar and saturated fats	steaming, or baking (never frying)
Sauces and gravies	Spices, herbs, lemon juice, wine, flavored wine vinegars
Salad dressings containing cream, cheeses, or mayonnaise	

TABLE 2-3   Guidelines for a Diet Low in Saturated Fat

Foods to avoid	Foods to choose
Red meat, especially when highly "marbled"; salami, sausages, bacon	Lean cuts of meat, fresh fish, poultry with skin removed before cooking, grilled meats
Whole milk, whipping cream	Low-fat or skim milk
Tropical oils (coconut, palm oils; cocoa butter)	Monosaturated cooking oils (e.g., olive or canola oil)
Candy	Fresh fruits, vegetables
Sweet rolls, donuts	Whole grain breads, cereals
Ice cream	Nonfat yogurt, sherbet
Salad dressings	Vinegar, lemon juice
Peanut butter, peanuts, hot dogs, potato chips	Unbuttered popcorn
Butter	Margarine (safflower oil listed as the first ingredient)

- Monitor for presence of headache and hypotension after administering NTG. Keep patient recumbent during angina and NTG administration.
- Administer O_2 as prescribed to increase O_2 supply to the myocardium. Deliver O_2 with humidity to help prevent its drying effects on oral and nasal mucosa.

- Emphasize to patient the importance of immediately reporting angina to health care team.
- Instruct the patient to avoid activities and factors that are known to cause stress and that may precipitate angina.
- Discuss the value of relaxation techniques, including tapes, soothing music, biofeedback, meditation, or yoga. See **Health-seeking behaviors,** p. 59.
- Administer β-blockers and calcium channel blockers as prescribed to decrease cardiac workload and O_2 demand.
- Administer long-acting and/or topical nitrates to decrease O_2 demand and likelihood of angina.

NIC: Cardiac Precautions; Energy Management; Medication Administration; Oxygen Therapy; Pain Management; Surveillance

Activity intolerance related to generalized weakness and imbalance between oxygen supply and demand secondary to tissue ischemia (MI)
Desired outcome: During activity, patient rates perceived exertion at ≤3 on a 0-10 scale and exhibits cardiac tolerance to activity as evidenced by RR ≤20 breaths/min, HR ≤120 bpm (or within 20 bpm of resting HR), systolic BP within 20 mm Hg of patient's resting systolic BP, and absence of chest pain and new dysrhythmias.

- Observe for and report increasing frequency of angina, angina that occurs at rest, angina that is unrelieved by NTG, or decreased exercise tolerance without angina. See Table 2-1 for classifications of angina.
- Assess patient's response to activity. Be alert to chest pain, increase in HR (>20 bpm), change in systolic BP (20 mm Hg over or under resting BP), excessive fatigue, and SOB. Ask patient to rate perceived exertion (see p. 739 for details).
- Assist patient with recognizing and limiting activities that increase O_2 demands, such as exercise and anxiety.
- Administer O_2 as prescribed for angina episodes. Deliver O_2 with humidity to help prevent its drying effects on oral and nasal mucosa.
- Have patient perform ROM exercises, depending on tolerance and prescribed activity limitations. Because cardiac intolerance to activity can be further aggravated by prolonged bedrest, consult health care provider about in-bed exercises and activities that can be performed by the patient as the condition improves.
- For further interventions, see Appendix One, "Caring for Patients on Prolonged Bedrest," **Risk for activity intolerance,** p. 738, and **Risk for disuse syndrome,** p. 740.

NIC: Activity Therapy; Cardiac Care; Energy Management; Environmental Management; Exercise Promotion; Surveillance; Teaching: Prescribed Activity/Exercise

Altered nutrition: More than body requirements of calories, sodium, or fats
Desired outcome: Within the 24-hr period before hospital discharge, patient demonstrates knowledge of the dietary regimen by planning a 3-day menu that includes and excludes appropriate foods.

- If patient is over ideal body weight, explain that a low-calorie diet is necessary.
- Show patient how to decrease dietary intake of saturated (animal) fats and increase intake of polyunsaturated (vegetable oil) fats (see Table 2-3).
- Teach patient to limit dietary intake of cholesterol to <300 mg/day (see Table 2-2). Encourage patients to use food labels to determine the cholesterol content of foods.
- Teach patient to limit dietary intake of refined/processed sugar.
- Teach patient to limit dietary intake of sodium chloride (NaCl) to <4 g/day (mild restriction). Encourage patients to use food labels to determine the Na^+ content of foods (see Table 3-2, p. 133).

- Instruct patient and significant other in the use of "Nutrition Facts" (federally mandated public information on all food product labels) to determine the amount of calories, total fat, saturated fat, cholesterol, and sodium in foods. Teach patient and significant other to be especially aware of the serving size listed for the respective nutrients; that is, a serving size listed as 4 oz on a package containing 12 oz would mean the patient would get three times the amount of each ingredient if the patient eats the entire contents of the container!
- Encourage intake of fresh fruits, natural (unrefined or unprocessed) carbohydrates, fish, poultry, legumes, fresh vegetables, and grains for a healthy, balanced diet.

NIC: Nutrition Management; Nutritional Counseling; Teaching: Individual; Teaching: Prescribed Diet; Weight Reduction Assistance

Health-seeking behaviors: Relaxation technique effective for stress reduction
Desired outcome: Patient reports subjective relief of stress after using relaxation technique.
- Discuss with patient the importance of relaxation for decreasing nervous system tone (sympathetic), energy requirements, and O_2 consumption.
- Many techniques use breathing, concentration, or imagery to promote relaxation and decrease energy requirements. The following technique can be used easily by anyone. Speaking slowly and softly, give patient the following guidelines:
  —Find a comfortable position. Close your eyes.
  —Go through the following relaxation exercise. Begin by concentrating on your feet and toes; tighten the muscles in your feet and toes, and hold this tightness for a count of three. Now slowly relax your feet and toes. Feel or imagine the tension flowing out of your feet and toes. Now concentrate on your lower legs. Tense the muscles of your lower legs for a count of three. Now slowly release this tightness and feel the tension drain from your lower legs. Continue with this purposeful tightening and relaxation with each successive major body part, moving up the body, until finally you reach your facial muscles. When you reach your face, tighten the muscles of your face for a count of three. When you go to relax the muscles in your face, take a deep breath and exhale. As you breathe out, imagine that you are blowing all the tension of your body out and away from you, leaving you totally relaxed and calm.
  —Now breathe through your nose. Concentrate on feeling the air move in and out. As you exhale, say the word *one* silently to yourself. Again continue feeling the air move in and out of your lungs. Continue for approximately 20 min.
  —Try to clear your mind of worries; be passive. Let relaxation occur. If distractions appear, gently push them away. Continue breathing through your nose, repeating *one* silently.
  —After approximately 20 min, slowly begin to allow yourself to become aware of your surroundings. Keep your eyes closed for a few moments.
  —Open your eyes.
- Encourage patient to practice this technique 2-3 ×/day or whenever feeling stressed or tense. Acknowledge that this technique may feel strange at first but that it becomes easier and more effective with each practice.
- Explain that baroque or new age music, played softly, helps many individuals achieve an even greater state of relaxation.

NIC: Anxiety Reduction; Calming Technique; Meditation; Music Therapy; Simple Guided Imagery; Simple Relaxation Therapy; Teaching: Prescribed Activity/Exercise

Knowledge deficit: Precautions and side effects of nitrates
Desired outcome: Within the 24-hr period before hospital discharge, patient verbalizes understanding of the precautions and side effects of the prescribed medication.

- Instruct patient to report to health care provider or staff the presence of a headache associated with NTG, in which case the health care provider may alter the dose.
- Teach patient to assume a recumbent position if a headache occurs. Explain that the vasodilation effect of the drug can result in transient headache.
- Explain that the vasodilation from nitrates may also decrease BP, which may result in orthostatic hypotension. Instruct the patient to rise slowly from a sitting or lying position and to remain by the chair or bed for 1 min after standing to be assured that he or she is not going to experience orthostatic changes.

NIC: Activity Therapy; Fall Prevention; Risk Identification; Surveillance: Safety; Teaching: Prescribed Medication

Knowledge deficit: Precautions and side effects of β-blockers
Desired outcome: Within the 24-hr period before hospital discharge, patient verbalizes understanding of the precautions and side effects of β-blockers.

- Instruct patient to be alert to depression, fatigue, dizziness, erythematous rash, respiratory distress, and sexual dysfunction, which can occur as side effects of β-blockers. Explain the importance of notifying health care provider promptly if these side effects occur.
- Explain that weight gain and peripheral and sacral edema can occur as side effects of β-blockers. Teach patient how to assess for edema and the importance of reporting signs and symptoms promptly if they occur.
- Explain that BP and heart rate (HR) are assessed before administration of β-blockers because these drugs can cause hypotension and excessive slowing of the heart.
- Caution patient not to omit or abruptly stop taking β-blockers, because this can result in rebound angina or even MI.

NIC: Surveillance; Teaching: Individual; Teaching: Prescribed Medication; Vital Signs Monitoring

Knowledge deficit: Disease process and life-style implications of CAD
Desired outcome: Within the 24-hr period before hospital discharge, patient verbalizes knowledge about the disease process of CAD and the concomitant life-style implications.

- Teach patient about CAD, including the pathophysiologic processes of cardiac ischemia, angina, and infarction.
- Assist patient with identifying risk factors for CAD and risk factor modification as follows:
  —Diet low in cholesterol and saturated fat
  —Smoking cessation
  —Regular activity/exercise programs
- Discuss symptoms that necessitate medical attention, such as chest pain unrelieved by NTG.
- Discuss guidelines for sexual activity, such as resting before intercourse, finding a comfortable position, taking prophylactic NTG, and postponing intercourse for 1-1½ hr after a heavy meal.
- Discuss medical procedures, such as cardiac catheterization, and surgical procedures, such as PTCA and CABG, if appropriate.

PATIENT-FAMILY TEACHING AND DISCHARGE PLANNING

When providing patient-family teaching, focus on sensory information; avoid giving excessive information; and initiate a visiting nurse referral for necessary

follow-up teaching. Consider including verbal and written information about the following:

- Medications, including drug name, dosage, purpose, schedule, precautions, drug/drug and food/drug interactions, and potential side effects. Discuss the potential for headache and dizziness after NTG administration. Caution patient about using NTG more frequently than prescribed and notifying health care provider if three tablets do not relieve angina.
- Importance of reducing or eliminating intake of caffeine, which causes vasoconstriction and increases HR.
- Dietary changes: low saturated fat (see Table 2-3), low Na^+ (see Table 3-2, p. 133), low cholesterol (see Table 2-2), and the need for weight loss if appropriate. Encourage patients to use food labels to determine the caloric, cholesterol, fat, and Na^+ content of foods.
- Pulse monitoring: how to self-measure pulse, including parameters for target heart rates and limits.
- Prescribed exercise program and importance of maintaining a regular exercise schedule. Remind patient of the need to measure pulse, stop if pain occurs, and stay within prescribed exercise limits. See Table 2-4 for a progressive at-home walking program. Caution patient not to exercise during extremes of weather (hot or cold), which can place an additional strain on the heart.
- Indicators that necessitate medical attention: progression to unstable angina, loss of consciousness, decreased exercise tolerance, unrelieved pain, angina that is unrelieved by NTG, increasing frequency of angina, and need to increase the number of NTG tablets to relieve angina.
- Elimination of smoking; refer patient to a "stop smoking" program as appropriate. The following free brochures outline ways to help patients stop smoking:

  How to Help Your Patients Stop Using Tobacco: A National Cancer Institute Manual for the Oral Health Team, from the Smoking and Tobacco Control Program of the National Cancer Institute; call 1-800-4-CANCER.

  Clinical Practice Guideline: A Quick Reference Guide for Smoking Cessation Specialists, from the Agency for Health Care Policy and Research (AHCPR); call 1-800-358-9295.

- Importance of involvement and support of significant others in patient's life-style changes.
- Importance of getting BP checked at regular intervals (at least monthly if the patient is hypertensive).
- Importance of avoiding strenuous activity for at least 1 hr after meals to avoid excessive O_2 demands.

TABLE 2-4   Guidelines for a Progressive At-Home Walking Program

Week	Distance	Time
1	100-200 ft	2 ×/day
2	200-400 ft	2 ×/day
3	¼ mi	8-10 min
4	½ mi	15 min
5	1 mi	30 min
6	1¾ mi	30 min
7	2 mi	40 min

- Importance of reporting to health care provider any change in the pattern or frequency of angina.
- Availability of community and medical support, such as American Heart Association. Either provide the address or phone number for the local chapter, or encourage the patient to write for information to the following address:

  American Heart Association
  7320 Greenville Avenue
  Dallas, TX 75231   (800) 242-8721
  WWW address: *http://occ.com/amerh*

- Phone numbers to call should questions or concerns arise about therapy or this condition after discharge. Additional general information can be obtained by contacting the following organization:

  National Center for Cardiac Information
  8180 Greensboro Drive #1070
  McLean, VA 22102   (703) 356-6568

- Sexual activity guidelines:
  —Rest is beneficial before sexual activity.
  —Medications such as NTG may be taken prophylactically if pain occurs with activity.
  —Postpone sexual activity for 1-1½ hr after a meal.

Myocardial infarction

Ischemic heart disease accounts for approximately one third of all deaths in the United States, and of patients with ischemic heart disease, half die because of MI. Most MIs are caused by critical narrowing of the coronary arteries as a result of atherosclerosis (see "Coronary Artery Disease"). Occlusion also can be caused by thrombus formation or coronary artery spasm. When ischemia is prolonged and unrelieved, irreversible damage (infarction) occurs. MI can occur in various areas of the heart, depending on the location of the coronary artery occlusion and distribution of blood supply.

ASSESSMENT

Signs and symptoms: Chest pain, substernal pressure and burning, pain that radiates to the jaw, shoulder, or arm. Weakness, diaphoresis, nausea, vomiting, and acute anxiety also can occur. Heart rate (HR) can be abnormally slow (bradycardia) or rapid (tachycardia).

Physical assessment: Possible minor hypotension, increasing respiratory rate (RR), and crackles (rales) if ventricular failure occurs. Temperature elevations to 39.4° C (104° F) can occur secondary to the inflammatory process. Intensity of S_1 and S_2 heart sounds may be decreased, and pulmonary congestion will occur if papillary muscle rupture has occurred. S_3 and S_4 sounds may be present if heart failure has occurred.

History of: Sudden onset of intense chest pain that is unrelieved by stopping activity or taking nitroglycerin (NTG), positive family history, cigarette smoking, hypercholesterolemia, obesity, diabetes mellitus, stressful or sedentary life-style.

DIAGNOSTIC TESTS

Serum enzymes: Will reveal myocardial muscle damage. The following enzyme levels will increase: creatinine phosphokinase (CPK or CK), the MB isoenzyme (CPK-MB), serum glutamic-oxaloacetic transaminase (SGOT or AST [aspartate aminotransferase]), and lactic dehydrogenase (LDH). Serial examination (q6hr × 3) of the CPK-MB isoenzyme is useful to quantify the amount of myocardial infarction and to time the onset of infarction. The CPK-MB isoenzyme is used to determine the appropriateness of thrombolytic therapy (see p. 64); that is, a high CPK-MB level on admission suggests significant infarction has already occurred and precludes use of thrombolytic therapy.

Serial ECGs: For comparison with the baseline. Lead changes, including ST-segment elevation, T-wave inversion, and formation of Q waves, identify the area of infarct.

Chest x-ray: Usually reveals cardiomegaly and signs of left ventricular failure.

Radionuclide studies: May help localize area of infarct and examine myocardial ejection fraction.

Technetium-99m pyrophosphate: Taken up by infarcted myocardial tissue and thus the acute MI will show up as a "hot spot" on the scan.

Technetium-99m sestamibi: Provides more clear imaging with information similar to that of angiocardiography, allowing collection of information on myocardial tissue perfusion, ventricular function, and gated-pool ejection fractions (GPEFs).

Gated-pool ejection fraction: Evaluates left ventricular and right ejection fractions, detects aneurysms, and identifies wall motion abnormalities. Using a computer-assisted gated (synchronized) scan allows recording of the myocardial wall during contractions; the computer collects information over several cardiac cycles to allow determination of cardiac contractility. This also permits calculation of the amount of blood ejected with ventricular contraction (systole) and is called gated pool ejection or *multiple-gated acquisition (MUGA) scan,* for the computer originally required.

Thallium-201: Taken up by normal myocardial cells, with ischemic cells showing up as "cold spots" on the scan. A **thallium stress test** may be used to identify areas of myocardium that are underperfused during exercise; the test is performed with the patient at rest and during exercise to allow comparison. Thallium stress testing is used to detect coronary occlusive disease and to assess patency of grafts following coronary artery bypass grafts (CABGs).

Dipyridamole–thallium-201: Used when exercise testing is not possible, such as for patients with arthritic, neurologic, pulmonary, or similar restrictions to exercise. Dipyridamole is a coronary vasodilator that simulates exercise's effect on the heart, allowing for scanning to identify decreased coronary artery blood flow.

> **Caution:** This test may result in angina or MI and should be performed with a cardiologist present. Aminophylline is used to reverse the effect of dipyridamole.

Single-photon emission computed tomography (SPECT): Identifies three-dimensional views of cardiac processes and cellular level metabolism by viewing the heart from several different angles and using tomography methods to reconstruct the image. Allows clearer resolution of myocardial ischemia and better quantification of cardiac damage.

Echocardiography: Detects abnormalities of left ventricular wall motion, which usually correspond to the ECG site of infarction.

Dobutamine stress echocardiogram: Uses progressively larger doses of dobutamine every 3 min with continued echocardiography to identify cardiac wall movement changes.

Transesophageal echocardiography (TEE):   Provides clearer ultrasonic images of the heart by avoiding interposition of subcutaneous tissues, bony thorax, and lungs. A high-frequency transducer on an endoscope is placed in the esophagus behind the heart or advanced to the stomach to allow an inferior view of the heart.

Hemodynamic monitoring in the coronary care unit (CCU):   Measures cardiac output and pulmonary artery pressures, which may reflect significant myocardial injury and dysfunction.

Angiocardiography: Determines areas of stenosis or occlusion and suitability for CABG or percutaneous transluminal coronary angioplasty (PTCA). This test remains the gold standard for assessing cardiac perfusion. See also "Cardiac Catheterization, Angioplasty, and Atherectomy," p. 109.

ABG analysis: May reveal hypoxemia (decreased partial pressure of dissolved oxygen in arterial blood [Pao_2]) and hyperventilation (decreased partial pressure of dissolved carbon dioxide in arterial blood [$Paco_2$]).

CBC: May reveal leukocytosis secondary to the inflammatory process.

Erythrocyte sedimentation rate (ESR):   Increased in the presence of an inflammatory process.

Indium-111 antimyosin antibody imaging: A diagnostic tool that is showing promise for detecting infarcted cells and tissue. The antibody is injected and taken up by damaged but not intact cells.

COLLABORATIVE MANAGEMENT

Relief of acute pain: NTG by IV drip until pain is relieved or IV morphine sulfate in small increments (2 mg).

O_2:   Usually 2-4 L/min by nasal cannula or mask for 2-3 days to increase the patient's O_2 supply. Hypoxia is common and adds stress to the compromised myocardium.

Transfer to CCU: For close monitoring if needed.

Limiting infarct size by decreasing cardiac workload: β-Blockade, controlled exercise program, risk-factor management, bedrest with commode privileges.

Treatment and prevention of dysrhythmias: Antidysrhythmic agents (e.g., lidocaine) for premature ventricular beats; atropine for bradycardia.

Magnesium supplementation: Magnesium has been used to treat muscular excitability and to decrease dysrhythmias and resultant mortality and improve left ventricular function when given in the first 24 hr following MI.

Management of fluid imbalance: Oral or IV fluids for dehydration; diuretics for fluid overload.

Treatment of ventricular failure: See "Heart Failure."

Dietary management: Low-cholesterol (see Table 2-2), low-fat (see Table 2-3), low-Na^+ (see Table 3-2, p. 133) diet as indicated.

Medical reperfusion to limit infarct size

Thrombolytic therapy with streptokinase, tissue plasminogen activator (TPA), anisoylated plasminogen streptokinase activator complex (APSAC), or the thrombolytic agent, alteplase (Activase), a recombinant tissue plasminogen activator: To lyse (break down) the fibrin clot. Usually, it is done in the cardiac catheterization laboratory, ICU, or emergency room.

Heparin therapy: Used along with or following thrombolytic therapy to inhibit further clotting and prevent recurring coronary artery occlusion. Recombinant desulfatohirudin (Hirudin) is a direct-action antithrombin agent for the patient receiving thrombolytic agents; it is available for patients with heparin sensitivity.

Antiplatelet agents (abciximab, aspirin, dipyridamole, sulfinpyrazone, ticlopidine (Ticlid):   To inhibit platelet aggregation and prolong bleeding time. Used as adjunctive therapy for PTCA or atherectomy, for the prevention of acute MI, and following cardiac surgery.

PTCA: To compress plaque in the coronary artery. See "Cardiac Catheterization, Angioplasty, and Atherectomy," p. 109.

Surgical reperfusion: CABG. (See "Cardiac Surgery," p. 113).

NURSING DIAGNOSES AND INTERVENTIONS

Pain related to ischemia and infarction of myocardial tissue

Desired outcomes: Patient's subjective perception of pain decreases within 30 min of onset as documented by a pain scale. Objective indicators, such as grimacing and diaphoresis, are absent.

- Assess location, character, duration, and intensity of pain, using a pain scale of 0 (no pain) to 10 (worst pain). Assess associated symptoms, such as nausea and diaphoresis.
- If the patient is on telemetry, use the telemetry device's notification button or call the telemetry monitoring station with the patient's bedside phone to notify the telemetry nurse that the patient is experiencing chest pain. The telemetry nurse will run a rhythm strip from the monitor to allow the health care provider to assess the patient's ECG reading during the episode.
- Use the "PQRST" mnemonic to assess chest pain and quickly rule out other noncardiac pain:
  —**P** = Provoked/palliative: Was the pain provoked by activity, or what preceded the pain?
  —**Q** = Quality: Ask the patient to describe the characteristics of the pain (e.g., burning, crushing, stabbing).
  —**R** = Region/radiation: Where did the pain start; does the pain radiate anywhere (e.g., jaw, arm, shoulder)?
  —**S** = Severity: Rate the pain on a scale of 0-10 (0 being no pain and 10 being most painful).
  —**T** = Timing: Describe the duration of the pain and what time of day the symptoms began.
- Assess and document BP and HR with episodes of pain. BP and HR may increase because of sympathetic stimulation or decrease because of ischemia and decreased cardiac function.
- Administer prescribed pain medications (usually morphine sulfate), and document quality of relief obtained, using the pain scale, and the time interval from administration to expressed relief.
- Provide reassurance during episodes of pain; stay with patient if possible.
- Observe for and report side effects of pain medications, such as hypotension, slowed RR, and difficulty with urination.
- Administer O_2 as prescribed, usually 2-4 L/min per nasal cannula. Deliver O_2 with humidity to help prevent its drying effects on oral and nasal mucosa.
- Position the patient in semi-Fowler's position to reduce cardiac workload.
- If appropriate, prepare patient for transport to CCU.

NIC: Analgesic Administration; Anxiety Reduction; Calming Technique; Cardiac Care: Acute; Cardiac Precautions; Oxygen Therapy; Teaching: Individual

Decreased cardiac output related to negative inotropic changes (decreased cardiac contractility) secondary to ischemia and infarction

Desired outcome: Patient has adequate cardiac output within 1 hr of treatment/intervention as evidenced by systolic BP ≥90 mm Hg, HR ≤100 bpm, urinary output ≥30 ml/hr, RR 12-20 breaths/min with normal depth and pattern (eupnea), O_2 saturation ≥92%, absence of crackles (rales), and edema ≤1+ on a 0-4+ scale.

- Assess for and document the following as indicators of decreased cardiac output: restlessness and/or change in mental status or level of consciousness (LOC), extra heart sounds (e.g., S_3), systolic BP <90 mm Hg, HR >100 bpm, and O_2 saturation (via oximetry readings) <92%.
- Observe for and report any indicators of fluid accumulation in the lungs, such as dyspnea, crackles (rales), and shortness of breath (SOB).
- Administer O_2 as prescribed, usually 2-4 L/min per nasal cannula. Deliver O_2 with humidity to help prevent its drying effects on oral and nasal mucosa.
- Position the patient in semi-Fowler's position to reduce cardiac workload.
- Be alert to and report decreasing urine output (particularly <30 ml/hr) and increasing specific gravity (>1.030).
- Assess for peripheral (sacral, pedal) edema.
- Maintain IV infusion as prescribed. Usually fluids are monitored closely to prevent failure and circulatory overload.
- As prescribed, administer medications, such as β-blockers and vasodilators, to decrease cardiac workload and prevent a decrease in cardiac output.
- Prepare patient for possible transfer to CCU.

NIC: Cardiac Care: Acute; Fluid/Electrolyte Management; Hemodynamic Regulation; Medication Management; Oxygen Therapy; Vital Signs Monitoring

Activity intolerance related to imbalance between oxygen supply and demand secondary to decreased strength of cardiac contraction and decreased cardiac output

Desired outcome: During exercise/activity, patient rates perceived exertion at ≤3 on a 0-10 scale and exhibits cardiac tolerance to activity as evidenced by systolic BP within 20 mm Hg of resting systolic BP, RR ≤20 breaths/min, and HR ≤120 bpm (or ≤20 bpm over resting HR).

- Ask patient to rate perceived exertion during activity, and monitor for evidence of activity intolerance. For details, see **Risk for activity intolerance** in Appendix One, "Caring for Patients on Prolonged Bedrest," p. 739. Notify health care provider of significant findings.
- Observe for and report any symptoms of decreased cardiac output or cardiac failure, such as decreasing BP, pale and cold extremities, oliguria, decreased peripheral pulses, and increased HR.
- Monitor I&O, and be alert to urinary output <30 ml/hr.
- Auscultate lung fields q2hr for presence of crackles (rales), which can occur with fluid retention and cardiac failure.
- Palpate peripheral pulses at frequent intervals. Be alert to irregularities and decreased amplitude, which can signal cardiac failure.
- Administer O_2 and medications as prescribed. Deliver O_2 with humidity to help prevent its drying effects on oral and nasal mucosa.
- During acute periods of decreased cardiac output and as prescribed, support patient in maintaining bedrest by keeping personal articles within reach, providing a calm and quiet atmosphere, and limiting visitors to ensure periods of undisturbed rest.
- Assist patient to commode when bathroom privileges are allowed.
- Assist patient with passive or assistive ROM exercises, as determined by activity tolerance and activity limitations. Consult health care provider about the type and amount of in-bed exercises the patient can perform as the condition improves. Also discuss with health care provider patient's participation in an exercise program after hospital discharge.
- As appropriate, teach patient self-measurement of HR for gauging exercise tolerance.

- Facilitate coordination of health care providers to provide rest periods between care activities to decrease cardiac workload. Ensure 90 min for undisturbed rest.
- For further interventions, see Appendix One, "Caring for Patients on Prolonged Bedrest," **Risk for activity intolerance,** p. 738, and **Risk for disuse syndrome,** p. 740.

NIC: Activity Therapy; Cardiac Care; Energy Management; Environmental Management; Exercise Promotion; Respiratory Monitoring; Surveillance; Teaching: Prescribed Activity/Exercise

Impaired gas exchange related to alveolar-capillary membrane changes secondary to fluid accumulation in the lungs
Desired outcome: Patient has adequate gas exchange within 30 min of treatment/intervention as evidenced by a state of eupnea. For at least 24 hr before hospital discharge, patient's Pao_2 is ≥80 mm Hg, $Paco_2$ is 35-45 mm Hg, and O_2 saturation is ≥92%.
- Assess ABG levels, and be alert to evidence of hypoxemia (decreased Pao_2) or hyperventilation (decreased $Paco_2$).
- Monitor O_2 saturation via oximetry; report O_2 saturation <92% to the health care provider.
- Auscultate lung fields q2hr for presence of crackles (rales), which occur with fluid accumulation.
- Monitor for sudden changes in respiratory pattern (increased dyspnea or decreased RR), which can occur with an extension of the infarction and decreased cardiac output; report immediately if they occur.
- Monitor BP. In the absence of marked hypotension, place patient in semi-Fowler's position (head of bed [HOB] up 30-45 degrees) to ease dyspnea.
- Administer O_2 as prescribed. Deliver O_2 with humidity to help prevent its drying effects on oral and nasal mucosa.
- Administer prescribed analgesics (usually morphine sulfate) to decrease cardiac workload by vasodilation and ease respiratory effort.

NIC: Acid-Base Monitoring; Airway Management; Analgesic Administration; Laboratory Data Interpretation; Oxygen Therapy; Respiratory Monitoring; Vital Signs Monitoring

See Also: "Coronary Artery Disease" for **Health-seeking behaviors:** Relaxation technique effective for stress reduction, p. 59; **Knowledge deficit:** Disease process and life-style implications of CAD, p. 60; Appendix One, "Caring for Preoperative and Postoperative Patients," p. 717; psychosocial nursing diagnoses and interventions in "Caring for Patients With Cancer and Other Life-disrupting Illnesses," p. 791.

PATIENT-FAMILY TEACHING AND DISCHARGE PLANNING

When providing patient-family teaching, focus on sensory information; avoid giving excessive information; and initiate a visiting nurse referral for necessary follow-up teaching. Consider including verbal and written information about the following:
- Process of MI and extent of the patient's injury.
- Indicators that necessitate immediate medical attention: unrelieved pain, decreased activity tolerance, sudden onset of SOB, weight gain.
- Medications, including drug name, purpose, dosage, schedule, precautions, drug/drug and food/drug interactions, and potential side effects. Provide instructions for taking prophylactic NTG before activities, such as sexual activity.

- Exercise program specific to patient's condition. Guidelines for walking are provided in Table 2-4. Caution patient to start slowly, walk 3-5 times/wk, warm up and cool down with stretching exercises, notify health care provider of any change in exercise tolerance, avoid overexertion, and stop when tired.
- Importance of avoiding overexertion and getting rest when tired.
- Resumption of sexual activity as directed, usually after 2-4 wk, but will vary with each patient.
- Diet regimen as prescribed. See Tables 2-2, 2-3, and 3-2, p. 133, for descriptions of low-cholesterol, low-fat, and low-Na^+ diets. Encourage patients to use food labels to determine the cholesterol, fat, and Na^+ content of foods.
- Cessation of smoking. Refer patient to a "stop smoking" program as appropriate. The following free brochures outline ways to help patients stop smoking:

  How to Help Your Patients Stop Using Tobacco: A National Cancer Institute Manual for the Oral Health Team, from the Smoking and Tobacco Control Program of the National Cancer Institute; call 1-800-4-CANCER.

  Clinical Practice Guideline: A Quick Reference Guide for Smoking Cessation Specialists, from the Agency for Health Care Policy and Research (AHCPR); call 1-800-358-9295.

- Phone number and address of local American Heart Association branch, local heart rehabilitation programs, family health care provider, and primary nurse. Either provide the address or phone number for the local chapter or encourage the patient to write for information to the following address:

  American Heart Association
  7320 Greenville Avenue
  Dallas, TX 75231   (800) 242-8721
  WWW address: *http://occ.com/amerh*

- Additional general information can be obtained by contacting the following organization:

  National Center for Cardiac Information
  8180 Greensboro Drive #1070
  McLean, VA 22102   (703) 356-6568

- Referral to stress management programs if appropriate.
- For further interventions, see "Coronary Artery Disease," **Health-seeking behaviors:** Relaxation technique effective for stress reduction, p. 59.

Heart failure

Heart (cardiac) failure is not a disease in and of itself, but rather, it is the end product of a variety of insults to the heart that result in its failure as a pump. Heart failure is the state in which the heart is unable to pump blood at a rate sufficient to meet metabolic requirements of the tissues. Heart failure can occur as a result of myocardial or cardiac muscle damage, such as after large infarcts, or when an adequate cardiac muscle is stressed or forced to work harder over a period of time. When the heart is unable to pump sufficient blood to meet metabolic demands, it relies on three main compensatory mechanisms:

Increasing cardiac fluid to increase fiber length and subsequent force of contraction (Frank-Starling law). The fluid that fills the ventricles before systole is termed *preload,* and it is a critical factor in patients with cardiac failure. It is important to have enough volume to stretch the fibers, but not so much of a stretch that decreased contractility and decreased cardiac output occur.

Increasing catecholamine discharge (epinephrine and norepinephrine) to increase contractility. This causes systemic vasoconstriction, which in turn increases workload of the heart by increasing resistance. This is called *afterload.*

Myocardial hypertrophy to increase the mass of working contractile tissue. The hypertrophy will be either right sided, left sided, or both, depending on the cause of failure. Conditions that can result in primary right-sided heart failure include right ventricular MI, COPD, left-to-right shunts, and pulmonary valve stenosis. Primary left-sided heart failure is caused by conditions such as left ventricular MI, aortic valve stenosis, mitral regurgitation, and hypertension. Over time, left-sided failure can result in the involvement of both sides of the heart.

ASSESSMENT

Signs and symptoms: Orthopnea, nocturnal dyspnea, dyspnea on exertion (DOE), fatigue, weakness, nocturia, cardiac cachexia (malnutrition/wasting), and confusion, which can occur late in the disease. In addition, decreased right ventricular output can cause increased CVP, distended neck veins, and peripheral edema; decreased left ventricular output can cause dyspnea and SOB, as well as other indicators of pulmonary edema.

Physical assessment: Decreased BP, dysrhythmias, tachycardia, tachypnea, increased venous pulsations and pressure, crackles (rales), pitting edema, ascites, galloping heart sounds, and pulsus alternans (alternating strong and weak heart beats). Hepatomegaly may occur in the presence of right-sided or left-sided heart failure.

History of: Noncompliance with medication or diet regimen, sleeping on extra pillows to enhance respirations, decreased exercise tolerance, increasing SOB, coronary artery disease (CAD), and risk factors for CAD (see p. 55).

DIAGNOSTIC TESTS

Chest x-ray: Will show cardiomegaly and engorged pulmonary vasculature.

Serum electrolytes: May reveal hyponatremia (dilutional); hyperkalemia if glomerular filtration is decreased; or hypokalemia, which can result from some diuretics.

Serum enzymes: May reveal an elevated serum glutamic-oxaloacetic transaminase (SGOT or AST [aspartate aminotransferase]) level with hepatic congestion and decreased liver function.

Serum bilirubin: May reveal hyperbilirubinemia in the presence of liver dysfunction following hepatomegaly with right-sided failure.

CBC: May reveal decreased Hgb and Hct levels in the presence of anemia.

Ejection fraction (EF): Provides an indirect measure of the effectiveness of the heart as a pump. EF is the fraction (proportion) of the blood ejected from the left ventricle during systole. This may be determined via cardiac catheterization or echocardiogram.

COLLABORATIVE MANAGEMENT

Treatment of underlying cause

Surgical repair of abnormalities such as valvular lesions or treatment of conditions such as hypertension or endocarditis

Cardiomyoplasty: An investigational surgical technique that involves a muscle transfer of the latissimus dorsi around the heart where it acts to supplement myocardial tissue. It takes approximately 2 mo for this muscle to respond similarly to myocardial tissues. Cardiomyoplasty is an option for patients who are not candidates for heart transplantation.

Heart transplantation: May be an option for some patients with end-stage (New York Heart Association [NYHA] class IV) heart failure (Table 2-5).

Treatment of precipitating factors: Such as infection or dysrhythmias.

T A B L E 2 - 5   New York Heart Association (NYHA) Functional Classification of Persons With Heart Failure

Class	Definition
1	No limitation of physical activity; ordinary physical activity does not result in symptoms
2	Slight limitation on physical activity; no symptoms at rest, but symptoms possible with ordinary physical activity
3	More severe limitations; patient usually comfortable at rest; clinical manifestations with unusual physical activity
4	Inability to carry on any physical activity without producing symptoms; symptoms possible at rest

Physical and emotional rest

Low-Na$^+$ diet: In less severe disease states, this may mean elimination of table salt only. See Table 3-2, p. 133.

Weight control: If appropriate.

Pharmacotherapy

Diuretics (amiloride, bumetanide, furosemide): To control fluid accumulation and reduce blood volume.

Vasodilators: To decrease cardiac workload by decreasing sympathetic nervous system vasoconstriction. Although there is some controversy about when to initiate vasodilator therapy, it is believed that it is appropriate when patients develop symptoms with light activity or when they are being treated with digitalis. This provides a combination of increased contractility (digitalis) and decreased afterload (vasodilator). The administration of IV vasodilators such as sodium nitroprusside and nitroglycerin (NTG) necessitates the patient's transfer to the CCU.

Inotropic drugs (usually digitalis): Administered during acute exacerbation to increase the strength of contractions. Administration of inotropic drugs may necessitate the patient's transfer to the CCU for close monitoring of vasoactive effects.

Angiotensin-converting enzyme (ACE) inhibitors (benazepril, captopril, enalapril, fosinopril, lisinopril, moexipril , quinapril, ramipril): To inhibit the conversion of circulating angiotensin II and thus reduce preload and afterload; decrease the work of the left ventricle; and increase cardiac output and perfusion.

NURSING DIAGNOSES AND INTERVENTIONS

Fluid volume excess related to compromised regulatory mechanisms secondary to decreased cardiac output

Desired outcome: For at least 24 hr before hospital discharge, patient is normovolemic as evidenced by urinary output ≥30 ml/hr, balanced I&O, stable weight (or weight loss attributable to fluid loss), edema ≤1+ on a 0-4+ scale, HR ≤100 bpm, and absence of crackles (rales).

- Auscultate lung fields at least q8hr; report presence of crackles (rales), which occur with fluid volume excess and heart failure.
- Monitor and document I&O at least q8hr. Report imbalances, including urinary output <30 ml/hr, which can occur with decreased renal blood flow.
- Monitor weight daily, and report unusual gains. Be alert to the presence of pitting edema. To assess for pitting edema, apply firm pressure to the edematous area with a finger. If the indentation remains after the finger has been removed, pitting edema is present.

- Auscultate heart sounds; be alert to S_3 gallop, an early sign of heart failure.
- Administer diuretics as prescribed. Observe for indicators of decreased effective circulating volume, such as hypotension, decreased CVP (<5 cm H_2O), and tachycardia. Monitor potassium (K^+) levels, and notify health care provider of levels <3.5 mEq/L.
- If appropriate, teach patient the importance of decreasing intake of Na^+ (or table salt). See Table 3-2, p. 133, for a list of foods high in Na^+.
- If fluids are limited, help relieve patient's thirst by offering ice chips or popsicles. Record the amount of intake on the I&O record.

NIC: Fluid/Electrolyte Management; Invasive Hemodynamic Monitoring; Medication Management; Nutrition Counseling; Surveillance; Teaching: Disease Process

Knowledge deficit: Precautions and side effects of diuretic therapy
Desired outcome: Within the 24-hr period before hospital discharge, patient verbalizes knowledge of the precautions and side effects of diuretic therapy.
- Depending on type of diuretic used, teach patient to report signs and symptoms of the following:
  —*Hypokalemia:* anorexia, irregular pulse, nausea, apathy, and muscle cramps.
  —*Hyperkalemia:* muscle weakness, hyporeflexia, and irregular HR, which can occur with K^+-sparing diuretics.
  —*Hyponatremia:* fatigue, weakness, and edema (caused by fluid extravasation).
- For patients on long-term diuretic therapy, explain the importance of follow-up monitoring of blood levels of Na^+ and K^+.
- For patients receiving K^+-wasting diuretics (e.g., furosemide), instruct patients in the need to take in supplemental high-potassium foods, such as apricots, bananas, oranges, raisins.
- As appropriate, instruct patient to use care when rising from a sitting or recumbent position to prevent injury from orthostatic hypotension.

NIC: Learning Facilitation; Learning Readiness Enhancement; Nutrition Counseling; Teaching: Individual; Teaching: Prescribed Medication

Knowledge deficit: Precautions and side effects of digitalis therapy
Desired outcome: Within the 24-hr period before hospital discharge, patient verbalizes understanding of the precautions and side effects associated with digitalis therapy.
- Teach patient the technique and importance of assessing HR before taking digitalis. Explain that he or she should obtain HR parameters from the health care provider but that digitalis is usually withheld when HR is <60 bpm (unless the patient's usual HR before digitalis administration is <60 bpm). Also instruct the patient to hold the dose if there is a ≥20 bpm change from his or her normal rate. Teach patient to notify health care provider if he or she has omitted a dose because of a slow or significantly changed HR.
- Explain that serum K^+ levels are monitored routinely because low levels can potentiate digitalis toxicity.
- Explain that the apical HR and peripheral pulses are assessed for irregularity, which is a sign of digitalis toxicity.
- Teach patient to be alert to other indicators of digitalis toxicity, including nausea, vomiting, anorexia, headache, diarrhea, blurred vision, yellow-haze vision, and mental confusion. Explain the importance of reporting signs and symptoms promptly to health care provider or staff if they occur.

NIC: Learning Facilitation; Learning Readiness Enhancement; Teaching: Individual; Teaching: Prescribed Medication; Teaching: Psychomotor Skill

Knowledge deficit: Precautions and side effects of vasodilators

Desired outcome: Within the 24-hr period before hospital discharge, patient verbalizes knowledge of the precautions and side effects associated with vasodilators.

- Explain that a headache can occur after administration of a vasodilator and that lying down will help alleviate the pain.
- Teach the importance of assessment for weight gain and signs of peripheral or sacral edema, any of which can occur as side effects of vasodilator therapy.
- For patients on long-term ACE inhibitor therapy, explain the importance of follow-up monitoring of blood levels of serum creatinine because ACE inhibitors may decrease creatinine clearance.
- For patients receiving ACE inhibitors, instruct patient to use care when rising from a sitting or recumbent position to prevent injury from orthostatic hypotension.
- Teach patient receiving ACE inhibitors the technique and importance of assessing BP before taking medication. It is possible to purchase automatic BP machines from local pharmacies. If necessary, seek reimbursement or funding information from a social worker. Explain that patient should obtain BP parameters from the health care provider but that ACE inhibitor is usually withheld when BP is <110/60. Teach patient to notify health care provider if he or she has omitted a dose because of a low or significantly changed BP.
- Instruct patient to alert health care provider to side effects of this therapy.

NIC: Learning Facilitation; Learning Readiness Enhancement; Teaching: Individual; Teaching: Prescribed Medication; Teaching: Psychomotor Skill

---

See Also: "Coronary Artery Disease" for **Altered nutrition,** p. 58; **Knowledge deficit:** Precautions and side effects of β-blockers, p. 60; "Myocardial Infarction" for **Impaired gas exchange,** p. 67; Appendix One, "Caring for Patients on Prolonged Bedrest," p. 738; psychosocial nursing diagnoses in "Caring for Patients With Cancer and Other Life-disrupting Illnesses," p. 791.

PATIENT-FAMILY TEACHING AND DISCHARGE PLANNING

When providing patient-family teaching, focus on sensory information; avoid giving excessive information; and initiate a visiting nurse referral for necessary follow-up teaching. Consider including verbal and written information about the following:

- Medications, including drug name, purpose, dosage, schedule, precautions, drug/drug and food/drug interactions, and potential side effects. Stress the importance of taking medications regularly and not stopping them without health care provider consultation. Teach patient and significant other how to measure HR for digitalis therapy and/or BP for ACE inhibitor therapy.
- Diet: Advise patient that Na^+ restriction may be lessened as cardiac function improves. Assist patient with diet planning or refer to a nutrition specialist if major dietary changes are necessary. Low-Na^+ guidelines are found in Table 3-2, p. 133. Encourage patients to use food labels to determine the Na^+ content of foods.
- Signs and symptoms that necessitate medical attention: irregular pulse, bradycardia, unusual SOB, increased orthopnea, decreased exercise tolerance, and unusual or steady weight gain.
- Importance of quitting smoking, which causes vasoconstriction and increases cardiac workload. Refer patient to a "stop smoking" program as appro-

priate. The following free brochures outline ways to help patients stop smoking:

> *How to Help Your Patients Stop Using Tobacco: A National Cancer Institute Manual for the Oral Health Team,* from the Smoking and Tobacco Control Program of the National Cancer Institute; call 1-800-4-CANCER.

> *Clinical Practice Guideline: A Quick Reference Guide for Smoking Cessation Specialists,* from the Agency for Health Care Policy and Research (AHCPR); call 1-800-358-9295.

- Importance of limiting exertional activities at home (e.g., minimize bending and lifting and avoid stair climbing). However, stress the importance of a progressive increase in activity.
- Emergency phone numbers to call if needed.
- Importance of follow-up care; confirm date and time of next medical appointment.

Pulmonary hypertension

As blood passes through the pulmonary vasculature, it exchanges CO_2 and particulate matter for O_2. Normally the pulmonary vascular bed offers little resistance to blood flow, but when resistance occurs, pulmonary hypertension results. Pulmonary hypertension can be primary (rare), which has a poor prognosis and affects primarily young and middle-age women, or it can be secondary (most common), which often responds to therapy and is found in a variety of medical conditions. The cause of primary pulmonary hypertension is unknown. Possible causes of secondary pulmonary hypertension include increased pulmonary blood flow from a ventricular or atrial shunt, left ventricular failure, chronic hypoxia related to COPD, pulmonary embolus, pulmonary stenosis, or any physiologic occurrence that increases pulmonary vascular resistance or constriction of the vessels in the pulmonary tree.

ASSESSMENT

Acute indicators: Exertional dyspnea, syncope, and precordial chest pain, all of which result from low cardiac output or hypoxia. Cough and palpitations also can occur.

Chronic indicators: Signs of right or left ventricular failure:

Right ventricular failure: Peripheral edema, increased venous pressure and pulsations, liver engorgement, distended neck veins.

Left ventricular failure: Dyspnea; shortness of breath (SOB), particularly on exertion; decreased BP; oliguria; orthopnea; anorexia.

Physical assessment: Cyanosis from decreased cardiac output and subsequent systemic vasoconstriction, systolic murmur caused by tricuspid regurgitation or pulmonary stenosis, diastolic murmur caused by pulmonary valvular incompetence, and accentuated S_2 heart sound.

DIAGNOSTIC TESTS

Chest x-ray: Will show enlargement of the pulmonary artery and right atrium and ventricle. Pulmonary vasculature may appear engorged.

Echocardiography: Often valuable for showing increased right ventricular dimension, thickened right ventricular wall, and possible tricuspid or pulmonary valve dysfunction.

Radionuclide imaging: For example, equilibrium-gated blood pool imaging and thallium imaging to assess function of the right ventricle.

Cardiac catheterization with angiography: Necessary to confirm pulmonary hypertension. Pulmonary vascular resistance will be very high, and pulmonary artery and right ventricular pressures can approach or equal systemic arterial pressures. (See "Cardiac Catheterization, Angioplasty, and Atherectomy," p. 109, for further detail.)

Pulmonary perfusion scintigraphy (perfusion scan): A noninvasive way to assess pulmonary blood flow. This study involves IV injection of serum albumin tagged with trace amounts of a radioisotope, most often technetium. The particles pass through the circulation and lodge in the pulmonary vascular bed. Subsequent scanning reveals concentrations of particles in areas of adequate pulmonary blood flow.

ECG: Will show evidence of right atrial enlargement and right ventricular enlargement (evidenced by right axis deviation and tall, peaked P waves) secondary to the increased pressure needed to force blood through the hypertensive pulmonary vascular bed.

Pulmonary function test: Results are usually normal, although some individuals will have increased residual volume, reduced maximum voluntary ventilation, and decreased vital capacity.

ABG analysis: May show low partial pressure of dissolved carbon dioxide in arterial blood ($Paco_2$) and high pH, which occur with hyperventilation, or increased $Paco_2$ with decreased gas exchange.

Oximetry: May show decreased O_2 (e.g., <92%).

CBC: Polycythemia can occur in the presence of chronic hypoxemia as a result of compensation.

Liver function tests: May be abnormal if venous congestion is significant. Examples include increased serum glutamic-oxaloacetic transaminase (SGOT or AST [aspartate aminotransferase]), serum glutamic-pyruvic transaminase (SGPT or ALT [alanine aminotransferase]), and bilirubin.

Open lung biopsy: May be done to establish the type of disorder causing the hypertension.

COLLABORATIVE MANAGEMENT

O_2: Usually 2-5 L/min by nasal cannula. If hypoxia is severe, O_2 is administered by mask.

> **Caution:** Use care when administering O_2 to patients with a history of COPD.

Diet: Low in Na^+ (see Table 3-2, p. 133) if signs of heart failure are present. Encourage patients to use food labels to determine the Na^+ content of foods.

Pharmacotherapy

Diuretics: If indicators of right-sided or left-sided heart failure are present.

Anticoagulant (warfarin sodium): Although prophylactic use is controversial, it may be administered if pulmonary emboli are present.

Vasodilators and calcium antagonists: To decrease cardiac workload by vasodilation.

Inhaled nitrous oxide (NO): A selective pulmonary vasodilator used to decrease pulmonary vascular resistance (PVR) in patients with primary pulmonary hypertension.

Bronchodilators (aminophylline): Have been shown to reduce pulmonary artery and right ventricular pressures in some cases.

β-*Adrenergic agents (e.g., terbutaline):* To decrease pulmonary vascular resistance.

Treatment of causative factor if possible: For example, by surgically closing arteriovenous shunts or replacing defective valves.

Heart-lung transplantation: For advanced (end-stage) pulmonary vascular disease.

NURSING DIAGNOSES AND INTERVENTIONS

Impaired gas exchange related to altered blood flow secondary to pulmonary capillary constriction

Desired outcome: Patient has improved gas exchange by at least 24 hr before hospital discharge, as evidenced by O_2 saturation $\geq$92% and partial pressure of dissolved oxygen in arterial blood (Pao_2) $\geq$80 mm Hg.

- Monitor oximetry for low O_2 saturation; report O_2 saturation <92% to health care provider.
- Monitor ABG results for evidence of hypoventilation: decreased $Paco_2$, increased $Paco_2$, and decreased pH; and for evidence of hyperventilation: low $Paco_2$ and high pH. Report significant findings to the health care provider.
- Auscultate lung fields q4-8hr, or more frequently as indicated, to assess lung sounds. Note and report to health care provider the presence of adventitious sounds (especially rales), which can occur with fluid extravasation.
- Assess respiratory rate, pattern, and depth; chest excursion; and use of accessory muscles of respiration q4hr.
- Observe for and document presence of cyanosis or skin color change, which can occur with decreased gas exchange.
- Help patient into Fowler's position (HOB up 90 degrees), if possible, to reduce work of breathing (WOB) and maximize chest excursion.
- Teach patient to take slow, deep breaths to enhance gas exchange.
- Administer prescribed low-flow O_2 as indicated. Deliver O_2 with humidity to help prevent its drying effects on oral and nasal mucosa.
- Monitor mental status for and report changes in mental acuity or level of consciousness as indications of acid-base imbalance.

NIC: Acid-Base Monitoring; Neurologic Monitoring; Oxygen Therapy; Positioning; Respiratory Monitoring; Vital Signs Monitoring

Activity intolerance related to generalized weakness and imbalance between oxygen supply and demand secondary to right and left ventricular failure

Desired outcome: By at least 24 hr before hospital discharge, patient rates perceived exertion at $\leq$3 on a 0-10 scale and exhibits cardiac tolerance to activity as evidenced by RR $\leq$20 breaths/min, HR $\leq$20 bpm over resting HR, and systolic BP within 20 mm Hg of resting range.

- Ask patient to rate perceived exertion during activity, and monitor for evidence of activity intolerance. For details, see **Risk for activity intolerance** in Appendix One, "Caring for Patients on Prolonged Bedrest," p. 739. Notify health care provider of significant findings.
- Observe for and document any changes in VS. Monitor BP at least q4hr. Report drops >10-20 mm Hg, which can signal decompensation of the cardiac muscle. Also be alert to other signs of left ventricular failure, including dyspnea, SOB, crackles (rales), and decreased O_2 saturation (<92%) as determined by oximetry.
- Measure and document I&O and weight, reporting any steady gains or losses. Be alert to other signs of right ventricular failure, including peripheral edema, both pedal and sacral; ascites; distended neck veins; and increased CVP (>12 cm H_2O).
- Administer diuretics, vasodilators, and calcium channel blockers as prescribed.
- Facilitate coordination of health care providers to provide rest periods between care activities to decrease oxygen demand. Allow 90 min for undisturbed rest. If necessary, limit visitors to allow adequate rest.
- Keep frequently used items within patient's reach so that exertion can be avoided as much as possible.

- Assist patient with maintaining prescribed activity level and progress as tolerated. If activity intolerance is observed, stop the activity and have patient rest.
- Assist patient with ROM exercises at frequent intervals. To help prevent complications caused by immobility, plan progressive ambulation and exercise based on patient's tolerance and prescribed activity restrictions. See also Appendix One, "Caring for Patients on Prolonged Bedrest," **Risk for activity intolerance,** p. 738, and **Risk for disuse syndrome,** p. 740.

NIC: Activity Therapy; Cardiac Care; Energy Management; Environmental Management; Exercise Promotion; Surveillance

Knowledge deficit: Disease process and treatment
Desired outcome: Within 24 hr before hospital discharge, patient and significant other verbalize knowledge of the disease, its treatment, and measures that promote wellness.
- Assess the patient's level of knowledge of the disease process and its treatment.
- Discuss the purposes of the medications: to ease the workload of the heart (vasodilators); "relax" the heart (calcium antagonists); and prevent fluid accumulation (diuretics).
- Provide emotional support to the patient adapting to the concept of having a chronic disease.
- If the cause of pulmonary hypertension is known, reinforce explanations of the disease process and treatment.
- Discuss life-style changes that may be required to prevent future complications or control the disease process.
- Explain the value of relaxation techniques, including tapes, soothing music, meditation, and biofeedback. See "Coronary Artery Disease," **Health-seeking behaviors:** Relaxation technique effective for stress reduction, p. 59.
- If the patient smokes, explain that smoking increases the workload of the heart by causing vasoconstriction. Provide materials that explain the benefits of quitting smoking, such as pamphlets prepared by the American Heart Association. Either provide the address or phone number for the local chapter or encourage the patient to write for information to the following address:

American Heart Association
7320 Greenville Avenue
Dallas, TX 75231   (800) 242-8721
WWW address: *http://occ.com/amerh*

- Provide the phone number to find out about local smoking cessation programs.
- Confer with health care provider about type of exercise program that will benefit the patient; provide patient teaching as indicated.
- If appropriate, involve the dietitian to assist patient with planning low-sodium meals.

NIC: Coping Enhancement; Health Education; Simple Relaxation Therapy; Smoking Cessation; Teaching: Disease Process; Teaching: Prescribed Diet; Teaching: Prescribed Medication

---

See Also: "Heart Failure" for **Fluid volume excess,** p. 70; **Knowledge deficit:** Precautions and side effects of diuretic therapy, p. 71; **Knowledge deficit:** Precautions and side effects of vasodilators, p. 72; psychosocial nursing diagnoses in Appendix One, "Caring for Patients With Cancer and Other Life-disrupting Illnesses," p. 791.

PATIENT-FAMILY TEACHING AND DISCHARGE PLANNING

When providing patient-family teaching, focus on sensory information; avoid giving too much information; and initiate a visiting nurse referral for necessary follow-up teaching. Consider including verbal and written information about the following:

- Indicators that necessitate medical attention: decreased exercise tolerance, increasing SOB or dyspnea, swelling of ankles and legs, steady weight gain.
- Medications, including drug name, purpose, dosage, schedule, precautions, drug/drug and food/drug interactions, and potential side effects.
- Elimination of smoking; refer patient to a "stop smoking" program as appropriate. The following free brochures outline ways to help patients stop smoking:

    How to Help Your Patients Stop Using Tobacco: A National Cancer Institute Manual for the Oral Health Team, from the Smoking and Tobacco Control Program of the National Cancer Institute; call 1-800-4-CANCER.

    Clinical Practice Guideline: A Quick Reference Guide for Smoking Cessation Specialists, from the Agency for Health Care Policy and Research (AHCPR); call 1-800-358-9295.

- For additional information see **Knowledge deficit** on p. 76.

Section Two: Inflammatory Heart Disorders

The disorders described in this section are inflammations or infections involving mainly the heart muscle and its linings, the pericardium and endocardium. The inflammation can be acute or chronic, and prognosis usually depends on extent of the involvement, structures involved, and secondary disorders that occur.

Pericarditis

Pericarditis is an inflammation of the stiff, fibrous sac (pericardium) that surrounds, supports, and protects the heart. The pericardium is composed of a fibrous outer layer and a serous inner layer. The inflammatory condition produces friction between the layers during cardiac movement. Acute pericarditis causes exudate production and formation of chronic fibrinous adhesions. The inflammation accompanying pericarditis may allow formation of pericardial effusions. Pericarditis occurs in a large number of medical disorders. The most common causes are viral or bacterial infections, uremia, acute MI, neoplastic disease, and trauma.

ASSESSMENT

Chronic indicators: Elevated CVP and signs secondary to systemic venous congestion, including edema, ascites, and hepatic congestion. If fibrous constriction is severe, symptoms of left-sided heart failure may appear, such as dyspnea, cough, and orthopnea.

Acute indicators: Chest pain localized to the retrosternal and left precordial regions or pain that mimics acute abdominal pain or ischemic pain. The pain is described as sharp and may radiate to the back, neck, or left shoulder or arm. Unlike ischemic pain, however, it is often increased with coughing or deep inspirations (a pleuritic component is possible), movement, or lying down and eased by sitting up and leaning forward. Other indicators include dyspnea (may result from thoracic pain, splinting the chest, or cardiac compression by fluid), tachycardia, fever, and pulsus paradoxus (decrease in pulse volume and an abnormal fall in systolic BP ≥10 mm Hg during inspiration as compared with exhalation).

Physical assessment: Characteristic pericardial friction rub (a scratching, grating, high-pitched sound) heard on auscultation.

> **Note:** Cardiac tamponade may create compression of the heart by fluid accumulating in the pericardial sac. Cardiac tamponade is a potentially life-threatening condition. The presenting symptom is tachycardia, which occurs to maintain adequate cardiac output as the heart compensates for decreased ability of the ventricles to fill during diastole and provide adequate stroke volume. Additional symptoms may include anxiety, restlessness, dyspnea, feelings of fullness in the chest, distant heart sounds, narrowed pulse pressure, jugular venous distention, elevated CVP, and changes in mental status progressing to loss of consciousness. As decompensation progresses, cardiac output, and thus blood pressure, will fall, eventually creating a shocklike state. Treatment involves emergency pericardiocentesis (see below).

DIAGNOSTIC TESTS

Serial ECGs: Typically show widespread ST-segment elevation in most leads, unlike localized ischemic ST-segment elevation.

CBC and other hematologic studies: Often show presence of increased WBCs (leukocytosis) and increased erythrocyte sedimentation rate (ESR) in the presence of inflammation.

Cardiac enzymes: Probably will be normal, although the MB fraction of creatinine phosphokinase (CPK or CK) may increase with epicardial inflammation.

Chest x-ray: Often is normal, but with sufficient pericardial effusion the heart will appear more globe shaped; with chronic pericarditis the x-ray may reveal pericardial calcifications.

Echocardiogram: Reveals increase in pericardial fluid, which occurs with infection or irritation.

COLLABORATIVE MANAGEMENT

Treatment of underlying disorder

Bedrest: Until pain and fever are relieved.

Pharmacotherapy

Nonsteroidal antiinflammatory drugs (NSAIDs):   To combat fever, reduce inflammation, and control pain. See Table 8-1, p. 555.

Corticosteroids: (e.g., prednisone, 60-80 mg qd in divided doses for 5-7 days and tapered thereafter) if symptoms are unrelieved by NSAIDs.

Antibiotics: Given only in the presence of purulent pericarditis.

Emergency pericardiocentesis: If cardiac tamponade (accumulation of fluid that restricts ventricular filling and reduces cardiac output) develops. This procedure involves needle aspiration of the fluid in the pericardial sac to relieve pressure and allow for normal cardiac muscle contraction. Aspirated fluid may be sent for culture and sensitivity. Usually it is done with the patient under local anesthesia in the ICU, operating room, or cardiac catheterization laboratory.

Partial or total pericardiectomy: To allow normal cardiac movement and function if pericarditis is recurrent and has produced scar tissue and constriction. This procedure involves the removal of part (a pericardial "window") or all of the pericardium to prevent constriction by scar tissue, exudate, or bleeding.

NURSING DIAGNOSES AND INTERVENTIONS

Activity intolerance related to imbalance between oxygen supply and demand secondary to inflammation of the cardiac muscle and restriction of contraction
Desired outcome: During activity, patient rates perceived exertion at ≤3 on a 0-10 scale and exhibits cardiac tolerance to activity as evidenced by systolic BP within 20 mm Hg of resting systolic BP, RR ≤20 breaths/min, HR ≤20 bpm above resting HR, and absence of chest pain or new dysrhythmias.

- Ask patient to rate perceived exertion during activity, and monitor for evidence of activity intolerance. For details, see **Risk for activity intolerance** in Appendix One, "Caring for Patients on Prolonged Bedrest," p. 738. Notify health care provider of significant findings.
- Ensure that patient maintains bedrest during febrile period and understands the rationale for doing so.
- Anticipate patient's needs by placing personal articles within easy reach.
- Advise patient about the importance of frequent rest periods during convalescence.
- Monitor VS for changes indicative of cardiac or pulmonary decompensation, such as pallor, diaphoresis, dysrhythmia, decreasing BP, and increasing heart and respiratory rates.
- Assist patient with turning at least q2hr, and provide passive ROM exercises at frequent intervals to help prevent complications of immobility. As the patient's condition improves, consult health care provider about in-bed exercises that require more cardiac tolerance. Examples are found in Appendix One, **Risk for activity intolerance,** p. 738, and **Risk for disuse syndrome,** p. 740.

NIC: Activity Therapy; Cardiac Care; Energy Management; Environmental Management; Exercise Promotion; Surveillance

Altered peripheral, cardiopulmonary, cerebral, and renal tissue perfusion (or risk for same) related to interrupted blood flow secondary to dysfunctional cardiac muscle
Desired outcome: Within 24 hr of admission, patient has adequate tissue perfusion as evidenced by distal pulses >2+ on a 0-4+ scale; HR ≤100 bpm; BP ≥90/60 mm Hg; RR ≤20 breaths/min with normal depth and pattern (eupnea); normal heart sounds; absence of significant mental status changes and orientation to person, place, and time; and urinary output ≥30 ml/hr.

- Observe for and report increasing restlessness or anxiety and changes in mentation, which can occur with decreased cerebral perfusion.
- Palpate distal pulses at least q2-4hr to assess peripheral perfusion and dysrhythmias.
- Be alert to signs of cardiac tamponade, including anxiety, restlessness, dyspnea, feelings of fullness in the chest, distant heart sounds, narrowed pulse pressure, jugular venous distention, elevated CVP, and changes in mental status progressing to loss of consciousness. Report significant findings to health care provider, and prepare for emergency pericardiocentesis.
- Assess for pulsus paradoxus (decrease in pulse volume, and systolic BP >10 mm Hg during inhalation as compared with exhalation), which is produced by pericardial restriction and subsequent decreased ventricular filling. The assessment is performed as follows:
  —Apply BP cuff to the patient's arm; palpate the brachial pulse.
  —Place the stethoscope over the pulse point, and inflate the cuff to above the level of the patient's normal systolic BP.
  —Slowly deflate the cuff. Ask patient to exhale.
  —Listen for the first sound that occurs after the patient exhales. Note the manometer reading, and tell patient to breathe normally.

—Continue to deflate the BP cuff slowly until sounds are heard during inhalation and exhalation. Note the reading.

—Calculate the difference in mm Hg between the two readings. This is the measurement of pulsus paradoxus.

- Instruct patient to perform foot and leg exercises q4hr to enhance venous circulation. Consider use of antiembolism hose to reduce venostasis and sequential compression devices or pneumatic foot pumps to further enhance venous return. See Appendix One, p. 742, for a description of exercises.
- If patient exhibits signs of decreased cerebral perfusion, reorient and institute safety precautions as necessary. Notify the health care provider of significant or continued mental status changes.
- Monitor urinary output to determine renal perfusion. Be alert to output <30 ml/hr for 2 consecutive hr, and report findings to the health care provider if appropriate.

NIC: Cerebral Perfusion Promotion; Circulatory Care; Fluid Management; Neurologic Monitoring; Surveillance; Vital Signs Monitoring

Pain (friction rub) related to inflammatory process
Desired outcomes: Within 24 hr of initiation of antiinflammatory medication, patient's subjective perception of pain decreases, as documented by a pain scale. Objective indicators, such as grimacing, are absent.
- Auscultate heart sounds for the presence of friction rub as an indicator of pericardial inflammation.
- Assess and document character, intensity, and duration of pain. Establish a pain scale with the patient, rating the pain from 0 (no pain) to 10 (worst pain). Administer pain medications as prescribed, and document their effectiveness using the pain scale. Advise patient to request pain medication before pain becomes severe.
- Use the following interventions to enhance the effectiveness of the medication: support the patient in a side-lying position with pillows, or place the patient in Fowler's position (HOB up 90 degrees); pad an overbed table with pillows or bath blankets to support the patient; provide emotional support; and control environmental stimuli by limiting visitors (as necessary to ensure adequate rest), dimming lights, and maintaining quiet.
- Administer O_2 as prescribed, typically 2-3 L/min by nasal cannula. Deliver O_2 with humidity to help prevent its drying effects on oral and nasal mucosa.
- Administer NSAIDs, steroids, or antibiotics as prescribed to manage the pericardial inflammation.

NIC: Analgesic Administration; Emotional Support; Environmental Management: Comfort; Medication Management; Oxygen Therapy; Pain Management

Ineffective breathing pattern related to decreased lung expansion secondary to guarding because of pericardial pain
Desired outcome: Within 1 hr of the intervention(s), patient's RR is 12-20 breaths/min with normal depth and pattern (eupnea) and O_2 saturation is ≥92%.
- Assess breath sounds and respirations at least q4hr. Report the presence of crackles (rales) or areas of diminished breath sounds, which may occur as a result of atelectasis caused by decreased depth of respirations (guarding).
- Assess the breathing effort for adequate depth at least q2hr, and teach the patient to breathe deeply. Teach the use of an incentive spirometer.
- Monitor O_2 saturation; report saturation readings <92% to the health care provider. Provide supplemental O_2 as prescribed, typically 2-3 L/min by nasal cannula. Deliver O_2 with humidity to help prevent its drying effects on oral and nasal mucosa.

- Instruct the patient in use of a cascade cough to reduce stressful coughing, which increases pain. Cascade cough is a series (2-5) of small forceful exhalations used to mobilize secretions.
- Place the patient in semi-Fowler's (HOB up 30-45 degrees) or high Fowler's (HOB up 90 degrees) position to ease pressure on the heart, which will help decrease the effort of breathing.

NIC: Airway Management; Cough Enhancement; Oxygen Therapy; Respiratory Management; Teaching: Individual

---

See Also: Appendix One, "Caring for Patients on Prolonged Bedrest," p. 738.

PATIENT-FAMILY TEACHING AND DISCHARGE PLANNING

When providing patient-family teaching, focus on sensory information; avoid giving excessive information; and initiate a visiting nurse referral for necessary follow-up teaching. Consider including verbal and written information about the following:

- Importance of frequent rest periods during convalescence.
- Importance of prompt treatment if symptoms of pericarditis recur.
- Procedure for measuring temperature, which can be an indicator of recurring inflammation.
- Importance of avoiding individuals with upper respiratory infections (URIs) and promptly seeking medical attention if influenza or cold symptoms occur.
- Medications, including drug name, purpose, dosage, schedule, precautions, drug/drug and food/drug interactions, and potential side effects.
- Importance of understanding that feelings of wellness do not necessarily mean that the inflammation has completely resolved.

Infective endocarditis

Inflammation of the inner lining of the atria, ventricles, and covering of the heart valves is called *infective endocarditis*. This infection involves the left side of the heart more frequently than the right side and is characterized by vegetation (fibrous networks of platelets, blood cells, and pathogenic organisms) that are found most frequently on the mitral and aortic valves or around prosthetic valves. Vegetation on the valves can prevent adequate closure and adherence of the valve flaps, resulting in regurgitation or stenosis. When the vegetation affects the chamber lining, muscle fibers eventually undergo degenerative changes, and the patient becomes at risk for emboli because parts of the vegetation can break off. In addition, fibrin and platelets tend to deposit on the vegetation, and these may embolize as well. Endocarditis usually is classified as acute or subacute. Manifestations of infective endocarditis are the result of infection (systemic and local), the effects of emboli or valvular dysfunction, or antigen-antibody reactions and resultant complexes causing injury to the microvasculature. Endocarditis occurs most commonly in IV drug users or patients with recent cardiac surgery, prosthetic heart valves, or prolonged IV therapy.

ASSESSMENT

Chronic indicators: Murmurs (sign of valvular involvement); dyspnea, distended neck veins, peripheral edema, pulmonary congestion, splenomegaly, and activity intolerance (signs of heart failure).

Acute indicators: Temperature elevation (to 104° F [40° C]), chills, malaise, anorexia, weight loss, tachycardia, pallor, diaphoresis, night sweats, joint pain.

Physical assessment: Presence of a murmur. If heart failure has developed as a result of valvular dysfunction, the following may be present: crackles, SOB, edema, neck vein distention, hepatomegaly.

> **Note:** If embolization has occurred, signs may include evidence of decreased renal, cerebral, and peripheral perfusion.

History of: URI, influenza, or other infectious process; cardiac surgery or heart valve replacement; prolonged IV therapy; IV drug use.

DIAGNOSTIC TESTS

Blood cultures: To identify causative organism; should include aerobic and anaerobic cultures.

Erythrocyte sedimentation rate (ESR):   Usually elevated because of inflammatory process.

WBC count: May be normal in subacute forms and can range from 15,000-20,000/mm^3 in acute disease.

Chest x-ray: May reveal early findings of heart failure (e.g., vascular engorgement, increased heart size).

Two-dimensional echocardiography: May be used to detect intracardiac complications such as valvular disorders or wall motion abnormalities. This test uses sound waves (or echoes), which allow visualization of the cardiac wall and valvular movement.

Echo with Doppler: May be performed to evaluate valvular involvement. Adding the Doppler to the echocardiogram provides more or different information than would be found using the echo alone.

COLLABORATIVE MANAGEMENT

Specific antibiotic therapy: Will depend on the causative organism and its susceptibility or sensitivity to drugs. In the subacute form of the disorder, it is satisfactory to wait until the organism is identified, but with acute endocarditis, broad-spectrum antibiotic therapy is instituted immediately after blood cultures are drawn and then adjusted if necessary after organism identification. Intermittent IV antibiotics are given q4-6hr. The duration of therapy usually is 4-6 wk.

Bedrest

Well-balanced diet: To maintain resistance to infection.

Surgical repair or valve replacement: Performed when heart failure does not respond to medical management; when an infection does not respond to antimicrobial therapy within 1 wk; when repeated episodes of embolization occur, especially when vascular occlusions are found in the eyes, brain, coronary arteries, and kidneys; when repeated infections occur (e.g., relapse after 3 mo); and when fungal endocarditis is found. See discussion of mitral valve replacement in "Mitral Stenosis," p. 84.

Treatment of heart failure, if present: See "Heart Failure," p. 69.

NURSING DIAGNOSES AND INTERVENTIONS

Risk for infection with risk factors associated with invasive procedures and inadequate secondary defenses (decreased immune response) secondary to prolonged antibiotic therapy

Desired outcome: Patient is free of infection as evidenced by normothermia, normal skin temperature and color at IV sites, HR ≤100 bpm, and straw-colored, clear urine.

- Use sterile technique when working with IV lines, urinary catheters, and wounds.
- Monitor patient's body temperature and WBC count for increases from baseline assessment. Both already may be increased as a result of the primary infection, but unexplained increases may occur after resolution of the acute phase as a result of a secondary infection.
- For patients with indwelling urinary catheters, monitor urine for signs of infection, including cloudiness and foul odor. Cleanse the urethral meatus and surrounding area daily, using soap and water.
- Rotate IV sites and change tubing and dressings q48-72hr or per agency protocol.

NIC: Infection Control; Laboratory Data Interpretation; Surveillance; Tube Care: Urinary; Vital Signs Monitoring

Knowledge deficit: Disease process, therapeutic regimen, and assessment for infection
Desired outcome: Within the 24-hr period before hospital discharge, patient verbalizes understanding of the disease process and measures that prevent bacteremia.
- Assess patient's level of knowledge about the disease and therapy.
- As indicated, explain the disease process and the need for prolonged antibiotic therapy.
- Because of the increased risk of bacteremia, discuss the need for antibiotic prophylaxis before dental procedures and all major and minor surgical procedures and of early treatment of common infections (e.g., UTIs, URIs, and wound infection).
- Teach patient the early indicators of infection (see descriptions in "Care of the Renal Transplant Recipient," p. 161; Table 5-4, p. 382) and the importance of reporting indicators to health care provider promptly. Teach patient how to measure body temperature and the importance of monitoring temperature weekly if asymptomatic and more frequently if weakness, fatigue, or symptoms of a cold or influenza occur.

NIC: Learning Facilitation; Learning Readiness Enhancement; Teaching: Disease Process; Teaching: Prescribed Medication; Teaching: Psychomotor Skill

---

See Also: "Pulmonary Embolus" for **Altered protection** related to risk of prolonged bleeding or hemorrhage secondary to anticoagulation therapy, p. 18; "Myocardial Infarction" for **Impaired gas exchange,** p. 67; "Pericarditis" for **Activity intolerance,** p. 79; "Osteomyelitis" for **Knowledge deficit:** Side effects from prolonged use of potent antibiotics, p. 581; Appendix One, "Caring for Preoperative and Postoperative Patients," p. 717; "Caring for Patients on Prolonged Bedrest," p. 738.

PATIENT-FAMILY TEACHING AND DISCHARGE PLANNING

When providing patient-family teaching, focus on sensory information; avoid giving excessive information; and initiate a visiting nurse referral for necessary follow-up teaching. Consider including verbal and written information about the following:
- Need for prolonged antibiotic therapy, including prophylaxis before dental procedures (including teeth cleaning) and surgery.
- Other medications to be taken at home, including drug name, purpose, dosage, schedule, precautions, drug/drug and food/drug interactions, and potential side effects.

> **Note:** The patient may be required to self-administer IV antibiotics at home to decrease the length of hospital stay; teach the technique if indicated.

- Importance of medical follow-up to check valve function; confirm date and time of next medical appointment.
- Signs and symptoms of URI and other infections (see p. 161 and Table 5-4) that can precipitate recurrence of endocardial infection, indicators of recurrence of endocarditis, and the importance of getting prompt medical attention if they occur.
- Inform the patient of a booklet available from the American Heart Association entitled "Prevention of Endocarditis," which summarizes preventive procedures. The address is as follows:

  American Heart Association
  7320 Greenville Avenue
  Dallas, TX 75231   (800) 242-8721
  WWW address: *http://occ.com/amerh*

- Importance of reporting signs of increasing cardiac failure *stat*. These include steady weight gain, decreased exercise tolerance, fatigue, and dyspnea.
- Importance of regular temperature measurement (e.g., weekly if asymptomatic and more frequently if weakness, fatigue, or symptoms of a cold or influenza occur).

Section Three: Valvular Heart Disorders

Mitral stenosis

The most common cause of mitral valve stenosis is rheumatic heart disease, although it can be caused also by bacterial or viral endocarditis or malignancy. The mitral valve is composed of two leaflets, and obstruction occurs because of adhesions between the leaflets, calcifications and loss of leaflet mobility, or fibrosis of the chordae tendineae and associated papillary muscles.

Because the mitral valve is located between the left atrium and ventricle, stenosis results in decreased ventricular filling and increased left atrial and pulmonary pressures. As the severity of the stenosis increases, maintenance of cardiac output becomes more difficult. In addition, high pulmonary pressures cause fluid extravasation into the alveoli, which results in pulmonary edema.

Individuals with valvular disorders are predisposed to endocarditis. Bacteria in the bloodstream have a tendency to lodge in the malfunctioning valves because of calcium deposits or turbulent blood flow, so special care should be taken whenever a systemic infection is present or the patient is undergoing major or minor surgical procedures, such as dental work.

> **See Also:** "Infective Endocarditis," p. 81.

ASSESSMENT

Chronic indicators: Decreased exercise tolerance secondary to decreased cardiac output; increased pulmonary artery pressures.
Acute indicators: Dyspnea usually is the first symptom of worsening stenosis. Orthopnea, hemoptysis, thromboembolism, and chest pain with subsequent right ventricular failure may occur with elevated pulmonary pressure. In some patients, chest pain occurs secondary to decreased O_2 perfusion.

Physical assessment: Decreased arterial pulse volume, as determined by palpation or Doppler ultrasonic probe; increased venous pulsations; low-pitched diastolic murmur; elevated CVP; ascites; peripheral edema; hepatomegaly. Erythema of the cheeks, so-called *malar flush*, may also be present. Left ventricular impulse (the point of maximal impulse [PMI]) may be displaced by an enlarged right ventricle. Normally, it is best heard over the mitral area, fifth intercostal space, midclavicular line. A characteristic diastolic murmur is frequently audible at the cardiac apex; this is best heard with the patient in the left lateral position while listening with the bell of the stethoscope. With increasing obstruction there may also be a high-pitched "snap" as the mitral valve opens in the presence of increased atrial pressure.

DIAGNOSTIC TESTS

Chest x-ray: May reveal an enlarged left atrium and right ventricle.
Echocardiography: Can readily diagnose mitral stenosis by poor valve leaflet separation and thickened leaflets; also may demonstrate pulmonary hypertension.
ECG: Although not useful for a definitive diagnosis, it will demonstrate characteristic changes associated with left atrial and right ventricular enlargement, such as tall P waves and right axis deviation.
Cardiac catheterization: To assess pressures within each heart chamber and major vessels to determine extent of the stenosis. See "Cardiac Catheterization, Angioplasty, and Atherectomy," p. 109.

COLLABORATIVE MANAGEMENT

Restriction of physically strenuous activities
Antibiotic prophylaxis for endocarditis: Before and after invasive procedures, including dental work. See "Infective Endocarditis," p. 81.
Low-Na$^+$ diet: To reduce fluid retention. See Table 3-2, p. 133.
Pharmacotherapy
Diuretics (amiloride, bumetanide, furosemide): To control fluid accumulation and reduce blood volume to reduce pulmonary artery pressures and relieve dyspnea.
Positive inotropic drugs such as digitalis glycosides: To increase the strength of contraction for patients with ventricular failure.
Oral anticoagulants (warfarin sodium): May be prescribed to prevent thromboemboli.
Quinidine: To combat supraventricular dysrhythmias.
Mitral commissurotomy (mitral valvulotomy): To relieve stenosis by incising the valve leaflets. This procedure involves a heart-lung bypass. Usually the chest is entered through the left fifth intercostal space. The left atrial appendage is incised, and a dilator is inserted and guided through the mitral orifice.
Percutaneous mitral valve balloon valvuloplasty: An alternative to surgery for some patients, this procedure is done in the cardiac catheterization laboratory, using local anesthetic. A balloon dilating catheter is inserted into the valve and inflated across the area of stenosis.
Mitral valve replacement: Three types of valve replacements are currently in use: a bioprosthesis (porcine heterograft), tilting disk valve (Bjork-Shiley valve), or caged ball valve (Starr-Edwards prosthesis). The bioprosthesis has a relatively short longevity (6-10 yr), requiring periodic surgical replacement. The two mechanical prostheses have excellent longevity but may cause thrombus formation, necessitating lifelong antithrombotic therapy with sodium warfarin. The valves are placed via a midline sternotomy incision, whereas the prosthesis is inserted while the patient is on a heart-lung bypass machine. Usually the patient remains in the ICU for 24-48 hr after the procedure.

NURSING DIAGNOSES AND INTERVENTIONS

Activity intolerance related to generalized weakness and imbalance between oxygen supply and demand secondary to decreased left ventricular filling
Desired outcome: By at least 24 hr before hospital discharge, patient rates perceived exertion at ≤ 3 on a 0-10 scale and exhibits cardiac tolerance to activity as evidenced by HR ≤ 20 bpm over resting HR, systolic BP within 20 mm Hg of resting systolic BP, and RR ≤ 20 breaths/min with normal depth and pattern (eupnea).

- Monitor VS with patient activity, and report significant (20 mm Hg or more) decrease or increase in BP. Be alert to indicators of activity intolerance, including SOB, dyspnea, and fatigue. Ask patients about perceived exertion (see description, p. 739).
- Assess for orthostatic changes in BP that occur when the patient moves from supine to standing position.
- Assess peripheral pulses, capillary refill, and temperature and color of the extremities as indicators of cardiac output.
- Facilitate coordination of health care providers to provide rest periods between care activities to decrease cardiac workload. Ensure 90 min for undisturbed rest.
- Confer with health care provider about in-bed exercises that can be incorporated as the patient's condition improves. Increase ambulation progressively and to the patient's tolerance.
- For further interventions, see Appendix One, **Risk for activity intolerance,** p. 738, and **Risk for disuse syndrome,** p. 740, for examples of in-bed exercises.

NIC: Activity Therapy; Cardiac Care; Energy Management; Environmental Management; Exercise Promotion; Surveillance

Fluid volume excess related to compromised regulatory mechanisms secondary to right-sided heart failure
Desired outcome: Within 24 hr of treatment, patient is normovolemic as evidenced by CVP 5-12 cm H_2O, balanced I&O, stable weight, urine output ≥ 30 ml/hr, edema $\leq 1+$ on a 0-4+ scale, flattened neck veins, and lungs clear on auscultation.

- Observe for and report the following indicators of right-sided heart failure: increasing CVP (≥ 12 cm H_2O), peripheral edema, dyspnea, hepatic enlargement on palpation, and jugular vein distention.
- Monitor I&O and administer fluids only as prescribed to ensure that patient maintains adequate volume without overload. Weigh patient daily, and report significant I&O imbalance.
- If fluids are limited, offer ice chips and popsicles to help patient control thirst. Record the amount of intake. Offer frequent oral hygiene to reduce oral dryness.
- As prescribed, administer inotropic drugs, such as digitalis, to increase the strength of cardiac contraction.
- Administer diuretics as prescribed to decrease volume load.

NIC: Fluid Management; Invasive Hemodynamic Monitoring; Medication Management; Surveillance; Vital Signs Monitoring

Risk for infection (with concomitant endocarditis) with risk factors from tissue destruction and increased exposure secondary to lodging of bacteria in the malfunctioning valve
Desired outcome: Patient is free of infection as evidenced by normothermia, WBC count $\leq 11,000/mm^3$, and HR ≤ 100 bpm.

- Maintain sterile technique for all invasive procedures.
- Monitor temperature q4hr, and report significant increases.
- Be alert to rising HR, which can signal an infection.

- Administer prescribed antibiotics on time.
- Maintain hydration, as prescribed, through oral and prescribed IV fluids, making sure that patient has adequate volume without overload.

NIC: Fluid Management; Infection Protection; Intravenous (IV) Therapy; Medication Management; Vital Signs Monitoring

Knowledge deficit: Disease process and treatments/management
Desired outcome: Within the 24-hr period before hospital discharge, patient verbalizes knowledge of valvular disorder, its treatment/management, and the potential for developing endocarditis.
- Discuss patient's valve disorder and associated physiologic effects and symptoms. Describe treatment options, including commissurotomy, percutaneous balloon valvuloplasty, and valve replacement surgery.
- Assess patient's knowledge about the potential for endocarditis. As indicated, explain how endocarditis affects the heart and its valves and why individuals with valvular disorders are predisposed toward developing this disorder.
- Teach patient the following indicators of endocarditis: temperature increases, malaise, anorexia, tachycardia, pallor. Explain the importance of reporting the symptoms early.
- Teach patient the indicators of frequently encountered infections (e.g., upper respiratory, urinary tract, wound). For a description, see "Care of the Renal Transplant Recipient," p. 161; Table 5-4, "Infectious Processes Requiring Medical Intervention," p. 382. Stress the importance of reporting symptoms promptly should they occur, since a systemic infection can lead to endocarditis.
- Discuss the importance of antibiotic prophylaxis before and after any major or minor surgical procedures, including dental procedures.

NIC: Learning Facilitation; Learning Readiness Enhancement; Teaching: Disease Process; Teaching: Preoperative; Teaching: Prescribed Medication

> **See Also:**   "Pulmonary Embolus" for **Altered protection** related to risk of prolonged bleeding or hemorrhage secondary to anticoagulation therapy, p. 18; "Heart Failure" for **Knowledge deficit:** Precautions and side effects of diuretic therapy, p. 71; **Knowledge deficit:** Precautions and side effects of digitalis therapy, p. 71. As appropriate, nursing diagnoses and interventions in "Cardiac Catheterization, Angioplasty, and Atherectomy," p. 110; "Cardiac Surgery," p. 113. Also see Appendix One, "Caring for Preoperative and Postoperative Patients," p. 717.

PATIENT-FAMILY TEACHING AND DISCHARGE PLANNING

When providing patient-family teaching, focus on sensory information; avoid giving excessive information; and initiate a visiting nurse referral for necessary follow-up teaching. Consider including verbal and written information about the following:
- Medications, including drug name, purpose, dosage, schedule, precautions, drug/drug and food/drug interactions, and potential side effects.
- Gradually increasing exercise, avoiding heavy lifting (>10 lb), incorporating rest periods.
- Name and phone number of a resource person (e.g., health care provider, primary nurse) should questions arise after hospital discharge.
- Referral to cardiac rehabilitation program if appropriate.
- Resumption of sexual activity as directed by health care provider.
- Indicators that necessitate immediate medical attention: decreased exercise tolerance, signs of infection, SOB, bleeding.

- Importance of consulting health care provider before using over-the-counter (OTC) medications, especially aspirin products for individuals taking oral anticoagulants. Aspirin can prolong coagulation times.
- Importance of follow-up care; confirm date and time of next medical appointment.

Mitral regurgitation

Abnormalities of the mitral valve can cause mitral regurgitation (MR) (also known as *mitral insufficiency*). MR can be caused by a number of conditions, including myocardial infarction (MI), coronary artery disease (CAD), papillary muscle dysfunction, mitral valve prolapse, cardiomyopathy, or inflammatory heart disorders. The significant effects of MR occur during ventricular systole. Normally, the mitral valve is closed during ventricular systole, but with MR the valve allows approximately half the ventricular volume back into the left atrium rather than forcing it forward into the aorta. The heart may be able to compensate for a period of time, but eventually cardiac output decreases and heart failure occurs. In addition, the increase in pulmonary vascular volume causes pulmonary hypertension (see p. 73).

ASSESSMENT

Chronic indicators: A majority of patients with MR remain asymptomatic, although weakness and low exercise tolerance secondary to low cardiac output may be present. Anxiety, intermittent palpitations, and chest discomfort can also occur.

Acute indicators: Fatigue, exhaustion, dyspnea, palpitations, dyspnea on exertion, paroxysmal nocturnal dyspnea, and signs of pulmonary edema (see p. 103) and heart failure (see p. 69).

Physical assessment: Holosystolic murmur heard at the apex, radiating toward the axilla; possible presence of S_3 heart sounds; characteristic ejection click.

DIAGNOSTIC TESTS

ECG: Will show left atrial enlargement, possibly with atrial fibrillation.

Chest x-ray: Will demonstrate cardiomegaly with left ventricular and left atrial enlargement.

Echocardiography: Provides a definitive diagnosis and reveals severity of the disorder.

Radionuclide imaging: Often useful in follow-up; progressive increases in end-systolic or end-diastolic volumes can indicate a worsening condition.

Angiography and ventriculogram: Will show decreased contraction and dilation.

COLLABORATIVE MANAGEMENT

Endocarditis prophylaxis with antibiotics: Initiated before major or minor surgical procedures, dental procedures, or any activity that may result in bacteremia.

Pharmacotherapy

β-Blockade: To decrease cardiac workload and prevent chest pain and irregularities in rhythm.

Digitalis: To increase strength of contraction.

Vasodilators: To decrease afterload and increase cardiac output.

Diuretics: To control fluid accumulation and prevent pulmonary edema.

Anticoagulants (heparin or warfarin):   To prevent embolization.

Diet: Low in Na^+ (see Table 3-2, p. 133).

Mitral valve replacement: If necessary. See "Mitral Stenosis," p. 85.

Medical treatment for heart failure: As appropriate (see p. 69).

NURSING DIAGNOSES AND INTERVENTIONS

Activity intolerance related to generalized weakness and imbalance between oxygen supply and demand secondary to decreased cardiac output with valvular regurgitation

Desired outcome: By a minimum of 24 hr before hospital discharge, patient rates perceived exertion at ≤3 on a 0-10 scale and exhibits cardiac tolerance to activity as evidenced by HR ≤20 bpm over resting HR, systolic BP within 20 mm Hg of resting systolic BP, and RR ≤20 breaths/min with normal depth and pattern (eupnea).

- Assess patient's VS during activities, being alert to HR >20 bpm over resting HR, systolic BP >20 mm Hg over or under resting systolic BP, and RR >20 breaths/min. Ask patient to rate perceived exertion (see p. 739 for description).
- Facilitate coordination of health care providers to provide rest periods between care activities to decrease cardiac workload. Ensure 90 min for undisturbed rest.
- Encourage alternating activity and rest periods within the patient's cardiopulmonary tolerance.
- As necessary, assist patient with ADL to avoid SOB.
- Discuss ways to decrease energy output at home.
- Progressively increase ambulation to patient's tolerance. Be alert to dyspnea, fatigue, and SOB with activity. Modify or restrict activities as indicated.

See Also: Appendix One for **Risk for activity intolerance,** p. 738; **Risk for disuse syndrome,** p. 740; "Pulmonary Embolus" for **Altered protection** related to risk of prolonged bleeding or hemorrhage secondary to anticoagulation therapy, p. 18; "Coronary Artery Disease" for **Knowledge deficit:** Precautions and side effects of β-blockers, p. 60; "Heart Failure" for **Fluid volume excess,** p. 70; **Knowledge deficit:** Precautions and side effects of diuretic therapy, p. 71; **Knowledge deficit:** Precautions and side effects of digitalis therapy, p. 71; **Knowledge deficit:** Precautions and side effects of vasodilators, p. 72; "Mitral Stenosis" for **Risk for infection** (with concomitant endocarditis), p. 86; **Knowledge deficit:** Disease process and treatments/management, p. 87; "Cardiac Catheterization," p. 110; "Cardiac Surgery," p. 113; Appendix One, "Caring for Preoperative and Postoperative Patients," p. 717.

NIC: Activity Therapy; Cardiac Care; Energy Management; Environmental Management; Surveillance

PATIENT-FAMILY TEACHING AND DISCHARGE PLANNING

See "Heart Failure," p. 72; "Cardiac Surgery," p. 115, depending on patient's clinical course.

Aortic stenosis

Aortic stenosis is a condition that obstructs outflow from the left ventricle into the ascending aorta. It is either congenital or acquired (most commonly from degenerative changes of aging or rheumatic fever). Aortic stenosis results from adhesions and fusion of the valve cusps. Usually, normal left ventricular output can be maintained by compensatory left ventricular hypertrophy, but eventually progressive stenosis causes signs of low cardiac output, such as cool extremities, fluid accumulation, decreased urinary output, and cardiac failure.

ASSESSMENT

Signs and symptoms: Often patients are asymptomatic until approximately 60 yr of age, when angina, fatigue, palpitations, paroxysmal nocturnal dyspnea, orthostatic hypotension, syncope with exertion, orthopnea, signs of pulmonary edema, and cardiac failure are seen. Signs of left ventricular failure may also be present, including dyspnea and SOB. Thrombi created on damaged valve leaflets may break free and cause visual field deficits.

Physical assessment: Decreased systolic BP, decreased pulse pressure (the difference between systolic and diastolic pressures), increased left ventricular impulse (point of maximal impulse [PMI] palpable at fifth intercostal space, midclavicular line as a "lift" of the chest wall during ventricular systole), and systolic ejection murmur (best heard at the apex of the heart, second intercostal space).

DIAGNOSTIC TESTS

ECG: Will show presence of left ventricular hypertrophy as evidenced by left axis deviation and increased amplitude of QRS complexes.

Chest x-ray: May reveal aortic valve calcification.

Cardiac catheterization with angiography: Demonstrates degree of thickness of the stenotic valve and the pressure gradient across the valve.

Echocardiography: Allows visualization of the narrowed valve opening. Two-dimensional echocardiography can be helpful in determining severity of the stenosis.

COLLABORATIVE MANAGEMENT

Antibiotics: As a prophylaxis against endocarditis.

Treatment of heart failure: If present. See this section in "Heart Failure," p. 69.

Aortic valve replacement: Appropriate for patients with left ventricular dysfunction and symptoms of decreased cardiac output and functional disability. Aortic valve replacement is performed using heart-lung bypass, and the patient is in ICU for 2-3 days postoperatively.

> **Note:**   Artificial (prosthetic) mechanical valves, as well as those obtained from human donors (cadavers) and animals, may be used (see "Mitral Valve Replacement," p. 85). For specific information on allograft aortic valves, see *http://quality.redcross.org/tissue*. Patients with artificial valves are maintained on lifetime anticoagulant therapy.

Percutaneous aortic valve valvuloplasty: An alternative to surgery for some patients. The procedure uses a balloon dilating catheter, which is advanced to the stenotic valve and then inflated to dilate the valve. The procedure is performed with the patient under local anesthesia in the cardiac catheterization laboratory.

NURSING DIAGNOSES AND INTERVENTIONS

See "Pulmonary Embolus" for **Altered protection** related to risk of prolonged bleeding or hemorrhage secondary to anticoagulation therapy, p. 18; "Coronary Artery Disease" for **Knowledge deficit:** Precautions and side effects of β-blockers, p. 60; "Heart Failure" for **Fluid volume excess,** p. 70; **Knowledge deficit:** Precautions and side effects of diuretic therapy, p. 71; **Knowledge deficit:** Precautions and side effects of digitalis therapy, p. 71; **Knowledge deficit:** Precautions and side effects of vasodilators, p. 72; "Mitral Stenosis" for **Activity intolerance,** p. 86; **Risk for infection** (with concomitant endocarditis), p. 86; **Knowledge deficit:** Disease process and treatments/management, p. 87. As appropriate, see "Cardiac Catheterization,

Angioplasty, and Atherectomy," p. 110; "Cardiac Surgery," p. 113; Appendix One, "Caring for Preoperative and Postoperative Patients," p. 717.

Aortic regurgitation

Many disorders can cause aortic valve regurgitation (or insufficiency), but the most common are degenerative changes of aging or rheumatic fever. The cusps of the valve become fibrotic and retract, preventing valve closure during diastole. Incompetence of this valve allows backward flow, which results in a large ventricular volume. If the condition develops slowly, the patient remains asymptomatic longer because the left ventricle hypertrophies to accommodate a larger volume. Aortic regurgitation may result from an inherited disorder (Marfan's syndrome), rheumatic heart disease, trauma, syphilis, or bacterial endocarditis.

ASSESSMENT

Signs and symptoms: With slowly developing regurgitation, the patient can remain asymptomatic for years. When the heart begins to fail, signs associated with left ventricular failure develop, including dyspnea, dyspnea on exertion, orthopnea, decreasing BP, changes in mentation, peripheral vasoconstriction, and pulmonary edema.

Physical assessment: Widened aortic pulse pressure (the difference between systolic and diastolic pressures), low diastolic BP, high systolic BP until heart failure develops, low-pitched diastolic murmur located in the second intercostal space to the right of the sternum, tachycardia, crackles (rales), and increased pulmonary arterial pressures.

DIAGNOSTIC TESTS

ECG: Will demonstrate left axis deviation and left ventricular conduction defects with chronic aortic regurgitation. With acute regurgitation, nonspecific ST-segment changes or left ventricular hypertrophy will be seen.

Chest x-ray: Results depend on the severity and duration of the disorder, but it eventually demonstrates cardiac enlargement and left ventricular dilation.

Cardiac catheterization with angiography: Useful in determining severity of the regurgitation.

Echocardiography: May identify the cause of regurgitation by revealing damaged cusps or vegetation caused by endocarditis.

COLLABORATIVE MANAGEMENT

Pharmacotherapy

Positive inotropic agents, such as digitalis: To maintain ventricular function by increasing the strength of ventricular contractions.

Vasodilators: To decrease afterload.

Treatment of heart failure: See "Heart Failure," p. 69.

Surgical interventions: Heart failure is not uncommon in patients with aortic regurgitation, even with aggressive medical treatment. Therefore aortic valve replacement is usually recommended (see "Mitral Valve Replacement," p. 85). Indications for this surgery include chronic aortic regurgitation that has become symptomatic and ventricular dysfunction during exercise.

NURSING DIAGNOSES AND INTERVENTIONS

See "Pulmonary Embolus" for **Altered protection** related to risk of prolonged bleeding or hemorrhage secondary to anticoagulation therapy, p. 18; "Coronary Artery Disease" for **Knowledge deficit:** Precautions and side effects of β-blockers, p. 60; "Heart Failure" for **Fluid volume excess,** p. 70; **Knowledge deficit:** Precautions and side effects of diuretic therapy, p. 71;

Knowledge deficit: Precautions and side effects of digitalis therapy, p. 71; **Knowledge deficit:** Precautions and side effects of vasodilators, p. 72; "Mitral Stenosis" for **Risk for infection** (with concomitant endocarditis), p. 86; **Knowledge deficit:** Disease process and treatments/management, p. 87. As appropriate, see "Cardiac Catheterization, Angioplasty, and Atherectomy," p. 110; "Cardiac Surgery," p. 113; Appendix One, "Caring for Preoperative and Postoperative Patients," p. 717.

PATIENT-FAMILY TEACHING AND DISCHARGE PLANNING

See "Heart Failure," p. 72, and "Cardiac Surgery," p. 115, depending on patient's clinical course.

Section Four: Cardiovascular Conditions Secondary to Other Disease Processes

Cardiac and noncardiac shock (circulatory failure)

A shock state exists when tissue perfusion decreases to the point of cellular metabolic dysfunction. Shock is classified according to the causative event.

Hematogenic (hemorrhagic or hypovolemic) shock: Occurs when blood volume is insufficient to meet metabolic needs of the tissues, as with severe hemorrhage.

Cardiogenic shock: Occurs when cardiac failure results in decreased tissue perfusion, as in MI.

Distributive shock conditions: Characterized by displacement of a significant amount of vascular volume. The three types are described below.

Neurogenic shock: Resulting from a neurologic event (e.g., head injury) that causes massive vasodilation and decreased perfusion pressures.

Anaphylactic shock: Caused by a severe systemic response to an allergen (foreign protein), resulting in massive vasodilation, increased capillary permeability, decreased perfusion, decreased venous return, and subsequent decreased cardiac output.

Septic shock: Occurs when bacterial toxins cause an overwhelming systemic infection.

•   •   •

Regardless of the cause, shock results in cellular hypoxia secondary to decreased perfusion and ultimately in cellular, tissue, and organ dysfunction. A prolonged shock state can result in death, so early recognition and intervention are essential.

ASSESSMENT

Early signs and symptoms: Cool, pale, and clammy skin; decreased pulse strength; dry and pale mucous membranes; restlessness; hyperventilation; anxiety; nausea; thirst; weakness.

Physical assessment: Rapid HR; decreased systolic BP and increased diastolic BP secondary to catecholamine (sympathetic nervous system [SNS]) response.

Late signs and symptoms: Decreased urinary output, hypothermia, drowsiness, diaphoresis, confusion, and lethargy, all of which can progress to a comatose state.

Physical assessment: Irregular HR; continually decreasing BP, usually with systolic pressure palpable at 60 mm Hg or less; rapid and possibly irregular RR.

• • •

See Table 2-6 for a depiction of the clinical signs by shock type.

DIAGNOSTIC TESTS
Diagnosis is usually based on the presenting symptoms and clinical signs.
ABG values: Will reveal metabolic acidosis (bicarbonate [HCO_3^-] <22 mEq/L and pH <7.40) caused by anaerobic metabolism.
Serial measurement of urinary output: Less than 30 ml/hr indicates decreased perfusion and decreased renal function.
Blood urea nitrogen (BUN) and creatinine: Increase with decreased renal perfusion.
Blood glucose: Hyperglycemia may be present because of epinephrine-induced glycogenolysis.

For septic shock
Serial creatinine and BUN levels: To assess for potential renal complications and dysfunction.
Serum electrolyte levels: Identify renal complications and dysfunctions as evidenced by hyperkalemia and hypernatremia.
Blood culture: To identify the causative organism.
WBC count and erythrocyte sedimentation rate (ESR): Elevated in the presence of infection.

For hematogenic shock
CBC: Hct and Hgb will be decreased because of decreased blood volume.

For anaphylactic shock
WBC count: Will reveal increased eosinophils, a type of granulocyte that appears in the presence of allergic reaction.

COLLABORATIVE MANAGEMENT
Interventions are determined by clinical presentation and severity of the shock state. Patients are transferred to ICU to assess severity of the shock state and closely monitor status.

For cardiogenic shock
Vascular support: To reduce cardiac workload.
Intraaortic balloon counterpulsation: To augment perfusion pressures.
Ventricular assist devices: Used to bypass the ventricles, lowering myocardial oxygen requirements, reducing cardiac stress, and permitting cardiac muscle rest.
Optimization of blood volume: Either with volume expanders such as dextran or with diuretics if fluid overload is the problem.
Pharmacotherapy
Sympathomimetics: For example, dopamine infusion at low doses (2-5 µg/kg/min) to increase renal perfusion and decrease systemic vasoconstriction. Moderate doses (5-8 µg/kg/min) help strengthen cardiac contraction. Dopamine is administered via continuous infusion with an infusion control device; the rate is titrated based on the patient's response (e.g., blood pressure).
Vasopressors: To stimulate vasoconstriction. Usually they are used in conjunction with vasodilators to achieve the desired effect without the negative effects of one drug alone. Norepinephrine (Levophed), for example, may be used in combination with phentolamine (Regitine), which counteracts the severe end-organ and peripheral damage caused by the severe vasoconstriction

TABLE 2-6 Systemic Clinical Signs of Shock

	Cardiogenic	Septic	Hypovolemic	Neurogenic	Anaphylactic
Cardiovascular	↓ BP ↑ HR ↓ Pulses	*Early:* ↑ BP 　　　↑ Pulses *Late:* ↓ BP 　　　↓ Pulses	↓ BP ↑ HR Flat neck veins	*Early:* vasodilation, ↑ BP	↓ BP ↑ HR ↓ Pulses
Respiratory	Dyspnea, crackles	*Early:* ↑ RR *Late:* ↓ RR, crackles 　　　(rales)	Lungs clear	Lungs clear	Dyspnea to air hunger; wheezes and complete obstruction
Neurologic	Confusion, lethargy, drowsiness	↓ LOC	↓ LOC	Normal or ↓ LOC	↓ LOC
Renal	↓ Urinary output	↓ Urinary output	↓ Urinary output	Normal or ↓ urinary output	↓ Urinary output
Cutaneous	Cool skin	*Early:* warm *Late:* cool	Cool skin	Warm (because of vasodilation)	Urticaria, angioedema

BP, Blood pressure; *HR,* heart rate; *RR,* respiratory rate; *LOC,* level of consciousness.

associated with norepinephrine. Norepinephrine is administered via continuous infusion with an infusion control device; the rate is titrated based on the patient's response (e.g., blood pressure).

Vasodilators: To increase peripheral perfusion and reduce afterload vasoconstriction caused by the vasopressors (see above).

Osmotic diuretics: To increase renal blood flow.

O_2 support: As needed, to increase O_2 availability to the tissues.

Correction of acidosis and electrolyte imbalances

For anaphylactic shock
Pharmacotherapy

Epinephrine (0.5 ml, 1:1000 in 10 ml saline):   To promote vasoconstriction and decrease the allergic response by counteracting vasodilation caused by histamine release.

Bronchodilators: To relieve bronchospasm.

Antihistamines: To prevent relapse and relieve urticaria.

Hydrocortisone: For its antiinflammatory effects.

Vasopressors: May be necessary for reversing shock state.

O_2 and airway support: As needed.

For hemorrhagic shock
Control of hemorrhage: If possible, depending on the location and cause.

Fresh whole blood: To increase O_2 delivery at the tissue level when >2 L of blood has been lost. Often a combination of packed RBCs and a crystalloid solution is administered.

Albumin or dextran: Sometimes used to increase vascular volume.

Ringer's solution: Often used as an isotonic solution to replace electrolytes and ions lost with bleeding.

For septic shock
Antibiotic therapy: Specific to causative organism.

Fluid administration: To maintain adequate vascular volume.

Vasoactive drugs (α-, β-, or dopaminergic-receptor agents):   May be required to reverse vasodilation and maintain perfusion.

Positive inotropic drugs: To augment cardiac contractility.

NURSING DIAGNOSES AND INTERVENTIONS

Altered peripheral, cardiopulmonary, cerebral, and renal tissue perfusion related to decreased circulating blood volume

Desired outcome: Within 1 hr of treatment, patient has adequate perfusion as evidenced by peripheral pulse amplitude >2+ on a 0-4+ scale; brisk capillary refill (<2 sec); BP within patient's normal range; CVP ≥5 cm H_2O; HR regular and ≤100 bpm; no significant change in mental status and orientation to person, place, and time; and urine output ≥30 ml/hr.

- Assess and document peripheral perfusion status. Report significant findings, such as coolness and pallor of the extremities, decreased amplitude of pulses, and delayed capillary refill.

- Monitor BP at frequent intervals; be alert to readings >20 mm Hg below patient's normal range or to other indicators of hypotension, such as dizziness, altered mentation, or decreased urinary output.

- If hypotension is present, place patient in a supine position to promote venous return. Remember that BP must be ≥80/60 mm Hg for adequate coronary and renal artery perfusion.

- Monitor CVP (if line is inserted) to determine adequacy of venous return and blood volume; 5-10 cm H_2O usually is considered an adequate range. Values near zero can indicate hypovolemia, especially when associated with decreased urinary output, vasoconstriction, and increased HR, which are found with hypovolemia.

- Observe for indicators of decreased cerebral perfusion, such as restlessness, confusion, mental status changes, and decreased LOC. If positive indicators are present, protect patient from injury by raising side rails and placing bed in its lowest position. Reorient patient as indicated.
- Monitor for indicators of decreased coronary artery perfusion, such as chest pain and an irregular HR.
- Monitor urinary output hourly. Notify health care provider if it is <30 ml/hr in the presence of adequate intake. Check weight daily for evidence of gain.
- Monitor laboratory results for elevated BUN (>20 mg/dl) and creatinine (>1.5 mg/dl) levels; report increases.
- Monitor serum electrolyte values for evidence of imbalances, particularly Na^+ (>147 mEq/L) and K^+ (>5.0 mEq/L). Be alert to signs of hyperkalemia, such as muscle weakness, hyporeflexia, and irregular HR. Also monitor for signs of hypernatremia, such as fluid retention and edema.
- Administer fluids as prescribed to increase vascular volume. The type and amount of fluid depend on the type of shock and the patient's clinical situation. See Table 2-6 for a description of clinical signs associated with different types of shock.
  —*Cardiogenic shock:* fluids are probably limited to prevent overload, yet dehydration must be avoided to ensure support of vascular space and cardiac muscle.
  —*Hypovolemic shock:* the amount lost is replaced. Ringer's solution, as much as 1000 ml/hr, may be administered if volume loss is severe. Most often this includes blood replacement.
  —*Septic shock:* Ringer's solution, plasma, and blood are administered.
- Prepare for transfer of patient to ICU if appropriate.

NIC: Cerebral Perfusion Promotion; Circulatory Care; Fluid/Electrolyte Management; Invasive Hemodynamic Monitoring; Oxygen Therapy; Shock Management; Surveillance; Vital Signs Monitoring

Impaired gas exchange related to altered oxygen supply secondary to decreased respiratory muscle function occurring with altered metabolism
Desired outcome: Within 1 hr of intervention, patient has adequate gas exchange as evidenced by O_2 saturation ≥92%; partial pressure of dissolved oxygen in arterial blood (Pao_2) ≥80 mm Hg; partial pressure of dissolved carbon dioxide in arterial blood ($Paco_2$) ≤45 mm Hg; pH ≥7.35; presence of eupnea; and orientation to person, place, and time.
- Monitor ABG results. Be alert to and report presence of hypoxemia (decreased O_2 saturation, decreased Pao_2), hypercapnia (increased $Paco_2$), and acidosis (decreased pH, increased $Paco_2$). Report significant findings.
- Monitor oximetry readings; be alert for readings ≤92%. Report significant findings.
- Monitor respirations q30min; note and report presence of tachypnea or dyspnea. Be alert to mental status changes, restlessness, irritability, and confusion, which are indicators of hypoxia.
- Teach patient to breathe slowly and deeply to promote oxygenation.
- Ensure that the patient has a patent airway; suction secretions as needed to assist with gas exchange.
- Administer O_2 as prescribed. Deliver O_2 with humidity to help prevent its drying effects on oral and nasal mucosa.

NIC: Acid-Base Monitoring; Airway Management; Bedside Laboratory Testing; Oxygen Therapy; Respiratory Management

See Also: Psychosocial nursing diagnoses and interventions in Appendix One, "Caring for Patients With Cancer and Other Life-disrupting Illnesses," p. 791.

PATIENT-FAMILY TEACHING AND DISCHARGE PLANNING
For interventions, see discussion with patient's primary diagnosis.

Dysrhythmias and conduction disturbances

Dysrhythmias are abnormal rhythms of the heart's electrical system. They can originate in any part of the conduction system, such as the sinus node, atrium, atrioventricular (A-V) node, His-Purkinje system, bundle branches, and ventricular tissue. Although a variety of diseases may cause dysrhythmias, the most common are coronary artery disease (CAD) and myocardial infarction (MI). Other causes include electrolyte imbalance, changes in oxygenation, and drug toxicity. Cardiac dysrhythmias may result from the following mechanisms.

Disturbances in automaticity: May involve an increase or decrease in automaticity in the sinus node (i.e., sinus tachycardia or sinus bradycardia). Premature beats may arise via this mechanism from the atria, junction, or ventricles. Abnormal rhythms, such as atrial or ventricular tachycardia, also may occur.

Disturbances in conductivity: Conduction may be too rapid, as in conditions caused by an accessory pathway (e.g., Wolff-Parkinson-White syndrome), or too slow (e.g., A-V block). *Reentry* is a situation in which a stimulus reexcites a conduction pathway through which it already has passed. Once started, this impulse may circulate repeatedly. For reentry to occur, there must be two different pathways for conduction: one with slowed conduction and one with unidirectional block.

Combinations of altered automaticity and conductivity: Observed when several dysrhythmias are noted (e.g., first-degree A-V block, or a disturbance in conductivity; and premature atrial contractions, or a disturbance in automaticity).

ASSESSMENT
Signs and symptoms: Can vary on a continuum from absence of symptoms to complete cardiopulmonary collapse. General indicators include alterations in LOC, vertigo, syncope, seizures, weakness, fatigue, activity intolerance, SOB, dyspnea on exertion, chest pain, palpitations, sensation of "skipped beats," anxiety, and restlessness.

Physical assessment: Increases or decreases in HR, BP, and RR; dusky color or pallor; crackles (rales); cool skin; decreased urine output; and paradoxical pulse and abnormal heart sounds (e.g., paradoxical splitting of S_1 and S_2).

ECG: Some findings seen with various dysrhythmias include abnormalities in rate such as sinus bradycardia or sinus tachycardia, irregular rhythm such as atrial fibrillation, extra beats such as premature atrial contractions (PACs) and premature junctional contractions (PJCs), wide and bizarre-looking beats such as premature ventricular contractions (PVCs) and ventricular tachycardia (VT), a fibrillating baseline such as ventricular fibrillation (VF), and a straight line as with asystole.

History and risk factors: CAD, recent MI, electrolyte disturbances, drug toxicity.

DIAGNOSTIC TESTS

12-lead ECG: To detect dysrhythmias and identify possible cause.

Serum electrolyte levels: To identify electrolyte abnormalities, which can precipitate dysrhythmias. The most common are hyperkalemia and hypokalemia.

Drug levels: To identify toxicities (e.g., of digoxin, quinidine, procainamide, aminophylline) that can precipitate dysrhythmias.

Ambulatory monitoring (e.g., Holter monitor or cardiac event recorder): To identify subtle dysrhythmias and associate abnormal rhythms by means of the patient's symptoms.

Electrophysiologic study: Invasive test in which two to three catheters are placed into the heart, giving the heart a pacing stimulus at varying sites and of varying voltages. The test determines origin of dysrhythmia, inducibility, and effectiveness of drug therapy in dysrhythmia suppression.

Exercise stress testing: Used in conjunction with Holter monitoring to detect advanced grades of PVCs (those caused by ischemia) and to guide therapy. During the test, ECG and BP readings are taken while the patient walks on a treadmill or pedals a stationary bicycle; response to a constant or increasing workload is observed. The test continues until the patient reaches target heart rate or symptoms such as chest pain, severe fatigue, dysrhythmias, or abnormal BP occur.

Oximetry or ABG values: To document trend of hypoxemia.

COLLABORATIVE MANAGEMENT

Antidysrhythmic drugs: See Table 2-7.

Implantable cardioverter-defibrillator (ICD):   To treat lethal cardiac dysrhythmias. It is recommended for patients who have survived an episode of sudden cardiac death (cardiac arrest), for patients with CAD who have had a cardiac arrest, and for those in whom conventional antidysrhythmic therapy has failed. The pulse generator, which is powered by lithium batteries, is surgically inserted (in the OR or catheterization laboratory) into a "pocket" formed in the pectoral area. Leads are tunneled beneath the skin from the pocket to the subclavian vein through which they are advanced to the right ventricle. The ICD is programmed to deliver the electrical stimulus at a predetermined rate and/or after assessing the morphology of the ECG. First- and second-generation ICDs provide for only cardioversion or defibrillation; third-generation ICDs also provide overdrive pacing and backup ventricular pacing.

Postoperative complications include atelectasis, pneumonia, seroma at the generator "pocket," pneumothorax, and thrombosis. Lead migration and lead fracture are the two most common structural problems. Interference from unipolar pacemakers and "myopotentials" (electrical interference) are common mechanical complications. ICDs may need to be deactivated during surgical procedures, use of electrocautery, and MRI.

Radio frequency (RF) ablation: A procedure in which a catheter is placed in the heart via cardiac catheterization and radio frequency waves are applied to the area in which the dysrhythmia originates. The radio frequency waves cause controlled, localized necrosis of the area. This procedure is used for conduction disturbances such as Wolff-Parkinson-White syndrome and some forms of A-V block.

Dietary guidelines: Usually patients with recurrent dysrhythmias are placed on a diet that restricts or reduces caffeine and is low in cholesterol (see Table 2-2).

Surgical procedures

Left ventricular aneurysmectomy and infarctectomy: Excision of possible focal spots of ventricular dysrhythmias.

Cryoablation: Performed alone or in conjunction with electrophysiologic mapping, with excision of the dysrhythmia focus.

TABLE 2-7 Antidysrhythmic Drugs

Class I

Local anesthetics and other drugs that decrease automaticity of ventricular conduction, delay ventricular repolarization, decrease conduction velocity, increase conduction via A-V node, and suppress ventricular automaticity. Class IA decreases depolarization moderately and prolongs repolarization. Class IB decreases depolarization and shortens repolarization. Class IC significantly decreases depolarization with minimal effect on repolarization.

A	B	C
quinidine (PO, IV)	phenytoin (PO)	encainide (PO)
procainamide (PO, IV, IM)	mexiletine (PO)	
disopyramide (PO)	tocainide (PO)	

Class II

β-Blockers that slow sinus automaticity, slow conduction via A-V node, control ventricular response to supraventricular tachycardias, and shorten the action potential of Purkinje fibers.

propranolol (PO, IV)
metoprolol (PO, IV)
atenolol (PO)
acebutolol (PO)

Class III

Increase the action potential and refractory period of Purkinje fibers, increase ventricular fibrillation threshold, restore injured myocardial cell electrophysiology toward normal, and suppress reentrant dysrhythmias.

bretylium (IV, IM)
amiodarone (PO, IV)
sotalol (PO)

Class IV

Calcium channel blockers that depress automaticity in the S-A and A-V nodes, block the slow calcium current in the A-V junctional tissue, reduce conduction via the A-V node, and are useful in treating tachydysrhythmias because of A-V junction reentry.

verapamil (IV)
diltiazem (PO)
nifedipine (PO)

A-V, Atrioventricular; *PO,* by mouth; *IV,* intravenous; *IM,* intramuscular; *S-A,* sinoatrial.

NURSING DIAGNOSES AND INTERVENTIONS

Decreased cardiac output related to altered rate, rhythm, or conduction or negative inotropic changes secondary to cardiac disease

Desired outcome: Within 1 hr of treatment/intervention, patient has adequate cardiac output as evidenced by BP ≥90/60 mm Hg, HR 60-100 bpm, and normal sinus rhythm on ECG.

- Monitor patient's heart rhythm continuously; note BP and symptoms if dysrhythmias occur or increase in occurrence.
- If symptoms of decreased cardiac output occur, prepare to transfer patient to the coronary care unit (CCU).

- Document dysrhythmias with rhythm strip. Use a 12-lead ECG as necessary to identify the dysrhythmia.
- Monitor patient's laboratory data, particularly electrolyte and digoxin levels. Serum K^+ levels <3.5 mEq/L or >5.0 mEq/L can cause dysrhythmias.
- Administer antidysrhythmic agents as prescribed; note patient's response to therapy.
- Provide O_2 as prescribed. O_2 may be beneficial if dysrhythmias are related to ischemia. Deliver O_2 with humidity to help prevent its drying effects on oral and nasal mucosa.
- Maintain a quiet environment, and administer pain medications promptly. Both stress and pain can increase sympathetic tone and cause dysrhythmias.
- If life-threatening dysrhythmias occur, initiate emergency procedures and cardiopulmonary resuscitation (as indicated by advanced cardiac life support [ACLS] protocol).
- When dysrhythmias occur, stay with patient; provide support and reassurance while performing assessments and administering treatment.

NIC: Cardiac Care: Acute; Dysrhythmia Management; Environmental Management; Fluid/Electrolyte Monitoring; Invasive Hemodynamic Monitoring; Medication Administration; Surveillance

Knowledge deficit: Mechanism by which dysrhythmias occur and life-style implications
Desired outcome: Within the 24-hr period before hospital discharge, patient and significant other verbalize knowledge about causes of dysrhythmias and the implications for patient's life-style modifications.

- Discuss causal mechanisms for dysrhythmias, including resulting symptoms. Use a heart model or diagrams as necessary.
- Teach the signs and symptoms of dysrhythmias that necessitate medical attention: unrelieved and prolonged palpitations, chest pain, SOB, rapid pulse (>150 bpm), dizziness, and syncope.
- Teach patient and significant other how to check pulse rate for a full minute.
- Teach patient and significant other about medications that will be taken after hospital discharge, including drug name, purpose, dosage, schedule, precautions, drug/drug and food/drug interactions, and potential side effects. Stress that patient will be taking long-term antidysrhythmic therapy and that it could be life threatening to stop or skip these medications without health care provider approval because doing so may decrease blood levels effective for dysrhythmia suppression.
- Advise patient and significant other about the availability of support groups and counseling; provide appropriate community referrals. Patients who survive sudden cardiac arrest may experience nightmares or other sleep disturbances at home. Explain that anxiety and fear, along with periodic feelings of denial, depression, anger, and confusion, are normal following this experience.
- Stress the importance of leading a normal and productive life, even though patient may fear breakthrough of life-threatening dysrhythmias. If patient is going on vacation, advise him or her to take along sufficient medication and to investigate health care facilities in the vacation area.
- Advise patient and significant other to take CPR classes; provide addresses of community programs.
- Teach the importance of follow-up care; confirm date and time of next appointment if known. Explain that outpatient Holter monitoring is performed periodically.
- Explain dietary restrictions that individuals with recurrent dysrhythmias should follow. Discuss the need for reduced intake of products containing caffeine, including coffee, tea, chocolate, and colas. Because of the overlap

between dysrhythmias and CAD, provide instruction for a general low-cholesterol diet (see Table 2-2). Encourage patients to use food labels to determine the cholesterol content of foods.

- As indicated, teach patient relaxation techniques, which will reduce stress and enable patient to decrease sympathetic tone (see p. 59).

NIC: Learning Facilitation; Learning Readiness Enhancement; Risk Identification; Teaching: Disease Process; Teaching: Prescribed Medication; Teaching: Psychomotor Skill

PATIENT-FAMILY TEACHING AND DISCHARGE PLANNING
See patient's primary diagnosis.

Cardiac arrest

> **Note:** *This section is intended as an overview only. In the event of a cardiac arrest, the reader should refer to cardiac arrest procedures established by the institution, including ACLS guidelines.*

Cardiac arrest occurs when the heart stops beating or when the contraction is ineffective in maintaining cardiac output (as in ventricular tachycardia [VT] or ventricular fibrillation [VF]). Many conditions can precipitate cardiac arrest, including MI, heart failure, shock state, severe electrolyte disturbances, drowning, electrocution, drug overdose, and hypoxia. Often the events that precipitate cardiac arrest occur in a vicious cycle. For example, a cardiac rhythm disturbance leads to decreased cardiac output, which leads to decreased tissue perfusion, which results in hypoxia, which leads to more rhythm disturbances, and the cycle goes on. Management of the prearrest stage is directed toward breaking this cycle and correcting the condition to prevent cardiac arrest. To help prevent an arrest from occurring, accurate and prompt nursing assessment is crucial. However, an arrest can occur without prior warning. This is an emergency situation, which requires *immediate* medical intervention.

ASSESSMENT
Signs and symptoms: Loss of consciousness—inability to arouse the patient by shaking and shouting.
Physical assessment: Absence of carotid pulse, audible or palpable BP, and respirations.

COLLABORATIVE MANAGEMENT
Management of prearrest phase: Includes treatment for shock, O_2 therapy or airway support, transfer to ICU, antidysrhythmic drugs, and pain relief.
Basic life support: CPR to maintain ventilation and circulation until normal cardiac rhythm is restored.
Ventilation: To prevent hypoxia and subsequent anaerobic metabolism. The method depends on the patient's clinical presentation. Mouth-to-mask breathing, O_2 mask with 100% O_2 if the patient is breathing, oral or nasal airways, endotracheal intubation, and manual ventilation may be used.

> **Note:** Mouth-to-mask breathing is the preferred method of providing adjunct ventilation (rather than mouth-to-mouth). It is the nurse's responsibility to ensure availability of the mask before an emergency and know how to use it properly.

Closed chest compressions: An adjunct to circulation. If done properly, cardiac compression can provide 25%-30% of the normal cardiac output.

IV access line: In arrest situations, it is often difficult to establish a peripheral IV line because of vascular collapse or constriction. In addition, with decreased peripheral perfusion, absorption of drugs can be variable. The health care provider may instead insert a central venous catheter into the femoral, jugular, or subclavian vein.

Treatment of cardiac rhythm abnormalities: Lidocaine to suppress ventricular ectopic beats; atropine for bradycardia; defibrillation or epinephrine to combat ventricular fibrillation.

Stimulation of effective cardiac contractions

Inotropic drugs: To increase strength of cardiac contractions.

Maintenance of acid-base and electrolyte balance: Disorders such as acidosis, hyperkalemia, hypocalcemia, and hypomagnesemia are identified and corrected.

Restoration of effective ventilation and circulation and stable cardiac rhythm before transfer to ICU

NURSING DIAGNOSES AND INTERVENTIONS

Decreased cardiac output related to altered mechanical and electrical factors secondary to cardiac arrest

Desired outcome: Within 15 min of arrest, patient has adequate cardiac output as evidenced by systolic BP ≥90 mm Hg, HR 60-100 bpm with regular rhythm, peripheral pulse amplitude >2+ on a 0-4+ scale, equal radial/apical pulses, and RR 12-20 breaths/min with normal depth and pattern (eupnea).

- Ensure adequate oxygenation by maintaining a patent airway; provide O_2 support as prescribed.
- Maintain closed chest compressions until cardiac rhythm is restored.
- Maintain or establish an IV line. Typically, 5% dextrose in water (D_5W) is run at a rapid rate unless otherwise prescribed.
- Assess and document BP at frequent intervals (q5-15min), and report changes in pressure to health care provider immediately.
- Administer antidysrhythmic agents, such as lidocaine, bretylium, quinidine, and procainamide, and inotropic drugs, such as dopamine hydrochloride, as prescribed.
- Assess and document HR; report irregularities or apical/radial deficit (e.g., apical rate 80 bpm/radial rate 50 bpm).
- Monitor ventilatory status, and be alert to indicators of hypoxia or inadequate ventilation, such as changes in breathing rhythm, adventitious breath sounds, or breath sounds that are not equal in both lungs. Be alert to ABG results that signal hypoxemia, hypercapnia, or acidosis, such as low pH (<7.35), low partial pressure of dissolved oxygen in arterial blood (Pao_2) (<80 mm Hg), decreased O_2 saturation (≤92%), and high partial pressure of dissolved carbon dioxide in arterial blood ($Paco_2$) (>45 mm Hg). Report significant findings.
- Monitor femoral pulses for peripheral perfusion. Be alert to and report decreasing amplitude of pulse pressures.

NIC: Acid-Base Management; Circulatory Care: Mechanical Assist Device; Code Management; Dysrhythmia Management; Hemodynamic Regulation; Medication Management; Resuscitation

See Also: Psychosocial nursing diagnoses in Appendix One, "Caring for Patients With Cancer and Other Life-disrupting Illnesses," p. 791.

PATIENT-FAMILY TEACHING AND DISCHARGE PLANNING

See discussion under patient's primary diagnosis.

Pulmonary edema

Acute pulmonary edema is an emergency situation in which hydrostatic pressure in the pulmonary vessels is greater than the vascular colloid osmotic pressure that holds fluid in the vessels. As a result, fluid floods the alveoli. When the alveoli contain fluid, their ability to participate in gas exchange is reduced and hypoxia will occur. The most common cause or precipitating factor in acute pulmonary edema is acute left ventricular failure, or an acute exacerbation of heart failure. Other causes include hypertension, volume overload, or nervous system disorders such as head trauma and grand mal seizures, which result in sympathetic nervous system hyperactivity and produce shifts in blood volume to the pulmonary system to increase pulmonary capillary pressure. Pulmonary edema can develop suddenly, or it can develop slowly over a period of hours or days. Prompt determination of cause and treatment are critical.

ASSESSMENT

Signs and symptoms: Anxiety, restlessness, frothy and blood-tinged sputum, orthopnea, extreme dyspnea. The patient exhibits "air hunger" and may thrash about and describe a sensation of drowning.

Physical assessment: Crackles (rales), tachycardia, tachypnea, engorged neck veins, S_3 heart sound, and murmurs (with valve dysfunction, such as mitral regurgitation).

History of: Recent MI or "heart problems" in the past; hypertension; fluid overload, often from IV fluids.

DIAGNOSTIC TESTS

Oximetry or ABG values: Will reveal hypoxemia.

Chest x-ray: Will delineate vascular engorgement and interstitial fluid and may reveal an increased heart size or pericardial tamponade (fluid accumulation in the pericardial space, resulting in compression of the heart muscle and interference with normal cardiac function).

ECG: May reveal evidence of old or new MI.

COLLABORATIVE MANAGEMENT

Transfer to ICU

O_2:   High flow either by nonrebreathing mask or endotracheal intubation and mechanical ventilation. Deliver O_2 with humidity to help prevent its drying effects on oral and nasal mucosa.

High Fowler's position (HOB up 90 degrees):   To decrease venous return.

Morphine sulfate: In small increments (2-4 mg IV slowly) to decrease anxiety, work of breathing [WOB], and sympathetic vasoconstriction.

> **Note:**   Morphine is avoided when pulmonary edema is associated with bronchial asthma, COPD, or CO_2 retention.

Diuretics: To reduce fluid volume and decrease venous return to the heart. Usually they are injected over a 2-min period.

Other pharmacotherapy

Vasodilators, such as nitroprusside: May be used to reduce systemic and venous pressures. Nitroglycerin (0.3-0.6 mg sublingual or transdermal) may also be given for venous dilation and to decrease preload.

Digitalis: To decrease ventricular rate and strengthen contractions for patients who are not already using the drug.

Theophylline: To reduce bronchodilation if bronchospasm further complicates the pulmonary edema. The tachycardia caused by theophylline, however, may further decrease cardiac output, so the risk/benefit ratio must be considered.

Identification and treatment of precipitating factors

NURSING DIAGNOSES AND INTERVENTIONS

Impaired gas exchange related to alveolar-capillary membrane changes secondary to fluid accumulation in the alveoli

Desired outcome: Within 30 min of treatment/intervention, patient has adequate gas exchange as evidenced by normal breath sounds and skin color, presence of eupnea, HR ≤100 bpm, partial pressure of dissolved oxygen in arterial blood (Pao_2) ≥80 mm Hg, and partial pressure of dissolved carbon dioxide in arterial blood ($Paco_2$) ≤45 mm Hg.

- Auscultate lung fields for breath sounds; be alert to the presence of crackles (rales), which signal alveolar fluid congestion.
- Assist patient into high Fowler's position (HOB up 90 degrees) to decrease WOB and enhance gas exchange.
- Teach patient to take slow, deep breaths to increase oxygenation.
- Administer O_2 as prescribed. Deliver O_2 with humidity to help prevent its drying effects on oral and nasal mucosa.
- Monitor oximetry and report findings of ≤92% to the health care provider. If ABGs are tested, monitor the results for the presence of hypoxemia (decreased Pao_2) and hypercapnia (increased $Paco_2$).
- Be alert to signs of increasing respiratory distress: increased RR, mental status changes, gasping for air, cyanosis, or rapid HR.
- Administer diuretics as prescribed. Monitor K^+ levels because of the potential for hypokalemia (K^+ <3.5 mEq/L) in patients taking certain diuretics.
- Administer vasodilators such as nitrates as prescribed to increase venous capacitance (venous dilation) and decrease pulmonary congestion.
- As indicated, have emergency equipment (e.g., airway, manual resuscitation bag) available and functional.
- As indicated, prepare to transfer patient to ICU.

NIC: Airway Management; Anxiety Reduction; Cardiac Care: Acute; Medication Management; Oxygen Therapy; Respiratory Management

Fluid volume excess related to compromised regulatory mechanisms secondary to decreased cardiac output

Desired outcome: Within 2 hr of intervention/treatment, patient becomes normovolemic as evidenced by balanced I&O, normal breath sounds, and urine output ≥30 ml/hr. Within 1 day of treatment/intervention, edema is ≤1+ on a 0-4+ scale, and weight becomes stable within 2-3 days.

- Closely monitor I&O, including insensible losses from diaphoresis and respirations.
- Record weight daily, and report steady gains.
- Assess for edema (interstitial fluids), especially in dependent areas such as the ankles and sacrum.
- Assess the respiratory system for indicators of fluid extravasation, such as crackles (rales) or pink-tinged, frothy sputum.
- Monitor for indications of fluid overload, such as jugular vein distention, crackles (rales), elevated CVP, peripheral edema, and ascites.
- Monitor laboratory results for indications of fluid retention, such as increased urinary specific gravity, increased BUN, decreased hematocrit, and increased urine osmolality.

- Monitor IV rate of flow to prevent volume overload. Use an infusion control device.
- Unless contraindicated, provide ice chips or popsicles to help patient control thirst. Record the amount on the I&O record. Provide frequent mouth care to reduce dry mucous membranes.
- Administer diuretics as prescribed, and record patient's response.
- Administer morphine sulfate if prescribed to induce vasodilation and decrease venous return to the heart.

NIC: Fluid/Electrolyte Management; Intravenous (IV) Therapy; Medication Management; Oral Health Maintenance; Respiratory Monitoring; Urinary Catheterization

Altered cardiopulmonary, peripheral, and cerebral tissue perfusion related to interrupted blood flow secondary to decreased cardiac output
Desired outcome: Within 2 hr of intervention/treatment, patient has adequate tissue perfusion as evidenced by BP within 20 mm Hg of patient's baseline; HR ≤100 bpm with regular rhythm; RR ≤20 breaths/min with normal depth and pattern (eupnea); brisk capillary refill (<2 sec); and significant mental status change or orientation to person, place, and time.

- Monitor BP q15min or more frequently if unstable. Be alert to decreases >20 mm Hg over patient's baseline or associated changes, such as dizziness and altered mentation.
- Check pulse rate q15-30min. Monitor for irregularities, increased HR, or skipped beats, which can signal decompensation and decreased function.
- Monitor for indicators of peripheral vasoconstriction (from sympathetic nervous system compensation), such as cool extremities, pallor, and diaphoresis. Evaluate capillary refill. Optimally, pink color should return within 1-2 sec after applying pressure to nail beds.
- Monitor for indicators of decreased cerebral perfusion, such as restlessness, anxiety, mental status changes, confusion, lethargy, stupor, and coma. Institute safety precautions accordingly.
- Administer inotropic drugs, such as digitalis, as prescribed. Administer vasodilators as prescribed, and monitor the effects closely. Be alert to problems such as hypotension and irregular heartbeats.
- Implement measures for decreasing venous return (e.g., rotating tourniquets) and increasing peripheral perfusion, such as placing patient in high Fowler's position (HOB up 90 degrees).

NIC: Cardiac Precautions; Circulatory Care; Medication Management; Neurologic Monitoring; Respiratory Monitoring

Fear related to potentially life-threatening situation
Desired outcomes: Within 24 hr of this diagnosis, patient communicates fears and concerns and relates the attainment of increasing physical and psychologic comfort.

- Provide the opportunity for patient and significant other to express feelings and fears. Be reassuring and supportive.
- Help make patient as comfortable as possible with prompt pain relief and positioning, typically high Fowler's position (HOB up 90 degrees).
- Keep the environment as calm and quiet as possible.
- Explain all treatment modalities, especially those that may be uncomfortable (e.g., O₂ face mask and rotating tourniquets).
- Remain with patient if at all possible, providing emotional support for both the patient and significant other.
- For further interventions, see Appendix One, "Caring for Patients With Cancer and Other Life-disrupting Illnesses," **Fear,** p. 795.

NIC: Anxiety Reduction; Calming Technique; Environmental Management: Comfort; Meditation; Simple Guided Imagery

See Also: "Coronary Artery Disease" for **Knowledge deficit:** Precautions and side effects of nitrates, p. 60; "Heart Failure" for **Knowledge deficit:** Precautions and side effects of diuretic therapy, p. 71; **Knowledge deficit:** Precautions and side effects of digitalis therapy, p. 71; **Knowledge deficit:** Precautions and side effects of vasodilators, p. 72; psychosocial nursing diagnoses and interventions in Appendix One, "Caring for Patients With Cancer and Other Life-disrupting Illnesses," p. 791.

PATIENT-FAMILY TEACHING AND DISCHARGE PLANNING
See the patient's primary diagnosis.

Section Five: Special Cardiac Procedures

Pacemakers

A mechanical pacemaker delivers an electrical impulse to the heart to stimulate contraction when the heart's natural pacemakers fail to maintain normal rhythm. Patients for whom pacemakers are indicated have a history of syncopal episodes, dizziness, intolerance to exercise, blacking out, or an episode of cardiac arrest. When patients suffer from temporary or transient rhythm disturbances, such as severe bradycardia or a conduction block, a temporary pacemaker can be inserted. Temporary pacemakers are seen most often in ICUs and on an emergency basis. The lead wire is inserted through a central vein into the right side of the heart where it lodges in atrial or ventricular tissue to deliver the electrical impulse. An alternative method is transcutaneous pacing, which employs two large skin electrodes connected to a pulse generator.

Some patients who have had temporary pacemakers inserted are observed for the possibility of permanent pacing. Permanent pacemakers are indicated for patients with a complete or an incomplete conduction block that recurs or is not transient. Symptomatic bradycardia, or Stokes-Adams syncope (an intermittent heart block), is also an indication for permanent pacing. The pacemaker is implanted subcutaneously with the patient under local anesthesia and lead wires tunneled beneath the skin to the subclavian vein where they are threaded into the right atrium.

UNIVERSAL CODING
The increasing complexity of pacemakers has led to the development of a five-letter code for universal language by the Intersociety Commission on Heart Disease. However, the first three letters remain the basis for classification.
First letter: Chamber that is paced.
V: Ventricle.
A: Atrium.
D: Dual (both).
Second letter: Chamber that is sensed.
V: Ventricle.
A: Atrium.
D: Dual (both).
O: None.
Third letter: Mode of response.
T: Triggered by ventricular activity.
I: Inhibited by ventricular activity.
D: Dual (both)—atrial triggered, ventricular inhibited.
O: Neither (paces continuously).
R: Reverse (pacing occurs when tachycardia is sensed).

Fourth letter: Programmable functions.
P: Programmable.
M: Multiprogrammable.
O: None.
Fifth letter: Special antitachycardia functions.
B: Burst ventricular pacing to break ventricular tachycardia.
N: Silent during normal rates.
S: Scans and delivers progressive stimuli.
E: Externally activated.

PACEMAKER TYPES

Asynchronous or fixed rate: Discharges an impulse to the ventricle at a prescribed rate, without a sensing mechanism. Asynchronous or fixed-rate pacemakers can be VOO, AOO, or DOO.
Ventricular demand: Senses intrinsic cardiac function and discharges only when the ventricle fails to do so (at the prescribed rate). This type of pacemaker is coded VVI or VVT.
Synchronous: Senses the activity in the atrium and stimulates the ventricle. This type of pacemaker is coded VAT.
Sequential: Senses the activity in the atrium and ventricle and stimulates both sequentially if no intrinsic activity occurs. This type of pacemaker is coded DVI, VDD, or DDD.
Rate responsive: Increasing numbers of patients have this type of pacemaker, which is designed to increase rate in response to activity. For example, it "senses" changes in right ventricular blood temperature, cardiac output, O_2 saturation, or stroke volume and responds accordingly.

Temporary pacemakers often are inserted in the ICU where the patient can be monitored continuously. Permanent pacemakers are implanted in the operating room, after which the patient is transferred to the telemetry unit for 24-48 hr of close monitoring. After implantation, a sling or other immobilizer may be applied for 24 hr. Exercise is encouraged the day after insertion to prevent joint contractures.

NURSING DIAGNOSES AND INTERVENTIONS

Knowledge deficit: Pacemaker insertion procedure, pacemaker function, and precautions to take after hospital discharge
Desired outcomes: Before the procedure, patient verbalizes knowledge about the insertion procedure and the function of the pacemaker. Before hospital discharge, patient describes precautions to take after hospital discharge.

Before pacemaker insertion
- Assess patient's knowledge about the insertion procedure and function of the pacemaker. As appropriate, describe the procedure and explain that the pacemaker stimulates the patient's own heart to beat when the heart becomes "lazy" or slows down.
- Begin a teaching program specific to the patient's rhythm disorder and type of pacemaker inserted, including normal function of the heart, patient's disorder of rhythm that requires a pacemaker, and how the patient's pacemaker works.
- Reinforce explanation by health care provider about the length of time of the procedure, use of local anesthetic, and postprocedure care.
- Explain that after the procedure patient can expect the following: continuous ECG monitoring, stiffness and soreness at the insertion site, and no vigorous activity. Explain that patient should request pain medication before pain becomes severe. Some health care providers prescribe that ice be placed on the wound for the first 24 hr postoperatively to prevent edema formation and reduce pain.

After pacemaker insertion
- Explain activity restrictions as directed by health care provider, such as no heavy lifting, and give instructions about the amount and type of exercise allowed. Resumption of sexual activity probably will not be affected, but this will depend on patient's underlying condition.
- Teach patient the signs and symptoms that necessitate medical attention, such as decreasing pulse rate, irregular pulse, dizziness, SOB, ankle swelling, passing out, and signs of infection. Teach patient the technique for measuring radial pulse.
- Stress the necessity of follow-up care, usually at pacemaker clinic; confirm date of next appointment. Telephonic monitoring of pacemakers is used frequently as a method of assessing patients between visits. If this method is to be used, inform patient about this type of monitoring.
- Teach patient the expected life of the pacemaker battery, which is approximate and can vary from 5-10 yr, depending on the type of battery. It is important to know the manufacturer of the specific pacemaker because some start to show signs of battery failure 2 yr before absolute failure.
- Instruct patients on the need to carry their pacemaker identification card with them and to wear a Medic-Alert bracelet. The card contains information about the type of pacemaker for health care providers in case of emergency.

NIC: Heat/Cold Application; Learning Readiness Enhancement; Teaching: Preoperative; Teaching: Prescribed Activity/Exercise; Teaching: Psychomotor Skill

Altered cardiopulmonary and peripheral tissue perfusion (or risk of same) related to interrupted blood flow secondary to pacemaker malfunction
Desired outcome: On an ongoing basis, patient has adequate perfusion as evidenced by BP within 20 mm Hg of baseline BP, peripheral pulse amplitude >2+ on a 0-4+ scale, and apical/radial pulses regular, equal, and at rate ≥ that established for pacemaker.
- Monitor perfusion by assessing BP at frequent intervals.
- Assess rate and regularity of apical and radial pulses. At minimum, it should be the rate established for the pacemaker.
- Assess for apical/radial deficit, which if present indicates that the heart is mechanically contracting but that there is no peripheral perfusion (e.g., the apical pulse rate is 80 bpm with auscultation, but the palpable radial pulse is 42 bpm).
- Be alert to pulse irregularity, which can signal pacemaker malfunction or decreasing patient response.
- Ensure that patient maintains strict bedrest for the prescribed amount of time postoperatively to prevent pacemaker displacement.
- Most health care providers request that patient use a sling or other immobilizer to prevent pacemaker displacement caused by arm movement.
- Alert health care provider to significant findings.

NIC: Cardiac Care; Dysrhythmia Management; Vital Signs Monitoring

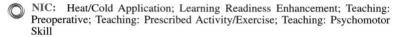

See Also: Appendix One, "Caring for Preoperative and Postoperative Patients," **Pain or chronic pain**: disease process, injury, or surgical procedure, p. 719.

PATIENT-FAMILY TEACHING AND DISCHARGE PLANNING

When providing patient-family teaching, focus on sensory information; avoid giving excessive information; and initiate a visiting nurse referral for necessary

follow-up teaching. Consider including verbal and written information about the following:

- Activity restrictions as directed by health care provider, such as no heavy lifting, and instructions about the amount and type of exercise allowed. Resumption of sexual activity probably will not be affected, but this will depend on patient's underlying condition.
- Technique for measuring radial pulse.
- Signs and symptoms that necessitate medical attention, such as decreasing pulse rate, irregular pulse, dizziness, passing out, and signs of infection.
- Necessity of follow-up care, usually at pacemaker clinic; confirm date of next appointment. Telephonic monitoring of pacemakers is used frequently as a method of assessing patients between visits. If this method is to be used, inform patient about this type of monitoring.
- Medications, including drug name, purpose, dosage, schedule, precautions, drug/drug and food/drug interactions, and potential side effects.
- Importance of using caution around strong magnetic fields, which can alter the function of the pacemaker. Strong magnetic fields can convert some pacemakers to a fixed-rate mode. Once the patient moves away from the magnetic field, the pacemaker will return to the normal programmed function.
- Expected life of the pacemaker battery, which is approximate and can vary from 5-10 yr, depending on the type of battery. It is important to know the manufacturer of the specific pacemaker because some start to show signs of battery failure 2 yr before absolute failure.

Cardiac catheterization, angioplasty, and atherectomy

Cardiac catheterization: Cardiac catheterization is an invasive diagnostic procedure used to assess the extent of coronary artery disease or valvular heart disease. It involves insertion of a radiopaque catheter through a peripheral vessel into the heart. With *left heart catheterization,* the catheter is advanced retrogradely, usually through the femoral artery, into the left ventricle and the coronary arteries. Subsequently, pressure measurements are made and the amount of cardiac output is determined to diagnose valvular stenosis and resistance to blood flow. Then dye is injected so that the heart structures, including ventricular chambers, coronary arteries, great vessels, and valves, can be visualized with fluoroscopy. *Right heart catheterization* involves advancement of a catheter from a peripheral vein into the right side of the heart to the pulmonary artery. This catheter measures pulmonary vascular pressures.

Associated procedures may include *electrophysiologic studies (EPS)* to assess conduction system abnormalities and ectopic (irregular) beats. If indicated, *transvenous intracardiac pacing wires* also may be inserted to assess conduction defects and determine the exact location of the disorder. Another procedure performed in the cardiac catheterization laboratory is the *intracoronary injection of streptokinase,* a therapeutic measure used to dissolve a clot or thrombus that is occluding a coronary artery. This procedure restores circulation to the myocardial muscle distal to the occlusion.

Patients are sedated before cardiac catheterization and given a local anesthetic so that they can be awake to alert the health care provider to any chest pain and cooperate with position changes. Usually cardiac catheterization is an elective, scheduled procedure, but it may be performed in emergency situations.

Percutaneous transluminal coronary angioplasty: Percutaneous transluminal coronary angioplasty (PTCA) is an invasive procedure for improving blood flow through stenotic coronary arteries. A balloon-tipped catheter is inserted into the coronary arterial lesion, and the balloon is inflated to compress the plaque material against the vessel wall, thereby opening the narrowed lumen. This is a nondebulking procedure; that is, the plaque is not removed—it is remodeled. PTCA is indicated for the surgical candidate whose angina is refractory to medical treatment. It also is being performed in individuals with postinfarction angina, postbypass angina, and chronic stable angina. The ideal candidate has single-vessel disease with a discrete, proximal, noncalcified lesion.

During the procedure the patient is sedated lightly and given a local anesthetic at the insertion site, usually the femoral artery; ECG electrodes are placed on the chest. A pulmonary artery catheter is passed through the vena cava and right atrium into the heart to measure heart pressure. A pacing wire may be inserted as well. An introducer sheath is inserted into the femoral artery, a guide wire is passed into the aorta and coronary artery, and the balloon catheter is passed over the guide wire to the stenotic site. The patient may be asked to take deep breaths and cough to facilitate passage of the catheter. Heparin is given to prevent clot formation, and intracoronary nitroglycerin (NTG) and sublingual nifedipine are administered to dilate coronary vessels and prevent spasm. The balloon is inflated repeatedly for 60-90 sec at a pressure of 4-11 atm. Subsequently, radiopaque dye is injected to determine whether the stenosis has been reduced to less than 50% of the vessel diameter, which is the goal of the procedure. The introducer sheath is left in the femoral artery for up to 12 hr after PTCA for heparin infusion or in case repeat angiography is needed, and the patient usually is in a special care unit.

Complications after PTCA include acute coronary artery occlusion, MI, coronary artery spasm, bleeding, circulatory insufficiency, renal hypersensitivity to contrast material, hypokalemia, vasovagal reaction, dysrhythmias, and hypotension. Restenosis can occur 6 wk to 6 mo after PTCA, although the patient may not experience angina.

Endovascular stent: In this procedure an endovascular stent is implanted within stenosed vessels to stretch them and improve blood flow. A variety of designs, materials, and deployment techniques have been developed. This procedure may be used for stenosed coronary arteries or to stretch anastomotic sites after coronary artery bypass grafts. It improves coronary artery blood flow in most patients with failed PTCA.

Laser angioplasty: Laser angioplasty is a treatment for some patients with coronary artery occlusions. It is similar to cardiac catheterization and involves application of a laser beam to the occlusion or lesion in the coronary artery to debulk the lesion and allow reperfusion.

Coronary artery atherectomy: Atherectomy is a debulking procedure that removes plaque from the intima of affected arteries.

Rotational atherectomy: Rotational atherectomy pulverizes plaque into microscopic particles, which then are dispersed by the circulation. A high-speed rotating burr is adapted to the tip of the cardiac catheter and advanced to the area of obstruction to rotoablate the plaque and reopen the clogged artery.

Transluminal extraction catheterization: Transluminal extraction catheterization (TEC) uses a specially adapted catheter to excise and aspirate the plaque to reopen coronary arteries.

Directional coronary atherectomy: Directional coronary atherectomy (DCA) uses a balloon on the side of the catheter to guide the plaque on the artery's intima into a shaver where it is cut up and aspirated into the tip of the catheter.

NURSING DIAGNOSES AND INTERVENTIONS

Knowledge deficit: Catheterization procedure and postcatheterization regimen
Desired outcome: Before the procedure, patient verbalizes knowledge about cardiac catheterization and the postcatheterization regimen.

- Assess patient's knowledge about the catheterization procedure. As appropriate, reinforce health care provider's explanation of the procedure, and answer any questions or concerns of the patient and significant other. If possible, arrange for an orientation visit to the catheterization laboratory before the procedure.

- Before the cardiac catheterization, have the patient practice techniques (e.g., Valsalva's maneuver, coughing, deep breathing) that will be used during the catheterization.
- Explain that after the procedure bedrest will be required and that VS, circulation, and the insertion site will be checked at frequent intervals to ensure integrity. In addition, explain that sandbags may be used over the insertion site and that flexing of the insertion site (arm or groin) is contraindicated to prevent bleeding.
- Stress the importance of promptly reporting signs and symptoms of hemorrhage, hematoma formation, or embolization.

◎ **NIC:** Learning Facilitation; Learning Readiness Enhancement; Teaching: Disease Process; Teaching: Preoperative; Teaching: Prescribed Medication

Altered cardiopulmonary, peripheral, and cerebral tissue perfusion related to interrupted arterial flow secondary to the catheterization procedure
Desired outcome: Within 1 hr after the procedure, patient has adequate perfusion as evidenced by HR regular and within 20 bpm of baseline HR; apical/radial pulse equality; BP within 20 mm Hg of baseline BP; peripheral pulse amplitude >2+ on a 0-4+ scale; warmth and normal color in the extremities; and no significant change in mental status and orientation to person, place, and time.
- Monitor BP q15min until stable on three successive checks, q2hr for the next 12 hr, and q4hr for 24 hr unless otherwise indicated. If the systolic pressure drops 20 mm Hg below previous recordings, lower HOB and notify health care provider.

> **Note:** If the insertion site was the antecubital space, measure BP in the unaffected arm.

- Be alert to and report indicators of decreased perfusion, including cool extremities, decreased amplitude of peripheral pulses, cyanosis, changes in mental status, decreased LOC, and SOB.
- Monitor patient's HR, and notify health care provider if dysrhythmias occur. If the patient is not on a cardiac monitor, auscultate apical and radial pulses with every BP check and report irregularities or apical/radial discrepancies.
- If the femoral artery was the insertion site, maintain HOB at a 30-degree elevation to prevent acute hip joint flexion.

◎ **NIC:** Bleeding Precautions; Cerebral Perfusion Promotion; Circulatory Care; Peripheral Sensation Management; Respiratory Monitoring; Shock Management; Vital Signs Monitoring

Risk for fluid volume deficit with risk factors from hemorrhage or hematoma formation caused by arterial puncture and/or osmotic diuresis from the dye
Desired outcomes: Patient remains normovolemic as evidenced by HR ≤100 bpm; BP ≥90/60 mm Hg (or within 20 mm Hg of baseline range); and no significant change in mental status and orientation to person, place, and time. The patient's dressing is dry, and there is no swelling at the puncture site.
- Be alert to indicators of shock or hemorrhage, such as a decrease in BP, increase in HR, and decreasing LOC.
- Inspect dressing on the groin or antecubital space for presence of frank bleeding or hematoma formation (fluctuating swelling).

- Monitor peripheral perfusion, and be alert to decreased amplitude or absence of distal pulses, delayed capillary refill, coolness of the extremities, and pallor, which can signal embolization or hemorrhagic shock.
- To minimize the risk of bleeding, caution patient about flexing the elbow or hip for 6-8 hr, or as prescribed.
- If bleeding occurs, maintain pressure at the insertion site as prescribed, usually 1 inch proximal to the puncture site or introducer insertion site. Typically this is done with a pressure dressing or a 2½- to 5-lb sandbag.

NIC: Bleeding Precautions; Bleeding Reduction; Fluid Management; Hypovolemia Management; Intravenous (IV) Therapy; Shock Management: Volume

Altered peripheral (involved limb) tissue perfusion (or risk of same) related to interrupted arterial flow secondary to embolization
Desired outcome: Patient has adequate perfusion in the involved limb as evidenced by peripheral pulse amplitude >2+ on a 0-4+ scale; normal color, sensation, and temperature; and brisk capillary refill (<2 sec).

- Assess peripheral perfusion by palpating peripheral pulses q15min for 30 min, then q30min for 1 hr, then hourly for 2 hr, or per protocol.
- Monitor for and report any indicators of embolization in the involved limb, such as faintness or absence of pulse, coolness of extremity, mottling, decreased capillary refill, cyanosis, and complaints of numbness, tingling, and pain at the insertion site. Instruct patient to report any of these indicators promptly.
- If there is *no* evidence of an embolus or thrombus formation, instruct patient to move fingers or toes and rotate wrist or ankle to promote circulation.
- Ensure that patient maintains bedrest for 4-6 hr or as prescribed.

NIC: Bleeding Precautions; Circulatory Care; Embolus Precautions; Peripheral Sensation Management; Surveillance

Altered renal tissue perfusion (or risk of same) related to interrupted blood flow secondary to decreased cardiac output or reaction to contrast dye
Desired outcome: Patient has adequate renal perfusion as evidenced by urinary output ≥30 ml/hr, specific gravity <1.030, good skin turgor, and moist mucous membranes.

- Because contrast dye for cardiac catheterization may cause osmotic diuresis, monitor for indicators of dehydration, such as poor skin turgor, dry mucous membranes, and high urine specific gravity (≥1.030).
- Monitor I&O. Notify health care provider if urinary output is <30 ml/hr in the presence of an adequate intake.
- If urinary output is insufficient despite adequate intake, restrict fluids. Be alert to and report indicators of fluid overload, such as crackles (rales) on auscultation of lung fields, distended neck veins, and SOB. Notify health care provider about significant findings.
- If patient does not exhibit signs of cardiac or renal failure, encourage daily intake of 2-3 L of fluids, or as prescribed, to flush the contrast dye out of the system.

NIC: Fluid Management; Fluid Monitoring; Surveillance

See Also: "Coronary Artery Disease" for **Pain,** p. 56; **Knowledge deficit:** Precautions and side effects of nitrates, p. 60; **Knowledge deficit:** Precautions and side effects of β- blockers, p. 60.

PATIENT-FAMILY TEACHING AND DISCHARGE PLANNING

When providing patient-family teaching, focus on sensory information; avoid giving excessive information; and initiate a visiting nurse referral for necessary

follow-up teaching. Consider including verbal and written information about the following:

- Use of NTG, including purpose, dosage, schedule, precautions, drug/drug and food/drug interactions, and potential side effects, such as headache and dizziness. Caution patient to avoid using NTG more frequently than prescribed and to notify health care provider if three tablets do not relieve pain.
- Use of calcium antagonists, β-blockers, antidysrhythmic agents, and antihypertensive agents, including the drug name, purpose, dosage, schedule, precautions, drug/drug and food/drug interactions, and potential side effects. Advise patient about the importance of taking the medications regularly and not discontinuing them without health care provider approval.
- Signs and symptoms necessitating immediate medical attention, including chest pain unrelieved by NTG, decreased exercise tolerance, increasing SOB, and loss of consciousness.
- Activity and dietary limitations as prescribed.
- Importance of follow-up with health care provider; confirm date and time of next appointment.

Cardiac surgery

Cardiac surgery is performed to correct a variety of heart disorders. For example, *coronary artery bypass grafting (CABG)* is a technique used to treat blocked coronary arteries; a portion of the saphenous vein or internal mammary artery is excised and anastomosed to coronary arteries to shunt blood around the blocked portions of arteries to maintain flow to the heart muscle. *Valve replacement,* another type of cardiac surgery, is performed for patients with valvular stenosis or valvular incompetence of the mitral, tricuspid, pulmonary, or aortic valve. Cardiac surgery is also performed to correct heart defects that are either acquired or congenital, such as ventricular aneurysm, ventricular or atrial septal defects, transposition of the great vessels, and tetralogy of Fallot. *Heart transplantation* has become an accepted treatment modality for some patients diagnosed with end-stage cardiac disease, most commonly idiopathic dilated cardiomyopathy or ischemic cardiomyopathy. The supply of donor organs is a major difficulty; donors should be men younger than 40 yr or women younger than 45 yr with established brain death. *Combined heart-lung transplantation* is used for patients with end-stage disease affecting both organs or where poor function in one organ has had adverse effects on the other organ.

Unless an emergency occurs, patients usually are admitted to the hospital the day of surgery. After surgery, most patients are in an ICU for 24-72 hr and then transferred to a special unit called *transitional care*, *special care*, or a *step-down* unit. Immunosuppressive treatment to prevent organ rejection after heart transplantation is similar to that of patients who receive a renal transplant. See "Care of the Renal Transplant Recipient," p. 161.

NURSING DIAGNOSES AND INTERVENTIONS

Knowledge deficit: Diagnosis, surgical procedure, preoperative routine, and postoperative course
Desired outcome: Before surgery, patient verbalizes knowledge about the diagnosis, surgical procedure, and preoperative and postoperative regimens.
- Assess patient's level of knowledge about the diagnosis and surgical procedure, and provide information where necessary. Encourage questions, and allow time for verbalization of concerns and fears.
- If appropriate for the patient, provide orientation to the ICU and equipment that will be used postoperatively.
- Provide instructions for deep breathing and coughing in the preoperative teaching.

- Reassure patient that postoperative discomfort will be relieved with medication.

Note: Pain after a midline sternotomy (the usual incision with cardiac surgery) usually is less than that with conventional thoracotomy because the somatic nerves are not divided by the surgical incision.

- Advise patient that in the immediate postoperative period, speaking will be impossible because of the presence of an endotracheal tube, which will assist with breathing. Introduce the patient to an alternative means of communication (paper and pencil, picture board, flash cards) that will be used while the endotracheal tube is in place.
- Explain to the patient that a chest tube will be present. Teach patient how he or she will move, deep breathe, and cough with a chest tube in place. (See pp. 23-25 for care considerations for patients with chest tubes.)

NIC: Communication Enhancement: Speech Deficit; Learning Facilitation; Learning Readiness Enhancement; Teaching: Disease Process; Teaching: Preoperative

Activity intolerance related to generalized weakness and bedrest secondary to cardiac surgery
Desired outcome: By a minimum of 24 hr before hospital discharge, patient rates perceived exertion at ≤3 on a 0-10 scale and exhibits cardiac tolerance to activity after cardiac surgery as evidenced by HR ≤120 bpm, systolic BP within 20 mm Hg of resting systolic BP, and RR ≤20 breaths/min with normal depth and pattern (eupnea).
- Ask patient to rate perceived exertion during activity, and monitor for evidence of activity intolerance. For details, see **Risk for activity intolerance** in Appendix One, "Caring for Patients on Prolonged Bedrest," p. 739. Notify health care provider of significant findings.
- Monitor VS at frequent intervals, and be alert to indicators of cardiac failure, including hypotension, tachycardia, crackles (rales), tachypnea, and decreased amplitude of peripheral pulses. Notify health care provider of significant findings.
- Monitor BP, and note a decrease >20 mm Hg of resting systolic BP.

Note: A mean BP of 50 mm Hg is required for adequate brain perfusion.

- Facilitate coordination of health care providers to provide rest periods between care activities to decrease cardiac workload. Ensure 90 min for undisturbed rest.
- As prescribed, administer medications that decrease myocardial O_2 consumption, such as β-blockers or calcium antagonists.
- Assist patient with ROM and other exercises, depending on tolerance and prescribed activity limitations. Consult health care provider about patient's readiness to participate in exercises that require increased cardiac tolerance.
- See Appendix One, **Risk for activity intolerance,** p. 738, and **Risk for disuse syndrome,** p. 740, for a discussion of in-bed exercises.

NIC: Activity Therapy; Cardiac Care: Rehabilitative; Energy Management; Environmental Management; Exercise Promotion; Surveillance

See Also: "Pulmonary Embolus" for **Altered protection** related to risk of prolonged bleeding or hemorrhage secondary to anticoagulation therapy, p. 18; "Coronary Artery Disease" for **Altered nutrition:** More than body requirements of calories, sodium, or fats, p. 58; **Health-seeking behaviors:** Relaxation technique effective for stress reduction, p. 59; "Atherosclerotic Arterial Occlusive Disease" for **Altered renal tissue perfusion,** p. 120; Appendix One, "Caring for Preoperative and Postoperative Patients," **Ineffective breathing pattern,** p. 729; **Risk for infection,** p. 732; Appendix One, "Caring for Patients on Prolonged Bedrest," **Altered peripheral tissue perfusion,** p. 742.

PATIENT-FAMILY TEACHING AND DISCHARGE PLANNING

When providing patient-family teaching, focus on sensory information; avoid giving excessive information; and initiate a visiting nurse referral for necessary follow-up teaching. Consider including verbal and written information about the following:

- Medications, including drug name, dosage, schedule, purpose, precautions, drug/drug and food/drug interactions, and potential side effects.
- Untoward symptoms requiring medical attention for patients taking warfarin, such as bleeding from the nose (epistaxis) or gums, hemoptysis, hematemesis, hematuria, melena, hematochezia, menometrorrhagia, and excessive bruising. In addition, stress the following: take warfarin at the same time every day; notify health care provider if *any* signs of bleeding occur; keep appointments for physical therapy (PT) checks; avoid over-the-counter (OTC) medications unless approved by health care provider; carry a Medic-Alert bracelet or card; avoid constrictive or restrictive clothing; and use soft-bristled toothbrush and electric razor.
- Maintenance of low-Na^+ (see Table 3-2, p. 133, for a list of high-Na^+ foods to avoid), low-fat (see Table 2-3), and low-cholesterol (see Table 2-2) diet. Encourage patients to use food labels to determine sodium, fat, and cholesterol content of foods.
- Importance of pacing activities at home and allowing frequent rest periods.
- Technique for assessing radial pulse, temperature, and weight, if these indicators require monitoring at home, and reporting significant changes to health care provider.
- Introduction to local American Heart Association activities. Either provide the address or phone number for the local chapter or encourage the patient to write for information to the following address:

American Heart Association
7320 Greenville Avenue
Dallas, TX 75231   (800) 242-8721
WWW address: *http://occ.com/amerh*

- For patients awaiting heart transplantation, provide the following information, as appropriate:

The United Network for Organ Sharing
UNOS Communication Department
P.O. Box 13770
Richmond, VA 23225   (804) 330-8561 or (800) 243-6667 (voice mail)
WWW address: *http://www.unos.org*

- Phone number of nurse available to discuss concerns and questions or clarify unclear instructions.

- Importance of follow-up visits with health care provider; confirm date and time of next appointment.
- Signs and symptoms that necessitate immediate medical attention: edema, chest pain, dyspnea, SOB, weight gain, and decrease in exercise tolerance.
- Activity restrictions (e.g., no heavy lifting [≥10-20 lb], pushing, or pulling for at least 6 wk); prescribed exercise program; and resumption of sexual activity, work, and driving a car, as directed.
- Care of the incision site; importance of assessing for signs of infection, such as drainage, swelling, fever, persistent redness, and local warmth and tenderness.
- Referral to a cardiac rehabilitation program.
- Discussion of the patient's home environment and the potential need for changes or adaptations (e.g., too many steps to climb, ADLs that are too strenuous).

Section Six: Disorders of the Peripheral Vascular System

Atherosclerotic arterial occlusive disease

Arteriosclerosis is a normal aging process resulting in changes in the arteries, including thickening of the walls, loss of elasticity, increase in calcium deposits, and, usually, an increase in external diameter and a decrease in internal diameter. In contrast, *atherosclerosis* refers to a pathologic process of focal changes in the arteries, usually involving the accumulation of lipids, carbohydrates, calcium, blood components, and fibrous tissue. Although the two processes differ, they usually occur simultaneously.

The process of atherosclerotic disease results in narrowing of the arterial lumen, which limits blood flow. Thrombosis or aneurysm can occur, depending on the reaction of the tissue that is supplied by the atherosclerotic vessels. Arterial occlusion and insufficiency are usually found in the lower extremities in patients older than 50 yr. *Raynaud's disease* is a type of impairment that tends to affect younger individuals and women. It is characterized by vasospasm of small arteries and arterioles in the extremities, particularly associated with an oversensitivity to the sympathetic nervous system (SNS) effects of cold and possibly stress. The cause of Raynaud's disease is unknown.

ASSESSMENT

Signs and symptoms: Severe, cramping pain (called *intermittent claudication*) that follows exercise and is relieved by rest. It is indicative of ischemia secondary to decreased blood flow. The patient also may have delayed healing, collapsed veins, decreased sensory or motor function, leg ulcers, or gangrene.

Physical assessment: Decreased pulse amplitude, decreased hair distribution, and bluish discoloration of the extremities and areas of decreased circulation. The skin may appear shiny and the nails thickened. Audible bruits may be assessed with a stethoscope over partially occluded vessels. Capillary filling will be ≥2 sec (with normal circulation, capillary filling occurs in <2 sec), and amplitude of peripheral pulses will be decreased.

Risk factors: Hypertension, cigarette smoking, diabetes mellitus, family history of atherosclerotic disease, and hyperlipoproteinemia. Use of β-blocker drugs can exacerbate patient's symptoms because of their peripheral vasoconstricting effect.

DIAGNOSTIC TESTS

Angiography of peripheral vasculature: Locates obstruction and reveals extent of vascular lesions. This invasive study usually is done only if surgery is planned.

Duplex imaging: Uses ultrasound to assess arteries for plaque formation and measurement of flow and pressure.

Doppler flow studies: Use a transducer that emits sound waves through a probe to determine the amount of blood flow in arteries in which palpable pulses are difficult to obtain.

Digital subtraction angiography (DSA):   Uses computerized tomography (CT) to visualize arteries radiologically and determine presence and extent of occlusion.

Exercise testing: Determines the amount of exercise that precipitates ischemia and claudication.

Oscillometry: Uses a BP cuff connected to a manometer to locate occlusive sites, as evidenced by decreased pressure readings.

Ankle-brachial index (ABI):   Determines the degree of ischemia. Blood pressure is determined at the ankle (using either posterior tibial or dorsalis pedis pulses) and at the brachial artery. The pressure obtained at the ankle is divided by that at the brachial artery. Normally the ABI is >1.0; resting pain occurs with an ABI ≤0.3.

COLLABORATIVE MANAGEMENT

Regular lower extremity exercise program: To increase circulation. This can include a walking program or Buerger-Allen exercises. Activity may be contraindicated for some patients with severe disease, who may instead require bedrest to decrease O_2 demands to the tissues. See also **Impaired tissue integrity** of extremity, p. 118.

Cessation of cigarette smoking: To prevent increased vasoconstriction and severity of the circulation deficit.

Control of hyperlipidemia and cholesterol levels: To help prevent progression of atherosclerosis. This is accomplished through a low-fat (see Table 2-3), low-cholesterol (see Table 2-2) diet or the controversial antilipemic drugs, which may be used if diet control is ineffective. Examples of these drugs include clofibrate and cholestyramine.

Control of hypertension: Administration of agents such as thiazide diuretics.

Provision of warmth: To promote arterial flow.

> **Caution:**   Care must be taken to avoid applying extreme heat, because the patient's sensitivity to temperature is often decreased and burns can result.

Pharmacotherapy

Mild analgesics: For relief of pain.

Antiplatelet agents (e.g., aspirin):   May be used to help prevent platelet adherence and thromboembolism. The use of anticoagulants, such as warfarin, to prevent thrombus formation is controversial.

Thrombolytics (e.g., streptokinase):   To lyse the clot.

Pentoxyphylline (Trental):   To increase flexibility of erythrocytes (which enhances their movement through the microcirculation), prevent aggregation of RBCs and platelets, and decrease blood viscosity. This has the potential to increase circulation at the capillary level.

Calcium channel blockers (e.g., diltiazem):   To reduce vasospasm.

Lovastatin (Mevacor):   To reduce serum cholesterol level.

Surgical management: For patients who are severely limited by the occlusion and for whom the occlusion is fairly localized.

Endarterectomy: Removal of the atheromatous obstruction via an arterial incision.

Bypass vascular grafting: Removal or bypass of the obstructed segment by suturing a graft proximally and distally to the obstruction. The most common procedures are aortofemoral, aortoiliac, and femoropopliteal bypasses. Graft material may be the patient's saphenous vein or prosthetic materials such as Gortex or Dacron.

Percutaneous transluminal angioplasty (PTA):   May be used to treat focal arterial obstruction. A balloon-tipped catheter is inserted through the vein or artery to the area of the occlusion. The balloon is gradually inflated to ablate the obstruction.

Laser angioplasty: Technique similar to PTA. A fiberoptic catheter is inserted and threaded to the area of occlusion. Energy from a laser is applied, and the occlusion is obliterated.

Endovascular stent: Implants a stent within stenosed vessels to stretch them and improve blood flow. A variety of designs, materials, and deployment techniques have been developed. This procedure may be used both for stenosed arteries or to stretch anastomotic sites after artery bypass grafts.

Rotational atherectomy: Pulverizes plaque into microscopic particles, which then are dispersed by the circulation. A high-speed rotating burr at the tip of the catheter is advanced to the area of obstruction to rotoablate the plaque and reopen the clogged artery.

Amputation: See discussion in Chapter 8.

NURSING DIAGNOSES AND INTERVENTIONS

Impaired tissue integrity of extremity (or risk of same) related to altered arterial circulation secondary to atherosclerotic process
Desired outcome: Patient's extremity tissue remains intact.

* Assess leg(s) for ulcerations that can occur with decreased arterial circulation.
* Teach patient to elevate HOB to increase circulation to the lower extremities. Explain that this can be accomplished at home by raising the HOB on 6-in blocks.
* Teach patient that walking and ROM exercises for the hip, knee, and ankle promote collateral circulation.
* Discuss an exercise program with health care provider, and describe the routine to the patient. Often this includes walking to the patient's tolerance (without pain).

Note: Bedrest without exercise may be prescribed to decrease O_2 demand in acute, severe cases.

---

* If prescribed, teach the patient Buerger-Allen exercises as follows:
  —Teach patient to lie flat in bed with the legs elevated above the level of the heart for 2-3 min.
  —Have the patient sit on the edge of the bed for 2-3 min with the legs relaxed and dependent.
  —Have the patient, in the same position, flex, extend, invert, and evert the feet, holding each position for 30 sec.
  —Finally, have the patient lie flat with the legs at heart level and covered with a warm blanket for approximately 5 min.
* Teach patient to assess peripheral pulses, warmth, color, hair distribution, and capillary filling. To check for capillary filling, teach the patient to press on a nail bed until blanching occurs and release the pressure. Explain that with normal capillary filling, color (pink) returns in 1-2 sec.
* As appropriate, teach patient that smoking results in a decrease in both blood flow to the extremities and extremity temperature, particularly to the fingers and toes.

- Discuss the importance of keeping warm by wearing socks when walking or in bed. Caution patient about using heating pads, which increase metabolism and may promote ischemia if circulation is limited.
- Caution patient to cover all exposed areas when going outside in cooler weather.
- Teach patient to maintain moderate room temperatures and avoid extremes.
- Administer antiplatelet agents as prescribed to help prevent platelet adherence.

NIC: Circulatory Care; Positioning; Pressure Management; Skin Care: Topical Treatments; Skin Surveillance

Chronic pain related to atherosclerotic obstructions
Desired outcomes: By hospital discharge, patient's subjective perception of chronic pain decreases as documented by a pain scale. Objective indicators, such as grimacing, are absent.
- Assess for the presence of pain, using a pain scale from 0 (no pain) to 10 (worst pain). Administer pain medications as prescribed; document effectiveness using the pain scale.
- Teach patient to rest and stop exercising before claudication (severe, cramping pain) occurs.
- Because the pain may be chronic and continuous, explore alternate methods of pain relief, such as visualization, guided imagery, biofeedback, meditation, and relaxation exercises or tapes. See "Coronary Heart Disease," **Health-seeking behaviors,** p. 59, for an example of a relaxation exercise.
- Institute measures to increase circulation to ischemic extremities, such as Buerger-Allen exercises (see **Impaired tissue integrity,** p. 118) and walking.
- Administer calcium channel blockers, such as diltiazem hydrochloride, as prescribed to reduce vasospasm.
- Advise patient about the possibility of "rest" pain, which occurs at night when recumbent and decreases when the legs are in a dependent position.

NIC: Biofeedback; Calming Technique; Cutaneous Stimulation; Distraction; Music Therapy; Simple Guided Imagery; Simple Relaxation Therapy

Knowledge deficit: Potential for infection and impaired tissue integrity caused by decreased arterial circulation
Desired outcome: By hospital discharge, patient verbalizes knowledge about the potential for infection and impaired tissue integrity, as well as measures to prevent these problems.
- Teach patient how to assess for signs of infection or problems with skin integrity and to report significant findings to health care provider.
- Caution patient about the increased potential for easily traumatizing the skin (e.g., from bumping the lower extremities).
- Instruct the patient to inspect both feet each day for any open wounds or bruises. If necessary, suggest the patient use a long-handled mirror to see the bottoms of the feet. Advise the patient to report any open areas to the health care provider.
- Stress the importance of wearing shoes or slippers that fit properly.
- Instruct patient to cut toenails straight across to prevent ingrown toenails.
- Advise patient to cover corns or calluses with pads to prevent further injury.
- Encourage patient to keep the feet clean and dry, using mild soap and warm water for cleansing, and apply a mild lotion to prevent dryness.
- Advise patient not to scratch or rub the skin on the feet because this can result in abrasions that easily can become infected.
- Suggest that patient keep the feet warm with loose-fitting socks and warm soaks. Caution patient to check the temperature of warm soaks and bath water carefully to protect the skin from burns.

- Discuss potential surgical interventions, such as endarterectomy, bypass vascular grafting, and angioplasty.

NIC: Learning Facilitation; Learning Readiness Enhancement; Self-Care Assistance: Bathing/Hygiene; Skin Surveillance; Teaching: Disease Process; Teaching: Psychomotor Skill

Altered peripheral tissue perfusion (or risk of same) related to interrupted arterial flow with postsurgical graft occlusion
Desired outcome: Patient has adequate peripheral perfusion as evidenced by peripheral pulse amplitude >2+ on a 0-4+ scale, BP within 20 mm Hg of baseline BP, and absence of the six *P*s (see below) in the involved extremities.

- Assess peripheral pulses and the involved extremity for the six *P*s: pain, pallor, pulselessness, paresthesia, polar (coolness), and paralysis. Sensory changes usually precede other symptoms of ischemia, that is, pain, loss of two-point discrimination, and paresthesias. Report significant findings.
- Monitor BP, another indicator of peripheral perfusion pressure. Report to health care provider any significant increase or decrease (>15-20 mm Hg, or as directed).
- If necessary, use the Doppler ultrasonic probe to check pulses, holding the probe to the skin at a 45-degree angle to the blood vessel. In the presence of blood flow, wavelike, whooshing sounds will be heard. Record the presence or absence of pulsations, as well as the rate, character, frequency, and intensity of the sounds.
- To prevent pressure on the tissue, use a foot cradle or foam protectors to keep sheets and blankets off the legs and feet.
- For the first 48-72 hr after surgery (or as directed), prevent acute joint flexion in the presence of a graft, which can occlude blood flow.

NIC: Circulatory Care; Embolus Care: Peripheral; Peripheral Sensation Management; Positioning; Surveillance

Altered renal tissue perfusion related to interrupted blood flow during surgery and potential embolization
Desired outcome: Within 1 hr after surgery, patient has adequate renal perfusion as evidenced by urinary output ≥30 ml/hr.

> **Note:** During many vascular surgical procedures, the aorta is clamped temporarily to facilitate endarterectomy and grafting. Although all body systems are affected to a degree, the renal system is especially sensitive to the lack of blood flow.

- Monitor I&O. Report output <30 ml/hr.
- Monitor results of renal function tests. Be alert to increases in serum creatinine (>1.5 mg/dl) and BUN (>20 mg/dl), which occur with decreasing renal function.
- Monitor for signs of fluid retention (e.g., distended neck veins, crackles [rales], peripheral edema).
- In the absence of acute cardiac or renal failure, encourage adequate fluid intake (2-3 L/day) to help maintain adequate renal blood flow and promote fluid balance.

NIC: Circulatory Care; Embolus Precautions; Fluid Monitoring; Surveillance

See Also: Appendix One, "Caring for Preoperative and Postoperative Patients," p. 717.

PATIENT-FAMILY TEACHING AND DISCHARGE PLANNING

When providing patient-family teaching, focus on sensory information; avoid giving excessive information; and initiate a visiting nurse referral for necessary follow-up teaching. Consider including verbal and written information about the following:

- Refer patient to a "stop smoking" program if appropriate. The following free brochures outline ways to help patients stop smoking:

  How to Help Your Patients Stop Using Tobacco: A National Cancer Institute Manual for the Oral Health Team, from the Smoking and Tobacco Control Program of the National Cancer Institute; call 1-800-4-CANCER.

  Clinical Practice Guideline: A Quick Reference Guide for Smoking Cessation Specialists, from the Agency for Health Care Policy and Research (AHCPR); call 1-800-358-9295.

- Importance of avoiding factors and activities that cause vasoconstriction (e.g., tight clothing and crossing the legs at the knee).
- Exercise program as prescribed by health care provider; importance of rest periods if claudication occurs.
- Skin and foot care.
- Measures that optimize arterial blood flow, such as keeping warm and raising HOB on blocks to promote circulation to the lower extremities.
- Medications, including drug name, purpose, dosage, schedule, precautions, drug/drug and food/drug interactions, and potential side effects.

Aneurysms: abdominal, thoracic, and femoral

An aneurysm is a localized, outpouching sac that is formed at a weak point in an arterial wall. The most likely cause of aneurysm is hereditary lack of elastin, although vessel wall trauma, congenital defect, infection, and atherosclerosis may be other causes. Loss of vessel wall elasticity and atherosclerotic deposits cause the vessel to weaken, resulting in gradual dilation. Unless this condition is recognized and surgically treated, rupture and exsanguination can occur. Although aneurysms can develop in any vessel, peripheral vessel aneurysms are most commonly found in the abdominal aorta, thoracic aorta, and femoral arteries. In *fusiform aneurysms* the weakened arterial wall allows dilation around the entire circumference of the vessel. In *saccular aneurysms* an isolated portion of the arterial wall weakens and a balloonlike deficit is created. *Dissecting aneurysms* occur in vessels that have atherosclerotic lesions and develop intimal tears, allowing bleeding into the layers of the vessel, which causes weakening and hematoma formation.

Until the aneurysm reaches sufficient size to press on adjacent organs, the individual may be asymptomatic. Complications include rupture and bleeding, exsanguination, and embolization. Most individuals with aneurysms are hypertensive.

ASSESSMENT

Chronic indicators

Abdominal aneurysm: Patient describes sensation of heartbeat in the abdomen. Chronic abdominal pain in the middle or lower abdomen also may be present. This form occurs more frequently in men and represents approximately 80% of all aneurysms.

Thoracic aneurysm: Patient may be asymptomatic for years. Pressure from the aneurysm on adjacent structures can result in dull pain in the upper back, dyspnea, cough, dysphagia, and hoarseness.

Femoral aneurysm: Signs of decreased distal arterial blood flow occur. See the indicators discussed under "Atherosclerotic Arterial Occlusive Disease." **Acute indicators (rupture or dissection):** Sudden onset of severe pain, often described as tearing or ripping; pallor; diaphoresis; and sudden loss of consciousness.

Pain with aneurysm at ascending aorta: Nonradiating, central chest pain.
Pain with aneurysm at distal aorta: Radiation to back, abdomen, and legs.
Physical assessment: Decreased BP and peripheral pulses, tachycardia, cyanosis, and cool, clammy skin. Patient may have pulsating abdominal mass or systolic bruit over the abdomen (abdominal aneurysm) or a diastolic murmur (thoracic aneurysm).

DIAGNOSTIC TESTS

Chest x-ray: May reveal the outline of an aneurysm, especially if there is calcification.
Aortography: Uses contrast dye to locate the lesion and identify its size as well as the condition of the proximal and distal vessels.
Ultrasound: May assist in diagnosis when x-ray and physical examination are inconclusive. The sound waves may help determine the size, shape, and location of the aneurysm.
Digital subtraction angiography (DSA): Confirms diagnosis via CT, which visualizes the arteries radiographically.
ECG: May help differentiate the pain of thoracic aneurysm from that of MI.
Transesophageal echocardiography: Provides clearer ultrasonic images of the heart by avoiding interposition of subcutaneous tissues, bony thorax, and lungs. A high-frequency transducer on an endoscope is placed in the esophagus behind the heart or advanced to the stomach to allow an inferior view of the heart to identify any associated aneurysms.
CT scan: Determines the site of the intimal tear and size of the aneurysm.
Arteriography: Important before surgery to identify proximal and distal blood vessels.

COLLABORATIVE MANAGEMENT

Decrease BP: Using antihypertensive agents, such as atenolol or hydralazine.
Decrease aortic pulsatile flow: Using medications that decrease myocardial contractility, such as propranolol.
Analgesics: For pain relief.
Surgical interventions: Indicated if the aneurysm is symptomatic, increasing in size over time, larger than 4 cm in diameter; if peripheral embolization has occurred; if there is rupture (a surgical emergency); or if a stable aneurysm suddenly becomes tender or causes severe pain. The most common procedure is reconstructive and involves resection of the aneurysm and restoration of vascular flow with an autogenous graft, such as the patient's saphenous vein or a synthetic graft.

NURSING DIAGNOSES AND INTERVENTIONS

Altered peripheral tissue perfusion (or risk of same) related to interrupted arterial flow secondary to postoperative embolization
Desired outcome: Patient has adequate peripheral perfusion as evidenced by peripheral pulse amplitude >2+ on a 0-4+ scale, brisk capillary refill (<2 sec), and baseline extremity sensation, motor function, color, and temperature.

- Assess peripheral pulses at least hourly, and report decreases in amplitude or absence of a pulse.
- Assess peripheral sensation with the vital signs, especially two-point discrimination and paresthesias. Instruct patient to report impaired sensation promptly to staff members. Report significant findings to the health care provider.

- Report to health care provider any changes in color, capillary refill, temperature, and motor function of the extremities.
- Maintain patient on bedrest until otherwise directed.
- Keep patient flat to maintain graft patency and ensure healing with decreased risk of embolization.
- For further interventions, see Appendix One, "Caring for Preoperative and Postoperative Patients," **Risk for fluid volume deficit:** Postoperative bleeding/hemorrhage, p. 729.

NIC: Circulatory Care; Embolus Care: Peripheral; Peripheral Sensation Management; Positioning; Surveillance

PATIENT-FAMILY TEACHING AND DISCHARGE PLANNING

When providing patient-family teaching, focus on sensory information; avoid giving excessive information; and initiate a visiting nurse referral for necessary follow-up teaching. Consider including verbal and written information about the following:

- Importance of regular medical follow-up to ensure graft patency and prompt identification of the development of a new aneurysm.
- Prevention of recurrence of aneurysm by avoiding factors that accelerate atherosclerosis, such as cigarette smoking, obesity, and hypertension.
- Necessity of a regularly scheduled exercise program that alternates exercise with rest.
- Indicators of wound infection and thrombus or embolus formation, and the need to report them promptly to health care provider should they occur.
- Medications, including drug name, purpose, dosage, schedule, precautions, drug/drug and food/drug interactions, and potential side effects.
- Phone number of nurse available to discuss concerns and questions or clarify unclear instructions.
- Importance of follow-up visits with health care provider; confirm date and time of next appointment.
- Potential for aneurysm rupture if surgery is not immediately planned.
- Symptoms of rupture, including sudden onset of severe pain, often described as tearing or ripping; pallor; diaphoresis; and sudden loss of consciousness.
- Importance of seeking immediate medical attention should any signs and symptoms of rupture occur. Provide numbers of emergency services in the area.
- Potential need for ultrasound for other family members to rule out aneurysm.

Arterial embolism

An embolus is a fragment of a thrombus, globule of fat, clump of tissue, fragment of an atherosclerotic lesion, bacteria, or a bubble of air that moves in the circulation, lodges in a vessel, and ultimately obstructs flow.

Emboli can be venous (see "Venous Thrombosis/Thrombophlebitis," p. 125) or arterial. An arterial embolism most commonly arises from thrombi that develop in the chambers of the heart secondary to valvular heart disease, atrial fibrillation (a dysrhythmia with ineffective atrial contraction), MI, acute or chronic heart failure, or vascular injury or disease. Emboli also can arise from atherosclerotic plaque lesions in any vessel. The clinical course after embolism depends on the size of the embolus, the vessel(s) affected, the degree of obstruction, and whether distal tissue is involved. Also see "Pulmonary Embolus," p. 14.

ASSESSMENT

Signs and symptoms: Sudden onset of severe pain and a gradual decrease in sensory and motor functioning. Changes in sensory function usually precede other indicators of ischemia, especially loss of two-point discrimination and paresthesias. Later findings include the six *P*s of arterial occlusion: pain, pulselessness, pallor, polar [coolness], paresthesia, and paralysis as early as 12-18 hr after occlusion.

Physical assessment: Possible presence of a darkened or mottled extremity; diminished or absent pulse(s). Necrosis or gangrene can occur if there is total occlusion and absence of collateral flow.

History of: Vascular injury or surgery, infection such as cellulitis, valvular heart disease, cardiac dysrhythmias.

DIAGNOSTIC TESTS

Ultrasonic Doppler flow studies: Will reveal decreased or absent arterial blood flow distal to the embolus.

Angiography: Provides visualization of the embolus in the arterial tree and collateral circulation.

COLLABORATIVE MANAGEMENT

Bedrest: To prevent further embolization.

Anticoagulation with oral anticoagulant or heparin via continuous IV drip: To prevent proximal and distal embolization.

Thrombolytic drugs (e.g., urokinase or streptokinase):   To speed up the process of clot lysis; used in individuals who are poor surgical risks or as an alternative to surgical procedures.

Analgesics: To relieve pain caused by distal vasospasm and ischemia.

Embolectomy: Surgical removal of the embolus. Embolectomy is most commonly done by performing a proximal arteriotomy (femoral or brachial). Through the arterial opening a special catheter with a balloon at the tip (Fogarty catheter) is advanced to the site of the embolus (may be facilitated with fluoroscope). The catheter is slid past the embolus, and its balloon is inflated; then the catheter is withdrawn, pulling the embolus and any associated thrombus out of the artery.

NURSING DIAGNOSES AND INTERVENTIONS

Altered peripheral tissue perfusion related to interrupted arterial flow secondary to embolization (preoperative period)

Desired outcome: Optimally, patient's peripheral perfusion is adequate as evidenced by peripheral pulse amplitude >2+ on a 0-4+ scale and normal extremity color, capillary refill, temperature, sensation, and motor function.

- Maintain patient on bedrest to prevent further embolization.
- Monitor peripheral circulation. Keep extremities warm (room temperature). Advise patient to avoid chilling by wearing socks or slippers.
- Protect extremities from trauma. Provide a foot cradle or foam protectors to keep the weight of sheets and blankets off tissue that has decreased circulation.
- If prescribed, keep the lower extremities slightly dependent (but not >45 degrees) to promote circulation.
- Teach patient and significant other signs and symptoms of embolization that necessitate immediate medical attention: sudden onset of severe pain and a gradual decrease in sensory and motor functioning; presence of tingling, numbness, coolness, and cyanosis.

NIC: Circulatory Care; Embolus Care: Peripheral; Peripheral Sensation Management; Positioning; Surveillance; Teaching: Individual

---

See Also: "Pulmonary Embolus" for **Altered protection** related to risk of prolonged bleeding or hemorrhage secondary to anticoagulation therapy, p. 18; Appendix One, "Caring for Preoperative and Postoperative Patients," p. 717, as appropriate.

PATIENT-FAMILY TEACHING AND DISCHARGE PLANNING

When providing patient-family teaching, focus on sensory information; avoid giving excessive information; and initiate a visiting nurse referral for necessary follow-up teaching. Consider including verbal and written information about the following:

- Prescribed exercise plan to prevent peripheral stasis of the blood.
- Signs and symptoms that necessitate immediate medical attention: extremity pain, changes in sensation, coolness, pallor, cyanosis.
- Indicators of wound infection, if surgery was performed.
- Oral anticoagulant therapy: need for regular medical checkups and immediate reporting of bleeding gums, epistaxis, ecchymosis, hemoptysis, hematemesis, hematochezia, melena, menometrorrhagia, or hematuria; administration at the same time every day; not changing regular dietary habits (e.g., becoming a vegetarian without first consulting health care provider or nurse; many green, leafy vegetables are high in vitamin K, which reverses the effect of warfarin; vegetarian diets may necessitate an increase in warfarin dosage to achieve therapeutic anticoagulation); importance of consulting health care provider before taking any over-the-counter (OTC) medications, especially aspirin products, which affect platelet aggregation and potentiate the anticoagulant effect of warfarin.
- Other medications, including drug name, purpose, dosage, schedule, precautions, drug/drug and food/drug interactions, and potential side effects.
- Risk factor modification, such as smoking cessation, control of hypertension, and dietary modifications to decrease the potential for atherosclerosis and acute arterial occlusion.

Venous thrombosis/Thrombophlebitis

Although venous thrombosis and thrombophlebitis are different disorders, clinically they are referred to as a single entity, and the terms are used interchangeably to refer to the development of a venous thrombus or thrombi, with associated inflammation. Disturbances in the venous system can have a variety of causes and precipitating factors, including stasis of blood, hemoconcentration, venous trauma, inflammation, or altered coagulation. Venous stasis can occur with heart failure, shock states, immobility from prolonged bedrest, or structural disorders of the veins or as a side effect of anesthesia. Hemoconcentration most commonly occurs with dehydration or inadequate fluid resuscitation after surgery. Vessel trauma can result from chemical irritation caused by IV solutions, direct trauma, or positioning. Altered coagulation states usually are related to liver disease or withdrawal from anticoagulants. Venous thrombosis and thrombophlebitis most often occur in the lower extremities, and the most serious complication is embolization. Emboli will most commonly travel through the right side of the heart to the lungs.

ASSESSMENT

Signs and symptoms: Assessments may be divided into those in the area of the thrombus (associated with inflammation) and those distal to the clot (associated with venous congestion). Over the site of thrombus the assessments include pain, tenderness, erythema, local warmth, and increased limb circumference. Distal to the area of thrombus the extremity will be cool, pale or cyanotic, and edematous and display prominent superficial veins. Additional findings include unilateral leg swelling, fever, and tachycardia. Sometimes the condition is clinically "silent," and the presenting sign is a pulmonary embolus (PE). See "Pulmonary Embolus," p. 14.

Physical assessment: A knot or bump occasionally can be felt on palpation. If patient is asymptomatic for deep vein thrombosis (DVT), assess for a positive

Homans' sign: flex the knee 30 degrees, and dorsiflex the foot. Pain elicited with the dorsiflexion may be a sign of DVT.

> **Caution:**   Because of the risk of embolization, never test for a positive Homans' sign in the presence of clinical indicators of venous thrombosis or thrombophlebitis.

Risk factors: Prolonged bedrest and immobility, leg trauma, recent surgery, use of oral contraceptives, obesity, varicose veins.

DIAGNOSTIC TESTS

Contrast phlebography (venography):   A contrast dye is injected into the venous system that is to be studied, allowing visualization of the veins by showing filling or absence of filling.

Doppler ultrasound: Identifies changes in blood flow secondary to presence of a thrombus.

Duplex imaging: Use of ultrasound to assess veins for flow and pressure.

α-fibrinogen injection test: Useful screening device for early detection of thrombosis because the isotope identifies clots that are forming.

Impedance plethysmography: Estimates blood flow using measures of resistance and normal changes that occur during pulsatile blood flow.

Elevated erythrocyte sedimentation rate (ESR):   Normal ESR (Westergren method) in males younger than 50 yr is 0-15 mm/hr and older than 50 yr is 0-20 mm/hr; in females younger than 50 yr it is 0-20 mm/hr and older than 50 yr is 0-30 mm/hr.

COLLABORATIVE MANAGEMENT

Prevention: Involves identifying patients at risk, increasing fluid intake to at least 2-3 L/day, promoting leg exercises to prevent stasis, prescribing elastic stockings and early ambulation, administering enoxaparin (Lovenox) or minidoses of heparin to prevent clot formation, and using sequential compression devices or pneumatic foot compression devices.

Therapeutic anticoagulation: Prevents development of a PE. Heparin is used during the acute phase, and long-term warfarin therapy is used after the acute phase.

Thrombolytic therapy: Instituted to lyse and digest the clot. Streptokinase or urokinase may be used.

Bedrest: During the acute phase, with support hose and leg elevation to decrease venous stasis.

Analgesics for pain: Usually acetaminophen.

Exercise regimen: Walking or leg exercises after the acute phase.

Warm moist packs: To reduce discomfort and pain.

Thrombectomy: Necessary when the danger of PE is extreme, the patient cannot tolerate anticoagulation, or extremity damage from the absence of venous drainage is imminent.

NURSING DIAGNOSES AND INTERVENTIONS

Altered peripheral and cardiopulmonary tissue perfusion (or risk of same) related to interrupted blood flow secondary to embolization from thrombus formation

Desired outcome: Patient has adequate peripheral and cardiopulmonary perfusion as evidenced by normal extremity color, temperature, and sensation; RR 12-20 breaths/min with normal depth and pattern (eupnea); HR ≤100 bpm; BP within 20 mm Hg of baseline BP; O$_2$ saturation ≥92%; and normal breath sounds.

• Be alert to and promptly report early indicators of peripheral thrombus formation: pain, erythema, increased limb girth, local warmth, distal

pale skin, edema, positive Homans' sign, and venous dilation. If indicators appear, maintain patient on bedrest and notify health care provider promptly.
- Monitor for and immediately report signs of PE: sudden onset of chest pain, dyspnea, tachypnea, tachycardia, hypotension, hemoptysis, shallow respirations, crackles (rales), O_2 saturation <92%, decreased breath sounds, and diaphoresis. Should they occur, prompt medical attention is crucial.
- Administer anticoagulants as prescribed. Double-check drip rates and doses with a colleague.
- Minimize the risk of PE by keeping patient on bedrest, providing ROM exercises, and applying support hose, sequential compression devices, or pneumatic foot compression devices as prescribed.

NIC: Bed Rest Care; Circulatory Care; Embolus Precautions; Exercise Therapy: Joint Mobility; Positioning; Surveillance

Pain related to inflammatory process caused by thrombus formation
Desired outcomes: Within 1 hr of intervention, patient's subjective perception of pain decreases, as documented by a pain scale. Objective indicators, such as grimacing, are absent.
- Monitor patient for the presence of pain. Document the degree of pain, using a pain scale from 0 (no pain) to 10 (worst pain). Administer analgesics as prescribed, and document relief obtained using the pain scale.
- Ensure that the patient maintains bedrest during the acute phase to minimize painful engorgement and the potential for embolization.
- If prescribed, apply warm, moist packs. Be sure that the packs are warm (but not extremely so) and not allowed to cool. If appropriate, use a Kock-Mason dressing (warm towel covered by plastic wrap and a K-pad) to provide continuous moist heat.
- To promote venous drainage and reduce engorgement, keep the legs elevated above heart level (but not >45 degrees).

NIC: Heat/Cold Application; Pain Management; Positioning; Teaching: Disease Process

Altered peripheral tissue perfusion (or risk of same) related to interrupted venous flow secondary to venous engorgement or edema
Desired outcome: Patient has adequate peripheral perfusion as evidenced by absence of discomfort and normal extremity temperature, color, sensation, and motor function.
- Assess for signs of inadequate peripheral perfusion, such as pain and changes in skin temperature, color, and motor or sensory function. Be alert to venous engorgement (prominence) in the lower extremities.
- Elevate patient's legs above heart level (but not >45 degrees) to promote venous drainage.
- As prescribed for patients without evidence of thrombus formation, apply antiembolic hose, which compress superficial veins to increase blood flow to the deeper veins. Remove the stockings for approximately 15 min q8hr. Inspect the skin for evidence of irritation.
- Apply sequential compression devices or pneumatic foot compression devices as prescribed. Remove these devices for 15 min q8hr, and inspect underlying skin for irritation. To reduce trapping heat and moisture, place a cloth sleeve (stockinette) beneath the plastic device.
- Encourage patient to perform ankle circling and active or assisted ROM exercises of the lower extremities to prevent venous stasis. Perform passive ROM exercises if patient cannot.

> **Caution:** If there are any signs of acute thrombus formation, such as calf hardness or tenderness, the exercises are contraindicated because of the risk of embolization. Notify health care provider.

- Encourage deep breathing, which creates increased negative pressure in the lungs and thorax, to assist in the emptying of large veins.
- Arterial circulation usually will not be impaired unless there is arterial disease or severe edema compressing arterial flow. Assess pulses regularly, however, to confirm the presence of good arterial flow.

NIC: Exercise Promotion; Positioning; Skin Surveillance; Teaching: Prescribed Activity/Exercise

Knowledge deficit: Disease process with venous thrombosis/thrombophlebitis and treatment/management measures after hospital discharge
Desired outcome: Before hospital discharge, patient verbalizes knowledge of the disease process and treatment/management measures that are to occur after hospital discharge.

- Discuss the process of venous thrombosis/thrombophlebitis and ways to prevent thrombosis and discomfort, such as avoiding restrictive clothing, avoiding prolonged periods of standing, and elevating legs above heart level when sitting.
- Teach patient the signs of venous stasis ulcers, such as redness and skin breakdown. Stress the importance of avoiding trauma to the extremities and keeping the skin clean and dry.
- Instruct the patient to inspect both feet each day for any open wounds or bruises. If necessary, suggest the patient use a long-handled mirror to see the bottoms of the feet. Advise the patient to report any open areas to the health care provider.
- Discuss the prescribed exercise program. Walking usually is considered the best exercise.
- Teach patient how to wear antiembolic hose if prescribed. The hose must fit properly without wrinkling and should be snug over the feet and progressively less snug as they reach the knee or thigh.
- Describe indicators that necessitate medical attention: persistent redness, swelling, tenderness, weak or absent pulses, and ulcerations in the extremities.

NIC: Learning Facilitation; Learning Readiness Enhancement; Self-Care Assistance: Bathing/Hygiene; Skin Surveillance; Teaching: Disease Process; Teaching: Psychomotor Skill

> **See Also:** "Pulmonary Embolus" for **Altered protection** related to prolonged bleeding or hemorrhage secondary to anticoagulation therapy, p. 18.

PATIENT-FAMILY TEACHING AND DISCHARGE PLANNING
- See **Knowledge deficit**, above, for topics to discuss (both verbally and through written information) with the patient and significant other.
- If the patient is discharged from the hospital on warfarin therapy, provide information about the following:
  —As directed, see health care provider for scheduled prothrombin time (PT) checks.
  —Take warfarin at same time each day; do not skip days unless directed to by the health care provider.
  —Wear a Medic-Alert bracelet.

—Avoid alcohol consumption and changes in diet (e.g., changing to a vegetarian diet), both of which can alter the body's response to warfarin.
—When making appointments with other health care providers and dentists, inform them that warfarin is being taken.
—Be alert to indicators that necessitate immediate medical attention: hematuria, hematemesis, menometrorrhagia, hematochezia, melena, epistaxis, bleeding gums, ecchymosis, hemoptysis, dizziness, and weakness.
—Avoid taking over-the-counter (OTC) medications (e.g., aspirin, which also prolongs coagulation time) without consulting health care provider or nurse.

Selected Bibliography

Ahrens SG: Managing heart failure: a blueprint for success, *Nursing* 25(12): 26-32, 1995.

Antman EM: Hirudin in acute myocardial infarction, *Circulation* 94(5):911-918, 1996.

Baas LS: Cardiovascular dysfunctions. In Swearingen PL, Keen JH, editors: *Manual of critical care: applying nursing diagnoses to adult critical illness,* ed 3, St Louis, 1995, Mosby.

Bower J: New therapy for ventricular arrhythmias, *AORN J* 59(5):985-996, 1994.

Burns WB, Davidson CJ: Thrombolysis or primary angioplasty? *Emerg Med Clin North Am* 28(10):18-33, 1995.

Chyun D: Nursing management of coronary heart disease in women: using research findings, *Crit Care Nurs* 17(2):10-14, 1997.

Dracup K et al: Rethinking heart failure, *Am J Nurs* 95(7):22-28, 1995.

Edelman ER, Rogers C: Hoop dreams, stents without restenosis, *Circulation* 94(6):1199-1202, 1996.

English MA: Advanced concepts in heart failure, *Crit Care Q* 18(1):1-84, 1995.

Fellows E: Abdominal-aortic aneurysm: warning flags to watch for, *Am J Nurs* 95(5):26-33, 1995.

Gossage JR: Acute myocardial infarction: reperfusion strategies, *Cardiopul Crit Care J* 106(6):1851-1863, 1994.

Hayes DD: Understanding coronary arthrectomy, *Am J Nurs* 96(12): 38-45, 1996.

Holcomb S: Sotalol, new weapon against ventricular arrhythmias, *Nursing* 25(12):240, 1995.

Horne MM, Heitz UE, Swearingen PL, editors: *Pocket guide to fluid, electrolyte, and acid-base balance,* ed 3, St Louis, 1997, Mosby.

Interqual: *The ISD-A review system with adult ISD criteria,* Northhampton, NH, and Marlboro, Mass, August 1992, Interqual.

Jackimczyk KC, Moore GP: Differential diagnosis of chest pain. I. Noncardiac causes, *Emerg Med* 28(9):14-30, 1995.

Jackimczyk KC, Moore GP: Differential diagnosis of chest pain. II. Diagnosing myocardial infarction, *Emerg Med* 28(9):50-60, 1995.

Jensen L, King KM: Women and heart disease: the issues, *Crit Care Nurs* 17(2):45-53, 1997.

Kim MJ et al: *Pocket guide to nursing diagnoses,* ed 7, St Louis, 1997, Mosby.

Lazzara D, Sellegren C: Chest pain emergencies: making the right call when the pressure is on, *Nursing* 26(11):42-53, 1996.

Lewandowski D, Jacobson C: AV blocks, are you up to date? *Am J Nurs* 95(12):26-33, 1995.

Mayer DM, Docktor WJ: Abciximab, a novel platelet-blocking drug: pharmacology and nursing implications, *Crit Care Nurs* 18(2):29-37, 1998.

McCloskey J, Bulechek G, editors: *Nursing Interventions Classification (NIC),* ed 2, St Louis, 1996, Mosby.

Merva JA: Providing electrical support for the heart: temporary pacemakers, *RN* 55(5):28-33, 1992.

Moreau D, editor: *Nursing 97 drug handbook*, Springhouse, Pa, 1997, Springhouse Co.

Moser DK: Correcting misconceptions about women and heart disease, *Am J Nurs* 97(4):26-33, 1997.

O'Donnell LO: Complications of MI: beyond the acute phase, *Am J Nurs* 96(9):25-31, 1996.

Pagana K, Pagana T: *Mosby's diagnostic and laboratory test reference,* ed 3, St Louis, 1996, Mosby.

Possanza CP: What you should know about coronary artery bypass graft surgery, *Nursing* 26(2):48-50, 1996.

Redeker NS, Sadowski AV: Update on cardiovascular drugs and elders, *Am J Nurs* 95(9):34-41, 1995.

Ruppert SD: Advances in transplantation, *Crit Care Nurs* 17(4):1-66, 1995.

Sherman A: Critical care management of the heart failure patient in the home, *Crit Care Nurs Q* 18(1):77-87, 1995.

Steuble BT: Cardiovascular dysfunctions. In Swearingen PL, Keen JH, editors: *Manual of critical care: applying nursing diagnoses to adult critical illness,* ed 3, St Louis, 1995, Mosby.

Steuble BT: Multi-system stressors. In Swearingen PL, Keen JH, editors: *Manual of critical care: applying nursing diagnoses to adult critical illness,* ed 3, St Louis, 1995, Mosby.

Steuble BT: Cardiovascular disorders. In Swearingen PL, editor: *Pocket guide to medical-surgical nursing: diagnoses and interventions,* ed 2, St Louis, 1996, Mosby.

Stimike C: Understanding ultrasound, *Am J Nurs* 96(6):40-44, 1996.

Williamson DJ et al: Acute hemodynamic responses to inhaled nitrous oxide in patients with limited scleroderma and isolated pulmonary hypertension, *Circulation* 94(3):477-481, 1996.

3 RENAL-URINARY DISORDERS

Section One: Renal Disorders

Glomerulonephritis

Glomerulonephritis (GN) is the name of a group of diseases that damage the renal glomeruli. When the glomerulus is injured, protein and RBCs are allowed to enter the renal tubule and be excreted in the urine. GN can be acute or chronic. Most individuals with acute GN improve dramatically within weeks and recover completely within 1 to 2 years, but renal damage continues to progress for those with chronic GN. Chronic GN is one of the most common causes of chronic renal failure. Most forms of GN are the result of immunologic processes (e.g., group A hemolytic streptococcal infection, systemic lupus erythematosus). This process also has been linked to recent use of penicillin or sulfonamide antibiotics. See "Acute Renal Failure," p. 144, and "Chronic Renal Failure," p. 150, as appropriate.

ASSESSMENT
Indicators usually follow the primary infection by about 2 weeks and can range from subtle to blatant, depending on the patient's level of renal function.
Acute indicators: Hematuria, proteinuria, oliguria, dull bilateral flank pain, headache, low-grade fever.
Chronic indicators: Fatigue, lethargy, malaise, anorexia, nausea, nocturia, headache, weakness.
Physical assessment: Presence of edema (peripheral, periorbital, sacral), crackles (rales), elevated BP, pallor, costovertebral angle (CVA) tenderness, oliguria.
History of: Recent URI or other infection; recent use of penicillin or sulfonamide antibiotics; systemic lupus erythematosus or other autoimmune disease; bloody urine (commonly reported as dark or rust-colored).

DIAGNOSTIC TESTS
Urinalysis and 24-hour urinary protein excretion: Hematuria with red cell casts and proteinuria are the cardinal findings. Hyaline and granular casts also may be noted.
BUN and serum creatinine: If elevated, may indicate decreased renal function.
Plasma complement, antinuclear antibody titer, antistreptolysin O titer, throat and blood cultures, hepatitis B antigen, and immunoelectrophoresis of the serum and urine: Optional tests to determine cause of GN.
Renal biopsy: Indicated when tissue diagnosis is needed to direct therapy or provide prognostic data. Usually a percutaneous (closed) renal biopsy is performed. Postbiopsy care includes keeping the patient supine with a rolled towel under the biopsy site (to apply direct pressure) for 12 hr and frequent

T A B L E   3 - 1   Diuretics

Generic name	Common brand names	Usual dosage/24 hr (mg)
Acetazolamide	Diamox	250-375 (qod)
Amiloride HCl*	Midamor	5-10
Chlorothiazide sodium	Diuril	250-1000
Chlorthalidone	Hygroton	25-100
Ethacrynic acid	Edecrin	25-200
Furosemide	Lasix	20-160
Hydrochlorothiazide	Esidrix	25-100
Metolazone	Zaroxolyn, Diulo	2.5-10
Spironolactone*	Aldactone	25-200
Torsemide	Demadox	5-200
Triamterene*	Dyrenium	50-300

*Although most diuretics can cause hypokalemia, these diuretics may cause hyperkalemia. For this reason they are often used in combination with thiazide diuretics.

monitoring of VS (q15min initially). Two possible complications of renal biopsy are bleeding and infection. Severe pain, hypotension, persistent gross hematuria, or fever should be reported to the health care provider immediately. Samples of urine from the first several voidings may be saved to assess for hematuria.

WBC count: To identify excessive immunosuppression in patients treated with cytotoxic agents.

COLLABORATIVE MANAGEMENT

Bedrest: For patients with acute GN. Limited activity may be necessary for weeks to months.

Pharmacotherapy

Corticosteroids and cytotoxic agents: To suppress the immune system and reduce antibody formation.

Anticoagulants: To reduce nonimmunologic mediators of glomerular damage.

Antibiotics: If causative factor is bacterial.

Diuretics: To remove excess fluid (Table 3-1).

Antihypertensives: To control BP.

Plasmapheresis: To remove immune complexes or antiglomerular basement antibodies. It is used only in patients with Goodpasture's syndrome and rapidly progressing GN.

Diet: Restriction of sodium (Na^+) (Table 3-2) and fluids if edema or hypertension is present. A high-carbohydrate diet is encouraged to maintain nutrition and prevent tissue catabolism that would further contribute to elevated BUN and creatinine. If renal function is markedly decreased, protein and phosphorus may be limited to prevent retention of excess nitrogenous wastes and hyperphosphatemia.

Peritoneal dialysis or hemodialysis: To maintain homeostasis or prevent uremic complications if renal function is markedly decreased (see "Renal Dialysis," p. 155).

NURSING DIAGNOSES AND INTERVENTIONS

Fluid volume excess related to compromised regulatory mechanisms secondary to decreased renal function

TABLE 3-2 Foods High in Sodium Content

Bouillon
Celery
Cheeses
Dried fruits
Frozen, canned, or packaged foods
Monosodium glutamate (MSG)
Mustard
Olives
Pickles
Preserved meat
Salad dressings and prepared sauces
Sauerkraut
Snack foods (e.g., crackers, chips, pretzels)
Soy sauce

Desired outcomes: With successful therapy, patient is normovolemic as evidenced by urine output of at least 30-60 ml/hr (or patient's normal range), stable weight, edema ≤1+ on a 0-4+ scale, and subjective statement that thirst is controlled. BP and HR are within patient's normal range, CVP is 5-12 cm H_2O, and RR is 12-20 breaths/min with normal depth and pattern (eupnea). Within the 24-hr period before hospital discharge, patient lists foods that are high in Na^+ and plans a 3-day menu that excludes foods high in Na^+.

- Monitor I&O closely. Notify health care provider about sudden changes in output.
- Monitor weight daily. Weigh patient at the same time each day, using the same scale and with the patient wearing the same amount of clothing. Report unusual or steady gains or losses (e.g., 0.5-1 kg/day).
- Observe for indicators of fluid overload: edema, hypertension, crackles (rales), tachycardia, lethargy, distended neck veins, SOB, and increased CVP. **Note:** Not all patients with edema are fluid-overloaded. Edema can occur also because of lowered serum colloidal osmotic pressure resulting from decreased serum albumin secondary to urinary losses.
- Offer ice chips or popsicles to minimize thirst in the fluid-restricted patient; be sure to record the amount on the intake record. Frequent mouth care also may help minimize thirst.
- Provide patient with data about foods high in Na^+ content (see Table 3-2), which should be avoided. Mustard and soy sauce, which traditionally are high in Na^+ content, are available in low-salt versions. Many over-the-counter preparations are high in Na^+ (e.g., mouthwashes, antacids). Advise patient and significant other to read all labels carefully.

You may also wish to refer to the following intervenitons from the Nursing Interventions Classification (NIC):

NIC: Electrolyte Management: Hypernatremia; Fluid/Electrolyte Management; Fluid Management; Vital Signs Monitoring

Knowledge deficit: Signs and symptoms of fluid and electrolyte imbalance (caused by decreased renal function or diuretic therapy)
Desired outcomes: Within 36 hr of admission, patient verbalizes knowledge about the signs and symptoms of fluid and electrolyte imbalance and the

importance of reporting them promptly to health care provider or staff if they occur.
- Alert patient and significant others to signs and symptoms of the following:
    —*Hypokalemia*: Muscle weakness, lethargy, dysrhythmias, nausea, and vomiting
    —*Hyperkalemia*: Abdominal cramping, diarrhea, irritability, and muscle weakness (if severe)
    —*Hypocalcemia:* Twitching, numbness and tingling of fingers and circumoral region, and muscle cramps
    —*Hyperphosphatemia:* Precipitation of calcium phosphate in the soft tissue (e.g., cornea, lungs, kidneys, gastric mucosa, heart, blood vessels) and periarticular region of the large joints (e.g., hips, shoulders, elbows)
    —*Uremia:* Anorexia, nausea, metallic taste in the mouth, irritability, confusion, lethargy, restlessness, and pruritus (itching)
- Instruct patient to report the above signs and symptoms to health care provider or staff promptly should they occur.

NIC: Discharge Planning; Teaching: Individual; Teaching: Disease Process; Teaching: Prescribed Medication; Teaching: Procedure/Treatment

Knowledge deficit: Side effects of corticosteroids and cytotoxic agents
Desired outcome: Within the 24-hr period before hospital discharge, patient verbalizes knowledge of the side effects of corticosteroids and cytotoxic agents and the importance of reporting them promptly to staff or health care provider should they occur.
- Corticosteroids and cytotoxic agents are potent medications with potentially serious side effects. They are used in GN to suppress the immune system and reduce antibody formation. Alert patient who is taking corticosteroids to the potential for the following, depending on dose and duration of therapy: poor resistance to infection, poor wound healing, increasing BP, mental changes, hyperglycemia, capillary fragility, and GI bleeding. Stress the importance of avoiding individuals known to have infections. If the patient has been taking corticosteroid therapy over a prolonged period, Na^+ and water retention, hypokalemia, and indicators similar to Cushing's syndrome can occur, as manifested by edema, buffalo hump, hirsutism, moon face, skin striae and thinning, weight gain, peptic ulcer, headache, osteoporosis, aseptic necrosis, nervousness, insomnia, and metabolic acidosis, in addition to the initial indicators described previously.
- If patient has been taking corticosteroids for 1 week or longer, caution against abrupt withdrawal, which can result in adrenal insufficiency. Therapy must be withdrawn with gradual reductions in dosage. Signs and symptoms that can occur with abrupt withdrawal include fever, malaise, fatigue, anorexia, orthostatic hypotension, dyspnea, muscle and joint pain, and hypoglycemia.
- Alert patient taking cytotoxic agents about the potential for the following: infection, cystitis with hematuria, and abnormal hair loss. See Appendix One, "Caring for Patients With Cancer and other Life-disrupting Illnesses," p.747, for additional information about cytotoxic agents. Resources include:

The American Cancer Society
1599 Clifton Road NE
Atlanta, GA 30329   (800) ACS-2345
WWW address: *http://www.cancer.org*

National Cancer Institute Information Service (CIS)
Bldg. 31, Room 10A16
9000 Rockville Pike
Bethesda, MD 20892   (800) 422-6237
WWW address: *http://www.meds.com/pdq/cancerlinks.html*

- Stress the importance of notifying health care provider or staff promptly if any of these symptoms occur.

◎ NIC: Discharge Planning; Teaching: Disease Process; Teaching: Individual; Teaching: Prescribed Medication; Teaching: Procedure/Treatment

Risk for infection with risk factors related to immunosuppression with corticosteroid therapy, immobility, invasive techniques, and impaired skin integrity
Desired outcomes: Patient is free of infection as evidenced by normothermia and absence of adventitious breath sounds. Respiratory secretions are of normal color, consistency, and quantity.

- Because the respiratory system is a common site for infection in the immunocompromised patient, be alert to indications of infection, such as increased body temperature, adventitious breath sounds, and increased, thickened, or colored airway secretions. If secretions are noted, encourage frequent deep breathing or coughing or provide suctioning at frequent intervals. **Note:** Individuals who are uremic and older adults tend to run subnormal temperatures, so even slight fevers can be significant. Remember that steroids may mask the signs and symptoms of infection.
- Use meticulous sterile technique when performing invasive procedures or manipulating urinary catheters, peripheral IV lines, or central venous catheters.
- Provide oral hygiene and skin care at frequent intervals. Edema, bedrest, and uremia all increase the potential for skin breakdown, which further increases the risk of infection.
- Teach patient the necessity of avoiding infections and seeking treatment promptly if infections occur after hospital discharge. Teach the signs and symptoms of URI, otitis media, UTI, and impetigo. (See **Risk for infection** in "Care of the Renal Transplant Recipient," p. 162.)

◎ NIC: Cough Enhancement; Environmental Management; Infection Protection; Medication Management; Positioning; Respiratory Monitoring; Surveillance; Teaching: Disease Process; Vital Signs Monitoring; Wound Care

---

See Also: "Pulmonary Embolus" for **Altered protection** related to risk of prolonged bleeding or hemorrhage secondary to anticoagulation therapy, p.18; **Activity intolerance** related to deconditioned status and other nursing diagnoses and interventions in Appendix One, "Caring for Patients on Prolonged Bedrest," p. 738.

PATIENT-FAMILY TEACHING AND DISCHARGE PLANNING

When providing patient-family teaching, focus on sensory information; avoid giving excessive information; and initiate a visiting nurse referral for necessary follow-up teaching. Consider including verbal and written information about the following:

- Medications, including drug name, purpose, dosage, schedule, drug/drug and food/drug interactions, precautions, and potential side effects.
- Diet, including fact sheet listing foods that should be avoided or limited. Inform patient that diet and fluid restrictions may be altered as renal function changes. Provide sample menus with examples of how dietary restrictions may be incorporated into daily meals.
- Indicators that require medical attention: irregular pulse, fever, unusual SOB or edema, sudden change in urine output, or unusual weakness.
- Technique for measuring temperature and pulse and recording I&O.
- Necessity for continued medical evaluation; confirm date and time of next health care provider appointment, if known.

- Importance of adjusting and gradually increasing activities to avoid fatigue.
- Necessity of avoiding infections and seeking treatment promptly should they occur. Teach the signs and symptoms of URI, otitis media, UTI, and impetigo. (See **Risk for infection** in "Care of the Renal Transplant Recipient," p. 162.)
- Phone numbers to call should questions or concerns arise about therapy or this condition after discharge. Additional general information can be obtained by contacting:

National Kidney and Urologic Diseases Information Clearinghouse
3 Information Way
Bethesda, MD 20892-3580 (301) 907-8906 FAX

National Kidney Foundation
30 E. 33rd Street, 11th Floor
New York, NY 10016   (800) 622-9010; (212) 689-9261 FAX
WWW address: *http://www.nephron.com/NKF.html*

In addition
- Coordinate family and social service support for the patient who must continue bedrest or restrict activity at home. Consider such factors as meals, loss of income, housework, childcare, and transportation.

Acute pyelonephritis

Acute pyelonephritis is an infection of the renal parenchyma and pelvis, which usually occurs secondary to an ascending UTI. UTIs typically result from anatomic or functional obstruction to urine flow (e.g., from prostatic hypertrophy, renal calculi, instrumentation such as catheterization or cystoscopy). Pathogenic organisms can ascend from the urinary bladder to the kidney via an incompetent ureterovesical junction. Hematogenous infection also can occur in acute pyelonephritis when bacteria reach the kidney via the bloodstream.

The incidence of acute pyelonephritis increases with advancing age. In the absence of anatomic obstruction or instrumentation, acute pyelonephritis is almost exclusively a disease of females. The infecting organism may be a type of fecal flora, such as *Escherichia* or *Klebsiella*, or normal flora from the periurethral skin (e.g., *Staphylococcus saprophyticus*). Recurrent infections are common; chronic renal failure is a rare complication.

ASSESSMENT

Signs and symptoms: Fever, chills, flank pain (may be unilateral or bilateral), nausea, vomiting, malaise, frequency and urgency of urination, dysuria, cloudy and foul-smelling urine, and nocturia. **Note:** These indicators can be nonspecific, especially in older persons. Severe infection may produce peripheral vasoconstriction, hypotension, and acute renal failure.
Physical assessment: Tender, enlarged kidneys; abdominal rigidity; and CVA tenderness.
History of: UTI or obstruction; recent urologic procedure; pregnancy.

DIAGNOSTIC TESTS

Unless an anatomic or preexisting renal disease is present, renal function should remain normal.
Urine culture: Should be positive for the causative organism. **Note:** Asymptomatic bacteriuria is common in older persons.
Urinalysis: Will reveal presence of WBCs, WBC casts, RBCs, and bacteria.

> **Caution:** All urine samples should be sent to the laboratory immediately after they are obtained, or they should be refrigerated if this is not possible. Urine left at room temperature has greater potential for bacterial growth, turbidity, and alkalinity, any of which can distort the test results. Urine cultures should *not* be refrigerated.

Blood culture: Positive for the causative organism in hematogenous infection. It is obtained from patients who appear septic or are hypotensive.
CBC: Demonstrates leukocytosis.
Radiographic studies
KUB, an abdominal flat plate film: May demonstrate renal or ureteral calculi.
Chest x-ray: May show pleural effusion.
IVP or retrograde pyelogram: May be performed if there are recurrent episodes or if obstruction is suspected.

COLLABORATIVE MANAGEMENT

Fluids: Oral fluids are encouraged or IV fluids are administered to replace losses and ensure adequate urinary output.
Pharmacotherapy
Antibiotics: For the infection; initially parenteral, then oral. Low-dose antimicrobial prophylaxis may be indicated for women with recurrent UTI.
ASA or acetaminophen: To control the fever and treat the discomfort.
Surgical intervention: May be necessary if an obstruction is present.

NURSING DIAGNOSES AND INTERVENTIONS

Pain related to dysuria and tissue inflammation secondary to infection
Desired outcomes: Within 1 hr of intervention, patient's subjective perception of discomfort decreases, as documented by a pain scale. Objective indicators, such as grimacing, are absent or diminished.
- Monitor patient for the presence of CVA pain and tenderness, abdominal pain, and dysuria. Devise a pain scale with patient, rating pain from 0 (absent) to 10 (worst pain).
- As appropriate, administer the prescribed analgesics, and document their effectiveness, using the pain scale. Encourage patient to request medication before discomfort becomes severe.
- If it is not contraindicated, increase the patient's fluid intake to help relieve dysuria.
- Notify health care provider about unrelieved or increasing flank pain.
- As appropriate, assist patient with repositioning if it is effective in relieving discomfort.
- Use nonpharmacologic interventions when possible (e.g., relaxation techniques, guided imagery, distraction).

NIC: Analgesic Administration; Coping Enhancement; Distraction; Meditation; Music Therapy; Pain Management; Progressive Muscle Relaxation; Simple Guided Imagery; Simple Relaxation Therapy; Sleep Enhancement

Risk for infection (or its recurrence) with risk factors associated with a chronic disease process
Desired outcomes: Patient is free of infection as evidenced by normothermia; urine clear and of normal odor; HR ≤100 bpm; BP ≥90/60 mm Hg (or within patient's normal range); absence of flank, CVA, low back, buttock, scrotal, or labial pain; and absence of dysuria, urgency, and frequency. Within the 24-hr period before hospital discharge, patient verbalizes knowledge about strategies for preventing recurrent infections and the signs and symptoms of infection and the importance of reporting them promptly if they occur.

- Monitor patient's temperature at least q4hr. Report temperature ≥38° C (100.4° F) to health care provider. Monitor for the presence of flank, CVA, low back, buttock, scrotal, or labial pain; foul-smelling or cloudy urine; malaise; headache; and frequency and urgency of urination. Teach these indicators to the patient, and stress the importance of reporting them promptly to health care provider or staff if they occur.
- Monitor BP, pulse, and indications of peripheral vasoconstriction at least q4hr. The presence of hypotension and tachycardia can be indicative of sepsis and bacteremic shock.
- Administer prescribed antibiotics as scheduled. Draw prescribed antibiotic serum levels at correct times to ensure reliable results. **Note:** Antibiotic serum concentrations are measured at peak (30-60 min after infusion) and trough (30-60 min before the next dose) levels.
- Use urinary catheters only when mandatory. Use sterile technique when inserting, irrigating, or obtaining specimens. Provide perineal care daily. For indwelling catheters, maintain unobstructed flow and always keep the urinary collection container below the level of the patient's bladder to prevent reflux of urine. Tape the catheter to the thigh or abdomen in males to decrease meatal irritation. **Note:** Intermittent catheterization carries less of a risk of UTI than indwelling catheterization.
- Offer cranberry, plum, or prune juices, which leave an acid ash in the urine and inhibit bacteriuria.
- Treat fever with prescribed antipyretics and tepid baths as needed.
- Because of CVA pain, these patients are prone to inadequate airway clearance and atelectasis. Be alert to indications of pulmonary infection, such as increased body temperature, adventitious breath sounds, and increased, thickened, or colored airway secretions. If secretions are noted, encourage frequent deep breathing or coughing or provide suctioning at frequent intervals.
- Teach female patients the importance of wiping the perianal area from front to back, wearing undergarments with cotton crotch, and voiding before and immediately after sexual intercourse to minimize the risk of introducing bacteria into the urinary tract.
- Stress the importance of emptying the bladder at least q3-4hr and once during the night to help prevent UTI caused by residual urine.

NIC: Infection Protection; Medication Management; Perineal Care; Respiratory Monitoring; Teaching: Disease Process; Tube Care: Urinary; Urinary Catheterization: Intermittent

Fluid volume deficit related to decreased intake secondary to anorexia or active loss secondary to vomiting and diaphoresis
Desired outcomes: Following treatment patient becomes normovolemic as evidenced by balanced I&O, urinary specific gravity 1.010-1.030, stable weight, urinary output ≥30-60 ml/hr, and BP and HR within patient's normal range. Within 24 hr of admission, patient verbalizes knowledge about the importance of a fluid intake of at least 2 to 3 L/day.
- Maintain adequate fluid intake to avoid fluid volume deficit. An intake of at least 2 to 3 L/day is usually indicated; however, the appropriate amount depends on the patient's output, which includes gastric, fecal, urinary, sensible, and insensible losses. Obtain guidelines from health care provider for the desired amount of fluid intake. Teach nonrestricted patients the importance of maintaining a fluid intake of at least 2 to 3 L/day.
- Monitor I&O, urinary specific gravity, and daily weight as indicators of hydration status. Weigh patient at the same time each day, using the same scale and with the patient wearing the same amount of clothing.
- Report indicators of volume deficit: poor skin turgor, thirst, dry mucous membranes, urinary specific gravity >1.030, tachycardia, or orthostatic hypotension.

◎ NIC: Fluid/Electrolyte Management; Teaching: Prescribed Diet; Surveillance; Vital Signs Monitoring

PATIENT-FAMILY TEACHING AND DISCHARGE PLANNING

When providing patient-family teaching, focus on sensory information; avoid giving excessive information; and initiate a visiting nurse referral for necessary follow-up teaching. Consider including verbal and written information about the following:

- Medications, including drug name, purpose, dosage, schedule, drug/drug and food/drug interactions, precautions, and potential side effects.
- Importance of taking medications for prescribed length of time, even if feeling "well."
- Necessity of reporting the following indicators of UTI to health care provider: chills; fever; hematuria; flank, CVA, suprapubic, low back, buttock, scrotal, or labial pain; cloudy and foul-smelling urine; frequency; urgency; dysuria; and increasing or recurring incontinence.
- Importance of perineal hygiene for female patients and the necessity of wiping from front to back, wearing undergarments with cotton crotch, and voiding before and after intercourse.
- Importance of emptying the bladder at least q3-4hr and once during the night to help prevent UTI caused by residual urine.
- Necessity of maintaining a fluid intake of at least 2 to 3 L/day and drinking fruit juices (cranberry, plum, prune) that leave an acid ash in the urine.
- Importance of continued medical follow-up because of the high incidence of recurrence.

Hydronephrosis

Hydronephrosis is the dilation of the renal pelvis and calyces secondary to the obstruction of urinary flow. It results from any condition or abnormality that causes urinary tract obstruction. If the obstruction is not corrected, the affected kidney eventually atrophies and fails. Obstruction in the urethra or bladder will affect both kidneys, whereas obstruction in a single ureter or kidney will affect only the involved kidney.

Dramatic postobstructive diuresis can occur after the release of the obstruction. Inappropriate loss of Na^+ and H_2O can in turn lead to volume depletion.

ASSESSMENT

Indicators are determined by the level, severity, and duration of obstruction. Onset of hydronephrosis usually is insidious.

Kidney/ureteral obstruction: Flank pain and abdominal tenderness, renal colic, gross hematuria.

Bladder neck/urethral obstruction: Frequency, hesitancy, dribbling, incontinence, nocturia, signs and symptoms of renal insufficiency, suprapubic pain, anuria.

Physical assessment: Enlarged kidney (s), distended bladder (if bladder neck obstruction is present), crackles (rales), and possibly hypertension and edema if patient has fluid overload from retention.

History of: UTI, nephrolithiasis, BPH, neurogenic bladder, or other obstruction.

DIAGNOSTIC TESTS

BUN and serum creatinine: To determine level of renal function.
Urinalysis: To determine the presence of stone formation or infection.

Renal ultrasound: Noninvasive technique that uses high-frequency sound waves to assess renal size, contour, and structural changes. Because it does not rely on dye uptake, it can be used to evaluate poorly functioning kidneys.
Abdominal x-ray, IVP, and retrograde pyelogram: To identify cause and location of obstruction.

COLLABORATIVE MANAGEMENT

Management of hydronephrosis depends on the cause and duration of the urinary tract obstruction. Major causes of obstruction in the pelvis and ureter are calculi (see "Ureteral Calculi," p. 165) and neoplasms. Major causes of obstruction in the bladder and urethra are neoplasms (see "Cancer of the Bladder," p. 172), neurogenic bladder (see "Neurogenic Bladder," p. 188), and prostatic hypertrophy (see "Benign Prostatic Hypertrophy," p. 656).

See Also: "Urinary Tract Obstruction," p. 169, for a general discussion of urinary tract obstruction; "Acute Renal Failure," p. 145, and "Chronic Renal Failure," p. 150, as appropriate.

Management of hydronephrosis might include the insertion of a nephrostomy tube into the renal pelvis to drain urine and relieve pressure. It is inserted percutaneously with the patient under local anesthesia, or it is inserted in an open surgical procedure. The tube may be permanent or temporary.

NURSING DIAGNOSES AND INTERVENTIONS

Risk for infection with risk factors associated with an invasive procedure (insertion/presence of nephrostomy tube)
Desired outcome: Patient is free of infection as evidenced by normothermia, BP and HR within patient's normal range, urine that is clear and normal in odor and color, and absence of dysuria.

* Maintain sterile technique when providing dressing changes and nephrostomy tube care.
* Observe for and report indicators of infection, such as fever, pain, purulent drainage, and tachycardia. Document changes in color, odor, or clarity of urine. Infection is common with hydronephrosis.
* Do not change, clamp, or irrigate the nephrostomy tube unless specifically prescribed by health care provider.

Caution: Because the renal pelvis is small and holds little volume, never insert more than 5 ml at one time into the tube unless a larger amount has been specifically prescribed by the health care provider.

* Keep the urine collection container and tubing in a dependent position to prevent reflux of the tube's contents into the renal pelvis. Avoid kinks in the tubing.
* Encourage fluid intake, unless contraindicated, to provide a physiologic flushing of the system and tubing.

NIC: Fluid Management; Teaching: Disease Process; Tube Care; Urinary Elimination Management; Wound Care: Closed Drainage

Risk for injury with risk factors associated with insertion/presence of nephrostomy tube
Desired outcome: Patient remains free of signs of nephrostomy tube complications as evidenced by urine that is clear and of normal color after the first 24 to 48 hr, a urine output of at least 30 to 60 ml/hr, and absence of discomfort/pain.

- Report gross hematuria (urine that is bright red, possibly with clots). Transient hematuria can be expected for 24-48 hr after tube insertion.
- Notify health care provider of leakage around the catheter, which can occur with blockage, as well as a sudden decrease in urine output, which can signal a dislodged or blocked catheter.
- Report a sudden onset of or increase in pain, which can indicate perforation of a body organ by the catheter.
- Keep the tube securely taped to the patient's flank with elastic tape. If the tube accidently becomes dislodged, cover the site with a sterile dressing; notify health care provider immediately.

Note: Before removing the nephrostomy tube, the health care provider may request that it be clamped for several hours at a time to evaluate patient tolerance. While the tube is clamped, monitor the patient for the following indications of ureteral obstruction: flank pain, diminished urinary output, and fever.

NIC: Fluid Monitoring; Surveillance; Urinary Elimination Management; Vital Signs Monitoring; Wound Care: Closed Drainage

PATIENT-FAMILY TEACHING AND DISCHARGE PLANNING

When providing patient-family teaching, focus on sensory information; avoid giving excessive information; and initiate a visiting nurse referral for necessary follow-up teaching. Consider including verbal and written information about the following:

- Medications, including drug name, purpose, dosage, schedule, drug/drug and food/drug interactions, precautions, and potential side effects.
- Care of the nephrostomy catheter, if discharged with one; procedure to follow should the catheter become dislodged.
- Frequency of and procedure for dressing changes. Patient or significant others should demonstrate safe dressing-change technique before hospital discharge or receive a referral for home health follow-up.
- Need for continued medical follow-up; confirm date and time of next health care provider appointment, if known.
- Signs and symptoms that necessitate medical attention: fever; cloudy or foul-smelling urine; flank, CVA, low back, buttock, scrotal, or labial pain; increased catheter drainage or drainage around the catheter site.

Renal artery stenosis

Stenosis of the renal artery or one of its main branches usually is the result of fibromuscular dysplasia or arteriosclerotic changes. A reduction in the lumen of the renal artery causes a decrease in blood flow to the affected kidney, which in turn stimulates the renin-angiotensin system, causing systemic hypertension. The elevation in blood pressure usually is proportional to the degree of ischemia in the affected kidney. If the hypertension is left untreated, the nonischemic kidney will develop arteriolar hyperplasia. When both kidneys are involved, renal failure can occur.

ASSESSMENT

Signs and symptoms: Headache, nose bleeds, tinnitus.
Physical assessment: Auscultation of a bruit in the mid-epigastric area. BP can be severely elevated.
History of: Accelerated hypertension with abrupt onset; hypertensive retinopathy.

DIAGNOSTIC TESTS

Intravenous pyelogram: Visualizes kidneys via excretion of iodine-containing contrast medium; will demonstrate an ischemic kidney.

Renal arteriography: Injection of contrast medium into the renal arteries to visualize renal vasculature. The arteriogram can be false-positive in the older adult. Complications include allergic reaction to the contrast medium, contrast medium–induced acute renal failure, hemorrhage, embolus, and infection.

Radioisotope renogram: Will demonstrate a delayed transit time of the radioisotope through the affected kidney; may be performed in combination with the captopril test (see *Captopril test*, below).

Renal vein renin levels: Will show a difference between the two kidneys in unilateral disease. The renin level from the ischemic kidney should be 1.5 times that of the nonischemic kidney.

Plasma renin level: Will be increased because of stimulation of the renin-angiotensin system.

Captopril test: A significant increase in plasma renin levels after a dose of captopril suggests renovascular hypertension. Captopril inhibits the enzyme that converts angiotensin I to angiotensin II. Individuals with hypertension caused by increased renin levels will respond to captopril by producing more renin.

BUN and serum creatinine: May be normal or increased and reflect the level of renal function.

Serum K^+ levels: Often decreased secondary to increased secretion of aldosterone.

COLLABORATIVE MANAGEMENT

Renovascular hypertension can be treated medically, invasively via percutaneous transluminal angioplasty, or surgically. Patients with diffuse arteriosclerotic vascular disease or bilateral renal artery lesions may be considered poor surgical risks. Type and duration of the disease are additional factors that can contribute to the decision to treat patients medically.

Invasive procedure

Percutaneous transluminal angioplasty: Performed if the patient is a suitable candidate and the necessary equipment and personnel are available. Angioplasty involves the insertion of a balloon-tipped catheter to dilate the narrowed vessel. It can be performed with the patient under local anesthesia and requires minimal hospitalization.

Surgical interventions

Arterial endarterectomy with follow-up anticoagulant therapy

Resection or bypass of the lesion (aortorenal bypass graft): Performed for those patients who are unsuitable candidates for endarterectomy or angioplasty or when angioplasty has been unsuccessful or is unavailable. Revascularization may be achieved using the patient's saphenous vein or internal iliac artery or a synthetic graft.

NURSING DIAGNOSES AND INTERVENTIONS

Knowledge deficit: Rationale for frequent assessments after aortorenal bypass graft, angioplasty, or endarterectomy and the technique for measuring BP

Desired outcome: Before the procedure, patient verbalizes knowledge about the renal procedure he or she will undergo and the rationale for frequent VS checks and demonstrates BP measurement technique before hospital discharge.

- Monitor BP frequently during the first 48 hr after aortorenal bypass graft. Explain to patient and significant other that hypertension during this period usually is temporary but may require treatment. When angioplasty is successful, hypertension should decrease within 4 to 6 hr postprocedure.

- Explain the rationale for measuring VS q15min immediately after angioplasty. Monitor the integrity of the pulses distal to the angioplasty site.
- Alert patient and significant other to the potential for bleeding and hematoma formation at the angioplasty site, as well as symptoms of hidden bleeding, including hypotension and tachycardia. Explain that if a hematoma is noted, it will be circled with ink and the time will be noted to detect further bleeding.
- Explain the rationale for measuring BP under the same conditions each day: sitting, standing, lying down. Teach the technique for measuring BP to the patient and significant other before hospital discharge.
- Explain that BP may remain elevated after the renal procedure and that antihypertensive medications still may be required. Review the purpose, action, dose, and potential side effects of all medications with patient and significant other before hospital discharge.
- Stress the need for continued medical evaluation of BP and renal function.

NIC: Bleeding Precautions; Circulatory Care; Health Education; Teaching: Disease Process; Teaching: Prescribed Medication

---

See Also: Nursing diagnoses and interventions in Appendix One, "Caring for Preoperative and Postoperative Patients," p. 717.

PATIENT-FAMILY TEACHING AND DISCHARGE PLANNING

When providing patient-family teaching, focus on sensory information; avoid giving excessive information; and initiate a visiting nurse referral for necessary follow-up teaching. Consider including verbal and written information about the following:

- Medications: include drug name, purpose, dosage, schedule, drug/drug and food/drug interactions, precautions, and potential side effects.
- Diet: low in Na^+ (see Table 3-2). Include lists of foods high in K^+ (see Table 3-4) if patient is taking diuretics that cause hypokalemia. Provide sample menus, and have the patient demonstrate understanding of the diet by planning meals for 3 days.
- Technique for measuring BP: patient or significant other should demonstrate proficiency before discharge.
- Care of incision or angioplasty site: teach patient the indicators of wound infection (e.g., erythema, purulent discharge, local warmth, fever) and the importance of reporting them promptly to the health care provider.
- Need for continued medical follow-up to evaluate effectiveness of the treatment.
- Importance of avoiding other risk factors for hypertension: obesity, smoking, stress, and poorly controlled diabetes mellitus.
- Phone numbers to call should questions or concerns arise about therapy or disease after discharge. Additional general information can be obtained by contacting:

National Kidney and Urologic Diseases Information Clearinghouse
3 Information Way
Bethesda, MD 20892-3580 (301) 907-8906 FAX

National Kidney Foundation
30 E. 33rd Street, 11th Floor
New York, NY 10016 (800) 622-9010; (212) 689-9261 FAX
WWW address: *http://www.nephron.com/NKF.html*

Section Two: Renal Failure

Acute renal failure

Acute renal failure (ARF) is a sudden loss of renal function, which may or may not be accompanied by oliguria. The kidneys lose the ability to maintain biochemical homeostasis, causing retention of metabolic wastes and dramatic alterations in fluid, electrolyte, and acid-base balance. Although the alteration in renal function usually is reversible, ARF may be associated with a mortality of 40%-80%. Mortality varies greatly with the cause of ARF, the patient's age, and co-morbid conditions.

The causes of ARF are classified according to development as prerenal, intrinsic, and postrenal. A decrease in renal function secondary to decreased renal perfusion but without renal parenchymal damage is called *prerenal failure*. Causes of prerenal failure include fluid volume deficit, shock, and decreased cardiac function. If hypoperfusion has not been prolonged, restoration of renal perfusion will restore normal renal function. A reduction in urine output because of obstruction to urine flow is called *postrenal failure*. Conditions causing postrenal failure can include neurogenic bladder, tumors, and urethral strictures. Early detection of prerenal and postrenal failure is essential since, if prolonged, they can lead to parenchymal damage.

The most common cause of *intrinsic renal failure*, or renal failure that develops secondary to renal parenchymal damage, is acute tubular necrosis (ATN). Although typically associated with prolonged ischemia (prerenal failure) or exposure to nephrotoxins (aminoglycoside antibiotics, heavy metals, radiographic contrast media), ATN can occur also after transfusion reactions, septic abortions, or crushing injuries. The clinical course of ATN can be divided into the following three phases: oliguric (lasting approximately 7-21 days), diuretic (7-14 days), and recovery (3-12 months). Causes of intrinsic renal failure other than ATN include acute GN, malignant hypertension, and hepatorenal syndrome. Additional medications associated with the development of ARF include NSAIDs, ACE-inhibitors, cyclosporine, cisplatin, and amphotericin B.

ASSESSMENT

Electrolyte disturbance: Muscle weakness and dysrhythmias.

Fluid volume excess: Oliguria, pitting edema, hypertension, pulmonary edema.

Metabolic acidosis: Kussmaul respirations (hyperventilation), lethargy, headache.

Uremia (retention of metabolic wastes):   Altered mental state, anorexia, nausea, diarrhea, pale and sallow skin, purpura, decreased resistance to infection, anemia, fatigue. **Note:** Uremia adversely affects all body systems.

Physical assessment: Pallor; edema (peripheral, periorbital, sacral); crackles (rales); and elevated BP in patient who has fluid overload.

History of: Exposure to nephrotoxic substances, recent blood transfusion, prolonged hypotensive episodes or decreased renal perfusion, sepsis, administration of radiolucent contrast media, or prostatic hypertrophy.

DIAGNOSTIC TESTS

BUN and serum creatinine: Assess the progression and management of ARF. Although both BUN and creatinine will increase as renal function decreases, creatinine is a better indicator of renal function because it is not affected by diet, hydration, or tissue catabolism.

Creatinine clearance: Measures the kidney's ability to clear the blood of creatinine and approximates the glomerular filtration rate. It will decrease as renal function decreases. Creatinine clearance is normally decreased in older persons. **Note:** Failure to collect all urine during the period of study can invalidate the test.

Urinalysis: Can provide information about the cause and location of renal disease as reflected by abnormal urinary sediment (renal tubular cell casts and renal tubular cells).

Urinary osmolality and urinary Na⁺ levels: To rule out renal perfusion problems (prerenal). In ATN the kidney loses the ability to adjust urine concentration and conserve Na^+, producing a urine sodium level >40 mEq/L (in prerenal azotemia the urine sodium is <20 mEq/L).

> **Caution:** All urine samples should be sent to the laboratory immediately after collection or refrigerated if this is not possible. Urine left at room temperature has greater potential for bacterial growth, turbidity, and alkalinity, any of which can distort the reading.

Renal ultrasound: Provides information about renal anatomy and pelvic structures, evaluates renal masses, and detects obstruction and hydronephrosis.

Renal scan: Provides information about the perfusion and function of the kidneys.

CT scan: Identifies dilation of renal calices in obstructive processes.

Retrograde urography: Assesses for postrenal causes, i.e., obstruction.

COLLABORATIVE MANAGEMENT

The goal is to remove the precipitating cause, maintain homeostatic balance, and prevent complications until the kidneys can resume function. Initially, prerenal or postrenal causes are ruled out or treated. A trial of fluid and diuretics may be used to rule out prerenal problems.

Restrict fluids: Replace losses plus 400 ml/24 hr. **Note:** Insensible fluid losses are only partially replaced to offset the water formed during the metabolism of protein, carbohydrates, and fats.

Pharmacotherapy

> **Caution:** Medications that are handled primarily by the kidney (Table 3-3) require modification of dosage or frequency to prevent medication toxicity. Renal failure also may decrease hepatic metabolism and protein binding of certain medications, resulting in increased medication effect.

Diuretics: In nonoliguric ARF for fluid removal (see Table 3-1).

Furosemide (Lasix) (100-200 mg) or mannitol (12.5 g): May be given early in ARF to limit or prevent the development of oliguria.

Antihypertensives: To control BP.

Aluminum hydroxide antacids, calcium carbonate, or calcium acetate: To control hyperphosphatemia.

Cation exchange resins (Kayexalate): To control hyperkalemia. Severe hyperkalemia may be treated also with *IV sodium bicarbonate*, which shifts K^+ into the cells temporarily, or *glucose and insulin.* Insulin also helps move K^+ into the cells, and glucose helps prevent dangerous hypoglycemia, which could result from the insulin. *IV calcium* is given to reverse the cardiac effects of life-threatening hyperkalemia.

Calcium or vitamin D supplements: For patients with hypocalcemia.

Sodium bicarbonate: To treat metabolic acidosis with a serum bicarbonate level <15 mmol/L. It is used cautiously in patients with hypocalcemia or fluid overload.

Vitamins B and C: To replace losses if patient is on dialysis.

Packed RBCs: For active bleeding or if anemia is poorly tolerated.

TABLE 3-3   Drug Usage in Renal Failure

Drugs handled primarily by the kidneys have an increased effect in patients with renal failure. Usually either the dosage or scheduling of these drugs must be modified.

Drugs that require modification of dosage or scheduling:

Antibiotics	*Antihypertensives*	*H₂-receptor blockers*

Antibiotics
   Carbenicillin*
   Cefazolin*
   Gentamicin*
   Kanamycin*
   Tobramycin*
   Vancomycin
Antidysrhythmics
   Digoxin
   Procainamide*

Antihypertensives
   Atenolol*
   Enalapril*
Hypoglycemic Agent
   Insulin
Sedative
   Phenobarbital*

H₂-receptor blockers
   Cimetidine
   Famotidine
   Ranitidine

Drugs that usually do not require modification of dosage or scheduling:

Antibiotics
   Chloramphenicol*
   Clindamycin
   Dicloxacillin
   Erythromycin
   Nafcillin sodium
Anticoagulant
   Heparin
Antidysrhythmics
   Propranolol
   Quinidine gluconate*

Antihypertensives
   Clonidine HCl
   Hydralazine
   Methyldopa*
   Minoxidil
   Prazosin HCl
Antiinflammatory agent
   Indomethacin
Diuretics
   Furosemide
   Metolazone

Hypoglycemic agent
   Glipizide
Narcotics
   Codeine
   Morphine
Sedatives
   Chlordiazepoxide HCl
   Diazepam

---

*Dialyzable drug, which may require increased dosage after dialysis.

TABLE 3-4   Foods High in Potassium

Apricots	Nuts
Artichokes	Oranges, orange juice
Avocados	Peanuts
Bananas	Potatoes
Cantaloupe	Prune juice
Carrots	Pumpkin
Cauliflower	Spinach
Chocolate	Sweet potatoes
Dried beans, peas	Swiss chard
Dried fruit	Tomatoes, tomato juice, tomato sauce
Mushrooms	Watermelon

Diet: High carbohydrate, low protein (high biologic value), low K$^+$ (Table 3-4), low Na$^+$ (see Table 3-2), and low phosphorus (Table 3-5). Carbohydrates are increased to provide adequate calories and limit protein catabolism. Na$^+$ is limited to prevent thirst and fluid retention. K$^+$ and phosphorus are limited because of the kidney's decreased ability to excrete

TABLE 3-5 Foods High in Phosphorus
Meats, especially organ meats (e.g., brain, liver, kidney)
Fish
Poultry
Milk and milk products (e.g., cheese, ice cream, cottage cheese)
Whole grains (e.g., oatmeal, bran, barley)
Seeds (e.g., pumpkin, sesame, sunflower)
Nuts (e.g., Brazil, peanuts)
Eggs and egg products (e.g., eggnog, souffles)
Dried beans and peas

From Horne MM, Heitz UE, Swearingen PL, editors: *Pocket guide to fluid, electrolyte, and acid-base balance,* ed 3, St Louis, 1996, Mosby.

them. Protein is limited to minimize retention of nitrogenous wastes. **Note:** Because of the loss of K^+ during the diuretic phase, K^+ might need to be increased during that time.

TPN: May be necessary for patients unable to maintain adequate oral/enteral intake.

Peritoneal dialysis or hemodialysis: The present trend is to use dialysis early (see "Renal Dialysis," p. 155). Dialysis is done every 1 to 3 days. Prophylactic use of dialysis has reduced the incidence of complications and rate of death in patients with ARF.

NURSING DIAGNOSES AND INTERVENTIONS

Fluid volume excess related to compromised regulatory mechanisms secondary to renal dysfunction: *Oliguric phase*

Desired outcome: Patient adheres to prescribed fluid restrictions and becomes normovolemic as evidenced by decreasing or stable weight, normal breath sounds, edema ≤1+ on a 0-4+ scale, CVP ≤12 cm H_2O, and BP and HR within patient's normal range.

- Closely monitor and document I&O.
- Monitor weight daily. The patient should lose 0.5 kg/day if not eating; a sudden weight gain suggests excessive fluid volume. Weigh patient at the same time each day, using the same scale and with the patient wearing the same amount of clothing.
- Observe for indicators of fluid volume excess, including edema, hypertension, crackles (rales), tachycardia, distended neck veins, SOB, and increased CVP.
- Carefully adhere to prescribed fluid restriction. Provide oral hygiene at frequent intervals, and offer fluids in the form of ice chips or popsicles to minimize thirst. Hard candies also may be given to decrease thirst. Spread allotted fluids evenly over a 24-hr period, and record the amount given. Instruct patient and significant others about the need for fluid restriction. **Note:** Patients nourished via TPN are at increased risk for fluid overload because of the necessary fluid volume involved and its hypertonicity.

NIC: Fluid/Electrolyte Management; Surveillance; Teaching: Prescribed Diet; Vital Signs Monitoring

Risk for fluid volume deficit with risk factors associated with active loss secondary to excessive urinary output: *Diuretic phase*

Desired outcome: Patient remains normovolemic as evidenced by stable weight, balanced I&O, good skin turgor, CVP ≥5 cm H_2O, and BP and HR within patient's normal range.

- Closely monitor and document I&O.
- Monitor weight daily. A weight loss ≥0.5 kg/day may reflect excessive volume loss. Weigh patient at the same time each day, using the same scale and with the patient wearing the same amount of clothing.
- Observe for indicators of volume depletion, including complaints of light-headedness, poor skin turgor, hypotension, tachycardia, and decreased CVP.
- As prescribed, encourage fluids in the dehydrated patient.
- Report significant findings to health care provider.

NIC: Electrolyte Monitoring; Fluid Management; Intravenous (IV) Therapy; Teaching: Disease Process; Vital Signs Monitoring

Altered nutrition: Less than body requirements related to nausea, vomiting, anorexia, and dietary restrictions
Desired outcome: Within 2 days of admission, patient has stable weight and demonstrates normal intake of food within restrictions, as indicated.

- The presence of nausea, vomiting, and anorexia may signal increased uremia. Alert health care providers to symptoms, and monitor BUN levels. BUN levels >80-100 mg/dl usually require dialytic therapy.
- Provide frequent, small meals in a pleasant atmosphere, especially controlling unpleasant odors.
- Administer prescribed antiemetics (e.g., hydroxyzine, ondansetron, prochlorperazine, promethazine) as necessary. Instruct patient to request medication before discomfort becomes severe.
- Coordinate meal planning and dietary teaching with patient, significant others, and renal dietitian. Dietary restriction may include reduced protein, Na^+, K^+, phosphorus, and fluid intake. Provide fact sheets that list foods to restrict. Demonstrate with sample menus with examples of how dietary restrictions may be incorporated into daily meals.

NIC: Diet Staging; Fluid/Electrolyte Management; Nutritional Counseling; Nutrition Therapy; Teaching: Prescribed Diet

Altered protection related to neurosensory, musculoskeletal, and cardiac changes secondary to uremia, electrolyte imbalance, and metabolic acidosis
Desired outcomes: After treatment, patient verbalizes orientation to person, place, and time and is free of injury caused by neurosensory, musculoskeletal, or cardiac disturbances. Within the 24-hr period before hospital discharge, patient verbalizes the signs and symptoms of electrolyte imbalance and metabolic acidosis and the importance of reporting them promptly should they occur.

- Assess for and alert patient to indicators of the following:
  - *Hypokalemia* (may occur during the diuretic phase): Muscle weakness, lethargy, dysrhythmias, and abdominal distention, nausea and vomiting (secondary to ileus).
  - *Hyperkalemia*: Muscle cramps, dysrhythmias, muscle weakness, peaked T waves on ECG.

> **Caution:** A normal serum K^+ level is necessary for normal cardiac function. Hyperkalemia is a common and potentially fatal complication of ARF during the oliguric phase.

  - *Hypocalcemia*: Neuromuscular irritability, e.g., positive Trousseau (carpopedal spasm) and Chvostek signs (facial muscle spasm), and paresthesias.
  - *Hyperphosphatemia*: Although usually asymptomatic, may cause soft tissue calcifications.
  - *Uremia*: Anorexia, nausea, metallic taste in the mouth, irritability, confusion, lethargy, restlessness, and itching.
  - *Metabolic acidosis*: Rapid, deep respirations; confusion.

- Avoid giving patient foods high in K^+ (see Table 3-4). Salt substitutes also contain K^+ and should be avoided.
- Minimize tissue catabolism by controlling fevers, maintaining adequate nutritional intake (especially calories), and preventing infections. If caloric intake is inadequate, body protein will be used for energy, resulting in increased end products of protein metabolism, i.e., nitrogenous wastes. A high-carbohydrate diet helps to minimize tissue catabolism and production of nitrogenous wastes.
- Medications that may cause an increase in serum K^+ should be avoided or used with caution (e.g., NSAIDs, ACE-inhibitors, and K^+-sparing diuretics).

> **Note:** Soon after renal disease is initially diagnosed, ACE-inhibitors may be prescribed for their renal protective effects. However, after chronic renal failure has developed, ACE-inhibitors may be contraindicated because of the risk of hyperkalemia.

- Prepare patient for the possibility of altered taste and smell.
- Patients with renal failure are at risk for increased magnesium levels because of decreased urinary excretion of dietary magnesium, and thus magnesium-containing medications should be avoided. Patients using magnesium-containing antacids such as Maalox typically are switched to aluminum hydroxide preparations such as AlternaGEL or Amphojel. Milk of Magnesia should be substituted with another, non-magnesium-containing, laxative, such as casanthranol.
- Administer aluminum hydroxide or calcium antacids as prescribed to control hyperphosphatemia. Experiment with different brands, or try capsules for patients who refuse certain liquid antacids. Phosphate binders vary in their aluminum or calcium content, however, and one may not be exchanged for another without first ensuring that the patient is receiving the same amount of elemental aluminum or calcium.
- Assure patient and his or her significant other that irritability, restlessness, and altered thinking are temporary. Facilitate orientation through calendars, radios, familiar objects, and frequent reorientation.
- Ensure safety measures (e.g., padded side rails, airway) for patients who are confused or severely hypocalcemic. For patients who exhibit signs of hyperkalemia, have emergency supplies (e.g., manual resuscitator bag, crash cart, and emergency drug tray) available.

NIC: Electrolyte Management; Infection Protection; Neurologic Monitoring; Peripheral Sensation Management; Respiratory Monitoring; Seizure Precautions

Risk for infection with risk factors associated with uremia
Desired outcome: Patient is free of infection as evidenced by normothermia, WBC count $\leq 11,000/mm^3$, urine that is clear and of normal odor, normal breath sounds, eupnea, and absence of erythema, warmth, tenderness, swelling, and drainage at the catheter or intravenous access sites.

> **Note:** One of the primary causes of death in ARF is sepsis.

- Monitor temperature and secretions for indicators of infection. Even minor increases in temperature can be significant because uremia masks the febrile response and inhibits the body's ability to fight infection.
- Use meticulous sterile technique when changing dressings or manipulating venous catheters, IV lines, or indwelling catheters.
- Avoid long-term use of indwelling urinary catheters because they are a common source of infection. Whenever possible, use intermittent catheterization instead.

- Provide oral hygiene and skin care at frequent intervals. Use emollients and gentle soap to avoid drying and cracking of skin, which can lead to breakdown and infection. Rinse off all soap when bathing patient because soap residue may further irritate skin.

○ NIC: Environmental Management; Infection Protection; Perineal Care; Pressure Management; Respiratory Monitoring; Urinary Catheterization: Intermittent

---

See Also: Nursing diagnoses and interventions in "Care of the Patient Undergoing Peritoneal Dialysis," p. 157, and "Care of the Patient Undergoing Hemodialysis," p. 159, as appropriate; Appendix One, "Caring for Patients on Prolonged Bedrest," **Constipation** related to less than adequate fluid or dietary intake and bulk, immobility, lack of privacy, positional restrictions, and use of narcotic analgesics, p. 743.

PATIENT-FAMILY TEACHING AND DISCHARGE PLANNING

When providing patient-family teaching, focus on sensory information; avoid giving excessive information; and initiate a visiting nurse referral for necessary follow-up teaching. Consider including verbal and written information about the following:

- Medications: Include drug name, purpose, dosage, schedule, drug/drug and food/drug interactions, precautions, and potential side effects.
- Diet: Include fact sheets that list foods to restrict. Provide sample menus with examples of how dietary restrictions may be incorporated into daily meals.
- Care and observation of the dialysis access if the patient is being discharged with one (see "Renal Dialysis," p. 160).
- Importance of continued medical follow-up of renal function.
- Signs and symptoms of potential complications. These should include indicators of infection (see **Risk for infection,** p. 149); electrolyte imbalance (see **Altered protection**, p. 148); **Fluid volume excess**, p. 147; and bleeding (especially from the GI tract for patients who are uremic).
- Phone numbers to call should questions or concerns arise about therapy or disease after discharge. Additional general information can be obtained by contacting:

National Kidney and Urologic Diseases Information Clearinghouse
3 Information Way
Bethesda, MD 20892-3580   (301) 907-8906 FAX

National Kidney Foundation
30 E. 33rd Street, 11th Floor
New York, NY 10016   (800) 622-9010; (212) 689-9261 FAX
WWW address: *http://www.nephron.com/NKF.html*

In addition
- If the patient requires dialysis after discharge, coordinate discharge planning with dialysis unit staff.

Chronic renal failure

Chronic renal failure (CRF) is a progressive, irreversible loss of kidney function that develops over days to years. Eventually it can progress to end-stage renal disease (ESRD), at which time renal replacement therapy (dialysis or transplantation) is required to sustain life. Before ESRD the individual with CRF can lead a relatively normal life managed by diet and medications. The length of this period varies, depending on the cause of renal disease and the patient's level of renal function at the time of diagnosis.

Of the many causes of CRF, some of the most common are glomerulonephritis (GN), diabetes mellitus, hypertension, and polycystic kidney disease. Regardless of the cause, the clinical presentation of CRF, particularly as the individual approaches ESRD, is similar. Retention of metabolic end products and accompanying fluid and electrolyte imbalances adversely affect all body systems. Alterations in neuromuscular, cardiovascular, and gastrointestinal function are common. Renal osteodystrophy is an early and frequent complication. The collective manifestations of CRF are termed *uremia*.

ASSESSMENT

Fluid volume abnormalities: Crackles (rales), hypertension, edema, oliguria, anuria.

Electrolyte disturbances: Muscle weakness, dysrhythmias, pruritus, neuromuscular irritability, tetany.

Uremia—retention of metabolic wastes: Weakness, malaise, anorexia, dry and discolored skin, peripheral neuropathy, irritability, clouded thinking, ammonia odor to breath. **Note:** Uremia adversely affects all body systems.

Metabolic acidosis: Deep respirations, lethargy, headache.

Potential acute complications

Heart failure: Crackles (rales), dyspnea, orthopnea.

Pericarditis: Chest pain, SOB.

Cardiac tamponade: Hypotension, distant heart sounds, pulsus paradoxus (exaggerated inspiratory drop in systolic BP).

Physical assessment: Pallor, dry and discolored skin, edema (peripheral, periorbital, sacral). With fluid overload, crackles and elevated BP may be present.

History of: GN, diabetes mellitus, polycystic kidney disease, hypertension, systemic lupus erythematosus, chronic pyelonephritis, and analgesic abuse, especially the combination of phenacetin and aspirin.

DIAGNOSTIC TESTS

BUN and serum creatinine: Both will be elevated. **Note:** Nonrenal problems, such as dehydration or GI bleeding, also can cause the BUN to increase, but there will not be a corresponding increase in creatinine.

Creatinine clearance: Measures the kidney's ability to clear the blood of creatinine and approximates the glomerular filtration rate. Creatinine clearance will decrease as renal function decreases. Dialysis is usually begun when the creatinine clearance is less than 10 ml/min. Creatinine clearance normally is decreased in older adults. **Note:** Failure to collect all urine specimens during the period of study will invalidate the test.

X-ray of the kidneys, ureters, and bladder (KUB): Documents the presence of two kidneys, changes in size or shape, and some forms of obstruction.

IVP, renal ultrasound, renal biopsy, renal scan (using radionuclides), and computerized axial tomography (CT) scan: Additional tests for determining the cause of renal insufficiency. Once the patient has reached ESRD, these tests are not performed.

Serum chemistries, chest and hand x-rays, and nerve conduction velocity test: To assess for development and progression of uremia and its complications.

COLLABORATIVE MANAGEMENT

Before ESRD, medical management is aimed at slowing the progression of CRF and avoiding complications. Diabetes and hypertension should be aggressively treated. Volume depletion, infection, and nephrotoxic agents must be rigorously avoided to prevent further deterioration of renal function. Once the patient reaches ESRD, management is aimed at alleviating uremic symptoms and providing dialysis or renal transplantation.

Diet: Protein and phosphorus (see Table 3-5) are initially restricted to slow progression of CRF and prevent early development of renal osteodystrophy. Carbohydrates are increased for patients on protein-restricted diets to ensure adequate caloric intake to prevent tissue catabolism (contributing to the buildup of nitrogenous wastes). As the patient approaches ESRD, Na^+ intake is limited to reduce thirst and fluid retention (see Table 3-2); K^+ intake is limited because of the kidneys' decreased ability to excrete this ion (see Table 3-4); and protein may be further restricted to limit the production of nitrogenous wastes. For patients on protein-restricted diets, protein intake should be restricted to protein sources primarily of high biologic value.

Fluid restriction: For patients at risk for developing fluid volume excess. For patients on hemodialysis, interdialytic fluid weight gain should be limited to 3%-4% of an individual's "dry" weight (i.e., weight with stable fluid balance).

Pharmacotherapy

Aluminum hydroxide, calcium carbonate, or calcium acetate: To control hyperphosphatemia. Use of aluminum-containing, phosphate-binding agents is limited because of the increased risk of renal osteodystrophy and encephalopathy caused by elevated tissue aluminum levels.

Antihypertensives: To control BP. Because increased release of angiotensin may occur with renal pathology, some patients require bilateral nephrectomies to control excessive hypertension.

Multivitamins and folic acid: For patients with dietary restrictions or who are on dialysis (water-soluble vitamins are lost during dialysis).

Parenteral iron, ferrous sulfate, recombinant human epoetin alfa (Epogen): To treat anemia. Epogen may be administered subcutaneously or intravenously.

Diphenhydramine: To treat pruritus.

Sodium bicarbonate: To treat acidosis.

Vitamin D preparations and calcium supplements: To treat hypocalcemia and prevent renal osteodystrophy. When the serum phosphorus level is near normal, calcitrol may be administered orally or intravenously to replace the kidney's lost ability to convert natural vitamin D and thus facilitate calcium absorption.

Deferoxamine: To treat iron or aluminum toxicity.

Caution: Medications that are excreted primarily by the kidney require modification of dosage or frequency. Of special concern are the digitalis preparations, which are 85% excreted by the kidneys. Use of digitalis preparations in elderly patients with CRF requires careful dosage titration to allow adequate therapeutic effect while avoiding toxicity. In addition, dialyzable medications may need to be increased or held and given postdialysis (see Table 3-3).

Packed red blood cells: To treat severe or symptomatic anemia.

Maintenance of homeostasis and prevention of complications by avoiding the following: Volume depletion, hypotension, use of radiopaque contrast medium, and nephrotoxic substances. Pregnancy is contraindicated.

Renal transplantation or dialysis: Patients with CRF with a glomerular filtration rate (GFR) >15 ml/min and a serum creatinine <6 mg/dl generally do not need maintenance dialysis. However, if the above therapies are inadequate and the GFR is <10 ml/min, intermittent dialysis is required.

NURSING DIAGNOSES AND INTERVENTIONS

Activity intolerance related to generalized weakness secondary to anemia and uremia

Desired outcome: Following treatment, patient rates perceived exertion at ≤3 on a 0-10 scale and exhibits improving endurance to activity as evidenced by HR ≤20 bpm over resting HR, systolic BP ≤20 mm Hg over or under resting systolic pressure, and RR ≤20 breaths/min with normal depth and pattern (eupnea).

> **Note:** Anemia is better tolerated in the uremic than in the nonuremic patient.

- Anemia is usually proportional to the degree of azotemia. In patients not treated with recombinant human erythropoietin (epoetin alfa [Epogen]), the Hct can be as low as 20% or less but usually stabilizes at around 20%-25%. Typically these patients are not transfused unless the Hct drops below 20% or anemia is poorly tolerated. The target Hct for patients receiving epoetin alfa is 30% or greater, depending on the individual's age and cardiovascular status. Epoetin alfa takes approximately 2-6 weeks to significantly affect the Hct. Epoetin alfa may be contraindicated in patients with uncontrolled hypertension or sensitivity to human albumin.
- Monitor patient during activity, and ask patient to rate perceived exertion (see **Risk for activity intolerance,** p. 739, in Appendix One, "Caring for Patients on Prolonged Bedrest," for details).
- Notify health care provider of increased weakness, fatigue, dyspnea, chest pain, or further decreases in Hct. In addition:
  —Provide and encourage optimal nutrition.
  —Administer epoetin alfa (Epogen), if prescribed. Gently mix the container (shaking may denature the glycoprotein); use only one dose per vial (do not re-enter used vials; discard unused portions). Monitor for dyspnea, chest pain, seizures, and severe headache.
  —Administer anabolic steroids (e.g., nandrolone) if prescribed. Prepare women patients for side effects, including increasing facial hair, deepening tone of voice, and menstrual irregularities.
  —Coordinate laboratory studies to minimize blood drawing.
  —Observe for and report evidence of occult blood and blood loss.
  —Report symptomatic anemia: weakness, SOB, chest pain.
  —Do not administer ferrous sulfate at the same time as antacids. The two medications should be given at least 1 hr apart to maximize absorption of the ferrous sulfate.
  —Administer parenteral iron if prescribed. Anaphylaxis is a possible complication.
  —Assist patient with identifying activities that cause increased fatigue and adjusting those activities accordingly.
  —Assist the patient with ADL while encouraging maximum independence to the patient's tolerance.
  —Establish with the patient realistic, progressive exercises and activity goals that are designed to increase endurance. Ensure that they are within the patient's prescribed limitations. Examples are found in **Risk for activity intolerance,** p. 738, and **Risk for disuse syndrome,** p. 740, in Appendix One, "Caring for Patients on Prolonged Bedrest."

NIC: Energy Management; Exercise Promotion; Medication Management; Mutual Goal Setting; Surveillance; Teaching: Prescribed Activity/Exercise

Impaired skin integrity related to pruritus and dry skin secondary to uremia and edema

Desired outcome: Patient's skin remains intact and free of erythema and abrasions.

- Because accumulating nitrogenous wastes begin to be excreted through the skin, pruritus is common in patients with uremia, causing frequent and intense scratching. Pruritus often decreases with a reduction in BUN and improved phosphorus control. Encourage use of phosphate binders and the reduction of dietary phosphorus if elevated phosphorus level is a problem (see Table 3-5). Give phosphate binders with meals for maximum effects. If necessary, administer antihistamines as prescribed. Keep patient's fingernails short.
- Because uremia retards wound healing, instruct the patient to monitor scratches for evidence of infection and seek early medical attention should signs and symptoms of infection appear.
- Uremic skin is often dry and scaly because of reduction in oil gland activity. Encourage use of skin emollients. Patients should avoid harsh soaps and excessive bathing. Advise patient to bathe every other day and use bath oils as needed if dry skin is a problem.
- Clotting abnormalities and capillary fragility place the patient with uremia at increased risk for bruising. Advise patient and significant others that this can occur.
- Provide scheduled skin care and position changes for individuals with edema.

◎ NIC: Bathing; Medication Administration: Topical; Nail Care; Nutrition Management; Skin Surveillance

Knowledge deficit: Need for frequent BP checks and adherence to antihypertensive therapy and the potential for change in insulin requirements for individuals who have diabetes
Desired outcomes: Within the 24-hr period before hospital discharge, patient verbalizes knowledge about the importance of frequent BP checks and adherence to antihypertensive therapy. The patient with diabetes mellitus (DM) verbalizes knowledge about the potential for change in insulin requirements.

> Note: Patients with CRF may experience hypertension because of fluid overload, excess renin secretion, or arteriosclerotic disease.

- Teach patient about the importance of getting BP checked at frequent intervals and adhering to the prescribed antihypertensive therapy. Control of hypertension may slow the progression of chronic renal insufficiency.
- Teach patients with DM that insulin requirements often decrease as renal function decreases. Instruct these patients to be alert to indicators of hypoglycemia, including weakness, blurred vision, headache, diaphoresis, and shaking.

◎ NIC: Teaching: Prescribed Activity/Exercise; Teaching: Prescribed Medication; Teaching: Procedure/Treatment

PATIENT-FAMILY TEACHING AND DISCHARGE PLANNING

When providing patient-family teaching, focus on sensory information; avoid giving excessive information; and initiate a visiting nurse referral for necessary follow-up teaching. Consider including verbal and written information about the following:

- Medications, including drug name, purpose, dosage, schedule, drug/drug and food/drug interactions, precautions, and potential side effects.
- For patients not on dialysis but requiring epoetin alfa, instruct patient and/or significant other in preparation of the medication and subcutaneous injections. Teach the patient and/or significant other to gently mix the container (shaking may denature the glycoprotein); use only one dose per vial (do not re-enter used vials, discard unused portions). Instruct the patient and/or significant other to monitor for and rapidly report to the health care provider any of the following: dyspnea, chest pain, seizures, and severe headache.
- Diet, including fact sheet listing foods that are to be restricted or limited. Inform patient that diet and fluid restrictions may be altered as renal function

decreases. Provide sample menus, and have the patient demonstrate understanding by preparing 3-day menus that incorporate dietary restrictions.
- Care and observation of dialysis access if the patient has one (see "Renal Dialysis," p. 160).
- Signs and symptoms that necessitate medical attention: irregular pulse, fever, unusual SOB or edema, sudden change in urine output, and unusual muscle weakness.
- Need for continued medical follow-up; confirm date and time of next health care provider appointment.
- Importance of avoiding infections and seeking treatment promptly should one develop. Instruct the patient in the indicators of frequently encountered infections, including URI, UTI, impetigo, and otitis media. For details, see **Risk for infection,** p. 162, in "Care of the Renal Transplant Recipient."
- Phone numbers to call should questions or concerns arise about therapy or disease after discharge. Additional general information can be obtained by contacting:

National Kidney and Urologic Diseases Information Clearinghouse
3 Information Way
Bethesda, MD 20892-3580   (301) 907-8906 FAX

National Kidney Foundation
30 E. 33rd Street, 11th Floor
New York, NY 10016   (800) 622-9010; (212) 689-9261 FAX
WWW address: *http://www.nephron.com/NKF.html*

In addition
- For the patient with or approaching end-stage renal disease (ESRD), provide data concerning the various treatment options and support groups. The local chapter of the National Kidney Foundation can be helpful in identifying support groups and organizations in the area. Patient and significant others should meet with the renal dietitian and social worker before discharge.
- Coordinate discharge planning and teaching with the dialysis unit or facility. If possible, have patient visit dialysis unit before discharge.
- For the individual with ESRD, the importance of coordinating all medical care through the nephrologist and the importance of alerting all medical and dental personnel to ESRD status, because of the increased risk of infection and the need to adjust medication dosages. In addition, dentists may want to premedicate ESRD patients with antibiotics before dental work and avoid scheduling dental work on the day of dialysis because of the heparinization that is used with dialytic therapy.

Section Three: Renal Dialysis

Note: The care of patients undergoing dialysis can be complex, and the actual dialysis (especially hemodialysis) is generally accomplished by nurses with specialized education and guided experience. This section does not focus on the specific care of the patient during dialysis but rather provides essential background data, especially the nursing care of the patient who will undergo peritoneal dialysis and special issues related to patients who are receiving hemodialysis.

Peritoneal dialysis and hemodialysis are lifesaving procedures used to treat severely decreased or absent renal function. Dialysis can be either temporary, until the kidneys can resume adequate function, or permanent. Dialysis is defined as the selective movement of water and solutes from one fluid compartment to another across a semipermeable membrane. The two fluid compartments are the patient's blood and the dialysate (electrolyte and glucose solution). With hemodialysis, the semipermeable membrane is an artificial one, whereas with peritoneal dialysis, the peritoneum serves as a natural dialysis membrane.

Indications for dialysis: Acute renal failure or acute episodes of renal insufficiency that cannot be managed by diet, medications, and fluid restriction; ESRD; drug overdose; hyperkalemia; fluid overload; or metabolic acidosis.

Functions of dialysis: Correction of electrolyte abnormalities; removal of excess fluid and metabolic wastes; correction of acid-base abnormalities. **Note:** Dialysis does not compensate completely for the lack of functioning kidneys. Medications and dietary and fluid restrictions are necessary to supplement dialysis.

Peritoneal dialysis: Slower; does not require heparinization; requires surgical placement of a peritoneal catheter; can be performed by trained medical-surgical nurses; requires a minimum of equipment.

Hemodialysis: Faster; requires heparinization, specially trained staff, expensive and complex equipment; patient must have adequate vasculature for access.

Continuous arteriovenous hemofiltration (CAVH):   One of the newest forms of renal replacement therapy, its use is currently limited to patients in critical-care settings because it requires continuous monitoring and cannulation of a high-flow vessel, usually the femoral artery. Blood flows from an arterial line through the hemofilter and returns to the patient's circulation via a venous access. Ultrafiltrate (fluid, metabolic wastes, and electrolytes) drains from the hemofilter into a collection device.

Care of the patient undergoing peritoneal dialysis

Peritoneal dialysis uses the peritoneum as the dialysis membrane. Dialysate is instilled into the peritoneal cavity via a catheter surgically placed in the abdominal wall. Once the dialysate is within the abdominal cavity, movement of solutes and fluid occurs between the patient's capillary blood and the dialysate. At set intervals the peritoneal cavity is drained and new dialysate is instilled.

COMPONENTS OF DIALYSIS

Catheter: Silastic tube that is either implanted using general anesthesia as a surgical procedure for patients who will have long-term treatment or inserted using local anesthesic at the bedside for short-term dialysis.

Dialysate: Sterile electrolyte solution similar in composition to normal plasma. The electrolyte composition of the dialysate can be adjusted according to individual need. The most commonly adjusted electrolyte is K^+. Glucose is added to the dialysate in varying concentrations to remove excess body fluid via osmosis. **Note:** Some glucose crosses the peritoneal membrane and enters the patient's blood. Patients with diabetes mellitus may require additional insulin. Observe for and report indicators of hyperglycemia (e.g., complaints of thirst, changes in sensorium).

TYPES OF DIALYSIS

Intermittent peritoneal dialysis (IPD):   The patient is dialyzed for periods of 8-10 hr, 4-5 times/wk. A predetermined amount of dialysate (usually 2 L) is instilled for a set length of time (usually 20-30 min). It is then allowed to drain by gravity, and the process is repeated. IPD can be performed manually with individual bags or mechanically using a proportioning machine or cycler. The patient is restricted to a chair or bed. Peritoneal dialysis can be performed also as an acute, temporary procedure. Continuous hourly exchanges are performed for 48-72 hr. The patient is restricted to bed.

Continuous ambulatory peritoneal dialysis (CAPD): The patient attaches a specialized bag of dialysate to the peritoneal catheter; allows the dialysate to drain in; clamps the catheter, leaving the bag attached; and goes about his or her daily routine. After 4 hr (8 hr at night) the clamp is opened and the dialysate is allowed to drain out. Using sterile technique, the patient attaches a new bag of dialysate and the process is repeated. Dialysis exchanges are done continuously, 7 days a week. CAPD is used primarily for ESRD.

Continuous cycling peritoneal dialysis (CCPD): This is a combination of IPD and CAPD. A cycler performs three dialysate exchanges at night. In the morning a fourth exchange is instilled and left in the peritoneal cavity for the entire day. At the end of the day, the fourth exchange is allowed to drain out and the process is repeated. The patient is ambulatory by day and restricted to bed at night. CCPD is commonly done every night or 4-5 nights/wk.

NURSING DIAGNOSES AND INTERVENTIONS

Risk for infection with risk factors associated with an invasive procedure (direct access of the catheter to the peritoneum)

Desired outcomes: Patient is free of infection as evidenced by normothermia and absence of the following: abdominal pain, cloudy outflow, nausea, malaise, erythema, edema, increased local warmth, drainage, and tenderness at the exit site. Before hospital discharge, patient verbalizes the signs and symptoms of infection and the need for sterile technique for bag, tubing, and dressing changes.

- The most common complication of peritoneal dialysis is peritonitis. Monitor for and report indications of peritonitis, including fever, abdominal pain, distention, abdominal wall rigidity, rebound tenderness, cloudy outflow, nausea, and malaise.

Caution: To minimize the risk of peritonitis, it is essential that sterile technique be used when connecting and disconnecting the catheter from the dialysis system.

- The dialysate must remain sterile because it is instilled directly into the body. Maintain sterile technique when adding medications to the dialysate.
- Follow agency policy for care of the catheter exit site.
- Observe for and report redness, local warmth, edema, drainage, or tenderness at exit site. Culture any exudate, and report the results to the health care provider.
- Report to health care provider if dialysate leaks around the catheter exit site. This can indicate an obstruction or the need for another purse-string suture around the catheter site. Continued leakage at the site can lead to peritonitis.
- Instruct the patient in the preceding interventions and observations if peritoneal dialysis will be performed after discharge.

NIC: Infection Protection; Peritoneal Dialysis Therapy; Teaching: Disease Process; Teaching: Psychomotor Skill

Risk for fluid volume deficit with risk factors associated with hypertonicity of the dialysate; *or*
Fluid volume excess related to inadequate exchange

Desired outcomes: Postdialysis the patient is normovolemic as evidenced by balanced I&O, stable weight, good skin turgor, CVP 5-12 cm H_2O, RR 12-20 breaths/min with normal depth and pattern (eupnea), and BP and HR within patient's normal range. The volume of dialysate outflow equals or exceeds inflow.

- Fluid retention can occur because of catheter complications that prevent adequate outflow or because of a severely scarred peritoneum that prevents adequate exchange. Observe for and report indicators of fluid overload, such as hypertension, dyspnea, tachycardia, distended neck veins, or increased CVP. Also be alert to incomplete dialysate returns. Accurate measurement and recording of outflow are critical.

- Outflow problems can occur because of the following:
  —*Full colon*: Use stool softeners, high-fiber diet, laxatives, or enemas if necessary.
  —*Catheter occlusion by fibrin* (usually occurs soon after insertion): Obtain prescription to irrigate with heparinized saline.
  —*Catheter obstruction by omentum*: Turn patient from side to side, elevate HOB or FOB, or apply firm pressure to the abdomen. **Note:** Notify health care provider for unresolved outflow problems.
- Monitor I&O and weight daily. A steady weight gain indicates fluid retention. Weigh patient at the same time each day, using the same scale and with the patient wearing the same amount of clothing (or with same items on the bed if using a bed scale).
- Respiratory distress can occur because of compression of the diaphragm by the dialysate. If this occurs, elevate the HOB, drain the dialysate, and notify health care provider.
- Bloody outflow may appear with initial exchanges. Report gross bloody outflow.
- Volume depletion can occur with excessive use of hypertonic dialysate. Observe for and report indicators of volume depletion, including poor skin turgor, hypotension, tachycardia, and decreased CVP.

NIC: Constipation/Impaction Management; Fluid/Electrolyte Management; Infection Protection; Peritoneal Dialysis Therapy; Surveillance; Tube Care

Altered nutrition: Less than body requirements related to protein loss in the dialysate

Desired outcomes: At a minimum of 24 hr before hospital discharge, patient exhibits adequate nutrition as evidenced by stable weight and serum albumin 3.5-5.5 g/dl. Patient's protein intake is 1.2-1.5 g/kg body weight/day.

- Protein crosses the peritoneum, and a significant amount is lost in the dialysate. An increased intake of protein is necessary to prevent excessive tissue catabolism. Protein loss increases with peritonitis. Ensure adequate dietary intake of protein: 1.2-1.5 g/kg body weight/day.
- Patients undergoing peritoneal dialysis typically have fewer dietary restrictions than those on hemodialysis. Ensure that a dietary evaluation and teaching program are performed when the patient changes from one type of dialysis to the other.
- Provide a list of restricted and encouraged foods with menus that illustrate their integration into the daily diet. Ensure patient's understanding by having him or her plan a 3-day menu that incorporates the appropriate foods and restrictions.

NIC: Fluid/Electrolyte Management; Nutritional Counseling; Nutrition Management; Peritoneal Dialysis Therapy; Teaching: Prescribed Diet

Care of the patient undergoing hemodialysis

During hemodialysis, blood is removed via a special vascular access, heparinized, pumped through an artificial kidney (dialyzer), and then returned to the patient's circulation. Hemodialysis is a temporary, acute procedure performed as needed, or it is performed long-term 2-4 times/wk for 3-5 hr each treatment.

COMPONENTS OF HEMODIALYSIS

Artificial kidney (dialyzer): Composed of a blood compartment and dialysate compartment, separated by a semipermeable membrane that allows the diffusion of solutes and the filtration of water. Protein and bacteria do not cross the artificial membrane.

Dialysate: An electrolyte solution similar in composition to normal plasma. Each of the constituents may be varied according to patient need. The most commonly altered component is K^+ and bicarbonate. Glucose may be added to prevent sudden drops in serum osmolality and serum glucose during dialysis.

Vascular access: Necessary to provide a blood flow rate of 200-500 ml/min for an effective dialysis. Vascular access sites may include an arteriovenous fistula; arteriovenous graft; arteriovenous shunt (less commonly used); subclavian or femoral vein catheterization.

NURSING DIAGNOSES AND INTERVENTIONS

Risk for fluid volume deficit with risk factors from excessive fluid removal from dialysis; *or*

Fluid volume excess related to compromised regulatory mechanism resulting in fluid retention secondary to renal failure

Desired outcomes: Postdialysis patient is normovolemic as evidenced by stable weight, RR 12-20 breaths/min with normal depth and pattern (eupnea), CVP 5-12 cm H_2O, HR and BP within patient's normal range, and absence of abnormal breath sounds and abnormal bleeding. After instruction, patient relates the signs and symptoms of fluid volume excess and deficit.

- Monitor I&O and daily weight as indicators of fluid status. A steady weight gain indicates retained fluid. The patient's weight is an important guideline for determining the quantity of fluid that needs to be removed during dialysis. Weigh patient at the same time each day, using the same scale and with the patient wearing the same amount of clothing (or with same items on the bed if using a bed scale).
- Instruct patient and staff to observe for and report indications of fluid volume excess: edema, hypertension, crackles (rales), tachycardia, distended neck veins, SOB, and increased CVP.
- After dialysis observe for and report indicators of fluid volume deficit, including hypotension, decreased CVP, tachycardia, and complaints of dizziness or light-headedness. Describe the signs and symptoms to the patient, and explain the importance of reporting them promptly should they occur. Be aware that because of autonomic neuropathy, the patient with uremia may not develop a compensatory tachycardia when hypovolemic. **Note:** Antihypertensive medications usually are held before and during dialysis to help prevent hypotension during dialysis. Clarify medication prescriptions with the health care provider.
- Monitor for postdialysis bleeding (needle sites, incisions), which can occur because of use of heparin during dialysis. Alert patient to the potential for bleeding from these areas.
- To prevent hematoma formation, do not give IM injection for at least 1 hr after dialysis.
- GI bleeding is common in patients with renal failure, especially after heparinization. Test all stools for the presence of blood. Report significant findings.

NIC: Bleeding Precautions; Fluid/Electrolyte Management; Infection Protection; Teaching: Individual; Teaching: Disease Process

Risk for fluid volume deficit with risk factors associated with bleeding/hemorrhage that can occur with vascular access puncture or disconnection

Risk of altered peripheral tissue perfusion with risk factors associated with interrupted blood flow that can occur with clotting in the vascular access; *and*

Risk for infection with risk factors associated with an invasive procedure (creation of the vascular access for hemodialysis)

Desired outcomes: Patient's vascular access remains intact and connected, and patient is normovolemic (see description in preceding nursing diagnosis). Patient has adequate tissue perfusion as evidenced by normal skin temperature and color and brisk capillary refill (<2 sec) distal to the vascular access. Patient's access is patent as evidenced by presence of bright red blood within shunt tubing or presence of thrill with palpation and bruit with auscultation of fistula or graft. Patient is free of infection as evidenced by normothermia and absence of erythema, local warmth, exudate, swelling, and tenderness at the access site.

- After the surgical creation of the vascular access, assess for patency, auscultate for bruit, and palpate for thrill. Report complaints of severe or unrelieved pain, numbness, and tingling of the area of vascular access or extremity distal to the access, any of which can signal impaired tissue perfusion. Expect postoperative swelling along the graft or fistula or area around the shunt; elevate the extremity accordingly.
- Notify health care provider if the extremity distal to vascular access becomes cool or swollen, has decreased capillary refill, or is discolored, because these problems can indicate occlusion of the vascular access.
- Follow the three principles of nursing care common to all types of vascular access: prevent bleeding, prevent clotting, and prevent infection. Explain the monitoring and care procedures to the patient. Remember that the vascular access is the patient's lifeline. Monitor it closely, and handle it with care. Vascular accesses include the following:
- **Subclavian or femoral lines:** External, temporary catheters inserted into a large vein.
  - —*Prevent bleeding*: Anchor catheter securely because it might not be sutured in. Tape all connections. Keep clamps at bedside in case line becomes disconnected. If the line is removed or accidently pulled out, apply firm pressure to site for at least 10 min.

> **Caution:** An air embolus can occur if a subclavian line accidently becomes pulled out or disconnected. If this occurs, immediately clamp the line. Turn the patient onto a left-side-lying position to help prevent the air from blocking the pulmonary artery, and lower the HOB into Trendelenburg position to increase intrathoracic pressure. This will decrease the flow of inspiratory air into the vein. Administer 100% oxygen by mask, and obtain VS. Notify health care provider stat!

  - —*Prevent clotting*: Keep line patent by priming with heparin or by constant infusion with a heparinized solution. Follow protocol, or obtain specific directions from health care provider. Attach a label to all lines that are primed with heparin to alert other personnel.
  - —*Prevent infection*: Perform sterile dressing changes according to agency protocol. Observe for and report indications of infection, including presence of erythema, local warmth, exudate, swelling, and tenderness at exit site. Report and culture any drainage.
- **Fistula or graft:** Internal, permanent connection between an artery and a vein, or the insertion of an internal graft that is joined to an artery and vein. Grafts can be straight or U-shaped. **Shunts** are similar to a fistula or graft, in that they are plastic tubes used to connect an artery and vein. However, they exit the skin and can be disconnected to allow connection to dialysis. Shunts are usually temporary. Shunts, grafts or fistula are located in the arm or thigh.
  - —*Prevent bleeding*: Inspect needle puncture sites for postdialysis bleeding. If bleeding occurs, apply just enough pressure over the site to stop it. Release the pressure, and check for bleeding q5-10min. Check shunt

connections postdialysis to ensure they are securely sealed. If a shunt becomes disconnected, clamp the ends and follow hospital protocol for cleansing the connections before reconnection.

—*Prevent clotting*: Do not take BP, start IV, or draw blood in the arm with the shunt, graft, or fistula. Have patient avoid tight clothing, jewelry, name bands, or restraint on affected extremity. Palpate for thrill and auscultate for bruit at least every shift and after hypotensive episodes. Notify health care provider *stat* if bruit or thrill has changed significantly or is absent.

—*Prevent infection*: Observe for and report indications of infection: presence of erythema, local warmth, swelling, exudate, and unusual tenderness at the graft, fistula, or shunt site. Culture and report any drainage. Follow hospital protocol for preparations for disconnecting and reconnecting the shunt.

NIC: Bleeding Precautions; Hemodialysis Therapy; Infection Protection; Peripheral Sensation Management; Teaching: Prescribed Activity/Exercise; Wound Care

Section Four: Care of the Renal Transplant Recipient

Annually, approximately 10,000 patients with end-stage renal disease (ESRD) receive a renal transplant. A small but increasing number of patients with ESRD and diabetes receive a combined kidney/pancreas transplant. Although patients receive transplants at major medical centers and are cared for postoperatively in specialized units, they may be admitted to any hospital for treatment of a rejection episode, medication complication, or unrelated illness. The majority of the transplanted kidneys come from cadavers, although living family members or friends also might donate. The organs for combined kidney/pancreas transplants come from a single cadaveric donor. Unless the graft is donated from an identical twin, transplant success depends on the suppression of graft rejection. This is accomplished by carefully matching donors to recipients through tissue typing before transplantation and immunosuppression after transplantation. Rejection is the major complication of renal transplant. Long-term complications occur secondary to the use of immunosuppressive agents and include infection, hypertension, cardiovascular disease, chronic liver disease, bone demineralization, cataracts, GI hemorrhage, and cancer. **Note:** For patients awaiting kidney transplantation with questions about organ procurement, provide the following information:

The United Network for Organ Sharing
UNOS Communication Department
P.O. Box 13770
Richmond, VA 23225 (804) 330-8561; or (800) 243-6667 (voice mail)
WWW address: *http://www.unos.org*

IMMUNOSUPPRESSION

Necessary for the life of the graft. Puts patient at increased risk for infection and development of malignancy in the long term.

Immunosuppressive medication management: Typically includes a combination of the following:

Azathioprine (Imuran): Dosage is adjusted based on the patient's WBC count. Maintenance is usually accomplished with 1 mg/kg or less daily. Side effects include decreased WBC and platelet counts and jaundice.

Prednisone: Initial maintenance dosages vary but usually are 0.5 mg/kg/day. Gradually the maintenance dose may be reduced to 10 mg/day. Side effects include increased susceptibility to infection, hypertension, capillary fragility and bruising, muscle wasting, aseptic necrosis of bone, cataracts, bleeding, Na^+ retention, altered carbohydrate metabolism, acne, mood and behavior changes, and cushingoid changes.

Cyclosporine (Sandimmune):   Initial posttransplant dosages are 15 mg/kg/ day, which are slowly tapered to a maintenance level of 5-10 mg/kg/day. Serum levels should be closely monitored to avoid side effects. Side effects include nephrotoxicity, hepatotoxicity, hirsutism, tremors, gum hyperplasia, hypertension, infection, and malignancy (especially lymphoma). Route is either PO or IV. If IV, administer slowly over a period of 2-4 hr and monitor for anaphylaxis. Although most commonly given as a capsule, if liquid oral form is required: use a glass container; mix with orange juice or chocolate milk to make it more palatable; do not allow solution to stand.

Tacrolimus (FK506, Prograf):   Dosage is 0.15-0.3 mg/kg/day; oral administration is preferred. Side effects may include hepatotoxicity, tremor, headache, insomnia, constipation, diarrhea, vomiting, and renal dysfunction.

REJECTION

Acute: 1 wk to 4 mo after surgery; potentially reversible; treated with increased immunosuppression.

Chronic: Months to years after transplant; irreversible; managed conservatively with diet and antihypertensives until dialysis is required.

Indicators of rejection: Oliguria, tenderness over graft site (located in iliac fossa), sudden weight gain (2-3 lb/day), fever, malaise, hypertension, and increased BUN and serum creatinine. In addition, hyperglycemia will develop with combined kidney/pancreas transplants.

Management of acute rejection

Antilymphocyte globulin (ALG):   Given IV in doses of 10-30 mg/kg/ day. Side effects include increased risk of infection and malignancy. In addition, immediate side effects include chills, fever, rash, joint pain, and anaphylaxis.

Monoclonal antibody (Orthoclone OKT3):   Given IV bolus in <1 min. Recommended to precede dosage with methylprednisolone 1 mg/kg IV and follow 30 min after the dosage with 100 mg of hydrocortisone. Side effects include increased risk of infection and malignancy. In addition, immediate side effects include fever, chills, tremor, headache, vomiting, nausea, dyspnea, and bronchospasm. Patients receiving initial doses require close monitoring because of the high incidence of side effects. **Note:** Respiratory side effects, especially pulmonary edema, are more likely to occur if the patient has fluid volume excess.

Prednisone: During acute rejection, dosage may be increased to 2-3 mg/kg/ day followed with gradually tapering the dose.

NURSING DIAGNOSES AND INTERVENTIONS

Risk for infection with risk factors from invasive procedures, exposure to infected individuals, and immunosuppression

Desired outcomes: Patient is free of infection as evidenced by normothermia, HR ≤100 bpm (or within patient's normal range), and absence of erythema, edema, increased local warmth, tenderness, or purulent drainage at wounds or catheter exit sites. Patient verbalizes the indicators of infection and the importance of reporting them promptly to health care provider or staff.

- Remember that these patients are taking large doses of immunosuppressive agents and that their immune response and thus response to infectious agents will be muted. When caring for these patients, increase your sensitivity to

any indicator of infection as a cue to increase the depth and frequency of assessments for infection.

- Be especially sensitive to low-grade temperature elevation, fever, and unexplained tachycardia.
- Instruct the patient to be alert to signs and symptoms of commonly encountered infections and the importance of reporting them promptly. These include *urinary tract infection* (UTI)—cloudy and malodorous urine; dysuria, frequency, and urgency; pain in the suprapubic area, buttock, thighs, labia, or scrotum; *upper respiratory tract infection* (URI)—productive cough, malodorous, purulent, colored, and copious secretions, chest pain or heaviness; *pharyngitis*—painful swallowing; *otitis media*—malaise, earache; *impetigo*—inflamed or draining areas on the skin.
- Because cytomegalovirus (CMV) is a common infectious agent among these patients, monitor for symptoms of CMV infection, including fever, malaise, fatigue, and muscle aches.
- Teach patient to avoid exposure to individuals known to have infections.
- Some health care providers encourage prophylactic antibiotics for any minor invasive procedures, including dental cleaning.
- Use sterile technique with all invasive procedures and dressing changes.

NIC: Cough Enhancement; Infection Protection; Medication Management; Respiratory Monitoring; Wound Care

Knowledge deficit: Signs and symptoms of rejection, side effects of immunosuppressive agents, transplantation complications, and importance of protecting the existing hemodialysis vascular access
Desired outcome: Within the 24-hr period before hospital discharge, patient verbalizes knowledge of the signs and symptoms of rejection, the side effects of immunosuppressive therapy, complications of transplantation, and the importance of protecting the hemodialysis vascular access.

- Explain the importance of renal function monitoring: I&O, daily weight, and BUN and serum creatinine values. As renal function decreases, BUN and creatinine values will increase.
- Alert patient to the following signs and symptoms of rejection: oliguria, tenderness over the transplanted kidney (located in the iliac fossa), sudden weight gain, fever, malaise, hypertension, and increased BUN (>20 mg/dl) and serum creatinine (>1.5 mg/dl). Provide patient with a notebook in which to record daily VS and weight measurements. Instruct patient to weigh himself or herself at the same time each day, using the same scale and wearing the same amount of clothing. Remind patient to bring the notebook to all out-patient visits and to report abnormal values promptly should they occur.
- Explain that significant decreases in WBC and platelet counts can be a side effect of immunosuppressive agents and therefore serial monitoring is essential.
- Explain that GI bleeding is a potential side effect of immunosuppressive agents. Alert patient to the signs and symptoms of GI bleeding (e.g., tarry stools, "coffee-ground" emesis, orthostatic changes, dizziness, tachycardia, increasing fatigue and weakness) and the importance of reporting them promptly should they occur.
- In the patient who has undergone renal transplantation, hypertension may develop for a variety of reasons, including cyclosporine or steroid use, rejection, or renal artery stenosis. Teach patient and/or significant others how to measure BP, and provide guidelines for values that would necessitate notification of health care provider or staff member.
- If the patient has a patent fistula, shunt, or graft (hemodialysis vascular access), explain that it must be handled with care because the patient will need it if a return to dialysis is indicated. Explain that taking BPs,

drawing blood, and starting IVs are contraindicated in the arm with the vascular access and therefore patient should warn others about these contraindications.

- Stress the need for continued medical evaluation of the transplant.

NIC: Circulatory Care; Fluid Monitoring; Health Education; Incision Site Care; Infection Protection; Surveillance

Section Five: Disorders of the Urinary Tract

Ureteral calculi

Ureteral calculi (stones) are a common urologic condition. Although the cause of stones is unknown in 50% of reported cases, it is believed that they originate in the kidney and are passed through the kidney to the ureter. About 90% of all stones pass from the ureter into the bladder and out of the urinary system spontaneously.

ASSESSMENT

Signs and symptoms: Pain that is sharp, sudden, and intense or dull and aching; located in the flank area; and frequently radiating toward the groin. Pain may be intermittent (colic) as the stone moves along the ureter and may subside when it enters the bladder. Nausea, vomiting, diarrhea, abdominal pain, and paralytic ileus may occur. Patient may experience urgency and frequency, void in small amounts, and have hematuria.

Physical assessment: Hypertension, pallor, diaphoresis, tachycardia, and tachypnea may be noted; chills and fever may be present in the acute stage. Costovertebral angle tenderness and guarding may be present. Bowel sounds may be absent secondary to ileus, and the abdomen may be distended and tympanic. The patient will be restless and unable to find a position of comfort.

History of: Sedentary life-style; residence in geographic area in which water supply is high in stone-forming minerals; vitamin A deficiency; vitamin D excess; hereditary cystinuria; treatment with acetazolamide, which is given for glaucoma; inflammatory bowel disease; recurrent urinary tract infections (UTI); prolonged periods of immobilization; gout or prophylactic therapy with allopurinol; decreased fluid intake; hyperparathyroidism; Paget's disease; sarcoidosis; and familial history of calculi or renal disease such as renal tubular acidosis.

DIAGNOSTIC TESTS

Serum tests: To assess calcium levels >5.3 mEq/L, phosphorus levels >2.6 mEq/L, and uric acid levels >7.5 mg/dl, which have been implicated in the formation of stones.

BUN and creatinine tests: To evaluate renal-urinary function. Abnormalities are reflected by high BUN and serum creatinine and low urine creatinine levels. **Note:** Be aware that BUN levels are affected by fluid volume excess and deficit. Volume excess will reduce BUN levels, whereas volume deficit will increase levels. For the older adult, serum creatinine level may not be a reliable measure of renal function because of reduced muscle mass and a decreased glomerular filtration rate. These tests must be evaluated based on an adjustment for the patient's age and hydration status and in comparison with other renal-urinary tests.

Urinalysis: To provide baseline data on the functioning of the urinary system, detect metabolic disease, and assess for the presence of UTI. A cloudy or hazy appearance, foul odor, pH >8.0, and the presence of RBCs, leukocyte esterase, WBCs, and WBC casts signal UTI. A pH <5 is associated with uric acid calculi, whereas a pH ≥7.5 may signal presence of urea-splitting organisms (responsible for magnesium-ammonium-phosphate or struvite calculi).

Urine culture: To determine the type of bacteria present in the genitourinary tract. To avoid contamination, a midstream specimen should be collected.

24-hr urine collection: To test for high levels of uric acid, cystine, oxalate, calcium, phosphorus, or creatinine.

Note: All urine samples should be sent to the laboratory immediately after they are obtained or refrigerated if this is not possible (specimens for culture are *not* refrigerated). Urine left at room temperature has greater potential for bacterial growth, turbidity, and alkaline pH, any of which can distort the reading.

Kidney, ureter, bladder (KUB) x-ray: To outline gross structural changes in the kidneys and urinary system. Typically, calcified calculi are seen (90% of urinary calculi are radiopaque, i.e., calcium or cystine) but not all calculi are radiopaque. Serial radiography monitors progressive movement of the stone. Plain x-rays of the skeletal system may reveal Paget's disease, sarcoidosis, or changes associated with prolonged immobilization.

Excretory urogram/intravenous pyelogram (IVP): Used to visualize the kidneys, renal pelvis, ureters, and bladder. This test also outlines nonradiopaque stones within the ureters; nonradiopaque stones (such as uric acid calculi) are seen as radiolucent defects in the contrast media.

Renal ultrasound: To identify ureteral dilation and presence of stones in the ureters.

CT scan with or without injection of contrast medium: To distinguish cysts, tumors, calculi, and other masses and determine presence of ureteral dilation and bladder distention.

COLLABORATIVE MANAGEMENT

Pharmacotherapy during the acute stage

Narcotic and antispasmodic agents: To relieve pain and ureteral spasms. **Note:** Morphine increases ureteral peristalsis, which aids in passage of the stone but also can increase pain in the process. Conservative therapy may consist of a 6-wk trial of analgesia and increased fluid intake to allow the calculus to pass through the ureter.

Antiemetics (e.g., hydroxyzine, ondansetron, prochlorperazine, promethazine): For nausea and vomiting.

Antibiotics: For infection.

Prophylactic pharmacotherapy

For uric acid stones: Allopurinol or sodium bicarbonate is given to reduce uric acid production or alkalinize the urine, keeping the pH at ≥6.5.

For calcium stones: Sodium cellulose phosphate, when used with a calcium-restricted diet, reduces risk of stone formation. **Note:** Sodium cellulose phosphate should be taken before meals; should not be taken at bedtime; and should be used with caution in postmenopausal women at risk for osteoporosis. Orthophosphates (potassium acid phosphate and disodium and dipotassium phosphates) are given to decrease urinary excretion of citrate and pyrophosphate and thus inhibit stone formation. Thiazides also reduce excretion of citrate and reduce urinary calcium.

For cystine stones: Sodium bicarbonate or sodium-potassium citrate solution is given to increase urinary pH (≥7.5). Penicillamine or tiopronin can be given to lower cystine levels in the urine.

IV therapy: For patients who are dehydrated or to provide increased hydration to facilitate stone passage.

Increase fluid intake: To help flush stone from the ureter to the bladder and out through the system.

Diet: Specific to patient's stone type. (See **Health-seeking behaviors,** p. 168, for detail.)

Endoscopic removal of calculi via cystoscope: A basket catheter is placed beyond the stone and rotated in a downward movement to capture and remove the stone.

Ureteral catheters (stents): Positioned above the stone to promote ureteral dilation, allowing the calculus to pass. These catheters also can be used for intermittent or continuous irrigation with an acidic solution to combat alkalinity. They may be placed temporarily after removal of the stone to allow for healing and promote patency of the ureter in the presence of edema.

Ureterolithotomy: Removal of calculi that cannot pass through the ureter. The ureter is surgically incised, and the stone is manually removed.

Extracorporeal shock wave lithotripsy (ESWL): The affected area is positioned under a membrane coupling device to generate shock waves, which shatter the calculi. May be done using general, regional, or, in selected patients, local anesthesic. Usually, 1000-2000 shock waves over a period of 30-45 min are adequate to break the calculi into fine particles. The fragments pass naturally in the patient's urine within a few days.

Chemolysis: Instillation of solutions (acids, alkaline agents, chelate, thiol) via nephrostomy and ureteral catheters to dissolve stones or stone fragments left by other treatments.

NURSING DIAGNOSES AND INTERVENTIONS

Pain related to presence of the calculus or the surgical procedure to remove it
Desired outcomes: Patient's subjective perception of pain decreases within 1 hr of intervention, as documented by a pain scale. Objective indicators, such as grimacing, are absent or diminished.

- Assess and document quality, location, intensity, and duration of pain. Devise a pain scale with the patient that ranges from 0 (no pain) to 10 (worst pain). Notify health care provider of sudden and/or severe pain.
- Notify health care provider of a sudden cessation of pain, which can signal the passage of the stone. (Strain all urine for solid matter, and send it to the laboratory for analysis.)
- Medicate patient with prescribed analgesics, narcotics, and antispasmodics; evaluate and document the response based on the pain scale. Encourage patients to request medication before discomfort becomes severe.
- Provide warm blankets, heating pad to affected area, or warm baths to increase regional circulation and relax tense muscles.
- Provide back rubs. These are especially helpful for postoperative patients who were in the lithotomy position during surgery.

NIC: Analgesic Administration; Coping Enhancement; Distraction; Heat/Cold Application; Pain Management; Progressive Muscle Relaxation; Simple Relaxation Therapy

Altered urinary elimination (dysuria, urgency, or frequency) related to obstruction caused by ureteral calculus
Desired outcomes: Patient relates the return of a normal voiding pattern within 2 days. Patient demonstrates the ability to record I&O and strain urine for stones.

- Determine and document patient's normal voiding pattern.
- Monitor quality and color of the urine. Optimally it is straw-colored and clear and has a characteristic urine odor. Dark urine is often indicative of dehydration, and blood-tinged urine can result from the rupture of ureteral capillaries as the calculus passes through the ureter.

- In patients for whom fluids are not restricted, encourage a fluid intake of at least 3 L/day to help flush calculus through ureter into the bladder and out through the system.
- Record accurate I&O; teach patient how to record I&O.
- Strain all urine for evidence of solid matter; teach patient the procedure.
- Send any solid matter to the laboratory for analysis.

NIC: Fluid Management; Teaching: Psychomotor Skill; Urinary Elimination Management

Altered urinary elimination related to obstruction or positional problems of the ureteral catheter
Desired outcome: Following intervention, patient has output from the ureteral catheter and is free of spasms or flank pain, which could signal obstruction or displacement.

- Occasionally patients return from surgery with a ureteral catheter. If patient has more than one catheter, label one *right* and the other *left*; keep all drainage records separate.
- Monitor output from ureteral catheter. Amount will vary with each patient and will depend on catheter dimension. If drainage is scanty or absent, milk the catheter and tubing gently to try to dislodge the obstruction. If this fails, notify health care provider.

Caution: Never irrigate the catheter without specific health care provider instructions to do so. If irrigation is prescribed, use gentle pressure and sterile technique. Always aspirate with sterile syringe before instillation to prevent ureteral damage from overdistention. Use another sterile syringe to insert amounts no greater than 3 ml per instillation.

- Typically patient will require bedrest if ureteral catheter is indwelling. Explain to patient that semi-Fowler's and side-lying positions are acceptable. Fowler's position should be avoided, however, because sutures are seldom used and gravity can cause catheter to move into the bladder.
- Ureteral catheters are often attached to the urethral catheter after placement in the ureters. Carefully monitor the urethral catheter for movement, and ensure that it is securely attached to the patient. **Note:** After the ureteral catheters have been removed (usually simultaneously with the urethral catheter), monitor for indicators of ureteral obstruction, including flank pain, CVA tenderness, nausea, and vomiting.

NIC: Fluid Management; Infection Protection; Perineal Care; Tube Care: Urinary; Urinary Catheterization

Risk for impaired skin integrity with risks associated with wound drainage after ureterolithotomy or procedures entering the ureter
Desired outcome: Patient's skin surrounding the wound site remains non-erythemic and intact.

- Monitor incisional dressings frequently during the first 24 hr, and change or reinforce as needed. Flank approaches to the ureter require muscle splitting incisions and result in significant postoperative oozing of blood. Because drainage will also include urine leaking from the entered ureter, excoriation can result from prolonged contact of urine with the skin.
- Note and document odor, consistency, and color of drainage. Immediately after surgery, drainage may be red.
- To facilitate frequent dressing changes, use Montgomery straps or net wraps (e.g., Surginet) rather than tape to secure dressing.
- If drainage is copious after drain removal, apply wound drainage or ostomy pouch with a skin barrier over the incision. Use a pouch with an antireflux valve to prevent contamination from reflux.

◎ NIC: Bathing; Bleeding Precautions; Incision Site Care; Ostomy Care; Skin Surveillance; Wound Care

Health-seeking behaviors: Dietary regimen and its relationship to calculus (stone) formation
Desired outcome: Within the 24-hr period before hospital discharge, patient verbalizes knowledge about foods and liquids to limit to prevent stone formation and demonstrates this knowledge by planning a 3-day menu that excludes or limits these foods.

- Assess patient's knowledge about diet and its relationship to stone formation.
- Advise patient to maintain a urine output of >3 L/day. Increasing the urine output reduces saturation of stone-forming solutes.
- Teach patient to maintain adequate hydration of at least 3 L/day. Good hydration after meals and exercise is important because the patient's solute load is highest at these times.

> **Caution:**   Persons with cardiac, liver, or renal disease require special fluid intake instructions from their health care provider.

- Teach patient the technique for measuring urine specific gravity via a hydrometer. Explain that to minimize stone formation, specific gravity should remain <1.010.
- As appropriate, provide the following information:
  - —*For uric acid* stones: Limit intake of foods high in purines, such as lean meat, legumes, whole grains. Limit protein intake to 1 g/kg/day.
  - —*For calcium stones*: Limit intake of foods high in calcium, such as milk, cheese, green leafy vegetables, yogurt. Limit Na^+ intake (see Table 3-2 for foods high in sodium). Explain to patient that a low-Na^+ diet helps reduce intestinal absorption of calcium. Limit intake of refined carbohydrates and animal proteins, which cause hypercalciuria. Encourage patient to eat foods high in natural fiber content (e.g., bran, prunes, apples). Foods high in natural fiber content provide phytic acid, which binds dietary calcium. Explain that sodium cellulose phosphate, 5 g tid, may be given to bind with intestinal calcium and thus increase the excretion of calcium.
  - —*For oxalate stones*: Limit intake of foods high in oxalate, such as chocolate, caffeine-containing drinks (including instant and decaffeinated coffees), beets, spinach, and peanuts. Large doses of pyridoxine may help with certain types of oxalate stones, and cholestyramine, 4 g qid, may be prescribed to bind with oxalate enterally. Explain that vitamin C supplements should be avoided because as much as half is converted to zoxalic acid.

◎ NIC: Fluid Management; Nutrition Management; Teaching: Prescribed Medication; Teaching: Psychomotor Skill; Urinary Elimination Management

> **See Also:**   Nursing diagnoses and interventions in Appendix One, "Caring for Preoperative and Postoperative Patients," p. 717.

PATIENT-FAMILY TEACHING AND DISCHARGE PLANNING

When providing patient-family teaching, focus on sensory information; avoid giving excessive information; and initiate a visiting nurse referral for necessary follow-up teaching. Consider including verbal and written information about the following:

- Medications, including drug name, purpose, dosage, schedule, drug/drug and food/drug interactions, precautions, and potential side effects.

- Indicators of UTI that necessitate medical attention: chills; fever; hematuria; flank, CVA, suprapubic, low back, buttock, scrotal, or labial pain; cloudy and foul-smelling urine; frequency; urgency; dysuria; and increasing or recurring incontinence.
- Care of incision, including cleansing and dressing. Teach patient signs and symptoms of local infection, including redness, swelling, local warmth, tenderness, and purulent drainage.
- Care of drains or catheters if patient is discharged with them.
- Importance of daily fluid intake of at least 3 L/day in nonrestricted patients.
- Dietary changes as specified by health care provider. Include fact sheets that list foods to restrict or add to the diet. Provide sample menus with examples of how dietary restrictions and requirements may be incorporated into daily meals.
- Activity restrictions as directed for patient who has had surgery: avoid lifting heavy objects (>10 lb) for the first 6 wk, be alert to fatigue, get maximum rest, increase activities gradually to tolerance.
- Use of nitrazine paper to assess pH of urine. Desired pH will be determined by type of stone formation to which the patient is prone. Instructions for use are on nitrazine container.
- When appropriate, teach patient the technique for measuring urine specific gravity via a hydrometer.
- Importance of walking or other exercise to decrease risk of stone formation.

Urinary tract obstruction

Urinary tract obstruction usually is the result of blockage from pelvic tumors, calculi, and urethral strictures. Additional causes include neoplasms, benign prostatic hypertrophy, ureteral or urethral trauma, inflammation of the urinary tract, pregnancy, and pelvic or colonic surgery in which ureteral damage has occurred. Obstructions can occur suddenly or slowly, over weeks to months. They can occur anywhere along the urinary tract, but the most common sites are the ureteropelvic and ureterovesical junctions, bladder neck, and urethral meatus. The obstruction acts like a dam, blocking the passage of urine. Muscles in the area contract to push urine around the obstruction, and the structures behind the obstruction begin to dilate. The smaller the site of obstruction, the greater the damage. Obstructions in the lower urinary structures, such as the bladder neck or urethra, can lead to urinary retention and urinary tract infection. Obstructions in the upper urinary tract can lead to bilateral involvement of the ureters and kidneys, leading to hydronephrosis, renal insufficiency, and kidney destruction. Hydrostatic pressure increases, and filtration and concentration processes in the tubules and glomerulus are compromised.

ASSESSMENT

Signs and symptoms: Anuria, nausea, vomiting, local abdominal tenderness, hesitancy, straining to start a stream, dribbling, decreased caliber and force of urinary stream, oliguria, and nocturia. Pain may be sharp and intense or dull and aching; localized or referred, e.g., flank, CVA, low back, buttock, scrotal, labial pain.

Physical assessment: Bladder distention and "kettle drum" sound over bladder with percussion (absent if obstruction is above the bladder); mass in flank area.

History of: Recent fever (possibly caused by the obstruction); hypertensive episodes (caused by increased renin production from the body's attempt to increase renal blood flow).

DIAGNOSTIC TESTS

Serum K$^+$ and Na$^+$ levels: To determine renal function. Normal range for K$^+$ is 3.5-5.0 mEq/L; normal range for Na$^+$ is 137-147 mEq/L.

BUN and creatinine: To evaluate renal-urinary status. Normally, their values will be elevated with decreased renal-urinary function. **Note:** These values must be considered based on the patient's age and hydration status. For the older adult, serum creatinine level may not be a reliable indicator, because of decreased muscle mass and a decreased glomerular filtration rate. Hydration status can affect BUN: fluid volume excess can result in reduced values, whereas volume deficit can cause higher values.

Urinalysis: To provide baseline data on the functioning of the urinary system, detect metabolic disease, and assess for the presence of urinary tract infection (UTI). A cloudy, hazy appearance; foul odor; pH >8.0; and presence of RBCs, leukocyte esterase, WBCs, and WBC casts are signals of a UTI.

Urine culture: To determine type of bacteria present in the genitourinary tract. To minimize contamination, a sample should be obtained from a midstream collection.

Hgb and Hct: To assess for anemia, which may be related to decreased renal secretion or erythropoietin.

Kidney, ureter, bladder (KUB) radiography: To identify the size, shape, and position of the kidneys, ureters, and bladder and abnormalities such as tumors, calculi, or malformations.

Imaging studies: A variety of imaging studies may be used to identify the area and cause of obstructions.

- Excretory urography/intravenous pyelogram: To evaluate the cause of urinary dysfunction by visualizing the kidneys, renal pelvis, ureters, and bladder.
- Antegrade urography: Involves placement of a percutaneous needle or tube nephrostomy through which radiopaque contrast is injected. Antegrade urography is indicated when the kidney does not concentrate or excrete intravenous dye.
- Retrograde urography: Radiopaque dye is injected through ureteral catheters placed during cystoscopy.
- Cystogram: Radiopaque dye is instilled via cystoscope or catheter. This allows visualization of the bladder and evaluation of the vesicoureteral reflex.
- CT scans: To identify the degree and location of obstruction, as well as the cause in many situations.

Cystoscopy: To determine degree of bladder outlet obstruction and facilitate visualization of any tumors or masses.

Ultrasonography: To reveal areas of ureteral dilation or distention from retained urine.

COLLABORATIVE MANAGEMENT

Catheterization: To establish drainage of urine; may include urethral, ureteral, suprapubic or percutaneous catheters placed in the renal pelvis.

Pharmacotherapy

Narcotics: For pain relief.

Antispasmodics: For relief of spasms.

Antibiotics: For bacterial infection.

Corticosteroids: For reduction of local swelling.

IV therapy: For acutely ill, dehydrated patients or to increase fluids in patients with calculi.

Surgically establish drainage: Via catheters or drains (ureteral, urethral, suprapubic or percutaneous) above point of obstruction.

Surgical removal of obstruction or dilation of strictures: Recurrent strictures may require dilation and placement of a stent or resection with end-to-end anastomosis.

NURSING DIAGNOSES AND INTERVENTIONS

Risk for fluid volume deficit with risk factors associated with postobstructive diuresis

Desired outcomes: Patient is normovolemic as evidenced by HR ≤100 bpm (or within patient's normal range), BP ≥90/60 mm Hg (or within patient's normal range), RR ≤20 breaths/min; no significant changes in mental status; and orientation to person, place, and time (within patient's normal range). Within 2 days after bladder decompression, output approximates input, patient's urinary output is normal for patient (or ≥30-60 ml/hr), and weight becomes stable.

- Using sterile technique, insert a urinary catheter to drain the patient's bladder. Monitor the patient carefully during catheterization; clamp the catheter if the patient complains of abdominal pain or has a symptomatic drop in systolic BP of ≥20 mm Hg. Research has demonstrated that rapid bladder decompression of >750-1000 ml does not result in shock syndrome as previously believed.
- Monitor I&O hourly for 4 hr and then q2hr for 4 hr after bladder decompression. Notify health care provider if output exceeds 200 ml/hr or 2 L over an 8-hr period. This can signal postobstructive diuresis, which can lead to major electrolyte imbalance. If this occurs, anticipate initiation of IV infusion.
- Monitor VS for signs of shock: decreasing BP, changes in LOC or mentation, tachycardia, tachypnea, thready pulse.
- Anticipate the need for urine specimens for analysis of electrolytes and osmolality and blood specimens for analysis of electrolytes.
- Observe for and report indicators of the following:
  —*Hypokalemia*: Abdominal cramps, lethargy, dysrhythmias.
  —*Hyperkalemia*: Diarrhea, colic, irritability, nausea, muscle cramps, weakness, irregular apical or radial pulses.
  —*Hypocalcemia*: Muscle weakness and cramps, complaints of tingling in fingers, positive Trousseau's and Chvostek's signs.
  —*Hyperphosphatemia*: Excessive itching.
- Monitor mentation, noting signs of disorientation, which can occur with electrolyte disturbance.
- Weigh patient daily using the same scale and at the same time of day (e.g., before breakfast). Weight fluctuations of 2-4 lb (0.9-1.8 kg) normally occur in a patient who is undergoing diuresis.

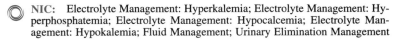 **NIC:** Electrolyte Management: Hyperkalemia; Electrolyte Management: Hyperphosphatemia; Electrolyte Management: Hypocalcemia; Electrolyte Management: Hypokalemia; Fluid Management; Urinary Elimination Management

Pain related to bladder spasms

Desired outcomes: Within 1 hr of intervention, patient's subjective perception of discomfort decreases, as documented by a pain scale. Objective indicators, such as grimacing, are absent or diminished.

- Assess for and document patient complaints of pain in the suprapubic or urethral area. Devise a pain scale with the patient, rating the pain from 0 (no pain) to 10 (worst pain). Reassure patient that spasms are normal with obstruction.
- Medicate with antispasmodics or analgesics as prescribed; belladonna and opium (B&O) suppositories may be specifically ordered for bladder spasms. Document the pain relief obtained, using the pain scale.
- If the patient is losing urine around the catheter and has a distended bladder (with or without bladder spasms), check the catheter and drainage tubing for evidence of obstruction. Inspect for kinks and obstructions in drainage tubing, compress and roll catheter gently between fingers to assess for gritty matter within catheter, milk drainage tubing to release obstructions, or

instruct patient to turn from side to side. Obtain prescription for catheter irrigation if these measures fail to relieve the obstruction.

- In nonrestricted patients, encourage intake of fluids to at least 2-3 L/day to help reduce frequency of spasms.
- Instruct patient in the use of nonpharmacologic methods of pain relief, such as guided imagery, relaxation techniques, and distraction. See relaxation technique described under "Coronary Artery Disease," **Health-seeking behaviors,** p. 59.

NIC: Analgesic Administration; Anxiety Reduction; Pain Management; Progressive Muscle Relaxation; Simple Relaxation Therapy; Urinary Elimination Management

---

See Also: " Hydronephrosis" for **Risk for injury** related to insertion/presence of nephrostomy tube, p. 140; "Ureteral Calculi" for **Risk for impaired skin integrity** related to wound drainage, p. 167; nursing diagnoses and interventions in Appendix One, "Caring for Preoperative and Postoperative Patients," p. 717.

PATIENT-FAMILY TEACHING AND DISCHARGE PLANNING

When providing patient-family teaching, focus on sensory information; avoid giving excessive information; and initiate a visiting nurse referral for necessary follow-up teaching. Consider including verbal and written information about the following:

- Medications, including drug name, dosage, purpose, schedule, drug/drug and food/drug interactions, precautions, and potential side effects.
- Indicators that signal recurrent obstruction and require prompt medical attention: pain, fever, decreased urinary output.
- Activity restrictions as directed for patient who has had surgery: avoid lifting heavy objects (>10 lb) for the first 6 wk, be alert to fatigue, get maximum rest, increase activities gradually to tolerance.
- Care of drains or catheters if patient is discharged with them; care of the surgical incision if present.
- Indicators of *wound infection*: persistent redness, local warmth, tenderness, drainage, swelling, and fever
- Indicators of UTI that necessitate medical attention: chills; fever; hematuria; flank, CVA, suprapubic, low back, buttock, scrotal, or labial pain; cloudy and foul-smelling urine; frequency; urgency; dysuria; and increasing or recurring incontinence.

Cancer of the bladder

Cancer of the bladder is the most common form of urinary system cancer, and it occurs most often in persons 50-70 years of age. Bladder cancer is more commonly seen in men; individuals with a history of occupational exposure to industrial dyes, solvents, or aromatic amines; individuals with a history of chronic urinary tract infections or acetaminophen or phenacetin overuse; and patients who have received cyclophosphamide or pelvic radiation therapy.

Bladder cancer can be classified as superficial or invasive. Superficial cancers are localized to the layers superficial to the bladder wall muscle. Superficial bladder cancers usually do not require aggressive therapy and reoccur. Invasive bladder cancer is defined as involving bladder wall muscle or deeper tissues and requires more radical and aggressive treatment.

Bladder cancer often begins in the bladder lumen, but the bladder neck wall and ureteral orifices also can be involved. Cancers from nearby sites, particularly the prostate and uterine cervix, as well as the sigmoid colon, rectum, or uterus, also can invade the bladder. Cellular proliferation can occur throughout the transitional epithelium, which lines the kidneys, ureters, and mucosa of the bladder. Metastasis most commonly occurs in the bones, liver, and lungs and spreads throughout the lymph nodes.

ASSESSMENT

Signs and symptoms: Painless and intermittent gross hematuria, dysuria, urgency, burning with urination, increased frequency, decreasing volumes of urine, and nocturia. Depending on tumor size, the patient may experience suprapubic pain. If the tumor causes urinary obstruction, see "Urinary Tract Obstruction," p. 169, for further data. In later stages, low back pain, pelvic pain, and leg edema can occur.

Physical assessment: Usually normal. A bladder tumor can be palpated through the abdominal wall only after the disease has become deeply invasive. Rectal examination may reveal large tumors.

DIAGNOSTIC TESTS

Urinalysis, urine culture: To check for RBCs, WBCs, WBC casts, and a pH >8.0, which occur with infection; culture is used to identify infecting organisms.

Urine cytology: To assess for cells that have been sloughed off from tumors/neoplasms. The urine sample is taken from a voided specimen.

CBC: To check for presence of infection (WBCs >11,000 mm^3) and anemia (RBCs, Hct, and Hgb less than normal).

Serum transaminase and alkaline phosphatase: May occur with liver metastasis.

Excretory urography/intravenous pyelogram (IVP):   Can reveal filling defects within the urinary tract and presence of obstruction by tumor.

Ultrasonography/magnetic resonance imaging (MRI):   These tests are used to diagnose the cancer. Ultrasonography, either external or transrectal, helps determine degree of tumor invasion in the bladder wall, and MRI can facilitate recognition of early bladder cancer and assist in staging of the bladder neoplasm.

Biopsy in conjunction with cystoscopy: A cystoscope is inserted through the urethra and into the bladder to visualize the structures. If abnormalities are seen, a section of the tissue is removed for examination (biopsy). Local, regional, or general anesthesia can be used.

Cystogram (cystography):   To outline tumors that are present in the bladder. A radiopaque medium is introduced into the bladder via a urethral catheter. X-rays are taken both before and after urination.

COLLABORATIVE MANAGEMENT

Grading and staging the disease: To formulate a prognosis and guide treatment using the TNM staging classification system. The degree of grading and staging is determined by the extent of metastasis and tissue involvement: the more tissue involved and the greater the metastasis, the higher the grade and stage.

Transurethral resection of the bladder and tumor (TURBT):   Removal of the tumor with electrocautery via cystoscope and rectoscope. Water is used as the irrigant during this procedure because it causes the tumor cells released by the procedure to swell and lyse. TURBT is used to treat superficial bladder tumors.

Photodynamic (laser) or electrical fulguration: Laser or electrical cauterization of small, well-delineated lesions. Usually it is followed by intravesical infusion of chemotherapy directly into the bladder. **Note:** Patients undergoing photodynamic therapy become photosensitive and should avoid any exposure to sunlight for 4-6 wk. Skin gradually can be exposed to sunlight after this period.

Intravesical chemotherapy: Delivers chemotherapeutic agents to topically act on bladder tumors. Agents are introduced into the bladder through an indwelling urethral catheter. Bacille Calmette-Guérin (BCG) is most commonly used, but thiotepa, mitomycin, or doxorubicin also can be used. These drugs are used to remove existing tumor or to reduce the recurrence rate of tumor growth in patients undergoing TURBT.

Intravenous chemotherapy: Provides systemic chemotherapy for more invasive tumors. Cisplatin and methotrexate may be used alone or in combination with vinblastine alone or vinblastine and doxorubicin. Intravenous chemotherapy is used to attempt to preserve the bladder or to arrest tumor growth and metastasis in patients who have had a cystectomy.

Palliative radiation therapy: Used primarily in the late stages for pain relief, but it can be used also early in treatment.

Radon seeds: May be implanted around the base of the tumor in an attempt to eradicate the bladder tumor and prevent regrowth. Typically, this is done after a transurethral resection (TUR) and fulguration of the bladder tumor. Severe cystitis is likely to occur from the irradiation.

Supervoltage radiation therapy: Often used in conjunction with surgery or chemotherapy to shrink very large tumors or for pain relief if the cancer has metastasized widely.

Pharmacotherapy
- *Analgesics and narcotics*: For pain relief.
- *Antibiotics*: For therapy-induced infections.

Partial cystectomy/segmental resection: Performed if the dome of the bladder is involved. The top half of the bladder is removed via an abdominal incision.

Cystectomy: Removal of the entire bladder. Radical cystectomy involves removal of the entire bladder, portions or all of the urethra, and the distal ends of both ureters. In addition, seminal vesicles and the prostate gland are removed in males and the ovaries, uterus, fallopian tubes, and anterior vaginal wall are removed in females.

Urinary diversion: See "Urinary Diversions," p. 193, for discussion.

NURSING DIAGNOSES AND INTERVENTIONS

Risk for fluid volume deficit with risk factors associated with postsurgical hemorrhage after TURBT or segmental resection; *or*

Fluid volume excess (or risk of same) related to excessive fluid intake secondary to irrigation with water during TURBT

Desired outcome: Patient is normovolemic as evidenced by BP ≥90/60 mm Hg (or within patient's normal range), HR ≤100 bpm (or within patient's normal range); no significant changes in mental status; and orientation to person, place, and time (within patient's normal range).

- Monitor and record VS and I&O; record color and consistency of catheter drainage at least q8hr. Drainage may be dark red after surgery, but it should lighten to pink or blood-tinged within 24 hr. **Note:** Patients who have undergone TURBT may have clots passing through the drainage tubing. Continuous bladder irrigation (CBI) is often used to flush bloody drainage from the bladder to prevent clot formation, which can occlude the urethral catheter. For more information about patient care of patients who have CBI, see "Benign Prostatic Hypertrophy," p. 656.
- Be alert to hypotension and rapid HR, and watch for bright red, thick drainage or drainage that does not lighten after irrigation, any of which can signal arterial bleeding within the operative area and necessitate immediate surgical intervention.
- Monitor TURBT patient's postoperative mental status, being alert to changes in mentation, such as confusion, which can denote a change in electrolyte balance and necessitate medical intervention. Water intoxication and

hyponatremia (as evidenced by headache, lassitude, apathy, confusion, weakness, hypertension, muscle spasms, convulsions, coma) can occur because of possible systemic absorption of the high volumes of irrigation water that are used with a TUR.

⊙ NIC: Bladder Irrigation; Bleeding Precautions; Circulatory Precautions; Fluid/Electrolyte Management; Urinary Elimination Management

Risk for infection with risk factors related to an invasive procedure (presence of ureteral, suprapubic, urethral catheter) or increased environmental exposure (opening of a closed drainage system)
Desired outcome: Patient is free of infection as evidenced by WBCs ≤11,000/mm^3; normothermia; no significant change in mental status; and orientation to person, place, and time (within patient's normal range).
- Using sterile technique, cleanse the area surrounding ureteral or suprapubic catheter with an antimicrobial solution, such as povidone-iodine. Apply one or more sterile 4 × 4 split gauze pads (drain sponges) over the catheter exit site, and tape securely. Change these dressings as soon as they become wet; use a pectin wafer skin barrier to protect insertion site if indicated. **Note:** If a trocar system is used, clean around the plastic cover and keep the area dry. Tape plastic edges securely to the skin to prevent accidental removal.
- Wash hands *before* and *after* manipulating the catheter, and use sterile technique when opening closed drainage systems, changing dressings, or irrigating the catheter.
- Irrigate the catheter *only* if an obstruction is present and with the prescription of the health care provider.
- Protect the catheter by keeping it securely taped to the patient's lateral abdomen or flank.
- If the catheter is accidently pulled out of the insertion site, immediately cover the site with a sterile 4 × 4 gauze pad and call the health care provider.
- To keep the urine dilute to help prevent UTI, encourage fluid intake of ≥3 L/day in nonrestricted patients.
- Keep drainage collection container below the level of the patient's bladder to prevent infection from reflux of urine.
- See also **Altered urinary elimination** related to obstruction or positional problems of the ureteral catheter, p. 167.

⊙ NIC: Teaching: Disease Process; Tube Care: Urinary; Urinary Elimination Management; Vital Signs Monitoring; Wound Care

Risk for infection with risk factors related to an invasive procedure or use of intravesical chemotherapy
Desired outcome: Patient is free of infection as evidenced by WBCs ≤11,000/mm^3, normothermia, and orientation to person, place, and time (within patient's normal range).
- Using sterile technique, insert a straight or indwelling catheter into the bladder.
- Slowly instill the ordered chemotherapy agent (usually over 30 minutes), and remove the catheter.
- Instruct the patient to remain flat in bed but to turn from side to side to ensure distribution of the chemotherapy drug over all of the surfaces of the bladder.
- Instruct the patient not to void—to hold the chemotherapeutic agent in the bladder—for as long as possible (at least for 2 hr).
- Frequently assess the patient for comfort needs, and provide emotional support.
- After 2 hr, request that the patient void; collect and dispose of the urine as per hospital protocol for the agent in use.

- To reduce bladder irritation after the chemotherapy agent has been voided, instruct the patient to drink as much fluid as possible (2.5-3 L/day) for 48 hr after the intravesical therapy.
- Instruct the patient about the side effects of medications:
  —BCG may cause influenza-like symptoms
  —Mitomycin, thiotepa, and doxorubicin may cause chemical cystitis with symptoms of frequency, urgency, and burning. In addition, mitomycin may cause a rash on the palms and genitals.
- Instruct the patient to notify the health care provider if the above symptoms do not resolve within 48 hr, if he or she develops a fever ($\geq 100°$ F) or symptoms of UTI (e.g., chills; fever; hematuria; flank, CVA, low back, buttock, scrotal, or labial pain; cloudy and foul-smelling urine; frequency; and urgency), or if hematuria is noted.
- Anticipate use of antispasmodics, NSAIDs, or urinary antiseptics to aid the patient in dealing with pain or discomfort.

NIC: Chemotherapy Management; Emotional Support; Teaching: Disease Process; Urinary Elimination Management; Vital Signs Monitoring

Altered urinary elimination related to obstruction of suprapubic catheter or anuria/dysuria secondary to removal of catheter
Desired outcome: Patient's urinary output is appropriate for the amount of intake within 3 days after surgery.
- Keep separate drainage records for all catheters and drains.
- Prevent external obstruction of the catheter, assessing frequently for patency. Irrigate *only* if catheter is internally obstructed and *only* with health care provider prescription.
- Before removal of suprapubic catheter, health care provider may request a 3- to 4-hr clamping routine to assess patient's ability to void normally. The catheter is clamped for 3-4 hr, and the patient is asked to void. After patient has voided, unclamp the catheter and measure the residual urine that flows into the drainage collection container. Once the residual urine is <100 ml after each of two successive voidings, notify health care provider. Usually the catheter can be removed at that time.
- After removal of the catheter, evaluate patient's ability to void by recording the time and amount during the first 24 hr. Patients with partial cystectomy will void frequently and in small amounts at first because the bladder capacity is approximately 60 ml. Explain to the patient that the bladder capacity will increase to 200-400 ml within a few months.
- If patient cannot void 8-12 hr after catheter removal and experiences abdominal pain or has a distended bladder, notify health care provider for intervention.
- Obtain specimen for urine culture as prescribed if patient complains of burning, urgency, or frequency. The culture will differentiate between sterile pyuria and bacterial cystitis.

NIC: Fluid Management; Teaching: Disease Process; Tube Care: Urinary; Urinary Habit Training

---

See Also: "Urinary Tract Obstruction" for **Pain** related to bladder spasms, p. 171; Appendix One, "Caring for Preoperative and Postoperative Patients," p. 717, and "Caring for Patients With Cancer and Other Life-disrupting Illnesses," p. 747 (in particular, **Altered urinary elimination** related to hemorrhagic cystitis secondary to cyclophosphamide treatment; oliguria or renal toxicity secondary to cisplatin or high-dose methotrexate administration; or dysuria secondary to cystitis, p. 790).

PATIENT-FAMILY TEACHING AND DISCHARGE PLANNING

When providing patient-family teaching, focus on sensory information; avoid giving excessive information; and initiate a visiting nurse referral for necessary follow-up teaching. Consider including verbal and written information about the following:

- Medications, including drug name, purpose, dosage, route, schedule, drug/drug and food/drug interactions, precautions, and potential side effects.
- Indicators of complications from photodynamic therapy, such as redness or swelling over areas exposed to sun, the importance of reporting them to health care provider, and the necessity of avoiding sun exposure for 4-6 wk after the last treatment.
- Expectations of severe urinary frequency and urgency, blood-tinged urine, and dysuria during the first week after cauterization or catheterization.
- Indicators of UTI that necessitate medical attention: chills; fever; hematuria; flank, CVA, low back, buttock, scrotal, or labial pain; cloudy and foul-smelling urine; frequency; and urgency.
- When appropriate, provide a referral to hospice or agency that provides home help. This should occur before discharge planning begins to ensure continuity of care between the hospital and home. Information on local support groups may be obtained from:

  The American Cancer Society
  1599 Clifton Road NE
  Atlanta, GA 30329   (800) ACS-2345
  WWW address: *http://www.cancer.org*

- Phone numbers to call should questions or concerns arise about hospice after discharge. Information for these patients can be obtained by contacting:

  National Hospice Association
  1901 North Moore St., Suite 901
  Arlington, VA 22209   (703) 243-5900; (703) 525-5762 FAX
  WWW address: http://www.nho.org/

- Phone numbers to call should questions or concerns arise about therapy or disease after discharge. Additional general information can be obtained by contacting:

  National Kidney and Urologic Diseases Information Clearinghouse
  3 Information Way,
  Bethesda, MD 20892-3580   (301) 907-8906 FAX

  National Kidney Foundation
  30 E. 33rd Street, 11th Floor
  New York, NY 10016   (800) 622-9010; (212) 689-9261 FAX
  WWW address: *http://www.nephron.com/NKF.html*

Section Six: Urinary Disorders Secondary to Other Disease Processes

Urinary incontinence

Urinary incontinence occurs when an individual experiences involuntary loss of urine. The ability to urinate requires complex interactions between nerve pathways, the detrusor muscle, the internal sphincter, the external sphincter, and a urethral pressure higher than bladder pressure. Because incontinence occurs when bladder pressure exceeds urethral resistance, structural or musculature weakness or damage places an individual at increased risk. A spinal cord lesion above S2 through S4 may result in loss of sensation or awareness of bladder filling because of interruption of the nerve pathways. Thus the bladder acts in response to bladder pressure, which becomes higher than that in the urethra. Urinary incontinence can be short term, caused by an acute illness, or it can be chronic. General causes can be classified as interference with neural control (e.g., cerebrovascular accident [CVA], spinal cord injury [SCI]); interference with bladder function (e.g., inflammatory states, loss of or increased contractility, constipation or impaction); interference with urethral sphincter mechanism (e.g., stress incontinence in women, posttransurethral resection of the prostate [TURP] incontinence in men); and environmental interferences (e.g., radiation therapy, medications such as diuretics or anticholinergics). These conditions manifest as stress, urge, overflow, or functional incontinence or as combinations of two factors.

ASSESSMENT

Signs and symptoms: Polyuria; dysuria; low back or flank pain; loss of urine with increased intraabdominal pressure, such as during laughing, sneezing, coughing, lifting; involuntary urination occurring soon after the urge to void is sensed; involuntary passage of urine occurring at predictable intervals; inability to reach the commode in time when environmental barriers exist or disorientation occurs; nocturia.

History of: Neurologic dysfunctions, such as Parkinson's disease, CVA, brain injury, normal pressure hydrocephalus, SCI or spinal cord lesions, multiple sclerosis (MS); acute or chronic diminishing of cerebral functioning; abdominal or bladder surgery; radiation therapy for bladder cancer; meningitis; impaired mobility; diabetes mellitus (as a result of autonomic neuropathy and decreased detrusor contractility); multiparity; fecal impaction; low back syndrome; and use of caffeine or alcohol. History should include investigating use of such medications as diuretics; anticholinergics and adrenergic agents; psychotropics, antidepressants, antiparkinsonian agents, phenothiazines, antispasmodics, narcotic analgesics, sedatives, hypnotics, and CNS depressants.

Voiding problems may be verified via use of a diary in which the patient documents and describes duration, frequency, volume, and type of incontinence as well as fluid intake. An evaluation is made of environmental and social factors that may affect continence, such as access to toilets, living arrangements, and caregiver availability.

Mental status examination: To assess cognitive ability and the ability to identify the need for toileting and the desire to self-toilet.

Functional assessment: To assess manual dexterity (ability to handle clothing fasteners), mobility (ability to get to a toilet), and ability to perform toileting behaviors unaided.

Social factors: To assess living and working conditions; or to assess caregiver-provided care for the patient.

DIAGNOSTIC TESTS

Urinalysis: To provide baseline data on the functioning of the urinary system, detect metabolic disease, and assess for the presence of urinary tract infection (UTI). A cloudy or hazy appearance, foul odor, pH >8.0, and presence of RBCs, leukocyte esterase, WBCs, and WBC casts are indicative of UTI. **Note:** Obtain urine sample before rectal or genital examination. Urine collected after either examination may be contaminated by vaginal or prostatic secretions.

Urine culture: To determine the type of bacteria present in the genitourinary tract. To minimize the risk of contamination, a specimen should be obtained from a midstream collection.

Urodynamic studies: To evaluate cause and extent of the incontinence.

Uroflowmetry: To provide information about bladder strength and the opening ability of the urethral sphincter. If detrusor muscle contraction is adequately coordinated with sphincter relaxation, resistance to outlet flow will decrease as the pressure within the bladder increases. A normal flow rate in males is 20-25 ml/sec, whereas in females the normal is 20-30 ml/sec. A flow rate ≤15 ml/sec indicates voiding dysfunction. The force of the urine stream is tested, using a specially designed commode.

Cystometry: To measure the pressure-volume relationship of the bladder. The bladder is filled at a rate of 50 ml/min to the maximum capacity of the bladder. In a normal individual the bladder will fill smoothly without contractions and empty when the individual desires. Cystometry provides information on the patient's bladder capacity, the bladder's ability to accommodate fluid, the patient's ability to sense bladder filling (and temperature of fluid instilled), and the presence of an appropriate detrusor muscle contraction.

Urethral pressure profile: Most helpful in detecting stress incontinence, this test identifies the amount of closing pressure the urethra can produce, via a dual-tip, microtip, pressure-sensitive catheter, which enables simultaneous measurement of the intraurethral and intravesical pressures. The urethral pressure profile identifies either weakness or excessive response in either the internal or external voluntary sphincter.

Sphincter electromyography: To evaluate the function of the striated urinary sphincter. Results of this test are compared with the results from cystometry to identify abnormalities in coordination between the bladder and sphincter function.

Postvoid residual: To measure amount of urine in the bladder after a normal voiding. Amounts >100 ml imply retention problems.

BUN and creatinine: Serum values increase as renal-urinary function declines. **Note:** These values can be affected by hydration status and age. Fluid volume deficit can falsely increase the values, whereas fluid volume excess can decrease the values. Creatinine values may be misleading in the older adult because of the loss of muscle mass and decreased glomerular filtration rate.

COLLABORATIVE MANAGEMENT

Behavioral interventions

Bladder training: Incorporation of a progressively increased time interval between voidings. The patient is taught to resist the urge to void and thus delay voiding until a set time. Intervals are set close together initially and then further apart. Fluid intake also is adjusted. The goal with bladder training is reduction of small voidings and thus more normal bladder function.

Habit training: The patient voids according to a set schedule on a planned basis. The schedule is set according to the patient's voiding habits. The goal is for the patient to remain dry. Habit training differs from bladder training in that there is no attempt to encourage the patient to resist or delay voiding, and the caregiver takes the initiative in maintaining the schedule and toileting the patient.

Prompted voidings: In addition to habit training, the caregiver checks the patient regularly, asks whether he or she is wet or dry, and then requests that the patient use the toilet. If successful, positive feedback about maintaining continence is given; if unsuccessful, the caregiver gives no feedback. This technique is used with cognitively impaired or dependent individuals. The goal is to have the patient recognize incontinent status and learn to ask for assistance when needed.

Catheter drainage of urine: Either intermittent or continuous.

Vaginal cones: Cone-shaped devices of varying weights may be used to improve pelvic muscle tone and strength in females. The cones are inserted intravaginally (light ones first), and the patient must retain the device for 15 min bid. The cone's weight may provide heightened proprioceptive information to achieve the desired pelvic muscle contraction as well as increase pelvic muscle strength.

Pelvic muscle (Kegel) exercise program: To increase strength of voluntary periurethral and pelvic muscles via exercise of the pubococcygeus muscle. These exercises, which must be performed frequently during the day (i.e., 100 times), are done by tightening the paravaginal muscles and anal sphincter as though controlling urination or defecation.

Fluid intake: At least 2-3 L/day in nonrestricted patients.

External (condom) catheter: For male patients, if appropriate.

Surgical procedures to restore bladder-urethral structure: Many surgical procedures may be employed to reestablish normal vesicourethral structure. Examples of the most common are the following:

Urethral suspension (Marshall-Marchetti-Krantz; Stamey) procedure: For stress incontinence. A retropubic urethrovesical resuspension is accomplished via suprapubic transverse incision to lengthen the urethra, thereby creating resistance in the urethral lumen. The *Pereyra* procedure uses both vaginal and suprapubic approaches. Use of Teflon paste injected into the periurethral tissues, to increase urethral resistance, also is being tried.

Pubovaginal sling urethropexy: After harvesting a small strip of rectus fascia through a small suprapubic incision, a transvaginal approach is used. The area lateral to the urethra is joined to the junction of the pelvic floor and overlying symphysis pubis.

Artificial urinary sphincter: See p. 189.

Medications used for urge incontinence: Anticholinergics or smooth muscle relaxants, such as Imipramine or oxybutynin, may be prescribed to inhibit uncontrolled bladder contractions and enhance functional bladder capacity. **Note:** Anticholinergics must be used cautiously in the older adult because they can increase the occurrence of acute confusion.

Medications used for stress incontinence: α-Adrenergic drugs, such as pseudoephedrine, ephedrine, or phenylpropanolamine, assist smooth muscle contraction of the bladder neck. Estrogen therapy, which decreases muscle atrophy, is given to improve urgency and frequency.

NURSING DIAGNOSES AND INTERVENTIONS

Note: Patients with urinary incontinence may have overlapping conditions. For example, they may experience functional incontinence, which is made more severe by UTI superimposed on urge incontinence.

Stress incontinence related to degenerative changes or weakness in pelvic muscles and structural supports secondary to menopause, childbirth, obesity, or surgical procedure interfering with normal vesicourethral structure

Desired outcome: After implementation of bladder training program, patient becomes continent.

Bladder training program

- Assess and document the patient's voiding pattern: time, amount voided, amount of fluid intake, timing of fluid intake followed by voiding, and related information such as the degree of wetness experienced (e.g., number of incontinence pads used in a day, degree of underwear dampness) and the exertion factor causing the wetness (e.g., laughing, sneezing, bending, lifting). Teach patient to keep a voiding diary that incorporates this information.
- Determine the amount of time between voidings to estimate how long the patient can hold urine. Establish a voiding schedule that does not exceed this time period.
- Assist patient with scheduling times for emptying the bladder, such as (initially) q1-2hr when awake and q4hr at night. If successful, attempt to

lengthen the time intervals between voiding. Provide patient and significant other with a written copy of the schedule. **Note:** Patients need to empty their bladders at least q4hr to reduce the risk of UTI caused by urinary stasis.

- Estimate and document urinary output when patient is incontinent in clothes or bed linens. For example, a wet spot of approximately 2 inches in diameter is equal to approximately 5 ml urine.
- Teach patient techniques that strengthen the sphincter and structural supports of the bladder, such as the Kegel exercises (see **Knowledge deficit,** p. 183).
- In nonrestricted patients, encourage a fluid intake of at least 2-3 L/day. Be aware that patients with urinary incontinence often will reduce their fluid intake to avoid incontinence at the risk of dehydration and UTI.
- Educate patient about dietary irritants (e.g., caffeine, alcoholic beverages) that may increase stress incontinence.

NIC: Fluid Management; Nutrition Management; Teaching: Prescribed Activity/Exercise; Urinary Bladder Training; Urinary Elimination Management

Urge incontinence related to bladder irritation or reduced bladder capacity secondary to radiation treatment for bladder cancer, UTI, increased urine concentration, use of caffeine or alcohol, or enlarged prostate
Desired outcome: After implementation of the toileting program, patient becomes continent.

- Assess and document patient's usual pattern of voiding, including frequency and timing of incontinent episodes.
- Adhere to the toileting program (see interventions with **Stress incontinence,** earlier).
- Teach nonrestricted patient to increase fluid intake to ≥3 L/day but to avoid caffeinated drinks or alcohol, which are natural diuretics and bladder irritants.
- Explain the types of fluids patient should drink that are not irritating to the bladder, such as water, fruit juices, herbal drinks, and decaffeinated sodas, teas, and coffees.
- Encourage intake of cranberry juice, prunes, and plums, which leave an acid ash in the urine to minimize the occurrence of UTI.
- Teach patient to keep a voiding record for at-home use, documenting accurate information about frequency and timing of incontinent episodes.
- Encourage patient to decrease fluid intake a few hours before bedtime and to void before sleep.
- Keep a urinal or bedpan at the bedside, and instruct patient in its use.
- Teach patient deep, slow breathing technique, which can be used when the urge to void occurs prematurely.
- If the patient is ambulatory but has a cognitive impairment, label the bathroom door with signs that denote *toilet* to the patient, such as a picture of a commode. Adhere closely to the toileting program, reminding patient to void at the scheduled intervals.
- Administer prescribed anticholinergics or smooth muscle relaxants, which inhibit detrusor contractions or decrease detrusor instability.

NIC: Fluid Management; Nutritional Counseling; Teaching: Prescribed Activity/Exercise; Urinary Bladder Training; Urinary Elimination Management

Functional incontinence related to sensory, cognitive, or mobility deficits or related to environmental changes
Desired outcome: After implementation of habit training program, the patient becomes continent.

- Assess and document patient's pattern of voiding: time, amount voided, amount of fluid intake, timing of fluid intake followed by voiding, and other related factors.
- Determine environmental obstacles that would prevent patient from toileting appropriately, and intervene accordingly. For example, remove obstacles

between the bed and bathroom, leave a light on in the bathroom, attach the call light to the bed sheet.

- Assess patient's bowel status for the potential for constipation, which causes straining and weakens sphincter tone.
- Monitor patient for the increased need to void after taking medications such as diuretics, which increase urine production or the sensation of urgency.

Habit training
- Based on the assessed pattern of incontinence, establish a planned schedule for voiding.
- Offer bedpan, urinal, or assistance to the bathroom at least q2hr.
- Maintain the planned schedule for voiding, and note the time of any incontinent episode that occurs between the scheduled voidings. If the patient's incontinence pattern consistently does not match the voiding schedule, change the voiding schedule.

In addition
- Administer diuretics in the morning or early afternoon to reduce the risk of nighttime incontinence.
- If the patient has an intravenous infusion, consult with health care provider about advisability of reducing the infusion rate at night.
- For bedridden patients, keep call light within patient's reach and answer call quickly.
- For confused patients, keep a clock and calendar in the room and remind patient of the time and date as appropriate. Toilet patient as described above. If the patient is acutely confused, calmly let the patient know that you do not see or hear what he or she does, but do not argue (e.g., if the patient cries, "Help, I'm in jail," you might say, "It must feel like jail being tied to all these tubes"). This approach, rather than constantly trying to reorient the patient, will minimize her or his agitation until the underlying cause of the disorientation has been resolved. When the patient is calm, you can reorient to the environment, but if he or she becomes agitated, stop the attempt to reorient.
- If the patient has permanent or severe cognitive impairment, reorient to his or her baseline and toilet the patient as described previously.
- Monitor patient's bowel function and status, because constipation or impaction can cause symptoms of incontinence (e.g., dribbling).

NIC: Constipation/Impaction Management; Delirium Management; Fluid Management; Medication Management; Nutritional Counseling; Urinary Habit Training

Risk for impaired skin integrity with risk factors associated with incontinence of urine
Desired outcome: Patient's perineal skin remains intact.
- Assess the patient for wetness of the perineal area at frequent intervals. Inform the patient that prolonged exposure to urine can cause maceration and to alert staff as soon as wetness occurs.
- Keep bed linen dry. As necessary, use and change absorbent materials, such as protective underwear or underpads.
- Keep the perineum clean with mild soap and water; dry it well.
- Expose the perineum to air whenever possible by using a sheet draped over a bed cradle; ensure the patient's privacy.
- Use sealants and moisture-barrier ointments to protect the patient's skin.
- Make sure that plastic pads or sheet protectors do not contact the patient's skin directly because maceration can result from the increased perspiration they cause. Cover these pads with pillow cases, or place them under the sheets.

- Educate patient in the use of containment devices, such as briefs with pads, adult absorptive briefs, and external catheters.
- Initiate habit or bladder training to reduce episodes of incontinence.

NIC: Perineal Care; Teaching: Disease Process; Urinary Bladder Training; Urinary Habit Training

Body image disturbance related to odor, discomfort, and embarrassment secondary to incontinence
Desired outcomes: After intervention(s), patient verbalizes feelings and frustrations without self-deprecating statements. Within the 24-hr period before hospital discharge, patient verbalizes knowledge about actions that will control either incontinence or odor and discomfort.
- Encourage patient to discuss feelings and frustrations.
- Offer reassurance and encouragement, and provide information about treatment, especially about those activities that are within the patient's own control.
- Be realistic with the patient; if incontinence cannot be controlled, reassure patient that odor and discomfort *can* be controlled.
- Explore with patient the methods for relief of discomfort and odor control: maintenance of good hygiene, frequent changes of undergarments, use and frequent changes of incontinence pads.
- Although fluid intake of at least 2-3 L/day is essential for minimizing the risk of UTI, suggest that patient limit fluids when away from the home environment and increase them on return. A decrease also should be incorporated into the evening hours to prevent nighttime incontinence.
- For additional information, see this nursing diagnosis in Appendix One, "Caring for Patients With Cancer and Other Life-disrupting Illnesses," p. 773. Additional resources include:

  The American Cancer Society
  1599 Clifton Road NE
  Atlanta, GA 30329   (800) ACS-2345
  WWW address: *http://www.cancer.org*

  National Cancer Institute Information Service (CIS)
  Bldg. 31, Room 10A16
  9000 Rockville Pike
  Bethesda, MD 20892   (800) 422-6237
  WWW address: *http://www.meds.com/pdq/cancerlinks.html/*

NIC: Body Image Enhancement; Counseling; Emotional Support; Support Group

Knowledge deficit: Pelvic muscle (Kegel) exercise program to strengthen perineal muscles (effective for individuals with mild to moderate stress incontinence or for those with functional incontinence who are able to participate)
Desired outcome: Within the 24-hr period before hospital discharge, patient verbalizes and demonstrates knowledge about the pelvic muscle (Kegel) exercise program.
- Explain that Kegel exercises will strengthen the pelvic area muscles, which will help regain bladder control.
- Assist patient with identifying the correct muscle group:
  —To strengthen the proximal muscle, instruct patient to attempt to shut off urinary flow after beginning urination, hold for a few seconds, and then start the stream again. Explain to patient that if this can be accomplished, the correct muscle is being exercised.
  —To strengthen the distal muscle, teach patient to contract the muscle around the anus as though to stop a bowel movement.

> Note: A common error when attempting to identify the correct muscle group is contraction of the buttocks, quadriceps, and abdominal muscles.

- For female patients it is possible to make a cast of the vagina from which an elastic mold can be created. This mold can be attached to a manometer and then allows the patient visual evidence of her ability to contract the muscles in the pelvic floor to compress the vagina. Using this device allows for quantitative feedback on the relative strength of the woman's muscle contraction and empiric evidence of progress in strengthening these muscles.
- Teach the patient to repeat these exercises 10-20 times, 4 times/day. Advise the patient that these exercises may need to be done for 2-9 mo before any benefit is obtained.

NIC: Exercise Promotion; Pelvic Floor Exercise; Teaching: Prescribed Activity/Exercise; Teaching: Psychomotor Skill

Knowledge deficit: Use of external (condom) catheter
Desired outcomes: Within the 24-hr period before hospital discharge, patient or significant other successfully returns demonstration of condom catheter application and verbalizes knowledge about the rationale for its use.

> Note: Both external and internal catheters should be used only if other methods of achieving urinary incontinence have failed, because both are associated with an increased incidence of UTI.

- Instruct male patients or significant other in the procedure for application of a condom catheter.
- Teach the importance of keeping pubic hair trimmed or moved away from the penis to avoid contact with the adhesive used with the catheter.
- Instruct patient to cleanse and dry the penis thoroughly before and after every condom application. With uncircumcised patients, the foreskin should be retracted to cleanse the area under the prepuce and then returned to its original position.
- Teach patient or significant other to monitor skin under the external device daily for redness, rashes, or open areas.
- For ambulatory patients, demonstrate connecting the condom catheter to a leg drainage bag; for patients on bedrest, demonstrate connecting the catheter to a bedside urinary collection container, such as that used with an indwelling catheter.
- Advise patient to remove and replace the catheter as directed. Most manufacturers recommend that external catheters be changed and replaced daily.
- If appropriate for the patient, suggest that the condom catheter be used only during the night.

NIC: Skin Surveillance; Teaching: Prescribed Activity/Exercise; Teaching: Psychomotor Skill

> See Also: "Neurogenic Bladder" for **Reflex incontinence,** p.189; for surgical patients, nursing diagnoses and interventions in Appendix One, "Caring for Preoperative and Postoperative Patients," p. 717; in particular, **Risk for infection** related to presence of indwelling urinary catheter, p. 732.

PATIENT-FAMILY TEACHING AND DISCHARGE PLANNING

When providing patient-family teaching, focus on sensory information; avoid giving excessive information; and initiate a visiting nurse referral for necessary

follow-up teaching. Consider including verbal and written information about the following:

- Medications, including drug name, dosage, purpose, schedule, drug/drug and food/drug interactions, precautions, and potential side effects.
- Diet, including importance of increasing dietary fiber to help prevent constipation and keep stools soft. Provide a fact sheet that lists foods high in fiber. Demonstrate with sample menus how dietary fiber may be incorporated into daily meals.
- Indicators of UTI that necessitate medical attention: chills; fever; hematuria; flank, CVA, low back, buttock, scrotal, or labial pain; cloudy and foul-smelling urine; frequency; urgency; dysuria; increasing or recurring incontinence.
- Care of catheters and drains if the patient is discharged with them.
- Importance of maintaining fluid intake of at least 3 L/day and avoiding caffeine and alcohol, which act as bladder irritants and increase the risk of urgency.
- Maintenance of schedule for bladder training program.
- Use of perineal muscles to improve bladder tone.
- Care of perineal skin.
- Phone numbers to call should questions or concerns arise about therapy after discharge.
- Refer patient to support groups (see **Body image disturbance,** p. 183) or:

> Help for Incontinent People (HIP)
> P.O. Box 544
> Union, SC 29379   (800) BLADDER
> WWW address: *http://www.modernmedicine.com/geri/pein*

> Simon Foundation
> Box 815
> Wilmette, IL 60091   (800) 23-SIMON.

For surgical patients
- Care of the incision, including cleansing and dressing; and indicators of infection: fever, tenderness, purulent drainage, persistent redness, swelling, warmth along incision line.
- Activity restrictions: no heavy lifting (>10 lb) and resting when fatigued. Explain that prolonged periods of sitting can cause relaxation of the musculature of the bladder and sphincter, leading to incontinence. Encourage mild activity, such as walking, to improve muscle tone.

Urinary retention

When urine is produced and accumulates in the bladder but is not released, the condition is called *urinary retention.* In the acute care setting, urinary retention is most commonly seen as a postoperative complication after surgical procedures using general or spinal anesthesia. Another major cause is obstruction (e.g., from benign prostatic hypertrophy, tumor, calculi, urethral stricture, fibrosis, meatal stenosis, or fecal impaction). Other causes include decreased sensory stimulation to the bladder, anxiety, or muscular tension. Medications such as opiates, sedatives, antihistamines, antispasmodics, major tranquilizers and antidepressants, and antidyskinetics also can interfere with the normal micturition reflex.

ASSESSMENT

Signs and symptoms: Sudden inability to void, intense suprapubic pain, restlessness, diaphoresis, voiding small amounts (20-50 ml) at frequent intervals.

Physical assessment: "Kettle drum" sound with bladder percussion, bladder distention, bladder displacement to one side of the abdomen.

DIAGNOSTIC TESTS

Urinalysis: Provides baseline data regarding urinary system function, detects metabolic disease, and evaluates for the presence of urinary tract infection (UTI). A cloudy or hazy appearance, foul odor, pH >8.0, and the presence of RBCs, leukocyte esterase, WBCs, and WBC casts are all signals of UTI.

Urine culture: To determine the type of bacteria present in the genitourinary tract. To minimize contamination, a midstream specimen should be collected.

BUN and creatinine: To evaluate renal-urinary function. Generally, serum values increase in the presence of dysfunction. **Note:** BUN values are affected by the patient's hydration status: fluid volume excess can result in decreased values, whereas volume deficit can result in increased values. Creatinine may not be a reliable indicator of renal function in the older adult because of decreased muscle mass and decreased glomerular filtration rate.

Urinary function tests: To evaluate cause of the urinary retention.

Cystoscopy: A lighted, tubular scope is inserted into the bladder to allow visualization of potential sources of obstruction, e.g., strictures, calculi, malformations, or masses.

Cystogram: Radiopaque dye is instilled into the bladder via cystoscope or catheter to enable visualization of the bladder and evaluation of the vesicoureteral reflex.

Cystometrogram: Water or saline is instilled into the bladder via a catheter to create pressure against the bladder wall to evaluate bladder tone.

Kidney, ureter, bladder (KUB) radiography: Used diagnostically, this x-ray identifies the size, shape, and position of the kidneys, ureters, and bladder and abnormalities such as tumors, calculi, or malformations.

Excretory urograms/intravenous pyelogram: To visualize the kidney, renal pelvis, ureters, and bladder to evaluate for the cause of urinary dysfunction.

COLLABORATIVE MANAGEMENT

Catheterization: To drain urine.

Pharmacotherapy

Cholinergics: To stimulate bladder contractions.

Analgesia: To relieve pain.

Antibiotics: If infection is present.

IV therapy: For hydration of the acutely ill patient.

Surgery: Performed if obstruction is the cause of the retention (see "Urinary Tract Obstruction," p. 170).

NURSING DIAGNOSES AND INTERVENTIONS

Urinary retention related to weak detrusor muscle, blockage, inhibition of reflex arc, or strong sphincter

Desired outcome: Patient reports a normal voiding pattern within 2 days; or, if appropriate, the patient demonstrates self-catheterization before hospital discharge.

- Assess the bladder for distention by inspection, percussion, and palpation; measure and document I&O.
- If appropriate, try noninvasive measures to aid the patient in voiding: position patient in a normal position for voiding; have patient listen to the sound of running water or place hands in a basin of warm water. If these measures are ineffective, try pouring warm water over the perineum (if monitoring output, measure the warm water first to be able to determine

the amount of voided urine). Avoid use of the Credé method (pressure applied from the umbilicus to the pubis) because of the potential for reflux up the ureters.

- Maintain privacy for patient who is trying to use the commode, bedpan, or urinal. Remember that cold bedpans can cause muscle tension, so use a plastic bedpan or warm a metal bedpan under warm running water before giving it to the patient. Encourage relaxation technique, such as deep breathing or visualization.
- Provide an adequate amount of time (up to 10 min) for the patient's urge to void to occur. Do not rush the patient.
- Notify health care provider if patient is unable to void, has bladder distention, or has suprapubic or urethral pain.
- Monitor the patient's bowel function and status, inasmuch as constipation or impaction can cause urinary retention.
- If catheterization is prescribed, monitor patient's BP and HR during the procedure. If the patient complains of abdominal pain or has a symptomatic drop of >20 mm Hg systolic BP, clamp the catheter until patient's BP returns to within normal limits. Research has demonstrated that rapid bladder decompression of >750-1000 ml does not result in shock syndrome as previously believed. For additional information see **Risk for fluid volume deficit** related to postobstructive diuresis in "Urinary Tract Obstruction," p. 171.
- Catheterization may be difficult through the donut-like prostate gland at the base of the bladder in men with benign prostatic hypertrophy (BPH) or in those over age 65, a large percentage of whom have undiagnosed BPH. For these patients, use a coudé (bent tip) catheter instead of a straight catheter. The tip on this catheter is stiff and does not bend against an obstacle. Lubricate the catheter tip generously with a minimum of 5 ml of lubricating jelly before insertion. Insert the catheter with the bent tip pointing up to aid its movement through the urethra.
- Teach patient the technique for intermittent self-catheterization, if appropriate. Catheterization should be accomplished on a set q4hr schedule to prevent bladder distention, which can injure the bladder mucosa and increase the risk of infection. Teach the patient clean technique for use at home.

NIC: Self-Care Assistance: Toileting; Teaching: Prescribed Activity/Exercise; Teaching: Psychomotor Skill; Urinary Catheterization: Intermittent; Urinary Retention Care

> **See Also:** "Urinary Tract Obstruction" for **Risk for fluid volume deficit** related to postobstructive diuresis, p. 171, and **Pain** related to bladder spasms, p. 171; "Neurogenic Bladder" for **Dysreflexia** related to distended bladder, p. 191.

PATIENT-FAMILY TEACHING AND DISCHARGE PLANNING

When providing patient-family teaching, focus on sensory information; avoid giving excessive information; and initiate a visiting nurse referral for necessary follow-up teaching. Consider including verbal and written information about the following:

- Medications, including drug name, purpose, dosage, schedule, drug/drug and food/drug interactions, precautions, and potential side effects.
- Indicators of UTI and recurrent retention that necessitate medical attention: chills; fever; hematuria; flank, CVA, suprapubic, low back, buttock, scrotal, or labial pain; cloudy and foul-smelling urine; frequency; urgency; dysuria; increasing or recurring incontinence; and recurring or increasing difficulty in voiding.
- Self-catheterization technique, if appropriate.

Neurogenic bladder

Neurogenic bladder, also known as *neuromuscular bladder dysfunction*, *neurologic bladder dysfunction*, or *neuropathic bladder disorder*, is a complex phenomenon resulting from disruption of nerve impulse transmission from the bladder to the brain. Caused by a myriad of diseases, injuries, or lesions, interruption of transmission can be found in the central nervous system within either the brain or spinal cord. Certain conditions leave the sacral reflex intact while affecting the brain's ability to receive or interpret the signal.

Conditions such as multiple sclerosis (MS), cerebrovascular accident (CVA), dementia, tumors, and spinal cord lesions above level T12 lead to reflex or uninhibited bladder control. Interruption of the signal at the spinal level leads to an autonomic neurogenic bladder, from which the patient has no sensation of the need to void and no micturition reflex. Voiding occurs irregularly and has no voluntary control. Lack of nerve impulse transmission for muscle control results in loss of bladder contraction, leading to overflow incontinence. Conditions leading to overflow incontinence include sacral cord trauma, tumors, transection of the pelvic parasympathetic nerves during abdominal surgery, and herniated intervertebral disk disease. Loss of the sensation to void results in atonic bladder as evidenced by dribbling, voiding in small amounts, or complaints of loss of sensation of bladder fullness. Atonic bladder occurs with damage to the posterior (sensory) nerve roots or neuropathy associated with diabetes mellitus.

ASSESSMENT

Upper motor neuron disturbance (spastic bladder):   Urinary frequency, residual urine, urinary retention, recurrent urinary tract infections (UTIs), spontaneous loss of urine, urge incontinence, and lack of urinary control.
Lower motor neuron disturbance (flaccid bladder):   Urinary retention, recurrent UTIs, inability to perceive the need to void.
History of: Spinal cord injury (SCI), spinal tumor, MS, diabetes mellitus, CVA, Parkinson's disease, Alzheimer's disease, herpes zoster.

DIAGNOSTIC TESTS

Urinalysis: To provide baseline data on the functioning of the urinary system, detect metabolic disease, and assess for the presence of UTI. A cloudy or hazy appearance, foul odor, pH >8.0, and presence of RBCs, leukocyte esterase, WBCs, and WBC casts are indicative of UTI.
Urine culture: To determine the type of bacteria present in the genitourinary tract. To minimize the risk of contamination, a specimen should be obtained from a midstream collection.
Urodynamic studies: To evaluate cause and extent of the incontinence.
Uroflowmetry: To provide information about bladder strength and the opening ability of the urethral sphincter. If detrusor muscle contraction is adequately coordinated with sphincter relaxation, resistance to outlet flow will decrease as the pressure within the bladder increases. A normal flow rate in males is 20-25 ml/sec, whereas in females the normal is 20-30 ml/sec. A flow rate ≤15 ml/sec indicates voiding dysfunction. The force of the urine stream is tested, using a specially designed commode.
Cystometry: To measure the pressure-volume relationship of the bladder. The bladder is filled at a rate of 50 ml/min to its maximum capacity. In a normal individual the bladder will fill smoothly without contractions and empty when the individual desires. Cystometry provides information on the patient's bladder capacity, the bladder's ability to accommodate fluid, the patient's ability to sense bladder filling (and temperature of fluid instilled), and the presence of an appropriate detrusor muscle contraction.
Urethral pressure profile: Most helpful in detecting stress incontinence, this test identifies the amount of closing urethral sphincteric pressure. The urethral

pressure profile identifies either weakness or excessive response in either the internal or external voluntary sphincter. For a description of this test, see "Urinary Incontinence," p. 179.

Sphincter electromyography: To evaluate the function of the striated urinary sphincter. Results of this test are compared with the results from cystometry to identify abnormalities in coordination between the bladder and sphincter function.

BUN and creatinine: Serum values increase as renal-urinary function declines. **Note:** These values can be affected by hydration status and age. Fluid volume deficit can falsely increase the values, whereas volume excess can decrease the values. Creatinine values may be misleading in the older adult because of the loss of muscle mass and decreased glomerular filtration rate.

Excretory urography/intravenous pyelogram (IVP): To enable visualization of the kidneys, renal pelvis, ureters, and bladder to determine cause of the dysfunction.

Postvoid residual: The patient is catheterized 15-20 min after voiding to assess for residual urine (amounts >100 ml imply urinary retention).

Cystoscopy: To determine loss of muscle fibers and elastic tissue.

COLLABORATIVE MANAGEMENT

Pharmacotherapy

Parasympatholytics or anticholinergics (e.g., propantheline bromide and oxybutynin chloride): To treat hyperreflexive neurologic conditions.

Parasympathomimetics (e.g., bethanechol chloride): To treat hypotonic bladders by increasing bladder tone.

Intravesicular oxybutynin chloride: To increase bladder capacity and decrease intravesicular pressure.

Antibiotics: For infection, if indicated.

Catheterization: Either intermittent or continuous.

Increase fluid intake: To prevent infection, minimize calcium concentration in urine, and prevent formation of urinary calculi (ideally, 3 L/day).

Increase patient mobility: To augment renal blood flow and minimize urinary stasis.

Low-calcium diet: To prevent calculus formation.

Neuroprosthetics (bladder pacemaker): Electrodes are implanted on the ventral (motor) nerve roots of the sacral nerves that will produce detrusor contraction when stimulated. These electrodes are then connected to a subcutaneous receiver that can be controlled from outside the body. The bladder can be controlled selectively by the external transmitter.

Continent vesicostomy: Surgical closure of urethral neck of the bladder to form an internal reservoir for urine and create an opening or valve in the bladder wall so that the patient can insert a catheter intermittently to remove urine.

Artificial urinary sphincter implantation: Surgical placement of a hydraulically activated sphincter mechanism around the bladder neck or urethra. To empty the bladder, patient activates the device by squeezing the bulbs, which are implanted under the labia or in the scrotum.

NURSING DIAGNOSES AND INTERVENTIONS

Reflex incontinence related to neurologic impairment secondary to injury or disease that affects the transmission of signals from the reflex arc in the lower spinal cord to the cerebral cortex

Desired outcomes: The patient or significant other participates in a habit training program. Patient experiences a decrease in or absence of incontinent episodes.

Habit training program

- Assess patient's voiding pattern: time, amount voided, amount of fluid intake, timing of fluid intake followed by voiding, and other related factors.

- Determine the amount of time between voidings to estimate the amount of time patient can hold urine. Establish a voiding schedule that does not exceed this period. Post the voiding schedule on the patient's care plan and, unobtrusively, at the patient's bedside.
- Regulate fluids to achieve adequate hydration and a desirable voiding pattern. For example, teach patient to drink measured amounts of fluids (e.g., 8 oz q2hr) and attempt to void 30 min later, based on voiding schedule.
- Teach patient to reduce fluid intake during the evening to reduce incontinence at night.
- Assist patient with scheduling times for emptying the bladder, such as q1-2hr when awake and q4hr at night. If successful, attempt to lengthen the time intervals between voidings. Provide patient and significant other with a written copy of the schedule.

In addition

- Monitor for bladder retention by assessing I&O, inspecting the suprapubic area, and percussing and palpating the bladder. Be alert to the presence of swelling proximal to the symphysis pubis, a "kettle drum" sound (or sound like tapping on the side of a plastic gallon container of milk) with percussion of the lower abdomen, and dribbling of urine.
- As appropriate, teach patient techniques that stimulate the voiding reflex. Examples include tapping the suprapubic area with the fingers, pulling the pubic hair, or digitally stretching the anal sphincter. The latter is effective because the rectal nerves follow basically the same path as the urethral nerves; however, this maneuver is contraindicated in patients with an SCI at or above T6 because it can cause autonomic dysreflexia (see next nursing diagnosis). The Valsalva maneuver also can be used to stimulate voiding: the patient bears down as though having a bowel movement to increase intrathoracic and intraabdominal pressure.
- If an artificial inflatable sphincter is used, instruct the patient to deflate the valve q4hr, which allows the bladder to empty. Remind the patient to wear a Medic-Alert tag or bracelet to alert emergency personnel to the presence and use of the device.
- If a condom catheter is used, see **Knowledge deficit:** Use of external (condom) catheter in "Urinary Incontinence," p. 184, for appropriate nursing interventions.
- For males with extensive sphincter damage, a penile clamp might be prescribed. Before and after use, instruct patient (or significant other) to cleanse the penis with soap and water, dry it thoroughly, and sprinkle powder along the shaft. Explain that the clamp is placed horizontally behind the glans after voiding, and removed q3hr. Stress the importance of inspecting the skin for redness along the area in which the clamp presses. If breakdown occurs (i.e., redness does not disappear after massage), the clamp must be discontinued. If swelling appears along the glans, advise patient to set the clamp at a looser setting. **Caution:** Minimize the potential for injury by alternating the penile clamp with a condom catheter.
- If intermittent catheterization is prescribed, teach the procedure to the patient or significant other. Emphasize the need to follow a routine (e.g., q4hr) to minimize the potential for UTI caused by stasis and bladder distention.
- In nonrestricted individuals, encourage a fluid intake of at least 3 L/day, which dilutes the urine and increases output, thereby minimizing the risk of developing an infection and calculi.
- To help prevent urinary stasis, which can lead to UTI, and to increase cardiac output, which nourishes the kidneys, encourage as much mobility as the patient can tolerate.
- If diuretics are prescribed, administer them in the morning or early afternoon to reduce the risk of nighttime incontinence.

- If the patient has an intravenous infusion, consult with health care provider about advisability of reducing infusion rate at night to minimize the risk of nighttime incontinence.
- If the patient has a permanent cognitive impairment, use visual clues, such as a sign on the bathroom door that says *toilet* or a picture of a toilet.

NIC: Skin Surveillance; Teaching: Psychomotor Skill; Urinary Catheterization: Intermittent; Urinary Habit Training; Urinary Retention Care

Dysreflexia (or risk for same) related to distended bladder
Desired outcomes: Patient is free of the indicators of autonomic dysreflexia (AD) as evidenced by HR ≥60 bpm, BP within patient's normal limits, skin dry and of normal color above the level of SCI (if appropriate), normal vision, and absence of headache, nausea, piloerection (goose bumps) below the level of injury (if appropriate), and nasal congestion. Patient/ significant other verbalize understanding of the indicators, prevention, and treatment of AD.

Caution: Autonomic dysreflexia is a life-threatening condition that can occur in patients with neurogenic bladder, especially those with SCI at or above level T8.

- Be alert to the following indicators of AD: headache, bradycardia, excessively high BP, blurred vision, flushing and sweating above the level of injury, piloerection and pallor below the level of injury, and nausea.
- If signs of AD occur, raise the HOB immediately to help lower the BP, and assess for bladder distention. Have the patient empty the bladder in the accustomed manner, or check for patency of the indwelling catheter. **Caution:** Irrigation of the urinary catheter can increase bladder pressure and intensify the AD. If the catheter is obstructed, either recatheterize the patient using liberal amounts of anesthetic jelly or irrigate the catheter gently, using ≤30 ml normal saline. Follow agency policy.
- Monitor patient's BP for trends. Be aware that continuing increases in BP can be life threatening, leading to CVA, status epilepticus, and death.
- Administer appropriate medications as prescribed, such as phenoxybenzamine hydrochloride, a long-acting vasodilator that increases blood flow to the skin, mucosa, and abdominal viscera and lowers both standing and supine BP. Notify health care provider if symptoms do not disappear after the bladder is emptied, if the bladder is full and cannot be emptied, or if the medication does not relieve symptoms.
- Encourage a fluid intake of at least 3 L/day, which dilutes the urine and increases output, thereby minimizing the risk of developing an infection, calculi, and associated AD.
- To help prevent urinary stasis, which can lead to UTI and consequently to AD, encourage as much mobility as the patient can tolerate.
- Monitor bowel elimination patterns to reduce risk of impaction; fecal impaction can cause AD itself or contribute to urinary retention leading to AD.
- Teach patient and significant others the indicators, prevention, and treatment of AD and the importance of seeking help immediately if indicators occur.
- For additional information about AD, see **Dysreflexia (or risk of same)** in "Spinal Cord Injury," p. 261.

NIC: Bowel Management; Dysreflexia Management; Neurologic Monitoring; Surveillance: Safety; Urinary Elimination Management

Total incontinence related to neuropathy preventing transmission of reflex indicating bladder fullness or related to lower motor neuron disturbance secondary to SCI below S3-S4

Desired outcomes: Patient or significant other follows habit training program; incontinent episodes decrease to less than 3/wk.

Habit training program
- Assess and document patient's voiding pattern: time, amount voided, amount of fluid intake, timing of fluid intake followed by voiding, and other related factors.
- Determine the amount of time between voidings to estimate how long the patient can hold urine. Establish a voiding schedule that does not exceed this time period.
- Assist patient with scheduling times for emptying the bladder, such as q1-2hr when awake and q4hr at night. If successful, attempt to lengthen the time intervals between voiding. Post schedules for nursing staff, and provide patient and significant other with a written copy of the schedule.
- If the patient takes fluids orally, provide the necessary amounts for optimal hydration (3 L/day) during the day and decrease the amount given during the evening and nighttime hours.
- Provide information about incontinence aids, such as incontinence pads and easy-to-remove clothing.
- For male patients, demonstrate use of external (condom) catheters for nighttime use (see p. 184).

In addition
- Administer diuretics in the morning or early afternoon to reduce the risk of nighttime incontinence.
- If the patient has an intravenous infusion, consult with health care provider about advisability of reducing the infusion rate at night.

NIC: Teaching: Prescribed Activity/Exercise; Teaching: Psychomotor Skill; Urinary Elimination Management; Urinary Habit Training

Knowledge deficit: Function and care of long-term indwelling catheters after continent vesicostomy (continent urinary reservoir)

Desired outcomes: Before continent vesicostomy, patient verbalizes rationale for the use of a suprapubic catheter and vesicostomy tube, including the approximate amount of time they will be indwelling. Within the 24-hr period before hospital discharge, patient or significant other demonstrates proficiency with intermittent catheterization, tube irrigation, and dressing changes.
- Preoperatively, explain that the patient will return from surgery with a suprapubic catheter and vesicostomy tube in place.
- Explain that the patient will be discharged with the catheter and readmitted for catheter removal in approximately 6 wk. After removal of the indwelling catheter, intermittent catheterization will be performed hourly, progressing to 2-4 hr and ultimately to 4-6 hr. Continuous drainage will be used overnight. After removing the indwelling catheter, ensure that the patient or significant other demonstrates proficiency with the following:
  —Washing hands with soap and water before catheterization.
  —Selecting a clean catheter, and placing it on a clear paper towel.
  —Cleaning the stoma site with warm water and removing mucus that has drained from the stoma.
  —Inserting the catheter carefully into the stoma, and draining the bladder of urine. Lubricants usually are not necessary. If lubrication is needed, however, teach patient to use one that is water soluble—*never* products made from petroleum jelly, which can damage the catheter.
  —If mucus clogs the catheter, removing the catheter from the stoma, rinsing it with hot water, and reinserting the catheter to continue the drainage.

- Encourage patient's participation in care, including tube irrigation, which removes mucus from the pouch, and dressing changes. When prescribed, demonstrate the procedure for irrigation. Typically, sterile normal saline (30-50 ml) is used for irrigation. Instruct the patient to wash hands before handling the catheters to help prevent contamination and to cleanse around the catheter site daily with warm water.

NIC: Teaching: Preoperative; Teaching: Prescribed Activity/Exercise; Teaching: Psychomotor Skill

> See Also: As appropriate, "Urinary Incontinence" for **Risk for impaired skin integrity,** p. 182, and **Body image disturbance,** p. 183.

PATIENT-FAMILY TEACHING AND DISCHARGE PLANNING

When providing patient-family teaching, focus on sensory information; avoid giving excessive information; and initiate a visiting nurse referral for necessary follow-up teaching. Consider including verbal and written information about the following:

- For patients with artificial sphincters, the indicators of UTI and erosion: pain, fever, swelling, urinary retention, or incontinence.
- Phone numbers to call should questions or concerns arise about therapy or this condition after discharge. Additional general information can be obtained by contacting:

National Kidney and Urologic Diseases Information Clearinghouse
3 Information Way
Bethesda, MD 20892-3580   (301) 907-8906 FAX

National Kidney Foundation
30 E. 33rd Street, 11th Floor
New York, NY 10016   (800) 622-9010; (212) 689-9261 FAX
WWW address: *http://www.nephron.com/NKF.html*

- For more information, see this discussion in "Urinary Incontinence," p. 184.

Section Seven: Urinary Diversions

When the bladder must be bypassed or is removed, a urinary diversion is created. Urinary diversions most commonly are created for individuals with bladder cancer. However, malignancies of the prostate, urethra, vagina, uterus, or cervix may require the creation of a urinary diversion if anterior, posterior, or total pelvic exenteration must be done. Individuals with severe, nonmalignant urinary problems, such as radiation damage to the bladder, vesicovaginal fistula, urethrovaginal fistula, neurogenic bladder, radiation or interstitial cystitis, or urinary incontinence that cannot be managed conservatively, also are candidates for urinary diversion. A radical cystectomy may or may not accompany the placement of a urinary diversion. Although most urinary diversions are permanent, some act as a temporary bypass of urine, and undiversion (reversal) can be performed if the patient's condition changes.

The urinary stream may be diverted at multiple points: the renal pelvis (pyelostomy or nephrostomy); the ureter (ureterostomy); the bladder (vesicostomy); or via an intestinal "conduit." Cutaneous ureterostomy was the diversion most commonly performed in the past. Vesicostomies are most commonly performed in children as a temporary diversion. Construction of a small bowel pouch (Kock procedure) or ileocolonic pouch (Indiana or Mainz procedure) is now the most common type of urinary diversion. These procedures reconstruct a new bladder from intestinal segments, resulting in a more normal urinary pattern. In addition, because males have an external urinary sphincter that can be left in place when the bladder is removed, men may undergo attachment of a reconstructed bladder to the urethra, which will enable urination without the use of catheterization. However, there is a 5%-10% risk of urethral recurrence of neoplasm with this procedure.

Intestinal (ileal) conduit: Any segment of bowel may be used to create a passageway for urine, but the ileum conduit is most commonly used. A 15-20 cm section of the ileum is resected from the intestine to form a passageway for the urine. The proximal end is closed, and the distal end is brought out through the abdomen, forming a stoma. The ureters are resected from the bladder and anastomosed to the ileal segment. The intestine is reanastomosed, and therefore bowel function is unaffected. Occasionally jejunum is used for the conduit. However, jejunal-conduit syndrome (hyperkalemia, hyponatremia, hypochloremia) frequently occurs.

Cutaneous ureterostomy: The ureters are resected from the bladder and brought out through the surface of the abdomen, either separately or with one attached to the other inside the body, resulting in only one abdominal stoma. Typically, the stoma is flush with the abdomen rather than protruding. Stenosis and ascending urinary tract infections (UTIs) are a common problem with this diversion.

Continent urinary diversion: There are several different continent procedures, but the two that are most commonly performed are the Indiana reservoir and the Kock continent urostomy. All continent urinary diversions are constructed with the following three components: a reservoir or reconstructed bladder, a continence mechanism, and an antireflux mechanism. For example, the Indiana reservoir uses 15-18 cm of the distal ileum and 20-24 cm of the cecum sutured together to create the pouch, which stores eventually up to 800 ml of urine. The antireflux mechanism is established via use of the ileocecal valve, which acts as a one-way valve keeping urine in the reservoir until a catheter is passed through the skin-level stoma. The presence of a tapered ileal segment further strengthens the continence mechanism by creating increased resistance to urine outflow pressures. The ureters are attached at an angle to the wall of the cecum, preventing reflux of urine to the kidneys.

Orthotopic urinary diversion: Creates a pseudobladder from the ileum to which the urethra is attached to reestablish lower urinary tract function. Because this procedure requires an intact and functional external urethral sphincter, it is possible more frequently in males.

NURSING DIAGNOSES AND INTERVENTIONS

Anxiety related to threat to self-concept, interaction patterns, or health status secondary to urinary diversion surgery

Desired outcome: Before surgery, patient communicates fears and concerns, relates the attainment of increased psychologic and physical comfort, and exhibits effective coping mechanisms.

- Assess patient's perceptions of his or her impending surgery and resulting body function changes. Provide opportunities for patient to express fears and concerns (e.g., "You seem very concerned about next week's surgery"). Listen actively to the patient. Recognize that anger, denial, withdrawal, and demanding behaviors may be coping responses.
- Acknowledge patient's fears and concerns.
- Provide brief, basic information regarding physiology of the procedure and the equipment that will be used after surgery, including tubes and drains.
- Show patient pouches that will be used after surgery. Assure patient that the pouch usually cannot be seen through clothing and that it is odor resistant.

- For patient about to undergo a continent urostomy, explain that a pouching system may be needed for a short time after surgery. Reassure patient that teaching about accessing the continent urostomy will be done before hospital discharge.
- Discuss ADL with patient. Inform patient that showers, baths, and swimming can continue and that diet is not affected after the early postoperative period.
- As appropriate, ask patient what information has been relayed by the surgeon about the sexual implications of the surgery. This will help establish an open relationship between the patient and primary nurse and inform the nurse if the patient has understood the information given by the surgeon. Some males undergoing radical cystectomy with urinary diversion may become impotent, but recent surgical advances have enabled preservation of potency for others. The pelvic plexus, which innervates the corpora cavernosa (allowing penile erection), may be damaged permanently. Autonomic nerve damage results in loss of erection and ejaculation; however, because sensation and orgasm are mediated by the pudendal nerve (sensorimotor), they are not affected.
- Arrange for a visit by the enterostomal therapy (ET) nurse during the preoperative period. Collaborate with the surgeon, ET nurse, and patient to identify and mark the most appropriate site for the stoma. Showing the patient the actual spot for placement may help alleviate anxiety by reinforcing that the impact on life-style and body image will be minimal.

NIC: Active Listening; Anxiety Reduction; Ostomy Care; Sexual Counseling; Teaching: Preoperative

Altered protection related to neurosensory, musculoskeletal, and cardiac changes secondary to hyperchloremic metabolic acidosis with hypokalemia (can occur secondary to reabsorption of Na^+ and Cl^- from the urine in the ileal segment, which results in compensatory loss of K^+ and HCO_3^-)

Desired outcomes: Patient verbalizes orientation to person, place, and time (within patient's normal range) and remains free of injury caused by neurosensory, musculoskeletal, and cardiac changes. Electrolytes remain within normal limits.

- For patients with ileal conduits, assess for indicators of hypokalemia and metabolic acidosis, including nausea and changes in LOC (ranging from sleepiness to combativeness), muscle tone (ranging from convulsions to flaccidity), and irregular HR. Monitor results of serum electrolyte studies.
- If patient is confused or exhibits signs of motor dysfunction, keep the bed in the lowest position and raise the side rails. If convulsions appear imminent, pad the side rails of the bed. Notify health care provider of significant findings.
- Encourage oral intake as directed, and assess for the need for IV management. The health care provider may prescribe IV fluids with K^+ supplements.
- If patient is hypokalemic and allowed to eat, encourage foods high in K^+, such as bananas, cantaloupes, and apricots. See Table 3-4 for other foods that are high in K^+.
- Encourage patient to ambulate by the second or third day after surgery. Mobility will help prevent urinary stasis, which increases the risk of electrolyte problems.

NIC: Electrolyte Management; Neurologic Monitoring; Peripheral Sensation Management; Respiratory Monitoring; Surveillance; Teaching: Prescribed Diet

Risk for impaired skin integrity with risk factors from the presence of urine or sensitivity to the appliance material

Desired outcome: Patient's peristomal skin remains nonerythematous and intact.

- For patient with significant allergy history, patch-test the skin for a 24-hr period, at least 24 hr before ostomy surgery, to assess for allergies to the different tapes that might be used on the postoperative appliance. If erythema, swelling, bleb formation, itching, weeping, or other indicators of tape allergy occur, document the type of tape that caused the reaction and note on the cover of the chart "Allergic to _____ tape."

- Inspect the integrity of the peristomal skin with each pouch change, and question the patient about the presence of itching or burning, which can signal leakage. Change the pouch routinely (per agency or surgeon preference) or immediately if leakage is suspected.
- Assess for inflamed hair follicles (folliculitis) or a reaction to the tape. Report the presence of a rash to the health care provider, since this often occurs with a yeast infection and will require topical medication.
- Assess the stoma, pouch, or skin for crystalline deposits, which are signals of alkaline urine.
  —Teach patient to monitor urine pH every week and to maintain pH <6.0.
  —Teach patient to decrease urine pH by drinking fluids that leave acid ash in the urine, such as cranberry or orange juice, or taking ascorbic acid in a dose consistent with patient's size.
  —Teach patient signs of ascorbic acid toxicity: nausea, vomiting, heartburn, diarrhea, flushing, and insomnia.
- When changing the pouch, measure the stoma with a measuring guide and ensure that the opening of the skin barrier is cut to the exact size of the stoma to protect the peristomal skin. Protect the skin from maceration caused by pooling of urine on the skin:
  —*For a patient using a two-piece system or pouch with a barrier*: Size the barrier to fit snugly around the stoma. If using a barrier and attaching an adhesive pouch, size the barrier to fit snugly around the stoma and size the pouch to clear the stoma by at least ⅛ inch.
  —*For a patient using a one-piece "adhesive-only" pouch*: If the pouch has an antireflux valve, size the pouch to clear the stoma and any peristomal creases so that the pouch adheres to a flat, dry surface. An antireflux valve prevents pooling of urine on the skin. If the pouch does not have an antireflux valve, size the pouch so that it clears the stoma by ⅛ inch to prevent stomal trauma while minimizing the amount of exposed skin. Use a copolymer film sealant wipe on peristomal skin before applying adhesive-only pouch. This will provide a moisture barrier and reduce epidermal trauma when the pouch is removed.
- Wash the peristomal skin with water or a special cleansing solution marketed by ostomy supply companies. Dry the skin thoroughly before applying the skin barrier and pouch.
- When changing the pouch, instruct the patient to hold a gauze pad on (but not in) the stoma to absorb the urine and keep the skin dry.
- After applying the pouch, connect it to the bedside drainage system if the patient is on bedrest. When the patient is no longer on bedrest, empty the pouch when it is one-third to one-half full by opening the spigot at the bottom of the pouch and draining the urine into the patient's measuring container. Do not allow the pouch to become too full, because this could break the seal of the appliance with the patient's skin. Instruct the patient accordingly.
- Change the incisional dressing as often as it becomes wet, using sterile technique.
- Teach patient to treat peristomal skin irritation in the following ways after hospital discharge:
  —Dry the skin with a hair dryer on a cool setting.
  —Dust the peristomal skin with an absorptive powder (e.g., karaya or Stomahesive).
  —If desired, blot the skin with water or a sealant wipe to seal in the powder.
  —Use a porous tape to prevent moisture trapping.
  —Notify health care provider or ET nurse of any severe or nonresponsive skin problems.

◎ NIC: Medication Administration: Topical; Ostomy Care; Skin Care: Topical Treatments; Skin Surveillance; Teaching: Psychomotor Skill

Impaired stomal tissue integrity (or risk of same) related to altered circulation
Desired outcome: Patient's stoma is pink or bright red and shiny. The stoma of a cutaneous urostomy is raised, moist, and red.
- Inspect the stoma at least q8hr and as indicated. The stoma of an ileal conduit will be edematous and should be pink or red in color with a shiny appearance. A stoma that is dusky or cyanotic in color is indicative of insufficient blood supply and impending necrosis and must be reported to the health care provider immediately.
- Also assess the degree of swelling, and inform the patient that the stoma will shrink considerably over the first 6-8 wk and less significantly over the next year. For patients with ileal conduit, evaluate stomal height and plan care accordingly (see **Risk for impaired skin integrity,** p. 195). The stoma formed by a cutaneous ureterostomy is usually raised during the first few weeks after surgery, red in color, and moist.

◎ NIC: Skin Surveillance; Teaching: Disease Process; Teaching: Individual

Altered urinary elimination related to postoperative use of ureteral stents, catheters, or drains and to urinary diversion surgery
Desired outcome: Patient's urinary output is $\geq$30 ml/hr, and the urine is clear, straw-colored, and with normal, characteristic odor.
- Monitor color, clarity, and volume of urine output via stoma, stents, and/or catheter.
    - —*Ureterostomy*: Urine drainage via stoma and/or ureteral stents.
    - —*Intestinal conduit*: Urine drainage via stoma. The patient also may have ureteral stents and/or conduit catheter/stent in the early postoperative period to stabilize the ureterointestinal anastomoses and maintain drainage from the conduit during early postoperative edema.
    - —*Continent urinary diversions or reservoirs*: The Kock urostomy usually has a reservoir catheter and also may have ureteral stents. The Indiana (ileocecal) reservoir usually has ureteral stents exiting from the stoma through which most of the urine drains and may have a reservoir catheter exiting from a stab wound, which serves as an overflow catheter. The continent urinary diversion with urethral anastomosis will have a urethral catheter in place that will drain urine, which initially will be light red to pink in color with mucus but should clear in 24-48 hr. This catheter generally remains in place for 21 days to ensure adequate healing of the anastomosis.
- Monitor for evidence of anastomotic breakdown/intraabdominal urine leakage, which may occur in an individual with intestinal conduit or continent diversion: decreasing urinary output from stoma or stents, flank or abdominal pain, increasing abdominal distention, and increasing drainage from wound drains.
- Monitor functioning of the ureteral stents, which exit from the stoma into the pouch. These stents maintain the patency of the ureters and assist in the healing of the anastomosis. Right stents usually are cut at a 90-degree angle, and left stents are cut at a 45-degree angle. Each usually produces approximately the same amount of urine, although the amount produced by each is not important as long as each drains adequately and total drainage from all sources is $\geq$30 ml/hr. Urine is usually red to pink for the first 24-48 hr and becomes straw-colored by the third postoperative day. Absent or lessening amounts of urine may indicate a blocked stent or problems with the ureter. **Note:** Stents may become blocked with mucus. As long as urine is draining adequately around the stent and the volume of output is adequate, this is not a problem.

- Monitor functioning of the stoma catheters. In continent urinary diversions, a catheter is placed in the reservoir to prevent distention and promote healing of the suture lines. This new reservoir (i.e., resected intestine) exudes large amounts of mucus, necessitating irrigation of the catheter with 30-50 ml of normal saline, which is instilled gently and allowed to empty via gravity. Expect the output to include pink or light red urine with mucus and small red clots for the first 24 hr. Urine should become amber colored with occasional clots within 3 postoperative days. Mucus production will continue but should decrease in volume.
- Monitor functioning of the drains. Any urinary diversion may have Penrose drains or closed drainage systems in place to facilitate healing of the ureterointestinal anastomosis. Excessive lymph fluid and urine can be removed via these drains to reduce pressure on the anastomotic suture lines. Drainage from drainage systems may be light red to pink in color for the first 24 hr and then lighten to amber color and decrease in amount. In a continent urinary diversion, an increase in drainage after amounts have been low might signal an anastomotic leak. Notify health care provider if this occurs.
- Monitor I&O, and record the total amount of urine output from the urinary diversion for the first 24 hr postoperatively. Differentiate and record separately amounts from all drains, stents, and catheters. Notify health care provider of an output <60 ml during a 2-hr period, because in the presence of adequate intake this can indicate a ureteral obstruction, a leak in one of the anastomotic sites, or impending renal failure. Assess for other indicators of ureteral obstruction: flank pain, costovertebral angle (CVA) tenderness, nausea, vomiting, and anuria.
- Monitor drainage from Foley catheter or urethral drain (if present). Patients who have had a cystectomy may have a urethral drain, whereas those with a partial cystectomy will have a Foley catheter in place. Note color, consistency, and volume of drainage, which may be red to pink with mucus. Report sudden increase (which would occur with hemorrhage) or decrease (which can signal blockage that can lead to infection or, with partial cystectomy, hydronephrosis). Report significant findings to health care provider.
- Advise patient who has had a cystectomy that after removal of urethral catheter or drain, mucus drainage will continue from the urethral meatus for several months.
- To keep the urinary tract well irrigated, encourage an intake of at least 2-3 L/day in the nonrestricted patient.

NIC: Bladder Irrigation; Bleeding Precautions; Tube Care: Urinary; Urinary Elimination Management; Wound Care: Closed Drainage

Risk for infection with risk factors related to an invasive surgical procedure and risk of ascending bacteriuria with urinary diversion
Desired outcome: Patient is free of infection as evidenced by normothermia, WBC count $\leq 11,000/mm^3$, and absence of purulent or excessive drainage, erythema, edema, warmth, and tenderness along the incision.

- Monitor the patient's temperature q4hr during the first 24-48 hr after surgery. Notify health care provider of fever (>101° F).
- Inspect the dressing frequently after surgery. Infection is most likely to become evident after the first 72 hr. Assess for the presence of purulent or excessive drainage on the dressing, and notify health care provider accordingly. Change the dressing when it becomes wet, using sterile technique. Use extra care to prevent disruption of the drains.
- Note the condition of the incision. Be alert to indicators of infection, including erythema, tenderness, local warmth, edema, and purulent or excessive drainage.
- Monitor and record the character of the urine at least q8hr. Mucus particles are normal in the urine of patients with ileal conduits and continent urinary

diversions because of the nature of the bowel segment used. Cloudy urine, however, is abnormal and can signal an infection. The urine should be yellow or pink-tinged during the first 24-48 hr after surgery. Assess for other indicators of UTI, including flank or CVA pain, malodorous urine, chills, and fever.

- Note the position of the stoma relative to the incision. If they are close together, apply the pouch first to avoid the overlap of the pouch with the suture line, which can increase the risk of infection. If necessary, cut the pouch down on one side or place it at an angle to avoid contact with drainage, which may loosen the adhesive. To help prevent contamination and cross-contamination, wash your hands before and after caring for the patient.
- Patients with cystectomies without anastomosis to the urethra may have an indwelling urethral catheter to drain serosanguineous fluid from the peritoneal cavity. **Caution:** Do not irrigate this catheter, because irrigation can result in peritonitis.
- Encourage a fluid intake of at least 2-3 L/day because this helps flush urine through the urinary tract, removing mucus shreds and preventing stasis.

NIC: Fluid Management; Infection Protection; Tube Care: Urinary; Urinary Catheterization; Wound Care

Knowledge deficit: Self-care regarding urinary diversion
Desired outcome: Patient or significant other demonstrates proper care of stoma and urinary diversion before hospital discharge.

- Assess patient's or significant other's readiness to participate in care.
- Involve ET nurse in patient teaching if available.
- Assist patient with organizing the equipment and materials that are needed to accomplish home care. Usually the patient is discharged with disposable pouching systems. Most of these patients continue using disposable systems for the long term. Those who will use reusable systems usually are not fitted for 6-8 wk after surgery.
- Teach patient how to remove and reapply pouch, how to empty it, and how to use gravity drainage system at night, including procedures for rinsing and cleansing the drainage system.
- Teach patient the signs and symptoms of UTI, peristomal skin breakdown, and the appropriate therapeutic responses, including maintenance of an acidic urine (if not contraindicated), the importance of adequate fluid intake, and techniques for checking urine pH, which should be assessed weekly. Explain that urine pH should remain ≤6.0. Persons with urinary diversion have a higher incidence of UTI than the general public, so it is important to keep their urinary pH acidic. If it is >6.0, advise patient to increase fluid intake and, with health care provider approval, to increase vitamin C intake to 500-1000 mg/day, which will increase urine acidity.
- Teach patient with continent diversion the technique for reservoir catheter irrigation.
- Teach patient with continent urinary diversion with urethral anastomosis the signals of the urge to void: (1) feeling of vague abdominal discomfort and (2) feeling of abdominal pressure or cramping.
- Instruct patient with continent urinary diversion with urethral anastomosis about the procedure to void: relax the perineal muscles and employ Valsalva's maneuver.
- Emphasize the importance of follow-up visits, particularly for those patients with continent urinary diversions, who will be taught how to catheterize the reservoir and use a small dressing over the stoma rather than an appliance.
- Provide patient with a list of ostomy support groups and ET nurses in the area for referral and assistance.

- Provide patient with enough equipment and materials for the first week after hospital discharge. Remind patient that proper cleansing of ostomy appliances will reduce the risk of bacterial growth and decrease the risk of UTI.

NIC: Discharge Planning; Skin Surveillance; Teaching: Prescribed Activity/ Exercise; Teaching: Prescribed Medication; Teaching: Psychomotor Skill

---

See Also: "Fecal Diversions" for **Body image disturbance,** p. 461; nursing diagnoses and interventions in Appendix One, "Caring for Preoperative and Postoperative Patients," p. 717; and "Caring for Patients With Cancer and Other Life-disrupting Illnesses," p. 747.

PATIENT-FAMILY TEACHING AND DISCHARGE PLANNING

When providing patient-family teaching, focus on sensory information; avoid giving excessive information; and initiate a visiting nurse referral for necessary follow-up teaching. Consider including verbal and written information about the following:

- Medications, including drug name, dosage, schedule, drug/drug and food/ drug interactions, precautions, and potential side effects.
- Indicators that necessitate medical intervention: fever or chills; nausea or vomiting; abdominal pain, cramping or distention; cloudy or malodorous urine; incisional drainage, edema, local warmth, pain or redness; peristomal skin irritation; or abnormal changes in stoma shape or color from the normal bright and shiny red.
- Maintenance of fluid intake at least 2-3 L/day to maintain adequate kidney function.
- Monitoring of urine pH, which should be checked weekly. Urine pH should remain at ≤6.0. Individuals with urinary diversions have a higher incidence of UTI than the general public, so it is important to keep their urinary pH acidic. If it is >6.0, advise patient to increase fluid intake and, with health care provider approval, to increase vitamin C intake to 500-1000 mg/day, which will increase urine acidity
- Care of stoma and application of urostomy appliances. The patient should be proficient in the application technique before hospital discharge.
- Care of urostomy appliances. Remind patient that proper cleansing will reduce the risk of bacterial growth, which would contaminate the urine and increase the risk of UTI.
- Importance of follow-up care with health care provider and ET nurse. Confirm date and time of next appointment.
- Phone numbers to call should questions or concerns arise about therapy after discharge. In addition, many cities have local support groups. Information for these patients can be obtained by contacting:

United Ostomy Association
19722 MacArthur Blvd., Suite 200
Irvine, CA 92612-2405   (800) 826-0826
WWW address: *http://www.uoa.org/*

The American Cancer Society
1599 Clifton Road NE
Atlanta, GA 30329   (800) ACS-2345
WWW address: *http://www.cancer.org*

National Cancer Institute Information Service (CIS)
Bldg. 31, Room 10A16
9000 Rockville Pike
Bethesda, MD 20892   (800) 422-6237

Selected Bibliography

Arieff AI: Renal disease & the surgical patient. In Way LW, editor: *Current surgical diagnosis and treatment*, ed 10, Norwalk, Conn, 1994, Appleton & Lange.

Ascher NL et al: Organ transplantation. In Way LW, editor: *Current surgical diagnosis and treatment*, ed 10, Norwalk, Conn, 1994, Appleton & Lange.

Bates P, Lewis S: Nursing management: renal and urological problems. In Lewis SM, Collier IC, Heitkemper MM, editors: *Medical-surgical nursing: assessment and management of clinical problems*, ed 4, St Louis, 1996, Mosby.

Cammu H, Van Nylen M: Pelvic floor muscle exercises: 5 years later, *Urology* 45(1):113-118, 1995.

Chan R, Michelis MF: Renal failure: why today's patients live better and longer, *Geriatrics* 51(1):37-40, 1996.

Courtel JV et al: Percutaneous transluminal angioplasty of renal artery stenosis in children, *Pediatr Radiol* 28(1):59-63, 1998.

Derby L, Jick H: Acetaminophen and renal and bladder cancer, *Epidemiology* 7(4):358-362, 1996.

Donovan JF, Williams RD: Urology. In Way LW, editor: *Current surgical diagnosis and treatment*, ed 10, Norwalk, Conn, 1994, Appleton & Lange.

Downie J, Trudel G: The neurogenic bladder: disordered autonomic control, *Phys Med Rehab: State of Art Reviews* 10(1):61-80, 1996.

Games J: Nursing implications in the management of superficial bladder cancer, *Semin Urol Oncol* 14 (1 suppl 1): 36-40, 1996.

Goshorn J: Clinical snapshot: kidney stones, *Am J Nurs* 96(9):40-41, 1996.

Gross J, Johnson B: *Handbook of oncology nursing*, ed 3, Boston, 1998, Jones & Bartlett.

Horne MM: Renal disorders and renal failure. In Swearingen PL, editor: *Pocket guide to medical-surgical nursing*, ed 2, St Louis, 1996, Mosby.

Horne MM, Heitz UE, Swearingen PL, editors: *Pocket guide to fluid, electrolyte, and acid-base balance*, ed 3, St Louis, 1996, Mosby.

Interqual: *The ISD—a review system with adult ISD criteria*, August 1992, Northhamptom, NH, and Marlboro, Mass, Interqual.

Isselbacher K et al, editors: *Harrison's principles of internal medicine*, ed 13, New York, 1995, McGraw-Hill.

Jassal SV, Opelz G, Cole E: Transplantation in the elderly: a review, *Geriatr Nephrol Urol* 7(3):157-165, 1997.

Kelly L, Miaskowski C: An overview of bladder cancer: treatment and nursing implications, *Oncol Nurs Forum* 23(3):459-470, 1996.

Kelly M: Chronic renal failure, *Am J Nurs* 96(1) 36-27, 1996.

Kim MJ, McFarland GK, McLane AM: *Pocket guide to nursing diagnoses*, ed 7, St Louis, 1997, Mosby.

Kurzrock E et al: Fluorourodynamic and clinical evaluation in males following construction of a Kock ileal-urethral reservoir, *Urology* 46(6):801-803, 1995.

Lederer JR et al: *Care planning pocket guide: a nursing diagnosis approach*, ed 5, Redwood City, Calif, 1993, Addison-Wesley.

Matteson M, McConnell E, Linton A: *Gerontological nursing concepts & practice*, ed 2, Philadelphia, 1996, Saunders.

McCloskey J, Bulechek G, editors: *Nursing Interventions Classification (NIC)*, ed 2, St Louis, 1996, Mosby.

Moore S et al: Treating bladder cancer: new methods, new management, *Am J Nurs* 93(5):32-39, 1993.

Morris PJ, editor: *Kidney transplantation: principles and practice*, ed 4, Philadelphia, 1994, Saunders.

Obrador GT, Pereira BJ: Early referral to the nephrologist and timely initiation of renal replacement therapy: a paradigm shift in the management of patients with chronic renal failure, *Am J Kidney Dis* 31(3):398-417, 1998.

Pagana K, Pagana T: *Mosby's diagnostic and laboratory test reference*, ed 3, St Louis, 1997, Mosby.

Peterson K: ACE inhibitors and renoprotection, *J Fam Pract* 42(5): 453, 1996.

Rakel R, editor: *Conn's current therapy: latest approved methods of treatment for the practicing physician*, Philadelphia, 1995, Saunders.

Rose BD: *Clinical physiology of acid-base and electrolyte disorders*, ed 4, New York, 1994, McGraw-Hill.

Seigne J, McDougal W: Urinary diversion, *Surg Oncol Clin North Am* 3(2):307-321, 1994.

Swearingen PL, Howard C: *Addison-Wesley photo-atlas of nursing procedures*, ed 3, Redwood City, Calif, 1996, Addison-Wesley.

Szollar S, Lee S: Intravesical oxybutynin for spinal cord injury patients, *Spinal Cord* 34(5):284-287, 1996.

Tanagho EA, McAninch JW, editors: *Smith's general urology*, ed 14, Norwalk, Conn, 1995, Appleton & Lange.

Tiernery L, McPhee S, Papadakis M, editors: *Current medical diagnosis and treatment*, ed 36, Stamford, Conn, 1997, Appleton & Lange.

US Department of Health and Human Services: *Quick reference guide for clinicians: managing acute and chronic incontinence*, Number 2, Update, Public Health Service, Agency for Health Care Policy and Research, Rockville, Md, March 1996.

US Department of Health and Human Services: *Urinary incontinence in adults: clinical practice guideline*, Public Health Service, Agency for Health Care Policy and Research, Rockville, Md, March 1992.

Weiskittel PD: Renal-urinary dysfunctions. In Swearingen PL, Keen JH, editors: *Manual of critical care: applying nursing diagnoses to adult critical illness*, ed 3, St Louis, 1995, Mosby.

4 NEUROLOGIC DISORDERS

Section One: Inflammatory Disorders of the Nervous System

Inflammation of nervous system tissue results from a wide variety of causes, including bacterial or viral infections, autoimmune processes, or chemical toxins. The inflammatory response may cause increased vascular permeability with exudation of fluids from the vessels, resulting in swelling. Inflammation involving the myelin nerve sheath can cause the destruction or stripping away of the myelin. The resulting demyelinization interferes with the conduction of electric nerve impulses. Inflammation of other brain tissue, such as may occur in acute infectious processes, usually results in swelling, which in turn can cause increased intracranial pressure (IICP) and the potential for brain herniation.

Multiple sclerosis

Multiple sclerosis (MS) was first delineated as an individual disease process by Charcot in the mid-1800s. MS is an inflammatory disorder causing scattered and sporadic demyelinization of the central nervous system (CNS). Myelin permits nerve impulses to travel quickly through the nerve pathways of the CNS. In response to the inflammation, the myelin nerve sheaths scar, degenerate, or separate from the axon cylinders. This demyelinization interrupts electrical nerve transmission and causes the wide variety of symptoms associated with MS. As less severe inflammation resolves, myelin function may regenerate, allowing electric nerve impulse transmission to be restored. If the inflammation is severe and causes irreversible destruction of myelin, the involved areas are replaced by dense glial scar tissue that forms areas of sclerotic plaque, which permanently damage the conductive pathways of the CNS. Nerve fibers may degenerate. Deficits present after 3 mo usually are permanent.

The course of MS is highly variable, with several general categories of progression. Motor or coordination symptoms from onset and/or frequent attacks during the first 2 yr of the disease usually indicate a poorer outlook. In the *benign* form of MS (20% of patients), attacks are few and mild. Complete or nearly complete clearing of symptoms occurs with little or no disability. In the *relapsing-remitting* form (45%), attacks (exacerbations) occur early in the illness and become increasingly frequent. Less complete clearing of symptoms occurs, and there may be relatively long periods of stability (remission). The *relapsing-progressive* form (15%) has fewer remissions, and symptom resolution is less complete after an exacerbation. An increasing number of symptoms occur with each exacerbation, and they become cumulative. In the *chronic-progressive* form (20%), onset usually is insidious and without remissions. A slow, progressive accumulation of symptoms and deficits occurs.

Although the cause of MS is unknown, autoimmune processes, slow-acting viral infections, and allergic reactions to infectious agents, such as viruses, are suspected causes. MS is more common among people living in cool, temperate climates in the United States and Europe. African-Americans have half the incidence of whites. More females than males are affected, sometimes reported as twice as many. Onset is usually between 10-50 yr with peak onset between 20 and 40 yr. It is 12-15 times more common among siblings of individuals who have the disease, suggesting a possible inherited trait or genetic susceptibility. Infection and trauma are common precipitating factors, as are episodes of fatigue and physical or emotional stress. Exacerbations may be fewer during pregnancy but increase immediately postpartum. Heat and fever tend to aggravate symptoms.

ASSESSMENT

Onset of MS can be extremely rapid, causing disability within days, or it can be insidious, with exacerbations and remissions. Signs and symptoms vary widely, depending on the site and extent of demyelinization, and they can change from day to day. Usually, early symptoms are mild.

Damage to motor nerve tracts: Weakness, paralysis, and spasticity. Fatigue is common. Diplopia may occur secondary to ocular muscle involvement.

Damage to cerebellar or brain stem regions: Intention tremor, nystagmus, or other tremors; incoordination, ataxia; weakness of facial and throat muscles resulting in difficulty chewing, dysphagia, and dysarthria. Slurred speech often occurs early, whereas scanning speech (slow speech with pauses between syllables) is usually seen in later stages.

Damage to sensory nerve tracts: Decreased perception of pain, touch, and temperature; paresthesias, such as numbness and tingling; decrease or loss of proprioception; and decrease or loss of vibratory sense. Optic neuritis is an early common symptom, which may cause partial or total loss of vision, visual clouding, and pain with eye movement.

Damage to cerebral cortex (especially frontal lobes):   Mood swings, inappropriate affect, euphoria, apathy, irritability, depression, and hyperexcitability.

Damage to motor and sensory control centers: Urinary frequency, urgency, or retention; urinary and fecal incontinence; constipation.

Sacral cord lesions: Impotence; diminished sensations that result in inhibited sexual response.

Physical assessment: Ophthalmoscopic inspection may reveal temporal pallor of optic disks. Reflex assessment may show increased deep tendon reflexes (DTRs) and diminished abdominal skin and cremasteric reflexes.

DIAGNOSTIC TESTS

Note: MS is sometimes called the "great masquerader." Diagnostic testing is often done to exclude disorders with similar symptoms. The diagnosis of MS usually will be made after other neurologic disorders have been ruled out, when the patient has experienced two or more exacerbations of neurologic symptoms, and when the patient has two or more areas of demyelinization or plaque formation throughout the CNS, as demonstrated by diagnostic tests, such as the MRI and evoked potential studies, or by the patient's clinical symptoms.

MRI: Reveals presence of plaques and demyelinization in the CNS. This is the test of choice when MS is suspected. Once MS has been diagnosed, MRI may be used to monitor response to immunotherapy.

Evoked potential studies: May be slow or absent because of interference of nerve transmission from demyelinization or plaque formation. Stimulation of a sensory organ, such as the eye or ear, or of a peripheral nerve triggers a measurable electrical response (evoked potential) along the visual, auditory, and somatosensory nerve pathways. Measuring these evoked potentials enables evaluation of the integrity of these nerve pathways.

Lumbar puncture (LP) and CSF analysis: Evaluates CSF levels of oligoclonal bands of immunoglobulin G (IgG), protein, γ-globulin, myelin basic protein, and lymphocytes, any of which may be elevated in the presence of MS. Increased γ-globulin levels indicate hyperactivity of the immune system as a result of chronic demyelinization. Oligoclonal bands of IgG are seen in 85%-95% of patients with MS. Although these bands can be elevated in some other inflammatory diseases, they help confirm the diagnosis of MS. Detecting oligoclonal bands of IgG requires examination of the CSF γ-globulin by electrophoresis. During acute MS attacks, destruction of the myelin sheath will release myelin basic protein into the CSF. Lymphocytes also increase during acute demyelinization.

CT scan: Demonstrates presence of plaques and rules out mass lesions. This scan is less effective than MRI in detecting areas of plaque and demyelinization.

Electroencephalogram (EEG): Shows abnormal slowing in one third of patients with MS because of altered nerve conduction.

Positron emission tomography (PET): May show altered locations and patterns of cerebral glucose metabolism.

See Also: "General Care of Patients With Neurologic Disorders," **Knowledge deficit:** Neurologic diagnostic tests, p. 346, for care considerations for patients undergoing MRI, evoked potential studies, LP, CT scan, EEG, and PET.

COLLABORATIVE MANAGEMENT

Generally, treatment is symptomatic and supportive. Various treatments slow the rate of exacerbation or hasten recovery from an exacerbation, but the general course of the disease process has not been positively affected.

Bedrest: During acute exacerbation.

Pharmacotherapy

Steroidal antiinflammatory agents (e.g., prednisone, adrenocorticotropic hormone [ACTH], dexamethasone): May be prescribed during an exacerbation in an attempt to reduce symptoms by decreasing inflammation and associated edema of the myelin, thereby hastening onset of remission. IV methylprednisolone has largely replaced ACTH or oral prednisone in the treatment of relapsing-remitting MS or associated optic neuritis. Dosage regimens usually include initial high-dose therapy with tapering over a period of 1 mo. Antacids, histamine H_2-receptor blockers, potassium (K^+) supplements, diuretics, blood pressure medications, and psychotropic agents may be given to combat side effects of steroids.

Cladribine (an antilymphocytic agent): May be prescribed in an attempt to retard chronic progression of MS.

Interferon beta-1B: May be prescribed for patients with relapsing-remitting MS to reduce the rate of exacerbation and aid in stabilizing the patient's clinical status. Benefits of this agent are thought to be its enhancement of the body's immune response rather than its antiviral action (see p. 749 for more information on interferon beta-1B).

Copolymer I (a random polymer-stimulating myelin basic protein): May decrease the number of exacerbations in patients with relapsing-remitting MS. These patients should be monitored for injection site reactions, chest pain, weakness, nausea, and joint pain.

Antispasmodics and muscle relaxants (e.g., baclofen or dantrolene sodium): May be given to decrease spasticity. Severe spasticity may be treated with intramuscular injections of botulinum toxin or intrathecal baclofen continually administered via a surgically implanted pump.

Smooth muscle relaxants (e.g., propantheline bromide, oxybutynin): To decrease urinary frequency and urgency.

Smooth muscle stimulants (e.g., bethanechol chloride): To help prevent urinary retention.

Stool softeners (e.g., docusate), laxatives (e.g., bisacodyl), and suppositories: To maintain a bowel program that prevents fecal impaction and minimizes incontinence.

Antidepressants (e.g., amitriptyline): May benefit depression related to cerebral lesions. These agents may also reduce patient complaints of paresthesia.

Tranquilizers (e.g., diazepam): May be given for both their anxiety-reducing and their muscle relaxant effects, which may help spasms and tremors.

Amantadine: This antiviral and antiparkinsonian agent has been effective in relieving fatigue associated with MS (see "Parkinsonism," p. 231, for side effects and precautions). Pemoline (Cylert), a central nervous system stimulant, has also proven effective in combating fatigue in MS.

Propranolol, clonazepam, or primidone: Have been used to decrease tremors.

Carbamazepine: Used to help control some types of neuritic pain (see "Seizure Disorders," p. 319, for side effects and precautions). Imipramine (Tofranil) has also been demonstrated to effectively reduce neuritic burning and pain.

Physical medicine: Physical therapy (PT), occupational therapy (OT), and assistive devices or braces may be prescribed so that patient can maintain mobility and independence with ADL. Muscle-strengthening and conditioning exercises and gait training (to develop alternative muscle groups not yet weakened by demyelination) as well as stretching exercises are also frequently indicated. Placing weights on the affected limbs may help with mild tremors.

ROM exercises: To maintain or increase joint function and prevent contractures.

Bowel and bladder program: To prevent incontinence, constipation, and urinary retention. This program may include bowel and bladder training, intermittent catheterization, and external drainage appliances. Urodynamic studies may be done to determine specific physiologic deficits to allow a bladder program tailored to meet the individual needs of the patient.

Speech therapy: To improve speech deficits using accessory respiratory muscles and tongue and facial muscles.

Counseling or psychotherapy: To help patient and significant other adapt to the disability and deal with emotions and feelings that are either a direct or an indirect result of the disease process. Sexual counseling also should be included.

Treatment of complications: Complications, such as respiratory infection or urinary tract infection (UTI), may require treatment with antibiotics or other measures.

Surgical interventions: To treat complications, such as contractures, spasticity, decreased mobility, and pain. Intrathecal phenol may give 3-12 mo of relief from spasms refractory to drug treatment, but it produces a flaccid paralysis with sensory loss and possibly bladder and bowel dysfunction. Other interventions may include peripheral nerve block with phenol, tenotomy, myotomy, peripheral neurectomy, rhizotomy, or stereotactic thalamotomy. A penile prosthesis may be performed for men whose impotence occurs secondary to MS. Patients with recurrent or chronic UTIs may be candidates for a urinary diversion procedure.

Controversial therapies

Immunosuppressive drug therapy: Agents such as cyclophosphamide (Cytoxan, see p. 753), azathioprine (Imuran, see p. 161), methotrexate (see p. 757), or cyclosporine (see p. 162) may decrease the number and severity of exacerbations.

Myelin bovine compound (Myloral): Appears to reduce exacerbations and increase patient tolerance.

Total lymphoid irradiation: Suppresses the body's immune system and slows down chronic progressive MS by reducing the immunoinflammatory response that leads to demyelinization of the nerve sheaths. This procedure is less commonly done now. For more information about radiation therapy, see Appendix One, "Caring for Patients With Cancer and Other Life-disrupting Illnesses," p. 747.

Monoclonal antibodies (4-aminopyridine): Provide symptomatic improvement in nerve conduction, vision deficits, strength, and coordination.

Plasmapheresis: Reduces the patient's antibodies to CNS tissue by removing the plasma portion of the blood, which contains circulating antibodies. This therapy usually involves several exchanges that provide short-term improvement only. Because of perceived limited benefit and usefulness, this procedure is now less frequently used.

NURSING DIAGNOSES AND INTERVENTIONS

Knowledge deficit: Factors that aggravate and exacerbate MS symptoms

Desired outcome: By day 3 (or before hospital discharge), patient and significant other verbalize factors that exacerbate, prevent, or ameliorate symptoms of MS.

- Inform patient and significant other that heat, both external (hot weather, bath) and internal (fever), tends to aggravate weakness and other symptoms of MS.
- Teach preventive measures, such as avoiding hot baths or showers and using acetaminophen or aspirin to reduce fever, if present. Also instruct the patient in use of fans or air conditioning to aid in reducing body temperature.
- Because infection often precedes exacerbations, caution patient to avoid exposure to persons known to have infections of any kind.
- Teach the indicators of common infections (see "Care of the Renal Transplant Recipient," p. 162; Table 5-4, p. 382) and the importance of seeking prompt medical treatment should they occur. For example, the patient with MS is susceptible to UTI because of urinary retention. Because of the disease process, the patient may not feel any pain with urination. Teach the patient to monitor for increased frequency, urgency, or incontinence and to check the urine for changes in odor or the presence of cloudiness or blood. Instruct patients to check body temperature periodically for fever and indications that a UTI has reached the kidneys (e.g., costovertebral angle [CVA] tenderness, chills, flank pain).
- Teach patient the relationship between stress and fatigue to the exacerbations. Encourage patient to get sufficient rest, stop activity short of fatigue, schedule activity and rest periods, and reduce factors that cause stress.
- To reduce fatigue, encourage the patient to conserve energy in ADL by sitting while getting dressed, rather than standing; by sliding heavy objects along work surfaces, rather than lifting them; by using a wheeled cart to transport items; and by having work surfaces at the proper height. Amantadine (see "Parkinsonism," p. 224) or pemoline may be prescribed to aid patients in compensating for fatigue. See "Coronary Artery Disease" for **Health-seeking behaviors:** Relaxation technique effective for stress reduction, p. 59.
- As appropriate, explain to the patient that there may be an increase in exacerbations postpartum. Provide information about birth control measures to female patients who desire counseling.
- As appropriate, reassure patient and significant other that most persons with MS do not become severely disabled. Encourage continued activity and normal life-style even when limitations are necessary.

You may also wish to refer to the following interventions from the Nursing Interventions Classification (NIC):

NIC: Environmental Management; Health Education; Infection Protection; Teaching: Disease Process; Temperature Regulation

Knowledge deficit: Precautions and potential side effects of prescribed medications

Desired outcome: By day 3 (or before hospital discharge), patient verbalizes accurate information about the prescribed medications.

- Provide patient with verbal instructions and written handouts that describe the name, purpose, dose, and schedule of the prescribed medications.
- For patients taking ACTH, prednisone, or dexamethasone, provide additional instructions for the following:
  —Common side effects: sodium (Na^+) and fluid retention, hypertension, gastric ulcers, stomach upset, weakness, hypokalemia, mood changes, impaired wound healing, and masking of infections.
  —Importance of monitoring weight and BP for evidence of fluid retention; taking the medication with food, milk, or buffering agents to help prevent gastric irritation; avoiding aspirin, indomethacin, caffeine, or other GI irritants while taking this medication; and tapering rather than abruptly stopping the drug when it is discontinued. Advise patient to report symptoms of K^+ deficiency, such as anorexia, nausea, and muscle weakness, and to eat foods high in K^+ (see Table 3-4, p. 146). Encourage a diet low in Na^+ content (see Table 3-2, p. 133) to minimize the potential for fluid retention. Monitor for and report black, tarry stools, which may signal occult blood. Health care provider follow-up is important while the patient is taking these drugs.
- If the patient is taking baclofen or dantrolene, provide additional instructions for the following:
  —Common side effects: drowsiness, dizziness, fatigue, and nausea. In addition, dantrolene can cause diarrhea, muscle weakness, hepatitis, and photosensitivity.
  —Importance of taking the medication with food, milk, or a buffering agent to reduce gastric upset or nausea. Explain that although drowsiness is usually transient, patient should avoid activities that require alertness until the drug's effect on the CNS is known. The patient also should avoid alcohol intake because of its additive CNS depression effects. Baclofen can lower a person's seizure threshold and should be used cautiously in susceptible patients. Baclofen also may raise blood glucose levels, and individuals with diabetes mellitus may need an insulin dose adjustment. Monitor patients during transfers/ambulation initially because some weak patients cannot tolerate the loss in spasticity that may be permitting them to bear weight. Patients taking dantrolene should monitor for and report fever, jaundice, dark urine, clay-colored stools, and itching (all of which signal hepatitis) or severe diarrhea; avoid exposure to the sun; and use sunscreens if exposure is unavoidable.
- If bethanechol chloride has been prescribed, provide additional instructions for the following:
  —Common side effects: hypotension, diarrhea, abdominal cramps, urinary urgency, and bronchoconstriction.
  —Importance of taking the drug on an empty stomach to avoid nausea and vomiting; notifying health care provider if lightheadedness occurs because this can signal hypotension; and seeking medical attention if an asthmatic attack occurs. Caution patient to make position changes slowly and in stages to prevent fainting caused by orthostatic hypotension.
- If the patient is taking propantheline bromide, provide additional instructions for the following:
  —Common side effects: dryness of the mouth, blurred vision, constipation, palpitations, tachycardia, decreased sweating, and urinary retention or overflow incontinence.
  —Measures that relieve constipation; measures for remaining cool in hot or humid weather because heat stroke is more likely to develop while taking the medication; importance of notifying health care provider immediately

if urinary retention or overflow incontinence occurs. In addition, if the patient can chew and swallow effectively, explain that sugarless gum, hard candy, or artificial saliva products may reduce mouth dryness. Encourage slow position changes and monitoring for dizziness because postural hypotension may occur when the drug is first started.

NIC: Teaching: Disease Process; Teaching: Individual; Teaching: Prescribed Medication

Chronic pain and spasms related to motor and sensory nerve tract damage
Desired outcomes: Within 1-2 hr of intervention, patient's subjective evaluation of pain and spasms improves, as documented by a pain scale. Objective indicators, such as grimacing, are absent or reduced.
- Because heat tends to aggravate MS symptoms, maintain a comfortable room temperature. Advise patient to keep environment cool in warm weather and avoid hot baths or showers.
- To reduce muscle tightness and spasms, provide passive, assisted, or active ROM q2hr and periodic stretching exercises. Teach these exercises to patient and significant other, and encourage their performance several times daily. Explain that sleeping in a prone position may help decrease flexor spasm of the hips and knees.
- Administer antispasmodics as prescribed.
- For other interventions, see "General Care of Patients with Neurologic Disorders," **Pain,** p. 343.

NIC: Environmental Management; Exercise Promotion: Stretching; Pain Management; Teaching: Individual

---

See Also: "Guillain-Barré Syndrome" for **Knowledge deficit:** Therapeutic plasma exchange procedure, p. 215, for patients undergoing plasmapheresis; "Spinal Cord Injury" for **Constipation,** p. 263; **Risk for disuse syndrome,** p. 265; **Urinary retention or Reflex incontinence,** p. 267; **Sexual dysfunction,** p. 271; "General Care of Patients With Neurologic Disorders" for **Risk for trauma** related to unsteady gait, p. 331; **Risk for injury** related to impaired pain, touch, and temperature sensations, p. 332; **Impaired corneal tissue integrity,** p. 333; **Altered nutrition:** Less than body requirements, p. 333; **Risk for fluid volume deficit** related to decreased intake, p. 335; **Risk for aspiration,** p. 335; **Self-care deficit** related to spasticity, tremors, weakness, paresis, paralysis, or decreasing LOC secondary to sensorimotor deficits, p. 336; **Impaired verbal communication,** p. 338; **Constipation,** p. 337; **Sensory/perceptual alterations** (visual), p. 342; **Impaired swallowing,** p. 344; **Knowledge deficit:** Neurologic diagnostic tests (for discussions of EEG, MRI, CT scan, evoked potential studies, PET, and LP), p. 346; "Providing Nutritional Support," p. 681, for patients with impaired nutrition; "Pressure Ulcers," p. 710, for patients who are immobile; Appendix One, "Caring for Patients on Prolonged Bedrest," p. 738; Appendix One, "Caring for Patients With Cancer and Other Life-disrupting Illnesses," p. 747, for patients undergoing immunosuppressive drug or radiation therapy; for related psychosocial nursing diagnoses, p. 791, as appropriate.

PATIENT-FAMILY TEACHING AND DISCHARGE PLANNING

The patient with MS may have a wide variety of symptoms that cause disability, ranging from mild to severe. When providing patient-family teaching, focus on sensory information; avoid giving excessive information; and initiate a visiting nurse referral for necessary follow-up teaching. Consider including verbal and written information about the following:

- Remission/exacerbation aspects of the disease process. Explain the effects of demyelinization on sensory and motor function and factors that aggravate symptoms.
- Safety measures relative to decreased sensation, visual disturbances, and motor deficits.
- Medications, including drug name, purpose, dosage, frequency, precautions, drug/drug and food/drug interactions, and potential side effects.
- Exercises that promote muscle strength and mobility; measures for preventing contractures and skin breakdown; transfer techniques and proper body mechanics; use of assistive devices and other measures to minimize neurologic deficits.
- Measures for relieving pain, muscle spasms, or other discomfort.
- Indications of constipation, urinary retention, or UTI; implementation of bowel and bladder training programs; self-catheterization technique or care of indwelling urinary catheters.
- Indications of upper respiratory infection; implementation of measures that help prevent regurgitation, aspiration, and respiratory infection.
- Dietary adjustments that may be appropriate for neurologic deficit (e.g., soft, semisolid foods for patients with chewing difficulties or a high-fiber diet for patients experiencing constipation).
- Importance of follow-up care, including visits to health care provider, physical therapist, and occupational therapist, as well as speech, sexual, or psychologic counseling.
- Referrals to community resources, such as local and national Multiple Sclerosis Society chapters, public health nurse, visiting nurse association, community support groups, social workers, psychologists, vocational rehabilitation agencies, home health agencies, extended and skilled care facilities, and financial counseling. Additional general information can be obtained by contacting the following organization:

National Multiple Sclerosis Society
205 East 42nd Street
New York, NY 10017   (800) 624-8236
WWW address: *http://www.nmss.org*

Guillain-Barré syndrome

Guillain-Barré syndrome (GBS) is a rapidly progressing polyneuritis of unknown cause. An inflammatory process causes lymphocytes to enter the perivascular spaces and destroy the myelin sheath covering the peripheral or cranial nerves. Posterior (sensory) and anterior (motor) nerve roots can be affected because of this segmental demyelinization, and the individual may experience both sensory and motor losses. There is relative sparing of the axon. Respiratory insufficiency may occur in as many as one half of the individuals affected. Life-threatening respiratory muscle weakness can develop as rapidly as 24-72 hr after onset of initial symptoms. In about 25% of cases, motor weakness progresses to total paralysis.

Peak severity of symptoms usually occurs within 1-3 wk after onset of symptoms. A plateau stage follows that usually lasts 1-2 wk. Remyelinization with return of function then occurs, but it may take months to years for a full recovery. Full neurologic recovery occurs in about 50% of patients. Residual neurologic deficits tend to be mild motor or reflex alterations in the feet or legs and are the result of axonal nerve degeneration.

GBS may follow a recent viral illness, such as upper respiratory infection or gastroenteritis, a rabies or influenza vaccination, lupus erythematosus, or Hodgkin's disease or other malignant process. Although the exact cause of GBS is unknown, it is believed to be an autoimmune response to a viral infection. *Campylobacter jejuni* enteritis has been identified as a trigger for GBS in some people.

ASSESSMENT

Weakness is the most common indicator. Typically, numbness and weakness begin in the legs and ascend symmetrically upward, progressing to the arms and facial nerves. Peak severity usually occurs within 10-14 days of onset. GBS does not affect LOC, cognitive function, or pupillary function.

Anterior (motor) nerve root involvement: Weakness or flaccid paralysis. Weakness or paralysis of respiratory muscles can be life threatening. There is a loss of reflexes, muscle tension, and tone, but muscle atrophy usually does not occur.

Autonomic nervous system involvement: Sinus tachycardia, bradycardia, hypertension, hypotension, cardiac dysrhythmias, facial flushing, diaphoresis, inability to perspire, loss of sphincter control, urinary retention, adynamic ileus, and increased pulmonary secretions may occur. Autonomic nervous system involvement may occur unexpectedly and can be life threatening. Autonomic disturbances usually do not persist for longer than 2 wk.

Cranial nerve involvement: Inability to chew, swallow, speak, or close the eyes.

Posterior (sensory) nerve root involvement: Paresthesias, such as numbness and tingling, which usually are minor compared with the degree of motor loss. Ascending sensory loss often precedes motor loss. The patient may experience muscle cramping, tenderness, or pain that may become severe.

Physical assessment: Symmetric motor weakness, impaired position and vibration sense, hypoactive or absent deep tendon reflexes, hypotonia in affected muscles, and decreased ventilatory capacity.

DIAGNOSTIC TESTS

Diagnostic tests are performed to rule out other diseases, such as acute poliomyelitis. The diagnosis of GBS is based on clinical presentation, history of recent viral illness, and CSF findings.

Lumbar puncture (LP) and CSF analysis: Usually show an elevated protein (especially immunoglobulin G [IgG]) without an increase in cell count. Although CSF pressure usually is normal, in severe disease it may be elevated.

Electromyography (EMG): Reveals slowed nerve conduction velocities soon after paralysis appears. Findings occur because of segmental demyelinization. Denervation potentials appear later.

Serum CBC: Will show presence of leukocytosis early in illness, possibly as a result of the inflammatory process associated with demyelinization.

Evoked potentials (auditory, visual, brain stem): May be used to distinguish GBS from other neuropathologic conditions.

See Also: "General Care of Patients With Neurologic Disorders" for **Knowledge deficit:** Neurologic diagnostic tests, p. 346, for care considerations for patients undergoing LP, EMG, and evoked potential studies.

COLLABORATIVE MANAGEMENT

The patient is likely to be in ICU when the neurologic deficit is progressing and is at risk for respiratory failure and autonomic dysfunction.

Respiratory support: Serial vital capacity measurements and ABG analysis to monitor for respiratory muscle weakness or paralysis. Endotracheal tube, tracheostomy, or mechanical ventilation is used as necessary, generally when vital capacity falls below a preset level.

Pharmacotherapy

IV immunoglobulins: Given in an attempt to positively affect the antibody response. If there is no response after 10 days, plasmapheresis may be added to treatment.

Glucocorticosteroids (e.g., prednisone, adrenocorticotropic hormone [ACTH]): May include a 1-wk trial to determine whether symptoms decrease (see "Steroidal antiinflammatory agents," p. 205). Methylprednisolone is often given along with the initial course of IV immunoglobulins.

Analgesia (e.g., acetaminophen, codeine, morphine): For muscle pain. Other medications that may be tried to relieve uncomfortable paresthesias include perphenazine, phenytoin, carbamazepine, or amitriptyline.

Stool softeners (e.g., docusate), laxatives (e.g., bisacodyl), and suppositories: Given to maintain a bowel program that prevents fecal impaction and minimizes incontinence.

Exercise and activity: Activity other than bedrest and passive ROM is restricted during the acute phase. After the patient stabilizes, active ROM or active assistive ROM is implemented, and PT and a rehabilitation program are initiated. OT and assistive devices or braces are employed so that patient can maintain mobility and independence with ADL. Muscle-strengthening exercises, conditioning exercises, and gait training also are frequently prescribed.

Antithrombus prophylaxis: May include antiembolism hose, sequential compression devices, pneumatic foot pumps, or pharmacotherapy (low-dose heparin, low-molecular-weight heparin, or warfarin).

Nutritional support: A high-fiber diet may be prescribed to help prevent constipation. If the patient cannot chew or swallow effectively because of cranial nerve involvement, gastric, gastrostomy, or parenteral feedings may be initiated. The patient is advanced to a solid diet upon return of the gag reflex and swallowing ability.

Management of bowel and bladder dysfunction: A regular bowel program should be started to prevent fecal impaction. Indwelling urinary catheters, intermittent catheterizations, or external urinary collection devices may be needed until strength and mobility return.

Management of acute autonomic dysfunction: Short-acting antihypertensive agents for hypertension; intravascular volume expanders or vasopressors for hypotension; cardiac monitoring of dysrhythmias; gastric suction, nutrition, and parenteral fluids for adynamic ileus; and catheterization and medications for urinary retention. Phenoxybenzamine may be used to help with paroxysmal hypertension, headache, sweating, anxiety, and fever. Diabetes insipidus (see p. 362) and syndrome of inappropriate antidiuretic hormone (SIADH, see p. 371) have been reported, so urine output, state of hydration, and serum and urine electrolytes should be monitored.

Plasmapheresis: To reduce the patient's antibodies to peripheral and cranial nerve tissue by removing the plasma portion of the blood, which contains the circulating antibodies. If performed within 7-14 days of the onset of symptoms, removal of these autoantibodies appears to lessen the duration and severity of the disease.

Treatment of complications: For example, antibiotic therapy for aspiration pneumonia, anticoagulant therapy for deep vein thrombosis (DVT) or emboli, or histamine H_2-receptor blockers to prevent stress ulcers.

Controversial therapies: Immunosuppressive drug therapy (e.g., cyclophosphamide [Cytoxan, see p. 753], azathioprine [Imuran, see p. 161]) may slow and stabilize disease progression, probably by suppressing the immunoinflammatory response that leads to demyelinization of the peripheral nerve sheath. High-dose γ-globulin also is being tried in severe cases to affect antibody response.

NURSING DIAGNOSES AND INTERVENTIONS

Ineffective breathing pattern related to neuromuscular weakness or paralysis of the facial, throat, and respiratory muscles (severity of symptoms peaks around wk 1-3)

Desired outcome: Deterioration in patient's breathing pattern (e.g., Pao_2 <80 mm Hg, vital capacity <1 L [or <12-15 ml/kg], tidal volume <75% of predicted value, or O_2 saturation <92% via oximetry) is detected and reported promptly, resulting in immediate and effective medical treatment.

- Test for ascending loss of sensation by touching patient lightly with a pin or fingers at frequent intervals (hourly or more frequently initially). Assess from the level of the iliac crest upward toward the shoulders. Measure the highest level at which decreased sensation occurs. Decreased sensation frequently precedes motor weakness, so if it ascends to the level of the T8 dermatome, anticipate that intercostal muscles (used with respirations) soon will be impaired. Also monitor for upper arm and shoulder weakness, which precedes respiratory failure, by checking patient for the presence of arm drift and the ability to shrug the shoulders. Arm drift is detected in the following way: have the patient hold both arms out in front of the body, level with the shoulders and with the palms up; instruct patient to close the eyes while holding this position. Weakness is present if one arm pronates or drifts down or out from its original position. Alert health care provider to significant findings.
- Assist patient with oral intake to detect changes or difficulties that may indicate ascending paralysis. Assess patient q8hr and before oral intake for cough reflexes, gag reflexes, and difficulty swallowing.
- Observe patient for changes in mental status, LOC, and orientation, which may signal reduced oxygenation to the brain. Monitor patient's respiratory rate, rhythm, and depth. Watch for accessory muscle use, nasal flaring, dyspnea, shallow respirations, apnea, and loss of abdominal breathing. Auscultate for diminished breath sounds. Monitor patient for breathlessness while speaking. To observe for breathlessness, ask patient to take a deep breath and slowly count as high as possible. A reduced ability to count to a higher number before breathlessness occurs may signal grossly reduced ventilatory function. Alert health care provider to significant findings.
- Monitor effectiveness of breathing by checking serial vital capacity results on pulmonary function tests. If the vital capacity is <1 L or is rapidly trending downward or if the patient exhibits signs of hypoxia such as tachycardia, increasing restlessness, mental dullness, or cyanosis, report findings immediately to health care provider.
- Monitor ABG levels and pulse oximetry to detect hypoxia or hypercapnia.
- Raise HOB to promote optimal chest excursion.
- The patient may require tracheostomy, endotracheal intubation, or mechanical ventilation to support respiratory function. Prepare patient emotionally for such procedures or for the eventual transfer to ICU or transition care unit for closer monitoring.
- For other interventions, see **Risk for aspiration** in "General Care of Patients With Neurologic Disorders, p. 335.

NIC: Airway Management; Aspiration Precautions; Mechanical Ventilation; Neurologic Monitoring; Oxygen Therapy; Positioning; Respiratory Monitoring

Pain related to muscle tenderness; hypersensitivity to touch; or discomfort in shoulders, thighs, and back

Desired outcomes: Within 1-2 hr of intervention, patient's subjective perception of discomfort decreases, as documented by a pain scale. Objective indicators, such as grimacing, are absent or diminished.

- For patients with muscle tenderness, consider use of massage, moist heat packs, cold application, or warm baths, which may be very soothing for the muscles.

- For patients with hypersensitivity, assess the amount of touch that can be tolerated and incorporate this information into the patient's plan of care.
- Reposition patient at frequent intervals to decrease muscle tension and fatigue. Some individuals find that a supine "frog-leg" position is particularly comfortable.
- Provide passive ROM to reduce joint stiffness.
- For other interventions, see **Pain,** p. 343, in "General Care of Patients With Neurologic Disorders."

NIC: Analgesic Administration; Exercise Therapy: Joint Mobility; Heat/Cold Application; Pain Management; Simple Massage

Altered cardiopulmonary and cerebral tissue perfusion (or risk of same) related to interrupted sympathetic outflow with concomitant BP fluctuations secondary to autonomic dysfunction
Desired outcomes: Patient has optimal cardiopulmonary and cerebral tissue perfusion as evidenced by systolic BP ≥90 mm Hg and ≤160 mm Hg, no significant mental status changes, and orientation to person, place, and time. BP fluctuations, if they occur, are detected and reported promptly.
- Monitor BP, noting wide fluctuations; report significant findings to health care provider. Changes in BP that result in severe hypotension or hypertension may occur because of unopposed sympathetic outflow or loss of outflow to the peripheral nervous system, causing changes in vascular tone. Short-acting hypertensive agents may be required for persistent hypertension.
- Monitor carefully for changes during activities such as coughing, suctioning, position changes, or straining at stool.
- For patients with hypotension or postural hypotension, see **Altered cardiopulmonary and cerebral tissue perfusion,** p. 269, in "Spinal Cord Injury."

NIC: Circulatory Precautions; Fall Prevention; Hemodynamic Regulation; Medication Administration; Surveillance: Safety; Vital Signs Monitoring

Altered nutrition: Less than body requirements related to adynamic ileus
Desired outcome: Patient has adequate nutrition as evidenced by maintenance of baseline body weight.
- Auscultate abdominal sounds, noting presence, absence, or changes that may signal onset of ileus. Be alert to abdominal distention or tenderness, nausea and vomiting, and absence of stool output. Notify health care provider of significant findings.
- Patients with adynamic ileus generally require gastric decompression with a nasogastric tube. Because these patients are unable to take foods orally, parenteral nutrition may be required (see "Providing Nutritional Support," p. 687).
- For general interventions, see **Altered nutrition,** p. 333, in "General Care of Patients With Neurologic Disorders."

NIC: Enteral Tube Feeding; Gastrointestinal Intubation; Nutrition Management; Total Parenteral Nutrition (TPN) Administration; Tube Care: Gastrointestinal

Anxiety related to threat to biologic integrity and loss of control
Desired outcome: Within 24 hr of this diagnosis, patient expresses concern regarding changes in life events, states anxiety is less or under control, and exhibits fewer symptoms of increased anxiety (e.g., less apprehension, decreased tension).
- For the patient in whom the neurologic deficit is still progressing, arrange for a transfer to a room close to the nurses' station to help alleviate the anxiety of being suddenly incapacitated and helpless.

- Be sure that patient's call light is within easy reach. Frequently assess patient's ability to use it.
- Provide continuity of patient care through assignment of staff and use of care plan.
- Perform assessments at frequent intervals, letting patient know you are there. Provide care in a calm and reassuring manner.
- Allow time for the patient to ventilate concerns and provide realistic feedback on what the patient may experience. Determine the patient's past effective coping behaviors and problem solve with the patient for ways these methods, or others, may prove useful in the current situation.
- For other interventions, see **Anxiety,** p. 791, and **Fear,** p. 795, in Appendix One, "Caring for Patients With Cancer and Other Life-Disrupting Illnesses."

NIC: Anticipatory Guidance; Anxiety Reduction; Calming Technique; Coping Enhancement; Emotional Support; Presence

Knowledge deficit: Therapeutic plasma exchange procedure
Desired outcome: Before scheduled date of each procedure, patient verbalizes accurate information about the plasma exchange procedure.
- Before the plasma exchange procedure, the patient's health care provider explains the reason for the procedure, its risks, and anticipated benefits or outcome. Determine patient's level of understanding of the health care provider's explanation, and clarify or reinforce information accordingly.
- Determine patient's experience with plasmapheresis, the positive or negative effects, and the nature of any fears or concerns. Document and communicate this information to other caregivers.
- Explain in words the patient can understand that the goal of plasma exchange is to remove autoimmune factors from the blood to decrease or eliminate the patient's symptoms. These antibodies to the patient's peripheral and cranial nerve tissue are reduced by the removal of the plasma portion of the blood, which contains the circulating antibodies. The procedure is similar to hemodialysis. Blood is removed from the patient and separated into its components. The patient's plasma is discarded; the other blood components (e.g., RBCs, WBCs, platelets) are saved and returned to the patient with donor plasma or replacement fluid. If started within 1-2 wk of GBS symptoms, the exchange process seems to decrease the duration and severity of the disease. Multiple exchanges over a period of weeks can be expected.
- The patient is at risk for the following complications during this procedure: fluid volume deficit, hypotension, hypokalemia, hypocalcemia, cardiac dysrhythmias, clotting disorders, anemia, phlebitis, infection, hypothermia, and air embolism. Answer any questions regarding these complications accordingly.
- This procedure requires good blood flow. Inform patient that the antecubital vein most often is used as the access site, but if the patient has poor peripheral veins, the health care provider may need to insert a central IV line or a femoral catheter. If the antecubital site is used, place a sign alerting others to avoid using this site for routine laboratory sticks.
- Explain that the patient can expect the procedure to take 2-4 hr, although it may take considerably longer, depending on condition of the patient's veins, blood flow, and hematocrit (Hct) level.
- Explain that the patient can expect preprocedure and postprocedure blood work for clotting factors and electrolyte levels. The patient may be placed on cardiac monitoring to assess for electrolyte imbalance, particularly if taking prednisone or digitalis. Weight and VS will be taken before and after the procedure, with frequent VS checks during the procedure. Calcium gluconate or potassium chloride (KCl) may be administered to correct electrolyte imbalances.

- Encourage patient to report any unusual feelings or symptoms during plasma exchange. For example:
  —Instruct patient to report chills, fever, hives, sweating, or lightheadedness, which may signal reaction to donor plasma.
  —Teach patient to report thirst, faintness, or dizziness, which can occur with hypotension or hypovolemia. The patient should take oral fluids during the procedure if possible.
  —Instruct patient to report numbness or tingling around the lips or in the hands, arms, and legs; muscle twitching; cramping; or tetany, which can occur with hypocalcemia. Fatigue, nausea, weakness, or cramping may signal hypokalemia.
- Inform patient that medications may be held until after the procedure to prevent their removal from the blood.
- If the patient does not have a urinary catheter, remind him or her to void before and during the procedure, if necessary, to avoid any mild hypotension caused by a full bladder. I&O will be monitored closely because decreased urine output may signal hypovolemia.
- Explain that the patient's temperature will be checked during the procedure and warm blankets will be provided to prevent hypothermia.
- Explain that the patient probably will feel fatigued 1-2 days after the procedure because of decreased plasma protein levels. Encourage extra rest and a high-protein diet during this time.
- Teach patient to monitor IV access site for signs of infection, such as warmth, redness, swelling, or drainage, and to report significant findings.
- Teach patient to monitor for signs of bruising or bleeding. The anticoagulant citrate dextrose is used in the extracorporeal machine circuitry to prevent clotting. This may cause excessive bleeding at the access site. A pressure dressing may be kept in place over the access site for 2-4 hr after the procedure. Caution patient about avoiding cutting self or bumping into objects and to sustain pressure over cuts. Inform patient that black, tarry stools usually signal the presence of blood and should be reported.

NIC: Cardiac Care; Intravenous (IV) Insertion; Teaching: Disease Process; Teaching: Individual; Teaching: Procedure/Treatment

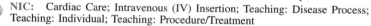

> **See Also:**   Related discussions in Chapter 3, for patients with urinary incontinence (p. 177), retention (p. 185), neurogenic bladder (p. 188), or urinary tract infection (UTI); "Spinal Cord Injury" for **Altered peripheral and cardiopulmonary tissue perfusion**, p. 269, for patients with auto-nomic dysfunction; "General Care of Patients With Neurologic Disorders" for **Risk for trauma** related to unsteady gait, p. 331; **Risk for injury** related to impaired pain, touch, and temperature sensations, p. 332; **Impaired corneal tissue integrity**, p. 333; **Risk for fluid volume deficit**, p. 335, **Self-care deficit**, p. 336; **Impaired verbal communication**, p. 338; **Constipation**, p. 339; **Impaired swallowing**, p. 344; **Altered body temperature**, p. 346; **Knowledge deficit:** Neurologic diagnostic tests, p. 346; related nursing diagnoses in "Pressure Ulcers," p. 710, for patients who are immobile; Appendix One, "Caring for Patients on Prolonged Bedrest" for **Risk for disuse syndrome:** Paralysis, mechanical immobili-zation, prescribed immobilization, severe pain or altered LOC, and other related nursing diagnoses, p. 740; Appendix One, "Caring for Patients With Cancer and Other Life-disrupting Illnesses" for care of patients undergoing immunosuppressive drug therapy, p. 749; patient and family psychosocial nursing diagnoses, p. 791, as appropriate.

PATIENT-FAMILY TEACHING AND DISCHARGE PLANNING

Most patients with GBS eventually recover fully, but because the recovery period can be prolonged, the patient often goes home with some degree of neurologic deficit. Discharge planning and teaching will vary according to the degree of disability. When providing patient-family teaching, focus on sensory information; avoid giving excessive information; and initiate a visiting nurse referral for necessary follow-up teaching. Consider including verbal and written information about the following:

- The disease process, expected improvement, and importance of continuing in the rehabilitation or PT program to promote as full a recovery as possible.
- Safety measures relative to the decreased sensorimotor deficit.
- Exercises that promote muscle strength and mobility; measures for preventing contractures and skin breakdown; transfer techniques and proper body mechanics; and use of assistive devices.
- Indications of constipation, urinary retention, or UTI; implementation of bowel and bladder training programs; and, if appropriate, care of indwelling catheters or self-catheterization technique.
- Indications of URI; measures for preventing regurgitation, aspiration, and respiratory infection.
- Medications, including drug name, purpose, dosage, schedule, precautions, drug/drug and food/drug interactions, and potential side effects.
- Importance of follow-up care, including visits to health care provider, physical therapist, and occupational therapist.
- Referrals to community resources, such as public health nurse, visiting nurse association, community support groups, social workers, psychologic therapy, home health agencies, and extended and skilled care facilities. Additional general information can be obtained by contacting the following organization:

  Guillain-Barré Syndrome Foundation International
  Box 262
  Wynnewood, PA 19096   (610) 667-0131 or (610) 667-7036 FAX
  WWW address: *http://www.webmaster.com/gbs/*

Bacterial meningitis

Bacterial meningitis is an infection that results in inflammation of the meningeal membranes covering the brain and spinal cord. Bacteria in the subarachnoid space multiply and cause an inflammatory reaction of the pia and arachnoid meninges. Purulent exudate is produced, and the inflammation and infection spread quickly through the CSF that circulates around the brain and spinal cord. Bacteria and exudate can create vascular congestion, plugging the arachnoid villi. This obstruction of CSF flow and decreased reabsorption of CSF can lead to increased intracranial pressure (IICP), brain herniation, and death.

Meningitis generally is transmitted in one of four ways: via airborne droplets or contact with oral secretions from infected individuals; from direct contamination (e.g., from a penetrating skull wound; a skull fracture, often basilar, causing a tear in the dura; lumbar puncture [LP]; ventricular shunt; or surgical procedure); via the bloodstream (e.g., pneumonia, endocarditis); or from direct contact with an infectious process that invades the meningeal membranes, as can occur with osteomyelitis, sinusitis, otitis media, mastoiditis, or brain abscess. In adults, pneumonococcal meningitis, caused by *Streptococcus pneumoniae,* is the most common bacterial meningitis. Meningococcal meningitis, caused by *Neisseria meningitidis,* is the next leading cause. In children the leading agent in infectious meningitis is *Haemophilus influenzae.* Any bacteria can cause a meningitis, and some, such as that caused by *Staphylococcus aureus*, can be difficult to treat because of their resistance to antibiotic therapy. Adhesions and fibrotic changes in the arachnoid layer and subspace may cause obstruction or reabsorption problems with CSF, resulting in hydrocephalus. The prognosis, however, is good and complete neurologic recovery is possible if the disorder is recognized early and antibiotic treatment is initiated promptly. However, if left untreated, mortality is 70%-100%.

ASSESSMENT

Infection: Fever, chills, malaise.

IICP and herniation: Decreased LOC (irritability, drowsiness, stupor, coma), nausea and vomiting, a decreasing Glasgow Coma Scale score (see p. 274), VS changes (increased BP, decreased HR, widening pulse pressure), changes in respiratory pattern, decreased pupillary reaction to light, pupillary dilation or inequality, severe headache.

Meningeal irritation: Back stiffness and pain, headache, nuchal rigidity.

Other: Generalized seizures and photophobia. In the presence of *H. influenzae,* deafness or joint pain may occur.

Physical assessment

- A positive Brudzinski's sign may be elicited because of meningeal irritation: when the neck is passively flexed forward, both legs flex involuntarily at the hip and knee.
- A positive Kernig's sign also may be found: when the thigh is flexed 90 degrees at the hip, the individual cannot extend the leg completely without pain.
- In the presence of meningococcal meningitis, a pink, macular rash, petechiae, ecchymoses, purpura, and increased deep tendon reflexes (DTRs) may occur.

DIAGNOSTIC TESTS

LP, CSF analysis, and Gram stain and culture: To identify causative organism. Glucose is generally decreased, and protein is usually increased. Typically, the CSF will be cloudy or milky because of increased WBCs, and CSF pressure will be increased because of the inflammation and exudate, causing an obstruction in outflow of CSF from the arachnoid villi. This test, in the presence of IICP, can cause brain herniation. If CSF pressure is elevated, check neurologic status and VS at frequent intervals for signs of brain herniation (decreased LOC; pupillary changes such as dilation, inequality, or decreased reaction; irregular respirations; hemiparesis).

Culture and sensitivity testing of blood, sputum, urine, and other body secretions: To identify infective organism and/or its source and determine appropriate antibiotic.

Coagglutination tests: To detect microbial antigens in CSF and allow identification of the causative organism. Coagglutination tests have generally replaced counterimmunoelectrophoresis because results are obtainable much more rapidly.

Counterimmunoelectrophoresis (CIE):   To detect bacterial antigens of pneumococci, meningococci, and *H. influenzae* in the CSF, blood, and urine.

Sinus, skull, and chest x-rays: Taken after treatment is started to rule out sinusitis, pneumonia, and cranial osteomyelitis.

Radioimmunoassay (RIA), latex particle agglutination (LPA), or enzyme-linked immunosorbent assay (ELISA):   To detect microbial antigens in the CSF to identify the causative organism.

CT scan with contrast: To rule out hydrocephalus or mass lesions such as brain abscess and detect exudate in the CSF spaces.

See Also: "General Care of Patient With Neurologic Disorders" for **Knowledge deficit:** Neurologic tests, p. 346, for care considerations for patients undergoing LP, CT scan, and MRI.

COLLABORATIVE MANAGEMENT

Respiratory precautions: Patients with *N. meningitidis,* with *H. influenzae,* or in whom the causative organism is in doubt require observation with special respiratory isolation precautions for 24 hr after initiation of the appropriate antibiotic therapy. The patient should be placed in a private room. Infection may be spread by contact with airborne droplets or oral secretions. Masks should be used, along with adherence to Standard Precautions (see p. 220).

Parenteral antibiotics: Because treatment cannot be delayed until the results of the culture are known, high doses are started immediately, based on Gram stain results. The antibiotic must penetrate the blood-brain barrier into the CSF. Adjustments in therapy can be made after coagglutination test, CIE, and culture and sensitivity test results are available. Antibiotics may include the following (usually in combination): cefotaxime, ceftriaxone, penicillin G, ampicillin, chloramphenicol, gentamicin, or vancomycin.

Prophylactic antibiotic treatment of significant other and close contacts: Rifampin is generally administered. Other antibiotics, such as sulfadiazine or minocycline, also may be used.

Other pharmacotherapy

Glucocorticosteroids (e.g., dexamethasone, prednisone):   High-dose therapy to stabilize the cell membrane and reduce inflammation and cerebral edema. Use is somewhat controversial because of the potential for depressed physiologic immune response to infection.

Osmotic diuretics (e.g., mannitol) and loop diuretics (e.g., furosemide):   To decrease cerebral edema in the presence of impending IICP.

Antiepilepsy drugs (e.g., carbamazepine, diazepam, phenytoin, phenobarbital, fosphenytoin):   To control seizures.

Analgesics (e.g., acetaminophen, codeine):   To relieve headache, myalgia, and other pain.

Antipyretics (e.g., acetaminophen):   For control of fever to reduce cerebral metabolism.

Mild sedatives (e.g., diphenhydramine):   To promote rest.

Antacids and histamine H_2-receptor blockers (e.g., ranitidine):   To reduce gastric acidity and prevent hemorrhage or ulcer formation.

Stool softeners and laxatives (e.g., docusate sodium, Milk of Magnesia):   To prevent constipation and straining at stool, which would increase ICP.

Tranquilizers (e.g., chlorpromazine):   To control shivering, which can increase ICP.

Support respirations: Via O_2, suctioning, airway maintenance, or intubation with ventilatory assistance as necessary.

Bedrest with elevation of HOB and seizure precautions: To promote venous drainage, help reduce cerebral congestion and edema, and prevent injury from possible seizure activity.

Fluid management: Traditionally, fluid therapy aimed at keeping the patient underhydrated to reduce cerebral edema and antidiuretic hormone (ADH) secretion. However, underhydration has been suspected to also reduce cerebral perfusion pressures and cerebral blood flow. *Current* therapy involves maintenance of normovolemia. I&O is monitored, and the patient usually has an indwelling urinary catheter. Hypotonic IV solutions, such as D_5W, may be avoided because they increase cerebral edema.

Nutritional support: Parenteral or enteral feedings or modified diet, depending on patient's LOC and ability to swallow.

Measures to reduce hyperthermia: Tepid sponges, cooling blankets, or convection blankets may assist in controlling hyperpyrexia.

Antithrombus therapy: Antiembolism hose, sequential compression devices, or pneumatic foot pumps may be prescribed to prevent thrombophlebitis in the legs from venous stasis.

Treatment of complications: Examples include disseminated intravascular coagulation, syndrome of inappropriate antidiuretic hormone (SIADH), IICP, respiratory or heart failure, and septic shock. A shunt may be needed if hydrocephalus from arachnoid adhesions and fibrotic changes persists.

Intrathecal antibiotics: Sometimes used if it is believed that systemic antibiotics alone will not be curative in the presence of particular bacteria (e.g., *Pseudomonas, Enterobacter, Staphylococcus*).

Physical medicine: Physical therapy (PT) and rehabilitation program may be needed, depending on neurologic deficits.

Vaccination: For people at increased risk (e.g., travelers to countries with endemic infections) a meningococcal vaccine (group A CY, W135) is available against some strains. *Haemophilus influenzae* group B vaccine should be incorporated as part of all routine childhood inoculations.

NURSING DIAGNOSES AND INTERVENTIONS

Knowledge deficit: Side effects and precautions for the prescribed antibiotics
Desired outcome: Before beginning the medication regimen, patient and significant other verbalize knowledge about the potential side effects and precautions for the prescribed antibiotics.

- For significant other and contacts taking prophylactic rifampin, explain the prescribed dose and schedule. Rifampin should be taken 1 hr before meals for maximum absorption. Emphasize the importance of taking this drug as a preventive measure against meningitis, and describe potential side effects, such as nausea, vomiting, diarrhea, orange urine, headache, and dizziness. Caution against wearing contact lenses, because the drug will permanently color them orange. In addition, rifampin reduces the effectiveness of oral contraceptives and is contraindicated during pregnancy.
- Instruct significant other and patient's other contacts who are taking rifampin to report the onset of jaundice (yellow skin or sclera), allergic reactions, and persistence of GI side effects.
- For other interventions, see **Knowledge deficit:** Adverse side effects from prolonged use of potent antibiotics, p. 581, in "Osteomyelitis."

NIC: Health Education; Teaching: Individual; Teaching: Prescribed Medication

Knowledge deficit: Rationale and procedure for Standard Precautions
Desired outcome: Before visitation, patient and significant other verbalize knowledge about the rationale for Standard Precautions and comply with the prescribed restrictions and precautionary measures.

> **Note:**   Patients with *N. meningitidis, H. influenzae,* or meningitis caused by an unidentified organism will be placed in a private room and will require special respiratory isolation precautions for 24 hr after initiation of appropriate antibiotic therapy. Masks should be worn and other Standard Precaution procedures observed.

- For patients with meningitis caused by *H. influenzae* or *N. meningitidis,* explain the method of disease transmission via airborne droplets and oral secretions and the rationale for private room and special precautions.
- Provide instructions for covering the mouth before coughing or sneezing and properly disposing of tissue.
- Instruct patients with specific respiratory precautions to stay in their rooms. If they must leave the room for a procedure or test, explain that a mask must be worn to protect others from contact with airborne droplets.
- For individuals in contact with the patient, explain the importance of wearing a surgical mask and using good hand-washing technique. Gloves should be worn when handling any body fluid, especially oral secretions. For more information, see Appendix Two, p. 817.

- Reassure patient that special respiratory precautions are temporary and will be discontinued once patient has been taking the appropriate antibiotic for 24-48 hr.
- Instruct individuals in contact with the patient that if the symptoms of meningitis develop (e.g., headache, fever, neck stiffness, photophobia), they should be reported rapidly to their health care provider.

NIC: Infection Control; Teaching: Disease Process; Teaching: Individual; Teaching: Procedure/Treatment

Pain related to headache, photophobia, and neck stiffness secondary to meningitis
Desired outcomes: Within 1-2 hr of intervention, patient's subjective perception of discomfort decreases, as documented by a pain scale. Objective indicators, such as grimacing, are absent or diminished.
- Provide a quiet environment and a darkened room. Restrict visitors as necessary to reduce noise. Sunglasses may promote comfort from photophobia.
- Promote bedrest and assist with ADL as needed to decrease movement that may cause pain.
- Apply an ice bag to the head or cool cloth to the eyes to help diminish the headache.
- Support patient in a position of comfort. Many persons with meningitis are comforted in a position with the head in extension and the body slightly curled. The HOB elevated to 30 degrees also may help. Keep the neck in alignment during position changes.
- Provide gentle passive ROM and massage to the neck and shoulder joints and muscles to help relieve stiffness. If the patient is afebrile, apply moist heat to the neck and back to promote muscle relaxation and decrease pain.
- Patients tend to be hyperirritable, with hyperalgesia. Sounds are loud. Keep communication simple and direct, in a soft, calm tone of voice. Touching startles the patient. Avoid needless stimulation. Consolidate activities. Loosen constricting bed clothing. Avoid restraining patient. Reduce stimulation to the minimal amount needed to accomplish required activity.
- For other interventions see **Pain** in "General Care of Patients With Neurologic Disorders," p. 343.

NIC: Analgesic Administration; Environmental Management: Comfort; Heat/Cold Application; Pain Management; Simple Massage

See Also: "Head Injury" for **Risk for disuse syndrome,** p. 282; **Fluid volume excess** related to SIADH, p. 283; "Seizure Disorders" for **Impaired tissue integrity** related to IV administration of phenytoin, p. 325; **Risk for trauma** with risk factors for oral, musculoskeletal, and airway vulnerability secondary to seizure activity, p. 324; Chapter 5 for **Fluid volume deficit,** p. 358; **Altered protection,** p. 369; "General Care of Patients With Neurologic Disorders" for **Risk for trauma** related to unsteady gait, p. 331; **Risk for injury** related to impaired pain, touch, and temperature sensations, p. 332; **Impaired corneal tissue integrity,** p. 333; **Altered nutrition:** Less than body requirements, p. 333; **Risk for fluid volume deficit,** p. 335; **Risk for aspiration,** p. 335; **Self-care deficit,** p. 336; **Constipation,** p. 339; **Decreased adaptive capacity:** intracranial, p. 340; **Impaired swallowing,** p. 344; **Altered body temperature,** p. 346; **Knowledge deficit:** Neurologic diagnostic tests, p. 346; nursing diagnoses in "Providing Nutritional Support," p. 687, for patients needing nutritional support; related nursing diagnoses in "Pressure Ulcers," p. 710, for patients who are immobile; Appendix One, "Caring for Patients on Prolonged Bedrest," p. 738; Appendix One, "Caring for Patients With Cancer and Other Life-disrupting Illnesses," p. 791, for appropriate patient and family psychosocial nursing diagnoses and interventions.

PATIENT-FAMILY TEACHING AND DISCHARGE PLANNING

The extent of teaching and discharge planning will depend on whether the patient has any residual damage. When providing patient-family teaching, focus on sensory information; avoid giving excessive information; and initiate a visiting nurse referral for necessary follow-up teaching. Consider including verbal and written information about the following:

- Referrals to community resources, such as public health nurse, visiting nurses association, community support groups, social workers, psychologic therapy, vocational rehabilitation agency, home health agencies, and extended and skilled care facilities.
- Medications, including drug name, purpose, dosage, schedule, precautions, drug/drug and food/drug interactions, and potential side effects for patient's medications, as well as those for the prophylactic antibiotics taken by family and significant other.
- For patients with residual neurologic deficits, teach the following as appropriate: exercises that promote muscle strength and mobility; measures for preventing contractures and skin breakdown; transfer techniques and proper body mechanics; safety measures if the patient has decreased pain and sensation or visual disturbances; use of assistive devices; indications of constipation, urinary retention, or urinary tract infection (UTI); bowel and bladder training programs; self-catheterization technique or care of indwelling catheters; and seizure precautions if indicated.

Section Two: Degenerative Disorders of the Nervous System

The central nervous system (CNS), peripheral nervous system, and autonomic nervous system are responsible for controlling and coordinating the functions of all body systems. With degenerative nerve disorders, the function of the nerve cells, dendrites, or axons is progressively altered or decreased. A variety of mechanisms, including outright destruction of the neurons and decreases in neurotransmitter synthesis uptake or release, account for this change in neuronal function.

Parkinsonism

Parkinson's disease is a slowly progressive degenerative disorder of the CNS affecting the brain centers that regulate movement. For unknown reasons, cell death occurs in the substantia nigra of the midbrain. When healthy, the substantia nigra projects dopaminergic neurons into the corpus striatum and releases the neurotransmitter dopamine in that area. Degeneration of these neurons leads to an abnormally low concentration of dopamine in the basal ganglia. The basal ganglia control muscle tone and voluntary motor movement via a balance between two main neurotransmitters, dopamine and acetylcholine. The deficit of dopamine, which has an inhibitory effect, allows the relative excess of acetylcholine. The excitatory effect of acetylcholine causes overactivity of the basal ganglia, which interferes with normal muscle tone and the control of smooth, purposeful movement, causing the characteristic symptoms of Parkinson's disease: muscle rigidity, tremors, and slowness of movement.

Possible causes include viral encephalitis, neurotoxins, cerebrovascular disease, head injury, phenothiazine use, and exposure to carbon monoxide. Improper synthesis of a heroin-like substance results in the product n-methyl 4-phenyl 1236 tetrahydropyridine (MPTP), which causes a severe form of Parkinson's disease in those who have taken this illegal recreational drug. The vast majority of Parkinson's disease occurs without an apparent or known cause, however. Approximately 1% of all individuals older than 50 yr have this disease. Parkinsonism is usually progressive, and death can result from aspiration pneumonia or choking. *Parkinsonian crisis*, a medical emergency, is usually precipitated by emotional trauma or failure to take the prescribed medications.

ASSESSMENT

Initially, symptoms are mild and include stiffness or slight hand tremors. They gradually increase and can become disabling. Cardinal features are tremors, rigidity, and bradykinesia. Assessment findings vary in degree and are highly individualized.

Bradykinesia: Slowness, stiffness, and difficulty initiating movement. The patient may have a masklike, blank facial expression; "unblinking" stare; difficulty chewing and swallowing; drooling caused by decreased frequency of swallowing; and a high-pitched, monotonal, weak voice. Speech may be slow and slurred. The patient also has loss of automatic associated movements, such as the ability to swing the arms when walking.

Loss of postural reflexes: Causes the typical stooped, forward-leaning, shuffling, propulsive gait with short, rapidly accelerating steps; stumbling; and difficulty maintaining or regaining balance, which makes the individual prone to stumbling and falling. Abnormal gait in which the body is bent backward (retropulsion) may also be present.

Increased muscle rigidity: Limb muscles become rigid on passive motion. Typically, this rigidity results in jerky ("cogwheel") motions or steady resistance to all movement ("lead-pipe" rigidity).

Tremors: Increase when the limb is at rest and stop with voluntary movement and during sleep (nonintentional tremor). "Pill-rolling" tremor of the hands and "to-and-fro" tremor of the head are typical.

Autonomic: Excessive diaphoresis, seborrhea, postural hypotension, decreased libido, hypomotility of the GI tract, and urinary hesitancy. Vision may blur as a result of lost accommodation.

Other: Dementia (e.g., forgetfulness, irritability, paranoia, hallucinations) commonly is associated with Parkinson's disease. However, not all patients develop impaired intellectual and mental functioning. Mental status testing may be complicated by the patient's movement disorder. Some patients may experience akathisia, a condition of motor restlessness in which the individual has a compelling need to walk about constantly. Handwriting becomes progressively smaller, cramped, and tremulous. Depression is common.

Physical assessment: Usually a positive blink reflex is elicited by tapping a finger between the patient's eyebrows. Blinking may occur 5-10 times/min instead of the normal 20 times/min. A positive palmomental (palm-chin) reflex can be elicited (muscles of the chin and corner of mouth contract when the patient's palm is stroked). Diminished postural reflexes are present on neurologic examination; however, there is risk of injury with this test because the patient may quickly lose balance and fall.

Parkinsonian crisis: This sudden and severe increase in bradykinesia, muscle rigidity, and tremors can lead to tachycardia, hyperpnea, hyperpyrexia, and muscle paralysis, causing an inability to swallow or maintain a patent airway.

Oculogyric crisis: Fixation of the eyes in one position, generally upward, sometimes for several hours. This is relatively rare.

DIAGNOSTIC TESTS

Diagnosis usually is made on the basis of physical assessment and characteristic symptoms and after other neurologic problems have been ruled out.

Urinalysis: May reveal decreased dopamine level, which supports the diagnosis.

Medication withdrawal: Long-term therapy with large doses of medications, such as haloperidol or phenothiazines, can produce extrapyramidal side effects known as pseudoparkinsonism. If caused by these medications, symptoms will disappear when the drug is discontinued.

Electroencephalogram (EEG):   Often shows abnormalities, such as diffuse, nonspecific slowing of θ-waves.

Lumbar puncture (LP) with CSF analysis: May show decreased levels of dopamine or its metabolite in the CSF.

Positron emission tomography (PET):   May reveal areas of decreased dopamine metabolism. PET can delineate physiologic metabolic processes by recording tracers of nuclear annihilation in body tissues. The nuclear tracers are specifically designed to match chemicals required for metabolic processes and thus be taken up by the body in its normal physiologic function.

Tremor studies: Serial measurements of functional activity will show decreased performance.

Cineradiographic study of swallowing: May show abnormal pattern and delayed relaxation of cricopharyngeal muscles.

See Also: "General Care of Patients With Neurologic Disorders," **Knowledge deficit:** Neurologic diagnostic tests, p. 346, for care considerations for patients undergoing EEG, LP, and PET.

COLLABORATIVE MANAGEMENT

Pharmacotherapy: See Table 4-1 for a description of the mechanisms, actions, and side effects of anti-Parkinson drugs.

Dopamine replacement (e.g., levodopa, levodopa-carbidopa or levodopa-benserazide combinations):   Given in increasing amounts until symptoms are reduced or patient's tolerance to side effects is reached. It may be used as initial therapy or later when other medications can no longer control Parkinson's symptoms.

Antiviral agents (e.g., amantadine):   Less effective than levodopa but with less severe side effects. May be used as the initial therapy or as an adjunct to anticholinergics or levodopa. Effects diminish in a few months, so this drug may be used intermittently.

Dopamine agonist (e.g., bromocriptine, pergolide):   Administered with a concomitant reduction of dopamine replacement dosage. It may be used to reduce levodopa-induced dyskinesia, such as involuntary movements and the frequency of "on-off" responses.

Monoamine oxidase (MAO) type B inhibitor (e.g., selegiline):   Used as an early intervention or as an adjunct with levodopa to inhibit the breakdown of levodopa, resulting in less fluctuation in blood levels.

Anticholinergics (e.g., ethopropazine, trihexyphenidyl, cycrimine, procyclidine, biperiden, benztropine mesylate):   Often used in conjunction with dopamine replacement therapy but may be used alone if the patient's symptoms are mild or if the patient cannot tolerate levodopa. Anticholinergics may improve tremor and rigidity but often do little for bradykinesia or balance problems.

Antihistamines (e.g., diphenhydramine, orphenadrine hydrochloride):   Usually given in conjunction with anticholinergic drugs but may be used alone if the patient's symptoms are mild.

Phenothiazine derivative (e.g., ethopropazine):   Generally used in combination with other anti-Parkinson drugs to reduce rigidity, tremors, and spasms.

Laxatives and stool softeners (e.g., docusate sodium, Milk of Magnesia):   Given to prevent constipation.

Antitremor medications (e.g., propranolol, primidone, clonazepam):   May be used to decrease tremors.

Antidepressants (e.g., nortriptyline, imipramine, amitriptyline): Used to treat depression as well as some parkinsonism symptoms; help to block reabsorption of dopamine and have some anticholinergic properties.

Antiemetics (e.g., trimethobenzamide, domperidone)

Physical medicine and exercise program: Massage; muscle stretching; active/passive ROM, especially on hands and feet; walking and gait training exercises; suggestions for maintaining mobility and initiating movements; occupational therapy (OT) evaluation for assistive devices to help in self-care with ADL.

Treatment of complications of dopamine replacement therapy

Choreiform or involuntary movements (e.g., facial grimacing, tongue protrusion, restlessness)

- Dose reduction or redistribution throughout the day.
- Drug "holiday": this treatment is controversial. After temporary withdrawal, levodopa is resumed at a much lower dose. Generally the patient can be maintained for several months to years at this much lower dose, with fewer drug-related adverse side effects and good mobility. This treatment requires hospitalization, because during withdrawal the patient may become completely immobile and dependent. Medications are tapered gradually. These individuals often need psychologic support because, without the drug's mitigating effects, this may be the first time they experience the full impact and immobility of their disease.

Severe mental status changes (e.g., agitation, confusion, psychosis)

- Dose reduction.
- Drug holiday.
- Clozapine for drug-related psychoses.

"End of dose" wearing-off phenomenon: Return of signs and symptoms before next dose is due.

- Administer smaller, more frequent doses.
- Use slow-release medication preparations.
- Encourage low-protein diet.

Vivid dreaming

- Reduce the last dose of levodopa given at night.

On-off response: This is a rapid fluctuation or change in the patient's condition. The individual is "on" one moment, in a state of relative mobility, and "off" the next, in a state of complete or nearly complete immobility. Attacks can occur over a 2- to 3-min period or may last several hours. Initially the attacks may occur 3-4 hr after anti-Parkinson medication is given. Later in the disease they may occur at any time. Cause is uncertain but appears to be related to fluctuating drug levels in the brain as loss of striatal ability to store dopamine progresses. Usually this response occurs after the patient has been on medication for several years and has not found relief through increasing levodopa dosages.

- Smaller, more frequent doses to titrate and space the levodopa doses during the 24-hr day.
- Combining levodopa with anticholinergic medications, dopamine agonists, or amantadine may be helpful.
- Use of sustained-release forms of levodopa.
- Administration of SC apomorphine. This dopamine agonist has been demonstrated in clinical trials to effectively counter the "on-off" response. Domperidone (a peripheral dopamine antagonist) is given before apomorphine to reduce emesis and orthostatic hypotension.
- Continuous enteral infusion of levodopa via gastric or jejunal (PEG or PEJ) tubes.
- Drug holiday. Not used too often since on-off response usually is very short-lived.

Treatment for parkinsonian crisis: This crisis necessitates respiratory and cardiac support. The patient is placed in a quiet, calm environment with

TABLE 4-1   Anti-Parkinson Drugs

Medication	Mechanism of action	Side effects
Dopamine replacements		
Levodopa	Levodopa, the metabolic precursor of dopamine, crosses the blood-brain barrier and restores dopamine levels in the brain. Before levodopa crosses the blood-brain barrier, much of it is converted into dopamine by the peripheral metabolism (GI tract and liver), causing many of the drug's side effects	Choreiform and involuntary movements (e.g., facial grimacing, tongue protusion); on-off response; severe depression with possible suicidal overtones; GI bleeding; orthostatic hypotension; blurred vision; anorexia; nausea and vomiting; dry mouth; constipation; urinary retention; confusion; agitation; hallucination
Carbidopa-levodopa, benserazide-levodopa	Carbidopa prevents peripheral metabolism of levodopa, thereby increasing the amount of levodopa available for transport to the brain. Carbidopa does not cross the blood-brain barrier and therefore does not affect the metabolism of levodopa in the brain. Carbidopa reduces the amount of levodopa needed	No reactions to carbidopa alone; adverse reactions are to levodopa
Antivirals		
Amantadine	Mechanism of action not understood; appears to increase the synthesis and release of dopamine from neuronal storage sites; has an anticholinergic effect as well	Most side effects are like those of levodopa but are milder and dose related; include insomnia, peripheral edema, heart failure, depression, nervousness, slurred speech, ataxia, orthostatic hypotension, blurred vision, anorexia, nausea, vomiting, dry mouth, constipation, urinary retention, confusion, irritability, hallucination

Dopamine agonists Bromocriptine, lisuride, pergolide	Have a direct stimulating effect on dopamine receptors, thereby enhancing their activity	Produce less nausea and vomiting than levodopa but otherwise have similar side effects, including orthostatic hypotension, blurred vision, nausea, vomiting, dry mouth, constipation, urinary retention, confusion, paranoia, insomnia, ataxia, digital vasospasm
Anticholinergics Ethopropazine, trihexy-phenidyl, cyrimine, procyclidine, biperiden, benztropine mesylate	Reduce the excitatory action of acetylcholine on cholinergic neuron receptors. In Parkinson's disease, because of the dopamine deficit, there is an imbalance between dopamine, with its inhibitory action, and acetylcholine, with its excitatory action. Anticholinergics reduce acetylcholine action and work to reestablish this balance	Side effects are dose related and include decreased sweating, orthostatic hypotension, tachycardia, dry mouth, blurred vision, photophobia, nausea, drowsiness, constipation, urinary retention or overflow incontinence, confusion, mental slowness, insomnia, nervousness, headache
Antihistamines Diphenhydramine, orphenadrine HCl	Have a central cholinergic blocking action, prolonging dopamine action by inhibiting its uptake and storage; used in conjunction with anticholinergics	GI effects are fairly minimal; other side effects include drowsiness, mild hypotension, dry mouth, anorexia, constipation, urinary retention
Phenothiazine derivative Ethopropazine	Has a central cholinergic blocking action; differs from other phenothiazines in that it is used to control extrapyramidal symptoms; used in conjunction with other anti-Parkinson drugs	Depression, drowsiness, hypotension, dizziness, ataxia, blurred vision, nausea, dry mouth, constipation
MAO B inhibitor Selegiline	Inhibits breakdown of levodopa	Nausea, lightheadedness, dizziness, abdominal pain, insomnia, confusion, dry mouth

GI, Gastrointestinal; *MAO,* monoamine oxidase.

subdued lighting. Sodium phenobarbital or sodium amobarbital is given IM or IV.

Speech therapy: Speech evaluation for patient with verbal deficits.

Antiembolism hose: To help prevent postural hypotension.

Counseling or psychotherapy: To help patient and significant other adapt to the disability and deal with emotions and feelings, such as depression, that are either a direct or an indirect result of the disease process or drug therapy. Occasionally, electroconvulsive therapy is used for persistent and serious depression.

Diet: A controlled, low-protein diet may be prescribed if the patient is receiving dopamine replacement therapy, because high-protein intake reduces the medication's effectiveness. A high-fiber diet may be given to prevent constipation. Because use of caffeine may increase patient's symptoms, a caffeine-free diet helps some patients.

Stereotactic pallidotomy surgery: Involves the use of electrical coagulation, freezing, radioactivity, or ultrasound to destroy portions of the globus pallidus of the ventrolateral nucleus of the thalamus to prevent involuntary movement and help relieve tremors and rigidity of the extremities. Stereotactic surgery is accomplished through a small incision with CT scanning across several viewing planes to aid the physician in directing specially designed probes. Bilateral chronic electrostimulation of the pallidum has also been demonstrated to reduce symptoms.

Adrenal transplant: Involves grafting one of the patient's own adrenal medullary glands to the caudate nucleus of the brain. The medullary portion of the adrenal gland produces dopamine for the peripheral nervous system. When grafted, the adrenal medullary may continue to produce dopamine in the CNS, reducing or eliminating Parkinson's disease symptoms and the need for medication. Postural problems causing falls often improve, but other benefits often are variable and minimal. This procedure involves three major surgeries: (1) stereotactic localization of the caudate nucleus, (2) craniotomy (see "Brain Tumors," p. 288), and (3) laparotomy for adrenalectomy.

Therapies undergoing clinical trials: Fetal neuronal tissue transplants (neonatal substantia nigra) produce dopamine in the CNS and reduce or alleviate symptoms. Continuous infusion of intracerebral and ventricular dopamine is also being investigated for effectiveness in controlling symptoms. Deep brain stimulation via surgically implanted electrodes to control severe tremors is undergoing clinical trials. New dopamine-agonist medications (pramipexole, cabergoline) aid in smoothing muscle action and function. A COMT (catechol-O-methyl-transferase) inhibitor (tolcapone) has been demonstrated to reduce levodopa degradation in the GI tract, kidneys, and liver to reduce fluctuation in serum levels. Additional pharmacologic research is being directed toward glutamate antagonists, glial cell line–derived neurotrophic factor (GDNF), and antioxidants.

NURSING DIAGNOSES AND INTERVENTIONS

Risk for trauma with risk factors from an unsteady gait secondary to bradykinesia, tremors, and rigidity

Desired outcome: Following instruction, patient demonstrates safe and effective ambulatory techniques and preventive measures and remains free of trauma.

- During ambulation, encourage patient to deliberately swing the arms to assist the gait and raise the feet to help prevent falls. Advise patient to step over an imaginary object or line, which will help raise the feet higher and increase the stride.
- Have patient practice movements that are especially difficult (e.g., turning). Teach patient to walk in a wide arc rather than pivot when turning to avoid crossing one leg over the other.
- Teach head and neck exercises to promote good posture. Remind patient repeatedly to maintain an upright posture, especially when walking.

- Advise patient to stop occasionally to slow down the walking speed. Teach patients to concentrate on listening to his or her feet as they touch the floor and count the cadence to prevent too fast a gait. Encourage patient to lift toes and to walk with the heel touching the floor first.
- Remind patient to maintain a wide-based gait.
- Provide a clear pathway while the patient is walking. Teach patient to avoid crowds, scatter rugs, uneven surfaces, fast turns, narrow doorways, and obstructions.
- Encourage patient to perform ROM exercises daily and to exercise for flexibility, strength, gait, and balance. Emphasize that routine exercises, along with prescribed medications, may prevent or delay disability.
- Advise the patient to wear leather-sole or smooth-sole shoes but to test the shoes to ensure they are not too slippery. Rubber-sole or crepe-sole shoes tend to catch on floors, especially carpeted floors, and may cause falls.
- Encourage patient not to hurry or rush because this may precipitate falls. Slowness of gait and inability to get to the bathroom fast enough may cause incontinence. Encourage males to keep a urinal at the bedside. A commode at the bedside may be helpful for females.
- For other interventions, see **Risk for trauma,** p. 331, in "General Care of Patients With Neurologic Disorders."

NIC: Activity Therapy; Environmental Management: Safety; Fall Prevention; Surveillance: Safety; Teaching: Individual

Impaired physical mobility related to difficulty initiating movement
Desired outcome: Following instruction, patient demonstrates measures that enhance the ability to initiate desired movement.
- Teach patient that rocking from side to side may help initiate leg movement. Marching in place a few steps before resuming forward motion also may be helpful. Other measures that may help the patient are relaxing back on the heels and raising the toes; tapping the hip of the leg to be moved; bending at the knees and straightening up; or raising the arms in a sudden, short motion. If the patient's feet remain "glued" to the floor despite these measures, suggest that he or she think of something else for a few moments and then try again.
- Teach patient to get out of a chair by getting to the edge of the seat, placing hands on the arm supports, bending forward slightly, moving feet back, and then rhythmically rocking in the chair a few times before trying to get up. Advise patient to sit in chairs with backs and arms and to purchase elevated toilet seats or sidebars in the bathroom to assist with rising and prevent falls.
- Teach patient measures that may help with getting out of bed: rocking to a sitting position, placing blocks under the legs of the head of the bed (HOB) to elevate it, and tying a rope or sheet to the foot of the bed to help the patient pull to a sitting position.
- "Freezing" is variable and can fluctuate with stress or the patient's emotional state. Teach patients and significant others to recognize situations that can cause freezing episodes so that they can anticipate and plan to avoid them. For example, attempting two movements simultaneously, such as trying to change direction quickly while walking, can cause freezing. Distracting environmental, visual, or auditory stimuli also can precipitate a freezing episode. Doorways; narrow passages; or a change in floor color, texture, or slope can pose problems for many patients.

NIC: Environmental Management: Safety; Exercise Therapy: Ambulation; Self-Care Assistance; Teaching: Individual; Teaching: Prescribed Activity/ Exercise

Knowledge deficit: Side effects of and precautionary measures for taking anti-Parkinson medications

Desired outcome: Following instruction and before hospital discharge, patient and significant other verbalize knowledge about the side effects of and necessary precautionary measures for taking anti-Parkinson medications.

Note: Teach patient and significant other to report adverse side effects promptly because many side effects are dose related and can be controlled by an adjustment in the dosage.

Side effects common to most anti-Parkinson medications

- Stress the importance of taking medication on schedule and not forgetting a dose. Missing a dose may adversely affect mobility. Patient and health care provider can adjust the dose schedule so that the medication peaks at mealtime or times when patient needs mobility most. To assist patient having difficulty with self-medication, premeasure doses in segmented or separate containers labeled with the date/time of the dose.
- Teach patient to take medications with meals to decrease the potential for nausea. Encourage the patient with anorexia to eat frequent, small nutritious snacks and meals.
- Advise patient to counteract orthostatic hypotension by making position changes slowly and in stages. Teach patient to dangle legs a few minutes before standing. Antiembolism hose may help some patients. Encourage male patients to urinate from a sitting rather than standing position if possible. Report dizziness to health care provider.
- To ease dry mouth and maintain the integrity of the oral mucous membrane, teach patient to use sugarless chewing gum or hard candy, frequent mouth rinses with water, or artificial saliva products.
- Advise patient to report any urinary hesitancy or incontinence because this may signal urinary retention. Individuals taking anticholinergics may find that voiding before taking the medication relieves this problem. See "Urinary Retention," p. 185, for additional measures.
- Constipation is a common problem with these medications. For interventions, see **Constipation,** p. 743, in Appendix One, "Caring for Patients on Prolonged Bedrest."
- Many of these drugs can cause or aggravate mental status changes, such as confusion, mental slowness or dullness, and even agitation, paranoia, and hallucinations. Teach patient to report these signs to the health care provider promptly for possible dose adjustment.
- For patient with blurred vision, orient to surroundings, identify self when entering the room, keep walkways unobstructed, and encourage patient to ask for assistance when ambulating.

Side effects specific to levodopa

- Teach the patient that levodopa should be taken with a full glass of water on an empty stomach to facilitate absorption. If nausea or GI upset occurs, suggest the patient eat 10-15 min after taking the medication. If the patient continues to experience GI upset or nausea, the medication may be taken with food.
- Teach patient to avoid vitamin preparations or fortified cereals that contain pyridoxine (vitamin B_6), which reduces the effectiveness of levodopa. The health care provider may limit the patient's intake of foods high in pyridoxine, such as wheat germ, whole grain cereals, legumes, and liver.
- Teach patient that a dietary intake high in protein may interfere with the effectiveness of levodopa. Although the diet should meet the recommended daily allowance of protein (i.e., 0.8 g/kg body weight), the patient should avoid excessive amounts of meat, eggs, dairy products, and legumes. If prescribed, dietary supplementation with l-tryptophan needs to be calculated

into the patient's total protein allotment. If possible, virtually all protein should be eaten at the evening meal to minimize interaction with levodopa.

- Instruct patient to report muscle twitching or spasmodic winking because these are early signs of overdose.
- Abnormal involuntary movements, such as facial grimacing and tongue protrusion, signal that an adjustment in dose may be needed. The health care provider may prescribe a reduced dose, redistribution throughout the day, or a medically supervised drug holiday.
- Explain signs and symptoms of parkinsonian crisis (i.e., sudden and severe increase in bradykinesia, muscle rigidity, tremors). Emphasize the need for immediate medical intervention with this crisis because respiratory and cardiac support may be necessary. Teach patient that to avoid this crisis, it is necessary to take levodopa as scheduled and not to stop the medication abruptly. Teach significant other to place patient in a quiet, calm environment with subdued lighting until medical help arrives if parkinsonian crisis occurs.
- Explain the signs of the on-off response (i.e., patient relatively mobile one moment and completely immobile the next) and the importance of seeking medical intervention should they occur. Titrating the dose, spacing the doses differently, using sustained-release forms of levodopa, and combining levodopa with other anti-Parkinson medications may be prescribed to counter the on-off effect.
- Monitor for behavioral changes. Severe depression with suicidal overtones can be caused by this drug and should be reported immediately. The health care provider may prescribe a dose reduction or, if this is ineffective, a medically supervised drug holiday.
- Explain that the patient's medication may cause dark-colored urine and sweat.
- Caution patient to avoid alcohol because it impairs levodopa's effectiveness.
- Explain the importance of medical follow-up while taking this drug to monitor for such problems as increased intraocular pressure and changes in glucose control.

Side effects specific to amantadine

- Teach patient that taking this drug earlier in the day may prevent insomnia.
- Teach patient and significant other to monitor for and report any SOB, peripheral edema, significant weight gain, or change in mental status because these signs often signal heart failure.
- Instruct patient not to stop taking this medication abruptly because doing so may precipitate parkinsonian crisis.
- A diffuse, rose-colored mottling of the skin, usually confined to the lower extremities, may develop. The condition may subside with continued therapy and will disappear in a few weeks to months after the drug is discontinued. Exposure to cold or standing may make the color more prominent. Teach patient to report this condition if it occurs, but reassure him or her that the condition is more cosmetic than serious.
- Patients with a history of seizures may have an increase in the number of seizures. Instruct patient to monitor and promptly report to health care provider a loss of seizure control.
- Caution patient to avoid alcohol and CNS depressants because these agents potentiate the effects of amantadine.
- Explain that most side effects of amantadine are dose related.

Side effects specific to dopamine agonists

- Caution patient to avoid alcohol when taking this medication because he or she will experience less tolerance.
- Bromocriptine can cause digital vasospasm. Teach patient to avoid exposure to cold and to report the onset of finger or toe pallor.

Side effects specific to anticholinergic medications
- Teach patient that this medication may decrease perspiration. Explain that patient should avoid strenuous exercise and keep cool during the summer to avoid heat stroke.
- Teach patient not to stop taking this medication abruptly because doing so can result in parkinsonian crisis.
- Teach patient to monitor for tachycardia or palpitation and to report either condition.

Side effects specific to selegiline hydrochloride (Eldepryl)
- Stress the importance of taking this medication only in the prescribed dose. Selegiline is a selective MAO type B inhibitor and in the recommended dose of ≤10 mg/day does not cause the hypertensive crisis that can occur when tyramine-containing foods (e.g., cheese, red wine, beer, yogurt) are eaten. Dosages >10 mg/day may result in hypertension if these foods are eaten. Usually, dietary modifications to reduce intake of tyramine-containing foods are recommended but they are not imperative.
- Avoidance of meperidine and other opioids is suggested. At recommended doses, no drug interactions have been noted. However, fatal drug interactions have occurred with patients taking other nonselective MAO inhibitors and could conceivably occur if higher-than-recommended doses were taken.
- Teach patient that taking the drug earlier in the day may prevent insomnia.

NIC: Nutritional Counseling; Teaching: Individual; Teaching: Prescribed Diet; Teaching: Prescribed Medication

Health-seeking behaviors: Facial and tongue exercises that enhance verbal communication and help prevent choking
Desired outcome: Following the demonstration and within the 24-hr period before hospital discharge, patient demonstrates facial and tongue exercises and states the rationale for their use.
- Explain to patient that special exercises can help strengthen and control facial and tongue muscles, which in turn will improve verbal communication and help prevent choking. Emphasize that routine exercises of the facial and tongue muscles, along with the prescribed medications, may prevent or delay disability.
- Teach the following exercises, and have patient return the demonstration: hold a sound for 5 sec, sing the scale, read aloud, and extend the tongue and try to touch the chin, nose, and cheek. Encourage patient to practice increasing voice volume.
- Provide a written handout that lists and describes the preceding exercises. Encourage patient to perform them hourly while awake.
- Teach patient the importance of stating feelings verbally because monotone speech and lack of facial expression impede nonverbal communication.

NIC: Exercise Promotion; Teaching: Individual; Teaching: Prescribed Activity/Exercise

See Also: "General Care of Patients With Neurologic Disorders" for **Impaired corneal tissue integrity,** p. 333; **Altered nutrition,** p. 333; **Risk for fluid volume deficit,** p. 335; **Risk for aspiration,** p. 335; **Self-care deficit,** p. 336; **Impaired verbal communication,** p. 338; **Constipation,** p. 339; **Impaired swallowing,** p. 344; **Knowledge deficit:** Neurologic diagnostic tests, p. 346; related nursing diagnoses in "Pressure Ulcers," p. 710; Appendix One, "Caring for Patients on Prolonged Bedrest," p. 738, for patients with varying degrees of immobility; Appendix One, "Caring for

Preoperative and Postoperative Patients," p. 717, for patients undergoing surgery; Appendix One, "Caring for Patients With Cancer and Other Life-disrupting Illnesses," p. 791, for psychosocial nursing diagnoses and interventions for patients and significant others as appropriate.

PATIENT-FAMILY TEACHING AND DISCHARGE PLANNING

When providing patient-family teaching, focus on sensory information; avoid giving excessive information; and initiate a visiting nurse referral for necessary follow-up teaching. Consider including verbal and written information about the following:

- Referrals to community resources, such as local and national Parkinson's Society chapters, public health nurse, visiting nurses association, community support groups, social workers, psychological therapy, vocational rehabilitation agency, home health agencies, and extended and skilled care facilities. Additional general information can be obtained by contacting the following organizations:

  American Parkinson Disease Association
  1250 Hylan Blvd., Suite 4B
  Staten Island, NY 10305   (800) 223-APDA

  United Parkinson's Foundation
  833 West Washington Blvd.
  Chicago, IL 60607   (312) 733-1893
  WWW address: *http://www.parkinsonsdisease.com/*

  Parkinson's Disease Foundation, Inc.
  Executive Director
  William Black Medical Research Building
  Columbia Presbyterian Medical Center
  650 West 168th Street
  New York, NY 10032   (212) 923-4700 or (800) 457-6676

  National Parkinson Foundation, Inc.
  1501 NW 9th Avenue
  Miami, FL 33136   (800) 327-4545
  WWW address: *http://www.parkinson.org/*

- Related safety measures for patients with bradykinesia, muscle rigidity, and tremors.
- Emphasis that disability may be prevented or delayed through exercises and medications.
- Techniques for unlocking a position (see p. 229).
- Evaluation of home environment and tips for home accident prevention.
- Measures to prevent or lessen postural hypotension.
- Signs and symptoms of parkinsonian crisis (see p. 223) and the need for immediate medical attention.
- For other interventions, see "Patient-Family Teaching and Discharge Planning" (third through tenth entries only), in "Multiple Sclerosis," p. 210.

Alzheimer's disease

Alzheimer's disease is a progressive disorder of the brain characterized by changes and degeneration of the cerebral cortical nerve cells and nerve endings, resulting in abnormal neurofibrillary tangles and neuritic plaques that affect nerve conduction between cells. This process causes irreversible impairment of memory and deterioration of intellectual functions. Genetics plays a role in some patients with Alzheimer's disease. Approximately 15% of these patients appear to have an autosomal dominantly inherited form. Accumulation of amyloid protein in the plaques may be pathogenic and is associated with a defect on chromosome 21. Presence of the *E4* allele of apolipoprotein E on chromosome 19 seems to be associated with increased susceptibility. Genetics as a factor seems to be more strongly linked if the time of onset is at a younger age. A neurotransmitter deficiency has also been speculated as a probable cause. The primary neurotransmitter that appears to be deficient is acetylcholine. Other neurotransmitters (e.g., somatostatin, norepinephrine, serotonin, dopamine) also may be reduced, but to a lesser degree. Male gender, postmenopausal estrogen therapy, and higher education have all been associated with decreased incidence of Alzheimer's disease. Endogenous toxins, such as glutamate, trauma, and aluminum poisoning, have all been speculated as playing a role in the pathogenesis of Alzheimer's disease. In other cases of Alzheimer's, the cause is unknown. The primary risk factor for Alzheimer's disease is age. Onset is insidious, and it can strike individuals as young as 40 yr. The disease progresses to total disability and eventually results in death from problems such as infection or aspiration, usually within 3-15 yr.

ASSESSMENT

The appearance and severity of signs and symptoms vary from individual to individual. Alzheimer's disease is characterized by progressive memory failure, intellectual deterioration, and personality change. It is classified into four stages: early, middle, late, and terminal, depending on the patient's degree of impairment. Initial indicators are mild, but short-term memory loss is a cardinal early sign. It may take several years before a definite diagnosis can be made. Often a diagnosis is not made until the middle stage, when the patient is having trouble recognizing objects or things, carrying out previously performed skills or activities, or communicating. By the late stage, memory and intellectual ability are absent. In the terminal stage, the individual is in both a mental and physical vegetative condition.

Memory: Initially, memory loss is slight, usually consisting of inability to retain recently acquired information. The individual may lose things and forget dates. The individual also may forget how to use common objects and tools, while retaining the power and coordination necessary for performing these activities. Long-term memory eventually is lost. The individual becomes lost in the home or other familiar surroundings. Gradually he or she loses the ability to recognize or name common objects and familiar people, including members of the immediate family.

Cognitive process: The individual demonstrates decreasing ability to think through problems, poor decision-making ability, shortened attention span, lack of insight, inability to perform arithmetic calculations, and loss of reading and writing capabilities. Gradually the ability to manage familiar activities, such as shopping or cooking, fails. The individual will become hesitant and reluctant to carry out minor and familiar tasks. As the ability to reason and abstract declines, the individual fails to recognize unsafe behaviors, resulting in a potential for injury. Hallucinations often occur because of misconceptions of the environment. Following even simple two- or three-step instructions is increasingly difficult. Eventually there is a total loss of intellectual ability and comprehension and an inability to participate in any activities. In the last stages, there may be instinctual and emotional awareness of family voices, touching, or presence, but there is no intellectual or conscious awareness or conscious interaction with the environment.

Personality changes: The realization that memory and intellect are deteriorating may result in depression, frustration, bitterness, anxiety, and apathy. Difficulty with tasks that are beyond the individual's capacity leads to easy frustration. As insight declines, depression becomes less of a problem. There is often emotional lability, panic, fear, bewilderment, and perplexity. As awareness of the environment declines, apathy may become more prominent. Symptoms of paranoia, delusion, agitation, and hallucination may appear, resulting in suspiciousness and accusing others of stealing things that have been misplaced. Previous psychotic traits are exaggerated. As the ability to communicate decreases and the world becomes more frightening, the potential for violence and agitation increases. The patient may have catastrophic reactions and emotional outbursts when faced with a complex task.

Social behavior: Decreased ability to handle social interaction, loss of social graces, loss of inhibitions (resulting in inappropriate language or acts), helplessness, dependency.

Communication patterns: Difficulty finding words, loss of spontaneity in speech, inability to express thoughts, incoherent speech. The individual gradually loses all language ability and becomes unable to communicate other than with such behaviors as yelling, noisiness, or striking out. Eventually, this limited ability may be lost and he or she may be able only to grunt or express pain by grimacing.

Sleep pattern: Restlessness, pacing, and wandering occur. Sleep/wake cycles are maintained, but generally the need for sleep decreases. Nocturnal awakenings and reversals of normal sleep patterns are common. Toward the final stages, the individual often sleeps excessively.

Self-care: Progressive neglect of routine tasks and personal hygiene; weight loss owing to refusal to eat and lack of awareness of the importance of nutrition; increasing inability to dress, bathe, toilet, and feed self or recognize the need to or where to urinate or defecate (resulting in incontinence). Eventually the individual becomes totally dependent on others for all self-care activities.

Mobility/posture: Stooped and shuffling gait; progressive balance and coordination problems; falling; inability to walk and use arms, hands, and legs for purposeful movement. The individual becomes bedridden. Joint contractures and muscle rigidity are common in the final stages.

Other: In the last stages of the disease, myoclonus and seizures can occur. Spontaneous involuntary movement occurs, but the ability to open the eyes and track is maintained. Brain stem reflexes are present, and grasping, snout (evidenced by tapping the nose, which results in a marked facial grimace), and sucking reflexes can be elicited. Control of sphincter muscles is gone, and the individual may be incontinent of stool and urine. Chewing and swallowing incoordination develops, and death usually occurs as a result of aspiration pneumonia.

DIAGNOSTIC TESTS

Many disorders that can cause a progressive dementia syndrome (e.g., head injuries, brain tumors, depression, arteriosclerosis, drug toxicity, metabolic disorders such as hypothyroidism, alcoholism) need to be ruled out. This is especially important because some dementias are reversible. The only definitive test for Alzheimer's is the brain biopsy, but usually this is done only after death. The diagnosis usually is made on the basis of the neurologic and mental status examination and after other causes have been ruled out.

Mental status examination: Tests orientation, memory, calculation, abstraction, judgment, and mood.

Neurologic examination: Indicators that may signal Alzheimer's disease: release signs, such as snout, grasp, and sucking reflexes; olfactory deficits; impaired stereognosis (inability to recognize the touch or smell of a familiar object when placed in the hand); short-stepped, bradykinetic gait; tremor; and abnormalities on cerebellar testing.

Positron emission tomography (PET): May show lower cerebral cortex metabolic rates for glucose, even in the early stages of the disease. PET is now considered the most definitive diagnostic procedure for Alzheimer's disease.

CT scan: May reveal brain atrophy and symmetric bilateral ventricular enlargement, which help support the diagnosis. It also helps rule out other neurologic problems, particularly mass lesions.

MRI: May reveal brain atrophy and symmetric bilateral ventricular enlargement, which help support the diagnosis. Because of its ability to detect both biochemical and anatomic changes, this test may identify Alzheimer's disease at a very early stage.

Tropicamide pupil dilation test: May allow earlier detection; dilation of the pupil is greater with Alzheimer's disease.

EEG: May reveal generalized slowed brain wave activity and reduced voltage, which support the diagnosis.

CSF: May show reduced acetylcholinesterase.

Brain biopsy: Will demonstrate the presence of neurofibrillary tangles and neuritic plaques.

Other tests: May be performed to rule out other causes of dementia: skull and chest x-rays, lumbar puncture (LP), serum tests (e.g., liver, thyroid, syphilis), urinalysis, arteriograms, drug screen, and brain scan.

See Also: "General Care of Patients With Neurologic Disorders," **Knowledge deficit,** p. 346, for care considerations for patients undergoing PET, MRI, CT scan, and EEG.

COLLABORATIVE MANAGEMENT

Generally, treatment is supportive only. No recognized treatment or cure exists at this time.

Pharmacotherapy: The following medications, if prescribed, are used to treat symptoms or behavioral manifestations.

Early stage

Tacrine: Improves some cognitive deficits in mild to moderate Alzheimer's but does not alter the course of the underlying dementia. The patient taking this medication should be monitored for nausea, vomiting, diarrhea, abdominal pain, anorexia, and liver toxicity.

Donepezil (Aricept):   Has recently been approved for use in improving mild to moderate memory deficit. The patient taking this medication should be monitored for nausea, diarrhea, fatigue, insomnia, and anorexia.

Ergoloid mesylate: Sometimes effective in improving cognitive performance in early stages of dementia. However, its effect is only temporary and declines as the disease advances. Side effects include postural hypotension, transient nausea, and GI disturbances.

Tricyclic or other antidepressants (e.g., desipramine, imipramine, trazodone, nortriptyline, amitriptyline):   May relieve depression and elevate mood. Side effects include drowsiness, dizziness, orthostatic hypotension, urinary retention, and lowered seizure threshold.

Stimulants (e.g., methylphenidate, dextroamphetamine):   May be given for loss of spontaneity or inattention.

Nonsteroidal antiinflammatory drugs (e.g., ASA, ibuprofen):   May play a role in reducing the risk of disease and in decreasing the severity and progression of Alzheimer's.

Investigational therapies: May be used in an attempt to improve cognitive function on a temporary basis. Xanomeline has been associated with a positive effect on memory and cognition in early stages. Combinations of high-dose vitamin E and selegiline are suspected to slow progression of Alzheimer's. Tenilsetam is suspected to reduce protein cross-linking and thus slow progression. Cholinergic therapy aims to correct the acetylcholine deficiency in the brain. Various drugs include choline derivatives (e.g., choline chloride, lecithin), anticholinesterase inhibitors (e.g., physostigmine, tetrahydroaminoacridine), and cholinergic receptor stimulants. Fetal neuronal tissue transplants are undergoing clinical trials to determine their effectiveness in reducing or alleviating symptoms. Gene therapy shows promise for future investigation once associated chromosomal sites have been clearly demarcated.

Middle stage

Antipsychotic agents (e.g., haloperidol):   Used for combative or extremely agitated patients.

Tranquilizers or sedatives (e.g., chloral hydrate, diphenhydramine, triazolam, oxazepam):   Used to control hyperactivity, restlessness, and sleep disturbances. Lorazepam and alpraxolam may be used for agitation.

Late stage

Antiepilepsy drugs (e.g., carbamazepine, phenobarbital, phenytoin, diazepam, fosphenytoin):   Used to control seizures.

Laxatives and stool softeners (e.g., psyllium, docusate):   For constipation.

Terminal stage

Oral morphine: May be given (in small doses) to patients who have developed hypersensitivity to touch or restlessness.

Atropine or scopolamine: May be given to decrease respiratory secretions and the need for frequent, uncomfortable suctioning.

Diet: A high-fiber diet may be given to prevent constipation. For restless, hyperactive patients, a high-calorie diet or supplements may be prescribed. Caffeine is avoided because of its stimulating effect. In later stages, tube feedings may be an option for some patients. Although vitamin (e.g., niacin, B_{12}), folate, zinc, and lecithin treatments have not been proven effective in treating Alzheimer's disease, they are relatively harmless and the family may find some consolation in their use.

Counseling or psychotherapy: Counseling focus generally is on the significant other to help him or her deal with the depression, grief, guilt, and emotions caused by the patient's progressive disability and behavior. In all but the early stages, patients with Alzheimer's disease quickly lose the insight and intellectual ability that would make counseling beneficial to them.

NURSING DIAGNOSES AND INTERVENTIONS

Risk for trauma with risk factors associated with lack of awareness of environmental hazards secondary to cognitive deficit

Desired outcomes: Patient is free of symptoms of physical trauma. At least 24 hr before patient's hospital discharge, significant other identifies and plans to eliminate or control potentially dangerous factors in the patient's home environment.

- Orient patient to new surroundings. Reorient as needed. Keep necessary items, including water, phone, and call light, within easy reach. Assess patient's ability to use these items. Keep bed in its lowest position. Side rail position (up or down) will vary with the patient. The patient may be at risk of falling from climbing over side rails.
- Maintain an uncluttered environment to minimize the risk of environmental confusion and tripping. Ensure adequate lighting to help prevent falls in the dark.
- Prevent exposure to hot food or equipment that can burn the skin. Discourage use of heating pads. Check temperature of heating device and bath water before patient is exposed to them.
- Encourage patient to use low-heel, nonskid shoes for walking. Teach the use of wide-based gait to give unsteady patients a broader base of support. Assess patient for the presence of ataxia, and assist with walking as necessary. Use

gestures or turn patient's body in the direction he or she is to go. Canes and walkers may be too complicated for patients with Alzheimer's disease.

- Request that significant other assists with watching restless patient. Provide attendant care if necessary. Avoid restraining patient because this usually increases agitation. If restraints must be used, reassure patient that he or she is not being punished, that you are trying to help him or her regain control, and the restraints will be removed when the staff is certain the patient will not cause self-injury. **Note:** For many persons with Alzheimer's disease, walking will reduce agitation.

- Check patient at frequent intervals. If necessary, move patient closer to the nursing station, away from stairways or unit exits, or seat patient in a chair at the nursing station. Consider obtaining a picture of the patient to assist in a search if necessary.

- Watch for nonverbal clues of pain or distress, such as restlessness, wincing, wrinkled brow, cautious breathing, rapid or shallow breathing, poor appetite, or crying. Report significant findings.

- Try to make tubes as unobtrusive as possible to prevent their removal. Place IV tubing high on the dominant arm. Dress patient in a long-sleeved gown with a cuff, with IV tubing going up the sleeve and out the neck opening of the gown. Place binders over the dressing to help prevent picking. Position hand splints to eliminate pincer grasp.

Suggestions for home safety
- Encourage significant other to evaluate the home environment carefully for potential safety hazards. Caution him or her to remove harmful objects (e.g., matches, scissors) from the bedside, and store medications and chemicals (e.g., insect spray, cleaning supplies, lighter fluid) in locked cabinets to prevent accidental ingestion, because these patients tend to put objects in their mouth. Remove plants that are toxic, plastic fruit, and toiletries because patient may attempt to eat them. The temperature of the home hot water heater should be turned down to prevent accidental scalding. Lock up hazardous power tools, lawn mowers, or kitchen appliances. Place gates or guard rails on porches and stairways as needed. Safety plugs should be placed in electrical outlets. Hand rails and grab bars also may be helpful. Remind significant other to check the house carefully before leaving because the patient may leave the stove on or water running. It may be necessary to remove knobs from stove burners and the oven or to disable the appliance with an override turn-off valve or switch.

- Advise significant other to dress the individual according to the physical environment and individual need. These patients may not know or be able to communicate if they are too cold or too warm.

- Advise significant other to keep the patient's home environment simple and familiar. Rearranging furniture can increase the patient's confusion and potential for falls. Encourage use of night lights in patient's home.

- If the patient tends to wander, encourage significant other to have an identification bracelet made with patient's name, phone number, and diagnosis. An identifying label can be sewn into clothes. Alert neighbors and local police to call if they notice the patient wandering. Keep a clear, current picture of patient available to help in searching in case he or she becomes lost. Covering door handles with cloth hangings or covering the door with a poster may be sufficient to prevent patient from exiting. Locks on doors to keep patient inside may be necessary but should not require a key, because this may hamper escape in case of a fire. A child-proof device mounted either high or very low on the door may be sufficient. Door or exit alarms can be installed on home doors; a mat alarm under a bedside rug or a motion detector may also help. Daily walks or exercise tends to decrease the amount of wandering. Exercise areas should be safe and securely enclosed. Register the patient with the "Safe Return" program

through the local Alzheimer's Association (see "Patient-Family Teaching and Discharge Planning," p. 246).
- Caution significant other that patient who is disoriented should be allowed to smoke only while being observed. Advise him or her to get a smoke detector and take control of matches (i.e., lock up matches and lighters).
- Advise significant other that patient should be restricted from driving. Document this advice. Significant other can inform the state automobile licensing bureau about the need for retesting to take the burden of restriction off the family. Suggest that significant other hide car keys and store them in a locked cabinet or disable the car if necessary to prevent patient from driving.

NIC: Area Restriction; Environmental Management: Safety; Fall Prevention; Fire-Setting Precautions; Physical Restraint; Risk Identification; Seclusion; Surveillance: Safety

Altered nutrition: Less than body requirements related to decreased intake secondary to cognitive and motor deficit and to increased nutritional needs secondary to constant pacing and restlessness
Desired outcome: Patient maintains baseline body weight.
- Because patient may not eat food that does not look familiar or is on hospital plate, request that significant other assist with menu planning or bring in meals and dishes the patient recognizes. These patients often are overwhelmed with choices and need help with menu selection.
- When patient is no longer able to handle a fork, knife, and spoon, cut up food for patient and/or provide finger foods.
- For the patient who is in constant motion, provide small snacks around the clock and a high-calorie diet unless contraindicated.
- Try to limit the number of foods on the plate or serve foods in courses because too many foods can be overwhelming for patient.
- If patient clenches teeth and refuses to eat, stimulate the oral suck reflex by stroking the cheeks or stimulating the mouth with a spoon. Use patient's forgetfulness to advantage by taking a short break from feeding and returning in a few moments when patient may be more receptive.
- Provide privacy. Accept eating with hands and whimsical food mixtures.
- Tolerate spills without scolding, and obtain unbreakable plates and nonspill cups when needed.
- Be creative. A punch card or ticket so that the patient can "pay for the meal" may persuade some patients to eat.
- For other interventions, see **Altered nutrition** in "General Care of Patients With Neurologic Disorders," p. 333.

NIC: Nutrition Management; Nutritional Monitoring

Impaired environmental interpretation syndrome related to chronic confusional state secondary to degeneration of neuronal functioning
Desired outcome: After intervention and on an ongoing basis, patient interacts appropriately with the environment.
- Monitor for and record short-term memory deficit. Once a level of comprehension has been determined, avoid repeatedly asking if the patient knows who and where he or she is and what time it is, because this may cause frustration and agitation. At frequent intervals, orient patient to reality, time, and place in the following ways: call patient by name; keep clocks and calendars in the room; inform patient of the day and time; correct patient gently; minimize disturbing noise; ensure adequate lighting to prevent shadows; request that significant other bring in familiar objects and family pictures; speak with patient about his or her interests, both present and past; allow patient to reminisce, and listen with tolerance to repeated stories; ensure that staff members show their name tags and identify themselves;

explain upcoming events; set up regular schedules for hygiene, eating, and waste elimination; do only one activity at a time.

- Approach the patient in a calm, slow, relaxed, nonthreatening, friendly manner. Treat the patient with dignity and respect. Remain calm and patient when repeating questions. Be nonjudgmental and objective when confronted with inappropriate behavior.
- Keep the patient's personal belongings where they can be used and seen.
- Evaluate the patient's cognitive impairment for any relation to medication use (e.g., sedatives, tranquilizers). Consult the health care provider if necessary.
- Provide a quiet, calm, pleasant environment. Simple, minimally decorated rooms are best. The patient may not recognize himself or herself in a mirror. Cover, or remove, artwork and mirrors if the patient misinterprets images (e.g., wallpaper patterns may be disturbing to some patients). Turning off the public address system in the patient's room may prevent patient stimulation and misinterpretation of the sound.
- Provide stimulation that the patient can handle. Soft music may be appropriate, but television may be too overwhelming because the images change quickly and may be misconceived (e.g., violence on TV may be confused with reality). Interpret strange noises for the patient.
- Limit visitors as appropriate because crowds and complex social interactions are often beyond the patient's ability to tolerate.
- Check to ensure that individuals who need eyeglasses or hearing aids wear them as appropriate. Eyeglasses should be clean and have the current prescription. Hearing aids should be functioning.
- If the patient becomes agitated, reduce environmental stimuli. Use a soft, reassuring voice and gentle touch. Avoid quick, unexpected movements.
- If the patient leaves the ward for testing or other procedures, communicate the patient's cognitive level to other caregivers (e.g., patient will wander).

NIC: Dementia Management; Environmental Management; Environmental Management: Safety; Hallucination Management; Reality Orientation; Risk Identification; Surveillance: Safety

Impaired environmental interpretation syndrome (urinating in inappropriate places) related to cognitive deficit
Desired outcome: Patient urinates in the toilet stool (commode) on an ongoing basis.

- Make sure patient knows location of the bathroom. If possible, locate patient within sight of the bathroom, ensure a clear path, and provide adequate light at night. Take patient to the bathroom q1-2hr; avoid a sense of hurry. Restrict fluids in the evenings to minimize the risk of enuresis.
- Identify bathroom door with a picture of a toilet to help patient locate the bathroom.
- Assess for nonverbal clues (e.g., restlessness, holding himself or herself) that can signal the need to void.
- As appropriate, provide disposable underpants. Indwelling and external catheters may increase confusion. Male patients may be able to accept condom catheters to help manage incontinence.
- Incontinence may signal a urinary tract infection (UTI). Investigate the cause of the incontinence to see whether it is treatable.
- After patient has voided, assess him or her for cleanliness and dryness of the perianal area; intervene accordingly to help ensure skin integrity.

NIC: Dementia Management; Environmental Management: Safety; Self-Care Assistance: Toileting; Surveillance: Safety; Urinary Bladder Training; Urinary Habit Training

Impaired environmental interpretation syndrome (defecating in inappropriate places) related to inability to find bathroom or decreased awareness or loss of sphincter control secondary to cognitive deficit
Desired outcome: Following intervention(s), patient has no or fewer episodes of defecating in inappropriate places.

- Show patient location of the bathroom. Identify the bathroom door with a picture of a toilet to help patient locate the bathroom.
- Assess patient's normal bowel habits. Take patient to the bathroom at the time of day patient normally has a bowel movement (e.g., first thing in the morning, following a cup of coffee, or after meals).
- Evaluate patient for nonverbal indications of the need to eliminate wastes (e.g., restlessness, picking at clothes, facial expressions or grunting sounds indicative of bearing down, passing flatus).
- As appropriate, provide disposable underpants.
- After bowel elimination, assess patient for cleanliness of perianal area to maintain skin integrity. The patient may forget to wipe the perianal area or clean the area only partially.
- For other suggestions, see **Constipation**, p. 743, in Appendix One, "Caring for Patients on Prolonged Bedrest."

NIC: Bowel Incontinence Care; Bowel Training; Dementia Management; Environmental Management: Safety; Self-Care Assistance: Toileting; Surveillance: Safety

Self-care deficit related to memory loss and coordination problems secondary to cognitive and motor deficits
Desired outcome: On an ongoing basis, patient's physical needs are met by self, staff, or significant other.

- Provide care for totally dependent patients, and assist those who are not totally dependent. Allow ample time to perform activities, encouraging patient's independence. Ask patient to perform only one task at a time; go through each step separately. Do not hurry patient. Involve significant other with care activities if he or she wishes to be involved. Ask significant other when patient normally bathes at home, and establish this as part of a daily routine. Provide a consistent caregiver. Use simple visual and verbal cues and gestures for self-care.
- Place a stool in the shower if sitting will enhance self-care. Use a hand-held shower head to prevent water from hitting patient's head, which can be frightening.
- To facilitate dressing and undressing, encourage significant other to buy shoes with elastic laces, without laces, or with Velcro fasteners and clothing that is loose fitting or has snaps, Velcro closures, or elastic waistbands. Offer clothing items one at a time, sequentially. Allow agitated patients for whom hygiene is not a problem to sleep in their shoes and clothing, and attempt a clothes change later.
- Provide a commode chair or elevated toilet seat as needed.
- If the patient becomes combative or agitated, postpone ADL and try again a short time later. The patient may forget the reason for the resistance.

NIC: Dementia Management; Dressing; Oral Health Maintenance; Self-Care Assistance: Bathing/Hygiene; Self-Care Assistance: Dressing/Grooming

Impaired verbal communication related to aphasia and altered sensory reception, transmission, and integration secondary to cognitive deficits
Desired outcome: Following the intervention(s), patient communicates needs to staff, follows instructions, and answers questions.

- Provide a supportive and relaxed environment for patients who are unable to form words or sentences or who are unable to speak clearly or appropriately.

Acknowledge patient's frustration about the inability to communicate. Maintain a calm, positive attitude; eliminate distracting noises, such as radio or television. Observe for nonverbal communication cues, such as gestures. Consider pain as a possible cause of restlessness, moaning, guarding, and yelling; provide analgesia as needed. Avoid meperidine, if possible, because of its common side effect of restlessness. Anticipate patient's needs.

- Explain activities in short, easily understood sentences. Use simple gestures, point to objects, or use demonstration if possible. When giving directions, be sure to break tasks into small, understandable units, using simple terms. Ask patient to do only one task at a time. Give patient time to accomplish one task before progressing to the next. Explain each procedure or task before initiating it.
- Be sure that you have the patient's attention. Repeat patient's name or gently touch patient to get his or her attention. Use touch to communicate if the patient is receptive to it. Speak slowly and calmly, using a clear, low-pitched voice. Use short, simple words and sentences, but speak as though patient understands you. Ask only one question at a time, and formulate questions that can be answered by "yes" or "no." Wait for a response. If patient does not respond (i.e., after 15 sec), repeat the question again, exactly as before, to help patient mentally process the question.
- Listen to and include patient in conversation.

NIC: Active Listening; Communication Enhancement: Speech Deficit; Reality Orientation; Surveillance: Safety

Anxiety related to actual or perceived threats or changes (e.g., from bewildering hospital environment, multiple tests and procedures)
Desired outcome: Within 1 hr of intervention, patient's anxiety is absent or reduced as evidenced by HR ≤100 bpm, RR ≤20 breaths/min with normal depth and pattern, and an absence of or decrease in irritability and restlessness.

- Remain calm with patient. Use slow, deliberate gestures. Patients with Alzheimer's disease frequently mirror the emotions of others. Use a low, soothing voice and a gentle touch. The tone of voice is often more important than the actual words used.
- Provide time for patient to verbalize feelings of fear, concern, and anxiety. Listen with regard. Alzheimer's patients often have trouble finding the correct words and may not be able to string more than a few words together. Provide calm and realistic assurance, and stay with patient during periods of acute anxiety.
- To help reduce anxiety and establish ongoing rapport, provide patient with a consistent caregiver. Avoid changing patient's room. Ask the patient's caregiver what the patient's normal routine is; document the patient's normal routine, and attempt to incorporate it whenever possible.
- Patients who still have reading capability may find reassurance with notes, orienting signs, or lists of names, phone numbers, or activities (e.g., the phone numbers of significant others or a written reminder of the reason they are in the hospital), which may reassure them that they are not lost or abandoned.
- Encourage significant others to bring in familiar items. Address patients with their preferred name.
- Permit patient to hoard inanimate objects because this may provide the individual with a sense of security. Enable patient to keep personal belongings (e.g., purse, wallet) in bed with patient.
- Assist with finding misplaced items. Label drawers and belongings.
- Refrain from forcing activities or giving patient too many choices.
- Encourage ambulation. Often, walking helps reduce anxiety and agitation.
- Encourage unlimited visiting hours for familiar significant others.
- Encourage patient to avoid caffeine, which has a stimulating effect.

NIC: Active Listening; Anxiety Reduction; Calming Technique; Dementia Management; Presence; Touch

Risk for violence with risk factors associated with irritability, frustration, and disorientation secondary to degeneration of cognitive thinking

Desired outcome: Patient demonstrates control of his or her behavior with absence of violence.

- Ask caregiver how patient usually acts when tired or overwhelmed, and ask what caregiver does to calm patient. Document this information.
- Monitor patient for signs of increasing anxiety, fright, or panic (e.g., inability to verbalize feelings, suspiciousness of others, fear of others or self, irritability, agitation), which can precede a violent act. Remove potential weapons (e.g., scissors) from the environment.
- Encourage verbalization of feelings rather than suppression because frustration can lead to violence. Avoid asking *why* the patient wants to do something because this may be overwhelming to the patient and increase frustration. Praise efforts at self-control.
- Try to identify what is immediately distressing to patient (e.g., full bladder, catheter, pain), and attempt to remedy it. Respond to the emotion. Respond to the patient's questions in simple, concrete replies that relate directly to the patient's questions, frustrations, or anger. Avoid making promises that cannot reasonably be kept. Do not confront or argue with patient and become authoritarian. If the situation cannot be remedied by calming the patient, use distraction and try to defuse the situation by redirecting attention away from the source of irritation. Talk about other topics, and vary the topics periodically. Provide diversional activities, offer juice, or walk with patient until the agitation has lessened. Use questions to interrupt a patient's repetitive or disturbing train of thought. A request for patient's help (e.g., with folding and unfolding towels, making a bed) may promote calm behavior by returning a sense of mastery or control.
- Remain calm, and keep gestures slow and deliberate. Keep your hands open and below your waist where they can be seen. Approach patient slowly in a confident, relaxed, open manner. Avoid sudden changes or surprises. Keep your voice low and soft, and smile. Humor and gentle laughter may help change the patient's mood. Some patients may respond positively to gentle touch (e.g., start with touching either a hand or arm because this is less threatening than touching other parts of the body).
- Reduce environmental stimuli, including people entering the room. Provide a private room if possible. Reduce noise level by turning the television volume down or off.
- Do not give routine care when patient is upset or agitated. Leave the room briefly, and return when the patient is calmer and more approachable. If the patient cannot be left alone, sit quietly with no talking except gentle reassurance. Use the patient's forgetfulness to your advantage.
- If patient is not combative unless approached, simply supervise from a safe distance. If you must approach patient, do so from the side rather than face-to-face. Stand off to one side, and maintain distance of at least one arm's length from the patient.
- If patient is upset or agitated, avoid turning your back on patient. Avoid cornering patient or being cornered. Think of escape routes for yourself, and be alert to potential weapons patient may use. Get help; protect yourself.
- Never attempt to deal with a physically aggressive patient by yourself. If other interventions fail, use physical or chemical restraints as necessary for your own or patient's safety.
- Document the signs and symptoms, precipitating factor, time of onset, duration, and successful interventions. Prevent further episodes by controlling precipitating stressors (e.g., controlling pain, simplifying schedule, limiting visitors).

NIC: Anxiety Reduction; Area Restriction; Calming Technique; Dementia Management; Elopement Precautions; Environmental Management: Violence Prevention; Physical Restraint; Seclusion

Sleep pattern disturbance related to restlessness and disorientation secondary to cognitive deficits
Desired outcome: Following the intervention(s), patient sleeps at least 6 hr per night or an amount of time appropriate for the patient.

- Space activities with quiet periods so that patient does not become excessively tired and require a daytime nap.
- Prevent patient from falling asleep during the day through such measures as periodic short walks, planned activities, and keeping him or her upright as much as possible. **Note:** If patient does nap during the day but also sleeps well at night, there is no need to impose a specific sleep schedule.
- Patients who nap should do so in an easy chair, if possible, rather than in bed. The easy chair may serve as a cue that the patient is just napping.
- Avoid continuous use of restraints because restraints often increase agitation and limit the patient's ability to rest.
- Adhere to regular bedtime schedules and rituals, such as a bedtime snack. Keep the room lighted until the patient is ready for sleep. Provide soft music, and tell patient that it is time for sleep.
- Administer tranquilizers and sedatives as prescribed to facilitate sleeping.
- Avoid turning on overhead light at night, which may cue patient to think it is time to get up.
- Try to schedule VS monitoring, medications, and treatments to allow uninterrupted sleep at night.

NIC: Dementia Management; Environmental Management: Comfort; Simple Relaxation Therapy; Sleep Enhancement

Altered family processes related to situational crisis (illness of family member)
Desired outcome: Within the 24-hr period before patient's hospital discharge, significant other verbalizes knowledge of measures that will assist with care of the patient after hospital discharge.

- Encourage significant other to interpret patient's behavior as a reflection of the disease process rather than a willful act. Advise significant other that generally another illness, surgery, or disease process will exaggerate the patient's disorientation. Once these problems are corrected, the patient usually returns to his or her previous cognitive level. Caregivers will eventually need to reduce their expectations of the patient's abilities as the disease process progresses.
- Encourage patient's major caregiver to have other family members or hired help take care of patient regularly so that he or she can have scheduled respites. Caregiver should schedule rest breaks for himself or herself throughout the day. A neighbor looking in or a home-health aide on a part-time, overnight, or live-in basis is another option. Local day-care or respite programs also are useful. If the patient is a veteran, he or she may be eligible for some respite programs offered by the Veterans Administration. Advise caregiver that some home health agencies or day-care programs have sliding payment scales for their services. Refer to community sources that supply equipment for home use. Encourage use of other support services, such as homemakers, chore workers, home-delivered food, and volunteer drivers. Support significant other in asking for help.
- If significant other is unaccustomed to handling finances, refer him or her to a place where help with financial management is available. Often, patients

with Alzheimer's disease lose the ability to manage finances and balance checkbooks and may give away money inappropriately. Eventually the patient's checkbook and credit cards will have to be taken away. Phone use may require monitoring because these patients cannot differentiate between local and long-distance calls. As appropriate, suggest that significant other posts important phone numbers and secures long-distance numbers to help prevent excessively high phone bills.

- Encourage early financial planning, and suggest professional financial counseling. Families should locate and identify the patient's various assets, sources of income, and liabilities and make arrangements for their security and daily management.
- Encourage early family legal planning and consultation. This is especially important because an individual must have mental capacity and competence to sign documents. Legal planning may involve wills, intervivos trusts, subpayee assignment for social security, traditional and durable power of attorney, guardianship, and conservatorship. Advise family that some free legal services are available to older persons in most areas.
- Explain to significant other that if patient refuses medication or is unable to swallow pills, obtaining a liquid form of the drug or crushing the pills and mixing them with soft food may help.
- Some individuals with this disease go through a phase in which, because of increased motor activity and lessening social inhibitions, they have increased sexual demands. This may result in increased sexual encounters. Be sure the family is aware that this is a symptom of the disease process. Further, the patient eventually will lose the ability to be intimate and tender. Sex will become a mindless act. Mates may feel rejected, frustrated, humiliated, or repulsed. Suggest that professional counseling be obtained to assist the patient's spouse or loved one in dealing with these feelings. Suggest that the use of gentle dissuasion or distraction may be effective with these patients. Remind patient that certain public behavior is unacceptable.
- Encourage caregivers to maintain their own friendships and attend social functions. The patient's embarrassing behaviors and the demands of giving care can lead to withdrawal from society.
- Encourage significant other to focus on specific problems as they occur and establish priorities (e.g., safety). Help him or her develop a plan of care and schedule of daily activities. Caregiver should focus on one difficult behavior at a time to target intervention strategies and prevent feeling overwhelmed. Note when behavior occurs and focus on stimuli that precede or trigger the behavior (e.g., overstimulation, noise). Consider other causes, such as a recent change in the environment.
- Encourage professional counseling and support so that significant other can work through feelings such as anger, guilt, embarrassment, and depression and develop effective coping strategies and mechanisms. Each new and subtle loss of patient function brings another round of grieving. Decisions about institutionalization and the extent of health care measures also are emotionally difficult. Behaviors such as hoarding, unjust accusations, angry outbursts, and clinging can precipitate burnout in the caregiver. Caregivers must be reassessed continually for their ability to care for patients at home.
- Encourage participation in local or national support groups, such as Alzheimer's Disease and Related Disorders Association (ADRDA) (see "Patient-Family Teaching and Discharge Planning," p. 246).
- For other interventions, see **Altered family processes** in Appendix One, "Caring for Patients With Cancer and other Life-disrupting Illnesses," p. 802.

NIC: Coping Enhancement; Family Support; Family Process Maintenance; Respite Care; Role Enhancement; Teaching: Disease Process

See Also: "Seizure Disorders," p. 319, for patients experiencing seizures; "General Care of Patients With Neurologic Disorders" for **Risk for fluid volume deficit,** p. 335; **Risk for aspiration,** p. 335; **Impaired swallowing,** p. 344; **Knowledge deficit:** Neurologic diagnostic tests, p. 346; related nursing diagnoses in "Pressure Ulcers," p. 710, for patients experiencing various degrees of immobility; Appendix One, "Caring for Patients on Prolonged Bedrest," p. 738; Appendix One, "Caring for Patients With Cancer and Other Life-disrupting Illnesses," p. 791, for psychosocial nursing diagnoses for patients and significant others, as appropriate.

PATIENT-FAMILY TEACHING AND DISCHARGE PLANNING

The degree and scope of discharge teaching and planning depend on the severity of the patient's condition. When providing patient-family teaching, focus on sensory information; avoid giving excessive information; and initiate a visiting nurse referral for necessary follow-up teaching. Consider including verbal and written information about the following:

- Referrals to community resources, local and national Alzheimer's disease chapters, public health nurse, visiting nurses association, community support groups, social workers, psychologic therapy, home health agencies, and extended and skilled care facilities. Additional general information can be obtained by contacting the following organizations:

  Alzheimer's Association
  919 N. Michigan Ave.
  Suite 1000
  Chicago, IL 60611   (800) 272-3900 or (312) 335-8700
  WWW address: *http://www.alz.org*

  Alzheimer's Disease Education and Referral Center
  National Institute on Aging
  Information Specialist
  P.O. Box 8250
  Silver Spring, MD 20907-8250   (800) 438-4380 or (301) 495- 3334 FAX
  WWW address: *http://www.alzheimers.org*

- Safety measures for preventing injury relative to cognitive deficits.
- Measures that assist in reorienting and communicating with patient in view of cognitive deficits.
- Importance of scheduled respites and involvement in support groups for significant other.
- Medications, including drug name, purpose, dosage, frequency, precautions, drug/drug and food/drug interactions, and potential side effects.
- Exercises that promote muscle strength and mobility; measures for preventing contractures and skin breakdown; transfer techniques and proper body mechanics; and use of assistive devices if appropriate.
- Techniques for dealing with incontinence; indications of constipation or infection; implementation of bowel and bladder training programs; and indwelling catheter care if appropriate.
- Indications of upper respiratory infection (URI) and measures that prevent regurgitation, aspiration, and infection.
- Techniques for encouraging adequate food and fluid intake and performance of ADL.
- Importance of seeking financial and legal counseling.

Section Three: Traumatic Disorders of the Nervous System

Intervertebral disk disease

The intervertebral disk is a semifluid-filled fibrous capsule that facilitates movement of the spine and acts as a shock absorber. The ability of the disk to withstand stressors is not unlimited and diminishes with aging. Pressure on the disk eventually may force elastic material from the center of the disk, called the nucleus pulposus, to break, or herniate, through the fibrous rim of the disk. Herniation usually occurs posteriorly because the posterior longitudinal ligament is inherently more weak than the anterior longitudinal ligament. The rupture or bulging of an intervertebral disk causes its typical symptoms by pressing on and irritating the spinal nerve roots or spinal cord itself. Herniated nucleus pulposus usually is the result of injury or a series of insults to the vertebral column from lifting or twisting. When the disk ruptures without a known discrete injury, it is believed to be caused by degenerative changes. Deterioration can occur suddenly, or it may happen gradually, with symptoms appearing months or years after the initial injury. Almost all herniated disks occur in the lumbar spine, with 90% of the problems occurring at L4-5 and L5-S1. Cervical disk problems most frequently occur at C5-6 and C6-7 and generally are caused by degenerative changes or trauma, such as whiplash or hyperextension. Thoracic disk problems are rare.

ASSESSMENT

General indicators: Onset can be sudden, with intense unilateral pain or with pain that is dull, diffuse, deep, and aching. Symptoms vary according to the level of injury and nerves involved. Usually, pain is increased with movement or activities that increase intraabdominal or intrathoracic pressure, such as sneezing, coughing, and straining. Often pain is improved by lying down. Immediate medical attention is essential if there is any paralysis, extreme sensory loss, or altered bowel or bladder function.

Cervical disk disease: Pain or numbness in the upper extremities, shoulders, thorax, occipital area, or back of the head or neck. Pain can radiate down the forearms and into the hands and fingers. Interscapular aching or suboccipital headaches are commonly associated with cervical disk disease. Usually the neck has restricted mobility, and there can be cervical muscle spasm and loss of the normal cervical lordosis. The patient may have upper extremity muscle weakness with diminished biceps or triceps reflexes.

Lumbar disk disease: Pain in the lumbosacral area with possible radiculopathy (sciatica) to the buttock, down the posterior surface of the thigh and calf, and to the lateral border of the foot. Sensory distribution for the L5 nerve root is the medial portion of the foot and the great toe, whereas sensory distribution for S1 is the lateral aspect of the foot, the fifth toe, and the sole of the foot. Frequently mobility is altered, as evidenced by decreased ability to stand upright, listing to one side, asymmetric gait, limited ability to flex forward, and restricted side movement caused by pain and muscle spasms. The individual walks cautiously, bearing little weight on the affected side, and often finds sitting or climbing stairs particularly painful. Reflex muscle spasms can cause bulging of the back with concomitant flattening of the lumbar curve and possible scoliosis at the level of the affected disk. Usually the patellar and Achilles tendon reflexes are depressed.

Physical assessment: Possible findings include depressed reflexes, muscle atrophy, paresthesias (described as "pins and needles"), or anesthesia (numbness) in the dermatome of the involved nerves. The following tests are two of several that are performed to confirm the presence of lumbar disk disease.

Straight leg raise test: Examiner extends and raises patient's leg. The test is positive if patient has pain on the posterior aspect of the leg. People without injury usually can have a leg raised to 90 degrees without significant discomfort.

Sciatic nerve test: Examiner extends and raises patient's leg until pain is elicited and then lowers the leg to a comfortable level. The examiner then dorsiflexes the foot to stretch the sciatic nerve. If this causes pain, the test is positive for sciatic nerve involvement.

Risk factors: Repetitive bending or lifting involving a twisting motion, continuous vibration, smoking, poor physical condition, obesity, above-average height, osteoporosis, prolonged sitting, depression, severe scoliosis, spondylolisthesis, or genetic predisposition.

DIAGNOSTIC TESTS

MRI: May reveal that the disk is impinging on the spinal cord or nerve root or may reveal a related pathologic condition, such as a tumor or spondylosis. MRI is rapidly replacing CT scan and myelogram as the test of choice in diagnosing herniated nucleus pulposus.

CT scan of the spine: May reveal disk protrusion/prolapse or a related pathologic condition, such as a tumor, spondylosis, or spinal stenosis.

Myelogram: May show characteristic deformity and filling defect or a related pathologic condition, such as a tumor, spondylolisthesis (forward displacement of one vertebra over the next), spondylosis (formation of bone spurs [osteophytes] around vertebral joints), spinal stenosis (narrowing of the spinal canal), or Paget's disease. Generally this test is performed only if surgery is considered.

X-ray of the spine: May show narrowing of the vertebral interspaces in affected areas, loss of curvature of the spine, and spondylosis.

Diskography: Identifies degenerated or extruded disks by means of contrast medium injected into the disk space, using fluoroscopy.

Electromyography (EMG): May show denervation patterns of specific nerve roots to indicate the level and site of injury.

Laboratory tests (serum alkaline and acid phosphatase, glucose, erythrocyte sedimentation rate [ESR], WBCs): Rules out metabolic bone disease, metastatic tumors, diabetic mononeuritis, and disk space infection.

See Also: "General Care of Patients With Neurologic Disorders," **Knowledge deficit:** Neurologic diagnostic tests, p. 346, for care considerations for patients undergoing MRI, CT scan, and myelography.

COLLABORATIVE MANAGEMENT

Bedrest: Has been used in the past with lumbar disk disease to limit motion of vertebral column, relieve nerve root compression, and enhance shrinkage of the disk. Current research has demonstrated no difference in the return-to-work time of patients maintained on bedrest, those doing graded exercise, and those doing ordinary activity.

Bedboards under the mattress: Support normal lumbar spine curvature and minimize spinal flexion.

Orthotics (e.g., splints, braces, girdles, cervical collars): Limit motion of the vertebral column. Generally, long-term use of braces is discouraged because it prohibits development of necessary supporting musculature. Soft or hard collars aid in immobilization of the cervical spine. Temporary use of a back brace or corset allows earlier return to activity with lumbar disk disease.

Pelvic/cervical skin traction: Reduces muscle spasm and distracts vertebral bodies to reduce bulging or rupture of the disk. **Note:** Controversy exists regarding whether traction actually provides any therapeutic benefit, especially for lumbar disk disease. However, it may be useful in enforcing decreased activity and some individuals find that it decreases pain.

Thermotherapy (heat): May reduce muscle spasm, whereas icing may prevent further inflammatory swelling and provide some topical anesthesia.

Other therapeutic modalities: Include hydrotherapy, massage, diathermy/ultrasound electrotherapy, transcutaneous electrical nerve stimulation (TENS), dorsal column stimulation, and stress reduction techniques.

Physical therapy and a graded exercise program: Strengthens the legs, back, and abdominal muscles and teaches correct body mechanics. It is initiated once acute symptoms subside. Physical therapy has become the mainstay of therapy for chronic low back pain.

Local injection of anesthetic (lidocaine or bupivacaine) and/or cortisone into paraspinal or paravertebral regions and epidural or subarachnoid spaces: Reduces pain and muscle spasms and increases function.

Antiembolism hose: Prevent thrombophlebitis while the patient is on bedrest. Hose should be worn until the amount of time out of bed ambulating is equal to the amount of time in bed.

Pharmacotherapy

Analgesics (e.g., aspirin, acetaminophen, narcotics): Administer sufficient medication to achieve pain relief or adequate pain reduction. Narcotics generally are used for acute pain episodes. Because of the potential for narcotics abuse, individuals with chronic back pain are usually discharged with nonnarcotic analgesia.

Muscle relaxants (e.g., carisoprodol, chlorzoxazone, cyclobenzaprine, metaxalone, methocarbamol, diazepam): Reduce muscle spasm. Common side effects are drowsiness, fatigue, dizziness, dry mouth, and GI upset.

Corticosteroids (e.g., dexamethasone): May be given for a short period to reduce cord edema if present.

Nonsteroidal antiinflammatory drugs: See Table 8-1, p. 555, for names and usual dosages.

Stool softeners or laxatives (e.g., docusate): Prevent constipation or straining that would be painful.

Note: Surgery is done without delay if signs of spinal cord compression are present, such as significant motor or sensory loss or loss of sphincter control. Otherwise, surgery is considered only after symptoms fail to respond to conservative therapy.

Diskectomy with laminectomy: An incision is made, allowing removal of part of the vertebra (laminectomy) so that the herniated portion of the disk can be removed (diskectomy). If multiple intervertebral disk spaces are explored, a wound drain may be present after surgery. Complications include paralytic ileus, urinary retention, CSF leakage, meningitis, hematoma at the operative site, nerve root injury causing wristdrop or footdrop, arachnoiditis, and postural deformity.

Microdiskectomy: The herniated portion of the disk and small parts of the lamina are removed, using microsurgical techniques. This surgery results in less tissue damage, less pain, fewer spasms, and increased postoperative spinal stability. Patients often are out of bed the first day and may be discharged in 1-3 days.

Percutaneous lumbar disk removal: An ultrasonic nucleotome cannula or fiberoptic arthroscopic cannula can be inserted in the intervertebral space via fluoroscopy to allow fragmentation of the disk and its aspiration. A laser may be used to aid in disk excision. This is a relatively less-invasive method of relieving pain from herniated disks. The procedure is done with the patient under local anesthesia and may be performed on an outpatient basis. Complications include back spasm or transient syncope.

Chemonucleolysis: Injection of enzymes (chymopapain, collagenase) directly into the disk has been used in the past to dissolve fibrocartilage or collagen materials of the nucleus pulposus in an attempt to relieve pressure on the spinal cord or nerve roots. Chemonucleolysis provides pain relief in 50%-80% of patients but may take as long as 3 mo to do so. Fluoroscopy is used to confirm proper position of the needle. There is a 1% incidence of allergic reaction and potential for severe anaphylaxis. Allergic reactions quickly can progress to laryngeal edema, laryngospasm, bronchospasm, and cardiac arrest if the patient is not treated promptly. Additional complications include nerve root injury, bowel or bladder dysfunction, transverse myelitis, and paraplegia. Chemonucleolysis is rarely used now because of these potential complications.

Spinal fusion: Fusion may be indicated for patients with recurrent low back pain, spondylolisthesis, or subluxation of the vertebrae. Some health care providers promote primary use of fusion for patients who have not responded to conservative therapy. Bone chips are harvested from the iliac crest or tibia and placed between the vertebrae in the prepared area of the unstable spine to fuse and stabilize the area. Internal fixation (e.g., rods, wiring, pedicle screws, fusion cages) may be necessary to provide added stability until the fusion has healed fully. If the patient's own bone quality or quantity is inadequate, allograft bone may be considered. Clinical trials are investigating use of a recombinant human osteogenic protein preparation as a bone graft substitute or supplement.

   Patients undergoing anterior cervical fusion may have difficulty swallowing or managing secretions because of postoperative edema and hematoma formation secondary to retraction of the trachea and esophagus during surgery. Hoarseness also can occur secondary to nerve irritation. Complaints of excessive pressure in the neck or severe, uncontrolled incisional pain may signal excessive bleeding.

Other surgical procedures: Foraminotomy involves surgical enlargement of the intravertebral foramen to reduce tension on the nerve root that traverses this area. Hemilaminectomy removes part of the lamina of a vertebra to reduce pressure on an adjacent nerve. Anterior cervical vertebrectomy with interbody fusion may be necessary for multilevel cervical disk disease. Implantable spinal cord stimulators have been placed to aid in the control of chronic pain when all other measures (e.g., physical therapy, medications, surgery) have failed.

NURSING DIAGNOSES AND INTERVENTIONS

Health-seeking behaviors: Proper body mechanics and other measures that prevent back injury

Desired outcome: Within the 24-hr period before hospital discharge, patient verbalizes knowledge of measures that prevent back injury and demonstrates proper body mechanics.

- Teach patient proper body mechanics: stand and sit straight with the chin and head up and the pelvis and back straight; bend at the knees and hips rather than at the waist (squat), keeping the back straight (not stooping forward); when carrying objects, hold them close to the body, avoiding twisting when lifting or reaching. Turn using the entire body. Do not strain to reach things. If an object is overhead, raise yourself to its level, or move things out of the way if they are obstructing the object. Avoid lifting anything heavier than 10-20 lb. Encourage use of long-handled pickup sticks to pick up small objects. Have patient demonstrate proper body mechanics, if possible, before hospital discharge.

- Teach patient about the following measures for keeping the body in alignment: sit close to the pedals when driving a car, and use a seat belt and firm back rest to support the back; support the feet on a footstool when sitting so that the knees are elevated to hip level or higher; obtain a firm mattress or bedboard; use a flat pillow when sleeping to avoid strain on the neck, arms, and shoulders; sleep in a side-lying position with the knees bent or in a supine position with the knees and legs supported on pillows; avoid sleeping in a prone position; avoid reaching or stretching to pick up objects. Avoid sitting on furniture that does not support the back.

- Encourage patient to perform the following measures to relieve pressure on the back: achieve and/or maintain proper weight for age, height, and gender; continue the exercise program prescribed by health care provider for strengthening abdominal, thoracic, and back muscles; use the thoracic and abdominal muscles when lifting to keep a significant portion of the weight off the vertebral disks.
- Teach patient the rationale and procedure for Williams' back exercises, which are performed while lying on the floor with the knees flexed.
  —*Pelvic tilt:* to strengthen the abdominal muscles. Stomach and buttock muscles are tightened, and the pelvis is tilted with the lower spine kept flat against the floor; that is, the hips and buttocks are kept on the floor.
  —*Knee-to-chest raise:* to help make a stiff back limber. Start with a pelvic tilt. Each knee is individually raised to the chest and returned to the starting position. Each knee is then individually raised to the chest and held there (both on the chest together).
  —*Nose-to-knee touch:* to stretch hip muscles and strengthen abdominal muscles. Raise the knee to the chest, and then pull the knee to the chest with the hands. Raise the head, and try to touch the nose to the knee. Keep the lower back flat on the floor.
  —*Half sit-ups:* to strengthen abdomen and back. Slowly raise the head and neck to the top of the chest. Reach both hands forward to knees, and hold for a count of 5. Repeat, keeping lower back flat on the floor.
- Instruct patient to wear supportive shoes with a moderate heel height for walking.
- Teach patient the following technique for sitting up at the bedside from a supine position: log-roll (see p. 253) to the side, and then raise to a sitting position by pushing against the mattress with the hands while swinging the legs over the side of the bed. Instruct patient to maintain alignment of the back during the procedure.
- Caution patient that pain is the signal to stop or change an activity or a position.
- Teach patient that the following indicators necessitate medical attention: increased sensory loss, increased motor loss/weakness, and loss of bowel and bladder function.

NIC: Activity Therapy; Coping Enhancement; Exercise Promotion; Health Education; Teaching: Prescribed Activity/Exercise

Health-seeking behaviors: Pain control measures
Desired outcome: Following instruction and within the 24-hr period before hospital discharge, patient verbalizes knowledge about pain control measures and demonstrates ability to initiate these measures when appropriate.

- Teach patient about the mechanisms of pain.
- Instruct patient about methods of controlling pain and their individual applications. Methods include distraction, use of counterirritants, massage, hydrotherapy, dorsal column stimulation, use of TENS, behavior modification, relaxation techniques, hypnosis, music therapy, imagery, biofeedback, and diathermy. In addition, suggest the application of local heat or cold massage to painful areas. The latter can be achieved by freezing water in a paper cup, tearing off the top of the cup to expose the ice, and massaging in a circular motion, using the remaining portion of the cup as a handle. A bag of frozen peas or corn may be used to apply continuous cold to the lower back.

- Suggest that patient use a stool to rest the affected leg when standing.
- Advise patient to sit in a straight-back chair that is high enough to get out of easily. Raised toilet seats also may be useful. Straddling a straight-back chair and resting the arms on the chair back are comfortable for many individuals.
- Encourage use of a firm mattress, to support normal spinal curvature, and extra pillows as needed for positioning. Some patients find the normal bed height too low and use blocks to raise it to a more comfortable height.
- Instruct patient on bedrest to roll rather than lift off the bedpan. The patient may find a fracture bedpan more comfortable than a regular bedpan.
- Caution patient to avoid sudden twisting or turning movements. Explain the importance of log-rolling when moving from side to side.
- Advise patient to avoid factors that enhance spasms, such as staying in one position too long, fatigue, chilling, and anxiety.
- Suggest positions of comfort, such as lying on the side with the knees bent or lying supine with the knees supported on pillows. A small pillow supporting the nape of the neck may be helpful with cervical pain. Usually the patient is on bedrest or limited activity during the period of acute pain. Once increased activity is allowed, teach patient to avoid prolonged periods of sitting, which stress the back.
- Inform patient that applying a heating pad to the back for 15-30 min before getting out of bed in the morning will help allay stiffness and discomfort. Heating pads should be used only for short intervals and only if patient's temperature sensations are intact. Remind patient to place a towel or cloth between heating pad and skin to prevent burns.

NIC: Pain Management; Progressive Muscle Relaxation; Teaching: Individual; Teaching: Procedure/Treatment

Knowledge deficit: Diskectomy with laminectomy or fusion procedure
Desired outcomes: Before surgery, patient verbalizes knowledge about the surgical procedure, preoperative routine, and postoperative regimen. Patient demonstrates activities and exercises correctly.
- Assess patient's knowledge about the surgical procedure, preoperative routine, and postoperative regimen. Provide ample time for instruction and clarification.
- Teach patient the technique for deep breathing, which will be performed immediately after surgery (coughing may be contraindicated in the immediate postoperative period to prevent disruption of the fusion or surgical repair). Also teach patient use of incentive spirometry.
- Document baseline neurovascular checks, including color, capillary refill, pulse, warmth, muscle strength, movement, and sensation. Explain that VS and neurologic status will be evaluated at frequent intervals after the surgery and compared with baseline. Reassure patient that this is normal and does not indicate that anything is wrong. Teach patient the following indicators of impairment, which necessitate immediate attention by the health care staff: paresthesias, weakness, paralysis, radiculopathy, and changes in bowel or bladder function. Patients undergoing fusion lose more blood during surgery than those undergoing laminectomy. Signs of hypovolemia, such as decreased BP, increased HR, and thirst, may be present. Teach patient to report faintness or dizziness.
- Explain that the surgical dressing will be inspected for excess drainage or oozing at frequent intervals. Bleeding with a laminectomy usually is minimal. Patients with fusion may have slight bloody oozing postoperatively. A closed wound drainage device may be present for 1-3 days postoperatively. Serous drainage usually is checked with a glucose reagent strip. The presence of glucose is a signal of CSF leakage. Bulging in the area of the wound may also signal CSF leakage or hematoma formation and should be reported. Lumbar dressings will be checked after each bedpan use. Wet or contami-

nated dressings require changing. Inform patients undergoing fusions that they will have a second dressing at the donor site.

- Instruct patient to report any nausea or vomiting, which is not uncommon, so that antiemetics can be given. Explain that the patient will be monitored for bowel and bladder dysfunction after the procedure. The abdomen will be checked for bowel sounds and distention. The patient may be asked to void within 8 hr of the procedure to check for urinary retention. Caution patient to avoid straining at stool.

- Explain that fever may occur during the first few days postoperatively but that this does not necessarily signal an infection. The patient will be assessed for other indicators of infection, such as heat, redness, irritation, swelling, or drainage at the wound site. Instruct patient to report headache, neck stiffness, or photophobia.

- Inform patient that postoperative pain or tingling (paresthesia) often is caused by nerve root irritation and edema. Spasms are common on the third or fourth postoperative day and should not discourage patient. Pain may take days or weeks to resolve and does not indicate that the surgery was unsuccessful. The patient should request medication for pain as needed and not let the pain get out of control. Patients who have had a fusion may expect significant pain from the bone graft donor site (commonly the iliac crest). The donor site may have extra padding. Muscle relaxants may be prescribed to supplement pain control. Patient-controlled analgesia (PCA) and nonsteroidal antiinflammatory drugs (NSAIDs) also may be used for postoperative pain control.

- Inform patient that in the immediate postoperative period he or she will probably be required to lie supine for several hours to minimize the possibility of wound hematoma formation. After this period, HOB of the laminectomy patient usually can be raised to 20 degrees to facilitate eating and bedpan use. The patient undergoing spinal fusion usually is kept flat and on bedrest considerably longer than the patient with laminectomy. Activity progression for the spinal fusion patient is usually more cautious and slower than for the laminectomy patient.

- Only the log-roll method is used for turning. Teach patient the following technique: position a pillow between the legs, cross the arms across the chest while turning, and contract the long back muscles to maintain the shoulders and pelvis in straight alignment. Explain that, initially, patient will be assisted in this procedure. Use a turning sheet and sufficient help when log-rolling patient.

- Teach patient the following technique for getting out of bed: log-roll to the side, splint the back, and rise to a sitting position by pushing against the mattress while swinging the legs over the side of the bed. While in the hospital with an electric bed, the HOB may be raised to facilitate a sitting position. Initially the patient will be helped to a sitting position and should not push against the mattress. Patients with a cervical laminectomy should not pull themselves up with their arms. When assisting patients with a cervical laminectomy to a sitting position, caution them not to put their arms on the nurse's shoulders.

- Explain that antiembolism hose and possibly sequential compression sleeves will be applied after surgery to prevent thrombus formation. Teach techniques for ankle circling and calf pumping to promote venous circulation in the legs. Teach patient to report calf pain, tenderness, or warmth.

- Advise patient that health care provider will prescribe certain postoperative activity restrictions. Sitting is commonly restricted or allowed for only limited, prescribed periods of time in a straight-back chair. Teach patient not to sit for long periods of time on the edge of the mattress because it does not provide enough support. Explain that weakness, dizziness, and lightheadedness may occur on a first walk. Patients are encouraged to walk progressively longer distances.

- Instruct patient to avoid stretching, twisting, flexing, or jarring the spine to prevent vertebral collapse, shifting of the bone graft, or a bleeding episode. Explain that the spine should be kept aligned and in a neutral position.
- If patient is scheduled for a cervical laminectomy, explain that a cervical collar will be worn postoperatively. Teach these patients not to pull with their arms on objects such as side rails.
- Instruct patient in use of braces or corsets if prescribed. Braces should be applied while in bed. Wearing cotton underwear under the brace, powdering the skin lightly with cornstarch, or providing additional padding will help protect the skin from irritation. The person undergoing a fusion procedure often wears a supportive brace or corset for ≤3 mo to keep the operative site immobile so that the graft will heal and not dislodge.
- Explain that the health care provider will give patient instructions for at-home activity restrictions, including driving or riding in the car, sexual activity, lifting and carrying objects, tub bathing (generally, soaking the incision is avoided until about 1 wk after the sutures are out), going up and down stairs, the amount of time to spend in and out of bed, back exercises, and expected time away from work.
- Teach patient the following symptoms of postoperative wound infection that require medical attention: swelling, discharge, persistent redness, local warmth, fever, and pain. The incision should be kept dry and open to the air.
- For additional interventions, see **Knowledge deficit:** Surgical procedure, preoperative routine, and postoperative care in Appendix One, "Caring for Preoperative and Postoperative Patients," p. 717.

NIC: Positioning: Neurologic; Preoperative Coordination; Preparatory Sensory Information; Surgical Preparation; Teaching: Preoperative; Teaching: Prescribed Activity/Exercise; Teaching: Psychomotor Skill

Impaired swallowing: (or risk of same) related to postoperative edema or hematoma formation secondary to anterior cervical fusion
Desired outcome: Patient regains uncompromised swallowing ability (usually by the third postoperative day) as evidenced by normal breath sounds and absence of food in the oral cavity or choking/coughing.
- As part of the preoperative teaching, instruct patient in the potential for difficulty with swallowing after anterior cervical fusion. Caution patient of the need to report promptly any significant postoperative difficulty with swallowing. A sore throat is not unexpected. A soft diet and throat lozenges may be prescribed for 2-3 days postoperatively.
- Monitor for edema of the face or neck or tracheal compression or deviation that could compromise respiratory function. Monitor and rapidly report stridor or respiratory distress.
- Listen for hoarseness, which can indicate laryngeal nerve irritation and signal an ineffective cough or swallowing difficulty in a particular patient. For patients with hoarseness, the voice will usually return to normal as inflammation around the laryngeal nerve subsides. Encourage voice rest, and facilitate alternative communication (e.g., story boards, pen and pencil, flash cards). Report immediately any respiratory distress, inability to speak, worsening hoarseness, or voice change.
- Monitor and report diminished breath sounds compared with the patient's normal or preoperative status.
- As indicated, monitor oximetry as a quantitative measure of systemic oxygenation.
- Monitor patient for complaints of excessive pressure in the neck or severe, uncontrolled incisional pain, which can signal excessive bleeding. Monitor closed suction devices, and recharge the suction device/chamber as indicated to facilitate wound drainage.

- Check for gag and swallowing reflexes before oral intake. Begin the postoperative diet with clear fluids, and progress to more solid foods only after patient demonstrates ability to ingest fluids safely.
- To minimize the risk of aspiration, position patient in Fowler's position, or semi-Fowler's position at minimum, when initiating fluid intake. If not prohibited by surgery, encourage use of the chin tuck to lessen potential for aspiration.
- Also see **Risk for aspiration,** p. 335, in "General Care of Patients With Neurologic Disorders."

NIC: Artificial Airway Management; Aspiration Precautions; Bleeding Precautions; Emotional Support; Respiratory Monitoring; Surveillance; Teaching: Individual

Knowledge deficit: Percutaneous lumbar disk removal
Desired outcome: Before the procedure, patient verbalizes information about percutaneous lumbar disk removal. After the procedure, the patient is able to resume normal activity pattern without symptoms of dizziness or lightheadedness.

- During the preoperative period, reinforce health care provider's explanation of the procedure, including its purpose, risks, and anticipated benefits and outcome.
- As indicated, explain that percutaneous lumbar disk removal involves injection of local anesthetic to allow percutaneous placement of an ultrasonic nucleotome or fiberoptic arthroscopic cannula into the intervertebral space. The procedure will be done using fluoroscopy and allows fragmentation of the disk and its aspiration to relieve pressure on the spinal cord or nerve roots.
- Document baseline distal neurologic status carefully, especially motor or sensory deficits of the legs and feet. Explain that VS and neurologic status will be monitored frequently after the procedure. IM injections (both before and after the procedure) are given in a site other than the patient's affected area to avoid confusing the patient's disk pathology with injection site pain. Instruct patient to report any numbness or weakness, especially if this is a change from baseline neurologic status, because this may signal nerve root injury.
- Explain that patient will be monitored for bowel and bladder dysfunction after the procedure. The abdomen will be checked for bowel sounds and distention. Patient should report any nausea or vomiting and may be asked to void within 8 hr of the procedure to check for urinary retention.
- Inform patient that he or she will be on bedrest for 2-24 hr after the procedure, depending on surgeon's preference.
- Explain that back stiffness, soreness, pain, or spasm may occur after the procedure and that patient should alert staff member so that analgesia can be given. Encourage patient to request medication before discomfort becomes severe.
- Be aware that transient syncope may occur after the procedure. When vital signs are stable, instruct patient to rise slowly to a sitting position and then to wait 1 min to assess for any lightheadedness or dizziness. If these occur, have patient lie down, assess VS, encourage lower extremity isometric exercises (to discourage venous pooling), and try mobilization again in 15-30 min. If there are no unusual findings, have the patient slowly stand, but stay by the bed until assured that patient is not dizzy or lightheaded.
- Instruct patient to report immediately any numbness, weakness, paraplegia, paraparesis, or change in bowel or bladder function after hospital discharge.
- For additional interventions, see **Knowledge deficit:** Surgical procedure, preoperative routine, and postoperative care in Appendix One, "Caring for Preoperative and Postoperative Patients," p. 717.

◎ NIC: Exercise Therapy: Ambulation; Pain Management; Surveillance; Teaching: Individual; Teaching: Preoperative; Teaching: Prescribed Activity/ Exercise

> See Also: "General Care of Patients With Neurologic Disorders" for **Risk for injury** related to impaired pain, touch, and temperature sensation, p. 332; **Knowledge deficit:** Neurologic diagnostic tests, p. 346; Appendix One, "Caring for Preoperative and Postoperative Patients," p. 717, for related nursing diagnoses and interventions; "Pressure Ulcers," p. 710, for patients experiencing various degrees of immobility; Appendix One, "Caring for Patients on Prolonged Bedrest," p. 738.

PATIENT-FAMILY TEACHING AND DISCHARGE PLANNING

When providing patient-family teaching, focus on sensory information; avoid giving excessive information; and initiate a visiting nurse referral for necessary follow-up teaching. Consider including verbal and written information about the following:

- Prescribed exercise regimen, including rationale for each exercise, technique for performing the exercise, number of repetitions of each, and frequency of the exercise periods. If possible, ensure that patient demonstrates understanding of the exercise regimen and proper body mechanics before hospital discharge.
- Wound incision care. Indicators of postoperative wound infection that necessitate medical attention include swelling, discharge, persistent redness, local warmth, fever, and pain.
- Review of use and application of cervical collar for patients who have had a cervical fusion. The cervical collar is worn at all times. The patient should be instructed to cleanse the neck 1-2 times/day, cleaning the incision with mild soap. To accomplish this, the patient should request help from a significant other. The patient should lie flat, open the front portion of the collar, keeping the head and neck still and straight while the collar is open. The incision should be cleansed and dried and the collar replaced and fastened. Then the patient should turn on one side with a thin pillow under the head. The posterior portion of the collar is opened; the back of the neck is washed and dried; and the posterior portion of the collar is replaced and fastened. Men should shave the chin and neck beneath the collar while lying flat. Whenever the collar is released and opened, the head and neck should be kept straight and not moved. A silk scarf worn beneath the collar may decrease discomfort. A small cervical pillow may be used. Patients should avoid watching wall-mounted television units because of the risk of extension, rotation, and flexion of the neck.
- Use and care of a brace or immobilizer if appropriate.
- Medications, including drug name, rationale, dosage, schedule, precautions, drug/drug and food/drug interactions, and potential side effects.
- Anticonstipation routine, which should be initiated during hospitalization.
- Pain control measures.
- Phone number of a resource person, should questions arise after hospital discharge.
- Postsurgical activity restrictions as directed by health care provider. These may affect the following: driving and riding in a car, returning to work, sexual activity, lifting and carrying, tub bathing, going up and down steps, and the amount of time spent in or out of bed.
- Signs and symptoms of worsening neurologic function and the importance of notifying health care provider immediately if they develop. These include numbness, weakness, paralysis, or bowel and bladder dysfunction.

Spinal cord injury

The spinal cord injuries (SCIs) discussed in this section are caused by vertebral fractures or dislocations that sever, lacerate, stretch, or compress the spinal cord and interrupt neuronal function and transmission of nerve impulses. Blood supply to the spinal cord also may be interrupted. The spinal cord swells in response to injury, and this, along with hemorrhage, can cause additional compression, ischemia, and compromised function. Neurologic deficits resulting from compression may be reversible if the resulting edema and ischemia do not lead to spinal cord degeneration and necrosis. Common causes of injury include motor vehicle accidents, diving or other sporting accidents, falls, and gunshot wounds. SCIs are classified in a number of different ways according to type (open, closed), cause, site (level of spinal cord involved), mechanism of injury (compression, hyperflexion, hyperextension, rotational, penetrating), stability, and degree of spinal cord function loss (complete, incomplete). A *spinal cord concussion* is a transient loss of cord function caused by a traumatic event and resulting in immediate flaccid paralysis that resolves completely in a matter of minutes or hours.

Prognosis: Any evidence of voluntary motor function, sensory function, or sacral sensation below the level of injury indicates an incomplete SCI, with the potential for partial or complete recovery. The level of injury is the lowest level in which motor function and sensation remain intact. After an acute injury, the spinal cord usually goes into a condition called *spinal shock*, in which there can be total loss of spinal cord function below the level of injury. During spinal shock there is no reflex activity. Resolution of spinal shock with return of reflexes usually occurs within 1-6 wk but may take 6 mo or more. If there is no evidence of returning motor function after local reflexes have returned, the spinal cord is considered irreversibly damaged. Generally, SCI does not cause immediate death unless it is at C1 through C3, which results in respiratory muscle paralysis. Individuals who survive these injuries require a ventilator for the rest of their lives. If the injury occurs at C4, respiratory difficulties may result in death, although some individuals who have survived the initial injury have been successfully weaned from the ventilator. Injuries below C4 also can be life threatening because of ascending cord edema, which can cause respiratory muscle paralysis. Immediately after injury, common complications that require treatment include hypotension (systolic BP <80 mm Hg), bradycardia, paralytic ileus, urinary retention, pneumonia, and stress ulcers. Other long-term, life-threatening, potential complications of SCI include autonomic dysreflexia, decubitus ulcers, pneumonia, sepsis, urinary calculi, and urinary tract infection (UTI).

ASSESSMENT

Acute indicators: Loss of sensation, weakness, or paralysis below the level of injury; localized pain or tenderness over the site of injury; headache; hypothermia or hyperthermia; and alterations in bowel and bladder function.

Cervical injury: Possible alterations in LOC, weakness or paralysis in all four extremities (quadriparesis or quadriplegia), paralysis of respiratory muscles or signs of respiratory problems, such as flaring nostrils and use of accessory muscles for respirations. Any cervical injury can result in a low body temperature (to 96° F [35.5° C]), slowed pulse rate (<60 bpm) caused by vagal stimulation of the heart, hypotension (systolic BP <80 mm Hg) caused by vasodilation, and decreased peristalsis.

Thoracic and lumbar injuries: Paraparesis/paraplegia or altered sensation in the legs; hand and arm involvement in upper thoracic injuries.

Acute spinal shock: Can last 2 days to 6 mo but usually resolves in 1-6 wk. Spinal shock results from a loss of sympathetic nerve outflow below the level of injury. Indicators depend on the severity of the injury and include total loss of spinal cord function, loss of skin sensation, flaccid paralysis or absence of reflexes below the level of injury, paralytic ileus and constipation second-ary to atonic bowel, bladder distention secondary to atonic bladder, brady-cardia, low/falling BP secondary to loss of vasomotor tone and decreased venous return, and anhidrosis (absence of sweating and loss of tempera-ture regulation) below the level of injury. Autonomic instability is more dramatic in higher (e.g., cervical) lesions. Resolution of spinal shock is indicated by the return of the bulbocavernosus reflex (slight muscle con-traction when the glans penis is squeezed or the urinary catheter is pulled) and the anal reflex (puckering of the anus on digital examination or gentle scratching around the anus). The remaining reflexes may take weeks to return.

Chronic indicators: As spinal shock resolves, muscle tone, reflexes, and some function may return, depending on severity and level of injury. The return of reflexes usually results in muscle spasticity. Chronic autonomic dysfunction may be manifested as fever; mild hypotension; anhidrosis; and alterations in bowel, bladder, and sexual function. Chronic neural pain may occur after SCI and tends to occur as either diffuse pain below the level of injury or pain adjacent to the level of injury. Injuries at or below L1 may result in permanent flaccid paralysis.

Upper motor neuron (UMN) involvement: UMNs are nerve cell bodies that originate in high levels of the CNS and transmit impulses from the brain down the spinal cord. Injury will interrupt this impulse transmission, causing muscle or organ dysfunction below the level of injury. However, since the injury does not interrupt reflex arcs coming from those muscles or organs to the spinal cord, hypertonic reflexes, clonus paralysis, and spastic paralysis are seen. The patient will have a positive Babinski reflex.

Lower motor neuron (LMN) involvement: LMNs are anterior horn cell bodies that originate in the spinal cord. LMNs transmit nerve impulses to muscles and organs and are involved in reflex arcs that control involuntary responses. Damage to LMNs will abolish voluntary and reflex responses of muscles and organs, resulting in flaccid paralysis, hypotonia, atrophy, and muscle fibrillations and fasciculations. The patient will have an absent Babinski reflex. The spinal cord ends at the T12-L1 level. Below that level, a bundle of nerve roots from the spinal cord, called the *cauda equina*, fills the spinal canal. Injuries at or below L1 that damage the nerve fiber after it leaves the spinal cord result in flaccid paralysis because of interrupted reflex arc activity.

Bowel and bladder dysfunction: Usually conscious sensation of the need to void or defecate is lost. UMN bowel and bladder involvement results in reflex incontinence. Flaccid LMN bladder involvement causes urinary retention with overflow incontinence. Flaccid LMN bowel involvement causes fecal retention/impaction.

Autonomic dysreflexia (AD): An uninhibited autonomic reflex response to stimuli can be life threatening as reflex activity returns. AD is seen most commonly in patients with injuries at or above T6, but it has been reported in patients with injuries as low as T8. Signs and symptoms include gross hypertension (up to 240-300/150 mm Hg), pounding headache, blurred vision, bradycardia, nausea, and nasal congestion. Above the level of the injury, flushing and sweating may occur. Below the level of injury, piloerection (goose bumps) and skin pallor, which signal vasoconstriction, often occur. Seizures, subarachnoid hemorrhage, cerebrovascular accident (CVA), or retinal hemor-rhage may occur.

Physical assessment

Acute (spinal shock): Absence of deep tendon reflexes (DTRs) below level of injury; absence of cremasteric reflex (scratching or light stroking of the inner thigh for male patients causes the testicle on that side to elevate) for T12 and L1 injuries; absence of penile or anal sphincter reflex.

Chronic: Generally, increased DTRs occur if the spinal cord lesion is of the UMN type.

DIAGNOSTIC TESTS

X-ray of spine: To delineate fracture, deformity, or displacement of vertebrae, as well as soft tissue masses, such as hematomas.

CT scan: To reveal changes in the spinal cord, vertebrae, and soft tissue surrounding the spine.

Myelography: To show blockage or disruption of the spinal canal; used if other diagnostic examinations are inconclusive. Radiopaque dye is injected into the subarachnoid space of the spine, using a lumbar or cervical puncture.

MRI: To reveal changes in the spinal cord and surrounding soft tissue. MRI evaluation is preferred for evaluation of the degree of injury in patients who can tolerate it.

ABG/pulmonary function tests: To assess effectiveness of respirations and detect the need for O_2 or mechanical ventilation.

Cystometry: To assess capacity and function of the bladder after resolution of spinal shock for the best type of bladder training program.

Pulmonary fluoroscopy: To evaluate the degree of diaphragm movement and effectiveness in individuals with high cervical injuries.

Evoked potential studies (e.g., somatosensory):   To help locate the level of spinal cord lesion by evaluating the integrity of the nervous system's anatomic pathways and connections. Stimulation of a peripheral nerve triggers a discrete electrical response along a neurologic pathway to the brain. Response or lack of response to stimulation is measured in this test.

> **See Also:**   "General Care of Patients With Neurologic Disorders" for **Knowledge deficit:** Neurologic diagnostic tests, p. 346, for care considerations for patients undergoing CT scan, myelography, MRI, and evoked potentials.

COLLABORATIVE MANAGEMENT

Acute care

Immobilization of injury site: Essential for preventing further damage. See "Surgery/immobilization," p. 260.

Bedrest on a firm surface: For example, Roto Rest Kinetic Treatment Table.

Pharmacotherapy

Corticosteroids (methylprednisolone):   Megadose given IV within 8 hr of injury to reduce damage and improve functional recovery by protecting the neuromembrane from further destruction. Dosage is IV bolus of 30 mg/kg followed by continuous IV infusion of 5.4 mg/kg/hr for a 48-hr period. If tirilazad mesylate (a nonglucocorticoid 21 aminosteroid) is used, it is administered as a 2.5 mg/kg bolus infusion q6hr for the first 48 hr.

Osmotic diuretics (e.g., mannitol):   Sometimes used for 10 days to reduce cord edema after the initial injury and minimize ascending cord edema.

Analgesics (e.g., acetaminophen, codeine) and sedatives: To decrease pain and anxiety.

Antacids; histamine H_2-receptor blockers (e.g., ranitidine):   To prevent gastric ulceration, which may occur because of increased production of gastric secretions with SCI and steroid use.

Anticoagulants (e.g., heparin, enoxaprin, warfarin):   To prevent thrombophlebitis and reduce the potential for pulmonary emboli.

Stool softeners (e.g., docusate sodium):   To keep stool soft and prevent fecal impaction while the bowel is atonic.

Vasopressors (e.g., dopamine):   To treat hypotension in the immediate postinjury stage caused by loss of vasomotor tone. *Fluid therapy* also may be given for hypotension. *Atropine* may be given for bradycardia. Typically, patient will be on a cardiac monitor and in ICU during this stage.

Aggressive respiratory therapy: For all patients with SCIs. Patients with injuries above C5 are intubated and put on a ventilator. Nasal intubation or tracheostomy may be used to prevent neck extension (and thus further damage) during intubation. Intermittent positive pressure breathing (IPPB) and chest physiotherapy are used to prevent and treat atelectasis. Respiratory therapy is ongoing past the acute stage.

Nasogastric decompression during spinal shock phase: To prevent aspiration of gastric contents and treat paralytic ileus.

Bladder decompression during spinal shock phase: Either intermittent catheterization or continuous drainage.

Surgery/immobilization: May include traction, fusion, laminectomy, and closed or open reduction of fractures. The surgical goal is to immobilize the spine and, if indicated, decompress the spinal cord or remove bone fragments as soon as possible after injury to help prevent additional neurologic deficit. The spine is surgically fused within 5-10 days of the injury. Complete healing may take 3-4 mo.

Cervical spine: Immobilized with devices such as Crutchfield tongs, Vinke-Gardner-Wells tongs, halo traction. Halo traction does not need to be removed for surgery; it enables early mobilization, and some types can be used in an MRI machine.

Thoracic spine: Immobilized with a surgical corset, plaster Minerva jacket, plastic body jacket, Harrington rods, Cotrel and DuBousset rods, or spinal fusion with bone graft, pedicle screws, fusion cages, or lamina hooks.

Lumbar spine injuries: Usually treated with closed reduction and hyperextension or extension with traction techniques, followed by immobilization in a plastic jacket or spica cast. If these interventions are unsuccessful or if neurologic symptoms occur, a laminectomy is usually performed. A halo type of device that provides femoral distraction has been developed for lumbar injuries.

Sacral (cauda equina) fracture: Usually treated with a laminectomy and spinal fusion.

Tracheostomy: If patient needs long-term ventilation.

Physical and occupational therapy: Passive ROM is started on all joints. After the injury is stabilized, an aggressive rehabilitation program is initiated, including muscle-strengthening and -conditioning exercises to develop alternative muscle groups needed for independence; a sitting program; massage; and instruction in adaptive devices, equipment, and transfer techniques as appropriate. Patients with sacral injuries have the potential to walk and should be instructed in the use of braces, crutches, or a cane as appropriate. Functional electrical stimulation of paralyzed muscles assists some paraplegic patients with walking. A therapy program is ongoing throughout the patient's rehabilitation.

Antiembolism hose or sequential compression devices: Prevent thrombophlebitis and reduce the effects of orthostatic hypotension.

Nutrition: Parenteral nutrition and fluids until the GI tract starts functioning and oral intake is possible. A diet high in calories, protein, and fiber usually is prescribed.

Bowel program during spinal shock: Usually consists of manual disimpaction and small-volume enemas while the bowel is atonic.

Counseling and psychotherapy: Helps patient and significant other adjust to the disability. This is ongoing and should address sexual functioning and vocational rehabilitation.

Investigational treatments

Monosialotetrahexosylgangliosides: GM-1 protein may be given to encourage axonal sprouting in the hope of enhancing neurologic function.

Endorphin-blocking agents: Used immediately after the injury to prevent the hypotensive action of endorphins that may contribute to cord ischemia.

Hyperbaric oxygen therapy: Used immediately after the injury to attempt to prevent ischemic cord destruction.

Spinal cord cooling: Used immediately after the injury to reduce edema, thus improving cord circulation. A small pad through which cool saline solution circulates is placed on the epidural layer of the cord for several hours. A major complication is infection caused by exposure of the cord during cooling.

Immunosuppressive therapy (e.g., cyclophosphamide):   Used to try to reduce cellular or immune responses after injury.

Functional electrical stimulation (FES):   Used to stimulate specific muscle groups to create contraction and relaxation for assisted ambulation.

Sacral anterior nerve root stimulator: Used to improve bladder continence.

Chronic care

Pharmacotherapy

Muscle relaxants (e.g., diazepam)

Antispasmodics (e.g., baclofen, dantrolene):   To decrease spasms. More severe spasticity may be treated with intramuscular injections of botulinum toxin.

Antibiotics (e.g., methenamine mandelate):   To prevent bladder infection.

Stool softeners (e.g., docusate sodium), laxatives (e.g., Milk of Magnesia, bisacodyl), and suppositories: To maintain a bowel program that prevents fecal impaction and minimizes incontinence. **Note:** Suppositories are avoided or used with caution in individuals at risk for AD.

Anticholinergics (e.g., oxybutynin, propantheline):   To reduce bladder spasms causing reflex incontinence.

Dietary management: Limiting milk and other dairy products to minimize the risk of renal calculi, and promoting juices (e.g., cranberry, plum, prune) that leave an acid ash in the urine and decrease urinary pH, thus reducing the potential for infection. Vitamin C also may be used to acidify the urine. An adequate diet also should include high roughage and fiber to promote soft stools. If not contraindicated, fluids are encouraged to promote adequate hydration.

Management of AD: AD is a medical emergency that can occur for patients with SCIs at or above T6. The noxious stimulus (e.g., a distended bladder) must be found and alleviated as quickly as possible. The following may be administered during crisis to control hypertension: vasodilators (e.g., hydralazine, nitroprusside, amyl nitrate), hypotensive nondiuretic thiazides (e.g., diazoxide), adrenergic blockers (e.g., IV phentolamine), ganglionic blocking agents (e.g., reserpine, guanethidine, mecamylamine), and fast-acting calcium channel blockers (e.g., nifedipine). Tetracaine or lidocaine may be instilled into the bladder to reduce bladder excitability. (For nursing interventions, see **Dysreflexia** below.)

Surgical interventions

Diaphragm pacer insertion: This is a phrenic nerve stimulator that may allow selected patients on the ventilator to be off the ventilator for short periods. Electrodes are implanted over the phrenic nerve and, when activated, cause the diaphragm to contract, generating a breath.

Intrathecal baclofen and clonidine: A programmable pump is implanted to deliver a continuous dose of baclofen into the sheath of the spinal canal to control spasticity.

Intrathecal clonidine: Clonidine may be administered to control chronic pain.

Tenotomies, myotomies, muscle transplants, peripheral neurectomies, and rhizotomy: These are some of the surgical approaches that may be used to treat spasticity that cannot be managed by medications or more conservative measures such as stretching or ROM.

Intrathecal injection of phenol: Phenol relieves muscle spasm for as long as 3-6 mo.

NURSING DIAGNOSES AND INTERVENTIONS

Dysreflexia (or risk of same) related to exaggerated unopposed autonomic response to noxious stimuli for individuals with SCI at or above T6.

> **Note:**   AD is seen most commonly in patients with injuries at or above T6, but cases have been reported in patients with injuries as low as T8.

Desired outcomes: On an ongoing basis, patient is free of symptoms of AD as evidenced by BP within patient's baseline range, HR 60-100 bpm, and absence of headache and other clinical indicators of AD. Following instruction, patient and significant other verbalize factors that cause AD, treatment and prevention, and when immediate emergency treatment is indicated.

- Monitor for indicators of AD, including hypertension (>20 mm Hg above baseline but may go as high as 240-300/150 mm Hg), pounding headache, bradycardia, blurred vision, nausea, nasal congestion, flushing and sweating above the level of injury, and piloerection (goose bumps) or pallor below the level of injury.
- If AD is suspected, raise HOB immediately to 90 degrees or assist patient into a sitting position to lower the BP.
- Call for someone to notify health care provider; stay with patient, and try to find and ameliorate the noxious stimulus. Speed is essential. Monitor BP q3-5min during the hypertensive episode. Remain calm and supportive of patient and significant other.
- Assess the following sites for causes, and implement measures for removing the noxious stimulus.

BLADDER (MOST LIKELY CAUSE):   Distention, UTI, calculus and other obstructions, bladder spasms, catheterization, or bladder irrigations performed too quickly or with too cold a liquid.

- Do not use Credé's method for a distended bladder.
- Catheterize patient (ideally using anesthetic jelly) if there is a possibility or question of bladder distention. Consult health care provider *stat.*
- If a catheter is already in place, check the tubing for kinks and lower the drainage bag. For obstruction, such as sediment in the tubing, irrigate the catheter as indicated, using no more than 30 ml of normal saline. If catheter patency is uncertain, recatheterize patient using anesthetic jelly.
- If the bladder is not distended, check for signs of UTI and/or urinary calculi, including cloudy urine, hematuria, and positive laboratory or x-ray results.
- Obtain urine specimen for culture and sensitivity studies as indicated.

BOWEL (SECOND MOST LIKELY CAUSE):   Constipation, impaction, insertion of suppository or enema, or rectal examination.

- Do not attempt rectal examination without first anesthetizing the rectal sphincter and anal canal with anesthetic jelly.
- Use large amounts of anesthetic jelly in the anus and rectum before disimpacting bowel to remove the potential stimulus. Allow 5 min for the anesthetic jelly to work, as manifested by lower BP, before disimpacting.

SKIN: Pressure, infection, injury, heat, pain, or cold.

- Loosen clothing and remove antiembolism hose, leg bandages, abdominal binder, or constrictive sheets as appropriate.
- For male patients, check for a pressure source on the penis, scrotum, or testicles and remove the pressure if present.
- Check the skin surface below level of injury. Monitor for the presence of a pressure area or sore, infection, laceration, rash, sunburn, ingrown toenail, or infected area. If indicated, apply a topical anesthetic.
- Observe for and remove the source of heat or cold (e.g., ice pack, heating pad).

ADDITIONAL CAUSES: Surgical manipulation, sexual activity, menstruation, or labor.

- Administer antihypertensive agents, such as hydralazine, diazoxide, or nifedipine, as prescribed.

- On resolution of the crisis, answer patient's and significant other's questions about AD. Discuss signs and symptoms, treatment, and methods of prevention. Encourage patient to wear a medical-alert type bracelet or tag.

Note: Prevention is the best way to deal with AD. A good bowel regimen and skin integrity program are key factors in preventing the noxious stimuli that constipation or pressure areas may cause. Loosen clothing, bed sheets, and constricting bands; turn patient off side to relieve other possible sources of pressure. Keep the bed free of sharp objects and wrinkles. Adhere to turning schedules. Institute measures to reduce the potential for UTI and urinary calculi, and teach the patient self-inspection of skin and urinary catheter and the importance of using anesthetic jelly for catheterization and disimpaction.

NIC: Anxiety Reduction; Bowel Management; Dysreflexia Management; Neurologic Monitoring; Positioning; Urinary Elimination Management; Vital Signs Monitoring

Constipation or fecal impaction related to immobility and decreased peristalsis, atonic bowel, and loss of sensation and voluntary sphincter control secondary to sensorimotor deficit

Desired outcome: Patient has bowel movements that are soft and formed every 2-3 days or within patient's preinjury pattern.

- During acute phase of spinal shock, assess patient's bowel function by auscultating for bowel sounds, inspecting for the presence of abdominal distention, and monitoring for nausea and vomiting and fecal impaction. Notify health care provider of significant findings. In the presence of fecal impaction, gentle manual removal or a small cleansing enema may be prescribed. Because the atonic intestine distends easily, administer small-volume enemas only. Avoid long-term use of enemas.
- Lesions above the conus medullaris (located at the lower two levels of the thoracic region where the cord begins to taper) generally leave the S3, S4, and S5 spinal cord nerve segments intact. If this spinal reflex arc is intact, the patient will have a UMN bowel and be capable of stimulating (training) the reflex evacuation of the bowel. Lesions below the conus medullaris (T12) may injure the S3, S4, and S5 nerve segments, resulting in disruption of the reflex arc and causing an LMN flaccid bowel and loss of anal tone. A flaccid bowel usually is managed with increased intraabdominal pressure techniques, manual disimpaction, and small-volume enemas.
- For the UMN reflex bowel, once bowel activity returns, teach patient to attempt bowel movement 30 min after a meal or warm drink. This regimen will allow patient's gastrocolic and duodenocolic mass peristalsis reflexes to assist with evacuation. Increasing intraabdominal pressure by bearing down, bending forward, or applying manual pressure to the abdomen also will help promote bowel evacuation. An abdominal belt may be used if the patient is unable to strain at stool. A prescribed, medicated suppository also may be used if necessary. If allowed, provide a bedside commode rather than a bedpan. Check patient's ability to maintain balance on a commode.

Caution: For patients with injuries at T8 or above, promote adequate fluid intake (>2500 ml/day) and use of stool softeners and high-fiber diet. Use suppositories and enemas only when essential and with extreme caution because they can precipitate AD. Use anesthetic jelly liberally when performing a rectal examination or inserting a suppository or an enema.

- For patients with hand mobility (who are not at risk for AD), teach the technique for suppository insertion and digital stimulation of the anus to promote reflex bowel evacuation. For digital stimulation, insert finger and gently rotate in a circular motion for about 30 sec (or longer) until the internal sphincter relaxes. Stop if sphincter spasms are felt or if signs of AD occur. Repeat q10min several times until adequate evacuation occurs. Suppository inserters and rectal stimulation devices are available for patients with limited hand mobility.
- For other interventions, see **Constipation** in Appendix One, "Caring for Patients on Prolonged Bedrest," p. 743.

⊚ NIC: Bowel Management; Bowel Training; Constipation/Impaction Management; Fluid Management; Nutritional Counseling

Ineffective airway clearance related to neuromuscular paralysis/weakness or restriction of chest expansion secondary to halo vest obstruction
Desired outcome: Following intervention, patient has a clear airway as evidenced by RR of 12-20 breaths/min with normal depth and pattern (eupnea) and absence of adventitious breath sounds.
- Monitor ventilation capability by checking vital capacity, tidal volume, and pulmonary function tests. Monitor serial ABG values and/or pulse oximetry readings. If vital capacity is less than 1 L or if patient exhibits signs of hypoxia (Pao_2 <80 mm Hg, O_2 saturation <92%, tachycardia, increased restlessness, mental status changes or dullness, cyanosis), notify health care provider immediately.
- Monitor for ascending cord edema, which may be signaled by increasing difficulty with secretions, coughing, respiratory difficulties, bradycardia, fluctuating BP, and increased motor and sensory losses at a higher level than baseline findings.
- Monitor for loss of previous ability to bend arms at the elbows (C5-6) or shrug shoulders (C3-4). If these findings are noted, notify health care provider immediately.
- Maintain patent airway. Keep patient's head in neutral position, and suction as necessary. Be aware that suctioning may cause severe bradycardia in the patient with AD. If indicated, prepare patient for a tracheostomy, endotracheal intubation, and/or mechanical ventilation to support respiratory function. If appropriate, arrange for a transfer to ICU for continuous monitoring.
- If patient is wearing halo vest traction, assess respiratory status at least q4hr or more frequently as indicated. Ensure that the vest is not restricting chest expansion. Teach the use of incentive spirometry. Be alert to the following indicators of pulmonary embolus (PE): SOB, hemoptysis, tachycardia, and diminished breath sounds. Pain may or may not be present with PE, depending on the level of SCI. Sudden shoulder pain may be referred pain from PE.
- If the patient's cough is ineffective, implement the following technique, known as "assisted coughing": place the palm of the hand under the patient's diaphragm (below the xiphoid process and above the naval). As the patient exhales forcibly, push up into diaphragm to assist in producing a more forceful cough. Assisted coughing may be contraindicated in patients with spinal instability.
- Feed patients in Stryker frames, Foster beds, or similar mechanical beds in the prone position to minimize the potential for aspiration. Raise stable patients in halo traction to high Fowler's position if it is not contraindicated.
- For additional information, see **Risk for aspiration,** p. 335, in "General Care of Patients with Neurologic Disorders."

NIC: Airway Management; Aspiration Precautions; Cough Enhancement; Neurologic Monitoring; Oxygen Therapy; Respiratory Monitoring

Risk for disuse syndrome with risk factors related to paralysis, immobilization, or spasticity secondary to SCI
Desired outcomes: After stabilization of the injury, patient exhibits complete ROM of all joints. By time of discharge, patient demonstrates measures that enhance mobility, reduce spasms, and prevent complications.
- Once the injury is stabilized, assist patient with position changes. For example, a prone position, if not contraindicated, helps prevent sacral decubiti and hip contractures. Assist patient into this position on a regular schedule.
- For patients with spasticity, use hand splints or cones to assist with maintaining a functional grasp.
- To help prevent foot contractures for patients with spasticity, it may be helpful to fit patient with splints or high-top tennis shoes that are cut off at the toes so that each shoe ends just proximal to the metatarsal head. These shoes help keep the feet dorsiflexed but prevent contact of the balls of the feet with a hard surface, which can cause spasticity. Avoid footboards for these patients because the hard surface may trigger spasticity and promote plantar flexion.
- Teach patient that some factors that trigger spasms are cold, anxiety, fatigue, emotional distress, infections, bowel or bladder distention, ulcers, pain, tight clothing, and lying too long in one position. Controlling these factors may reduce the number of spasms experienced.
- Teach patients with spasticity proper positioning, ROM, and daily sustained stretching exercises. Steady, continuous, directional stretching once or twice daily is especially important because it may decrease the amount of spasticity for several hours. Cooling and icing techniques, heat, vibration therapy, and transcutaneous electrical nerve stimulation (TENS) of the spastic muscles also may be helpful.
- Because tactile stimulation may trigger spasms, touch by caregivers should be limited. When touch is necessary, do it in a firm, gentle, steady manner.
- For additional interventions, see **Risk for disuse syndrome,** p. 740, in Appendix One, "Caring for Patients on Prolonged Bedrest."

NIC: Exercise Promotion: Stretching; Exercise Therapy: Joint Mobility; Peripheral Sensation Management; Positioning; Positioning: Neurologic

Risk for injury with risk factors related to incorrect neck position, irritation of cranial nerves, impaired lateral vision secondary to presence of halo vest traction, and lack of access for external cardiac compression
Desired outcome: At time of discharge (and ongoing during use of halo traction), patient exhibits no adverse changes in motor, sensory, or cranial nerve function and is free of symptoms of injury caused by impaired vision.
- Assess position of the patient's neck in relation to the body. Alert health care provider to the presence of flexion or hyperextension. Assess any difficulty with swallowing, because this may signal improper position of the neck and chin. Keep a torque screwdriver in a secure place so that health care provider can readily adjust tension on bars to return the patient's neck position to neutral.
- Evaluate degree of sensation and movement of the upper extremities, and assess cranial nerve function. Changes in cranial nerve function can occur if the cranial pins compress or irritate a nerve. Notify health care provider of sudden changes in motor, sensory, or cranial nerve function (e.g., weakness, paresthesias, ptosis, difficulty chewing or swallowing). Jaw pain may occur when chewing is attempted, and this needs to be differentiated from

cranial nerve problems. A diet of soft foods, cut into small pieces, will help jaw pain.

- Assess pins, bolts, and vest structure for looseness. Clicking sounds may signal a loose pin. Never use the superstructure of the halo traction in turning or moving patient. Notify health care provider if pins or vest becomes loose or dislodged. Stabilize patient's head as necessary.
- Instruct patient to avoid pulling clothes over the top of the halo apparatus because this may loosen pins. Patient should instead step into and pull clothes up over feet and legs. Advise patient to buy strapless bras, tube tops, or clothes that are several sizes larger or to modify neck openings (e.g., with Velcro closures, ties).
- Avoid loosening a buckle without health care provider's directive. Buckle holes should be marked so that they are always cinched correctly to the appropriate snugness.
- If patient is ambulatory, teach him or her how to survey the environment while walking, either by using a mirror, by turning the eyes to their extreme lateral positions, or by turning the entire body. A cane may help determine the height of curbs and detect unseen objects or uneven walking surfaces. Explain that trunk flexibility is limited and achieving balance can be difficult because of the top-heavy weight of the vest. Ambulating with a walker initially may help the patient learn to adjust. Abdominal- and back-strengthening exercises may aid balance and walking. Advise patient to walk only in low-heel shoes. Extra space allowance may be needed when passing through doorways and to avoid bumping into objects.
- Teach patient that bending over can be hazardous because of top-heaviness. A shower chair that rolls usually can fit over a toilet seat, providing an extra 3-6 inches in height. Slip-on shoes should be worn and long-handled assistive devices used to reach or pick up objects.
- To get out of bed, teach patients to roll onto their side at the edge of the bed and then drop their legs over the side of the bed while pushing up their trunk sideways.
- Recommend backing into the car seat with the body bent forward for getting into a car. Caution patient against driving because of the limited field of vision.
- Teach patient that a high table will help bring objects into view and that a swivel chair at home will permit easier visualization of the environment.
- Explain that the patient will need the assistance of another person to shampoo hair safely. Shampooing a short haircut is easiest, and hair should be blown dry because toweling the hair may loosen pins.
- Ensure that an open-end wrench is taped to the halo vest so that the bolts can be released and the vest removed promptly if external cardiac compression is needed. One type of halo vest permits the anterior vest to be lifted up after release of two side belts. Teach significant other how to release the vest in an emergency.

NIC: Environmental Management: Safety; Fall Prevention; Neurologic Monitoring; Teaching: Individual; Teaching: Psychomotor Skill

Risk for impaired skin integrity and/or **impaired tissue integrity** related to (or associated with risk factors from) altered circulation and mechanical factors secondary to presence of halo vest traction or tongs
Desired outcome: At time of discharge and on an ongoing basis, patient's skin is nonerythemic and unbroken; tissue underlying and surrounding the halo vest blanches appropriately.

- Inspect the skin around the vest edges for erythema and other signs of irritation. Massage nonerythematous areas routinely to promote circulation and help prevent breakdown. Teach skin inspection, which may require use of a mirror, flashlight, or another person. Teach patient to alert medical personnel if breakdown, sensitive spots, odor, dirty vest liner, or loose pins are present.

- Investigate complaints of discomfort or uncomfortable fit. A finger should be able to fit between the vest and patient's skin. Weight loss or gain can affect the fit. Pad the vest as needed until it can be properly adjusted or trimmed by health care provider. Protect the vest from moisture and soiling. Be alert to foul odor from in or around the cast openings, which can signal pressure necrosis beneath the vest. Serosanguineous drainage on a pillowcase slipped through the vest from one side to another may indicate an area of skin breakdown.

- Instruct/assist patient with changing body position q2hr. Support the vest while patient is in bed. Use pads to prevent pressure on prominent body areas such as the forehead or shoulder. Use a small pillow under the head for comfort at sleep time.

- Skin care should include cleansing with soap and warm water. Usually, releasing one vest belt at a time as the patient is lying down is allowed for washing. Avoid use of lotion and powder, which can cake under the vest. Replace soiled linens promptly. Patient's perspiration may be dried with a hair dryer on a cool setting.

- If a rash appears, consider that the patient may be allergic to the vest's lining. A synthetic liner, knitted body stockinette, or T-shirt may correct this problem.

- Provide oral care. A flexible disposable straw can be used both to sip clear water for rinsing teeth and to expel the rinse water into a sink or basin.

- In the event of skin breakdown, keep patient's skin cleansed, dried, and covered with a transparent dressing. Notify health care provider and orthotist accordingly because skin breakdown requires a brace adjustment.

- Place rubber corks over the tips of the halo device to diminish annoying sound vibrations if the apparatus is bumped and to prevent lacerations from possible sharp edges.

- Check tong placement. If slippage has occurred, immobilize patient's head with a sandbag and notify health care provider. Pain may signal erosion of bone and displacement into muscle. Check drainage for the presence of CSF (see pp. 281-282). Ensure that traction weights are hanging freely.

- Provide analgesia, as needed, for mild headache and discomfort.

- For a discussions of pin care, see "Fractures," p. 592, for **Knowledge deficit:** Function of external fixation, pin care, and signs and symptoms of pin site infection.

◎ NIC: Bathing; Positioning; Pressure Management; Teaching: Individual; Traction/Immobilization Care

Urinary retention or **reflex incontinence** related to neurologic impairment (spasticity or flaccidity occurring with SCI)
Desired outcomes: Patient has urinary output without incontinence. Patient empties bladder with residual volumes of <50 ml by time of discharge. Following instruction, patient demonstrates triggering mechanism and gains some control over voiding.

Note: Bladder dysfunction is complicated and should be assessed by cystometric testing to determine the best type of bladder program. Lesions above the conus medullaris (located at the lower two levels of the thoracic region where the cord begins to taper) generally leave the S2, S3, and S4 spinal cord nerve segments intact. If this spinal reflex arc is intact, the patient will have a UMN-involved bladder, resulting in a spastic bladder. This bladder has tone and occasional bladder contractions and periodically will empty on its own, resulting in reflex incontinence. The UMN-involved bladder is "trainable" with techniques that stimulate reflex voiding. Lesions below the conus medullaris (T12) may injure the S2, S3, and S4 nerve segments, which will disrupt the reflex arc, causing an LMN-involved flaccid bladder. This bladder has no tone and will distend until it overflows, resulting in overflow incontinence.

General guidelines for individuals with bladder dysfunction
- Initially patient will have an indwelling urinary catheter or scheduled intermittent catheterizations. If intermittent catheterization is used and episodes of incontinence occur or more than 500 ml of urine is obtained, catheterize the patient more often.
- Teach patient and significant other the procedure for intermittent catheterization, care of indwelling catheters, and indicators of UTI (e.g., fever, cloudy and/or foul-smelling urine, malaise, anorexia, restlessness, incontinence).
- Teach patient and significant other that the habit/bladder scheduling program consists of gradually increasing the time between catheterizations or periodically clamping indwelling catheters. The goal is a gradual increase in bladder tone. When the bladder can hold 300-400 ml of urine, measures to stimulate voiding are attempted.
- Make sure patient takes fluids at even intervals throughout the day. Restrict fluids before bedtime to prevent nighttime incontinence. Alcohol and caffeine-containing foods and beverages (e.g., cola, chocolate, coffee, tea) have a diuretic effect and may cause incontinence. In addition, caffeine-containing products may increase bladder spasms and reflex incontinence.
- Patients using bladder-emptying techniques should void at least q3hr. Wristwatches with timer alarms or an alarm clock can help the patient maintain this schedule. To obtain the postvoid residual urine, catheterize the patient after an attempt to empty the bladder. Residual amounts >100 ml usually indicate the need for a return to a scheduled intermittent catheterization program.

Guidelines for patients with UMN-involved spastic reflex bladder
- Explain to these patients that eventually they may be able to empty the bladder automatically and so may not require catheterization.
- Teach patient techniques that stimulate the voiding reflex, such as tapping the suprapubic area with the fingers, gently pulling the pubic hair, digitally stretching the anal sphincter, stroking the glans penis, stroking the inner thigh, or lightly punching the abdominal area just proximal to the inguinal ligaments. Perform the selected technique for 2-3 min or until a good urine stream has started. Wait 1 min before trying another stimulation technique.
  —*Bladder tapping:* position self in a half-sitting position. Tapping is performed over the suprapubic area, and the patient may shift the site of stimulation within that area to find the most effective site. Tapping is performed rapidly (7-8 times/sec) with one hand for approximately 50 single taps. Continue tapping until a good stream starts. When the stream stops, wait about 1 min and repeat tapping until the bladder is empty. One or two tapping attempts without response indicate that no more urine will be expelled.
  —*Anal stretch technique (contraindicated in individuals with lesions at T8 or above because of the potential for AD):* position self on commode or toilet. Lean forward on the thighs, and insert 1 or 2 lubricated fingers into the anus to the anal sphincter. Spread the anal sphincter gently by spreading the fingers apart or pulling in a posterior direction. Maintain the stretching position, take a deep breath, and hold breath while bearing down to void. Relax and repeat until the bladder is empty.

- Teach patients with abdominal muscle control to bear down using Valsalva's maneuver when attempting to trigger voiding.
- Be aware that stimulating the reflex trigger zones accidently may result in incontinence. Incontinence briefs will help control accidents. Avoid plastic or rubber sheets because these trap heat and moisture, promoting skin breakdown.
- Bacolfen may be prescribed, because it tends to promote more complete emptying of the bladder by reducing the tone of the external urinary sphincter.

Guidelines for patients with LMN-involved flaccid bladders
- Increasing intraabdominal pressure can overcome sphincter pressure, which may empty the bladder. This may be contraindicated, however, depending on the risk of ureteral reflux.
- Explain that occasionally these patients may be able to empty their bladders manually well enough to avoid catheterization. Need for catheterization can be determined by checking residual urine volume.
- Teach patient bladder-emptying techniques, such as straining or Valsalva's maneuver, to increase intraabdominal pressure. If Credé's method is prescribed, teach patient the following technique: place the ulnar surface of the hand horizontally along the umbilicus; while bearing down with the abdominal muscles, press the hand downward and toward the bladder in a kneading motion until urination is initiated; continue 30 sec or until urination ceases. For both these techniques, wait a few minutes and repeat the procedure to ensure complete emptying of the bladder. Use of Credé's method is controversial because of the potential for reflux past the vesicoureteral junction, thus increasing the potential for ascending UTIs.
- If the patient's bladder cannot be trained to empty completely, intermittent catheterization or external collection devices usually are indicated, and the patient may be a candidate for an artificial inflatable sphincter device or urinary diversion.

> See Also: "Urinary Incontinence," p. 177; "Urinary Retention," p. 185; "Neurogenic Bladder," p. 188.

NIC: Perineal Care; Self-Care Assistance: Toileting; Skin Surveillance; Urinary Bladder Training; Urinary Catheterization: Intermittent; Urinary Elimination Management; Urinary Incontinence Care; Urinary Retention Care

Altered cardiopulmonary and cerebral tissue perfusion related to relative hypovolemia secondary to decreased vasomotor tone with SCI
Desired outcomes: By at least 24 hr before hospital discharge (or as soon as vasomotor tone improves), patient has adequate cardiopulmonary and cerebral tissue perfusion as evidenced by systolic BP ≥90 mm Hg and orientation to person, place, and time. For a minimum of 48 hr before hospital discharge, patient is free of dysrhythmias.
- Monitor patient for hypotension (drop in systolic BP >20 mm Hg, systolic BP <90 mm Hg), lightheadedness, dizziness, fainting, and confusion.
- Monitor HR and rhythm. Sinus tachycardia/bradycardia may develop because of impaired sympathetic innervation or unopposed vagal stimulation. Document dysrhythmias.
- Monitor I&O. Give prescribed IV fluids cautiously because impaired vascular tone can make the patient sensitive to small increases in circulating volume. Intravascular volume expanders or vasopressors may be required for hypotension.

- Implement measures that prevent episodes of decreased cardiac output caused by postural hypotension:
  —Change position slowly.
  —Perform ROM exercises q2hr to prevent venous pooling.
  —Prevent patient's legs from crossing, especially when in a dependent position.
  —Patients with SCI at higher levels, especially above T6, may require abdominal binder in addition to antiembolic hose and sequential compression devices or pneumatic foot pumps because these individuals are prone to more severe hypotensive reactions, even with minor changes, such as raising the HOB.
  —Work with the physical therapist (PT) to implement a gradual sitting program that will help patient progress from a supine to an upright position. The goal is to increase the patient's ability to sit upright while avoiding adverse effects, such as hypertension, dizziness, and fainting. This may include a bed that can rotate gradually from a horizontal position to a vertical position or a chair that has multiple positions progressing from flat to sitting.
- For additional information, see **Decreased adaptive capacity:** Intracranial in Appendix One, "Caring for Patients on Prolonged Bedrest," p. 738.

◎ NIC: Cerebral Perfusion Promotion; Hemodynamic Regulation; Neurologic Monitoring; Surveillance; Vital Signs Monitoring

Altered peripheral and cardiopulmonary tissue perfusion related to interrupted blood flow (venous stasis) with corresponding risk of thrombophlebitis and pulmonary emboli (PE) secondary to immobility and decreased vasomotor tone

Desired outcome: For at least 24 hr before hospital discharge and on an ongoing basis, patient has adequate peripheral and cardiopulmonary tissue perfusion as evidenced by absence of heat, erythema, and swelling in calves and thighs; HR ≤100 bpm, RR ≤20 breaths/min with normal depth and pattern (eupnea), and Pao_2 ≥80 mm Hg or O_2 saturation ≥92%.

- Monitor for indicators of thrombophlebitis: erythema, warmth, decreased pulses, and swelling over the area of inflammation and venous dilation; coolness, paleness, and edema distal to the thrombus. Measure calves and thighs daily while the patient is supine or before activity, and monitor for increased circumference. An increase of ≥2 cm in 1 day is significant. The presence of pain or tenderness depends on the level of SCI. Low-grade fever may also signal thrombophlebitis. Notify health care provider about significant findings.
- Protect patient's legs from injury during transfers and turning. Avoid IM injections in the legs, and do not massage them.
- Provide ROM to legs qid. If not contraindicated, place patient in Trendelenburg position for 15 min q2hr to promote venous drainage or elevate the legs 10-15 degrees.
- Monitor for indicators of PE: tachycardia, SOB, hemoptysis, decrease in Pao_2, O_2 saturation <92%, and decreased or adventitious breath sounds. Presence of pain depends on the level of injury. Sudden shoulder pain may represent referred pain from PE. Notify health care provider about significant findings.
- Consult health care provider about use of antiembolism hose, sequential compression devices, pneumatic foot pumps, or prophylactic pharmacotherapy (e.g., ASA, warfarin, low-molecular-weight or low-dose heparin).
- For other interventions, see **Altered peripheral tissue perfusion** in Appendix One, "Caring for Patients on Prolonged Bedrest," p. 742.

NIC: Circulatory Care; Embolus Precautions; Positioning; Respiratory Monitoring; Surveillance; Vital Signs Monitoring

Sexual dysfunction related to altered body function secondary to SCI
Desired outcome: Within the 24-hr period before hospital discharge, patient discusses concerns about sexuality and verbalizes knowledge of alternative methods of sexual expression.

- Evaluate your own feelings about sexuality. Refer patient to someone (e.g., knowledgeable staff member, professional sexual therapy counselor) who can address patient's sexual concerns if you are uncomfortable discussing these issues with the patient.
- Provide a supportive environment that gives the patient permission to have and express sexual concerns. Sexuality can be discussed as it relates to an erection that occurs during a bath or to objective findings noted during a physical assessment. Elicit patient's knowledge, concerns, and questions. Expect acting-out behavior related to the patient's sexuality. This is a normal response to the patient's anxiety about his or her sexual response and prognosis.
- Provide limited information about normal sexual response and changes caused by SCI. Sexual functioning may be different but still possible with SCI. The general rule for men is the higher the lesion, the greater the chance of retaining the ability to have an erection but with less chance to ejaculate. Women may have problems with lubrication, and orgasm may be difficult to achieve because of decreased sensation. Women may also have a transient loss of ovulation. Ovulation usually returns, and women can become pregnant and deliver vaginally. Uterine contractions of labor in women with an SCI lesion at T8 or above, however, may cause AD. Provide information about birth control and oral contraception for women who desire it. Oral contraceptives may be contraindicated because of the risk of thrombophlebitis.
- Sexual activity may seem impossible to the SCI patient. Specific suggestions that may provide gratification include oral-genital sex, digital stimulation, cuddling, mutual masturbation, anal eroticism, and massage. Erection assistive techniques and devices (e.g., vacuum suction pump, prostaglandin penile injection, penile prosthesis or implant) may aid SCI men to attain erections. Specific suggestions for managing common problems include decreasing fluid intake 2-3 hr before sexual encounter, emptying the bladder and bowels (if necessary) before a sexual encounter, (for men) folding back indwelling catheter along the penis and holding it in place with a condom, (for women) taping the catheter to the abdomen and leaving it in place, taking a warm bath before sexual activity to reduce spasticity, planning sexual activity for a time of day in which both partners are rested, experimenting with a variety of positions, and applying topical anesthetics to areas that are hypersensitive to touch. Explain that water-soluble lubricants are useful, if needed, but that petroleum-based lubricants can cause UTI and should be avoided. Adductor spasms in women may pose a barrier but can be overcome if a rear entry is acceptable. Prolonged foreplay with stroking and light massage may also relax muscles. If AD occurs during sexual activity, suggest the patient consult a health care provider about preventive measures (e.g., taking a ganglionic blocking agent before having sexual intercourse or applying topical anesthetic).
- Nurses may not be able to answer all the patient's concerns and questions. When this occurs, acknowledge patient's concerns and refer to someone with more expertise.
- Suggest that patient's partner be included in discussion about sexual concerns. Explaining the physical condition caused by the SCI and preparing the partner for scars, lack of muscle tone, atrophy, and the presence of a

catheter are important and will provide the partner with an opportunity to discuss sexual concerns as well.

- For additional interventions, see **Altered sexuality pattern** in Appendix One, "Caring for Patients on Prolonged Bedrest," p. 745.

NIC: Active Listening; Family Process Maintenance; Sexual Counseling; Teaching: Sexuality

---

See Also: "Ureteral Calculi," p. 164, for nursing diagnoses for the prevention and treatment of renal or ureteral calculi; "Multiple Sclerosis" for **Knowledge deficit:** Precautions and potential side effects of prescribed medications, p. 208; **Knowledge deficit:** Diskectomy with laminectomy or fusion procedure, p. 252; **Impaired swallowing,** p. 254, for patients undergoing diskectomy with laminectomy or spinal fusion; "General Care of Patients With Neurologic Disorders" for **Risk for trauma** related to unsteady gait, p. 331; **Risk for injury** related to impaired pain, touch, and temperature sensations, p. 332; **Altered nutrition:** Less than body requirements, p. 333; **Risk for fluid volume deficit,** p. 335; **Self-care deficit,** p. 336; **Pain,** p. 343; **Altered body temperature,** p. 346; **Knowledge deficit:** Neurologic diagnostic tests, p. 346; "Peptic Ulcers," p. 409, for related nursing diagnoses and interventions; "Pressure Ulcers," p. 710; Appendix One, "Caring for Patients on Prolonged Bedrest," p. 738, for patients with varying degrees of immobility; Appendix One, "Caring for Preoperative and Postoperative Patients," p. 717, for individuals undergoing surgery; Appendix One, "Caring for Patients With Cancer and Other Life-disrupting Illnesses," p. 791, for psychosocial nursing diagnoses as appropriate.

PATIENT-FAMILY TEACHING AND DISCHARGE PLANNING

When providing patient-family teaching, focus on sensory information; avoid giving excessive information; and initiate a visiting nurse referral for necessary follow-up teaching. Consider including verbal and written information about the following:

- Spinal cord functioning and the effects trauma has on how the body works.
- Referrals to community resources, such as public health nurse, visiting nurses association, community support groups, social workers, psychologic therapy, vocational rehabilitation agency, home health agencies, and extended and skilled care facilities. Additional general information can be obtained by contacting the following organizations:

   National Spinal Cord Injury Association
   8300 Colesville Rd., Suite 551
   Silverspring, MD 20910   (800) 962-9629
   WWW address: *http://www.spinalcord.org/*

   American Paralysis Association
   500 Morris Avenue
   Springfield, NJ 07081   (800) 225-0292
   WWW address: *http://www.apacure.org/*

   Spinal Cord Injury Hotline: (800) 526-3456

- Safety measures relative to decreased sensation, motor deficits, and ortho-static hypotension, and the symptoms, preventive measures, and interventions for AD.
- Use and care of a brace or immobilizer as appropriate.
- What patient can expect if transferred to a rehabilitation center.
- Techniques and devices for performing ADL, including bathing, grooming,

turning, feeding, and other self-care activities to patient's maximum potential. The patient may need a home accessibility evaluation and a driving evaluation and training.

- Indicators of urinary calculi and dietary measures to prevent their formation (see p. 164).
- Indicators of deep vein thrombosis and measures to prevent it (see p. 125).
- For additional information, see teaching and discharge planning interventions (the fourth through tenth entries only) in "Multiple Sclerosis," p. 210, as appropriate.

Head injury

Head injuries (HIs) can cause varying degrees of damage to the skull and brain tissue. Primary injuries occur at the time of impact and include skull fracture, concussion, contusion, scalp laceration, brain tissue laceration, and tear or rupture of cerebral vessels. Problems that arise soon after the primary injury and are the result of that injury include hemorrhage and hematoma formation from the tear or rupture of vessels, ischemia from interrupted blood flow, cerebral swelling and edema, infection, and increased intracranial pressure (IICP) or herniation, any of which can interrupt neuronal function. These secondary injuries or events increase the extent of initial injury and result in poorer recovery and higher risk of death. Cervical neck injuries are commonly associated with HIs. Because of the potential for spinal cord injury, all HI patients should be assumed to have cervical neck injury until it is conclusively ruled out by cervical spine x-ray.

Most HIs result from a direct impact to the head. Depending on the force and angle of impact, the brain may suffer injury directly under the point of impact or in the region opposite the point of impact because of brain rebound action within the skull, or tissue tearing or shearing may occur elsewhere because of the rotational action of the brain within the cranial vault. HIs may be classified by location, severity, extent, or mechanism. Common causes include motor vehicle accidents, falls, and sports-related injuries, such as those occurring in football or boxing. Acts of violence often result in missile or implement HIs, such as gunshot or stab wounds.

ASSESSMENT

The Glasgow Coma Scale (Table 4-2) standardizes observations for objective assessment of a patient's LOC. This or some other objective scale should be used to prevent confusion with terminology and to detect changes or trends quickly in the patient's LOC. LOC is the most sensitive indicator of overall brain function. Consciousness has two components: awareness (occurring in the cerebral cortex) and arousal (occurring in the brain stem). Impaired awareness with intact arousal can result in a "vegetative state."

Concussion: Mild diffuse HI in which there is temporary, reversible neurologic impairment typically involving loss of consciousness and possible amnesia of the event. No damage to brain structure is visible on CT or MRI examination. After the concussion, the patient may have headache, dizziness, nausea, lethargy, and irritability. Although full recovery usually occurs in a few days, a postconcussion syndrome with headaches, dizziness, irritability, emotional lability, lethargy, and decreased judgment, concentration, and memory abilities may continue for several weeks or months.

Diffuse axonal injury (DAI): A diffuse brain injury caused by stretching and tearing of the neuronal projections because of a shearing type of injury. No distinct focal lesion, such as infarction, ischemia, contusion, or intracerebral bleeding, is noted, but the patient has an immediate and prolonged unconsciousness of at least 6-hr duration. CT scan may show small hemorrhagic areas in the corpus callosum, cerebral edema, and small midline ventricles. Brain stem

TABLE 4-2 Glasgow Coma Scale

Parameter	Patient response	Score
Best eye opening response (record "C" if eyes closed because of swelling)	Spontaneously	4
	To speech	3
	To pain	2
	No response	1
Best motor response (record best upper limb response to painful stimuli)	Obeys verbal command	6
	Localizes pain	5
	Flexion—withdrawal	4
	Flexion—abnormal	3
	Extension—abnormal	2
	No response (flaccid)	1
Best verbal response (record "E" if endotracheal tube is in place or "T" if tracheostomy tube is in place)	Conversation—oriented × 3	5
	Conversation—confused	4
	Speech—inappropriate	3
	Sounds—incomprehensible	2
	No response	1

Total score (sum of scores for each of the three groups)	Interpretation
15	Normal
13-15	Minor head injury
9-12	Moderate head injury
3-8	Severe head injury
≤7	Coma
3	Deep coma or brain death

injury may be associated with DAI, resulting in autonomic dysfunction. The injury may be quite mild with full recovery, or in severe cases the individual may be comatose for months, die, or be left in a vegetative state.

Contusion: Bruising of the brain tissue, which produces a longer-lasting neurologic deficit than concussion. The size and severity of bruising vary widely, and the bruise or small, diffuse venous hemorrhage usually is visible on CT scan. Traumatic amnesia often occurs, causing loss of memory not only of the trauma, but also of events occurring before the incident. Loss of consciousness is common, and it is generally more prolonged than that with concussion. Changes in behavior, such as agitation or confusion, can last for several hours to days. Headache, nausea, lethargy, motor paralysis, paresis, and possibly seizures can occur as well. Depending on the extent of damage, there is potential for either full recovery or permanent neurologic deficit, such as seizures, paralysis, paresis, or even coma and death.

Brain laceration: Actual tearing of the cortical surface of the brain, resulting in direct mechanical disruption of neural function, causing focal deficits. Blood vessel tearing causes hemorrhage, resulting in contusion, edema, or hematoma formation. Seizures often occur as well. Brain lacerations usually result from depressed skull fractures, penetrating injuries, missile or implement injuries, or rotational shearing injury within the skull. Shock waves from a bullet's high energy produce additional damage. A knife or other impalement object should be supported and left in the wound to control bleeding until it can be removed during surgery. Contusions and lacerations often are found together. The consequences of a laceration usually are more serious than those with a contusion because of the increased severity of trauma. Assessment findings are similar to those with contusion but generally are more pronounced.

Skull fracture: Can be *closed* (simple, with the skin intact) or *open* (compound), depending on whether the scalp is torn, thereby exposing the skull to the outside environment. Skull fractures are further classified as *linear* (hairline), *comminuted* (fragmented, splintered), or *depressed* (pushed inward toward the brain tissue). A blow forceful enough to break the skull is capable of causing significant brain tissue damage, and therefore close observation is essential. With a penetrating wound or basilar fracture (see below), there is potential for CSF leakage, meningitis, encephalitis, brain abscess, cellulitis, or osteomyelitis.

- *Basilar fractures:* fractures of the base of the skull do not show up easily on skull/cervical x-rays. Indicators include blood from the nose, throat, ears; serous or serosanguineous drainage from the nose (rhinorrhea), throat, ears (otorrhea), eyes; Battle's sign (bruising noted behind the ear); "raccoon's eyes" (bruising around the eyes in the absence of eye injury); and bleeding behind the tympanum (eardrum) noted on otoscopic examination. Glucose in serous drainage signals the presence of CSF. CSF leakage indicates a tear in the dura, making the patient particularly susceptible to meningitis. Basilar fractures may damage the internal carotid artery and the cranial nerves. Hearing loss also may occur.
- *Temporal fractures:* may result in deafness or facial paralysis.
- *Occipital fractures:* may cause visual field and gait disturbances.
- *Sphenoidal fractures:* may disrupt the optic nerve, possibly causing blindness.

Rupture of cerebral blood vessels

- *Epidural (extradural) hematoma or hemorrhage:* usually, bleeding between the dura mater (outer meninges) and skull causes hematoma formation. This creates pressure on the underlying brain and produces a local mass effect, causing IICP and shifting of tissue, which leads to brain stem compression and herniation. Indicators are primarily those of IICP: altered LOC, headache, vomiting, unilateral pupil dilation (on same side as the lesion), and possibly hemiparesis. Although some individuals never regain consciousness, most patients lose consciousness for a short period immediately after injury, regain consciousness, and have a lucid period lasting a few hours or 1-2 days. However, because arterial bleeding causes a rapid rise in ICP, a rapid decrease in LOC often ensues. The bleeding site often is the middle meningeal artery or vein because of temporal bone fracture. These patients are at risk for brain stem herniation. A unilateral dilated fixed pupil is a sign of impending herniation and is a neurosurgical emergency. The patient should not be left alone, because respiratory arrest may occur at any time.
- *Subdural hematoma or hemorrhage:* accumulation of venous blood between the dura mater (outer meninges) and arachnoid membrane (middle meninges) that is not reabsorbed. Hematoma formation creates pressure on the underlying brain and produces a local mass effect, causing IICP and shifting of tissue, leading to brain stem compression and herniation. This type of hematoma is classified as acute, subacute, or chronic depending on how quickly indicators arise. In acute subdural hematomas, indicators appear within 24-48 hr, resulting from focal neurologic deficit (hemiparesis, pupillary dilation) and IICP (decreased LOC, falling Glasgow Coma Scale score, nausea, vomiting, headache). When indicators occur 2-14 days later, the hematoma is considered subacute. When indicators occur ≥ 2 wk later, it is considered chronic. Early indicators can include headache, progressive personality changes, decreased intellectual functioning, and drowsiness. Later indicators may include unilateral weakness or paralysis and loss of consciousness and occasionally seizures. Patients with cerebral atrophy

(e.g., older persons, long-term alcohol users) are more prone to subdural hematoma formation.

- *Intracerebral hemorrhage:* arterial or venous bleeding into the white matter of the brain. Signs of IICP may develop early if the bleeding causes a rapidly expanding space-occupying lesion. If the bleeding is slower, signs of IICP can take 36-72 hr to develop. Indicators depend on location of the hematoma and can include altered LOC, headache, aphasia, hemiparesis, hemiplegia, hemisensory deficits, pupillary changes, and loss of consciousness.
- *Subarachnoid hemorrhage:* bleeding into the subarachnoid space below the arachnoid membrane (middle meninges) and above the pia mater (inner meninges next to brain). The patient often has a severe headache. Other general indicators include vomiting, restlessness, seizures, and loss of consciousness. Signs of meningeal irritation include nuchal rigidity and positive Kernig's and Brudzinski's signs (see p. 218). This patient may be a candidate for a shunt because of hemorrhagic interference with CSF circulation and reabsorption.

Indicators of IICP

- *Early indicators:* alteration in LOC ranging from irritability, restlessness, and confusion to lethargy; possible onset or worsening of headache; beginning pupillary dysfunction, such as sluggishness; visual disturbances, such as diplopia or blurred vision; onset of or increase in sensorimotor changes or deficits, such as weakness; onset or worsening of nausea.
- *Late indicators:* continued deterioration of LOC leading to stupor and coma; projectile vomiting; hemiplegia; posturing; alterations in VS (typically increased systolic BP, widening pulse pressure, decreased pulse rate); respiratory irregularities, such as Cheyne-Stokes breathing; pupillary changes, such as inequality, dilation, and nonreactivity to light; papilledema; and impaired brain stem reflexes (corneal, gag, swallowing).

> **Note:**   The single most important early indicator of IICP is a change in LOC. Late indicators of IICP usually signal impending or occurring brain stem herniation. Signs generally are related to brain stem compression and disruption of cranial nerves and vital centers. Hypotension and tachycardia in the absence of explainable causes, such as hypovolemia, usually are seen as a terminal event in HI. IICP usually peaks around 72 hr after the initial insult and then gradually subsides over 2-3 wk.

Brain herniation: Brain herniation occurs when IICP causes displacement of brain tissue from one cranial compartment to another. See late indicators of IICP, above, for signs of impending or initial herniation. In the presence of actual brain herniation, the patient is in a deep coma, pupils become fixed and dilated bilaterally, posturing may progress to bilateral flaccidity, brainstem reflexes generally are lost, and respirations and VS deteriorate and may cease.

Brain death: Universal criteria for determining brain death are not universally agreed upon. Check state and institutional guidelines. General criteria include absent brain stem reflexes (e.g., apnea, pupils nonreactive to light, no corneal reflex, no oculovestibular reflex to ice water calorics), absent cortical activity (e.g., several flat EEG tracings spaced over time), and coma irreversibility continued over a prescribed period of time (e.g., 24 hr). Brain stem auditory evoked responses and cerebral blood flow studies also may be used to help establish brain death.

DIAGNOSTIC TESTS

Cervical spine and skull x-rays: To locate neck and skull fractures. Because of the close association between head injuries and spinal or vertebral injuries, cervical immobilization is essential until cervical x-rays rule out fracture and potential spinal cord injury (SCI).

CT scan: Used with acute injury to identify type, location, and extent of injury, such as accumulation of blood or a shift of midline structure caused by IICP.

MRI: To identify the type, location, and extent of injury. Although not usually performed in acute, unstable patients, this test is the study of choice for subacute or chronic HI. It is superior to CT scan for detecting isodense chronic subdural hematomas or evaluating contusions and shearing injuries, especially in the brain stem area.

EEG: To reveal abnormal electrical activity indicating neuronal damage caused by ischemia or hemorrhage. EEG may be used to establish brain death in conjunction with other tests and may be done serially to assess development of pathologic waves.

Cerebral blood flow studies (xenon inhalation, transcranial Doppler [TCD]):   To determine focal areas of low blood flow or spasm, possibly indicating ischemic areas, by noninvasively measuring cerebral blood flow velocities.

Positron emission tomography (PET):   To evaluate tissue metabolism of glucose and oxygen.

Single photon emission computed tomography (SPECT):   To determine low cerebral blood flow and areas at risk for ischemic tissue perfusion.

Evoked response potentials: To evaluate the integrity of the brain's anatomic pathways and connections. Stimulation of a sense organ, such as an ear, triggers a discrete electrical response (i.e., evoked potential) along a neurologic pathway to the brain. Measurement of the brain's response to auditory, visual, and/or somatosensory stimulation also aids in predicting neurologic outcome.

Cerebral angiography: To reveal presence of a hematoma and status of blood vessels secondary to rupture or compression. Angiography usually is performed only if CT scan or MRI is unavailable or to evaluate possible carotid or vertebral artery dissection.

Infrared spectroscopy: To continuously and noninvasively assess cerebral O_2 saturation.

> **See Also:**   "General Care of Patients With Neurologic Disorders" for **Knowledge deficit:** Neurologic diagnostic tests, p. 346, for care considerations for patients undergoing CT scan, MRI, EEG, evoked potentials, cerebral angiography, and brain scan.

COLLABORATIVE MANAGEMENT

Maintenance of airway, respirations, and therapeutic O_2 levels: O_2 delivery, airway maintenance, intubation, and ventilation to prevent hypoxia. Hyperventilation may be used to reduce $Paco_2$ levels and promote cerebral vasoconstriction to reduce cerebral perfusion. Hyperventilation, while reducing intracranial cerebral perfusion, produces a varied response and may contribute to cerebral ischemia. The patient will require monitoring in an ICU. Ideally, cerebral blood flow measurements and continuous jugular venous oxygen saturation ($S_{jv}o_2$) monitoring should be considered. Nasal intubation or cricothyroidotomy may be performed to prevent neck hyperextension on patients in whom cervical neck injury has not yet been ruled out.

Monitoring of VS/neurologic status: Baseline assessment is established, and patient is monitored frequently for changes.

Positioning: Bedrest with HOB elevated (or as prescribed) to promote venous drainage and help reduce cerebral congestion and edema. If a subdural drain is placed, the HOB may be flat while the drain is in place and for 24 hr after removal to prevent air being pulled into the subdural space.

Fluids and electrolytes: NPO status for 8-24 hr (or longer if patient is unresponsive). IV fluids are given to maintain normovolemia and balanced electrolyte status. Fluid restrictions are avoided because resulting increased blood viscosity and decreased volume may lead to hypotension, decreasing cerebral perfusion pressure and increasing ischemia. I&O are monitored carefully, and the patient usually has an indwelling catheter. Supplementation of electrolytes is done in response to laboratory results. Hypotonic IV solutions, such as D_5W, are contraindicated because they increase cerebral edema.

Gastrointestinal decompression: Initially the patient may have a gastric tube for gastric decompression to prevent vomiting and aspiration. With basilar skull fractures the tube may be inserted through the mouth to avoid passing the tube via the nose through the fracture area and into the brain.

Nutritional support: Total parenteral nutrition (TPN), intralipids, tube feedings, or progressive diet, depending on patient's LOC, ability to swallow, and GI tract functioning. If aspiration is considered a risk, a barium swallow may be done to evaluate swallowing.

Treatment of secondary complications: Cerebral edema, IICP, syndrome of inappropriate antidiuretic hormone (SIADH), disseminated intravascular coagulation (DIC), adult respiratory distress syndrome (ARDS), diabetes insipidus, infection, and seizures. Hyperglycemia is avoided because it has been associated with less satisfactory neurologic outcomes.

Pharmacotherapy: Narcotics and other medications that alter mentation are generally avoided, with the possible exception of codeine for pain control.

Antiepilepsy drugs (e.g., carbamazepine, phenytoin, fosphenytoin, phenobarbital, diazepam): Prophylaxis for seizures with or following penetrating wounds.

Glucocorticosteroids (e.g., dexamethasone): To decrease cerebral edema. There is some controversy regarding effectiveness of glucocorticoids in reducing cerebral edema.

Osmotic diuretics (e.g., mannitol) and loop diuretics (e.g., furosemide): To decrease cerebral edema.

Antibiotics and tetanus prophylaxis: In the presence of penetrating wounds and basilar fractures.

Antipyretics (e.g., acetaminophen): To reduce fever, so that patient's metabolic needs are not increased.

Analgesics (e.g., acetaminophen, codeine): To decrease pain.

Mild sedatives (e.g., diphenhydramine): To decrease restlessness.

Blood pressure medications (e.g. dopamine, labetalol): To control hypertension and hypotension so that optimal cerebral blood flow is maintained and cerebral edema is reduced. Hypotension is especially not well tolerated by these patients.

Antacids and histamine H_2-receptor blockers (e.g., ranitidine, famotidine): To reduce gastric acidity and prevent gastric ulcer formation.

Stool softeners and laxatives (e.g., docusate sodium, Milk of Magnesia): To prevent constipation and straining at stool, which would increase ICP.

Tranquilizers (e.g., chlorpromazine): To control shivering, which can increase ICP.

Tricyclic antidepressants (e.g., amitriptyline, doxepin, imipramine, desipramine): To increase neurotransmitters in the CSF.

Skeletal muscle relaxants (e.g., atracurium, pancuronium): To decrease the skeletal muscle tension that is seen with abnormal flexion and extension posturing, which can increase ICP. This therapy requires transfer of patient to ICU for intubation and ventilation.

Tromethamine (THAM): IV infusion of this weak base has demonstrated ability to buffer cerebral acidosis and thereby reduce IICP.

Barbiturate coma therapy: To reduce cerebral metabolic rate during uncontrolled intracranial hypertension. This therapy requires transfer of patient to ICU for intubation and ventilation.

Antianxiety agents (haloperidol, lorazepam, midazolam, propofol): To decrease or control agitation.

Exogenous antidiuretic hormone (e.g., vasopressin, desmopressin): To treat diabetes insipidus.

Hypothermia: Hypothalamic dysfunction from swelling or injury may cause hyperthermia. Induced hypothermia via a cooling blanket is a controversial treatment used to obtain a subnormal body temperature and thereby minimize metabolic needs.

Antithrombus therapy (antiembolism hose, sequential compression devices, pneumatic foot pumps): To prevent thrombophlebitis and pulmonary emboli.

Bowel and bladder program: A bowel program is initiated to prevent straining at stool. Initially the patient usually has an indwelling urinary catheter. A bladder training program may be necessary, depending on the presence and type of neurologic deficit.

Physical medicine: Physical therapy, occupational therapy, and assistive devices or braces may be prescribed to promote mobility and independence with ADL, depending on presence and type of neurologic deficit.

Speech therapy: To evaluate and aid communication of aphasic or dysarthric patients.

Seizure precautions: To prevent injury in the event of seizure activity, especially for patients with penetrating head injuries.

Cognitive rehabilitation: To promote the highest level of cognitive functioning (Table 4-3). Start coma stimulation techniques (usually for short periods 2-4 times/day) on appropriate patients to increase the quantity, quality, and duration of responses. Most cognitive recovery occurs in the first 6 mo. Provide referrals, as appropriate, to cognitive retraining specialist.

Surgical procedures

Suturing: To repair superficial lacerations or dural tears.

Craniotomy, craniectomy: To evacuate hematomas, control hemorrhage, remove bone fragment or foreign objects, debride necrotic tissue, or elevate depressed fractures. (See "Brain Tumors," p. 288, for patient care.)

Trephination ("burr" holes): To evacuate hematomas or insert intracranial monitoring devices.

Cranioplasty: To repair traumatic or surgical defects in the skull.

Ventricular puncture, ventriculostomy: To remove excess CSF.

Ventricular shunt: To provide drainage of CSF and reduce ICP. (See "Brain Tumors," p. 288, for patient care.)

Placement of ICP monitoring device: To provide accurate and continual monitoring of patient's ICP. This necessitates transfer of patient to ICU for monitoring.

Repair of CSF leak: Most CSF leaks from dural tears heal themselves in 5-10 days. If they do not, serial lumbar punctures or a lumbar subarachnoid drain may be needed to drain CSF, reduce CSF pressure, and promote healing. Acetazolamide or dexamethasone may be given to decrease CSF production. Radionuclide-labeled materials may be injected into the subarachnoid space and pledgets placed in the nose and ears to find the site of the CSF leak. Surgical repair may be required if other methods prove ineffective. Basilar fractures are a common site of CSF leaks and make surgical repair difficult because of location inaccessibility.

With a lumbar drain the patient is on bedrest with HOB elevated up to 15-20 degrees and instructed not to cough, sneeze, or strain. Maintain HOB and collection container securely at prescribed levels. Maintain a sterile occlusive dressing. Possible complications include meningitis (see p. 217) or a tension pneumothorax (see p. 20) resulting from too rapid drainage of CSF, which causes air to siphon in through the dural tear, creating an intracranial mass effect. If neurologic signs deteriorate, clamp the lumbar drain tubing, place patient flat or in a slight Trendelenburg position, and

TABLE 4-3 Cognitive Rehabilitation Goals

Level	Response	Goal/Intervention
I	None	*Goal:* Provide sensory input to elicit responses of increased quality, frequency, duration, and variety.
II	Generalized	
III	Localized (purposeful)	*Intervention:* Give brief but frequent stimulation sessions and present stimuli in an organized manner, focusing on one sensory channel at a time, for example:
		Visual: Intermittent TV, family pictures, bright objects, mobiles (put object in visual field and move, turn light on/off)
		Auditory: Tape recordings of family or favorite song, talking to patient, intermittent TV or radio (change volume, location)
		Olfactory: Favorite perfume, shaving lotion, coffee, lemon, orange
		Cutaneous: Touch or rub skin with different degrees of pressures and textures, such as velvet, ice bag, warm cloth
		Movement: Turn, ROM exercises, raise/lower HOB, up in chair
		Oral: Oral care, lemon swabs, ice, sugar on tongue, peppermint, chocolate
IV	Confused, agitated	*Goal:* Reduce agitation and increase awareness of environment; this stage usually lasts 2-4 wk.
		Interventions: Remove offending devices (e.g., NG tube, restraints), if possible.
		Do not demand that patient follow through with task. Expect outbursts, acting out, and uninhibited behavior.
		Provide human contact unless this increases agitation.
		Provide a quiet, controlled, simplified environment.
		Use a calm, soft voice and manner around patient.
V	Confused, inappropriate	*Goal:* Reduce confusion and incorporate improved cognitive abilities into functional activity.
VI	Confused, appropriate	*Interventions:* Begin each interaction with introduction, orientation, and interaction purpose.
		List and number daily activities in the sequence in which they will be done throughout the day.
		Give patient plenty of time, and use simple, staged directions.
		Maintain a consistent environment.
		Provide memory aids (e.g., calendar, clock).
		Use gentle repetition, which aids learning.
		Provide supervision and structure.
		Reorient as needed.
VII	Automatic, appropriate	*Goal:* Integrate increased cognitive function into functional community activities with minimal structuring.
VIII	Purposeful	*Interventions:* Enable practicing of activities.
		Reduce supervision and environmental structure.
		Help patient plan adaptation of ADL and home living skills to home environment.
		Encourage completion of tasks.

Modified from Rancho Los Amigos Hospital, Inc, Levels of Cognitive Functioning (scale based on behavioral descriptions or responses to stimuli).
ROM, Range of motion; *HOB,* head of bed; *NG,* nasogastric; *ADL,* activities of daily living.

provide supplemental O_2, which will promote absorption of intracranial air and relieve IICP.

NURSING DIAGNOSES AND INTERVENTIONS

Knowledge deficit: Caretaker's responsibilities for observing the patient who is sent home with a concussion

Desired outcomes: Following instruction, caretaker verbalizes knowledge about the observation regimen. Caretaker returns patient to the hospital if neurologic deficits are noted.

If patient goes home for observation, provide caretaker with the following verbal and written instructions:

- Do not give patient anything stronger than acetaminophen to relieve headache. Aspirin is usually contraindicated because it can prolong bleeding, if it occurs.
- Assess patient at least q1-2hr for the first 24 hr as follows: awaken patient; ask patient's name, location, and caretaker's name; monitor for twitching or seizure activity. Return patient to the hospital immediately if he or she becomes increasingly difficult to awaken; cannot answer questions appropriately; cannot answer at all; becomes confused, restless, or agitated; develops slurred speech; develops twitching or seizures; develops or reports worsening headache or nausea/vomiting; has visual disturbances (e.g., blurred or double vision); develops weakness, numbness, or clumsiness or has difficulty walking; has clear or bloody drainage from the nose or ear; or develops a stiff neck.
- Ensure that patient rests and eats lightly for the first day or so after the concussion or until he or she feels well. Over the next 2-3 days, patient should avoid alcohol, driving, contact sports, swimming, using power tools, and taking medication for headache or nausea without calling the health care provider.
- Inform patient and significant other that some individuals may have a postconcussion syndrome in which they continue to have headaches, dizziness, or lethargy for several weeks or months after a concussion. Patient also may experience sleep disturbance, difficulty concentrating, poor memory, irritability, emotional lability, and difficulty with judgment or abstract thinking. Explain the importance of reporting these problems to the health care provider, especially if they worsen.

◎ **NIC:** Environmental Management: Comfort; Neurologic Monitoring; Surveillance; Teaching: Disease Process; Teaching: Individual

Risk for infection with risk factors related to inadequate primary defenses secondary to basilar skull fractures, penetrating or open head injuries, or surgical wounds

Desired outcomes: Patient is free of symptoms of infection as evidenced by normothermia, stable or improving LOC, and absence of headache, photophobia, or neck stiffness. Patient verbalizes knowledge about the signs and symptoms of infection and the importance of reporting them promptly.

- Monitor injury site or surgical wounds for indicators of infection, such as persistent erythema, local warmth, pain, hardness, and purulent drainage. Notify health care provider of significant findings.
- Be alert to indicators of meningitis or encephalitis (fever, chills, malaise, back stiffness and pain, nuchal rigidity, photophobia, seizures, ataxia, sensorimotor deficits), which can occur after a penetrating, open head injury or cerebral surgical wound.
- When examining scalp lacerations and assessing for foreign bodies or palpable fractures, wear sterile gloves and follow sterile technique. Cleanse the area gently, and cover scalp wounds with sterile dressings.

- Document drainage and its amount, color, and odor. If the patient has clear or bloody drainage from the nose, throat, or ears, notify health care provider of findings and assume that the patient has a dural tear with CSF leakage until proven otherwise. Complaints of a salty taste or frequent swallowing may signal CSF dripping down the back of the throat. Bending forward may produce nasal drainage that can be tested for CSF. Inspect the dressing and pillowcases for the presence of a halo ring, which may indicate CSF drainage. Clear drainage may be tested with a glucose reagent strip. Drainage may also be sent to the laboratory to test for Cl⁻. The presence of glucose and Cl⁻ (CSF Cl⁻ is > serum Cl⁻) in nonsanguineous drainage indicates that the drainage is CSF rather than mucus or saliva.
- If CSF leakage occurs, do not clean the ears or nose unless prescribed by health care provider. Place a sterile pad over the affected ear or under the nose to catch drainage, but do not pack them. Position patient so that fluids can drain. Change dressings when they become damp, using sterile technique.
- Avoid excessive movement. If not contraindicated, place the patient on bedrest with the HOB in semi-Fowler's position.
- With CSF leakage or possible basilar fracture, avoid nasal suction to prevent introduction of bacteria into the nervous system. Instruct the patient to avoid Valsalva's maneuver, straining with a bowel movement, and vigorous coughing, which may tear the dura and increase CSF flow. The patient should also know not to blow the nose, sneeze, or sniff in nasal drainage.
- If the patient is intubated, the tube for gastric decompression may be placed orally rather than nasally. If the nasogastric tube is placed nasally, the health care provider usually performs the intubation. Check placement of the tube, preferably by x-ray, before applying suction. Nasogastric (NG) tubes have been known to enter the fracture site and curl up into the patient's cranial vault during insertion attempts. Visually check the back of the patient's throat for the NG tube to help confirm placement.
- Individuals with basilar skull fractures generally are placed flat in bed on complete bedrest. This position helps decrease pressure and the amount of CSF draining from a dural tear. Patients are given antibiotics to prevent infection and observed for healing and sealing of the dural tear within 7-10 days.
- Teach patient to report any indicators of infection promptly.

NIC: Infection Protection; Positioning: Neurologic; Neurologic Monitoring; Surveillance; Tube Care: Ventriculostomy/Lumbar Drain; Wound Care; Vital Signs Monitoring

Risk for disuse syndrome with risk factors related to prescribed immobility and/or decreased LOC
Desired outcome: Patient exhibits full ROM of all joints.
- For patients at risk of IICP, perform passive ROM exercises rather than allow active or assisted ROM exercises, which can increase intraabdominal or intrathoracic pressure and hence ICP. For the same reason, avoid using the prone position.
- Once the risk of IICP is no longer significant, additional measures to enhance mobility and strength may be implemented. For discussion, see **Risk for activity intolerance,** p. 738, and **Risk for disuse syndrome,** p. 740, in Appendix One, "Caring for Patients on Prolonged Bedrest"
- See Table 4-3 for interventions for patients with varying responses to stimuli.

NIC: Exercise Therapy: Joint Mobility; Positioning: Neurologic; Teaching: Prescribed Activity/Exercise

Pain related to headaches secondary to head injury
Desired outcome: Within 1 hr of intervention, patient's subjective perception of pain decreases, as documented by a pain scale.

- Monitor and document the duration and character of the patient's pain, rating it on a scale of 0 (no pain) to 10 (worst pain).
- Administer analgesics as prescribed. Patients with head injuries generally do not have much pain, and the pain is usually relieved by analgesics, such as acetaminophen. Sometimes codeine is prescribed, but as a rule, other narcotics are contraindicated because they can mask neurologic indicators of IICP and cause respiratory depression.
- For additional interventions, see **Pain,** p. 343, in "General Care of Patients with Neurologic Disorders."

NIC: Analgesic Administration; Medication Management; Neurologic Monitoring; Pain Management; Simple Relaxation Therapy

Fluid volume excess related to compromised regulatory mechanisms with increased ADH and increased renal resorption secondary to SIADH
Desired outcomes: By hospital discharge (or within 3 days of injury), patient is normovolemic as evidenced by stable weight, balanced I&O, urinary output ≥30 ml/hr, urine specific gravity 1.010-1.030, BP within patient's baseline limits, absence of fingerprint edema over the sternum, and orientation to person, place, and time.

- Monitor I&O, daily weight, VS, urine specific gravity, and electrolyte and serum osmolarity studies. Sudden and significant weight gain, urine output <500 ml/24 hr, urine specific gravity >1.030, and hypertension occur with SIADH. SIADH creates a dilutional hyponatremia; therefore also be alert to serum Na^+ levels <137 mEq/L, serum osmolality <280 mOsm/kg, low BUN, and increased urine Na^+ and osmolality. Notify health care provider of significant changes.
- Monitor patient for changes in orientation and LOC (e.g., apprehension, irritability, confusion), incoordination, headache, anorexia, muscle cramps, and fatigue. These are mild symptoms of SIADH. As SIADH progresses, expect nausea, vomiting, and abdominal cramps. Symptoms of severe SIADH include weakness, lethargy, confusion, muscle twitching, and seizures. Expect seizure activity when serum Na^+ level drops below 118 mEq/L. Serum Na^+ level ≤115 mEq/L may result in loss of reflexes, coma, and death. Notify health care provider of significant findings. See "Syndrome of Inappropriate Antidiuretic Hormone," p. 371, for more information.
- Monitor patient for symptoms of IICP, and institute measures for its prevention (see **Decreased adaptive capacity:** Intracranial, p. 340).
- Assess for fingerprint edema over the sternum, which reflects cellular edema. Because fluid is not retained in the interstitium with SIADH, peripheral edema will not necessarily occur.
- Maintain fluid restriction as prescribed. Depending on the serum Na^+ value, fluids may be restricted to an amount as low as 500 ml/24 hr. Remove water or ice chips from the bedside. Hypotonic solutions such as D_5W usually are contraindicated because of their conversion to free H_2O.
- As appropriate, provide measured ice chips and frequent mouth care for thirst.
- Administer hypertonic saline (3%) as prescribed.
- As prescribed, give furosemide (Lasix) to promote diuresis; demeclocycline (Declomycin), which acts as an ADH inhibitor; and lithium, which interferes with the action of aldosterone.
- Ensure that HOB is elevated ≤10-20 degrees to promote venous return and left atrial filling pressure, thereby reducing release of ADH.
- Institute seizure precautions (see "Seizure Disorders," p. 324).

> **Caution:** Credé's method and other measures that can increase intraabdominal and intrathoracic pressure are contraindicated for patients who are at risk of IICP.

◎ NIC: Cerebral Edema Management; Electrolyte Management: Hyponatremia; Fluid/Electrolyte Management; Neurologic Monitoring

See Also: Chapter 3 for related discussions if the patient has urinary incontinence (p. 177), retention (p. 185), or neurogenic bladder (p. 188). See also: "Alzheimer's Disease" for **Impaired environmental interpretation syndrome**, p. 239; **Risk for violence**, p. 243; "Brain Tumors" for **Knowledge deficit:** Ventricular shunt procedure, p. 290; **Knowledge deficit:** Craniotomy procedure, p. 290; "Cerebrovascular Accident" for **Impaired verbal communication**, p. 314; **Impaired physical mobility**, p. 312; **Sensory/perceptual alterations**, p. 312; "Seizure Disorders," p. 324, for seizure-related nursing diagnoses; "General Care of Patients With Neurologic Disorders" for **Risk for trauma**, p. 331; **Risk for injury** related to impaired pain, touch, and temperature sensation, p. 332; **Impaired corneal tissue integrity**, p. 333; **Altered nutrition**, p. 333; **Risk for fluid volume deficit**, p. 335; **Risk for aspiration**, p. 335; **Self-care deficit**, p. 336; **Constipation**, p. 339; **Decreased adaptive capacity:** Intracranial, p. 340; **Sensory/perceptual alterations**, p. 342; **Impaired swallowing**, p. 344; **Altered body temperature**, p. 346; **Knowledge deficit:** Neurologic diagnostic tests, p. 346; nursing diagnoses in "Diabetes Insipidus," p. 362, for patients with diabetes insipidus; "Syndrome of Antidiuretic Hormone," p. 371, for patients with SIADH; Appendix One, "Caring for Preoperative and Postoperative Patients," p. 717, for patients undergoing surgical procedures; "Pressure Ulcers," p. 710; Appendix One, "Caring for Patients on Prolonged Bedrest," p. 738, for patients with varying degrees of immobility; Appendix One, "Caring for Patients With Cancer and Other Life-disrupting Illnesses," p. 791, for appropriate psychosocial nursing diagnoses and interventions.

PATIENT-FAMILY TEACHING AND DISCHARGE PLANNING

The head-injured patient can have varying degrees of neurologic deficit, ranging from mild to severe. When providing patient-family teaching, focus on sensory information; avoid giving excessive information; and initiate a visiting nurse referral for necessary follow-up teaching. Consider including verbal and written information about the following:

- Referrals to community resources, such as cognitive retraining specialist, head injury rehabilitation centers, visiting nurses association, community support groups, social workers, psychologic therapy, vocational rehabilitation agency, home health agencies, and extended and skilled care facilities. Additional general information can be obtained by contacting the following organization:

   Brain Injury Association, Inc.
   1776 Massachusetts Avenue NW, Suite 100
   Washington, DC 20036-1904   (202) 296-6443 or (800) 444-6443
   WWW address: *http://www.biausa.org/*

- Safety measures related to decreased sensation, visual disturbances, motor deficits, and seizure activity.
- Measures that promote communication in the presence of aphasia.
- Wound care and indicators of infection.
- Measures that deal with cognitive or behavioral problems. As appropriate, include home evaluation for safety. Caution significant other that personality can change drastically after HI. The patient may demonstrate inappropriate

social behavior, inappropriate affect, hallucination, delusion, and altered
sleep pattern.
- If patient had a concussion, a description of problems that may occur at home
and necessitate prompt medical attention (see **Knowledge deficit**, p. 281).
- For other information, see teaching and discharge planning interventions (the
fourth through tenth entries only) in "Multiple Sclerosis," p. 210, as
appropriate.

Section Four: Nervous System Tumors

Brain tumors

The abnormal and uncontrolled cell growth of neoplastic or benign tumors can
have a wide variety of effects on the brain. Most significant is the disruption of
neuronal function caused by infiltration of the tissue, compression of brain
tissue and blood vessels, or obstruction of normal flow of CSF. The increase in
ICP from tumor growth and other factors, such as cerebral edema, will cause
brain structures to shift, eventually leading to brain herniation and death.
Primary brain tumors, composed of nervous system tissue, rarely metastasize
outside the CNS. It is not uncommon, however, for primary brain tumors to
metastasize to other parts of the CNS. *Secondary brain tumors* arise from cells
that have metastasized from other parts of the body, such as the lung, breast, and
skin. Although benign tumors tend to be more treatable than neoplastic tumors,
they are considered serious because they are equally capable of destroying
adjacent nerves through compression and increasing ICP, which in turn
compromises vital centers.

Tumor classification: Generally, brain tumors are classified according to
their cell of origin. They may be further classified by cell differentiation (e.g.,
benign, malignant, grades I-IV) and by their location.

- *Gliomas:* comprise 45% of all brain tumors and arise from brain connective
tissue. Generally, they infiltrate surrounding tissues and cannot be removed
totally by surgery. As a group, gliomas usually are considered neoplastic.
  —Astrocytoma: the most common glioma, graded from I-IV, with grade I
  cytologically (but not necessarily biologically) benign and grade IV the
  most malignant. Glioblastoma multiforme is a grade III-IV astrocytoma; it
  is the most common (20% of all brain tumors) and is a highly malignant
  glioma with <20% survival rate at 12 mo. It is usually found in the cerebral
  hemisphere and may metastasize to other parts of the CNS.
  —Oligodendroglioma: the next most common glioma, arising out of cells
  involved in the process of myelination. Generally, they are slow-growing,
  often encapsulated tumors that are cytologically (but not necessarily
  biologically) benign.
  —Medulloblastoma: a relatively rare glioma that is highly malignant; often
  obstructs CSF flow and metastasizes to the spinal cord. It is found
  primarily in children.
  —Ependymoma: glioma that arises out of the cells that line the cavities of
  the CNS, such as the ventricles, and usually obstructs CSF flow. These
  rare tumors are quite invasive and are found primarily in children and
  young adults.
- *Meningiomas:* originate from pia or arachnoid membranes and make up
about 15% of all brain tumors. They are slow growing and, although
technically benign, can invade the skull and cause brain tissue compression. Surgical cures are possible with complete surgical excision of the
tumor.

- *Schwannomas (e.g., acoustic neuroma):* account for about 10% of brain tumors, affect the craniospinal nerve sheath, and are slow growing and commonly encapsulated. Although these tumors are cytologically benign, they may not be diagnosed until they are large in size and compressing sensitive brain stem centers. A surgical cure is possible with complete surgical excision, and early surgical intervention may preserve hearing and facial nerve function.
- *Pituitary tumors:* see "Pituitary and Hypothalamic Tumors," p. 367.
- *Secondary (metastatic) tumors:* most often occur in the cerebrum, may be multiple because of the "seeding" effect, and resemble the primary neoplasm histologically. Lung and breast carcinomas are the lesions that most frequently result in metastases to the brain.

ASSESSMENT

Onset of signs and symptoms usually is insidious and progressive, although seizure activity may be the first sign in 15% of cases.

General indicators: Headache (especially in the morning), nausea, projectile vomiting, lethargy, forgetfulness, disorientation, personality changes, and seizure activity.

Focal symptoms

- *Frontal lobe:* personality/mood changes, impaired judgment, weakness or paralysis (usually unilateral), apraxia, aphasia.
- *Parietal lobe:* visual field deficit, sensory disturbance, impaired position sense, perceptual problems, such as altered stereognosis and dyslexia.
- *Temporal lobe:* auditory changes, tinnitus, visual field deficit, sensory aphasia, impaired memory, personality changes, psychomotor seizures.
- *Occipital lobe:* seizures, visual agnosia (loss), visual field deficit.
- *Cerebellar:* tremors, nystagmus, incoordination, loss of balance, gait disturbances, nuchal headache.
- *Ventricular or hypothalamic:* diabetes insipidus, weight gain, somnolence, headache, disturbance of temperature regulation.
- *Cranial nerve:* sense of smell alterations, ptosis, diplopia, alterations in ocular movement, drooping of facial muscles on the same side as the tumor, difficulty swallowing, loss of cough/gag reflex, loss of corneal reflex, protrusion of the tongue toward the side of the tumor.
- *Schwannoma:* unilateral hearing loss with or without tinnitus, stiff neck. Other symptoms may include decreased facial sensation, facial muscle weakness or paralysis on same side as the hearing loss, and diplopia. Late symptoms include ataxia and arm coordination problems secondary to brain stem and cerebellar compression.

Indicators of IICP: See discussion in "Head Injury," p. 276.

Indicators of brain stem herniation: See discussion in "Head Injury," p. 276.

Physical assessment: Ophthalmoscopic examination may reveal papilledema if ICP is increased; visual field examination may reveal impairment such as hemianopia (blindness in part of the field of vision); and audiometry or vestibular function studies may show abnormalities such as hearing loss, especially with acoustic neuromas.

DIAGNOSTIC TESTS

Diagnostic tests are done to rule out vascular causes, such as hemorrhage, abscess, and trauma, as well as to diagnose brain tumor. Any one or a combination of the following tests may be performed.

MRI: May reveal presence of tumor, tissue shift, and hydrocephalus. This diagnostic tool, because of its ability to detect biochemical changes, can help diagnose tumors at an early stage. It is the imaging procedure of choice to visualize brain stem and posterior fossa structures.

CT scan: May detect tumor mass, tissue shift, and hydrocephalus. Serial screens may be done to track the tumor's response to therapy.

X-rays of the skull and spinal cord: May reveal tumors that contain calcium or cause bony erosion.

Positron emission tomography (PET):   May distinguish tumor tissue from normal brain tissue by identifying abnormal metabolic activity of the tumor tissue.

EEG: May localize abnormal brain wave activity, which may suggest tumor growth.

Brain scan: May demonstrate presence of a space-occupying lesion via uptake of radioisotope. This test is helpful in localizing certain tumors, such as meningiomas.

Cerebral angiography: May show abnormal perfusion patterns, which suggest tumor location; also may reveal alterations in the position of vessels caused by the tumor and may even outline the tumor via its circulation. The test may be performed preoperatively to plan surgical strategy.

Lumbar puncture (LP) and CSF analysis: May be performed in the absence of any indicators of IICP. CSF may be clear to bloody; protein values and WBC count may be increased; glucose values may be decreased; and cytology may reveal the presence of cancer cells. This test usually is done when there is concern about the possibility of an infectious process.

Lesion biopsy: Identifies pathologic cells and confirms diagnosis. Clonogenic assay may be done on tumor tissues grown in cultures to select the most appropriate cytotoxic agent.

Endocrine studies: May show abnormal hormonal levels that may signal a pituitary tumor. See "Pituitary and Hypothalamic Tumors," p. 366.

Evoked potentials: May show reduced brain stem auditory evoked response as a result of acoustic neuromas.

Stapedius reflex study: Measures the contraction of the stapedius muscle with high-intensity sound. The muscle should stay contracted as long as sound is present. With acoustic neuroma, the muscle initially may contract but then relax.

Electronystagmography: May show a reduced caloric response caused by acoustic neuroma.

Tumor markers: Measures presence of substances that are unique or very specific to a class of tumor. This test will aid in the diagnosis of the tumor type and measure response to therapy.

Other studies (e.g., chest x-rays):   Determine primary site(s) of metastatic brain tumors.

> **See Also:**   "General Care of Patients With Neurologic Disorders" for **Knowledge deficit:** Neurologic diagnostic tests, p. 346, for care considerations for patients undergoing MRI, CT scan, PET, EEG, brain scan, cerebral angiography, LP, and evoked potentials.

COLLABORATIVE MANAGEMENT

The mode of treatment depends on the tumor's histologic type, anatomic location, and sensitivity to radiation. Treatment usually includes surgery, often in combination with radiation or chemotherapy. Immune therapy also is being evaluated as a treatment modality. The location and accessibility of the tumor determine whether surgery can be performed. Tumors of the brain stem, medulla, pons, and corpus callosum tend to be inaccessible. Partial surgical resection may be done to debulk the tumor, decompress the brain, and relieve pressure-related symptoms temporarily.

Craniotomy/craniectomy: A surgical opening is made into the skull. The bone flap may be left open postoperatively to accommodate cerebral edema and prevent compression.

Surgical techniques: Laser neurosurgery has proven useful in certain types of tumor removal, such as meningiomas. *Laser neurosurgery* tends to be more precise than conventional dissection, resulting in less tissue damage and less postoperative swelling. Drugs such as hematoporphyrin may be given to photosensitize tumor cells selectively to increase their precise destruction. *Stereotactic neurosurgery* techniques using the CT scan and computer processing of stereoactive data allow the precise guidance of a surgical probe to the tumor for biopsy, ablative procedures, or radiation implants. Some deep tumors now can be removed or debulked without extensive damage to surrounding brain tissue. Sometimes ultrasound can be used during surgery to locate the tumor diagnostically and then remove the tumor layer by layer by fragmenting the tissue with an ultrasonic vibrating tip. Microsurgical techniques and intraoperative monitoring of the facial and cochlear nerves have improved outcomes with resection of acoustic neuromas.

Transsphenoidal hypophysectomy: Transsphenoidal hypophysectomy is used for pituitary tumors (see "Pituitary and Hypothalamic Tumors," p. 366).

Ventricular shunt for ventricular drainage: A ventricular shunt may be inserted to allow drainage of CSF. This procedure is usually performed if the brain tumor is inoperable and obstructs the flow of CSF, causing IICP. The shunt mechanically may carry CSF from the ventricles to another body part, such as the left atrium of the heart or peritoneal cavity. A surgical procedure called a *third ventriculostomy* produces an exit for ventricular fluid without tubes or synthetic materials by using a probe to create another drainage canal in the brain.

Supportive pharmacotherapy

Antiepilepsy agents (e.g., carbamazepine, phenytoin, fosphenytoin, phenobarbital, diazepam): Prophylaxis for seizures.

Osmotic diuretics (e.g., mannitol) and loop diuretics (e.g., furosemide): To decrease cerebral edema and IICP.

Glucocorticosteroids (e.g., dexamethasone): To help reduce tumor-associated cerebral edema. May be used after radiotherapy to decrease radiation-induced edema.

Antacids and histamine H_2-receptor blockers (e.g., ranitidine): To prevent/treat stress ulcers by reducing gastric acidity.

Analgesics (e.g., acetaminophen, codeine): To treat headaches.

Antipyretics (e.g., acetaminophen): To reduce fever so that cerebral metabolic needs are not increased.

Stool softeners and laxatives (e.g., docusate): To prevent constipation and straining at stool, which would increase ICP.

Radiation therapy: To destroy remaining tumor cells or treat inaccessible tumors. External beam radiation is frequently begun as soon as the surgical incision has healed. It can be localized or include the entire brain and part of the spinal cord, depending on the type, location, and extent of the tumor. Hyperfractionation radiation therapy (e.g., 2-3 treatments per day with 4-hr intervals between treatments) has increased "cell kill" while conserving normal tissue.

Radiation can cause inflammation of the brain, which in turn increases ICP and neurologic symptoms. A cerebral radiation necrosis with symptoms similar to tumor recurrence may occur 6-36 mo after treatment. MRI, CT scan, or PET will distinguish radiation necrosis from tumor recurrence. Treatment is surgical removal of the necrotic mass and high-dose steroids.

With inoperable tumors, radiation therapy often becomes the primary modality. Proton beam irradiation seems effective against certain tumor types. Stereotactic radiotherapy with a gamma knife is believed to be capable of destroying deep and inaccessible lesions in a single treatment. Multiple beams are focused at the tumor with such precision that surrounding tissue is spared. This irradiation is very useful with acoustic neuromas. Maximal shrinkage of tumors may take 1-4 yr. Other techniques include the placement of radionuclide seeds into the tumors of patients with recurrent malignant gliomas. Placement of the seeds requires either a stereotactic procedure or a craniotomy. Techniques being used to increase tumor cell sensitivity to radiation include localized tumor tissue heating (with an implanted microwave probe or electrode) and hyperbaric O_2 therapy. For more information about radiation therapy, see Appendix One, "Caring for Patients with Cancer and Other Life-disrupting Illnesses," p. 771.

Chemotherapy: Nitrosourea agents, such as carmustine (BCNU), lomustine (CCNU), and methyl-CCNU, cross the blood-brain barrier and because of this are useful for patients with brain tumors. Other drugs used include cisplatin, methotrexate, 5-fluorouracil, procarbazine, and etoposide. Generally, chemotherapy is used only as an adjunct to surgery and radiation therapy. Chemotherapy on some tumors is used only after tumor regrowth or when the tumor is not sensitive to radiation therapy. Implantation of biodegradable wafers allows release of chemotherapy in the area of the tumor over a period of several weeks. Intraarterial (carotid), intrathecal, and intraventricular (Ommaya reservoir) delivery of chemotherapeutic agents such as methotrexate to the brain is being investigated in the hope of getting higher drug doses to the tumor while limiting the degree of systemic side effects. Bone marrow sometimes is harvested and then returned to the patient to protect against bone marrow suppression. Immune therapy using biologic response modifiers (BRMs), such as interferons, interleukins, *Corynebacterium parvum,* tumor necrosis factor, and ImuVert, strives to act on the host immune system to improve antitumor response or increase antitumor defenses. See Appendix One, "Caring for Patients With Cancer and Other Life-disrupting Illnesses," p. 749, for more information about chemotherapy and immunotherapy.

Conductive hyperthermia: This investigational technique to destroy brain tumors is based on the fact that the cancer cell is heat sensitive and may be damaged by temperatures that do not harm normal cells. Hyperthermia catheters are inserted into the entire tumor mass using a stereotactic CT-guided technique. The tumor is then heated for a period of 3-4 days. Activity is restricted during this time, and the patient may have a headache. The catheters are removed before hospital discharge. The patient usually has three hyperthermia cycles at 6- to 8-wk intervals.

Investigational therapies: Investigational therapies include monoclonal antibody injections, antiangiogenesis drugs to reduce blood supply to the tumor, autologous lymphocytes, active immunization with irradiated autologous tumor cells, and genetically engineered viruses to control tumor cells.

Depending on the presence and severity of neurologic deficits, the patient also may need the following:

Respiratory support and intubation: To maintain the airway and supply O_2 as needed.

Fluid and nutritional support: The patient may require high-calorie, high-protein supplements and enteral feedings or parenteral nutrition because of swallowing/chewing deficits or side effects of radiation and chemotherapy and IV fluids to prevent dehydration. See "Providing Nutritional Therapy," p. 687, for more information.

Physical medicine: Physical therapy (PT), occupational therapy (OT), and assistive devices or braces help the patient maintain mobility and independence with ADL. Muscle-strengthening exercises, conditioning exercises, and gait training are also frequently prescribed.

ROM exercises: To maintain or increase joint function and prevent contractures. While the patient is at risk of IICP, the exercises are passive only. Once the risk of IICP is minimized, active or active-assistive ROM is employed.

Bowel and bladder program: To prevent incontinence and constipation.

Treatment of secondary complications: Complications include cerebral edema, IICP, SIADH, and diabetes insipidus.

NURSING DIAGNOSES AND INTERVENTIONS

Knowledge deficit: Ventricular shunt procedure

Desired outcome: Following the explanation, patient verbalizes accurate information about the ventricular shunt procedure, including presurgical and postsurgical care.

- Determine patient's understanding of the procedure after health care provider's explanation, including purpose, risks, and anticipated benefits or outcome. Intervene accordingly.
- Explain that the procedure is performed to enable drainage of CSF when flow is obstructed (e.g., because of the presence of a tumor or blood). Shunt types vary but can extend from the lateral ventricle of the brain to one of the following: subarachnoid space of the spinal canal, right atrium of the heart, a large vein, or the peritoneal cavity. The patient may have a cranial dressing as well as a dressing on the neck, chest, or abdomen.
- Explain that it is important to avoid lying on the insertion site after the procedure to prevent putting pressure on the shunt mechanism. The head and neck are kept in alignment to prevent kinking and compression of the shunt catheter. Explain that the shunt site will be monitored for redness, tenderness, bulging, or fluid collection, and swelling will be assessed along the shunt's course.
- If the shunt has a valve for controlling CSF drainage or reflux, explain that the valve will be pumped or compressed a certain number of times at prescribed intervals to flush the system of exudate and prevent plugging. Explain that the valve, which is usually located behind or above the ear and is the approximate diameter of a pencil, can be felt to empty and then refill. Malfunction may be noted by either deterioration in neurologic status or failure of the reservoir to refill when pumped.
- Reassure patient and significant other that before hospital discharge, specific instructions will be given about shunt care, recognition of shunt site infection and malfunction, and steps to take should they occur. Other complications that may occur include movement of the cannula (resulting in inadequate drainage of ventricles) or subdural hematoma formation. Teach signs and symptoms of IICP (i.e., headache, change in LOC such as drowsiness, lethargy, irritability, nausea, personality changes) that should be reported to the health care provider. For ventriculoatrial shunts, emboli or endocarditis may occur. For ventriculoperitoneal shunts, ascites or ruptured viscus may occur.
- For additional interventions, see **Risk for infection,** p. 281, in "Head Injury" and **Knowledge deficit:** Surgical procedure, p. 717, in Appendix One, "Caring for Preoperative and Postoperative Patients."

NIC: Cerebral Edema Management; Neurologic Monitoring; Teaching: Individual; Teaching: Preoperative; Teaching: Procedure/Treatment

Knowledge deficit: Craniotomy procedure

Desired outcome: Following the explanation, patient verbalizes accurate understanding of the craniotomy procedure, including presurgical and postsurgical care.

- After health care provider's explanation of the procedure, determine patient's level of understanding of the purpose, risks, and anticipated benefits or outcome. Intervene accordingly, or reinforce health care provider's explanation as appropriate.
- Explain that a craniotomy is a surgical opening into the skull to remove a hematoma or tumor, repair a ruptured aneurysm, or apply arterial clips or wrap the involved vessel to prevent future rupture. As appropriate, explain

that the bone flap may be left open postoperatively to accommodate cerebral edema and prevent compression. When the bone is removed, the procedure is called a craniectomy.

- Explain that before surgery, antiseptic shampoos may be given and the patient may be started on corticosteroids, such as dexamethasone, and antiepilepsy drugs. Explain that a baseline neurologic assessment will provide a basis for comparison with postoperative neurologic checks.
- During the immediate postoperative period, the patient is in the ICU. Explain the following considerations and interventions that are likely to occur.
  —Assessment of VS and neurologic status at least hourly. Patient will be asked to perform a variety of assessment measures, including squeezing tester's hand, moving extremities, extending the tongue, and answering questions. Emphasize the importance of performing these tasks to the best of the patient's ability.
  —Changes in body image that can occur because of loss of hair, presence of a head dressing, and the potential for and expected duration of facial edema.
  —Possible need for respiratory and airway support, including O_2, intubation, or ventilation. Typically patients are on a cardiac monitor for 24-48 hr because dysrhythmias are not unusual after posterior fossa surgery or when blood is in the CSF.
  —Presence of large head dressing and drains, which will be inspected periodically for bleeding or CSF leakage, which will be reported to the health care provider. Stress the importance of not pulling or tugging on the dressing or drains.
  —NPO status for the first 24-48 hr because of the risk of vomiting and choking. Explain that once fluids are allowed, they may be limited to minimize cerebral edema. The patient may experience a dry throat at this time.
  —Periorbital swelling, which usually occurs within 24-48 hr of supratentorial surgery. Explain that relief is obtained with applications of cold or warm compresses around the eyes. Having the HOB up with the patient lying on the nonoperative side also may help reduce edema.
  —Insertion of indwelling urinary catheter to enable accurate measurement of I&O and monitor for problems such as diabetes insipidus.
  —Measurement of core temperature (e.g., rectal, tympanic, bladder) at frequent intervals. A rectal probe or bladder catheter temperature probe may be used for continuous monitoring. Oral temperatures are avoided during the period while cognitive function is decreased.
- Teach patient that postsurgical positioning is a key factor during recovery.
  —*Supratentorial craniotomy:* patient maintained with HOB elevated to 30 degrees or as prescribed. The patient will be assisted with turning and usually will be kept off the operative site, especially if the lesion was large. The head and neck will be kept in good alignment.
  —*Infratentorial craniotomy* (for cerebellar or brain stem surgery): HOB is kept flat or as prescribed. Sitting may increase the risk of venous air embolus with posterior fossa surgery. Pressure usually is kept off the operative site, especially with a craniectomy, so these patients are kept off their backs for 48 hr. In posterior fossa surgery, the supporting neck muscles are altered. Log-roll patient to alternate sides, keeping the head in good alignment. A soft cervical collar may be used to prevent anterior or lateral angulation of the neck. A small pillow may be used for comfort.
- Explain that bedrest will be enforced immediately after surgery.
- Teach patients undergoing infratentorial surgery that they are likely to experience the following:
  —Dizziness and hypotension, necessitating a longer period of bedrest.
  —Nausea, which should be reported so that antiemetics (e.g., metochlorpramide, trimethobenzamide) can be given.

—Cranial nerve edema, which may result in swallowing difficulties, extraocular movements, or nystagmus, any of which should be reported promptly.
- Teach patient the following precautions that are taken to prevent increased intraabdominal and intrathoracic pressure, which can cause IICP:
  —Exhaling when being turned.
  —Not straining at stool.
  —Not moving self in bed, but rather letting staff members do all moving.
  —Importance of deep breathing and avoiding coughing and sneezing. If coughing and sneezing are unavoidable, they must be done with an opened mouth to minimize pressure buildup.
  —Avoiding hip flexion and lying prone.
- For additional precautions against IICP, see **Decreased adaptive capacity:** Intracranial, p. 340.
- Teach patient that precautions are taken for seizures (see **Risk for trauma** related to oral, musculoskeletal, and airway vulnerability secondary to seizure activity, p. 324).
- Teach patient wound care and indicators of infection. Generally, a surgical cap is worn after removal of the head dressing. The patient must avoid scratching the wound, staples, or sutures and must keep the incision dry. When the sutures or staples are removed, the hair can be shampooed, being careful not to scrub around the incision line. Hair dryers are avoided until the hair is regrown. For more information, see **Risk for infection,** p. 281, in "Head Injury."
- Explain that patients undergoing acoustic neuroma excision may have nausea, hearing loss, facial weakness or paralysis, diminished or absent blinking, eye dryness, tinnitus, vertigo, headache, and occasionally swallowing, throat, taste, or voice problems. Nausea and dizziness may be profound problems after surgery. Provide prescribed antiemetics, and turn and move the patient slowly. Speak to the patient on unaffected side for best hearing, and place phone and call light on that side of the bed. Contralateral routing of signal hearing aids may improve hearing by directing the sound from the deaf ear to the hearing ear via a tiny microphone and transmitter. Background music or other white noise may mask tinnitus. Awareness of tinnitus eventually should lessen. Balance exercises and walking with assistance will start the process of compensation by the functioning vestibular system. Because of vertigo, watching television or reading may be difficult; suggest books on tape, listening to the radio, or music as alternatives. Eye dryness, from impaired eyelid function, may require use of eye drops or ointment.
- For additional interventions, see **Knowledge deficit:** Surgical procedure, p. 290, and Appendix One, "Caring for Preoperative and Postoperative Patients."

NIC: Cerebral Edema Management; Cerebral Perfusion Promotion; Intracranial Pressure (ICP) Monitoring; Neurologic Monitoring; Positioning: Neurologic; Teaching: Preoperative; Teaching: Procedure/Treatment

See Also: Related discussions in Chapter 3 if patient has urinary incontinence (p. 177), retention (p. 185), or neurogenic bladder (p. 188); "Alzheimer's Disease" for **Impaired environmental interpretation syndrome,** p. 239; **Risk for violence,** p. 243; "Head Injury" for **Risk for disuse syndrome,** p. 282; **Fluid volume excess,** p. 283, if the patient has SIADH; "Cerebrovascular Accient" for **Impaired verbal communication,** p. 314; **Impaired physical mobility,** p. 312; **Sensory/perceptual alterations,** p. 312; "Seizure Disorders," p. 324, for nursing diagnoses related to seizures; "General Care of Patients With Neurologic Disorders," p. 331, for related diagnoses; related nursing diagnoses in "Diabetes

Insipidus," p. 366, if patient has diabetes insipidus; related nursing diagnoses in "Syndrome of Inappropriate Antidiuretic Hormone," p. 372, if patient has SIADH; related nursing diagnoses in "Pituitary and Hypothalamic Tumors," p. 369, if patient has a pituitary tumor; related nursing diagnoses in "Pressure Ulcers," p. 710, for patients with varying degrees of immobility; Appendix One, "Caring for Patients on Prolonged Bedrest," p. 738; Appendix One, "Caring for Preoperative and Postoperative Patients," p. 717; Appendix One, "Caring for Patients With Cancer and Other Life-disrupting Illnesses," p. 747.

PATIENT-FAMILY TEACHING AND DISCHARGE PLANNING

When providing patient-family teaching, focus on sensory information; avoid giving excessive information; and initiate a visiting nurse referral for necessary follow-up teaching. Consider including verbal and written information about the following:

- Safety measures specific to sensory deficits, motor deficits, incoordination, cognitive deficits, and seizures.
- Measures to promote communication in the presence of aphasia.
- Appropriate referrals to community resources, such as public health nurse, visiting nurses association, community support groups, social workers, psychologic therapy, vocational rehabilitation agency, home health agencies, and extended and skilled care facilities. Additional general information can be obtained by contacting the following organizations:

  American Cancer Society
  1599 Clifton Road NE
  Atlanta, GA 30329   (800) ACS-2345
  WWW address: *http://www.cancer.org/*

  National Cancer Institute Information Service (CIS)
  Bldg. 31, Room 10A16
  9000 Rockville Pike
  Bethesda, MD 20892   (800) 422-6237
  WWW address: *http://wwwicic.nic.nih.gov/*

  American Brain Tumor Association (ABTA)
  2720 River Road, Suite 146
  Des Plaines, IL 60018   (800) 886-2282
  WWW address: *http://www.abta.org/*

  National Brain Tumor Foundation
  785 Market St.
  Suite 1600
  San Francisco, CA 94103   (800) 934-CURE; (415) 284-0209 FAX
  WWW address: *http://www.braintumor.org/*

- Provide the following address for patients with acoustic neuroma:

  Acoustic Neuroma Association
  P.O. Box 12402
  Atlanta, GA 30355   (404) 237-8023
  WWW address: *http://neurosurgery.mgh.harvard.edu/ana/*

- Care of postoperative or postprocedure wounds and indicators of infection.
- Potential side effects and precautions for patients undergoing radiation therapy.
- Medications, including drug name, purpose, dosage, frequency, precautions, drug/drug and food/drug interactions, and potential side effects, especially for chemotherapeutic agents.

- Exercises that promote muscle strength and mobility, measures for preventing contractures and skin breakdown, transfer techniques and proper body mechanics, use of assistive devices, and other measures that promote independence with ADL.
- Measures for relieving pain, nausea, or other discomfort.
- Indications of constipation, urinary retention, or urinary tract infection; implementation of bowel and bladder training programs; and if appropriate, care of indwelling catheters.
- Indications of upper respiratory infections and measures to prevent regurgitation, aspiration, and respiratory infection.
- Importance of follow-up care, including visits to health care provider, PT, OT, speech therapy, psychologic counseling, and laboratory monitoring for side effects of radiation/chemotherapy.
- First aid measures for seizures.
- Causes of IICP and measures to prevent it.
- Care of ventricular shunt if present. Include specific instructions for shunt care and information about how to identify shunt infection or malfunction and steps to take if they occur.
- Measures that assist with reorientation, dealing with behavioral or cognitive problems, and communicating with patient in view of cognitive deficits.
- Referral to hospice or agency that provides home help. This should occur before discharge planning begins to ensure continuity of care between the hospital and home or hospice.
- Phone numbers to call should questions or concerns arise about hospice after discharge. Information for these patients can be obtained by contacting the following organization:

National Hospice Association
1901 North Moore St., Suite 901
Arlington, VA 22209   (703) 243-5900; (703) 525-5762 FAX
WWW address: *http://www.nho.org*

Spinal cord tumors

The majority of spinal cord tumors interrupt neuronal function and nerve impulse transmission by compressing the spinal cord, its roots, or its blood supply and eventually cause cord degeneration. Spinal cord tumors can occur anywhere along the length of the spinal cord, may obstruct or block CSF flow, and, if untreated, can lead to paralysis and sensory deficits. Cervical tumors may cause respiratory muscle weakness or paralysis. *Intramedullary tumors* occur within the cord itself and are fairly rare. Symptoms of cord dysfunction may occur from onset as cord function is interrupted by direct invasion and compression. *Extramedullary tumors* occur outside the spinal cord, and symptoms are related to compression of the spinal cord or destruction of nerve roots. Extramedullary tumors are further classified as intradural or extradural. *Intradural tumors,* such as meningiomas and schwannomas, arise from the membrane covering the spinal cord and nerve roots and account for the majority of all primary spinal cord tumors. Intradural tumors occur in the space between the cord and the dura. Intradural and intramedullary tumors usually are slow growing and cytologically benign but still can be extremely disabling. *Extradural tumors* usually are secondary (metastatic) tumors that have been seeded from other sites in the body, such as the prostate, bone marrow, lymph tissue, breast, or lungs. They occur in the epidural space or in the vertebrae that surround the spinal cord and related tissue. Tumors may be classified according to their anatomic locations, their cellular origin, their location in relation to the vertebral column, and whether they are primary or secondary.

ASSESSMENT

Indicators vary according to tumor site. Severity of symptoms generally depends on the rate of growth and degree of compression. Typically, pain or radiculopathy in the back precedes compression signs of motor, sensory, and bowel or bladder dysfunction by weeks or months. Compression signs initially may be quite subtle but may rapidly progress to complete paralysis in a few days.

Motor involvement: Weakness or paralysis of one or more body parts with the potential for spasticity below the level of the tumor. If the tumor interrupts the spinal cord reflex arc (e.g., a tumor at the level of the cauda equina), decreased or lost reflexes, flaccidity, muscle atrophy, and fasciculations can occur.

Sensory involvement: Decreased sensation to pain, touch, and temperature with potential loss of position and vibration sense.

Pain: Neck or back pain that persists despite bedrest, is most severe over the tumor site, and potentially radiates around the trunk or down the affected side because of nerve root irritation. The spinal processes can be quite tender to the touch. Pain often is aggravated by moving, straining, coughing, and sneezing. Pain may increase when the individual is recumbent.

Bladder and bowel dysfunction: Initially, the patient may have difficulty starting a stream or may empty the bladder incompletely. The patient may have a spastic bladder, causing urinary retention; a flaccid bladder, causing incontinence; or bowel incontinence from loss of control. The patient also may be constipated.

Physical assessment: Depending on location of the tumor, patient may exhibit increased, decreased, or absent deep tendon reflexes (DTRs).

DIAGNOSTIC TESTS

X-ray: May show changes in vertebrae such as destruction and collapse of bony matrix.

MRI: Is the procedure of choice to show tumor location and the presence of cord compression and rule out spinal abscess or syringomyelia. Because it can detect biochemical abnormalities, it may detect the tumor at a very early stage. MRI is of particular value in evaluating high cervical lesions, where the presence of bone makes the CT scan less effective.

Spinal CT scan: Reveals tumor location and presence of cord compression.

Bone scan: Shows increased radioactive tracer uptake where there is metastatic invasion of the vertebrae causing increased osteoblastic activity. **Note:** Check for pregnancy in appropriate patients, and notify health care provider accordingly. After procedure, patient should drink several glasses of water to facilitate clearance of free-circulating isotope.

Lumbar puncture (LP) and CSF analysis: May show malignant cells in CSF. With partial blockage, there may be slightly increased levels of protein and a yellow tinge to the fluid; with complete blockage, there are definite increases in protein and the fluid is yellow below the blockage.

Queckenstedt's test: Performed by compressing the jugular vein for 10 sec during the LP. Normally, a rise in CSF pressure occurs. For patients in whom a tumor is partially blocking the spinal cord above the level of the LP, the test may cause a sluggish rise in CSF. With complete blockage, there will be no rise in CSF pressure.

Myelography (sometimes with CT scan):   Shows boundaries and level at which the tumor is located if the spinal canal is not totally obstructed. This procedure can be dangerous because withdrawal of CSF may cause increased compression of the cord by the tumor.

Tissue biopsy: Confirms presence of a tumor.

Positron emission tomography (PET):   Will identify tumor location by showing abnormal metabolic activity.

See Also: "General Care of Patients with Neurologic Disorders" for **Knowledge deficit:** Neurologic diagnostic tests, p. 346, for care considerations for patients undergoing MRI, CT scan, LP, myelography, and PET.

COLLABORATIVE MANAGEMENT

Bedrest: For patients with cancer that has invaded the bony vertebral body. Body weight alone can cause vertebral collapse, resulting in possible cord laceration or compression.

Pharmacotherapy

Glucocorticoids (e.g., dexamethasone):   Often given in very high doses to decrease compression caused by cord edema. They are also given to reduce radiation-induced cord edema.

Hormone therapy: For hormone-mediated metastatic tumor.

Analgesics (e.g., acetaminophen, codeine, morphine):   For pain, which can be quite severe.

Stool softeners and laxatives (e.g., docusate):   To prevent constipation and straining at stool.

Antacids and histamine H_2-receptor blockers (e.g., ranitidine):   To reduce gastric acidity and prevent ulcer formation during steroid use.

Transcutaneous electrical nerve stimulation (TENS):   Battery-operated device that delivers electrical impulses to the body to relieve pain.

Surgery: Treatment of choice and may include a laminectomy or decompression or excision of primary tumors. Microsurgery techniques and the use of spinal cord evoked potentials during surgery have helped surgeons protect cord function. New surgical techniques permitting an anterior approach to the cord may enable better cord decompression and tumor excision. Generally, surgery is not indicated for metastatic tumors. Emergency surgical decompression of the spinal cord may save function in instances of sudden onset of partial paralysis or bowel or bladder dysfunction. Best surgical results occur when surgery is performed before neurologic deficits occur. (See "Intervertebral Disk Disease," p. 247, for care of patient with a laminectomy.) A cordotomy or palliative section of the sensory roots is sometimes done for intractable pain.

Radiation therapy: May be performed preoperatively and postoperatively to reduce tumor mass and symptoms and help prevent recurrence. Radiation therapy is the primary treatment modality for secondary metastatic tumors and those tumors that cannot be removed totally. Cord inflammation and edema caused by radiation therapy can result in an increase in the neurologic deficit. The patient also is at risk of developing radiation necrosis 6-36 mo (average 14 mo) after therapy. Onset usually is insidious and may progress to complete motor and sensory loss. MRI will rule out tumor recurrence and may show a swollen cord. There is no effective treatment, although high-dose corticosteroids may be used.

Chemotherapy: May be used for some lymphomas and myelomas. Usually it is not used with other types of tumors. A variety of immune therapies are being investigated for their potential efficacy in treating spinal cord tumors.

Physical medicine: May include physical therapy (PT), occupational therapy (OT), and assistive devices or braces so that the patient can maintain mobility and independence with ADL. Muscle-strengthening exercises, conditioning exercises, and gait training also are frequently prescribed.

ROM exercises: To maintain or increase joint function and prevent contractures.

Bowel and bladder program: To prevent incontinence and constipation and to retrain the bowel and bladder, depending on the neurologic deficit.

NURSING DIAGNOSES AND INTERVENTIONS

Pain (acute or chronic) related to tissue compression secondary to tumor growth
Desired outcomes: Within 1 hr of intervention, patient's subjective perception of pain decreases, as documented by a pain scale. Objective indicators, such as grimacing, are absent or diminished.

Note: Symptoms of primary tumors usually develop slowly, whereas with metastatic tumors they develop rapidly. Intense localized pain generally is the first symptom, with localized tenderness over the spine.

- Assess patient's character and degree of pain, using a pain scale. Rate pain from 0 (no pain) to 10 (worst pain). Pain may signal the need for immediate medical treatment (e.g., corticosteroids, radiation therapy, decompressive laminectomy) to help prevent or minimize neurologic deficits that may be permanently disabling. Have patient alert staff members or health care provider to the following: backache; sensations of heaviness or weakness in the arms or legs; any incoordination; loss of sensations of light touch, pain, and temperature; incontinence or difficulty urinating or defecating; and sexual impotence.
- Advise patient that moving slowly with good body alignment may help minimize pain. A soft cervical collar may help neck alignment.
- Suggest that keeping knees and hips slightly flexed when in bed will help reduce pain by preventing traction on nerve roots caused by full extension of the spinal cord.
- Inform patient that sneezing and straining can cause pain.
- For other interventions, see **Pain** in "General Care of Patients with Neurologic Disorders," p. 343.

NIC: Analgesic Administration; Cutaneous Stimulation; Pain Management; Patient-Controlled Analgesia (PCA) Assistance; Transcutaneous Electrical Nerve Stimulation (TENS)

See Also: Chapter 3 if patient has urinary incontinence (p. 177), retention (p. 185), or neurogenic bladder (p. 188); "Intervertebral Disk Disease" for **Knowledge deficit:** Diskectomy with laminectomy or fusion procedure, p. 252; "Spinal Cord Injury," p. 261, for nursing diagnoses and interventions related to the care of patients with disorders of the spinal cord; "General Care of Patients With Neurologic Disorders" for **Knowledge deficit:** Neurologic diagnostic tests, p. 346; "Pressure Ulcers," p. 710; Appendix One, "Caring for Patients on Prolonged Bedrest," p. 738, for nursing diagnoses and interventions for patients who are immobile; Appendix One, "Caring for Preoperative and Postoperative Patients," p. 717; Appendix One, "Caring for Patients With Cancer and Other Life-disrupting Illnesses," p. 747.

PATIENT-FAMILY TEACHING AND DISCHARGE PLANNING

When providing patient-family teaching, focus on sensory information; avoid giving excessive information; and initiate a visiting nurse referral for necessary follow-up teaching. Consider including verbal and written information about the following:
- Safety measures relative to sensorimotor deficits.
- For more information, see third through eleventh entries in "Brain tumor," p. 293.

Section Five: Vascular Disorders of the Nervous System

Cerebral aneurysm

An aneurysm is a localized weakness and dilation of an artery. With cerebral aneurysms, this dilation generally takes one of two forms: *fusiform*, in which the entire circumference of a vessel section is dilated; or *saccular*, in which the side of a vessel is dilated. Saccular aneurysms, also called berry aneurysms, are the most common. Depending on their size and location, unruptured aneurysms can produce neurologic symptoms by compressing brain tissue or cranial nerves. Usually, however, the aneurysm causes no symptoms until it ruptures. When this occurs, the hemorrhage usually bleeds into the subarachnoid space, although occasionally it may bleed directly into the intracranial tissue, causing direct neuronal damage. Rupture causes a sudden increase in ICP and a loss of cerebral perfusion pressure. Brain tissue may be compressed by the expanding mass effect of the bleeding. Cranial nerves and brain tissue are irritated by the presence of blood, and the brain begins to swell. Blood in the subarachnoid space prevents adequate circulation and reabsorption of CSF, which increases ICP further. In addition, interruption of blood flow to the areas supplied by the ruptured artery can cause brain ischemia and possibly infarction. The patient may experience permanent neurologic deficits, depending on the size and site of the bleed and the development of complications.

Aneurysms can be caused by a congenital defect in the arterial wall, degenerative processes, such as hypertension or atherosclerosis, or vessel trauma. Prognosis depends on the site and size of the ruptured aneurysm, but 45%-50% of affected individuals die immediately.

Common causes of death for individuals who survive the initial rupture include IICP, rebleeding, and vasospasm of the blood vessels. The patient is at greatest risk of rebleeding within the first 24-48 hr after the initial rupture. Rebleeding, however, is a significant risk for the first 2 wk because of the body's normal process of clot lysis at the rupture site. Approximately 20% of patients will rebleed within 2 wk. Nearly two thirds of patients experiencing rebleeding will die. Rebleeding may occur up to 6 mo after the initial rupture.

The patient also is at risk of experiencing cerebral vasospasm, which decreases cerebral blood flow, leading to cerebral ischemia. The cerebral ischemia can increase the patient's neurologic deficits and may cause cerebral infarct and death. Vasospasm seems to be directly related to the amount of blood present in the subarachnoid space after rupture. Vasospasm usually starts within 3-4 days after the subarachnoid hemorrhage, peaks in 7-10 days, and usually resolves in about 3 wk.

After rupture, 20%-25% of patients may develop acute or chronic hydrocephalus. The presence of blood in the subarachnoid space appears to damage the arachnoid villi and decrease or prevent CSF reabsorption. This will increase ICP, leading to possible brain herniation. Other complications the patient may be at risk for are diabetes insipidus, syndrome of inappropriate antidiuretic hormone (SIADH) because of pituitary gland or hypothalamus compression or damage, and cerebral salt-wasting syndrome.

ASSESSMENT

Indicators vary, depending on the site and amount of bleeding. Rupture often occurs with exertion, excitement, or a sudden rise in BP.

Signs and symptoms

- *Prodromal (as the aneurysm enlarges but before it ruptures):* periodic headaches, transitory weakness, numbness, tingling on one side, transitory diplopia, blurred vision, ptosis, and transitory speech disturbances.

- *Acute (with leakage and rupture):* sudden and severe headache, nausea and/or vomiting, loss of consciousness, and neck stiffness are among the most common symptoms.

IICP and herniation: Sudden, severe headache; nausea and vomiting; changes or alteration in LOC ranging from confusion, irritability, and restlessness to coma; a falling score on the Glasgow Coma Scale (see Table 4-2); pupillary dilation and changes in their size and reaction to light; VS changes, such as increasing BP with widening pulse pressure and decreased pulse rate; irregular respiratory pattern.

Meningeal irritation (caused by blood in the subarachnoid space): Neck stiffness; neck, back, and leg pain; fever; photophobia; seizures.

Cranial nerve irritation/compression: Blurred vision and other visual disturbances, ptosis, inability to rotate the eyes, difficulty with swallowing or speaking, tinnitus.

Focal symptoms: Sensory loss, motor weakness, or paralysis on one side of the body.

Autonomic disturbance (from increased catecholamines immediately following rupture): ECG changes, flushing, sweating, dilated pupils, hypertension, tachycardia, increased blood sugar, increased temperature, ileus.

Physical assessment: Positive Kernig's and Brudzinski's signs confirm presence of meningeal irritation. (See description with "Bacterial Meningitis," p. 218.)

Grading: Individuals with ruptured aneurysms are often graded according to the severity of the bleeding or injury:

- *Grade 1:* patient alert with no neurologic deficit; slight neck stiffness; minimal headache, if present.
- *Grade 2:* patient alert with mild to severe headache; presence of stiff neck; may have minimal neurologic deficit, such as third cranial nerve palsies.
- *Grade 3:* patient drowsy or confused; presence of stiff neck and headache; may have mild focal neurologic deficits.
- *Grade 4:* patient stuporous, semicomatose; presence of stiff neck; may have neurologic deficits, such as hemiparesis.
- *Grade 5:* patient comatose and posturing.

DIAGNOSTIC TESTS

CT scan: To reveal presence of aneurysm(s) and the site, size, and amount of bleeding from the subarachnoid or intracerebral hemorrhage. The scan also may reveal the presence of hydrocephalus. The scan may not identify small aneurysms or those in vasospasm. CT scan may be used 1-2 days after rupture to assess the amount of bleeding to predict risk of vasospasm. Spiral CT angiography may be used to detect unruptured aneurysms or monitor for vasospasm.

Cerebral angiography: To pinpoint site, structure, and size of aneurysm(s) and presence of vasospasm. This test provides the definitive diagnosis of aneurysm, and it usually is performed before surgery to exclude the presence of vasospasm and review accessibility. Small aneurysms may be missed.

MRI: To reveal presence of even small amounts of blood or small aneurysms that are not visualized with the CT scan or angiography. Magnetic resonance angiography is being used in some areas to highlight cerebral vascularity.

Lumbar puncture (LP) and CSF analysis: To reveal presence of bloody CSF, increased CSF pressure, and increased protein. Blood in the CSF indicates that a subarachnoid hemorrhage has occurred. This procedure is contraindicated for patients with IICP because of the risk of herniation. The LP usually is done only when CT scan is not diagnostic or unavailable.

Skull x-ray: To reveal calcification in the wall of a large aneurysm.

Cerebral blood flow studies (e.g., transcranial Doppler sonography): To monitor for cerebral vasospasms, changes in blood flow states, loss of autoregulation, IICP, and brain death.

See Also: "General Care of Patients With Neurologic Disorders" for **Knowledge deficit:** Neurologic diagnostic tests, p. 346, for care considerations for patients undergoing CT scan, angiography, MRI, and LP.

COLLABORATIVE MANAGEMENT

Respiratory support: Airway maintenance, intubation, and ventilation as necessary. ABG values are often monitored for evidence of hypoxia. If indicated, O_2 is administered to prevent hypoxia and carbon dioxide retention, which can cause vasodilation of the cerebral arteries and cerebral edema.

Activity restrictions: Strict bedrest in a quiet, dark room; limitation of visitors; restriction of ADL. Although active ROM is occasionally permitted, even the alert patient is usually limited to passive ROM. Restraints are avoided because they can result in IICP if the patient struggles against them.

Elevation of HOB: To 30 degrees or as prescribed to reduce cerebral congestion.

Pharmacotherapy

Corticosteroids (e.g., dexamethasone): To help decrease cerebral edema and ICP. Antacids and histamine H_2-receptor blockers, such as ranitidine, may be given concurrently to inhibit gastric secretions and reduce GI irritation.

Antihypertensives (e.g., hydralazine): If indicated, to treat underlying hypertension.

Laxatives and stool softeners (e.g., docusate sodium, Milk of Magnesia): To prevent straining with bowel movements.

Sedatives/tranquilizers (e.g., phenobarbital): To reduce stress and restlessness and promote rest.

Osmotic diuretics (e.g., mannitol): To reduce severe cerebral edema.

Loop diuretics (e.g., furosemide): Used by some health care providers because they appear to decrease cerebral edema without causing the increase in intracranial blood volume that occurs with mannitol.

Antiepilepsy drugs (e.g., carbamazepine, phenytoin, fosphenytoin, phenobarbital, diazepam): To control or prevent seizures.

Antipyretics (e.g., acetaminophen): To control fever, which increases the brain's metabolic activity. Aspirin is avoided because it prevents platelet adhesion.

Analgesics (e.g., acetaminophen, codeine): To manage pain. Aspirin is contraindicated because it prevents platelet adhesion.

Antifibrinolytic agents (e.g., aminocaproic acid): To decrease the risk of rebleeding at the site of aneurysm by delaying the body's lysis of the blood clot. Use of this drug is controversial because although it reduces the risk of rebleeding, it appears to increase the risk of vasospasm. Use of antifibrinolytic agents has decreased in favor of early surgery to clip the aneurysm before development of vasospasm. If used, an IV loading dose of 5 g is generally given over 1 hr followed by a continuous infusion of ≥30 g/day for 3 wk or until the patient goes for surgical repair. Rapid IV infusion may cause hypotension, bradycardia, or dysrhythmias. The IV drug route is preferred over the oral route. The drug should be diluted 1 g/50 ml D_5W or other compatible solution. Side effects include phlebitis at the insertion site (IV route) and nausea and diarrhea (oral route). Other side effects include headache, tinnitus, dizziness, fatigue, and generalized thrombosis.

Fluid: Initially fluids are given to keep the patient normovolemic. Fluid restriction has generally been abandoned because the resultant increased blood viscosity has been suspected to result in increased risk of vasospasm. Later, after aneurysm clipping, the patient may be kept hypervolemic to reduce vasospasm.

Nutrition: Coffee and other stimulants are restricted. Very hot and very cold liquids also may be restricted. A high-fiber diet may be prescribed to prevent constipation. For patients with dysphagia, enteral or parenteral feedings may be necessary. A low-Na⁺ (see Table 3-2, p. 133), low-cholesterol (see Table 2-2, p. 57) diet is often prescribed to control hypertension and atherosclerosis.

Antiembolism hose or sequential compression devices: To help prevent thrombophlebitis and deep vein thrombosis.

Avoiding rectal stimulation: Rectal suppositories, thermometers, enemas, and digital examinations are contraindicated because they can stimulate a type of Valsalva's maneuver in the patient, causing increased intrathoracic pressure and IICP, resulting in rupture or rebleeding.

Seizure precautions: To prevent patient injury in the event of seizure.

Cardiac monitoring: May be done to assess and treat cardiac dysrhythmias, which are common immediately following subarachnoid hemorrhage.

ICU monitoring: May be necessary, particularly if the patient develops cerebral vasospasm or IICP.

Surgical management/interventional neuroradiology: The patient's surgical candidacy depends on LOC, extent of neurologic deficit, nature and location of the aneurysm, and presence of vasospasm. The timing of the surgery is based on the patient's status and surgeon's preference. Usually, it is performed within 24-48 hr of the initial bleed. The surgical site is thoroughly irrigated to reduce the amount of blood present that might result in vasospasm. Surgery is not performed in the presence of vasospasm. Patients graded 1 or 2 are the best surgical candidates, and the trend is for them to have surgery within 1-3 days of the initial bleed. Computerized EEG may be used in the OR during the procedure for continuous monitoring of neuronal integrity. Brain activity as recorded on an EEG correlates with cerebral blood flow and can be used to identify ischemia in the anesthetized patient and thereby signal for interventions to prevent brain damage.

Surgical repair with craniotomy: To isolate the aneurysm and prevent rebleeding, a craniotomy is performed and the aneurysm is repaired by clipping, ligating, coagulating, wrapping the aneurysm neck with muscle, or encasing the aneurysmal sac in plastic or surgical gauze. (For information on craniotomy patient care considerations, see "Brain Tumors," p. 288.)

Carotid artery clamping: For internal carotid artery aneurysms, and sometimes for other inaccessible aneurysms, a carotid artery clamp may be used to reduce blood flow and blood pressure. After surgery, the carotid artery clamp is tightened slowly over several days, which allows time for collateral circulation to take over in the brain.

Endovascular balloon occlusion of aneurysm or parent vessel: A small and extremely flexible catheter is threaded through the femoral artery at the groin and advanced up to the aneurysm or parent vessel. The balloon can be inflated with a liquid that solidifies within 45 min. Balloon occlusion within the aneurysm is ideal, but sometimes the parent vessel (usually the carotid) must be occluded. A test occlusion is done to see if the patient can tolerate the parent vessel occlusion. If signs of ischemia occur, the balloon procedure is stopped. A bypass is done, if possible, and the balloon occlusion usually is performed a few days later. (See "Cerebrovascular Accident," p. 310, for cerebral artery bypass patient care considerations.)

Ventriculostomy: Ventriculostomy permits temporary ventricular drainage for acute hydrocephalus.

Daily lumbar punctures (LPs) or lumbar drain: LPs or lumbar drains provide temporary CSF drainage and restore the reabsorptive ability of the arachnoid villi by removing blood from the CSF.

Ventricular shunt for ventricular drainage: A ventricular shunt allows long-term drainage of CSF in patients who develop chronic hydrocephalus after a subarachnoid hemorrhage. (See discussion of ventricular shunt in "Brain Tumors," p. 288.)

Embolization of surgically inaccessible aneurysms: Endovascular techniques are used to place a metal coil in the area of the aneurysm to cause a thrombus to form that obliterates the aneurysm.

Proton beam: A proton beam is used to sclerose inoperable aneurysms.

Management of SIADH vs. cerebral salt-wasting syndrome: Hyponatremia and decreased fluid volume increase the risk of vasospasm. It is critical to distinguish correctly between these two types of hyponatremia and fluid imbalance because their treatment is so different. SIADH (characterized by dilutional hyponatremia with increased plasma volume, weight gain, low BUN, decreased serum osmolality) is treated with fluid restriction (see "Syndrome of Inappropriate Antidiuretic Hormone," p. 372, for more information). Cerebral salt-wasting syndrome (characterized by hyponatremia with decreased plasma volume, weight loss, high BUN, decreased serum osmolality, hypernatriuria) is treated with fluid replacement, volume expanders, and occasionally fludrocortisone to inhibit Na^+ excretion and induce Na^+ retention to counteract hyponatremia and volume depletion.

Treatments for cerebral vasospasm: There is no completely effective treatment for cerebral vasospasm, but some techniques seem to reduce its incidence or severity. Vasospasm is related to the amount of blood in basal cisterns or cerebral fissures. The following treatments necessitate ICU monitoring.

Craniotomy: Done within 48 hr to remove any blood clot that may aggravate vasospasm.

Hypervolemic, hypertensive, hemodilution therapy (HHHT) (e.g., albumin, crystalloid fluid): The patient is kept well hydrated with IV fluids or volume expanders to decrease blood viscosity (e.g., a hematocrit of 30%-34%) to improve cerebral blood flow through narrowed arteries.

Hypervolemic (e.g., plasma protein fraction, saline, albumin, hetastarch) and hypertensive (e.g., dopamine, phenylephrine) therapy: To achieve a mean arterial pressure (MAP) of 100-110. Usually performed only following aneurysm repair to increase cerebral perfusion pressure via increased blood volume and arterial pressure to reduce the ischemia and resulting neurologic deficits during vasospasm.

Calcium channel blockers (e.g., nicardipine, nimodipine): Suspected to cause vasodilation via smooth muscle relaxation and promote collateral circulation via dilation of small pia arteries.

Balloon angioplasty: To dilate arteries that are in vasospasm.

Tissue plasminogen activator instillation: Accomplished during aneurysm clipping into the basal cisterns to dissolve any clots to prevent or reduce vasospasm.

Treatments under investigation
- Nitroglycerin, isoproterenol, nitroprusside: to increase cerebral perfusion through smooth muscle dilation.
- Barbiturate coma: to decrease cerebral metabolic needs so that injury will be minimized until vasospasm subsides and cerebral blood flow improves.

NURSING DIAGNOSES AND INTERVENTIONS

The priorities of care for these patients revolve around maintenance of adequate cerebral perfusion, prevention of rebleeding, and prevention and treatment of vasospasm. See "Cerebrovascular Accident," p. 306, for a discussion of these issues. The following nursing diagnoses relate primarily to the patient whose aneurysm is graded 1-3. If the patient's aneurysm is graded 4 or 5, see nursing diagnoses in "Cerebrovascular Accident," p. 310, for patient care.

Knowledge deficit: Aneurysms and the potential for rebleeding, rupture, or vasospasm

Desired outcome: Following instruction and on an ongoing basis, patient verbalizes knowledge about the potential for rebleeding or vasospasm, measures to prevent their occurrence, and symptoms to report to the health care staff.

- Assess patient for sensorimotor deficits, such as decreased or absent vision, impaired temperature and pain sensation, unsteady gait, weakness, or paralysis. Document baseline neurologic and physical assessments so that changes in patient status are detected promptly. Teach patient and significant other these indicators, and explain the importance of reporting them to the staff promptly.
- Teach these patients the importance of reducing activity level to avoid rebleeding or rupture. Strict bedrest may be prescribed. Emphasize the necessity of allowing others to help them with moving, ADL, and passive ROM, even though they may feel capable of self-care. Explain that the number and frequency of visitors will be limited and that individuals whose presence is stressful to the patient should not be allowed to visit. The phone will be removed from the room, and television, radio, and reading may be restricted or limited to programs and books that are not overstimulating. The room will be darkened to promote rest, and sedatives and tranquilizers may be offered. Caffeine and other stimulants will be restricted, as well as nicotine, which can increase the risk of vasospasm.
- Teach patient measures that will prevent a sudden increase in ICP:
  —Avoid coughing and sneezing; if they are unavoidable, do so with an open mouth.
  —Exhale when being turned.
  —Avoid straining with bowel movements.
  —Avoid extreme hip flexion or lying prone.
  —Avoid moving self up in bed because this requires a pushing movement. Do not grip, push, or pull on side rails or push feet against the mattress or foot of bed. Request help from staff member for all moving and turning movements.
- Explain that the HOB may be maintained at 30 degrees and the patient may be asked to keep head and neck in good alignment to promote venous return to the heart and reduce cerebral congestion and ICP.
- Explain that the patient may be given a high-fiber diet and stool softeners to promote bowel elimination without straining.
- Describe, as appropriate, the following preventive measures: corticosteroids to prevent or reduce cerebral edema, antiepilepsy medications to prevent seizures, antihypertensive medications to keep BP within defined parameters, and a low-Na^+, low-cholesterol diet to help control BP.
- Teach patient to avoid taking aspirin or aspirin-containing products, which increase the risk of hemorrhage.

NIC: Environmental Management; Teaching: Disease Process; Teaching: Individual; Teaching: Prescribed Activity/Exercise

Knowledge deficit: Effects of aminocaproic acid drug therapy
Desired outcome: Following instruction and on an ongoing basis, patient verbalizes knowledge about the side effects of aminocaproic therapy, the measures to prevent complications from the drug therapy, and signs and symptoms that should be reported immediately to health care staff if they occur.

- Teach patients receiving aminocaproic acid therapy the indicators of pulmonary embolus, including SOB, chest pain (especially that which increases with inspiration), and blood-tinged sputum, as well as indicators of deep vein thrombosis, such as calf pain or tenderness and increased local warmth, swelling, or redness of the leg and coolness, pallor, venous dilation, and edema more distally. Stress the importance of notifying staff

immediately if they occur. Encourage patient to wear antiembolism hose and, if prescribed, to use sequential compression devices or pneumatic foot pumps.
- Monitor patient's IV site for signs of phlebitis. Instruct patient to report any tenderness, stiffness, or swelling at the site.
- Alert patient to the potential for loose stools, frequent stools (more than 3/day), cramps, and weakness with aminocaproic therapy. Instruct patient to report these problems promptly because, if the diarrhea is a side effect of oral aminocaproic therapy, the health care provider may switch patient to IV medication.
- Inform patient that because the drug may cause postural hypotension, he or she should make position changes very slowly and in stages. Faintness or dizziness should be reported promptly.
- Instruct patient to report any muscle weakness, muscle pain, sweating, fever, or myeloglobinuria (reddish brown urine) because these may be signs of myopathy caused by this drug therapy.
- Teach patient to report nausea, tinnitus, nasal stuffiness, or fatigue, which are other side effects of aminocaproic drug therapy.

NIC: Circulatory Care; Medication Management; Teaching: Disease Process; Teaching: Individual; Teaching: Prescribed Medication

Ineffective airway clearance (or risk of same) related to imposed inactivity secondary to the risk of aneurysm rupture or rebleeding
Desired outcomes: Following intervention and on an ongoing basis, patient's lungs are clear to auscultation. Secretions are thin and clear, and the patient remains normothermic.
- Assess patient for increased SOB or a change in the rate or depth of respirations. Auscultate lung fields for breath sounds, noting presence of crackles (rales), rhonchi, and diminished sounds. Assess for fever, purulent or discolored sputum, and cyanosis.
- Monitor patient's oximetry readings for an O_2 saturation <92% or ABG values for hypoxemia (Pao_2 <80 mm Hg) or hypercapnia ($Paco_2$ >45 mm Hg). Notify health care provider of significant findings.
- Encourage patient to breath deeply and change positions q2hr to help expand the lungs. Instruct patient to avoid coughing or sneezing because these activities increase intraabdominal and intrathoracic pressure, which in turn increase ICP and the risk of aneurysm rupture. Explain that if sneezing is unavoidable, it should be done with an open mouth.
- Maintain patient on oxygen as prescribed.
- Assist patient with using incentive spirometry if prescribed.

NIC: Airway Management; Oxygen Therapy; Respiratory Monitoring; Surveillance

Risk for disuse syndrome with risk factors related to prescribed immobilization secondary to risk of aneurysm rupture or rebleeding
Desired outcome: Patient exhibits complete ROM.
- To maintain joint mobility, perform passive ROM exercises during the period of activity restriction. Even if the patient feels well enough to perform assisted or active ROM, these activities are contraindicated because they increase ICP and the risk of rupture or rebleeding. Explain to patient the rationale for activity limitation.
- Maintain joint alignment, and provide support to the joints and extremities with pillows, trochanter rolls, sandbags, and other positioning devices.
- When the patient is no longer on bedrest and activity restrictions, additional strengthening and conditioning exercises may be necessary to counteract the effects of prolonged bedrest. In addition, the patient may have residual neurologic deficits that necessitate gait training or the use of assistive

devices to promote mobility. Obtain a physical therapy or occupational therapy referral as appropriate. For additional interventions, see **Risk for disuse syndrome** in Appendix One, Caring for Patients on Prolonged Bedrest," p. 740.

NIC: Activity Therapy; Exercise Promotion; Exercise Therapy: Joint Mobility; Exercise Therapy: Muscle Control; Positioning: Neurologic

Self care deficit related to imposed activity restrictions secondary to risk of aneurysm rupture or rebleeding
Desired outcome: Patient's care activities are completed for him or her during the period of strict bedrest.
- During the period of strict bedrest and activity restrictions, perform care activities, even for patients who do not exhibit signs of neurologic deficit. Explain the reason for patient's activity restrictions.
- If patient has bathroom privileges, provide a commode as appropriate and assist patient with transferring as necessary.

NIC: Bathing; Perineal Care; Self-Care Assistance: Bathing/Hygiene; Self-Care Assistance: Toileting

See Also: "Head Injury" for **Fluid volume excess** related to SIADH, p. 283; "Brain Tumors" for **Knowledge deficit:** Ventricular shunt procedure, p. 290, for surgical patients; **Knowledge deficit:** Craniotomy procedure, p. 290, for surgical patients; "Cerebrovascular Accident" for **Knowledge deficit:** Cerebral artery bypass surgery, p. 316; "Seizure Disorders," p. 324, for related nursing diagnoses; "General Care of Patients With Neurologic Disorders" for **Risk for fluid volume deficit,** p. 335; **Constipation,** p. 339; **Pain,** p. 343; **Knowledge deficit:** Neurologic diagnostic tests, p. 346; "Diabetes Insipidus" for **Altered protection** related to side effects of vasopressin, p. 367; "Pressure Ulcers," p. 710, for patients with varying degrees of immobility; Appendix One, "Caring for Patients on Prolonged Bedrest," p. 738; Appendix One, "Caring for Patients With Cancer and Other Life-disrupting Illnesses," p. 791, as appropriate, for psychosocial interventions.

PATIENT-FAMILY TEACHING AND DISCHARGE PLANNING

When providing patient-family teaching, focus on sensory information; avoid giving excessive information; and initiate a visiting nurse referral for necessary follow-up teaching. Consider including verbal and written information about the following:
- Wound care and indicators of wound infection for patients who have undergone surgery.
- Importance of avoiding strenuous physical activity. Check with health care provider regarding activity restrictions and limitations; instruct patient accordingly.
- Low-Na^+ (see Table 3-2, p. 133), low-cholesterol (see Table 2-2, p. 57) diet if prescribed to control hypertension and atherosclerosis.
- Medications, including drug name, rationale, schedule, dosage, precautions, drug/drug and food/drug interactions, and potential side effects.
- Signs and symptoms of rupture and rebleeding; patient is at risk for 6 mo after the initial bleed.
- Care of the ventricular shunt, if present. Instructions should include indicators of shunt infection and steps to take in the event of shunt infection or malfunction.

In addition:
- See the teaching and discharge planning section in "Cerebrovascular Accident," p. 318, for additional interventions for patients who have residual neurologic deficits.

Cerebrovascular accident

A cerebrovascular accident (CVA) is the sudden disruption of O_2 supply to the nerve cells, generally caused by obstruction or rupture in one or more of the blood vessels that supply the brain. *Ischemic CVA* has three main mechanisms: thrombosis, embolism, and systemic hypoperfusion. Thrombosis or embolism results in a blockage of blood supply to the brain tissue. The resulting ischemia, if prolonged, causes brain tissue necrosis (infarction), cerebral edema, and IICP. Most thrombotic strokes are caused by blockage as a result of atherosclerosis. Most embolic strokes are the result of emboli produced during atrial fibrillation of the heart. Ischemic stroke caused by systemic hypoperfusion usually is the result of decreased cerebral blood flow owing to circulatory failure. Circulatory failure results from too little blood, too low BP, or failure of the heart to pump blood adequately. Hypoxia from any cause also can produce this syndrome.

A transient ischemic attack (TIA), which is a temporary (<24 hr) neurologic deficit that resolves completely without permanent damage, occurs when the artery cannot deliver enough blood to meet the brain's O_2 requirement. TIAs usually are associated with thrombosis but may be caused by any of the ischemic mechanisms just mentioned. TIAs may precede a permanent ischemic CVA by hours, days, months, or years. TIAs are a warning sign, and treatment may prevent a stroke. Most TIAs last an average of 5-10 min. A reversible ischemic neurologic deficit (RIND) lasts longer than 24 hr but otherwise is similar to a TIA.

Hemorrhagic CVA causes neural tissue destruction because of the infiltration and accumulation of blood. Ischemia and infarction may occur distal to the hemorrhage because of interrupted blood supply. Although a cerebral hemorrhage usually results from hypertension or an aneurysm, trauma also can cause hemorrhagic CVA. Bleeding may spread into the brain tissue itself, causing an intracerebral hemorrhage, or into the subarachnoid space. Usually there is a large rise in ICP with a hemorrhagic stroke because of cerebral edema and the mass effect of blood (see "Cerebral Aneurysm," p. 298, for discussion of subarachnoid hemorrhage).

A CVA may be classified as a *progressive stroke in evolution,* in which deficits continue to worsen over time, or as a *completed stroke,* in which maximum deficit has been acquired and has persisted for longer than 24 hr. Progressive strokes usually are the result of a thrombus formation and often take 1-3 days to become "completed." CVA is the third most common cause of death and the most common cause of neurologic disability. Half the survivors are left permanently disabled or experience another CVA. Improvement may continue for 1-2 yr, but deficits at 6 mo usually are considered permanent.

ASSESSMENT

General findings: Classically, symptoms appear on the side of the body opposite the damaged site. For example, a CVA in the left hemisphere of the brain will produce symptoms in the right arm and leg. However, when the CVA affects the cranial nerves, the symptoms of cranial nerve deficit will appear on the same side as the site of injury. Similarly, an obstruction of an anterior cerebral artery can produce bilateral symptoms, as will severe bleeding or multiple emboli. Hemiplegia is fairly common. Initially, the patient usually has flaccid paralysis. As spinal cord depression resolves, more normal tone is seen and hyperactive reflexes occur.

Signs and symptoms: Vary with the size and site of injury and may improve in 2-3 days as the cerebral edema decreases. Changes in mentation, including apathy, irritability, disorientation, memory loss, withdrawal, drowsiness, stupor, or coma; bowel and bladder incontinence; numbness or loss of sensation; weakness or paralysis on part or one side of the body; aphasia; headache; neck stiffness and rigidity; vomiting; seizures; dizziness or syncope; and fever may occur. A brain stem infarct leaving the patient completely paralyzed with intact cortical function is called *locked-in syndrome.*

With *cranial nerve involvement,* visual disturbances include diplopia, blindness, and hemianopia; inequality or fixation of the pupils, nystagmus, tinnitus, and difficulty chewing and swallowing also occur.

Physical assessment: Papilledema, arteriosclerotic retinal changes, or hemorrhagic retinal areas on ophthalmic examination. Hyperactive deep tendon reflexes (DTRs), decreased superficial reflexes, and positive Babinski's sign also may be present. To check for Babinski's response, stroke the lateral aspect of the sole of the foot (from the heel to the ball of the foot) with a hard object. Dorsiflexion of the great toe with fanning of the other toes is a positive sign. Positive Kernig's or Brudzinski's sign (see "Bacterial Meningitis," p. 218) indicates meningeal irritation.

TIAs: Typical symptoms include temporal episodes of slurred speech, weakness, numbness or tingling, blindness in one eye, blurred or double vision, dizziness or ataxia, and confusion.

History of: TIAs; hypertension; atherosclerosis; high serum cholesterol or triglycerides; diabetes mellitus; gout; smoking; cardiac valve diseases, such as those that may result from rheumatic fever, valve prosthesis, and atrial fibrillation; cardiac surgery; blood dyscrasia; anticoagulant therapy; neck vessel trauma; oral contraceptive use; family predisposition for arteriovenous malformation (AVM); aneurysm; or previous CVA.

DIAGNOSTIC TESTS

The CT scan or MRI is the test most likely to be obtained for every patient with a suspected stroke. However, technologic advances have provided numerous diagnostic tests for CVA. The selection, sequence, and urgency of these tests will be determined by the patient's history and symptoms. For example, the patient who has a TIA will have a different set or sequence of tests than the patient who is in coma.

CT scan: To reveal site of infarction, hematoma, and shift of brain structures. CT scan is of particular value in identifying blood released early during hemorrhagic strokes. CT scan is the test of choice for unstable patients. Generally, identifying ischemic areas is difficult until they start to necrose at around 48-72 hr.

MRI: To reveal site of infarction, hematoma, shift of brain structure, and cerebral edema. MRI is of particular value in identifying ischemic strokes early.

Phonoangiography/Doppler ultrasonography: To identify presence of bruits if the carotid blood vessels are partially occluded.

Oculoplethysmography: To obtain indirect measurement of carotid blood flow by determining intraocular ophthalmic systolic pressure. Reduced pressure may signal carotid stenosis.

Transcranial Doppler ultrasound: To provide information (noninvasively) about pressure and flow in the intracranial arteries.

Positron emission tomography (PET): To provide information on cerebral metabolism and blood flow characteristics. This test is useful in identifying ischemic stroke by showing areas of reduced glucose metabolism.

Single photon emission computed tomography (SPECT): To identify cerebral blood flow.

EEG: To show abnormal nerve impulse transmission, such as focal slowing, which will help locate the lesion and/or indicate the amount of brain wave activity present.

Lumbar puncture (LP) and CSF analysis: Not done routinely, especially in the presence of IICP, but may reveal increase in CSF pressure; clear to bloody CSF, depending on the type of stroke; and presence of infection or other nonvascular cause for bleeding. CSF glutamic oxaloacetic transaminase (GOT) will be increased for 10 days after injury. Blood in the CSF signals that a subarachnoid hemorrhage has occurred.

Cerebral angiography: If surgery is comtemplated, this procedure is done to pinpoint site of rupture or occlusion and identify collateral blood circulation, aneurysms, or AVM.

Digital subtraction angiography (DSA):   To visualize cerebral blood flow and detect vascular abnormalities, such as stenosis, aneurysm, and hematomas.

Echocardiography: To evaluate valvular heart structures for thrombus and myocardial walls for mural thrombi that may provide a source of emboli.

Laboratory tests: To detect and monitor for clotting abnormalities as a source of hemorrhagic stroke; monitoring serum or capillary glucose to avoid hyperglycemia (hyperglycemia has been associated with poor outcomes).

> **See Also:**   **Knowledge deficit:** Neurologic diagnostic tests, p. 346, for care considerations for patients undergoing CT scan, MRI, oculoplethysmography, PET, EEG, LP, cerebral angiography, SPECT, and DSA.

COLLABORATIVE MANAGEMENT

Respiratory support: Maintenance of airway and delivery of O_2, as needed. IPPB and chest physiotherapy also may be prescribed. Mechanical ventilation occasionally may be used.

IV fluids: Maintenance of electrolyte balance and normovolemia. IV solutions should be saline rather than glucose. Hyperglycemia >150 mg/dl may increase size of the infarct. Fluid restrictions are avoided because resulting increased blood viscosity and decreased volume may lead to hypotension, decreasing cerebral perfusion pressure.

Positioning: Bedrest during acute stage. Activity level is increased as patient's condition improves. Maintain HOB as prescribed. HOB may be down or flat with thrombotic or embolic strokes to increase cerebral perfusion. HOB may be kept up with hemorrhagic strokes or patients at risk of IICP to decrease cerebral edema and improve venous outflow.

Diet: NPO status and possible gastric tube if swallow and gag reflexes are diminished or if patient has decreased LOC. A low-Na^+ (see Table 3-2, p. 133) and/or low-fat (see Table 2-3, p. 57), low-cholesterol (see Table 2-2, p. 57) diet may be prescribed to minimize other risk factors. Diet may consist of fluids and pureed, soft, or chopped foods, or tube feedings, depending on patient's LOC and ability to chew and swallow. A gastrostomy (percutaneous endoscopic gastrostomy [PEG], percutaneous endoscopic jejunostomy [PEJ]) tube may be required for nutrition, especially in aspiration-prone patients.

Pharmacotherapy

Thrombolytic enzymes (e.g., tissue plasminogen activator):   To cause lysis of thrombus or embolus obstructing cerebral arteries in an acute, nonhemorrhagic CVA. This agent is administered intravenously and must be given within 1-6 hr to restore circulation and save brain tissue. Intraarterial urokinase and streptokinase have also been used to restore blood flow.

Anticoagulants: To treat patients with thrombotic CVAs or TIAs. Medications include heparin sodium, enoxaparin, and warfarin sodium to help prevent further thrombosis. If the stroke or neurologic deficit is in evolution (still progressing), anticoagulants may be useful for 24-72 hr. Once the stroke is completed and neurologic status is stable, anticoagulants are no longer useful. Anticoagulants are contraindicated with hemorrhagic CVA. Anticoagulants may be continued if the stroke was caused by emboli.

Antihypertensive agents (e.g., nifedipine): To control very high BP, which may cause cerebral edema and IICP. Mild to moderate hypertension may be needed to maintain cerebral perfusion and prevent further ischemia, so BP may not be substantially lowered initially.

Antiplatelet medications (e.g., ticlopidine, aspirin in conjunction with dipyridamole or sulfinpyrazone): To prevent platelet aggregation that may lead to thrombus formation. Patients with TIAs or those at risk for additional thrombotic strokes may be started on this therapy to prevent future ischemic strokes from thrombosis. **Caution:** These medications should not be used in the presence of hemorrhagic CVA.

Vasopressors (e.g., dopamine): To treat low BP, which may increase ischemia.

Glucocorticosteroids (e.g., dexamethasone) and osmotic diuretics (e.g., mannitol): To prevent or reduce cerebral edema. Use is controversial.

Antacids and histamine H₂-receptor blockers (e.g., ranitidine): To reduce the risk of GI hemorrhage from gastric ulcer caused by stress or corticosteroid therapy.

Antiepilepsy drugs (e.g., carbamazepine, phenytoin, fosphenytoin, phenobarbital, diazepam): To control and prevent seizures if present.

Sedatives/tranquilizers (e.g., diphenhydramine): To promote rest. These are used cautiously to avoid further impairment of neurologic function.

Analgesics (e.g., acetaminophen): To control headache. If CVA is hemorrhagic, aspirin is avoided because it can increase bleeding.

Stool softeners (e.g., docusate): To prevent straining, which can result in IICP.

Antipyretics (e.g., acetaminophen): To reduce fever, which increases cerebral metabolic needs. During the acute phase, the patient may be kept mildly hypothermic with antipyretics and cooling measures (e.g., lowered room temperature, cooling blankets, convection devices) since cooling appears to be neuroprotective.

Hemodilution (e.g., albumin, crystalloid fluids): To promote hydration via IV fluids and volume expanders to decrease blood viscosity (hematocrit to 30%-33%) to improve cerebral blood flow through narrowed arteries.

Hypervolemic (e.g., plasma protein fraction, whole blood, saline, albumin, hetastarch): To increase cerebral perfusion pressure via increased blood volume.

Medications under investigation

- Calcium channel blockers (e.g., nimodipine): may reduce deficit by promoting collateral circulation via vasodilation and thereby decrease cerebral ischemia.
- Ancrod: a purified protein fraction of venom from the Malayan pit viper, which rapidly decreases circulating fibrinogen. The reduction in blood viscosity from this defibrinogenation produces a hemodilutional state, which increases cerebral blood flow to the ischemic brain. Impending infarction may be reversed with early intervention (e.g., ideally within 1-2 hr but no more than 6 hr from onset).
- Neural protectants: some classes of these drugs are glutamate inhibitors and antagonists, N-methyl-d-aspartate (NMDA) antagonists, free radical scavengers, and gangliosides.

Physical medicine and rehabilitation: To help patient maintain mobility and independence with ADL; may include physical therapy (PT), occupational therapy (OT), and assistive devices or braces. Muscle-strengthening exercises, conditioning exercises, swallowing facilitation exercises, and gait training are also frequently prescribed. Reinforce special mobilization techniques, such as Bobath method, which focuses on restoring bilateral function and incorporating affected side into weight bearing, or proprioceptive neuromuscular facilitation (PNF), which focuses on using reflex and patterning techniques.

ROM: To maintain or increase joint function and prevent contractures. Exercises may include passive ROM, active ROM, or active-assistive ROM. Passive ROM is started immediately for all joints.

Functional electrical stimulation (FES): To improve arm function and reduce shoulder subluxation in the hemiplegic patient.

Speech therapy: To help aphasic and dysarthric patients.

Antiembolism hose or sequential compression sleeves: To help prevent thrombophlebitis and deep vein thrombosis.

Bowel and bladder programs: A bowel program should be initiated to prevent constipation and incontinence. The patient initially may have an indwelling catheter but should soon start a bladder program to prevent incontinence or retention.

Typically, patients are placed in ICU in the immediate postoperative period for the following surgeries:

Carotid endarterectomy: Surgical removal of plaque in the obstructed artery to increase blood supply to the brain. The carotid is clamped while the artery is opened, the plaque removed, and the artery sutured or patched. Cerebral blood flow studies and EEG monitoring may be done during the procedure. A shunt is sometimes done while the carotid is occluded. This is treatment of choice for patients with TIAs or RINDs or asymptomatic patients with stenosis >70% when a lesion lies at or near the carotid bifurcation. This procedure is not generally done for patients who have experienced a CVA unless it is performed to correct a stenosis to the unaffected hemisphere.

Cerebral artery bypass surgery: Anastomosis of an extracranial vessel to an intracranial vessel to increase blood flow to the brain. The patient typically has an occlusion in the internal carotid artery that is not accessible through the neck. Most commonly, the superficial temporal artery is anastomosed to the middle cerebral artery to provide collateral circulation to the area distal to the stenosis. Another frequent bypass is the subclavian artery to the external carotid artery (ECA). Difficult posterior circulation bypasses also are being attempted and include anastomosis of the occipital branch of the ECA to the posterior inferior cerebellar artery. These procedures usually are limited to patients with TIAs and RINDs. The recipient artery also must be clamped 20-30 min to obtain a satisfactory anastomosis.

Craniotomy: To evacuate a hematoma, repair a ruptured aneurysm, or apply arterial clips or plastic spray to the involved vessel to prevent further rupture. Craniotomy may be performed also to do an embolectomy. This is a controversial procedure. If done, it must be performed within 6-12 hr of the occlusion. (See "Brain Tumors," p. 288, for patient care.)

Balloon angioplasty and intraarterial stent: Used, on a trial basis, to correct stenosed vessels. Endovascular laser and ultrasound probes are also undergoing trials as methods to open blockages in intracranial vessels.

NURSING DIAGNOSES AND INTERVENTIONS

Unilateral neglect related to disturbed perceptual ability secondary to neurologic insult

Desired outcome: Following intervention and on an ongoing basis, patient scans the environment and responds to stimuli on the affected side.

- Assess patient's ability to recognize objects to the right or left of his or her visual midline; perceive body parts as his or her own; perceive pain, touch, and temperature sensations; judge distances; orient self to changes in the environment; differentiate left from right; maintain posture sense; and identify objects by sight, hearing, or touch. Document specific deficits.
- Neglect of and inattention to stimuli on the affected side occur more often with right hemisphere injury. Neglect cannot be totally explained on the basis of loss of physical senses (e.g., both ears are used in hearing, but

with auditory neglect, patient may ignore conversation or noises that occur on the affected side). Assess patient for neglect of the affected side as follows:

—*Visual neglect:* patient does not turn his or her head to see all parts of an object (e.g., may read only half of a page or eat from only one side of the plate). When the patient exhibits signs of visual neglect, continue to place objects necessary for ADL and call bells on the unaffected side and approach patient from that side, but gradually increase stimuli on the affected side (e.g., while communicating with patient, physically move across her or his visual boundary and stand on that side to shift the patient's attention to the neglected side; encourage patient to turn his or her head past the midline and scan the entire environment; place patient's food on the neglected side, and encourage patient to look to the neglected side and name the food before eating; place a bright red tape or ribbon on the affected side, and encourage patient to scan and find it). Continuously clue patient to the environment. Initially place patient's unaffected side toward the most active part of the room, but as compensation occurs, reverse this. As the patient begins to compensate, place additional items out of his or her visual field.

—*Self-neglect:* patient does not perceive his or her arm or leg as being a part of the body. For example, when combing or brushing the hair, patient attends to only one (the unaffected) side of the head. Inadequate self-care and injury may occur. Encourage patients to touch or massage and look at their affected sides and make a conscious effort to care for neglected body parts; also, check them for proper position to ensure against contractures and skin breakdown. To enhance patient's self-recognition, periodically refer to the patient's body parts on the neglected side. When patient is in bed or up in a chair, provide safety measures, such as side rails and restraints, to prevent patient from attempting to get up, which can occur because of unawareness of the affected side. Teach patient to use unaffected arm to perform ROM exercises on the affected side. Integrate patient's neglected arm into activities. Position arm on the bedside table or wheelchair lap board with the hand or arm past the midline, where patient can see it. Teach patient to attend to the affected side first when performing ADL, consciously look for the affected side, monitor its position, and check for exposure to sharp objects and irritants. Provide a mirror so that patients can watch themselves shave or brush their teeth and hair. Instruct patient to take precautions with hot or cold items or when around moving machinery. Teach the use of an arm sling to support the affected arm when patient is out of bed and when in bed to elevate the affected arm. Stand on patient's affected side when ambulating with patient.

—*Auditory neglect:* patient ignores individuals who approach and speak from his or her affected side but communicates with those who approach or speak from the unaffected side. To stimulate patient's attention to the affected side, move across the auditory boundary while speaking, and continue speaking from the patient's neglected side to bring patient's attention to that area.

• Arrange the environment to maximize performance of ADL by keeping necessary objects, such as the call light, on patient's unaffected side. If possible, move the bed so that the patient's unaffected side faces the largest section of the room. Approach and speak to the patient from the unaffected side. If you must approach the affected side, announce yourself, to avoid startling the patient. Perform activities on the unaffected side unless you are specifically attempting to stimulate the neglected side. After attempting to stimulate the neglected side, return to patient's unaffected side for activities and communication. Inform significant other about patient's deficit and compensatory interventions.

◎ NIC: Environmental Management: Safety; Peripheral Sensation Management; Positioning; Unilateral Neglect Management

Impaired physical mobility related to neuromuscular impairment with limited use of the upper and/or lower limbs secondary to CVA
Desired outcome: By at least 24 hr before hospital discharge, patient and significant other demonstrate techniques that promote ambulating and transferring.

- Teach patient methods for turning and moving, using the stronger extremity to move the weaker extremity. For example, to move the affected leg in bed or when changing from a lying to a sitting position, slide the unaffected foot under the affected ankle to lift, support, and bring the affected leg along in the desired movement.
- Encourage patient to make a conscious attempt to look at the extremities and check position before moving. Remind patient to make a conscious effort to lift and then extend the foot when ambulating.
- Instruct patient with impaired sense of balance to compensate by leaning toward the stronger side. (The tendency is to lean toward the weaker or paralyzed side.) As necessary, remind patient to keep body weight forward over the feet when standing.
- Protect impaired arm with a sling to support the arm and shoulder when the patient is up to help maintain anatomic position. Position patient in correct alignment, and provide a pillow or lap board for support. Encourage active/passive ROM to improve muscle tone. Avoid pulling on the patient's shoulders or arms; use a lift sheet to reposition in bed. Monitor for subluxation of the shoulder (e.g., shoulder pain and tenderness, swelling, decreased ROM, altered appearance of bony prominences).
- General principles when transferring include:
  —Encourage weight bearing on patient's stronger side. Use a transfer belt to safely support the patient during transfers without excessive stress on upper extremities.
  —Instruct patient to pivot on the stronger side and use the stronger arm for support.
  —Teach patient that transferring toward the unaffected side is generally easiest and safest.
  —Instruct patient to place the unaffected side closest to the bed or chair he or she wishes to transfer to.
  —Explain that when transferring, the affected leg should be under the patient with the foot flat on the ground.
  —Position a braced chair or locked wheelchair close to patient's stronger side. If patient requires assistance from staff member, teach patient not to support self by pulling on or placing hands around assistant's neck. Staff members should use their own knees and feet to brace the feet and knees of patients who are very weak.
- Obtain PT and OT referrals as appropriate. Reinforce special mobilization techniques (e.g., Bobath, PNF) per patient's individualized rehabilitation program. These techniques may vary from the above general principles (e.g., Bobath focuses on the use of the affected side in mobility training).

◎ NIC: Exercise Therapy: Ambulation; Exercise Therapy: Balance; Exercise Therapy: Muscle Control; Positioning: Neurologic; Positioning: Wheelchair; Teaching: Prescribed Activity/Exercise

Sensory/perceptual alterations related to altered sensory reception, transmission, and/or integration secondary to neurologic damage
Desired outcome: Following intervention and on an ongoing basis, patient interacts appropriately with his or her environment and does not exhibit evidence of injury caused by sensory/perceptual deficit.

- Patients who have a dominant (left) hemisphere injury usually have normal awareness of their body and spatial orientation despite possible lack of or decreased pain sensation, position sense, and visual field deficit on the right side of the body. These patients may need reminders to scan their environment but usually do not exhibit unilateral neglect. They tend to be slow, cautious, and disorganized when approaching an unfamiliar problem and benefit from frequent, accurate, and immediate feedback on their performance. They may respond well to nonverbal encouragement, such as a pat on the back. Because of a short attention span and impaired logical reasoning, the patient is easily distracted, so give short, simple messages or questions and step-by-step directions. Because the patient may have poor abstract thinking, keep conversation on a concrete level (e.g., say "water," not "fluid"; "leg," not "limb"). These patients may have difficulty recognizing items by touch and benefit from touching them (e.g., washcloth, comb) and having caretaker name them.
- Patients with nondominant (right) hemisphere injury also may have decreased pain sensation, pain sense, and visual field deficit but typically are unaware of or deny their deficits or lost abilities. They tend to be impulsive and too quick with movements. Typically, they have impaired judgment about what they can or cannot do and often overestimate their abilities. Encourage these patients to slow down and check each step or task as it is completed. These individuals are at risk for burns, bruises, cuts, and falls and may need to be restrained from attempting unsafe activities. They also are more likely to have unilateral neglect (see **Unilateral neglect,** p. 310). The patient generally retains the ability to think logically but sees specifics rather than the global picture (i.e., can see the trees but not the forest). Be careful what you say because it may be taken literally (e.g., if you say "ate the lion's share," the patient may think that someone literally ate the lion's portion of the meal). Impaired ability to recognize subtle distinctions may occur (e.g., the difference between a fork and spoon may become too subtle to detect).
- Patients with apraxia have an inability to carry out previously learned motor tasks, although they may be able to describe them in detail. Have these patients return your demonstration of the task. They may be able to be talked through a task or may be able to talk themselves through a task step-by-step.
- Patients may have visual field deficits in which they can physically see only a portion of the normal visual field. Encourage making a conscious effort to scan the rest of the environment by turning the head from side to side.
- Patients with nondominant (right) hemisphere injury also may have the following sensory/perceptual alterations:
  - —Impaired ability to recognize, associate, or interpret sounds (e.g., voice quality, animal noises, musical pieces, types of instruments): direct patient's attention to a particular sound (e.g., if a cat meows on the television, state that it is the sound a cat makes and point to the cat on the screen).
  - —Visual-spatial misconception: for example, patient may underestimate distances and bump into doors or confuse the inside and outside of an object, such as an article of clothing. These patients may lose their place when reading or adding up numbers and therefore never complete the task. Marking the outer aspects of their shoes or tagging the inside sleeve of a sweater or pair of pants with an "L" and "R" may help self-dressing efforts. They will benefit from a structured, consistent environment.
  - —Difficulty recognizing and associating familiar objects: these patients may not recognize dangerous or hazardous objects because they do not know the purpose of the object. Assist these individuals with eating because they may not know the purpose of silverware. Monitor the environment for safety hazards, and remove unsafe objects, such as scissors, from the bedside.

—Inability to orient self in space: these patients may require a restraint or wheelchair belt for support because they may not know if they are standing, sitting, or leaning.

—Misconception of own body and body parts: these patients may not perceive their foot or arm as being a part of their body. Teach them to concentrate on their body parts (e.g., by watching their feet carefully while walking).

—Impaired ability to recognize objects by means of the senses of hearing, vibration, or touch: these patients rely more on visual cues. Keep their environment simple to reduce sensory overload and enable concentration on visual cues. Remove distracting stimuli.

NIC: Activity Therapy; Peripheral Sensation Management; Surveillance; Teaching: Individual

Impaired verbal communication related to aphasia secondary to cerebrovascular insult
Desired outcome: At least 24 hr before hospital discharge, patient demonstrates improved self-expression and relates decreased frustration with communication.

Note: Aphasia is the partial or complete inability to use or comprehend language and symbols and may occur with dominant (left) hemisphere damage. It is not the result of impaired hearing or intelligence. There are many different types of aphasia. Generally the patient has a combination of types, which vary in severity. *Receptive aphasia* (e.g., Wernicke's, sensory, or "nonfluent" aphasia) is characterized by inability to recognize or comprehend spoken words. It is as if a foreign language were being spoken or the patient has word deafness. The patient often is good at responding to nonverbal cues. *Expressive aphasia* (e.g., Broca's, motor, or "fluent" aphasia) is characterized by difficulty expressing words or naming objects. Gestures, groans, swearing, or nonsense words may be used.

- Evaluate the nature and severity of the patient's aphasia. When doing so, avoid giving nonverbal cues. Assess patient's ability to point or look toward a specific object, follow simple directions, understand yes/no questions, understand complex questions, repeat both simple and complex words, repeat sentences, name objects that are shown, demonstrate or relate the purpose or action of the object, fulfill written requests, write requests, and read. When evaluating patient for aphasia, be aware that patient may be responding to nonverbal cues and may understand less than you think. Document this assessment with simple descriptions and specific examples of patient's aphasia symptoms. Use it as the basis for a communication plan.
- Obtain a referral to a speech therapist or pathologist as needed. Provide therapist with a list of words that would enhance patient's independence and/or care. In addition, ask for tips that will help improve communication with patient.
- When communicating with patient, try to reduce distractions in the environment, such as television or others' conversations. Because fatigue affects a person's ability to communicate, try to ensure that patient is well rested.
- Communicate with patient as much as possible. General principles for patients who may not recognize or comprehend the spoken word include the following: face patient and establish eye contact, speak slowly and clearly, give patient time to process your communication and answer, keep messages short and simple, stay with one clearly defined subject, avoid questions with multiple choices but rather phrase questions so that they can be

answered "yes" or "no," and use the same words each time you repeat a statement or question (e.g., pill vs. medication, bathroom vs. toilet). If patient does not understand after repetition, try different words. Use gestures, facial expressions, and pantomime to supplement and reinforce your message. Give short, simple directions, and repeat as needed to ensure understanding. Use concrete terms (e.g., water instead of fluid, leg instead of limb).

- When helping patients regain use of symbolic language, start with nouns first and progress to more complex statements as indicated, using verbs, pronouns, and adjectives. For continuity, keep a record at the bedside of words to be used (e.g., pill rather than medication).
- Treat patient as an adult. It is not necessary to raise the volume of your voice unless patient is hard of hearing. Be respectful.
- When patients have difficulty expressing words or naming objects, encourage them to repeat words after you for practice in verbal expression. Begin with simple words such as "yes" or "no," and progress to others, such as "cup." Progress to more complex statements as indicated. Listen and respond to patient's communication efforts; otherwise patient may give up. Praise accomplishments. Be prepared for labile emotions because these patients become frustrated and emotional when faced with their impaired speech.
- When improvement is noted, let patient complete your sentence (e.g., "This is a _____."). Keep a list of words patient can say, and add to the list as appropriate. Use this list when forming questions patient can answer. Avoid finishing patient's sentences.
- Patients who have lost the ability to monitor their verbal output may not produce sensible language but may think they are making sense and not understand why others do not comprehend or respond appropriately to them. Avoid labeling patient as belligerent or confused when the problem is aphasia and frustration. Listen for errors in conversation, and provide feedback.
- Patients who have lost the ability to recognize number symbols or relationships will have difficulty understanding time concepts or telling time. Avoid instructing patient to "wait 5 min" because this may not be meaningful.
- Give practice in receiving word images by pointing to an object and clearly stating its name. Watch signals patient gives you.
- Patients with nondominant (right) hemisphere damage often have no difficulty speaking; however, they may use excessive detail, give irrelevant information, and get off on a tangent. Bring patients back to the subject by saying, "Let's go back to what we were talking about." These patients tend to respond better to verbal, rather than nonverbal, encouragement.
- Provide a supportive and relaxed environment for those patients who are unable to form words or sentences or speak clearly or appropriately. If patient makes an error, do not criticize patient's effort but rather compliment it by saying, "That was a good try." Do not react negatively to patient's emotional displays. Address and acknowledge patient's frustration over the inability to communicate. Maintain a calm and positive attitude. If you do not understand patient, say so. Ask patient to repeat unclear words, ask for more clues, ask patient to use another word, or have patient point to the object. Observe for nonverbal cues, and anticipate patient's needs. Allow time to listen if patient speaks slowly. To validate patient's message, repeat or rephrase it aloud.
- Ensure that the call light is available and patient knows how to use it.
- Dysarthria can complicate aphasia. For additional interventions for patients with dysarthria, see **Impaired verbal communication** in "General Care of Patients With Neurologic Disorders," p. 338.

NIC: Active Listening; Communication Enhancement: Speech Deficit; Surveillance: Safety; Teaching: Individual

Knowledge deficit: Cerebral artery bypass surgery

Desired outcome: Before the procedure, patient verbalizes understanding about the surgical procedure, including the purpose, risks, and anticipated benefits or outcome.

- After health care provider has explained the cerebral artery bypass surgery to the patient, determine patient's level of understanding. Reinforce information or clarify as indicated.
- As indicated, explain that cerebral artery bypass surgery connects an extracranial vessel to an intracranial vessel to bypass an obstruction and increase blood flow to the brain.
- Describe the following postoperative interventions that may occur in the ICU during the immediate postoperative period:
  —VS and neurologic status checks are performed at least hourly: patient will be asked to squeeze the examiner's hands, move extremities, answer questions, and extend the tongue. Emphasize the importance of performing these activities to the best of patient's ability and reporting any numbness, tingling, or weakness. Neurologic deficits, especially differences on either side of the body or face or indicators of IICP, will be reported to health care provider.
  —Inform patient that he or she will probably have a mild headache.
  —BP will be monitored frequently, and patient may require vasoactive medications to keep BP within prescribed parameters. Hypertension can cause bypass stretching and bleeding, with loss of anastomosis and graft. Hypotension may promote thrombosis, with loss of graft.
  —Strict bedrest usually is enforced for 24-48 hr.
  —For patients with bypass surgery involving the temporal artery, prevention of impaired perfusion to the temporal area graft site is a key consideration. HOB probably will be elevated 30 degrees, and the head, neck, and body will be kept in good alignment to prevent neck flexion or hyperextension. It is critical that there be no pressure on the graft site. Explain that the patient will be positioned away from the operative side. Dressings will be kept loose to prevent constriction of the graft site. The patient can expect the elastic bands on nasal cannulas or O_2 masks to be taped to the face to ensure they do not constrict the head, neck, and graft. Eyeglasses are contraindicated unless the earpiece on the operative side is removed. These precautions with eyeglasses and other constrictive gear usually are in effect for 3 mo after surgery.
  —The head dressing will be checked at frequent intervals for drainage and tightness. The scalp may swell after surgery, causing the dressing to tighten. The dressing should be loose enough to slip a finger beneath. Instruct patient to report any burning sensation on the scalp, which may indicate ischemia.
  —Graft patency will be assessed periodically either by palpation or using a Doppler probe on the temporal pulse.
  —The patient can expect anticoagulant and/or antiplatelet therapy for 3-6 mo after the procedure.
  —Precautions are taken against IICP (see "General Care of Patients with Neurologic Disorders" for **Decreased adaptive capacity:** Intracranial related to risk of IICP, p. 340). Teach these precautions to patient and significant other.

Caution: Credé's method and other interventions that increase intrathoracic or intraabdominal pressure are contraindicated until the risk of IICP is no longer a factor.

- For additional interventions, see **Knowledge deficit**: Surgical procedure, p. 717, in Appendix One, "Caring for Preoperative and Postoperative Patients."

◎ **NIC:** Circulatory Precautions; Teaching: Individual; Teaching: Preoperative; Teaching: Prescribed Activity/Exercise; Teaching: Procedure/Treatment

Knowledge deficit: Carotid endarterectomy procedure
Desired outcome: Before surgery, patient verbalizes understanding of the carotid endarterectomy procedure, including the purpose, risks, expected benefits or outcome, and postsurgical care.

- After health care provider has explained the procedure to the patient, determine patient's level of understanding and reinforce or clarify information as needed.
- As indicated, explain that carotid endarterectomy is the removal of plaque in the obstructed artery to increase blood supply to the brain.
- Describe the following postsurgical assessments that usually will occur in the ICU during the immediate postsurgical period:
  —Monitoring of VS and neurologic status at least hourly. Explain that the patient may be asked to swallow, move the tongue, smile, speak, and shrug shoulders to determine facial drooping, tongue weakness, hoarseness, dysphagia, shoulder weakness, or loss of facial sensation, which are signs of cranial nerve impairment. Stretching of the cranial nerves during surgery can occur, causing edema, and may leave a temporary deficit. The patient should report any numbness, tingling, or weakness, which may indicate occlusion of the carotid. In addition, the superficial temporal and facial pulses will be palpated for strength, quality, and symmetry to evaluate the patency of the external carotid artery.
  —Periodic assessment of the neck for edema, hematoma, bleeding, or tracheal deviation. Explain that the patient should report immediately any respiratory distress, difficulty managing secretions, or sensation of neck tightness. Additional O_2 will most likely be supplied, even without respiratory distress or airway compromise, because manipulation of the carotid sinus may cause temporary loss of normal physiologic response to hypoxia.
  —Pulse oximetry may be continuously monitored. Report readings <92% to health care providers.
  —Frequent BP checks may be performed because temporary carotid sinus dysfunction may cause BP problems (usually hypertension). The patient may need vasoactive medications to keep BP within a specified range to maintain cerebral perfusion while preventing disruption of graft or sutures.
  —HOB must be maintained in prescribed position (flat or elevated), and patient generally is positioned off the operative side.
  —A closed drainage system with suction may be left in the neck for a few days. Ice packs may be prescribed for the incision to reduce edema formation and pain.
  —Anticoagulant/antiplatelet therapy (e.g., aspirin, warfarin) is usually instituted for 3-6 mo after the procedure.
- For additional interventions, see **Knowledge deficit:** Surgical procedure, p. 717, in Appendix One, "Caring for Preoperative and Postoperative Patients."

◎ **NIC:** Circulatory Precautions; Teaching: Individual; Teaching: Preoperative; Teaching: Prescribed Activity/Exercise; Teaching: Procedure/Treatment

See Also: "Pulmonary Embolus" for **Altered protection** related to risk of prolonged bleeding or hemorrhage secondary to anticoagulant therapy, p. 18; Chapter 3 for related diagnoses for incontinence (p. 177), retention (p. 185), and neurogenic bladder (p. 188); "Alzheimer's Disease" for **Impaired environmental interpretation syndrome**, p. 239; "Head Injury" for **Risk for disuse syndrome** related to prolonged inactivity, p. 282; **Fluid volume excess** (related to SIADH), p. 283; "Brain Tumors" for **Knowledge deficit:** Craniotomy procedure, p. 290, for patients undergoing surgery; "Seizure Disorders," p. 324, for related nursing diagnoses; "General Care of Patients With Neurologic Disorders" for **Risk for trauma** related to unsteady gait, p. 331; **Risk for injury** related to impaired pain, touch, and temperature sensations, p. 332; **Impaired corneal tissue integrity**, p. 333; **Altered nutrition:** Less than body requirements, p. 333; **Risk for fluid volume deficit**, p. 335; **Risk for aspiration**, p. 335; **Self-care deficit**, p. 336; **Constipation**, p. 339; **Decreased adaptive capacity:** Intracranial, p. 336; **Impaired swallowing**, p. 344; **Sensory/perceptual alterations** (visual), p. 342; **Knowledge deficit:** Neurologic diagnostic tests, p. 346; "Diabetes Insipidus," p. 362, for patients with this disorder or who are at risk; "Pressure Ulcers," p. 710; Appendix One, "Caring for Patients on Prolonged Bedrest," p. 738, for nursing diagnoses and interventions related to immobility (adjust interventions accordingly if patient has IICP or is at risk for this problem); Appendix One, "Caring for Patients With Cancer and Other Life-disrupting Illnesses," p. 791, for appropriate psychosocial nursing diagnoses.

PATIENT-FAMILY TEACHING AND DISCHARGE PLANNING

When providing patient-family teaching, focus on sensory information; avoid giving excessive information; and initiate a visiting nurse referral for necessary follow-up teaching. Consider including verbal and written information about the following:

- Importance of minimizing or treating the following risk factors: diabetes mellitus, hypertension, high cholesterol, high Na^+ intake, obesity, inactivity, smoking, prolonged bedrest, and stressful life-style.
- Interventions that increase effective communication in the presence of aphasia or dysarthria. Additional patient information can be obtained by contacting the following organization:

  National Aphasia Association
  156 Fifth Ave., Suite 707
  New York, NY 10010   (800) 922-4622
  WWW address: *http://www.aphasia.org/*

- Referrals to the following as appropriate: public health nurse, visiting nurses association, psychologic therapy, vocational rehabilitation agency, home health agencies, and extended and skilled care facilities. Also provide the following address:

  National Stroke Association
  96 Inverness Drive East, Suite I
  Englewood, CO 80112   (303) 649-9229 or (800) 787-6537
  WWW address: *http://www.stroke.org/*

- For patient information pamphlets, contact the following organization:

  National Institute of Neurological Disorders and Stroke (NINDS)
  Box 5801 Bethesda, MD 20892   (800) 352-9424
  WWW address: *http://www.ninds.nih.gov/*

- Additional general information can be obtained by contacting the following organizations:

  National Center for Cardiac Information
  8180 Greensboro Drive #1070
  McLean, VA 22102   (703) 356-6568

  Stroke Connection/American Heart Association
  Manager
  7272 Greenville Avenue
  Dallas, TX 75231   (800) 553-6321
  WWW address: *http://www.amhrt.org/*

See Also: Teaching and discharge planning (third through tenth entries only) under "Multiple Sclerosis," p. 209.

Section Six: Seizure Disorders

Seizures result from an abnormal, uncontrolled, electrical discharge from the neurons of the cerebral cortex in response to a stimulus. If the activity is localized in one portion of the brain, the individual will have a partial seizure, but when it is widespread and diffuse, a generalized seizure occurs. Symptoms vary widely, depending on the involved area of the cerebral cortex. Seizures are generally manifested as an alteration in sensation, behavior, movement, perception, or consciousness lasting from seconds to several minutes. *Epilepsy* is a term used for recurrent seizures.

Seizure threshold refers to the amount of stimulation needed to cause the neural activity. Although anyone can have a seizure if the stimulus is sufficient, the seizure threshold is lowered in some individuals and this may result in spontaneous seizures. Potential causes for lowered seizure threshold include congenital defects; head injury, particularly that from a penetrating wound; subarachnoid hemorrhage; intracranial tumors; infections, such as meningitis or encephalitis; exposure to toxins, such as lead; hypoxia; drug withdrawal; and metabolic and endocrine disorders, such as hypoglycemia, hypocalcemia, uremia, hypoparathyroidism, excessive hydration, and fever. Phenothiazine, tricyclic antidepressants, and alcohol usage increase the risk of seizure by lowering the seizure threshold. For susceptible individuals, triggers may include emotional tension or stress; physical stimulation, such as loud music or bright, flashing lights; lack of sleep or food; fatigue; menses or pregnancy; and excessive drug/alcohol use. If a trigger stimulus is identified, the individual has what is termed *reflex epilepsy.*

Although a seizure itself generally is not fatal, individuals can be injured by hitting their head or breaking bones if they lose consciousness and fall to the ground. Seizure activity increases cerebral O_2 consumption by 60% and cerebral blood flow by 250%. Instances of prolonged and repeated generalized seizures, *status epilepticus,* can be life threatening because exhaustion, anoxia, respiratory arrest, and cardiovascular collapse can occur.

ASSESSMENT

There are many kinds of seizures (Table 4-4), but the following are the most serious or common.

Generalized tonic-clonic (grand mal):   Possible prodromal phase of increased irritability, tension, mood changes, or headache preceding the seizure

T A B L E 4 - 4   International Classification of Epileptic Seizures

I. Partial (seizure began in a local area)
   A. Simple (consciousness not impaired)
      1. Motor (with or without jacksonian march)
      2. Sensory or somatosensory
      3. Autonomic
      4. Psychic
   B. Complex (consciousness is impaired; may occur with or without automatisms)
      1. Simple partial onset—progresses to impaired consciousness
      2. Consciousness impaired at onset
   C. Secondarily generalized
      1. Simple partial onset—progresses to generalized seizure
      2. Complex partial onset—progresses to generalized seizure
      3. Simple partial to complex partial to generalized seizure
II. Generalized (associated with loss of consciousness; may be convulsive or nonconvulsive, bilateral without focal onset)
   A. Absence (petit mal)
   B. Myoclonic
   C. Clonic
   D. Tonic
   E. Tonic-clonic (grand mal)
   F. Atonic (drop attacks)
III. Unclassified (because of inadequate or incomplete data)

Modified from Commission on Classification and Terminology of the International League Against Epilepsy, 1981.

by hours or days. Patient may experience an aura (a sensory warning, such as a sound, odor, or flash of light) immediately preceding the seizure by seconds or minutes. The seizure usually does not last more than 2-6 min and includes the following phases.

Tonic (rigid/contracted):   Often lasts only 15 sec, usually subsiding in less than 1 min. Symptoms include loss of consciousness, clenched jaws (potential for tongue to be bitten), apnea (may hear a cry as air is forced out of the lungs), and cyanosis. The patient may be incontinent, and the pupils may dilate and become nonreactive to light.

Clonic (rhythmic contraction and relaxation of the extremities and muscles): May subside in 30 sec but can last 2-5 min. The eyes roll upward, and excessive salivation results in foaming at the mouth. During this phase, the potential is greatest for biting the tongue.

Stupor: May last 5 min. The individual is limp and unresponsive. The pupils begin to react to light and return to their normal size.

Postictal: In the period immediately after the seizure, the patient may be sleepy, semiconscious, confused, unable to speak clearly, and uncoordinated, have a headache, complain of muscle aches, and have no recollection of the seizure event. Temporary weakness, dysphasia, or hemianopia lasting up to 24 hr after the seizure may be experienced.

Generalized absence (petit mal):   Patient has momentary loss of awareness with an abrupt cessation of voluntary muscle activity. The patient may appear to be daydreaming with a vacant stare. Patient may experience facial, eyelid, or hand twitching. The patient usually does not lose general body muscle tone and so does not fall. The individual resumes previous activity when the seizure ends. There is usually no memory of the seizure, and the patient may have difficulty reorienting after the seizure event. This type of seizure can last 1-10 sec and may occur up to 100 times/day. This type of seizure usually resolves by puberty.

Generalized myoclonic: Sudden, very brief contraction or jerking of muscles or muscle groups. The individual may have a very brief, momentary loss of consciousness with some postictal confusion.

Partial simple motor (focal motor seizures):   An irritative focus located in the motor cortex of the frontal lobe causes clonic movement in a particular part of the body, such as the hands or face. If the seizure activity spreads or marches in an orderly fashion to an adjacent area (e.g., the hands to the arms to the shoulders), the seizure is termed a *focal motor seizure with jacksonian march*. The seizure usually lasts several seconds to minutes. There is no loss of consciousness. Other simple, partial seizures with somatosensory symptoms (e.g., smells, sounds), autonomic symptoms (e.g., tachycardia, tachypnea, diaphoresis, goose bumps [piloerection], pallor, flushing), or psychic symptoms (e.g., fear, déja vu) may be experienced.

Partial complex seizure (psychomotor):   Generally lasts 1-4 min. Usually there is loss of consciousness and a postictal state of confusion lasting several minutes. However, the individual does not fall to the ground. The patient is able to interact with the environment, exhibits purposeful but inappropriate movements or behavior, and has no memory of the event. The individual will perform such automatisms as lip smacking, chewing, facial grimacing, picking, or swallowing movements. These patients may experience and remember various sensory or emotional hallucinations or sensations that occur immediately before the seizure, such as smells, ringing or hissing sounds, or feelings of déja vu, fear, or pleasure.

Status epilepticus: State of continuous or rapidly recurring seizures in which the individual does not completely recover baseline neurologic functioning between seizures. Individuals who suddenly stop taking their antiepilepsy medication are likely to develop this condition. This is a medical emergency, resulting in potential complications, such as cerebral anoxia and edema, aspiration, hyperthermia, and exhaustion. Irreversible damage may occur in 60 min. Death may result.

DIAGNOSTIC TESTS

Because a variety of problems can precipitate seizures, testing may be extensive. Common tests include the following:

Serum electrolytes: To rule out metabolic causes, such as hypoglycemia, hyponatremia, or hypocalcemia.

EEG—both sleeping and awake: To reveal abnormal patterns of electrical activity, particularly with such stimuli as flashing lights or hyperventilation. Telemetry EEGs may also be performed. Generalized tonic-clonic seizures show up as high, fast-voltage spikes in all leads.

MRI: To show structural lesions causing partial seizures; also may reveal a space-occupying lesion such as a tumor or hematoma.

Positron emission tomography (PET):   To check for areas of cerebral glucose hypometabolism that correlate with the irritative seizure-causing focus. This test is useful in partial seizures.

CT scan: To check for presence of a space-occupying lesion, such as a tumor or hematoma.

Skull x-rays: To reveal fractures, tumors, calcifications, or congenital anomalies (pineal shift, ventricular deformity).

Lumbar puncture (LP) and CSF analysis: To rule out IICP or infection, such as meningitis, as the source of the seizures.

Single photon emission computerized tomography (SPECT):   To measure cerebral blood flow; may be used to evaluate patients for surgery.

> **See Also:** "General Care of Patients With Neurologic Disorders" for
> **Knowledge deficit:** Neurologic diagnostic tests, p. 346, for care consider-
> ations for patients undergoing EEG, PET, MRI, CT scan, and LP.

COLLABORATIVE MANAGEMENT

Antiepilepsy drugs: To help prevent seizure activity. Monotherapy is usually
indicated until either lack of seizure control is evident or toxicity occurs, at
which time additional medications are added to the regimen.
Hydantoin derivatives (e.g., phenytoin, mephenytoin, ethotoin):   For tonic-
clonic, partial simple, and partial complex seizures.
Carbamazepine: For tonic-clonic, partial simple, and partial complex
seizures.
Valproic acid: For absence, tonic-clonic, and mixed seizure types.
Succinimide derivatives (e.g., ethosuximide):   For absence seizures.
Barbiturate derivatives (e.g., phenobarbital, primidone):   May be used in
conjunction with one of the antiepilepsy drugs listed above or as monotherapy
for tonic-clonic or partial seizures. Other agents used to treat partial seizures
include gabapentin, lamotrigine, felbamate, or topiramate.

> **Note:**   If the patient is seizure free for 2-5 yr, medication tapering over
> several months and then discontinuation may be attempted under health care
> provider supervision.

Treatment of underlying causes: Such as metabolic disorder or infectious
process.
Stress management: Progressive relaxation training, diaphragmatic respiratory training, and biofeedback are used to reduce seizure frequency and severity
by controlling stress or hyperventilation trigger stimulation.
Nutrition: A balanced diet spaced evenly throughout the day is recommended to avoid hypoglycemia, which may trigger seizures. Patients are
advised to avoid caffeine and alcohol products and to prevent overhydration,
which also can precipitate seizure activity.
Counseling or psychotherapy: For patients with poor self-concept or coping
difficulties related to the diagnosis.
Surgery
Excision or evacuation of tumors or hematomas: Brain tumors or hematomas may be excised or evacuated if they are the source of seizure activity.
Excision of epileptogenic areas: For medically intractable seizures, excision
of known epileptogenic areas may be attempted to obtain seizure control.
Excision or evacuation may include cortical resection (e.g., temporal lobectomy
for partial seizures) and corpus callostomy (for generalized seizures). Corpus
callostomy is considered palliative and used to partially or completely
disconnect the cerebral hemispheres from one another to limit seizure spread
from one hemisphere to the other. To prevent increased or new neurologic
deficits, extensive presurgical testing is done, possibly including CT scan and
MRI to find structural abnormalities, angiograms to detect vascular abnormalities, 24-hr EEG monitoring (e.g., telemetry scalp EEG and video recording),
invasive intracranial EEG monitoring with depth or subdural "grid" electrodes,
and intracarotid sodium amytal test to determine hemispheric dominance and
function. Intraoperative mapping by electrocorticography also may be done.
Surgical procedures require a craniotomy (see "Brain Tumors," p. 288).
Implanted vagus nerve stimulation: May have an anticonvulsant effect on
partial seizures.

Management of status epilepticus
Respiratory management: O$_2$ therapy, oral airway suctioning, and intubation as needed to maintain airway and prevent hypoxia.
Assessment of blood glucose and administration of IV glucose: If indicated, to reverse hypoglycemia.
Serum laboratory studies: To evaluate for electrolyte (e.g., hyponatremia, hypocalcemia) or metabolic imbalances that may be causing seizures. Serum drug screens are performed to assess serum antiepilepsy drug level and determine the presence of alcohol or other drugs that may be causing the seizures.
Slow administration of IV diazepam or lorazepam, 2 mg/min: Initially given bolus. If seizures continue, diazepam occasionally is given in a continuous IV drip (10-15 mg/hr). **Note:** Monitor for signs of respiratory depression and hypotension.
Administration of IV phenytoin or fosphenytoin (Cerebyx): If diazepam is unsuccessful.

Note: Do not mix phenytoin with other medications and most IV fluids; give it slowly, undiluted, IV push, at no more than 50 mg/min. It should be given only with normal saline IV fluids because it will precipitate in the presence of D$_5$W. Monitor for hypotension, apnea, and cardiac dysrhythmias.

Note: Fosphenytoin is a water-soluble precursor of phenytoin that is rapidly converted to phenytoin in tissue and blood. Because this is a pro-drug, an equimolar dose of fosphenytoin, 1.5 mg, is required to yield 1 mg of phenytoin. Dosage of fosphenytoin is prescribed in phenytoin equivalents (PE). A vial of 750-mg PE fosphenytoin will provide an equivalent dose of 500 mg of phenytoin. This agent may be given IV or IM and has minimal local tissue irritation. IV dosage is 15-20 mg PE/kg (e.g., a 75-kg man would require 1125-1500 mg). Fosphenytoin should be diluted in D$_5$W or NS to a minimum of 25 mg PE/ml. Because hypotension can occur with too rapid IV administration, the infusion rate should not exceed 150 mg PE/min (infusion should take 7.5-10 min for a 75-kg man). Continuous ECG, BP, and respiration monitoring should be done when providing IV loading of this agent. Fosphenytoin must be refrigerated and has side effects similar to phenytoin with the exception of decreased local tissue irritation. Unique side effects include paresthesia and pruritus. This agent is contraindicated in patients with serious renal disease, renal failure, sinus bradycardia, or atrioventricular (A-V) block.

Administration of IV phenobarbital: If diazepam and phenytoin are unsuccessful. **Note:** Monitor for signs of respiratory depression.
Administration of thiamine: If alcohol withdrawal occurs or is suspected. Thiamine should be given before dextrose to protect against an exacerbation of Wernicke's encephalopathy.
Administration of glucocorticosteroids (e.g., dexamethasone): To relieve cerebral edema.
Administration of paraldehyde: If other medications are unsuccessful. **Note:** Because the solution reacts negatively with plastic, use a glass syringe for IM

and IV routes or a rubber catheter if it is given via retention enema. Occasionally lidocaine is administered.

Intubation and general anesthesia with large doses of short-acting barbiturate (e.g., phenobarbital) or neuromuscular blocking agent: For severe cases. Neuromuscular blocking agents may stop the movement but will not stop brain activity.

Search for the underlying cause: May include a wide variety of diagnostic tests (see diagnostic test section, p. 321). Patients in status epilepticus typically are transferred to ICU.

NURSING DIAGNOSES AND INTERVENTIONS

Risk for trauma with risk factors related to oral, musculoskeletal, and airway vulnerability secondary to seizure activity

Desired outcomes: Patient exhibits no signs of oral or musculoskeletal tissue injury or airway compromise after the seizure. Before hospital discharge, patient's significant other verbalizes knowledge of actions necessary during seizure activity.

Seizure precautions

- Pad side rails with blankets or pillows. Keep side rails up and the bed in its lowest position when the patient is in bed. Keep bed, wheelchair, or stretcher brakes locked.
- Tape a soft rubber oral airway to the bedside. Remove wooden tongue depressors (if used, they may splinter). Keep suction and oxygen equipment readily available. Consider a heparin lock for IV access for high-risk patient.
- Avoid using glass or other breakable oral thermometers when taking patient's temperature. If only breakable thermometers are available, take temperature via axillary or rectal route. Electronic tympanic thermometers are preferred for patients at high risk for seizure.
- Caution patients to lie down and push the call button if they experience a prodromal or aural warning. Encourage patient to empty the mouth of dentures or foreign objects. Keep call light within reach.
- Do not allow unsupervised smoking.
- Evaluate need for and provide protective headgear as indicated.

During the seizure

- Remain with patient. Observe for, record, and report type, duration, and characteristics of seizure activity and any postseizure response. This should include, as appropriate, precipitating event, aura, initial location and progression, automatisms, type and duration of movement, changes in LOC, eye movement (e.g., deviation, nystagmus), pupil size and reaction, bowel and bladder incontinence, head deviation, tongue deviation, or teeth clenching.
- Prevent or break the fall and ease patient to the floor if the seizure occurs while patient is out of bed. Keep patient in bed if the seizure occurs while there, and lower HOB to a flat position.
- If the patient's jaws are clenched, do not force an object between the teeth, because this can break teeth or lacerate oral mucous membranes. If able to do so safely and without damage to oral tissue, insert an airway. Tongue depressors should not be used, because they may splinter. A rolled washcloth may be used as an alternative. Never put your fingers in the patient's mouth.
- Protect patient's head from injury during seizure activity. A towel folded flat may be used to cushion the head from striking the ground. Be sure the head's position does not occlude the airway. Remove from the environment objects (e.g., chairs) that the patient may strike. Pad the floors to protect the patient's arms and legs. Remove patient's glasses.
- Do not restrain patient but rather guide the patient's movements gently to prevent injury.

- Roll patient into a side-lying position to promote drainage of secretions and maintain a patent airway. Use the head-tilt/chin-lift maneuver. Provide O_2 and suction as needed.
- Loosen tight clothing, collar, or belt.
- Maintain patient's privacy. Clear nonessential people from the room.
- Administer antiepilepsy drugs as prescribed.

After the seizure
- Reassure and gently reorient patient. Check neurologic status and VS; ask patient if an aura preceded the seizure activity. Record this information and postictal characteristics.
- Provide a quiet, calm environment because sounds and stimuli can be confusing to the awakening patient. Keep talk simple and to a minimum. Speak slowly and with pauses between sentences. Repeating may be necessary. Use room light that is behind, not above, patient to prevent additional seizures and for patient comfort. Do not offer food or drink until patient is fully awake.
- Check patient's tongue for lacerations and body for injuries. Monitor urine for red or cola color, which may signal rhabdomyolysis or myoglobinuria from muscle damage. Monitor for weakness or paralysis, dysphasia, or visual disturbances. If the patient vomited during the seizure, notify the health care provider because of the increased potential for aspiration.
- Check fingerstick blood glucose and obtain serum laboratory tests as prescribed. Administer antiepilepsy medication as prescribed.
- Monitor for status epilepticus (i.e., state of continuous or rapidly recurring seizures in which the individual does not completely recover baseline neurologic functioning). This condition is life threatening and can cause cerebral anoxia and edema, aspiration, hyperthermia, and exhaustion. Notify health care provider immediately.
- Provide significant other with verbal and written information for the preceding interventions.

NIC: Environmental Management: Safety; Positioning; Seizure Management; Seizure Precautions; Surveillance: Safety; Teaching: Disease Process; Teaching: Individual

Impaired tissue integrity (or risk of same) related to chemical irritation from IV phenytoin administration
Desired outcome: Patient's tissue surrounding the IV site remains undamaged as evidenced by absence of swelling, discoloration, discomfort, and blistering.
- If possible, avoid administering IV phenytoin through an insertion site in the wrist, hand, or foot. Ideally, IV phenytoin is administered through a central line. If a central line is not present, administer the drug through the largest-gauge needle possible.
- Monitor the insertion site for inflammation or infiltration before administering the drug. Check for line patency periodically during administration. Stop the injection immediately if there are any indicators of infiltration or inflammation.
- Flush the line with 0.9% NaCl before and after giving the drug to decrease the likelihood of irritation and prevent precipitation. Flush with enough solution to clear the line and tubing completely. Do not mix phenytoin with other medications. Phenytoin will precipitate in the presence of D_5W.
- Administer the drug undiluted and at a rate ≤50 mg/min. A more rapid administration rate will irritate the vein and also can cause hypotension, apnea, and cardiac dysrhythmias. For the older adult or a person with cardiovascular disease, a slower rate of 25 mg/min is recommended.

- After administration, inspect the insertion site often, for several hours. Monitor for swelling or discoloration. Instruct patient to report any pain at the site.
- Report any swelling or discoloration to the health care provider, and remove the vascular access device. Monitor for worsening discoloration, blistering, edema, or tissue sloughing. To control swelling, elevate patient's arm above the chest and, if prescribed, wrap the arm in warm compresses. Check circulation, sensation, and movement in the affected arm and hand, and report significant findings. Protect blisters with a sterile dressing.

NIC: Intravenous (IV) Therapy; Medication Administration; Medication Administration: Parenteral; Skin Surveillance

Knowledge deficit: Life-threatening environmental factors and preventive measures for seizures

Desired outcomes: Before hospital discharge, patient verbalizes accurate information about measures that may prevent seizures and environmental factors that can be life threatening in the presence of seizures. Patient exhibits health care measures that reflect this knowledge.

- Assess patient's knowledge of measures that can prevent seizures and environmental hazards that can be life threatening in the presence of seizure activity. Provide or clarify information as indicated.
- Advise patient to check into state regulations about automobile operation. Most states require 1-3 seizure-free years before an individual can obtain a driver's license.
- Caution patient to refrain from operating heavy or dangerous equipment, swimming, climbing excessive heights, and possibly even tub bathing until he or she is seizure free for the amount of time specified by health care provider. Teach patient never to swim alone, regardless of the amount of time he or she has been seizure free. Caution patient to swim only in shallow water and in the company of a strong swimmer, to make rescue easier if a seizure occurs.
- Advise patient to turn the temperature of hot water heaters down to prevent scalding if a seizure occurs in the shower.
- Encourage stress management, progressive relaxation techniques, and diaphragmatic respiratory training to control emotional stress and hyperventilation, which often trigger seizures.
- Advise patient that some activities, such as climbing or bicycle riding, require careful risk/benefit evaluation. The patient who decides to ride a bike should wear a helmet and avoid heavy traffic.
- Encourage vocational assessment and counseling. The patient's epilepsy may place others at risk in some occupations, such as bus driver or airline pilot.
- Advise female patients that seizure activity may change (increase or decrease) during menses or pregnancy. Tonic-clonic seizures have caused fetal death. Antiepilepsy drugs are associated with birth defects; however, 90% of women have normal pregnancies and healthy children. Provide birth control information if requested.
- Teach patient that use of stimulants (e.g., caffeine) and depressants (e.g., alcohol) should be avoided. Withdrawal from stimulants and depressants can increase the likelihood of seizures.
- Teach patient that getting adequate amounts of rest, avoiding physical and emotional stress, and maintaining a nutritious diet may help prevent seizure activity. Meals should be spaced throughout the day to prevent hypoglycemia. Overhydration may precipitate seizure activity. If stimuli such as flashing lights, video or computer games, or loud music appear to trigger seizures, advise patient to avoid environments that are likely to have these

stimuli. Poorly adjusted TVs may trigger seizures and should be fixed. Patients should monitor for and treat fever early during an illness.
- Encourage individuals who have seizures that occur without warning to avoid chewing gum or sucking on lozenges, which may be aspirated during a seizure.
- Encourage patient to wear a Medic-Alert bracelet or similar identification or to carry a medical information card.

NIC: Seizure Management; Seizure Precautions; Teaching: Disease Process; Teaching: Individual

Knowledge deficit: Purpose, precautions, and side effects of antiepilepsy medications
Desired outcome: Before hospital discharge, patient verbalizes accurate information about the prescribed antiepilepsy medication.
- Stress the importance of taking the prescribed medication regularly and on schedule and not discontinuing the medication without health care provider guidance. Explain that missing a scheduled dose can precipitate a seizure several days later. Stress that abrupt withdrawal of any antiepilepsy medication can precipitate seizures and that discontinuing these medications is the most common cause of status epilepticus. Assist patients in finding methods that will help them remember to take the medication and monitor their drug supply to avoid running out. Drugs may be necessary for the rest of the patient's life. Medications cannot be taken prn, and lack of seizures does not mean the drug is unnecessary. Explain the concept of drug half-lives and steady blood levels. Patients should consult their health care provider before changing from a trade name to a generic medication because of possible differences in bioavailability.
- Reinforce prescribed drug dose instructions.
- Stress the importance of informing health care provider about side effects and keeping appointments for periodic laboratory work, which determines whether blood levels are therapeutic and assesses for side effects. Many antiepilepsy medications can cause blood dyscrasia or liver damage. Teach patient to report immediately any bruising, bleeding, or jaundice. Vitamin D, vitamin K, and folic acid supplements may be prescribed.
- Explain that antiepilepsy medications may make people drowsy. Advise patient to avoid activities that require alertness until his or her CNS response to the medication has been determined.
- Nausea and vomiting are common side effects of most antiepilepsy medications. Teach patient to take the drug with food or large amounts of liquid to minimize gastric upset. Patients taking valproic acid (Depakote) should not chew the medication, because it may irritate the oral mucous membrane. Also advise patients taking valproic acid that this drug may produce a false-positive test for urine ketones and that any visual change should be reported immediately because it may signal ocular toxicity.
- Instruct patient to notify health care provider if a significant weight gain or weight loss occurs because it may necessitate a change in dose or scheduling.
- Teach patient to avoid alcoholic beverages and over-the-counter (OTC) medications containing alcohol. Long-term alcohol use stimulates the body to metabolize phenytoin (Dilantin) more quickly, thus lowering the seizure threshold because of the decreased plasma phenytoin levels. Patients taking phenobarbital (Luminal) or primidone (Mysoline) should avoid alcohol, which potentiates CNS depressant effects. Anticonvulsant agents are potentiated or inhibited by many other drugs, including aspirin and antihistamines, and may affect potency of other medications as well. Caution patient to avoid OTC medications.

- Other side effects common to antiepilepsy medications are ataxia, diplopia, nystagmus, and dizziness. Instruct patient to report these symptoms.
- Teach patients who take carbamazepine (Tegretol) or ethosuximide (Zarontin) to report immediately fever, mouth ulcers, sore throat, peripheral edema, dark urine, bruising, or bleeding.
- Advise patients taking phenytoin that this drug can cause gingival hypertrophy. The patient should perform frequent oral hygiene with gum massage and gentle flossing and brush teeth 3-4 times/day with a soft toothbrush. These patients also should report immediately any measlelike rash.
- Caution patients taking phenytoin that there are two types of this drug. Dilantin Kapseal is absorbed more slowly and is longer acting. It is important not to confuse this extended-release phenytoin with prompt-release phenytoin. Doing so may cause dangerous underdose or overdose. Generic phenytoin should not be substituted for Dilantin Kapseal.

NIC: Medication Management; Teaching: Individual; Teaching: Prescribed Medication

Noncompliance with the therapy related to denial of the illness or perceived negative consequences of the treatment regimen secondary to social stigma, negative side effects of antiepilepsy medications, or difficulty with making necessary life-style changes

Desired outcome: Before hospital discharge, patient verbalizes knowledge about the disease process and treatment plan, acknowledges consequences of continued noncompliant behavior, explains the experience that caused patient to alter the prescribed behavior, describes the appropriate treatment of side effects or the appropriate alternatives, and exhibits health care measures that reflect this knowledge, following an agreed-on plan of care.

- Assess patient's understanding of the disease process, medical management, and treatment plan. Explain or clarify information as indicated.
- Assess for causes of noncompliance, such as financial constraints, inconvenience, forgetfulness, medication side effects, or difficulty making significant life-style changes or following the medication schedule.
- Ensure awareness that stopping medications can be life threatening (e.g., status epilepticus). Explain drug half-life and the concept of a steady blood level. Intermittent medication use may be informal experimentation or an effort to gain control. Explain the importance of health care provider guidance if medication is stopped for any reason. Instruct and provide written instructions for the patient in how to contact his or her health care provider and the importance of health care provider and laboratory follow-up. Explain what to do if a dose is missed and how to refill a prescription if medication is lost or depleted.
- Evaluate patient's perception of his or her vulnerability to the disease process, and be alert to signs of denial of the illness. In addition, evaluate patient's perception of the effectiveness or noneffectiveness of treatment. Stress the importance of expressing feelings (e.g., dependence, powerlessness, embarrassment, being different).
- Determine if a value, cultural, or spiritual conflict is causing noncompliance. Confront myths and stigmas. Provide realistic assessment of risks, and counter misconceptions.
- Discuss methods of dealing with common problems, such as obtaining insurance and job or workplace discrimination.
- Assess patient's support systems. Determine whether the presence of a family disruption pattern (whether or not it is caused by the patient's illness) is making compliance difficult and "not worth it."

- After the reason for noncompliance is found, intervene accordingly to ensure compliance. If it appears that changing the medical treatment plan (e.g., in scheduling medications) may promote compliance, discuss this possibility with health care provider. Provide patient with information about interventions that can minimize the drug's side effects (e.g., taking the drug with food or large amounts of liquid to minimize gastric distress).
- Encourage involvement with support systems, such as local epilepsy centers and national organizations.

NIC: Coping Enhancement; Counseling; Teaching: Disease Process; Teaching: Individual; Teaching: Prescribed Medication

> **See Also:**   "General Care of Patients With Neurologic Disorders" for **Knowledge deficit:** Neurologic diagnostic tests, p. 346; Appendix One, "Caring for Patients With Cancer and Other Life-disrupting Illnesses" for **Body image disturbance,** p. 799; **Ineffective individual coping,** p. 795; **Altered family processes,** p. 802.

PATIENT-FAMILY TEACHING AND DISCHARGE PLANNING

When providing patient-family teaching, focus on sensory information; avoid giving excessive information; and initiate a visiting nurse referral for necessary follow-up teaching. Consider including verbal and written information about the following:

- Reinforcement of knowledge of the disease process, pathophysiology, symptoms, and the precipitating or aggravating factors.
- Medications, including drug name, purpose, dosage, schedule, precautions, drug/drug and food/drug interactions, and potential side effects (Table 4-5).
- Importance of follow-up care and keeping medical appointments. Stress that use of antiepilepsy drugs necessitates periodic monitoring of blood levels to ensure therapeutic medication levels and assessment for side effects. Instruct patient to keep emergency contact numbers for the health care provider.
- An uncomplicated convulsive seizure in an individual known to have epilepsy is not necessarily a medical emergency. On average, these people can continue about their business after a rest period. An ambulance should be called or medical attention sought if the seizure happens in water; if there is any question of the seizure being caused by epilepsy; if the individual is injured, pregnant, or diabetic; if the seizure lasts longer than 5 min; if a second seizure starts; or if consciousness does not begin to return.
- Environmental factors that can be life threatening in the presence of seizures, measures that may help prevent seizures, and safety interventions during seizures. Review state and local laws that apply to individuals with seizure disorders.
- Employment or vocational counseling as needed. Discuss the need to avoid overprotection and maintain, as possible, normal work and recreation.
- Risks of antiepilepsy drugs during pregnancy. Provide birth control information or genetic counseling referral as requested.
- Provide the following address as appropriate:

Epilepsy Foundation of America
4351 Garden City Drive, Suite 406
Landover, MD 20785   (301) 459-3700 or (800) 332-1000
WWW address: *http://www.efa.org/*

T A B L E 4 - 5   Common Antiepilepsy Drugs

Name	Side effects	Precautions
Phenytoin (Dilantin)	Drowsiness, gingival hypertrophy, nausea, vomiting, increased body hair, rash, or blood dyscrasias; signs of overdose; nystagmus, ataxia, slurred speech, confusion, diplopia	Ensure frequent oral hygiene, gum massage, and gentle flossing. Take drug with food or large amounts of liquid to decrease gastric upset. Periodic blood counts are necessary. Call health care provider if rash or jaundice appears. Vitamin K may be given to pregnant women 1 mo before and during delivery to prevent neonatal hemorrhage. If prescribed, supplement with vitamins K and D and folic acid.
Carbamazepine (Tegretol)	Blood dyscrasias, ataxia, rash, nystagmus, diplopia, nausea, vomiting, liver damage, drowsiness, dizziness, dry mouth	Check CBC frequently. Patient should report fever, mouth ulcers, sore throat, edema, dark urine, bruising, or bleeding immediately. Take drug with food. Liver and renal function tests should be performed periodically. Report jaundice to health care provider.
Phenobarbital (Luminal)	Drowsiness, lethargy, dizziness, nausea, vomiting, constipation, ataxia, anemia, mild rash, depression	Do not stop abruptly; this may cause withdrawal seizures. Avoid alcohol, which would potentiate CNS depressant effects. Vitamin D supplements are usually advised. Take with foods to prevent stomach upset. Vitamin K is usually given to pregnant women 1 mo before and during labor to prevent neonatal hemorrhage.
Primidone (Mysoline)	Drowsiness, emotional changes including depression and irritability, anemia, rash, nausea, vomiting, impotence; early signs of overdose: incoordination, slurred speech, blurred vision	Do not stop abruptly; it may cause withdrawal seizures. Take with food or large amounts of fluid. See information with phenobarbital above regarding alcohol avoidance and vitamin K.
Ethosuximide (Zarontin)	Gastric distress, nausea, vomiting, dizziness, drowsiness, aplastic anemia, vaginal bleeding, ataxia	Take with food or large amounts of fluid. Follow-up laboratory studies are important for detecting anemia. Patient should immediately report fever, mouth ulcers, sore throat, bruising, and bleeding.

CBC, Complete blood count; *CNS,* central nervous system; *GI,* gastrointestinal; *IV,* intravenously.

TABLE 4-5   Common Antiepilepsy Drugs—cont'd

Name	Side effects	Precautions
Valproic acid (Depakote)	Sedation, dizziness, nausea, vomiting, anorexia, liver damage, transient alopecia, ataxia, thrombocytopenia; any visual change may signal ocular toxicity	Do not chew; it may irritate mucous membranes. Take with food to prevent gastric upset. Patient should report any bleeding, bruising, or visual change immediately and monitor liver function studies via periodic laboratory tests. This drug may produce false-positive test for ketones in the urine.
Fosphenytoin (Cerebyx)	Fever, injection site reaction, facial edema, chills, high blood pressure, constipation, hypokalemia, myasthenia, hypesthesia, increased reflexes, dysarthria, rash, ataxia, headache, nystagmus	Monitor phosphate levels in patients with phosphate restriction. Contraindicated in patients with hydantoin sensitivity. Monitor serum values to ensure therapeutic levels (10-20 µg/ml). Severe hypotension can occur if administered rapidly IV.
Gabapentin (Neurontin)	Dizziness, somnolence, ataxia, GI upset, leukopenia, headache, fatigue	Periodically monitor CBC and hepatic function.
Lamotrigine	Rash, nausea, dizziness, somnolence, ataxia, diplopia, headache	Monitor hepatic and renal function before and periodically during therapy. Taper drug slowly over 2 weeks when discontinuing.
Felbamate	Anorexia, vomiting, headache, dizziness, fatigue, aplastic anemia, liver failure	Frequently monitor CBC and liver enzymes.

Section Seven: General Care of Patients With Neurologic Disorders

Risk for trauma with risk factors related to weakness, difficulties with balance, or unsteady gait secondary to sensorimotor deficit

Desired outcomes: Patient is free of trauma caused by gait unsteadiness. Before hospital discharge, patient demonstrates proficiency with assistive devices if appropriate.

- Evaluate patient's gait, and assess for motor deficits such as weakness, difficulty with balance, tremors, spasticity, or paralysis. Document baseline assessments so that changes in status can be detected promptly.
- To minimize the risk of injury, assist patient as needed when unsteady gait, weakness, or paralysis is noted. Instruct patient to ask or call for assistance with ambulation. Check frequently on patients who may forget to call for assistance. Stand on patient's weak side to assist with balance and support.

Use transfer belt for safety. Instruct patient to use stronger side for gripping railing when stair climbing or using a cane.

- Orient patient to new surroundings. Keep necessary items (including water, snacks, phone, call light) within easy reach. Assess patient's ability to use these items. The patient who is very weak or partially paralyzed may require a tap bell or specially adapted call light.
- Maintain an uncluttered environment with unobstructed walkways to minimize the risk of tripping. Ensure adequate lighting at night (e.g., a night light) to help prevent falls in the dark. In addition, keep side rails up and the bed in its lowest position with bed brakes on. Encourage patient to use any needed hearing aids and corrective lenses when ambulating.
- For unsteady, weak, or partially paralyzed patient, encourage use of low-heel, nonskid, supportive shoes for walking. Teach the use of a wide-based gait to provide a broader base of support. Instruct patient to note foot placement when ambulating or transferring to ensure that the foot is flat and in a position of support. Teach, reinforce, and encourage use of assistive device, such as a cane, walker, or crutches, that provides patient with added stability. Teach exercises that strengthen arm and shoulder muscles for using walkers and crutches. Teach safe use of transfer or sliding boards. Teach patients in wheelchairs how and when to lock and unlock the wheels. Demonstrate how to secure and support weak or paralyzed arms to prevent subluxation and injury from falling into wheelchair spokes or wheels. Patients with poor sitting balance may need a seat or chest belt, H-straps for leg positioning, and a wheelchair with an antitip device. Show how to get on and off elevators to prevent wheels from catching in the gaps between the elevator and floor. Keep wheelchair close to bed. Teach proper use of recliner mechanism or battery precautions on appropriate wheelchairs.
- Teach patients to maintain a sitting position for a few minutes before assuming a standing position for ambulating. This procedure gives patients time to get their feet flat and under them for balance and minimizes any dizziness that may occur because of rapid position changes.
- Monitor spasticity, antispasmodic medications, and their effect on physical function. Uncontrolled or severe spasms may cause falls, whereas mild to moderate spasms can be useful in ADL and transfers if the patient learns to control and trigger them.
- Review with patient and significant other potential safety needs at home, such as safety appliances (wall, bath, toilet hand rails; elevated toilet seat; nonslip surface in bathtub or shower). Loose rugs should be removed to prevent slipping and falling. Temperatures on hot water heaters should be turned down to prevent scalding in the event of a fall in the shower or tub. Furniture in the home may need to be moved to provide clear, safe pathways that avoid sharp corners on furniture, glass cabinets, or large windows that the patient might fall against. Strategically placed additional lighting also may be needed. The edges of steps in the home may require taping with a bright color strip to provide sufficient contrast so that the edges can be recognized and more safely negotiated. Beds should be modified to prevent rolling. Activity should be balanced with rest periods because fatigue tends to increase unsteadiness and the potential for falls.
- Seek referral for physical therapist (PT) as appropriate.

NIC: Environmental Management: Safety; Positioning: Neurologic; Positioning: Wheelchair; Skin Surveillance; Teaching: Individual

Risk for injury with risk factors related to impaired pain, touch, and temperature sensations secondary to sensory deficit or decreased LOC
Desired outcomes: Patient is free of symptoms of injury caused by impaired pain, touch, and temperature sensations. Before hospital discharge, patient and significant other identify factors that increase the potential for injury.

- Assess patient for indicators of sensory deficits, such as decreased or absent vision and impaired temperature and pain sensation. Document baseline neurologic and physical assessments so that changes in status can be detected promptly.
- Protect patient from exposure to hot food or equipment that can burn the skin. Avoid use of heating pads. Encourage use of sunscreen when outside.
- Always check the temperature of heating devices and bath water before patient is exposed to them. Teach patient and significant other about these precautions.
- Inspect patient's skin twice daily for evidence of irritation. Teach the coherent patient to perform self-inspection, and provide a mirror for inspecting posterior aspects of the body. Keep the skin soft and pliable with emollient lotion.
- Teach patient to inspect placement of limbs with altered sensation to ensure that they are in a safe and supported position and to avoid placing ankles directly on top of each other. Pad the wheelchair seat, preferably with a gel pad, to evenly distribute the patient's weight. Teach patient to change position q15-30min by lifting self and shifting position side to side and forward to backward. Encourage frequent turning while in bed and, if tolerated and not contraindicated, periodic movement into the prone position. Have patient lift, not drag, self during transfers to prevent shearing damage.
- Give injections in muscles with tone, for better absorption and less risk of sterile abscess formation. Avoid injecting ≥1 ml into a flaccid muscle.

NIC: Medication Administration; Positioning: Neurologic; Positioning: Wheelchair; Pressure Ulcer Prevention; Surveillance: Skin; Teaching: Individual

Impaired corneal tissue integrity related to irritation secondary to diminished blink reflex or inability to close the eyes
Desired outcome: Patient's corneas remain clear and intact.
- Normally, blinking occurs every 5-6 sec. If patient has a diminished blink reflex or is stuporous or comatose, assess the eyes for irritation or the presence of foreign objects. Instill prescribed eye drops or ointment to prevent corneal irritation. Instruct coherent patients to make a conscious effort to blink the eyes several times each minute to help prevent corneal irritation. Indicators of corneal irritation include red, itchy, scratchy, or painful eye; sensation of foreign object in eye; scleral edema; blurred vision; or mucus discharge. Apply eye patches or warm, sterile compresses over closed eyes for relief.
- If the eyes cannot be completely closed, use caution in applying an eye shield or taping the eyes shut. Semiconscious patients may open eyes underneath and injure their corneas. Consider use of moisture chambers (plastic eye bubbles), protective glasses, soft contacts, or humidifiers.
- For chronic eye closure problems, special springs or weights on the upper lids may ensure closure. Surgical closure (tarsorrhaphy) may also be necessary.
- Teach patient to avoid exposing eyes to irritants such as talc or baby powder, wind, cold air, smoke, dust, sand, or bright sunlight. Instruct patient not to rub eyes; restrain patients who may be incoherent. Patients should be taught to wear glasses to protect against wind and dust and tight-fitting goggles when swimming.

NIC: Eye Care; Health Education

Altered nutrition: Less than body requirements related to inability to ingest food secondary to chewing and swallowing deficits, fatigue, weakness, paresis, paralysis, visual neglect, or decreased LOC

Desired outcome: Patient experiences adequate nutrition as evidenced by maintenance of or return to baseline body weight by hospital discharge.

- Assess patient's alertness, ability to cough, and swallow and gag reflexes before all meals. Keep suction equipment at the bedside if indicated.
- Assess patient for type of diet that can be eaten safely. Request soft, semisolid, or chopped foods as indicated. Although a pureed diet may be needed eventually, pureed food can be unappealing and may have a negative impact on patient's self-concept.
- To help patient focus on eating, reduce other stimuli in the room (e.g., turn off the TV or radio). Minimize conversation and other disruptions such as phone calls. If patient wears glasses, put them on the patient; ensure adequate lighting.
- Provide analgesics, if appropriate, before meals so that patient is comfortable and can concentrate on eating.
- Evaluate patient's food preferences and offer small, frequent servings of nutritious food. Encourage significant other to bring in patient's favorite foods if not contraindicated. Plan meals for times when the patient is rested; use a warming tray or microwave oven to keep the food warm and appetizing until the patient is able to eat. Serve cold foods while they are cold.
- Provide oral care before feeding to enhance the patient's ability to taste. Clean and insert dentures before each meal.
- Encourage liquid nutritional supplements. Try different methods to make them more palatable (e.g., making a milkshake, serving it over ice, or diluting with carbonated beverages).
- Cut up foods, unwrap silverware, and otherwise prepare the food tray so that patients with a weak or paralyzed arm can manage the tray one-handed.
- For patient with visual neglect, place food within patient's unaffected visual field. Return during the meal to make sure he or she has eaten from both sides of the plate. Turn the plate around so that any remaining food is in patient's visual field.
- Feed or assist very weak or paralyzed patients. If not contraindicated, position patient in a chair or elevate HOB as high as possible. Ensure that patient's head is flexed slightly forward to close the airway. Begin with small amounts of food. Do not hurry patient. Be sure that each bite is completely swallowed before giving another. Encourage patients with hemiplegia to consciously sweep the paralyzed side of their mouth with their tongue to clear it.
- If appropriate, provide assistive devices, such as built-up utensil handles, broad-handled spoons, spill-proof cups, rocker knife for cutting, wrist or hand splints with clamps to hold utensils, stabilized plates, sectioned plates, and other devices that promote self-feeding and independence. Encourage eating of finger foods to promote independence and oral intake.
- Provide materials for oral hygiene after meals to minimize risk of aspiration of food particles. Good oral hygiene will also help maintain integrity of the mucous membranes to minimize risk of stomatitis, which may prevent adequate oral intake. Provide oral care for patients unable to do so for themselves.
- Document your assessment of the patient's appetite. Weigh patient regularly (at least weekly) to assess for loss or gain. If indicated, notify health care provider of the potential need for high-protein or high-calorie supplements. Obtain dietitian consultation. Patients may need enteral or parenteral nutrition. For additional information, see "Providing Nutritional Support," p. 687.
- For the weak, debilitated, or partially paralyzed patient, assess support systems, such as family or friends, who can assist patient with meals. Consider referral to an organization that will deliver a daily meal to patient's home.
- If appropriate for patient's diagnosis (e.g., multiple sclerosis [MS]) consider referral to a speech pathologist for exercises that enhance the ability to swallow.

- For patients with visual problems, assess their ability to see their food. Identify utensils and foods, and describe their location. Arrange foods in an established pattern to promote independence.
- For patients with chewing or swallowing difficulties, see interventions under **Impaired swallowing,** p. 344.

NIC: Aspiration Precautions; Nutrition Management; Nutrition Therapy; Swallowing Therapy; Weight Gain Assistance

Risk for fluid volume deficit with risk factors related to facial and throat muscle weakness, depressed gag or cough reflex, impaired swallowing, or decreased LOC affecting access to and intake of fluids
Desired outcome: Patient is normovolemic as evidenced by balanced I&O, stable weight, good skin turgor, moist mucous membranes, BP within patient's normal range, HR ≤100 bpm, normothermia, and urinary output ≥30 ml/hr with a specific gravity <1.030.

- Assess patient's gag reflex, alertness, and ability to cough and swallow before offering fluids. Keep suction equipment at the bedside if indicated.
- Monitor I&O to assess for fluid volume imbalance. Involve patient or significant other with keeping fluid intake records. Perform daily weights if patient is at risk for sudden fluid shifts or imbalances. Patients with neurologic deficits may have great difficulty attaining adequate intake of fluids. Alert health care provider to a significant I&O imbalance, which may signal the need for enteral or IV therapy to prevent dehydration.
- Assess for and teach patient and significant other the indicators of dehydration, including thirst, poor skin turgor, decreased BP, increased pulse rate, dry skin and mucous membranes, increased body temperature, concentrated urine (specific gravity >1.030), and decreased urinary output. Advise them that conditions such as fever or diarrhea increase fluid loss and increase the risk of dehydration.
- Evaluate fluid preferences (type and temperature). Offer fluids q1-2hr. For nonrestricted patients, encourage a fluid intake of at least 2-3 L/day.
- Feed or assist very weak or paralyzed patients. If not contraindicated, assist patient into a high Fowler's position to facilitate oral fluid intake. Instruct patient to flex the head slightly forward, which closes the airway and helps prevent aspiration. Begin with small amounts of liquid. Instruct patient to sip rather than gulp fluids. Do not hurry patient. In patients at risk for aspiration, use thickened fluids to facilitate patients' ability to swallow the fluid.
- Provide periods of rest to prevent fatigue, which can contribute to decreased oral intake. Provide oral care as needed to enhance taste perception and prevent stomatitis, which may decrease oral intake.
- If appropriate, provide assistive devices (e.g., plastic, unbreakable, special-handled, spill-proof cups or straws) to promote independence. Teach patient with hemiparalysis or paresis to tilt the head toward the unaffected side to facilitate intake. The individual who is paralyzed (e.g., with spinal cord injury [SCI]) may be able to drink independently via an extra-long tubing or straw connected to a water pitcher.
- For patients at risk for increased intracranial pressure (IICP), maintain fluid restrictions.
- For patients with chewing or swallowing difficulties, see interventions under **Impaired swallowing**, p. 344.

NIC: Airway Suctioning; Aspiration Precautions; Neurologic Monitoring; Respiratory Monitoring; Surveillance; Swallowing Therapy; Vital Signs Monitoring

Risk for aspiration with risk factors related to facial and throat muscle weakness, depressed gag or cough reflex, impaired swallowing, or decreased LOC
Desired outcomes: Patient is free of the signs of aspiration as evidenced by RR 12-20 breaths/min with normal depth and pattern (eupnea), O_2 saturation

≥92%, normal color, normal breath sounds, normothermia, and absence of adventitious breath sounds. Following instruction on an ongoing basis, patient or significant other relates measures that prevent aspiration.

- Monitor patient for the presence of dyspnea, pallor, restlessness, diaphoresis, and a change in the rate or depth of respirations. Auscultate lung fields for breath sounds. Note the presence of crackles (rales), rhonchi, or wheezes and diminished breath sounds. Assess effectiveness of patient's cough and the quality, amount, and color of the sputum. Measure body temperature q4hr. Often a low-grade fever (≤100° F, or 37.7° C) indicates the need for aggressive pulmonary hygiene. As indicated, monitor patient's O_2 saturation; report O_2 saturation <92%.

- Teach patient to use an incentive spirometer, deep breathe, and cough. Assist with repositioning at least q2hr. If it is not contraindicated, maintain patient in a side-lying position with HOB elevated. **Caution:** Instruct patients at risk of IICP not to cough, because it increases intraabdominal and intrathoracic pressure, which in turn increases ICP. If sneezing is unavoidable, teach the patient that it should be done with an open mouth to minimize the increase in ICP.

- Assess swallow and gag reflexes. If poor or absent, withhold oral fluids and foods and inform health care provider of the possible need for IV therapy or enteral or parenteral nutrition. Maintain adequate hydration to keep secretions thin.

- Keep HOB elevated after meals or assist patient into a right side-lying position to minimize the potential for regurgitation and aspiration. Provide small, frequent meals. Consult health care provider for an upper GI stimulant (e.g., metoclopramide) to reduce potential for regurgitation. Provide oral hygiene after meals to prevent aspiration of food particles.

- For patients not at risk for IICP, assist with prescribed postural drainage, chest physiotherapy, and IPPB.

- Keep O_2 and suction apparatus available as indicated. Assess patient frequently for the presence of obstructive material or secretions in the throat or mouth, and suction as needed. Turn patient on one side to facilitate secretion drainage. Anticipate the need for an artificial airway if secretions cannot be cleared. Teach significant other the Heimlich maneuver.

NIC: Airway Suctioning; Aspiration Precautions; Nutrition Management; Nutrition Therapy; Respiratory Monitoring; Surveillance; Swallowing Therapy; Vital Signs Monitoring

Self-care deficit related to spasticity, tremors, weakness, paresis, paralysis, or decreasing LOC secondary to sensorimotor deficits
Desired outcome: At least 24 hr before hospital discharge, patient performs care activities independently and demonstrates the ability to use adaptive devices for successful completion of ADL. (Totally dependent patients express satisfaction with activities that are completed for them.)

- Assess patient's ability to perform ADL.

- As appropriate, demonstrate use of adaptive devices, such as long- or broad-handled combs, long-handled pickup sticks, brushes, and eating utensils, dressing sticks, stocking helpers, Velcro fasteners, elastic waste bands, nonspill cups, and stabilized plates, all of which may assist the patient in maintaining independent care. A flexor-hinge splint or universal cuff may aid in brushing teeth and combing hair.

- Set short-range, realistic goals with patient to decrease frustration and improve learning. Acknowledge progress. Encourage continued effort and involvement (e.g., in selection of meals, clothing).

- Provide care to the totally dependent patient. Assist those who are not totally dependent according to degree of disability. Encourage patient to perform self-care to the maximum ability as defined by the patient. Encourage autonomy. Allow sufficient time for task performance; do not hurry the patient. Involve significant other with care activities if he or she is comfortable doing so. Ask for patient's input in planning schedules. Supervise activity until patient can safely perform the task without help.

- To improve mobility, encourage use of electronically controlled wheelchair and other technical advances (e.g., environmental control system) that may allow independent operation of electronic devices such as lights, radio, door openers, and window shade openers.
- Provide privacy and a nondistracting environment. Place patient's belongings within reach. Set out items needed to complete self-care tasks in the order they are to be used. Apply any needed adaptive devices such as hand splints.
- Encourage patient to wear any prescribed corrective eye lenses or hearing aids.
- Provide analgesics to relieve pain, which can hinder self-care activity.
- Provide a rest period before self-care activity, or plan activity for a time when patient is rested, because fatigue reduces self-care ability.
- To facilitate dressing and undressing, encourage patient or significant other to buy shoes without laces, long-handled shoe horns, loose-fitting clothing, wide-legged pants, and clothing with front fasteners, zipper pulls, or Velcro closures. Avoid items with small buttons or tight buttonholes. Lay out clothing in the order it will be put on.
- Place a stool in the shower if sitting down will enhance self-care with bathing. Bathrooms should have nonslip mats and grab bars for safety. Hand-held shower spray, long-handled bath sponge, or a washer mitt with a pocket that holds soap may promote autonomy.
- Provide a commode chair or elevated toilet seat or male or female urinal if it will facilitate self-care with elimination. Teach self-transfer techniques that will enable patient to get to the commode or toilet. Keep the call light within patient's reach. Instruct patient to call as early as possible so that the staff will have time to respond and the patient will not have to rush because of urgency. Offer toileting reminders q2hr, after meals, and before bedtime.
- Some patients with limited hand or arm mobility may have difficulty with perineal care after elimination. A long-handled grasper that can hold tissues or washcloth may help maintain independence with perineal care.
- For patient with hemiparesis or hemiparalysis, teach use of the stronger or unaffected hand and arm for dressing, eating, bathing, and grooming. Instruct patient to dress the weaker side first.
- For patients with visual field deficit, avoid placing items on their blind side. Encourage patients to scan their environment for needed items by turning the head.
- Patients with tremors may find splints, weighted utensils, or wrist weights helpful. Resting the head against a high-backed chair may reduce head tremors.
- Obtain a referral for occupational therapist (OT) if indicated to determine the best method for performing activity.
- Individuals with cognitive defects need simple visual or verbal cues, increased gesture use, demonstration, reminders of the next step, and gentle repetition. Provide a consistent caregiver and ADL routine.
- If indicated, teach patient self-catheterization or teach the technique to the caregiver. At-home intermittent catheterization usually is done with clean, not sterile, technique and equipment. The catheter is washed after use in warm, soapy water, rinsed, and placed in a clean plastic sack. Catheter insertion guides are available commercially for females with limited upper arm mobility. Crusted catheters are soaked in a solution of half distilled vinegar and half water. Teach patient to monitor and notify health professional of cloudy, foul-smelling, or bloody urine; urine with sediment; chills or fever; pain in the lower back or abdomen; or a red or swollen urethral meatus.
- Discuss, as appropriate, changing the home environment to improve ADL and independence (e.g., with extended sinks, lower closet hooks, wheelchair-

accessible shower, modified phones, lowered mirrors, and lever door handles that operate with reduced hand pressure).

- Listen and provide opportunities for patient to express self, and communicate that it is normal to have negative feelings about changes in autonomy. Discuss with the health care team ways to provide consistent and positive encouragement and strategies that increase independence progressively.

NIC: Active Listening; Coping Enhancement; Self-Care Assistance; Self-Care Assistance: Bathing/Hygiene; Self-Care Assistance: Feeding; Self-Care Assistance: Toileting; Support System Enhancement; Teaching: Individual; Urinary Catheterization: Intermittent

Self-care deficit (oral hygiene) related to sensorimotor deficit or decreased LOC

Desired outcome: Before hospital discharge, patient or significant other demonstrates ability to perform patient's oral care.

- Assess patient's ability to perform mouth care. Identify performance barriers (e.g., sensorimotor or cognitive deficits).
- If patient has decreased LOC or is at risk for aspiration, remove dentures and store them in a water-filled denture cup.
- If patient cannot perform mouth care, clean teeth, tongue, and mouth at least twice daily with a soft-bristled toothbrush and nonabrasive toothpaste. If patient is unconscious or at risk for aspiration, turn him or her to a side-lying position. Swab the mouth and teeth with a sponge-tipped applicator (toothette) moistened with diluted (half strength) mouthwash solution, and irrigate the mouth with a large syringe. If the patient cannot self-manage secretions, use only a small amount of liquid for irrigation each time, and, using a suction catheter or Yankauer tonsil suction tip, remove secretions. Perform this oral hygiene regimen at least q4hr. As appropriate, teach procedure to significant other.
- For patients with physical disabilities, the following toothbrush adaptations can be made:
  —*For patients with limited hand mobility:* enlarge toothbrush handle by covering it with a sponge hair roller or aluminum foil, attaching with an elastic band, or by attaching a bicycle handle grip with plaster of Paris.
  —*For patients with limited arm mobility:* extend toothbrush handle by overlapping another handle or rod over it and taping them together.

NIC: Oral Health Maintenance; Self-Care Assistance

Impaired verbal communication related to facial/throat muscle weakness, intubation, or tracheostomy

Desired outcome: Following intervention and on an ongoing basis, patient communicates effectively, either verbally or nonverbally, and relates decreasing frustration with communication.

- Assess patient's ability to speak, read, write, and comprehend.
- If appropriate, obtain referral to a speech therapist or pathologist to assist patient in strengthening muscles used in speech. Encourage patient to perform exercises that increase the ability to control the facial muscles and tongue. These exercises may include holding a sound for 5 sec, singing the scale, reading aloud, and extending the tongue and trying to touch the chin, nose, or cheek.
- Provide a supportive and relaxed environment for those patients who are unable to form words or sentences or who are unable to speak clearly or appropriately. Acknowledge patient's frustration over the inability to communicate. Explain that patience is needed for both the patient and caregiver. Maintain a calm, positive, reassuring attitude. Continue to speak to the patient using normal volume unless the patient's hearing is impaired. Maintain eye contact to promote focus. Provide enough time for the patient to articulate. Ask patient to repeat unclear words. Observe for nonverbal

cues; watch patient's lips closely. Do not interrupt or finish sentences. Anticipate needs and phrase questions to allow simple answers, such as "yes" or "no." Provide continuity of care to decrease patient's frustration.

- Provide alternative methods of communication if patient is unable to speak (e.g., a language board, alphabet cards, picture or letter-number board, flash cards, pad and pencil). Other alternatives are systems that use eye blinks, tongue clicks, or hand squeezes, bell signal taps, or gestures, such as hand signals, head nods, pantomime, or pointing. Use communication board for urgent situations. Document method of communication used.
- If patient's voice is weak and difficult to hear, reduce environmental noise to enhance listener's ability to hear words. Suggest that patient take a deep breath before speaking; provide a voice amplifier if appropriate for patient. Encourage patients to organize thoughts and plan what they will say before speaking. Encourage patients to express ideas in short, simple phrases or sentences. Remind patients to speak slowly, exaggerate pronunciation, and use facial expressions.
- If patient has swallowing difficulties that result in the accumulation of saliva, suction the mouth to promote clearer speech.
- For a patient with muscle rigidity or spasm, massage the facial and neck muscles before he or she attempts to communicate.
- If patient has a tracheostomy, ensure that a tap bell is within reach. Reassure the patient with a temporary tracheostomy that the ability to speak will return. For the patient with permanent tracheostomy, discuss learning alternate communication systems, such as sign language or esophageal speech. Fenestrated tubes or covering the tracheostomy tube opening with a finger will enable speech.
- Establish a method of calling for assistance, and ensure that the patient knows how to use it. Keep the calling device where the patient can activate it (e.g., place call bell on nonparalyzed side). Depending on the deficit, use a tap bell for weak patients, a pillow pad call light (triggered by arm or head movement), or a sip and puff device (triggered by mouth).
- Encourage patients with the ability to write to keep a diary or write letters as a means of ventilating feelings and expressing concerns. If patient has a weak writing arm, evaluate the need for a splint that will enable patient to hold a pen or pencil. Felt-tip markers also are useful because they require minimal pressure for writing.

NIC: Active Listening; Communication Enhancement: Speech Deficit; Socialization Enhancement

Constipation related to inability to chew and swallow a high-roughage diet, side effects of medications, immobility, and spinal cord involvement
Desired outcome: Within 2-3 days of intervention, patient passes soft, formed stools and regains and maintains his or her normal bowel pattern.

- Although a high-roughage diet is ideal for the patient who is immobilized or on prolonged bedrest, the individual with chewing and swallowing difficulties may be unable to consume such a diet. For these patients, consuming 1 or 2 servings of applesauce with added bran, prune juice, or cooked bran cereal each day may be effective. Otherwise encourage use of natural fiber laxatives such as psyllium (e.g., Metamucil).
- A bowel elimination program may include the following elements: setting a regular time of day for attempting a bowel movement, preferably 30 min after eating a meal or drinking a hot beverage; using a commode instead of a bedpan for more natural positioning during elimination; using a medicated suppository 15-30 min before a scheduled attempt; bearing down by contracting the abdominal muscles or applying manual pressure to the abdomen to help increase intraabdominal pressure; and drinking 4 oz of prune juice nightly. Abdominal and pelvic exercise also may be included in patient's morning and evening routine. Keep a call bell within patient's reach.

Assess patient's sitting balance to ensure safety while on commode. **Caution:** Spinal cord injury (SCI) patients with involvement at T8 and above should use *extreme* caution if use of an enema or suppository is unavoidable, because either can precipitate life-threatening autonomic dysreflexia (AD). Liberal application of anesthetic jelly into the rectum should precede their use. In addition, instruct patient at risk of IICP not to bear down with bowel movements because this action can cause increased intraabdominal pressure, which in turn increases ICP.

- Unless contraindicated, encourage fluid intake to >2500 ml/day, including liberal amounts of fresh fruit juices.
- If indicated by patient's diagnosis (e.g., MS), provide instructions for digital stimulation of the anus to promote reflex bowel evacuation. **Caution:** This intervention is contraindicated for SCI patients with involvement at T8 or above because it can precipitate life-threatening AD.
- For other interventions, see **Constipation**, p. 793, in Appendix One, "Caring for Patients on Prolonged Bedrest."

NIC: Bowel Management; Bowel Training; Constipation/Impaction Management; Fluid Monitoring; Nutritional Counseling

Decreased adaptive capacity: Intracranial related to altered blood flow with risk of IICP and herniation secondary to positional factors, increased intrathoracic or intraabdominal pressure, fluid volume excess, hyperthermia, or discomfort secondary to brain injury

Desired outcomes: Patient is free of symptoms of IICP and herniation as evidenced by stable or improving Glasgow Coma Scale score (see Table 4-2); stable or improving sensorimotor functioning; BP within patient's normal range; HR 60-100 bpm; pulse pressure 30-40 mm Hg (the difference between the systolic and diastolic BPs); orientation to person, place, and time; normal vision; bilaterally equal and normoreactive pupils; RR 12-20 breaths/min with normal depth and pattern (eupnea); normal gag, corneal, and swallowing reflexes; and absence of headache, nausea, nuchal rigidity, posturing, and seizure activity.

> **Note:**   ICP is the pressure exerted by brain tissue, CSF, and cerebral blood volume within the rigid, unyielding skull. An increase in any one of these components without a corresponding decrease in another will increase ICP. Normal ICP is 0-10 mm Hg; IICP is >15 mm Hg. Cerebral perfusion pressure (CPP) is the difference between systemic arterial pressure and ICP. As ICP rises, CPP may decrease. Normal CPP is 80-100 mm Hg. If CPP falls below 60 mm Hg, ischemia occurs. When CPP falls to 0, cerebral blood flow ceases. Cerebral edema and IICP usually peak 2-3 days after an injury and then decrease over 1-2 weeks.

- Monitor for and report any of the following indicators of IICP or impending/occurring herniation:
  —*Early indicators of IICP:* declining Glasgow Coma Scale score, alterations in LOC ranging from irritability, restlessness, and confusion to lethargy; possible onset of or worsening of headache; beginning pupillary dysfunction, such as sluggishness; visual disturbances, such as diplopia or blurred vision; onset of or increase in sensorimotor changes or deficits, such as weakness; onset of or worsening of nausea. **Note:** The single most important indicator of early IICP is a change in LOC.
  —*Late indicators of IICP* (generally related to brain stem compression and disruption of cranial nerves and vital centers): continuing decline in Glasgow Coma Scale score; continued deterioration in LOC leading to stupor and coma; projectile vomiting; hemiplegia; posturing; widening

pulse pressure, decreased HR, and increased systolic BP; Cheyne-Stokes breathing or other respiratory irregularity; pupillary changes, such as oval-shaped, inequality, dilation, and nonreactivity to light; papilledema; and impaired brain stem reflexes (corneal, gag, swallowing).

—*Brain herniation:* deep coma, fixed and dilated pupils (first unilateral and then bilateral), posturing progressing to bilateral flaccidity, lost brain stem reflexes, and continuing deterioration in VS and respirations.

- If changes occur, prepare for possible transfer of patient to ICU. Insertion of ICP sensors for continuous ICP monitoring, continuous bedside cerebral blood flow (CBF) monitoring, CSF ventricular drainage, intubation, mechanical ventilation, neuromuscular blocking, or barbiturate coma therapy may be necessary. Continuous cardiac monitoring for dysrhythmia will also be done.

- For patients at risk for IICP, prevention of hypoxia and CO_2 retention is essential for preventing vasodilation of cerebral arteries. Preventive measures include ensuring a patent airway, delivering O_2 as prescribed, and limiting suctioning to 10-15 sec. Monitor patient's ABG or pulse oximetry values. Regulate the ventilator, if present, to keep $Paco_2$ within prescribed parameters. Hyperventilation, through reduced $Paco_2$ levels and cerebral vasoconstriction, will reduce ICP, but hyperventilation produces a varied blood flow response and may cause cerebral ischemia. Ideally, CBF measurements and continuous jugular venous oxygen saturation should be considered if hyperventilation is used as a treatment.

- Promote venous blood return to the heart to reduce cerebral congestion by keeping HOB elevated at 15-30 degrees (unless otherwise directed); maintaining head and neck alignment to avoid hyperextension, flexion, or rotation; ensuring that tracheostomy, endotracheal tube ties, or O_2 tubing does not compress the jugular vein; and avoiding Trendelenburg position for any reason. Ensure that pillows under the patient's head are flat so that the head is in a neutral rather than flexed position.

- Take precautions against increased intraabdominal and intrathoracic pressure in the following ways: teach patient to exhale when turning. Provide passive ROM exercises rather than allow active or assistive exercises. Administer prescribed stool softeners or laxatives to prevent straining at stool; avoid enemas and suppositories because they can cause straining. Instruct patient not to move self in bed, because it requires a pushing movement; allow only passive turning; use a pull sheet. Instruct patient to avoid pushing against the foot of the bed or pulling against side rails. Avoid footboards; use high-top tennis shoes with toes removed to the level of the metatarsal heads instead. Assist patient with sitting up and turning. Instruct patient to avoid coughing and sneezing or, if unavoidable, to do so with an open mouth; provide antitussive for cough as prescribed and antiemetic for vomiting. Instruct patient to avoid hip flexion (increases intraabdominal pressure). Do not place patient in a prone position, and avoid using restraints (straining against them increases ICP). Rather than have patient perform Valsalva's maneuver to prevent an air embolism during insertion of a central venous catheter, health care provider should use a syringe to aspirate air from the catheter lumen.

- IV fluids are given to maintain normovolemia and balanced electrolyte status. Fluid restrictions are avoided because resulting increased blood viscosity and decreased volume may lead to hypotension, decreasing cerebral perfusion pressure. Administer IV fluids only with an infusion control device to prevent fluid overload. Keep accurate I&O records. When administering additional IV fluids (e.g., IV drugs) avoid using D_5W because its hypotonicity can increase cerebral edema and hyperglycemia that has been associated with inferior neurologic outcomes.

- Because fever increases metabolic requirements (10% for each 1° C) and aggravates hypoxia, help maintain patient's body temperature within normal limits by giving prescribed antipyretics, regulating temperature of the environment, limiting use of blankets, keeping patient's trunk warm to prevent shivering, and administering tepid sponge baths or using hypothermia blanket or convection cooling units to reduce fever. When using a hypothermia blanket, wrap the patient's extremities in blankets or towels to prevent shivering. If prescribed, administer chlorpromazine to prevent shivering, which would increase ICP.

- Administer prescribed osmotic and loop diuretics to reduce cerebral edema and reduce blood volume. Administer glucocorticosteroids to reduce edema and inflammation. Administer BP medications as prescribed to keep BP within prescribed limits that will promote optimal CBF without increasing cerebral edema. Because pain can increase BP and consequently increase ICP, administer prescribed analgesics promptly and as necessary. Barbiturates and narcotics are usually contraindicated because of the potential for masking the signs of IICP and causing respiratory depression. However, intubated, restless patients are usually sedated. A continuous midazolam drip has been demonstrated to decrease IICP. Lidocaine is sometimes used to block coughing before suctioning an endotracheal tube.
- Administer antiepilepsy drugs as prescribed to prevent or control seizures, which would increase cerebral metabolism, hypoxia, and CO_2 retention, thereby increasing cerebral edema and ICP.
- Monitor bladder drainage tubes for obstruction or kinks because a distended bladder can increase ICP.
- Provide a quiet and soothing environment. Control noise and other environmental stimuli. Speak softly, use a gentle touch, and avoid jarring the bed. Try to limit painful procedures; avoid tension on tubes (e.g., urinary catheter); and consider limiting pain-stimulation testing. Avoid unnecessary touch (e.g., leave BP cuff in place for frequent VS; use automatic recycling blood pressure monitoring devices); and talk softly, explaining procedures before touching to avoid startling patient. Try to avoid situations in which the patient may become emotionally upset. Do not say anything in the presence of the patient that you would not say if he or she were awake. Family discussions should take place outside the room. Limit visitors as necessary. Encourage significant other to speak quietly to patient because hearing a familiar voice may promote relaxation and decrease ICP. Listening to soft favorite music with earphones also may decrease ICP.
- Multiple procedures and nursing care activities can increase ICP. Individualize care to ensure rest periods and optimal spacing of activities; avoid turning, suctioning, and taking VS all at one time. Rousing patients from sleep has been shown to increase ICP. Plan activities and treatments accordingly so that patient can sleep undisturbed as often as possible.

NIC: Analgesic Administration; Anxiety Reduction; Cerebral Edema Management; Cerebral Perfusion Promotion; Environmental Management; Hemodynamic Regulation

Sensory/perceptual alterations: Visual related to diplopia secondary to neurologic deficit

Desired outcome: Following intervention, patient verbalizes that vision has improved.

- Assess patient for diplopia.
- If patient has diplopia, provide an eye patch or eyeglasses with a frosted lens, which is a temporary means of eliminating this condition. Alternate the eye patch q4hr.
- Orient the patient to the environment as needed.
- Advise patient of the availability of "talking books" (tapes) and large-type reading materials.
- Place a sign over patient's bed that indicates patient's visual impairment.
- Teach patient that depth perception will be altered and to use visual cues and scanning.

NIC: Communication Enhancement: Visual Deficit; Environmental Management; Eye Care

Pain related to spasms, headache, and photophobia secondary to neurologic dysfunction

Desired outcomes: Within 1 hr of intervention, patient's subjective perception of discomfort decreases, as documented by a pain scale. Objective indicators, such as grimacing, are absent or diminished.

- Assess characteristics (e.g., quality, severity, location, onset, duration, precipitating factors) of patient's pain or spasms. Devise a pain scale with patient, and document discomfort on a scale of 0 (no pain) to 10 (worst pain).
- Respond immediately to patient's complaints of pain. Administer analgesics and antispasmodics as prescribed. Consider scheduling doses of analgesia. Document effectiveness of the medication, using the pain scale. Monitor for untoward effects. Consult health care provider if dose or interval change seems necessary. Teach patient and significant other about the importance of timing the pain medication so that it is taken before the pain becomes too severe and before major moves.
- Teach patient about the relationship between anxiety and pain, as well as other factors that enhance pain and spasms (e.g., staying in one position for too long, fatigue, chilling).
- Instruct patient and significant other in the use of nonpharmacologic pain management techniques, such as repositioning; ROM; supporting painful extremity or part; back rubs, acupressure, massage, warm baths, and other tactile distraction; auditory distraction such as listening to soothing music; visual distraction such as television; heat applications such as warm blankets or moist compresses; cold applications such as ice massage; guided imagery; breathing exercises; relaxation tapes and techniques; biofeedback; and a transcutaneous electrical nerve stimulation (TENS) device, as appropriate. See **Health-seeking behaviors:** Relaxation technique effective for stress reduction, p. 59.
- Encourage rest periods to facilitate sleep and relaxation. Fatigue tends to exacerbate the pain experience. Pain may result in fatigue, which in turn may cause exaggerated pain and further exhaustion. Try to provide uninterrupted sleep time at night.
- If patient has photophobia, provide a quiet and dark environment. Close the door and curtains; provide sunglasses; avoid artificial lights whenever possible.
- Pain in the SCI patient often is poorly localized and may be referred. Intrascapular pain may be from the stomach, duodenum, or gallbladder. Umbilical pain may be from the appendix. Testicular or inner thigh pain may be from the kidneys (e.g., pyelonephritis). Evaluate patient for signs of infection or inflammatory process (e.g., tachycardia, restlessness, urinary incontinence when it was previously controlled, fever).
- If patient's present complaint of pain varies significantly from previous pain or if interventions are ineffective, notify health care provider.

NIC: Acupressure; Analgesic Administration; Anxiety Reduction; Autogenic Training; Biofeedback; Cutaneous Stimulation; Distraction; Environmental Management: Comfort; Heat/Cold Application; Medication Management; Meditation; Pain Management; Positioning; Progressive Muscle Relaxation; Simple Guided Imagery; Simple Massage; Simple Relaxation Therapy; Transcutaneous Electrical Nerve Stimulation (TENS)

Impaired swallowing related to neuromuscular impairment (e.g., decreased or absent gag reflex, decreased strength or excursion of muscles involved in mastication, perceptual impairment, facial paralysis)

Desired outcome: Before oral foods and fluids are reintroduced, patient exhibits ability to swallow safely without aspirating.

- Assess patient for factors that affect the ability to swallow safely, including LOC, gag and cough reflexes, and strength and symmetry of tongue, lip, and facial muscles. Monitor for signs of impaired swallowing, including regurgitation of food and fluid through the nares, drooling, food oozing from the lips, and food trapped in buccal spaces. The development of a weak or hoarse voice during or after eating may signal the potential for impaired swallowing. Check the swallow reflex by first asking patient to swallow his or her own saliva. If the larynx elevates with the attempt, a sign that the swallow reflex is intact, next ask the patient to swallow 3-5 ml of plain water. Document your findings.

Caution: The presence of the cough reflex is essential for the patient to relearn swallowing safely.

- Obtain a referral to a speech therapist for patients with a swallowing dysfunction. The act of swallowing is complex, and interventions vary according to the phase of swallowing that is dysfunctional. Video fluoroscopy may be used to evaluate swallowing. Encourage patient to practice any prescribed exercises (e.g., tongue and jaw ROM, sound phonation such as "gah-gah-gah" to promote elevation of the soft palate).
- Enteral or parenteral nutrition may be necessary for the patient who cannot chew or swallow effectively or safely. Alert health care provider to your findings. Be aware that an NG tube may desensitize the patient and impair the reflexive response to food bolus stimulus, thereby hindering the ability to relearn to swallow.
- Keep suction equipment and a manual resuscitation bag with face mask at patient's bedside. Suction secretions in the patient's mouth as necessary.
- Ensure that the patient is alert and responsive to verbal stimuli before attempting to swallow. Patients who are drowsy, inattentive, or fatigued have difficulty cooperating and are at risk of aspirating. To help minimize fatigue, provide a rest period before meals or swallowing attempts. Provide oral hygiene to enhance taste (see **Self-care deficit** [oral hygiene]), p. 338.
- Initial swallowing attempts should be made with plain water (see above) because of the risk of aspiration. Progressively add easy-to-swallow food and liquids as the patient's ability to swallow improves. Determine which foods and liquids are easiest for the patient to swallow. Generally, semisolid foods of medium consistency, such as puddings, hot cereals, and casseroles, tend to be easiest to swallow. Thicker liquids, such as nectars, tend to be better tolerated than thin liquids. Commercially available powders (e.g., Thicket) may be added to liquids to increase their viscosity and make them more easily swallowed. Gravy or sauce added to dry foods often facilitates swallowing. Sticky, mucus-producing foods, such as peanut butter, chocolate, or milk, are often restricted or limited. Avoid nuts, hard candies, or popcorn, which may be aspirated.
- To help the patient focus on swallowing, reduce stimuli in the room (e.g., turn off the television, lower the radio volume, minimize conversation, and limit disruptions from phone calls). Caution patient not to talk while eating.
- Most patients will swallow best when in an upright position. Sitting in a straight-back chair with feet on the floor is ideal. If the patient must remain in bed, use high Fowler's position if possible. Support the shoulders and neck with pillows. Ensure that the head is erect and flexed forward slightly, with the chin at the midline and pointing toward the chest (i.e., the "chin tuck," which is the *opposite* of the chin thrust maneuver used to open the airway), to promote movement of the food and fluid into the esophagus and minimize the risk that it will go into the airway. Stroking the anterior neck lightly may help some patients swallow. Maintain patient in an upright position for at least 30-60 min after eating to prevent regurgitation and aspiration.

- Teach patient to break down the act of chewing and swallowing. Encourage concentration and taking adequate time. Talk patient through the following steps:
  - —Take small bites or sips (approximately 5 ml each).
  - —Place food on the tongue.
  - —Use the tongue to transfer food so that it is directly under the teeth on the unaffected side of the mouth.
  - —Chew the food thoroughly.
  - —Move the food to the middle of the tongue, and hold it there.
  - —Flex the neck, and tuck the chin against the chest.
  - —Hold the breath, and think about swallowing.
  - —Without breathing, raise the tongue to the roof of the mouth and swallow.
  - —Swallow several times if necessary.
  - —When the mouth is empty, raise the chin and clear the throat or cough purposefully once or twice.
- Start with small amounts of food or liquid. Each bite should not exceed 5 ml (1 tsp). Feed slowly. Ensure that each previous bite has been swallowed. Check the mouth for pockets of food. After every few bites of solid food, provide a liquid to help clear the mouth. Avoid using a syringe because the force of the fluid, if sprayed, may cause aspiration. Avoid use of drinking straws.
- Teach patient who has food pockets in the buccal spaces to periodically sweep the mouth with the tongue or finger or to clean these areas with a napkin.
- Teach patients who have a weak or paralyzed side to place food on the side of the face they can control. Tilting the head toward the stronger side will allow gravity to help keep the food or liquid on the side of the mouth they can manipulate. Some patients may find that rotating the head to the weak side will close the damaged side of the pharynx and facilitate more effective swallowing.
- Patients with loss of oral sensation may be unable to identify foods or fluids of tepid temperature by their tongue or oral mucosa, potentially resulting in tissue injury. Serve only warm or cool foods to these individuals. Verbal cues and use of a mirror may help ensure that these patients keep their mouths clear after swallowing.
- Patients with a rigid tongue (e.g., with parkinsonism) have difficulty getting the tongue to move the bolus of food into the pharynx for swallowing. Encourage repeated swallowing attempts to facilitate movement of the food. Evaluate patient's swallowing ability at different times of the day. Reschedule mealtimes to times of the day when patient has improved swallowing, or, as appropriate, discuss with health care provider the possibility of changing the dose schedule of the patient's anti-Parkinson medication.
- If decreased salivation is contributing to the patient's swallowing difficulties, perform one of the following before feeding to stimulate salivation: swab the patient's mouth with a lemon-glycerin sponge; have the patient suck on a tart-flavored hard candy, dill pickle, or lemon slice; teach the patient to move the tongue in a circular motion against the inside of the cheek; or use artificial saliva. Moisten food with melted butter, broth or other soup, or gravy. Dip dry foods such as toast into coffee or other liquid to soften them. Rinse the patient's mouth as needed to remove particles and lubricate the mouth. Investigate medications the patient is taking for the potential side effect of decreased salivation (e.g., anti-parkinsonian medications or those with extrapyramidal side effects).
- Tablets or capsules may be swallowed more easily when added to foods such as puddings or ice cream. Crushed tablets or opened capsules also mix easily into these types of foods. However, check with the pharmacist to ensure that crushing a tablet or opening a capsule does not adversely affect its absorption

or duration (i.e., slow-release medications should *not* be crushed). Liquid forms of medications may also be available through the pharmacy.

- Teach significant other the Heimlich or abdominal thrust maneuver so that he or she can intervene in the event of choking.

NIC: Artificial Airway Management; Aspiration Precautions; Emotional Support; Respiratory Monitoring; Surveillance; Swallowing Therapy; Teaching: Psychomotor Skill

Altered body temperature related to illness or trauma affecting temperature regulation and inability or decreased ability to perspire, shiver, or vasoconstrict
Desired outcome: Following the intervention(s), patient is normothermic with core temperatures between 36.5° and 37.7° C (97.8° and 100° F).

> **Note:** Infection and hypothalamic dysfunction as a result of cerebral insult (trauma, edema) are two common causes of hyperthermia. The rapid development of spinal lesions (e.g., in SCI) breaks the connection between the hypothalamus and the sympathetic nervous system (SNS), causing an inability to adapt to environmental temperature. In spinal cord shock, temperatures tend to lower toward the ambient temperature. Inability to vasoconstrict and shiver makes heat conservation difficult; the inability to perspire prevents normal cooling.

- Monitor rectal, tympanic, or bladder core temperature q4hr or, if patient is in spinal shock, q2hr. Observe for signs of hypothermia: impaired ability to think, disorientation, confusion, drowsiness, apathy, and reduced HR and RR. Monitor for complaints of being too cold, goose bumps (piloerection), and cool skin (in SCI patients, above the level of injury). Observe for signs of hyperthermia: flushed face, malaise, rash, respiratory distress, tachycardia, weakness, headache, and irritability. Monitor for complaints of being too warm, sweating, or hot and dry skin (in SCI patients, above the level of injury). Observe for signs of dehydration: parched mouth, furrowed tongue, dry lips, poor skin turgor, decreased urine output, increased concentration of urine (specific gravity >1.030), and weak, fast pulse.
- *For hyperthermia:* maintain a cool room temperature (20° C [68° F]). Provide a fan or air conditioning to prevent overheating. Remove excess bedding, and cover patient with a thin sheet. Give tepid sponge baths. Place cool, wet cloths at patient's head, neck, axilla, and groin. Administer antipyretic agent as prescribed. Use a padded hypothermia blanket (wrap hands and feet in towels or blankets to prevent shivering) or convection cooling device if prescribed. Provide cool drinks. Evaluate for potential infectious cause.
- *For hypothermia:* increase environmental temperature. Protect patient from drafts. Provide warm drinks. Provide extra blankets. Provide warming (hyperthermia) blanket or convection warming device.
- Keep feverish patient dry. Change bed linens after diaphoresis. Provide careful skin care when patient is on a hypothermia or hyperthermia blanket. Maintain adequate hydration. Consider insensible water loss from fever, which may affect total hydration, when measuring I&O. Unless contraindicated, encourage increased fluid intake in febrile patients (e.g., >3000 ml/day). Increase caloric intake because of increased metabolic needs. Remember that steroids may mask fever or infection.

NIC: Cerebral Edema Management; Fever Treatment; Fluid Monitoring; Hypothermia Treatment; Teaching: Disease Process; Temperature Regulation

Knowledge deficit: Neurologic diagnostic tests (electroencephalogram [EEG], positron emission tomography [PET], MRI, CT scan, lumbar puncture [LP], myelography, digital subtraction angiography [DSA], cerebral angiography, oculoplethysmography, electromyography [EMG], nerve conduction velocity

[NCV], evoked potentials [EP], single photon emission computerized tomography [SPECT]) related to new treatment experience

Desired outcome: Following explanation and before the procedure, patient verbalizes understanding about the prescribed diagnostic test, including purpose, risks, anticipated benefits, and expectations for the patient before, during, and after the test.

- After the health care provider has explained the diagnostic study to the patient, reinforce or clarify information as indicated. Tell the patient who will perform the test, where it will be done, and to report any possible adverse reactions. Adjust and simplify the information to what the patient can understand, and repeat several times, as appropriate to the patient's cognitive dysfunction.

- If an **EEG** has been prescribed, explain that this test will indicate the amount of brain activity present and may reveal abnormal patterns of electrical activity, particularly with such stimuli as flashing lights or hyperventilation. Explain that an EEG may be performed while the patient is either asleep or awake and sometimes by telemetry. Cooperation is important, and the test may take 40-60 min. Alert EEG staff to medications the patient is taking. In addition, discuss the following as appropriate:

  —*Before the test:* antiepilepsy medications, sedatives, and tranquilizers may be withheld 24-48 hr before the test. The patient's hair should be thoroughly washed and dried, but sprays, creams, and oils must be avoided. If a sleep EEG has been prescribed, the patient will need to stay awake the night before the test. The patient usually is allowed a normal diet the morning of the test to prevent hypoglycemia, but caffeine-containing foods (e.g., chocolate) and beverages (e.g., coffee, tea, colas) are restricted.

  —*During the test:* small electrode patches are attached to the patient's head. The skin may be lightly abraded to ensure good contact. Reassure patient that he or she will not receive any electric shocks. The patient is requested to lie very still during the test and may be asked to watch flashing lights or to hyperventilate to elicit electrical activity patterns in the brain.

  —*After the test:* hair washing or acetone swabs will be provided to remove the paste used for attaching the electrodes. Medications probably will be reinstated at this time. If needle electrodes were used, avoid washing hair for 24 hr.

- If **PET** has been prescribed, explain that this test measures how rapidly tissue consumes or uses a radioisotope and may locate areas of cerebral glucose metabolism that correspond to the seizure-causing focus, distinguish tumor tissue from normal tissue by identifying abnormal metabolic activity of the tumor tissue, or identify areas of ischemia or low metabolism (e.g., Alzheimer's disease). In addition, discuss the following as appropriate:

  —*Before the test:* the procedure is contraindicated during pregnancy. Alcohol, caffeine, and tobacco may be restricted for 24 hr to prevent skewing of test results. Because the test is based on tissue glucose metabolism, the patient should eat a meal 3-4 hr before the test. If the patient has diabetes mellitus, the health care provider may give special instructions about insulin administration because insulin alters glucose metabolism. Generally, the patient will be allowed to take insulin before the pretest meal.

  —*During the test:* explain that the test takes 60-90 min and the patient is required to be still during that time. Tranquilizers are contraindicated, however, because they alter glucose metabolism. The patient is given radioisotope by injection or inhalation. If given by inhalation, a dome-shaped hood will be placed over the patient's head to prevent the exhaled tracer from circulating in the room.

  —*After the test:* encourage fluids if not contraindicated.

- If **MRI** has been prescribed, explain that this test may reveal biochemical changes caused by hypoxia or necrosis, by degenerative disease, or by a mass such as a tumor, hemorrhage, tissue shift, or hydrocephalus. This test also may show structural lesions that may be responsible for symptoms such as seizures. MRI is more useful than CT scanning in evaluating pituitary tumors, acoustic neuromas, posterior fossa tumors, spinal cord tumors and trauma, demyelinating disease, cerebral atrophy, and situations in which the patient is allergic to contrast medium. Expansion of magnetic resonance technology is increasing its usefulness. This technology is getting faster (i.e., MRI with FLAIR [fluid attenuated inversion recovery]) and has found broader applications (e.g., magnetic resonance spectroscopy to detect changes in tissue metabolism; magnetic source imaging to measure electrical activity in the brain; magnetic resonance angiography to create a subtraction angiogram). In addition, discuss the following as appropriate:

—*Before the test:* confirm with patients that they do not have a pacemaker, surgical aneurysm clip, prosthetic heart valve, or umbrella filter for emboli and are not pregnant. Ask about the presence of fractures that were treated with metal rods, other implants (cochlear, insulin pumps), or shrapnel or gunshot wounds. Explain that the MRI is contraindicated during pregnancy and can deactivate pacemakers and that the strong magnetic field can move ferrous metal aneurysm clips, valves, and umbrella filters within the body, putting the patient at obvious risk. The presence of these internal items makes the patient ineligible for MRI. The MRI also is not used on critically ill or unstable patients, because it is impossible to monitor cardiac rhythm and VS inside the scanner. Explain that the patient is not exposed to radiation during the test. The patient should void before the test and remove such items as jewelry, hair clips, clothing with metal fasteners, and glasses before entering the scanner.

—*During the test:* the patient must be able to cope with confined spaces and the ability to lie motionless throughout the 30- to 90-min test. A soft, humming sound and "knocking" on-off pulses will be heard. The health care provider may prescribe a sedative. The patient's head, chest, and arms may be restrained to help him or her lie still. The patient may be injected with an IV contrast medium, such as gadolinium, a paramagnetic agent that enhances tumor images.

• If a **CT scan** has been prescribed, explain that the test may detect masses from tumors, hemorrhage, tissue shift, and hydrocephalus. Serial scans may be performed to determine a tumor's response to therapy and detect a resolution or increase in a hemorrhage. CT scanning is more useful than MRI in evaluating acute trauma or hemorrhage, supratentorial enhancing tumors, and hydrocephalus; in predicting vasospasm; and when the patient has a pacemaker or internal ferrous metal objects or is uncooperative. If contrast agents are not used, there are no known complications from CT scans. If a contrast agent is used, discuss the following with the patient as indicated:

—*Before the test:* allergies to iodine or iodine-containing substances such as shellfish or contrast medium must be reported to the health care provider. Food and fluids may be restricted 4 hr before the test. Remove hair pins. The test usually lasts 15-60 min, and the patient can expect to hear a clicking noise as the machine moves. The patient must lie flat and still, the head may be immobilized, and sedation may be prescribed. Explain to the patient that the room will be cool (to protect the equipment).

—*During the test:* a warm flushed feeling or burning sensation is normal and may be felt with administration of the dye. The patient also may experience a salty taste with dye injection, nausea, vomiting, or a headache during or after the test. The patient may be asked to take and hold several deep breaths during the scanning.

—*After the test:* if it is not contraindicated, fluids are increased to ensure elimination of the contrast dye via the kidneys. The patient will be monitored for hives, rash, and itching, which may be delayed allergic reactions to the dye.

- If an **LP** has been prescribed, explain that it is performed to remove a sample of CSF for analysis, to determine CSF pressure, or to administer medication. Typically, the CSF is evaluated for microorganisms, blood cells, tumor markers, and chemical analysis. Skin or bone infection at the puncture site is a contraindication. This procedure is performed with great caution in the presence of IICP. Inability of the patient to cooperate, severe degenerative joint disease, and anticoagulant therapy also may preclude its use. Also discuss the following as indicated:
  - —*Before the test:* assure patient that the needle will not enter the spinal cord. Explain that the patient should empty bladder at this time.
  - —*During the test:* the patient will be assisted into a side-lying position, with the chin tucked into the chest and the knees drawn up to the abdomen. This position curves the spine and widens the intervertebral space for easier insertion of the spinal needle. The patient must lie still during the procedure, and a nurse will assist patient with maintaining the position. An alternate position is sitting flexed over an over-the-bed table with the patient's head and arms resting on a pillow. The patient should breathe normally during the test. There may be a short burning sensation when the local anesthetic is injected and some local transient pain when the spinal needle is inserted. The patient will feel pressure as the needle is advanced to the spinal canal. The patient should report any pain or sensations that continue after or differ from these expected discomforts. The patient will be monitored for discomfort, elevated HR, pallor, and clammy skin during the procedure. During the test, the health care provider may ask the patient to breathe deeply or may apply jugular pressure.
  - —*After the test:* the patient will remain in bed with the HOB flat or raised slightly for a prescribed period of time, usually no more than 8 hr; may turn from side to side during this time period; and should drink a large amount of fluids (1500-2000 ml) unless contraindicated. These measures will help prevent or minimize any postprocedure headache, which is the most common adverse effect of an LP. The patient should report any headache to the nurse so that analgesia, if prescribed, can be administered. The nurse will check the LP site periodically for redness, swelling, and drainage. The nurse also will check VS and neurologic status. The patient should report any neck stiffness, pain, numbness, or weakness.
- If **myelography** has been prescribed, explain that it is performed when other diagnostic tests are inconclusive to delineate or rule out blockage or disruption of the spinal cord. Radiopaque dye is injected into the subarachnoid space of the spine using a lumbar or cervical puncture. Discuss the following with the patient as indicated:
  - —*Before the test:* allergies or sensitivity to iodine, shellfish, and contrast medium; history of medications that could lower the seizure threshold (e.g., phenothiazines, neuroleptics [tricyclics, antidepressants], amphetamines) and epilepsy medication must be reported to the radiologist. Foods and fluids are withheld for a period of time, usually 4-8 hr, before the test.
  - —*During the test:* the patient may feel transient burning when the contrast dye is injected and a salty taste, headache, or nausea after the injection. With oil-based dyes, the table will tilt to facilitate flow of contrast dye to different parts of the spinal canal. With water-based dyes the patient will need to sit quietly to enable the controlled upward dispersion of the dye. The patient may feel some discomfort during the procedure because of needle insertion, positions used, and removal of contrast dye (oil-based dyes) at the end of the procedure. Explain the importance of lying quietly during the 60-min procedure.
  - —*After the test:* VS and peripheral neurologic status should be routinely assessed and changes from pretest assessments promptly reported to the health care provider. The patient should be instructed to report any increased motor or sensory deficit from pretest status, chills, fever, neck

stiffness, and redness or swelling at the puncture site. Headache (occurs in 25%-50%), nausea (15%-40%), and vomiting (25%) are frequent side effects and should be reported so that comfort measures can be taken. Nonrestricted persons should drink extra fluids, especially caffeinated drinks, to replace the CSF lost during the test. The following postmyelogram positions may be used:

—If an oil-based dye was used (e.g., isophendylate): patient must remain flat 6-24 hr or as prescribed. This agent has been almost completely replaced with the water-based dyes and thus is infrequently used.

—If a water-based dye was used (e.g., iohexol, iopamidol, metrizamide): HOB will be elevated to 60 degrees for 6-8 hr to minimize irritation to the cranial nerves and structures. Bathroom privileges are permitted, but minimal activity is permitted for 24 hr after the myelogram. Seizures, hallucination, depression, confusion, speech problems, chest pain, and dysrhythmia may occur if metrizamide reaches the cranial vault. Because phenothiazines and neuroleptics lower the seizure threshold, they should be held for 24 hr after myelograms done using water-based dyes.

- If **DSA** has been prescribed, explain that it is performed to help visualize cerebral blood flow and detect vascular abnormalities such as stenosis, aneurysm, and hematoma. Patients are expected to lie still for the 30- to 60-min procedure and hold their breath on command; minor movements such as swallowing can distort the results. This test is considered safer than angiography. Vein injection carries no risk of embolus and can be done on an outpatient basis. Vein injection (vs. arterial injection) requires more dye and carries an increased risk of kidney damage. This test consists of two scans: one scan without contrast and the other with. The two images are then digitally subtracted from one another. Also discuss the following as indicated:

—*Before the test*: patient will be assessed for adequate cardiac output to disperse the dye and adequate kidney function to excrete the dye. Allergies to iodine, shellfish, or radiopaque dye must be reported to the health care provider. Food and fluids usually are withheld 3-4 hr before the procedure, although clear liquids sometimes are allowed. The patient may feel transient discomfort with insertion of the needle or catheter, as well as a headache, warm sensation, or metallic taste when the dye is injected.

—*After the test:* the patient will be required to drink large amounts of fluid, if not contraindicated, to promote dye excretion by the kidneys. Nurses will check the venipuncture site for bleeding, redness, and swelling. The patient should be instructed to report itching, rash, hives, or dyspnea, which may signal delayed dye reaction 2-6 hr after the test. If an arterial route was used for injection, see the discussion of cerebral angiography, which follows.

- If **cerebral angiography** has been prescribed, explain that it enables visualization of the cerebral vasculature after injection of a contrast medium and determines the site, structure, and size of an aneurysm or arteriovenous malformation, the presence of vasospasm, and the site of rupture or obstructed blood flow. It also may show an abnormal perfusion pattern, which suggests presence of a tumor. Severe kidney, liver, or thyroid disease may contraindicate this test. Also discuss the following as indicated:

—*Before the test:* allergies to iodine, shellfish, or radiopaque dyes must be reported to the health care provider. Foods and fluids are withheld for 8-10 hr or as prescribed. Local anesthetic is used at the puncture site. Patient will feel a warm or burning sensation when the dye is administered and have a transient headache or metallic taste sensation. The proposed site may be shaved. If the femoral approach is used, pedal pulses will be checked and their location marked. If the carotid approach is used, the patient's neck circumference will be measured, marked, and recorded. Baseline neurologic status is checked and recorded for postprocedure comparison so that small changes can be detected early. Dentures and eyeglasses usually are removed.

—*During the test:* patient is expected to lie flat and still for the 60- to 120-min procedure. The patient's extremities or head may be immobilized with tape or straps.

—*After the test:* patient will be on strict bedrest for 6-8 hr, followed by a specified period of bathroom privileges only. Patient's VS and pulse quality will be checked frequently. Patient should notify staff if signs of reaction to the dye occur, including respiratory distress, lightheadedness (hypotension), hives, or itching. Fluids will be encouraged to eliminate dye and protect from kidney damage. The puncture site will be checked frequently for bleeding or hematoma. The patient should not be alarmed if bleeding occurs. Manual pressure will be maintained until the bleeding stops. A pressure dressing may then be applied and the health care provider notified. The quality of distal pulses and the temperature, color, capillary refill, motor function, and sensation in the extremity will be monitored at frequent intervals. Any weakening pulses, pallor, coolness, extremity pain, delayed capillary refill (≥ 3 sec), or cyanosis may signal thrombus formation and artery obstruction and should be promptly reported to the health care provider. Because of proximity to nerves, nerve injury during insertion of the needle/catheter is also possible; any paresthesia or weakness should be reported to the health care provider.

—If the femoral approach was used, patient should keep the leg straight for the prescribed amount of time (usually 6-8 hr) to minimize the risk of bleeding. Patients will use a bedpan or urinal and eat on their side during this time.

—If the brachial approach was used, the patient's arm will be immobilized for 6-8 hr or as prescribed. A sign will be posted over patient's bed that cautions against measuring BP or drawing blood in this arm.

—If the carotid artery was the puncture site, the patient should report any difficulty swallowing or breathing or any weakness or numbness. The neck will be checked for increasing circumference (comparing current measurements with preprocedural measurements) or tracheal displacement, which may signal hematoma formation. Changes in LOC or neurologic deficits may indicate thrombus formation and arterial obstruction.

• If **oculoplethysmography** has been prescribed, explain that it will help detect and evaluate carotid occlusive disease by the indirect measurement of blood flow in the ophthalmic artery, which is the first major branch of the internal carotid artery. Also discuss the following as indicated:

—*Before the test:* a history of recent eye surgery (within 6 mo), retinal detachment, or lens implantation, allergic reaction to local anesthetics, and current anticoagulant surgery should be reported to the health care provider. Contact lenses will be removed. Patients with glaucoma may take their usual eye medication. Anesthetic drops are instilled, and the patient's eyes may burn slightly for a short time after instillation.

—*During the test:* small eye cups that resemble contact lenses are applied to the corneas, and suction is applied. The patient will experience a transient loss of vision as the suction is applied. The patient must be able to lie very still and resist blinking because constant blinking or nystagmus may cause an artifact, making the results difficult to interpret.

—*After the test:* patient should not rub the eyes for at least 2 hr because the eyes are susceptible to corneal abrasion from the local anesthetic. Patient should report symptoms of corneal abrasion, including pain and photophobia. As the eye drops wear off, the patient probably will experience mild burning. Patient should report the presence of severe burning. Patients who wear contact lenses should leave them out for 2 hr to allow the anesthetic eye drops to wear off. A darkened room and sterile normal saline may sooth irritated eyes. A conjunctival hemorrhage may occur but will fade with time.

- **EMG** and **NCV** studies usually are performed together to diagnose and differentiate between peripheral nerve and muscle disorders.
  - —*Before the test:* bleeding disorders, use of anticoagulants, or extensive skin infection may contraindicate the test. Explain that patient cooperation will be necessary during the 20- to 30-min test.
  - —*During the test:* there will be some discomfort as small needles are inserted into muscle. The muscle will twitch when electrical stimulus is applied, but this is not painful.
  - —*After the test:* needle sites will be monitored to determine presence of hematomas or inflammation.
- **EPs** measure changes in the brain's electrical activity in response to sensory stimulation. Shampooing hair before the procedure is desired to remove oil and lotions from hair. Postprocedure shampooing is done to remove electrode paste. Also discuss the following:
  - —*Visual evoked response:* Cooperation is needed. Electrodes are placed over the occipital region. Prescription glasses should be worn. Patterned and flashing lights will provide retinal stimulation. This test is good for diagnosing optic neuritis with MS.
  - —*Somatosensory evoked response:* peripheral nerve responses in upper or lower extremities help evaluate spinal cord function, sensory dysfunction with MS, and nerve root compression.
  - —*Brain stem auditory evoked responses:* used to evaluate brain stem function. Auditory stimulation via headphone is provided. A series of clicks will be heard, varying in rate, intensity, and duration. This test does not require patient cooperation. It can help diagnose brain stem lesion in MS, acoustic neuroma, brain stem lesions related to coma, and hearing loss. It also may be used to monitor cranial nerve VIII for surgical injury.
- If **SPECT** has been prescribed, explain that this test provides a 3-day study of cerebral blood flow.
  - —*During the test:* the patient will receive a dose of a salty-tasting solution and an injection with an IV tracer. It is important to lie still during the 60-min scanning. During the test, the table will move and a large disk-shaped machine will rotate around the patient's head.
- After teaching, evaluate patient's level of understanding of the diagnostic test.

◎ **NIC:** Anxiety Reduction; Circulatory Precautions; Embolus Precautions; Positioning; Teaching: Disease Process; Teaching: Individual; Teaching: Preoperative; Teaching: Procedure/Treatment

Selected Bibliography

Adams RD, Victor M, Ropper AH: *Principles of neurology*, ed 6, New York, 1996, McGraw-Hill.

Banazak DA: Difficult dementia: six steps to control problem behaviors, *Geriatrics* 51(2):36-42, 1996.

Barker E: *Neuroscience nursing*, St Louis, 1994, Mosby.

Bell TE, Kongable GL: Innovations in aneurysmal subarachnoid hemorrhage: intracisternal t-pa for the prevention of vasospasm, *J Neurosci Nurs* 28(2):107-113, 1996.

Bracken MB et al: Administration of methylprednisolone for 24 or 48 hours or tirilazad mesylate for 48 hours in the treatment of acute spinal cord injury. Results of the Third National Acute Spinal Cord Injury Randomized Controlled Trial. National Acute Spinal Cord Injury Study, *J Am Med Assoc* 277(20):1597-1604, 1997.

Chisholm AH: Fetal tissue transplantation for the treatment of Parkinson's disease: a review of the literature, *J Neurosci Nurs* 28(5):329-337, 1996.

Eisenhart K: New perspectives in the management of adults with severe head injury, *Crit Care Nurs Q* 17(2):1-12, 1994.

Geraci E, Geraci T: A look at recent hyperventilation studies: outcomes and recommendations for early use in the head-injured patient, *J Neurosci Nurs* 28(1):222-233, 1996.

Gilbert M et al: Pallidotomy: a surgical intervention for control of Parkinson's disease, *J Neurosci Nurs* 28(1):215-221, 1996.

Guberman A: *An introduction to clinical neurology: pathophysiology, diagnosis and treatment*, Boston, 1994, Little Brown.

Hickey JV: *The clinical practice of neurological and neurosurgical nursing*, ed 3, Philadelphia, 1992, Lippincott.

Interqual: *The ISD-A review system with adult ISD criteria*, Northhampton, NH, and Marlboro, Mass, August 1992, Interqual.

Kelly CL: The role of interferons in the treatment of multiple sclerosis, *J Neurosci Nurs* 28(2):114-120, 1996.

Kim MJ et al: *Pocket guide to nursing diagnoses*, ed 7, St Louis, 1997, Mosby.

Lach HW et al: Alzheimer's disease: assessing safety problems in the home, *Geriatr Nurs* 16(4):160-164, 1995.

Lilly LL, Guanci R: Equivalence dosing, *Am J Nurs* 97(3):12, 1997.

Lugger KE: Dysphagia in the elderly stroke patient, *J Neurosci Nurs* 26(2):78-84, 1994.

Macabasco AC, Hickman JL: Thrombolytic therapy for brain attack, *J Neurosci Nurs* 27(3):138-149, 1995.

McCloskey JC, Bulechek GM, editors: *Nursing Interventions Classification (NIC)*, ed 2, St Louis, 1996, Mosby.

Meythaler JM et al: Prospective study on the use of bolus intrathecal baclofen for spastic hypertonia due to acquired brain injury, *Arch Phys Med Rehabil* 77(5):461-466, 1996.

Moreau D, editor: *Nursing 97 drug handbook*, Springhouse, Pa, 1997, Springhouse.

Ozer MN et al: *Management of persons with stroke*, St Louis, 1994, Mosby.

Pendlebury WW, Solomon PR: Alzheimer's disease, *Clin Symp* 48(3):1-32, 1996.

Ribby KJ, Cox KR: Development, implementation and evaluation of a confusion protocol, *Clin Nurs Specialist* 10(5):241-247, 1996.

Samuels MA, editor: *Manual of neurologic therapeutics*, ed 5, Boston, 1995, Little, Brown.

Samuels MA et al, editors: *Office practice of neurology*, New York, 1996, Churchill Livingstone.

Scheer SJ et al: Randomized controlled trials in industrial low back pain relating to return to work. II. Discogenic low back pain, *Arch Phys Med Rehabil* 77(11):1189-1197, 1996.

Schultz DL: The role of the neuroscience nurse in lumbar fusion, *J Neurosci Nurs* 27(2):90-95, 1995.

Schwartzer A et al: The prevalence and clinical features of internal disc disruption in patients with chronic low back pain, *Spine* 20(17):1878-1883, 1995.

Sosnowski C, Ustik M: Early intervention: coma stimulation in the intensive care unit, *J Neurosci Nurs* 26(2):336-341, 1994.

Stamatos CA et al: Meeting the challenge of the older trauma patient, *Am J Nurs* 96(5):40-47, 1996.

Swearingen PL, Keen JH, editors: *Manual of critical care: applying nursing diagnoses to adult critical illness*, ed 3, St Louis, 1995, Mosby.

Tierney LM et al, editors: *Current medical diagnosis & treatment*, ed 35, Stamford, Conn, 1996, Appleton & Lange.

Weiner WJ, Goetz CG: *Neurology for the non-neurologist*, ed 3, Philadelphia, 1994, Lippincott.

Whitney F: Drug therapy for acute stroke, *J Neurosci Nurs* 26(2):111-117, 1994.

5 ENDOCRINE DISORDERS

Section One: Disorders of the Adrenal Glands

The adrenal glands are found at the superior end of each kidney. Each adrenal gland is composed of two distinct parts: the adrenal cortex and the medulla.

In general, the adrenocortical hormones are released in response to serum levels of adrenocorticotropic hormone (ACTH), which functions via a negative-feedback mechanism: when serum cortisol levels decrease, ACTH release increases. The adrenal cortex is divided into three zones.

The *zona glomerulosa* (outer layer) secretes aldosterone, a major mineralo-corticoid hormone that stimulates the renal tubule to resorb Na^+ and Cl^- while excreting K^+ as protection against hypovolemia and hyperkalemia. When hypovolemia occurs, the kidneys secrete renin, which, among other things, results in the peripheral conversion of angiotensin I to angiotensin II, which in turn stimulates adrenal secretion of aldosterone. Aldosterone results in Na^+ and water retention and increased renal excretion of K^+.

The *zona fasiculata* (middle layer) and *zona reticularis* (inner layer) secrete cortisol, a major glucocorticoid hormone. Cortisol is secreted diurnally with a peak on awakening and a trough around bedtime. Cortisol aids regulation of carbohydrate, protein, and fat metabolism while inhibiting the production and action of mediators of inflammation and immunity (e.g., histamine, lympho-kines, prostaglandin). Increased cortisol secretion occurs with physiologic stressors, such as infection, trauma, and exercise.

The *zona reticularis* also secretes androgens (testosterone, androstenedi-one), which aid in sexual maturation.

The adrenal medulla secretes the catecholamines epinephrine and norepi-nephrine, which are released in response to sympathetic nervous system stimulation.

Addison's disease

Addison's disease is a deficiency of adrenocortical hormones following destruction of the adrenal cortex, which can occur suddenly as a result of such stressors as trauma, infection, or surgery but more commonly occurs gradually. As many as 80% of reported cases involve an autoimmune factor, such as polyglandular autoimmune syndrome. *Primary Addison's disease* is a patho-logic condition of the adrenal glands themselves, whereas *secondary Addison's disease* is often caused by prior treatment with glucocorticoids or other diseases of the pituitary gland that inhibit pituitary ACTH release.

Deficiency of glucocorticoids retards the mobilization of tissue protein and inhibits the ability of the liver to store glycogen, which causes muscle weakness and hypoglycemia to occur. Wound healing is slowed, and these individuals become particularly susceptible to infection. There is a loss of vascular tone in the periphery as well as decreased vascular response to the

354

catecholamines epinephrine and norepinephrine. Decreased secretion of aldosterone causes Na^+, Cl^-, and water loss from the kidneys and increased reabsorption of K^+.

Acute adrenal insufficiency, or *addisonian crisis,* is a life-threatening emergency caused by insufficient cortisol. Crisis occurs in patients with acute adrenal insufficiency (Addison's disease) or as the indication of adrenal insufficiency. Crisis usually follows stress (trauma, infection, prolonged fasting); sudden withdrawal of exogenous steroid therapy; bilateral adrenalectomy or removal of an adrenal tumor; sudden destruction of the pituitary gland; or injury to both adrenal glands.

ASSESSMENT

Signs and symptoms: Weakness, fatigue, anorexia, nausea, vomiting, abdominal pain, fever, restlessness, emotional instability, and confusion. More acutely ill patients may experience dizziness, postural hypotension, weight loss, arthralgia, and amenorrhea.

Physical assessment: Increased skin pigmentation (especially in skin creases, pressure areas, mucous membranes, nipples), small heart size, weakened pulse, sparse axillary hair growth, weight loss, emaciation, dehydration; also, in crisis, cyanosis may occur.

Acute adrenal insufficiency crisis: Weakness, headache, nausea, vomiting, fever, intractable abdominal pain, and severe hypotension, which can lead to vascular collapse and shock.

History of: Familial tendency, bilateral adrenalectomy, major trauma or infection, damage to the pituitary gland, or sudden withdrawal of exogenous steroids after long-term use.

DIAGNOSTIC TESTS

Cosyntropin (synthetic $ACTH_{1-24}$) stimulation test: Initially a blood sample is drawn to determine the baseline level of serum cortisol. Then 0.25 mg cosyntropin is given by IV push, at which time the patient may experience nausea and have a sudden urge to urinate, but these side effects resolve quickly. Additional blood samples are drawn 30-60 min later to determine serum cortisol levels. Individuals with adrenal insufficiency will demonstrate a slight rise in serum cortisol but not the peak values that would occur in individuals without adrenal insufficiency.

Other blood studies

Serum electrolyte studies: K^+ will be elevated; Na^+ and Cl^- decreased; glucose decreased; and Ca^{++} elevated.

Plasma ACTH: Markedly increased with primary adrenal disease (>200 pg/ml if patient is in, or approaching, crisis); decreased in secondary Addison's disease.

Cultures: When the patient is in addisonian crisis, blood, urine, or sputum cultures may be positive if the cause of the crisis is major infection. Meningococcal infections may result in associated Waterhouse-Friderichsen syndrome.

CBC with differential: In crisis there may be associated neutropenia (5000 cells/μl), lymphocytosis (35%-50%), and elevated eosinophils (>300 million/L).

Plasma cortisol: Low (<5 mg/dl) at 7-8 AM can be diagnostic of adrenal insufficiency or crisis, especially when accompanied by elevated plasma ACTH.

Urine Na^+ levels: Increased because of renal Na^+ wasting.

CT scan or MRI: May show a decrease in adrenal or pituitary size, which signals glandular destruction from an autoimmune process. Adrenal glands are enlarged in 85% of patients with granulomatous or metastatic disease. Calcification may be seen in TB, hemorrhage, pheochromocytoma, melanoma, and fungal infection.

Chest x-ray: May reveal underlying TB, fungal infection, or cancer in non-addisonian patients.

COLLABORATIVE MANAGEMENT

Pharmacotherapy

Hydrocortisone: For addisonian patients, 15-30 mg is given in twice-daily doses—two thirds in the morning and one third at night.

Prednisone: Used if hydrocortisone is ineffective; 3 mg in the morning and 2 mg at night.

Fludrocortisone acetate (Florinef acetate):   Because of sodium-retention properties, used in patients receiving hydrocortisone or prednisone who continue to excessively excrete sodium. If postural hypotension, weakness, or hyperkalemia occurs, the dose is increased; if hypertension, edema, or hypokalemia occurs, the dose is decreased.

Antibiotics or anti-TB therapy: If infection or TB is the cause.

Diet: High in calories, carbohydrates, proteins, and vitamins and provided in small, frequent feedings to enhance nutritional state for these patients, who tend to be anorectic.

For adrenal crisis

IV fluids: Rapid administration of 1-2 L of saline may be provided over 2 hours to correct dehydration or hypovolemic shock.

Pharmacotherapy

Hydrocortisone: 100-300 mg IV, in a saline infusion, given rapidly without awaiting serum cortisol level. The initial dosage may also be prescribed IV push over 1 min. Follow-up IV dosage of 50-100 mg is provided q6hr for the first day and then q8hr on the second day. When the patient is able to resume oral intake, hydrocortisone may be given orally q6hr and gradually reduced.

Vasopressors: To maintain adequate BP >90 mm Hg (e.g., norepinephrine [Levophed], dopamine).

Broad-spectrum antibiotics: Administered prophylactically until infecting organisms are identified (bacterial infection frequently precipitates acute adrenal crisis).

Dextrose 50%:   Administered IV to rapidly correct hypoglycemic reactions.

Continuous cardiac monitoring: For prompt identification of life-threatening dysrhythmias associated with hypotension and electrolyte imbalances.

Serum electrolyte monitoring: Serial monitoring of Na^+, Cl^-, K^+, glucose, CO_2^-, BUN, and creatinine to assess the patient's return to homeodynamism.

NURSING DIAGNOSES AND INTERVENTIONS

Risk for infection with risks related to compromised immunologic status secondary to decreased adrenal function

Desired outcome: Patient is free of infection as evidenced by normothermia, WBC count ≤11,000/mm^3, clear and straw-colored urine, well-healing wounds, negative culture results, and absence of adventitious breath sounds and sore throat.

- Monitor for and report early signs of infection, including fever; leukocytosis; frequency, urgency, dysuria, and cloudy or malodorous urine; persistent erythema, pain, local warmth, swelling, or purulent discharge from wounds or the IV site; and complaints of sore throat and pharyngitis. Teach patient these indicators and the importance of reporting them to health care provider or staff promptly. As directed, culture any drainage.
- Monitor temperature q2-4hr, and report significant elevation to health care provider.
- Use meticulous sterile technique for all invasive procedures and when changing dressings. Ensure meticulous indwelling catheter care to help

prevent urinary tract infection (UTI). Perform stringent hand-washing technique before caring for these patients.
- Caution visitors who have contracted or been exposed to a communicable disease to stay out of the room or to wear surgical mask when visiting patient.

You may also wish to refer to the following interventions from the Nursing Interventions Classification (NIC):

NIC: Infection Protection; Perineal Care; Surveillance; Tube Care: Urinary; Venous Access Devices (VAD) Maintenance

Altered protection related to potential for addisonian crisis
Desired outcomes: Patient is free of symptoms of addisonian crisis as evidenced by normothermia; BP ≥90/60 mm Hg (or within patient's baseline range); HR ≤100 bpm; RR 12-20 breaths/min with normal depth and pattern (eupnea); no significant change in mental status and orientation to person, place, and time; and absence of abdominal pain, nausea, vomiting, and headache. If addisonian crisis occurs, however, it is detected and reported promptly.
- Be alert to the following indicators of addisonian crisis: headache, nausea, vomiting, fever, abdominal pain, and severe hypotension. Be aware that profound hypotension can lead to vascular collapse and shock.
- Place patient in a quiet room away from loud noises and excessive activity. Caution staff and visitors not to discuss stress-provoking topics with patient.
- As prescribed, administer corticosteroids and prophylactic antibiotics, which help prevent addisonian crisis.
- If addisonian crisis is diagnosed, implement the following:
  —As prescribed, administer vasopressors to maintain BP and hydrocortisone preparations to replace cortisol.
  —Administer IV fluids as prescribed to prevent circulatory collapse.
  —Monitor VS q15min until stable and then as prescribed. Report significant changes in BP, HR, or respiratory rate or pattern to health care provider.
  —Monitor oximetry, report O_2 saturation ≤92%, and administer oxygen as prescribed.
  —Usually a continuous cardiac monitor is used if addisonian crisis is diagnosed. Monitor for signs of hypokalemia (increased premature ventricular contractions, depressed T waves) or hyperkalemia (peaked T waves).
  —As indicated, monitor capillary glucose levels, report capillary glucose ≤80 mg/dl, and administer glucose replacement as prescribed.
- Monitor for and report signs of Na^+ retention and fluid volume excess (peripheral, pulmonary, and cerebral edema) caused by excessive doses of medications used to treat or prevent addisonian crisis, including corticosteroids, Na^+, and fluids. Be alert to dependent jugular distention, edema, crackles (rales), weight gain, severe headache, irritability, mental status changes, and confusion. Teach these symptoms to patient and significant other, and stress the importance of reporting them promptly to health care provider or staff member.

NIC: Cardiac Care: Acute; Fluid/Electrolyte Management; Hypoglycemia Management; Neurologic Monitoring; Respiratory Monitoring; Resuscitation; Teaching: Disease Process; Vital Signs Monitoring

Activity intolerance related to generalized weakness and fatigue secondary to decreased cardiac output
Desired outcome: During activity, patient rates perceived exertion at ≤3 on a 0-10 scale and exhibits cardiac tolerance to activity as evidenced by HR ≤20 bpm over resting HR, systolic BP ≤20 mm Hg over or under resting systolic BP, RR ≤20 breaths/min with normal depth and pattern (eupnea), warm and dry skin, and absence of crackles (rales), murmurs, chest pain, and new dysrhythmias.

- Monitor VS for evidence of activity intolerance, and ask patient to rate perceived exertion (see **Activity intolerance**, p. 738, in Appendix One for detail). Also observe for and report indicators of impending circulatory collapse, such as hypotension, tachycardia, weak and thready pulse, pallor, and cyanosis.
- Gear activities to patient's tolerance. Provide frequent rest periods.
- To prevent complications of immobility, assist patient with ROM and other in-bed exercises. For details, see Appendix One for **Risk for activity intolerance**, p. 738, and **Risk for disuse syndrome**, p. 740.

NIC: Cardiac Precautions; Energy Management; Exercise Therapy: Joint Mobility; Fall Prevention; Hypovolemia Management; Self-Care Assistance

Fluid volume deficit related to active loss secondary to diuresis
Desired outcome: Patient becomes normovolemic within 24 hr of hospital admission, as evidenced by balanced I&O, urinary output ≥30 ml/hr, adequate skin turgor, stable weight, and moist tongue and oral mucous membranes.
- Monitor I&O, and be alert to indicators of fluid volume deficit, including thirst, poor skin turgor, and furrowed tongue.
- If deficit is noted, report findings to the health care provider and encourage oral fluids.
- Administer maintenance doses of mineralocorticoid as prescribed to promote salt and water retention.
- If prescribed, administer supplementary Na^+ to correct hyponatremia. As appropriate, advise patient to add salt to foods or eat foods relatively high in Na^+, such as meat, fish, poultry, eggs, and milk. See Table 3-2, p. 133, for a list of foods high in Na^+.

NIC: Fluid/Electrolyte Management; Hypovolemia Management; Medication Management; Nutritional Counseling; Skin Surveillance

> **Note:** If the patient experiences addisonian crisis, see psychosocial nursing diagnoses and interventions in Appendix One, "Caring for Patients With Cancer and Other Life-disrupting Illnesses," p. 791.

PATIENT-FAMILY TEACHING AND DISCHARGE PLANNING

When providing patient-family teaching, focus on sensory information; avoid giving excessive information; and initiate a visiting nurse referral for necessary follow-up teaching. Consider including verbal and written information about the following:
- Medications, including drug name, purpose, dosage, schedule, precautions, drug/drug and food/drug interactions, and potential side effects. Ensure that patient understands the necessity of lifetime hormone replacement.
- Diet (e.g., foods to increase, such as those high in Na^+ [see Table 3-2, p. 133]).
- Relationship between hormonal levels and stress. Instruct patient to seek medical help during periods of emotional or physical stress so that medication dosages can be adjusted accordingly.
- Signs and symptoms that necessitate medical attention. These include indicators of excessive adrenal hormones (e.g., weight gain, moon face, dependent edema, headache, weakness, irritability), adrenal insufficiency (e.g., progressive fatigue, nausea, vomiting, weakness, postural hypotension), and infections (e.g., URI, wound, UTI, oral).
- Methods for maximizing coping mechanisms to deal with stress, such as diversional activities and relaxation exercises. Explain the importance of avoiding physical or emotional stress. See **Health-seeking behaviors:** Relaxation technique effective for stress reduction, p. 59.
- Need for continued medical follow-up.

- Phone numbers to call should questions or concerns arise about therapy or disease after discharge. Additional general information can be obtained by contacting the following organization:

  National Adrenal Diseases Foundation
  505 Northern Blvd., Suite 200
  Great Neck, NY 11021 (516) 487-4992
  WWW address: *http://medhelp.netusa.net/*

- Obtaining a Medic-Alert bracelet and identification card outlining the diagnosis and emergency treatment from the following organization:

  Medic Alert
  2323 Colorado Ave.
  Turlock, CA 95382 (209) 668-3333

In addition
- Prepare an emergency kit, including alcohol sponges and syringes with 100 mg of hydrocortisone, to be carried and used for addisonian crisis. Teach technique for IM administration of the medication to patient and significant other.

Cushing's disease

Cushing's disease (hypercortisolism) is a spectrum of symptoms associated with prolonged elevated plasma concentration of adrenal glucocorticoids (e.g., cortisol). In individuals with normal functioning, the pituitary gland secretes adrenocorticotropic hormone (ACTH), which stimulates the adrenal glands to release the adrenal glucocorticoid hormones and mineralocorticoid. This is regulated by a negative-feedback mechanism in which increasing levels of plasma cortisol suppress ACTH. In pituitary pathologic conditions, the anterior pituitary gland fails to sense the plasma cortisol level, resulting in constant secretion of ACTH and resultant abnormally high levels of glucocorticoid hormones. This accounts for approximately 70% of reported cases and is termed *Cushing's disease.* Approximately 90% of patients with Cushing's disease have a pituitary adenoma. *Cushing's syndrome,* on the other hand, is caused by autonomous adrenal tumors (adenomas or carcinomas), ACTH-secreting tumors outside the pituitary, or iatrogenic causes, such as long-term administration of corticotropin (ACTH) or cortisol (steroids).

Actions of excessive glucocorticoid (cortisol) secretion include the following: increased protein catabolism; increased production of glucose and glycogen, with resultant hyperglycemia; a rise in plasma lipid levels causing atherosclerotic changes in blood vessels; decreased bone formation and increased bone resorption resulting in osteoporosis; and inhibition of the inflammatory response to tissue injury. Actions of excessive mineralocorticoid (aldosterone) include the following: Na^+ and water retention and increased renal excretion of K^+.

ASSESSMENT

Signs and symptoms: Weight gain; muscle weakness; kyphosis and back pain; generalized osteoporosis, especially in the vertebrae; pathologic fractures of the long bones; aseptic necrosis (especially of the femoral head); mental and emotional disturbances (mood lability to psychosis); capillary fragility and easy bruising; arteriosclerotic changes in the heart, brain, and kidney; renal calculi; thirst and polyuria; and impotence.
Physical assessment: Patients exhibit central obesity with pendulous abdomens and thin legs and arms; moon face (cushingoid faces); fat deposits on the neck and supraclavicular area (buffalo hump); edema; hypertension; and thin,

transparent skin with multiple ecchymoses. Androgen excess is most noticeable in females, as evidenced by changes in menstruation, as well as virilism and hirsutism. Patients frequently have stretch marks (abdominal striae) with red and purple lines showing through the stretched skin. Patients with Cushing's syndrome have hyperpigmentation of facial skin secondary to ectopic ACTH-secreting tumors.

History of: Excessive or chronic exogenous steroid ingestion, pituitary tumor.

DIAGNOSTIC TESTS

24-Hr urine sample for free cortisol or 17-hydroxycorticosteroid levels: Highly accurate; elevated in the presence of Cushing's disease.

Overnight dexamethasone suppression test: The patient is given a 1-mg tablet of dexamethasone at 11 PM the evening before the test. For patients without Cushing's disease this dose should suppress plasma cortisol levels at 8 AM the following morning to <50% of baseline. This test excludes Cushing's syndrome with 98% certainty. False-positive results are possible with concurrent administration of phenytoin, phenobarbital, and primidone.

Serum electrolyte studies: Blood glucose levels drawn after meals will be elevated in 80%-90% of patients with Cushing's disease. Serum K^+ levels will be decreased.

CT scan or MRI: May show adrenal masses or abnormalities in the sella turcica, which indicate pituitary dysfunction or pituitary adenoma.

COLLABORATIVE MANAGEMENT

Transsphenoidal pituitary surgery: Selective resection of pituitary adenoma is the preferred treatment because of low morbidity and few postsurgical complications (although around 20% of patients develop diabetes insipidus; see p. 362). CT-guided stereotactic surgery is also an option in some medical centers. After surgery, hydrocortisone replacement therapy is needed for 6-36 mo until normal corticotropic function resumes.

Bilateral adrenalectomy: If selective pituitary resection does not remit symptoms, removal of the adrenal glands may be necessary. Laparoscopic resection is used whenever possible; open resection may be necessary when adrenal neoplasm is suspected.

Adrenocortical inhibitors (e.g., metapyrone, ketoconazole, aminoglutethimide, cyproheptadine): To inhibit production of adrenocortical hormones. Exogenous steroids also may be given in conjunction with the adrenocortical inhibitors to prevent hypocortisolism. Adrenocortical inhibitors are used only for short periods, however, because increased ACTH production quickly overcomes their effect.

Irradiation of the pituitary gland: To decrease pituitary production of ACTH. It is used only in patients with a mild form of the disease or in those who are poor surgical candidates.

Diet: Low in calories and carbohydrates to reduce hyperglycemia. Salt is restricted to reduce BP, and foods high in K^+ (see Table 3-4, p. 146) are given to raise serum K^+ levels.

NURSING DIAGNOSES AND INTERVENTIONS

Body image disturbance related to hyperpigmentation, hair loss, and other physical changes associated with increased ACTH production

Desired outcome: Within the 24-hr period before hospital discharge, patient relates attaining self-acceptance and verbalizes knowledge that symptoms will abate with treatment.

- Budget time to spend with patient, and encourage patient to verbalize feelings and frustrations.
- Reassure patient that symptoms should subside with adequate treatment of the disorder.

- Assist patient with measures to improve appearance, such as keeping hair well groomed, wearing own gown or pajamas if possible, and performing personal hygiene (e.g., bathing, brushing teeth). Encourage use of cosmetics and toiletries as patient desires.
- See **Body image disturbance,** p. 799, in Appendix One for additional information.

NIC: Anxiety Reduction; Body Image Enhancement; Coping Enhancement; Emotional Support; Socialization Enhancement; Teaching: Disease Process

Risk for impaired skin integrity with risk factors related to thinning skin and fragile capillaries secondary to increased cortisol production
Desired outcome: Patient's skin remains intact and nonerythematous.
- Ensure that patient on bedrest turns q2hr. Establish and post a turning schedule. Provide gentle massage with nonirritating, nonalcohol lotions to help prevent pressure ulcers.
- Place alternating air pressure mattress or other pressure-relief mattress or pad on the bed.
- Position foot cradle over the bed to prevent pressure areas on lower extremities by keeping bed linen off the feet.
- To protect the skin of confused patients, pad the side rails of the bed.

NIC: Positioning; Pressure Management; Pressure Ulcer Prevention; Skin Surveillance

---

See Also: "Addison's Disease" for **Risk for infection,** p. 356; "Pituitary and Hypothalamic Tumors" for **Altered protection** (IICP, CSF leak, diabetes insipidus) secondary to transsphenoidal hypophysectomy, p. 369; Appendix One for nursing diagnoses and interventions in "Caring for Preoperative and Postoperative Patients," p. 717; "Caring for Patients With Cancer and Other Life-disrupting Illnesses," p. 747.

PATIENT-FAMILY TEACHING AND DISCHARGE PLANNING

When providing patient-family teaching, focus on sensory information; avoid giving excessive information; and initiate a visiting nurse referral for necessary follow-up teaching. Consider including verbal and written information about the following:

- Diet, including foods to increase, such as those high in K^+ (see Table 3-4, p. 146), and foods to restrict, including those high in Na^+ (see Table 3-2, p. 133) or carbohydrates. Arrange for a dietary consultation to help patient with meal planning and integration of individual restrictions into family diet.
- Medications, including drug name, purpose, dosage, schedule, precautions, drug/drug and food/drug interactions, and potential side effects. Advise patient with bilateral adrenalectomy of the necessity for lifetime hormone replacement therapy.
- Importance of continued medical follow-up; confirm date and time of next medical appointment.
- Relationship between hormone levels and stress. Advise patient to seek medical assistance during periods of emotional or physical stress so that medications can be adjusted accordingly. Provide suggestions for patient to maximize coping mechanisms, such as relaxation exercises or diversional activities. See **Health-seeking behaviors:** Relaxation technique effective for stress reduction, p. 59.
- Indicators of *excessive adrenal hormone:* weight gain, thirst, polyuria, easy bruising, and muscle weakness; or *adrenal insufficiency:* easy fatigability, weight loss, and abdominal pain. Any of these indicators necessitates medical attention.

- Signs and symptoms of UTI, URI, and wound and oral infections and the importance of seeking medical care if they occur.
- Phone numbers to call if questions or concerns arise about therapy or disease after discharge. Additional general information can be obtained by contacting the following organization:

  National Adrenal Diseases Foundation
  505 Northern Blvd., Suite 200
  Great Neck, NY 11021   (516) 487-4992
  WWW address: *http://medhelp.netusa.net/*

- Obtaining a Medic-Alert bracelet and identification card outlining the diagnosis and emergency treatment from the following organization:

  Medic Alert
  2323 Colorado Ave.
  Turlock, CA 95382   (209) 668-3333

In addition
- For patients with bilateral adrenalectomy, provide an emergency kit with alcohol sponges and syringes filled with 100 mg of hydrocortisone for episodes of acute adrenal insufficiency. Teach patient and significant other the technique for IM administration of the medication for emergency treatment.

Section Two: Disorders of the Pituitary Gland

The pituitary (hypophysis) is composed of two lobes—the anterior pituitary (adenohypophysis) and posterior pituitary (neurohypophysis). The anterior lobe is larger, and its secretory activities are controlled by tropic hormones produced by and transmitted from the hypothalamus in response to negative-feedback mechanisms. It secretes seven of the nine pituitary hormones: (1) adrenocorticotropic hormone (ACTH), which stimulates adrenocortical growth and secretion of adrenocortical hormones; (2) thyroid-stimulating hormone (TSH), or thyrotropic hormone, which stimulates thyroid growth and secretion of thyroid hormones; (3) follicle-stimulating hormone (FSH), which stimulates ovulation in females and sperm production in males; (4) luteinizing hormone (LH), called the *interstitial cell stimulating hormone (ICSH)* in males, in whom it stimulates production of testosterone; in females it stimulates ovulation and development of ovarian follicles; (5) melanocyte-stimulating hormone (MSH), which causes pigmentation; (6) luteotropic hormone (LTH), also called *prolactin*, which stimulates secretion of milk in females; and (7) growth hormone (GH), or somatotropic hormone (STH), which accelerates body growth.

Posterior pituitary secretion is regulated by nerve impulses originating in the hypothalamus in response to stimuli from other parts of the body. It produces two hormones: antidiuretic hormone (ADH), or vasopressin, which acts on the renal tubules to increase reabsorption of water; and oxytocin, which stimulates milk "letdown" and contraction of the uterus. These hormones are synthesized in the hypothalamus and stored in secretory granules located in the nerve terminals of the posterior pituitary.

Diabetes insipidus

Diabetes insipidus (DI) is a relatively uncommon disease that results from a defect in the synthesis of ADH by the hypothalamus or release from the posterior pituitary (neurogenic, or central, DI) or in the renal tubular response to ADH (nephrogenic DI) causing impaired renal conservation of water.

Neurogenic DI may be the result of primary DI (i.e., a hypothalamic or pituitary lesion or dominant familial trait), secondary DI (following injury to the hypothalamus or pituitary stalk), or vassopressinase-induced DI, which is seen in the last trimester of pregnancy (caused by a circulating enzyme that destroys vasopressin). Nephrogenic DI either occurs as a familial X-linked trait or is associated with pyelonephritis, renal amyloidosis, Sjogren's syndrome, sickle cell anemia, myeloma, potassium depletion, or chronic hypercalcemia. A rare form of DI, termed *psychogenic diabetes insipidus*, is associated with compulsive water drinking.

Except for DI following infection or trauma, the onset of DI is usually insidious, with progressively increasing polydipsia and polyuria. DI following trauma or infection has three phases. The first phase, of polydipsia and polyuria, immediately follows the injury and lasts 4-5 days. In the second phase, which lasts about 6 days, the symptoms disappear; and in the third phase, the patient experiences continued polydipsia and polyuria. Depending on the degree of injury, the condition can be either temporary or permanent.

The chief danger to patients with DI is dehydration from the inability to take in adequate fluids to balance the excessive output of urine. DI must be differentiated from other syndromes resulting in polyuria. History, physical, and simple laboratory procedures assist in diagnosis. Other causes of polyuria include recent lithium or mannitol administration, renal transplantation, renal disease, hyperglycemia, hyperosmolality (early), hypercalcemia, or K^+ depletion, including primary aldosteronism.

ASSESSMENT

Signs and symptoms: Polydipsia, polyuria (2-20 L/day) with dilute urine (specific gravity <1.007).

Physical assessment: Usually within normal limits, but patient may show signs of dehydration if fluid intake is inadequate. Individuals with cranial injury, disease, or trauma may exhibit impairment of neurologic status, including altered LOC and sensory or motor deficits.

History of: Cranial injury, especially basilar skull fracture; meningitis; primary or metastatic brain tumor; surgery in the pituitary area; cerebral hemorrhage; encephalitis; syphilis; or tuberculosis. Familial incidence rarely is a factor.

DIAGNOSTIC TESTS

Urine osmolality: Decreased (<50-200 mOsm/kg) in the presence of disease.

Specific gravity: Decreased (<1.007) in the presence of disease.

Serum osmolality: Increased (≥300 mOsm/kg) in the presence of disease.

Vasopressin challenge test: After administration of vasopressin SC or desmopressin nasal spray (Table 5-1), urine is collected q15min for 2 hr. Quantity and specific gravity are then measured. Normally, individuals will show a concentration of urine but not as pronounced as that of persons with DI; a person with kidney disease will have a lesser response to vasopressin.

Note: One serious side effect of this test is precipitation of heart failure in susceptible individuals.

Hypertonic saline infusions: Three percent sodium chloride (NaCl) solution is infused IV to assess for subsequent water conservation. Although this test seldom is necessary for a diagnosis of DI, it does assist in documentation of changes in the osmotic threshold for ADH release.

Water deprivation test: Although less frequently used, this test may still be used by some health care providers. Baseline measurements of body weight, serum and urine osmolalities, and urine specific gravity are obtained. Fluids are not permitted, and the above measurements are repeated q1hr. The

TABLE 5-1   Vasopressin Preparations

Generic name	Brand name	Onset	Duration (hr)	Usual dose	Advantages/ disadvantages	Comments
Nasal						
Vasopressin	Pitressin (20 pressor U/ml)	Within 1 hr	4-8	5-10 U bid or tid	Action decreased by nasal congestion or discharge or atrophy of nasal mucosa	Administer by spray, cotton pledget, or dropper
Desmopressin acetate	DDAVP (0.1 mg/ml)	Within ½ hr	8-20	0.1-0.4 ml qd in 1-3 doses (10-40 μg)	See vasopressin above	Administer by spray or nasal tube system; store in refrigerator at 4° C (39.2° F)
Lypressin	Diapid (0.185 mg/ml)	Within ½ hr	3-8	7-14 μg qid (1 or 2 sprays into each nostril)	See vasopressin above	Administer by spray
Subcutaneous						
Vasopressin	Pitressin (20 pressor U/ml)	½-1 hr	2-8	0.25-0.5 ml (5-10 U) q3-4hr prn for increased thirst or increased urine output	May be used as an alternative in patients for whom nasal route is contraindicated	Carbamazepine and chlorpropamide may potentiate antidiuretic effects of all forms of vasopressin
Desmopressin acetate	DDAVP	Within ½ hr	1½-4	0.5-1 ml (2-4 μg) qd in 2 divided doses		Keep refrigerated at 4° C (39.2° F)

Intramuscular						
Vasopressin tannate in oil	Pitressin tannate in oil (5 pressor U/ml)	Within 1-2 hr	36-48	0.3-1 ml (1.5-5 U) q2-3 days for increased thirst or increased urine output	Longer duration of action and slower absorption than SC route; response cumulative over 2-3 days	Store at 13°-18° C (55.4°-65.4° F); roll vial between hands before withdrawing solution; can warm vial by immersing in warm water
Vasopressin	Pitressin (20 pressor U/ml)	½-1 hr	2-8	0.25-0.5 ml (5-10 U) q3-4hr for increased thirst or increased urine output		
Intravenous						
Desmopressin acetate	DDAVP (4 µg/ml)	Within ½ hr	1½-4	0.5-1 ml (2-4 µg) qd in 2 divided doses	Generally not for home use	Keep refrigerated at 4° C (39.2° F); dilute in 10-50 ml 0.9% NaCl, and infuse over 15-30 min

SC, Subcutaneous; *NaCl,* sodium chloride.

test is terminated when urine specific gravity exceeds 1.020 and osmolality exceeds 800 mOsm/kg (normal responses), urine specific gravity does not increase for 3 hr (a positive result), or 5% of body weight is lost. The latter is, in itself, an abnormal response, and the corresponding urine osmolality will be <400 mOsm/kg, which is diagnostic of DI. Because the most serious side effect of this test is severe dehydration, the test should be performed early in the day so the patient can be more closely monitored. Before a firm diagnosis of DI can be made from an abnormal water deprivation test, it is also necessary to demonstrate that the kidneys can respond to vasopressin (see below).

COLLABORATIVE MANAGEMENT

For central, or neurogenic, DI

Rehydration: Lost water is replaced with IV hypotonic (e.g., 0.45% NaCl) solution. The initial replacement is rapid, necessitating close monitoring of BP, HR, and urine output.

Administration of exogenous vasopressin (Pitressin):   Replacement therapy for ADH. Several preparations are available (Table 5-1), and it is important to read the package insert carefully to ensure proper administration. Potential side effects include hypertension secondary to vasoconstriction, myocardial infarction secondary to constriction of coronary vessels, uterine cramps, and increased peristalsis of the GI tract.

Achieving a mild antidiuretic effect: For example, with hydrochlorothiazide, chlorpropamide, clofibrate, carbamazepine, or other medication that increases the action or release of ADH.

For nephrogenic DI

Indomethacin therapy: Short-term treatment is begun with 50 mg q8hr. May be combined with thiazide diuretics, desmopressin, or amiloride.

Therapy with thiazide diuretics (e.g., hydrochlorothiazide, 50-100 mg daily, or chlorthalidone, 50 mg daily):   Although it may seem antithetical to treat diuresis with a diuretic, one of the side effects of the thiazide diuretics is blocking of the kidneys' ability to excrete free water, which is the primary problem with DI.

For psychogenic DI

Psychotherapy: Necessary for patients with compulsive water drinking. Thioridazine and lithium should be avoided because they cause polyuria.

NURSING DIAGNOSES AND INTERVENTIONS

Fluid volume deficit related to active loss secondary to polyuria

Desired outcomes: Patient becomes normovolemic within 7 days of onset of symptoms as evidenced by stable weight, balanced I&O, good skin turgor, moist tongue and oral mucous membrane, BP ≥90/60 mm Hg (or within patient's normal range), HR ≤100 bpm, specific gravity >1.010, and CVP 2-6 mm Hg (or 5-12 cm H_2O).

- Monitor I&O, specific gravity, daily weight, and VS closely. Be alert to evidence of hypovolemia, including weight loss, inadequate fluid intake to balance output, thirst, poor skin turgor, decreased specific gravity, furrowed tongue, hypotension, and tachycardia. If available, monitor CVP for evidence of hypotension. Notify health care provider if any of the following occurs: (1) urinary output >200 ml in each of 2 consecutive hr, (2) urinary output >500 ml in any 2-hr period, or (3) urine specific gravity <1.002.
- Provide unrestricted fluids. Keep water pitcher full and within easy reach of patient. Explain the importance of consuming as much fluid as can be tolerated.
- Administer vasopressin and antidiuretic agents (or thiazide diuretic for patient with nephrogenic DI) as prescribed.

- For unconscious patients, administer IV fluids as prescribed. Unless otherwise directed, for every milliliter of urine output, deliver 1 ml of IV fluid.

○ NIC: Fluid/Electrolyte Management; Hypovolemia Management; Intravenous (IV) Therapy; Shock Management: Volume

Altered protection related to potential for side effects of vasopressin
Desired outcomes: Optimally, patient demonstrates normal mental acuity; verbalizes orientation to person, place, and time; and is free of signs of injury caused by side effects of vasopressin. As appropriate, patient or significant other demonstrates administration of coronary artery vasodilators by hospital discharge.

- Monitor VS and report significant changes, such as systolic BP elevated >20 mm Hg over baseline systolic BP or HR increased >20 bpm over baseline HR.
- Be alert to indicators of water intoxication, including changes in mental status or LOC, confusion, weight gain, headache, convulsions, and coma. If these develop, stop the medication, restrict fluids, and notify health care provider. Institute safety measures accordingly, and reorient patient as needed.
- For the older adult or person with vascular disease, keep prescribed coronary artery vasodilators (i.e., nitroglycerin) at the bedside for use if angina occurs. Teach patient and significant other how to administer these medications.

○ NIC: Cardiac Care: Acute; Neurologic Monitoring; Risk Identification; Seizure Precautions; Surveillance: Safety

PATIENT-FAMILY TEACHING AND DISCHARGE PLANNING

When providing patient-family teaching, focus on sensory information; avoid giving excessive information; and initiate a visiting nurse referral for necessary follow-up teaching. Consider including verbal and written information about the following:

- Importance of continued medical follow-up; confirm date and time of next appointment.
- Medications, including drug name, purpose, dosage, schedule, precautions, drug/drug and food/drug interactions, and potential side effects.
- Indicators that necessitate medical attention (e.g., signs of dehydration or water intoxication).

Pituitary and hypothalamic tumors

Lesions affecting pituitary function may be located in either the pituitary gland or the adjacent hypothalamus and include pituitary adenomas, craniopharyngiomas, metastatic tumors, primary pituitary cancer, and meningiomas. Undiagnosed, small pituitary adenomas have been reported in approximately 20%-30% of autopsies. Adenomas generally do not secrete anterior pituitary hormones, and patients manifest symptoms of hypopituitarism. Secreting tumors may produce any anterior pituitary hormone, but prolactin, adrenocorticotropic hormone (ACTH), and growth hormone (GH) secretions are found more often than thyroid-stimulating hormone (TSH) and gonadotropin secretions.

Hypopituitarism may result from primary pituitary disease or abnormal secretion of hormones by the hypothalamus and may be permanent or reversible. Gonadotropin and GH secretions generally are lost earlier in the disease process, followed by loss of TSH, ACTH, and prolactin at later stages. Loss of TSH secretion results in hypothyroidism, whereas loss of ACTH prompts adrenocortical insufficiency or Addison's disease (see p. 354). A small percentage of patients experience a mixture of both hypersecretion of some anterior pituitary hormones and hyposecretion of others.

ASSESSMENT

Altered neurologic status: Headache (dull, generalized) often unrelieved by analgesics, visual field changes (loss of peripheral vision, occasional double vision), and seizures and hydrocephalus (rare).

Hypopituitarism: Delayed puberty and short stature (in pre-adolescents and adolescents); loss of libido and sexual characteristics; impotence; apathy; mental slowing; weakness; mild anemia; dry and scaly skin with pale, waxy complexion; increased wrinkling around the mouth and eyes; hypotension; orthostatic hypotension; occasional hypoglycemia; myxedema; sparse body hair; generalized sensitivity to cold; decreased perspiration; and decreased resistance to colds, stress, and infections.

Excessive prolactin (hyperprolactinemia):   Males often present with impotence, decreased libido, infertility, and hypogonadism. Females often have amenorrhea, infertility, galactorrhea, reduced vaginal lubrication, dyspareunia, osteoporosis, and occasionally hirsutism.

Excessive GH: In growing children, excessive GH results in gigantism, and in adults, acromegaly. Symptoms of acromegaly include coarse facial features (i.e., large nose, thick lips), enlargement of hands and feet, oily skin, malodorous perspiration, chewing problems, need to change or refit dentures frequently, hoarseness, joint pain or deformities, cardiac enlargement, carpal tunnel syndrome, insulin resistance/hyperglycemia, headache, hypopituitarism, and salivary and thyroid gland enlargement.

Excessive ACTH: See "Cushing's Disease," p. 356.

Excessive TSH: May result in thyrotoxicosis. The most severe form is thyrotoxic crisis, or thyroid storm, which results from a sudden surge of large amounts of thyroid hormones into the bloodstream, causing an even greater increase in body metabolism. This is a medical emergency. Precipitating factors include infection, trauma, and emotional stress, all of which increase demands on body metabolism. Thyrotoxic crisis also can occur following subtotal thyroidectomy because of manipulation of the gland during surgery. Despite vigorous treatment, thyroid storm causes death in approximately 20% of affected patients.

Excessive gonadotropin (luteinizing hormone [LH]/follicle-stimulating hormone [FSH]):   Found most frequently in middle-age men. Indicators include visual field changes, LH secretion alteration causing low testosterone level, or marked elevation in FSH.

DIAGNOSTIC TESTS

General

X-ray of skull: Will show enlarged pituitary gland, thickened skull, and distorted, enlarged pituitary fossa or sella turcica.

CT scan or MRI: May reveal an abnormality of the sella turcica or extrasellar extension of the tumor.

Skeletal x-rays: Will show thickening of long bones.

Cerebral angiography: Used to exclude presence of aneurysm, extension of suprasellar and/or parasellar tumor, blood vessel involvement, and tumor blushes.

Serum tests (in hyperpituitarism):   May reveal elevated phosphate and postprandial blood glucose, prolactin, GH, ACTH, TSH, LH, and FSH levels.

Insulin tolerance test and metapyrone test: Measures the ability of pituitary ACTH to increase in response to stress. These tests may be dangerous in older persons and in individuals who are cardiac impaired or prone to seizures.

Rapid ACTH stimulation test: Measures adrenal response to exogenous ACTH administration.

For hypopituitarism

Urinary 17-ketosteroids, 17-hydroxycorticosteroids, and plasma cortisol levels: Are decreased but will rise slowly after administration of ACTH.

Urinary and serum gonadotropin levels: Are decreased.

Plasma testosterone and estradiol levels: Are decreased.

Serum levels of ACTH, TSH, LH, FSH, and GH: Are decreased; may be manifested as single or multiple hormonal deficiencies.

COLLABORATIVE MANAGEMENT

Exogenous hormone replacements: As appropriate for syndromes of insufficiency secondary to hypopituitarism.

Hormone suppression therapy: For hormone-secreting tumors. Dopamine agonists, such as bromocriptine (Parlodel), are used to inhibit synthesis and release anterior pituitary hormones by the gland or adenoma. This therapy has proven effective in prolactin- , GH- , and ACTH-secreting tumors.

X-ray and heavy-particle radiation therapy: For hormone-secreting tumors. Typically, the response with a return to normal is slow, but tumor progression is halted in most patients. Side effects can include malaise, nausea, serous otitis media, and hypopituitarism. For more information, see Appendix One, "Caring for Patients With Cancer and Other Life-Disrupting Illnesses," p. 747. Currently no chemotherapeutic agents cure pituitary adenomas.

Transsphenoidal hypophysectomy: Treatment of choice because it offers a more rapid cure with a low morbidity. An incision is made in the inner aspect of the upper lip, and the sella turcica is entered through the sphenoid process. Because an opening is created between the nose and upper airway, the patient is at increased risk for postoperative infection, necessitating preoperative use of nasal antibiotics. Postoperatively the patient will have periorbital ecchymosis. The pituitary is a highly vascular gland; therefore hemorrhage at the operative site is a potential risk. Diabetes insipidus (DI) can result from pituitary destruction and removal. For larger tumors, a frontal craniotomy may be necessary. (See "Brain Tumors," p. 288.)

NURSING DIAGNOSES AND INTERVENTIONS

Altered protection related to potential for increased intracranial pressure (IICP), DI, cerebrospinal fluid (CSF) leak, hemorrhage, and infection secondary to transsphenoidal hypophysectomy

Desired outcomes: Optimally, patient demonstrates normal level of mental acuity; verbalizes orientation to person, place, and time; and is free of indicators of injury caused by complications of transsphenoidal hypophysectomy. Immediately after instruction, patient and significant other verbalize understanding of the importance of avoiding Valsalva type of maneuvers; describe the signs and symptoms of IICP, DI, and infection; and verbalize the importance of notifying staff of postnasal drip or excessive swallowing.

- Be alert to indicators of IICP, such as a change in mental status or LOC, sluggish or unequal pupils, and changes in respiratory rate or pattern. Monitor patient for decreased vision, eye muscle weakness, abnormal extraocular eye movement, double vision, and airway obstruction. Report significant findings to health care provider. A change in vision may necessitate a CT scan.
- Measure I&O hourly for 24 hr, and monitor urine specific gravity q1-2hr. Report an output >200 ml/hr for 2 consecutive hr or a total of 500 ml/hr. Specific gravity <1.007 is found with DI. Monitor weight daily for evidence of loss. Explain the signs of DI (see p. 363). DI often occurs as a result of the edema caused by manipulating the pituitary stalk and usually is transitory.
- Inspect nasal packing at frequent intervals for the presence of frank bleeding or CSF leakage. Note the number of times the mustache dressing is changed. Expect nasal packing removal in about 3-4 days. Test *non*sanguineous drainage for the presence of CSF fluid using a glucose reagent strip. If the

drainage contains CSF, the test will be positive for the presence of glucose. Monitor patient for complaints of postnasal drip or excessive swallowing, which may signal CSF drainage down the back of patient's throat.

> **Caution:** Because the presence of CSF represents a serious breach in the integrity of the cranium, elevate the HOB to minimize the potential for bacteria entering the brain, and immediately report any suspicious drainage.

- Elevate the HOB 30 degrees to decrease ICP and swelling. Dexamethasone may be prescribed to reduce cerebral swelling.
- Explain to patient that coughing, sneezing, and other Valsalva type of maneuvers must be avoided because these actions can stress the operative site and increase ICP, causing CSF leakage. Teach patient to cough or sneeze with an open mouth if either is unavoidable. Remind patient that nose blowing should be avoided until the nasal mucosa is healed (about 1 mo). Advise patient about the importance of mouth breathing and the possibility of having a soft nasal airway. Obtain a prescription for a mild cathartic or stool softener to prevent straining with bowel movements if indicated.
- To prevent disturbance in the integrity of the operative site, do not allow patient to brush teeth. Provide mouthwash (e.g., hydrogen peroxide diluted with water to half strength) and sponge-tipped applicator for oral hygiene. Monitor for extreme erythema or swelling at the suture line. Remind patient that the front teeth should not be brushed until the incision has healed (about 10 days). Advise patient that the diet will be liquid initially but quickly will progress to soft.
- The patient may have periorbital edema, headache, and tenderness over the sinuses for 2-3 days, which may be helped with cold compresses to the eyes. The transsphenoidal donor site for fat or muscle packing usually is taken from the thigh or abdomen, and the patient should expect a small dressing there. Advise patient that the sense of smell usually returns in about 2-3 wk.
- Be alert to and teach patient the following signs and symptoms of infection, which necessitate medical attention: fever, nuchal rigidity, headache, and photophobia.

NIC: Infection Protection; Neurologic Monitoring; Self-Care Assistance; Surgical Precautions; Teaching: Disease Process; Wound Care

Sexual dysfunction related to physiologic changes secondary to abnormal hormone levels
Desired outcome: As appropriate, patient relates the attainment of satisfying sexual activity within 1 mo after hospital discharge.
- Encourage patient to express feelings of anger and frustration and to communicate feelings to significant other.
- If appropriate, suggest alternatives other than sexual intercourse for pleasuring partner and self.
- Administer testosterone or estrogens as prescribed.
- Provide instruction in the administration of alprostadil or sildenafil (Viagra) for impotence.
- Support health care provider's referral or suggest referral for psychotherapy related to loss of libido, sterility, impotence, or loss of self-esteem.

NIC: Anxiety Reduction; Coping Enhancement; Counseling; Self-Esteem Enhancement; Sexual Counseling; Teaching: Sexuality

> **See Also:** Appendix One, "Caring for Preoperative and Postoperative Patients," p. 717, for nursing diagnoses and interventions.

PATIENT-FAMILY TEACHING AND DISCHARGE PLANNING

When providing patient-family teaching, focus on sensory information; avoid giving excessive information; and initiate a visiting nurse referral for necessary follow-up teaching. Consider including verbal and written information about the following:

- Medications, including drug name, purpose, dosage, schedule, precautions, drug/drug and food/drug interactions, and potential side effects. Reinforce that after hypophysectomy, patient will be on lifetime hormone replacement therapy.
- Relationship between hormone levels and stress. Advise patient to seek medical help during times of emotional or physical stress so that dosages of medications can be adjusted accordingly.
- Measures for maximizing coping mechanisms to deal with stress, such as relaxation tapes, meditation, diversional activities. See **Health-seeking behaviors:** Relaxation technique effective for stress reduction, p. 59.
- Importance of continued medical follow-up; confirm time and date of next appointment.
- Indicators of: *adrenal hormone excess*—weight gain, easy bruising, muscle weakness, moon face, thirst, and polyuria; *adrenal hormone insufficiency*—weight loss, easy fatigue, and abdominal pain; *hypothyroidism*—weight gain, anorexia, apathy, slowed mentation, and cold intolerance; and *thyrotoxicosis*—tachycardia, diaphoresis, and heat intolerance. All these signs and symptoms necessitate medical attention.
- For patients requiring permanent vasopressin replacement therapy, the importance of obtaining a Medic-Alert bracelet and identification card outlining diagnosis and emergency treatment. Contact the following organization:

Medic Alert
2323 Colorado Ave.
Turlock, CA 95382   (209) 668-3333

For patients found to be acromegalic during hospitalization for another illness
- Role of GH excess in the development of hyperglycemia, diabetes mellitus, arthralgia, osteoarthritis, cardiac enlargement, headaches, sexual/reproductive dysfunction, dental problems, and change in physical appearance.
- Anatomy and physiology of the pituitary gland and hypothalamus, along with changes prompted by pituitary tumors.
- Management of pituitary tumors, including medical and surgical modalities.

Syndrome of inappropriate antidiuretic hormone

Syndrome of inappropriate antidiuretic hormone (SIADH) is caused by release of antidiuretic hormone (ADH) from the pituitary gland without regard to serum osmolality, resulting in excessive water retention and hyponatremia. The action of ADH increases reabsorption of water in the last segment of the distal tubules and collecting ducts of the kidney. ADH secretion usually is stimulated by one of three mechanisms: (1) increased plasma osmolality, (2) decreased plasma volume, or (3) decreased BP. SIADH is a rare disorder that requires differential diagnosis from other problems that prompt elevation of vasopressin and resultant hyponatremia because of an appropriate response to hypovolemic or hypotensive stimuli.

In the presence of excessive ADH, water that normally would be excreted is reabsorbed into the circulation, resulting in water retention and eventually water intoxication. The retained water expands extracellular fluid volume, causing serum osmolality and Na^+ to decrease because of dilutional effects. Decreased serum osmolality causes movement of water into the cells, which can result in cerebral edema. Further water retention results in an increased glomerular filtration rate and decreased aldosterone secretion, and more Na^+ is filtered out into the urine.

Water intoxication, cerebral edema, and severe hyponatremia cause altered neurologic/mental status, which if untreated may lead to death.

ASSESSMENT

Signs and symptoms: Decreased urine output with concentrated urine. Signs of water intoxication may appear, including altered LOC, fatigue, headache, diarrhea, anorexia, nausea, vomiting, and seizures.

> **Note:**   Because of the loss of Na^+, edema will not accompany the fluid volume excess.

Physical assessment: Weight gain without edema, elevated BP, altered mental status.

History of: Cancers of the lung, pancreas, duodenum, and prostate, which can secrete a biologically active form of ADH. Other common causes include pulmonary disease (e.g., tuberculosis, pneumonia, chronic obstructive pulmonary disease, empyema), AIDS, head trauma, brain tumor, intracerebral hemorrhage, meningitis, and encephalitis. Positive-pressure ventilation, physiologic stress, chronic metabolic illness, and a wide variety of medications (chlorpropamide, acetaminophen, oxytocin, narcotics, general anesthetic, carbamazepine, thiazide diuretics, tricyclic antidepressants, neuroleptics, ACE inhibitors, cancer chemotherapy agents) all have been linked to SIADH.

DIAGNOSTIC TESTS

Serum Na^+ level: Decreased to <137 mEq/L.
Plasma osmolality: Decreased to <275 mOsm/kg.
Urine osmolality: Elevated disproportionately relative to plasma osmolality.
Urine Na^+ level: Increased to >200 mEq/L. Urine Na^+ level (e.g., increased) is best evaluated in comparison with serum Na^+ level (e.g., decreased).
Urine specific gravity: >1.030.
Plasma ADH level: Elevated.

COLLABORATIVE MANAGEMENT

Fluid restriction: Based on urine output plus insensible losses. Restricting fluids to the amount manageable by the kidneys will allow restoration of normal serum Na^+ levels and osmolality without complications from drug therapy.

Isotonic (0.9%) or hypertonic (3%) NaCl: May be given if the patient has severe hyponatremia. Supplemental Na^+ solutions may be administered with IV furosemide (Lasix) or bumetanide (Bumex) or osmotic diuretics, such as mannitol, to promote water excretion.

Lithium or demeclocycline: Inhibits action of ADH on the distal renal tubules to promote water excretion.

Treatment of underlying cause: SIADH associated with surgery, trauma, or drugs usually is temporary and self-limiting. In chronic situations the focus is on treating the underlying cause with surgery (i.e., transsphenoidal hypophysectomy, craniotomy, thoracotomy), radiation therapy, or chemotherapy.

NURSING DIAGNOSES AND INTERVENTIONS

Fluid volume excess related to compromised regulatory mechanisms resulting in increased serum ADH level, renal water reabsorption, and renal Na^+ excretion

Desired outcome: Patient becomes normovolemic (and normonatremic) within 7 days of onset of symptoms, as evidenced by orientation to person, place, and time; intake that approximates output plus insensible losses; stable weight; CVP 2-6 mm Hg; BP within patient's normal range; and HR 60-100 bpm.

- Assess LOC, VS, and I&O at least q4hr; measure weight daily. Be alert to decreasing LOC, elevated BP and CVP, urine output <30 ml/hr, and weight gain. Promptly report significant findings or changes to health care provider.
- Monitor laboratory results, including those for serum Na^+, urine and serum osmolality, and urine specific gravity. Be alert to decreased serum Na^+ and plasma osmolality, urine osmolality elevated disproportionately in relation to plasma osmolality, and increased urine Na^+. Normal values are as follows: urine specific gravity, 1.010-1.020; serum Na^+, 137-147 mEq/L; urine osmolality, 300-1090 mOsm/kg; and serum osmolality, 280-300 mOsm/kg. Report significant findings to health care provider.
- Maintain fluid restriction as prescribed. Explain necessity of this treatment to patient and significant other. Do not keep water or ice chips at the bedside. Ensure precise delivery of fluid administered IV by using a monitoring device.
- Elevate HOB no more than 10-20 degrees to enhance venous return and thus reduce ADH release.
- Administer demeclocycline, lithium, furosemide, or bumetanide as prescribed; carefully observe and document patient's response.
- Administer hypertonic NaCl as prescribed. Rate of administration usually is based on serial serum Na^+ levels. To minimize the risk of hypernatremia, make sure that specimens for laboratory tests are drawn on time and that results are reported to health care provider promptly.
- Institute seizure precautions to prevent patient injury in the event of seizure. These include padded side rails, supplemental oxygen, and oral airway at the bedside, as well as side rails up at all times when staff member is not present.

NIC: Dysrhythmia Management; Electrolyte Management: Hyponatremia; Fluid/Electrolyte Management; Medication Management; Neurologic Management; Seizure Precautions

---

See Also: "Diabetic Ketoacidosis" for **Risk for injury** related to altered cerebral function, p. 391; "Pituitary and Hypothalamic Tumors" for **Altered protection** related to risk of IICP, DI, CSF leak, hemorrhage, and infection, p. 369, for the patient who has undergone a transsphenoidal hypophysectomy.

PATIENT-FAMILY TEACHING AND DISCHARGE PLANNING

When providing patient-family teaching, focus on sensory information; avoid giving excessive information; and initiate a visiting nurse referral for necessary follow-up teaching. Consider including verbal and written information about the following:

- Importance of fluid restriction for the prescribed period. Assist patient with planning permitted fluid intake (e.g., by saving liquids for social and recreational situations as indicated).
- How to safely enrich the diet with Na^+ and K^+ salts, particularly if ongoing diuretic use is prescribed.
- Obtaining daily weight measurements as an indicator of hydration status.
- Indicators of water intoxication and hyponatremia, including altered LOC, fatigue, headache, nausea, vomiting, and anorexia, any of which should be reported promptly to health care provider.
- Medications, including drug name, dosage, route, purpose, precautions, drug/drug and food/drug interactions, and potential side effects.
- Importance of continued medical follow-up; confirm date and time of next medical appointment.

- Importance of obtaining a Medic-Alert bracelet and identification card outlining diagnosis and emergency treatment. Contact the following organization:

  Medic Alert
  2323 Colorado Ave.
  Turlock, CA 95382   (209) 668-3333

Section Three: Diabetes Mellitus

General discussion

Diabetes mellitus (DM) is a chronic disease affecting 5% of the total U.S. population (9 million Americans) with metabolic, vascular, and neurologic disorders resulting from dysfunctional glucose transport into body cells. Insulin facilitates glucose transport into cells for oxidation and energy production. Food intake, glycogen breakdown, and gluconeogenesis increase the serum glucose level, which stimulates the beta islet cells of the pancreas to release the needed insulin for transport of glucose from the bloodstream into the cells. As glucose leaves the blood, serum levels return to normal (60-120 mg/dl).

Individuals with DM have impaired glucose transport because of decreased or absent insulin secretion and/or ineffective insulin action. Carbohydrate, fat, and protein metabolism are abnormal, and patients are unable to store glucose in the liver and muscle as glycogen, store fatty acids and triglycerides in adipose tissue, and transport amino acids into cells normally. DM is classified into the following five types of disorders.

Insulin-dependent diabetes mellitus (IDDM)/type 1:   Complete lack of effective endogenous insulin, causing hyperglycemia and ketosis. Previously this was termed *juvenile*, or *growth onset*, diabetes because a majority of those affected are <30 yr of age. This type of DM is precipitated by altered immune responses, genetic factors, and environmental stressors. Certain human leuko-cyte antigens (HLAs) have been strongly associated with type I DM, and immunoassay diagnostic kits are undergoing clinical trials. IDDM accounts for 10% of all DM. These individuals depend on insulin for survival and prevention of life-threatening diabetic ketoacidosis (DKA).

Non-insulin-dependent diabetes mellitus (NIDDM)/type 2:   Moderate to severe lack of effective endogenous insulin, causing severe hyperglycemia without ketosis. Previously it was termed *adult*, or *maturity onset*, diabetes, and it is precipitated by obesity and aging. Two subgroups of patients with type 2 DM are distinguished by the presence or absence of obesity. Approximately 25% of individuals with type 2 require periodic to regular insulin administration for blood glucose control. Oral hypoglycemic agents are used by 50% of these patients, whereas 25% control their blood glucose using only a structured American Diabetes Association (ADA) diet for maintenance of ideal body weight. This type accounts for 80%-90% of individuals with DM. Untreated hyperglycemia can result in hyperosmolar hyperglycemic nonketotic (HHNK) syndrome.

Other types: Formerly termed *secondary diabetes*, these include the following:

- *Pancreatic diseases that destroy the beta islet cells*: e.g., pancreatitis, cystic fibrosis, hemochromatosis.
- *Liver disease*: e.g., cirrhosis, hemochromatosis.
- *Muscle disorders*: e.g., myotonic dystrophies.
- *Adipose tissue disorders*: e.g., lipoatrophy, lipodystrophy, truncal obesity.

- *Drug-induced by insulin antagonists*: e.g., phenytoin (Dilantin), steroids (hydrocortisone, dexamethasone), hormones (estrogen).
- *Endocrine dysfunction/hormonal diseases*: e.g., acromegaly, Cushing's syndrome, pheochromocytoma.
- *Insulin resistance*: caused by dysfunctional insulin receptors.
- *Genetic syndromes*: those that predispose individuals to DM (e.g., HLA genetic system defects).
- *Defective insulin molecule production*: caused by mutation of the insulin gene.

Many of the above "secondary" causes have recently become subclassified under type 1 and type 2 DM as possible primary causes of these diseases.

Gestational diabetes: Intolerance to glucose, which develops during pregnancy in 2%-3% of pregnant women, resulting in increased perinatal risk to the child and increased risk of the mother developing chronic DM during the next 10-15 yr. This type does not include *previously* diabetic pregnant women.

Malnutrition-related diabetes: Type of DM added by the World Health Organization (WHO) for a syndrome with onset in individuals 10-40 yr of age in underdeveloped countries. This type requires insulin for control of blood glucose. Ketosis does not occur. The role of malnutrition as a cause currently is unknown.

• • •

Certain individuals may manifest chronic hyperglycemia without meeting other criteria for DM and are classified as having impaired glucose tolerance (IGT). IGT was formerly termed *borderline, chemical, latent, subclinical,* or *asymptomatic* diabetes. Of Americans >65 yr of age, 10%-30% have IGT, and 1%-5% of individuals with IGT progress to DM annually. Other individuals may have a higher probability of developing glucose intolerance because of previous abnormality or genetic predisposition. Genetically high-risk individuals often have never exhibited IGT and are classified as having potential abnormality of glucose tolerance.

ASSESSMENT

Metabolic: Fatigue, weakness, weight loss, paresthesias, mild dehydration, and symptoms of hyperglycemia (polyuria, polydipsia, polyphagia). These indicators are seen in the early stages of illness.

Impending type 1 (IDDM) crisis: Profound dehydration and hyperglycemia, electrolyte imbalance, metabolic acidosis caused by ketosis, altered mental status, Kussmaul's respirations (paroxysmal dyspnea), acetone breath, possible hypovolemic shock (hypotension, weak and rapid pulse), abdominal pain, and possible strokelike symptoms.

Impending type 2 (NIDDM) crisis: Severe dehydration, hypovolemic shock (hypotension, weak and rapid pulse), severe hyperglycemia, shallow respirations, altered mental status, slight lactic acidosis or normal pH, possible strokelike symptoms.

COMPLICATIONS

Potential for acute crisis: *For type 1,* include DKA and hypoglycemia; *for type 2,* include HHNK and hypoglycemia. These complications should be preventable in individuals diagnosed with DM and are discussed later in this section.

Long-term complications: The most important factor in delaying progression to long-term complications is the stabilization of blood glucose levels to normal range.

Macroangiopathy: Vascular disease affecting the coronary arteries and the larger vessels of the brain and lower extremities. Risk factors are hyperglycemia, hypertension, hypercholesterolemia, smoking, aging, and extended duration of DM. Macroangiopathy may result in myocardial infarction, cerebrovascular accident, and peripheral vascular disease.

Microangiopathy: Thickening of capillary basement membranes resulting in retinopathy and nephropathy. Early symptoms include increased leakage of retinal vessels and microalbuminuria. Late manifestations are blindness and renal failure.

Neuropathy: Affects the peripheral and autonomic nervous systems, resulting in impaired or slowed nerve transmission, for example, numbness or lack of sensation, particularly in the feet (peripheral), and orthostatic hypotension, neurogenic bladder, and impaired gastric emptying (autonomic).

Morning hyperglycemia: Blood glucose elevation found on awakening. Causes include each of the following or a combination of the effects of their interactions.

Insufficient insulin: The most common cause of hyperglycemia before breakfast is probably inadequate levels of circulating insulin. The patient may need a higher dosage, a mixture of insulins, or longer-acting insulin.

Dawn phenomenon: Glucose remains normal until approximately 3 am, when the effect of nocturnal growth hormone may elevate glucose in type 1 diabetes. It may be corrected by changing the time of the evening dose of intermediate-acting insulin injection to bedtime instead of dinnertime.

Somogyi phenomenon: The patient becomes hypoglycemic during the night. Compensatory mechanisms to raise glucose levels are activated and result in overcompensation. It may be corrected by decreasing the evening dose of intermediate-acting insulin and/or eating a more substantial bedtime snack.

Problems with insulin

Insulin resistance: A problem experienced by most individuals with DM and other diseases at some point in the illness, when the daily insulin requirement to control hyperglycemia and prevent ketosis exceeds 200 U. Typically, it results from profound or complete insulin deficiency in type 1 DM and obesity in type 2 DM. It is characterized as one of the following anomalies:

- Prereceptor: insulin abnormal or insulin antibodies present.
- Receptor: number of insulin receptors decreased or insulin binding to the receptors diminished.
- Postreceptor: receptors not appropriately activated by insulin. This condition is treated by changing the insulin to a purer preparation or changing from an animal source (beef, pork) to human insulin.

Local allergic reactions: Soreness, erythema, or induration at the insulin injection site within 2 hr after injection. Reactions are decreasing in frequency with the evolution of more purified insulins.

Systemic allergic reactions: Rare occurrence that begins with a localized skin reaction, which evolves into generalized urticaria or anaphylaxis. Patients must be desensitized to insulin by progression from minuscule to more normal doses over the course of 1 day, using a series of SC injections.

Lipodystrophy: Local disturbance in fat metabolism resulting in loss of fat (lipoatrophy) or development of abnormal fatty masses at the injection sites (lipohypertrophy). Lipoatrophy rarely has been seen since the development of 100U and human source insulins. Rotation of injection sites helps to prevent lipohypertrophy. Individuals experiencing lipohypertrophy should use alternate injection sites until the condition resolves. Treatment of lipoatrophy involves changing to 100U human source insulin and injecting subsequent scheduled doses into the periphery of the affected area(s).

DIAGNOSTIC TESTS

WHO defines the following diagnostic criteria for DM in nonpregnant adults.

Fasting blood sugar: A value >126 mg/dl is indicative of glucose intolerance if found on at least 2 occasions.

Oral glucose tolerance test: The 2-hr sample during the test is >200 mg/dl on at least 2 occasions.

Random plasma glucose: Measurement is >200 mg/dl on at least 2 occasions.

Glycosylated hemoglobin (Hgb): Normal range is 4%-7%. Individuals with DM will have values >7%. This value is measured to assess control of blood glucose over a preceding 2- to 3-mo period. The larger the percentage of glycosylated Hgb, the poorer the blood glucose control. Kits are now available to monitor this value in the home.

• • •

Diagnostic procedures under investigation

Immunoassay for islet cell antibodies: Kits to detect these antibodies are undergoing clinical trials. Islet cell antibodies have been identified in 85% of patients within the first few weeks after DM was diagnosed.

Serum fructosamine: Fructosamine is used to reflect glycemic control over the previous 2 weeks before the testing. Normal value is 1.5-2.4 mmol/L when albumin is 5 g/dl. Because this test is not affected by abnormal hemoglobin or hemolytic conditions, it may be used in place of glycohemoglobin, which is unreliable in these conditions.

COLLABORATIVE MANAGEMENT

Diet: The exchange programs of the ADA are the most commonly used methods of diet calculation and patient education. Dietary management is individually based on ideal body weight and adjusted to metabolic and activity needs. Typically, the patient is put on a fixed ADA diet that is composed of 50%-60% carbohydrates, 12%-20% protein, and 20%-30% fat. The focus on weight reduction for individuals with type 2 DM necessitates significant carbohydrate restriction if they are treated by diet alone. When treatment also includes oral hypoglycemic medications or insulin, increased amounts of carbohydrates are required to offset the hypoglycemic effects of these medications. Individuals with type 1 DM require day-to-day consistency in diet and exercise to prevent hypoglycemia. Typically, three daily meals and an evening snack are prescribed. Some fat and protein should be present in all meals and snacks to slow down the elevation of postprandial blood glucose. Adding 10-15 g of fiber will slow the digestion of monosaccharides and disaccharides. For all types of diabetes, refined and simple sugars should be reduced and complex carbohydrates (breads, cereals, pasta, beans) should be encouraged. Various artificial sweeteners are used in "diet" products. Some contribute calories, which must be accounted for in a calorie-restricted diet. Exchange lists commonly are used for meal planning.

Monitoring of blood glucose: Control of blood glucose is facilitated by a glycohemoglobin monitoring device, which is designed to provide timely measurement of the glucose level from a small drop of blood obtained by fingerstick. This simple technology affords the opportunity for closer monitoring and stabilization of glucose levels, which have been shown to decrease both the incidence and severity of long-term complications. Self-monitoring by patients has proven extremely useful in reducing complications, especially in IDDM (type 1) patients who require more stringent control of their serum glucose levels.

Oral hypoglycemic medications (sulfonylureas, biguanides): Hypoglycemics are used in individuals with type 2 DM for whom diet alone cannot control hyperglycemia (Table 5-2). Their primary action is to increase insulin production by affecting existing beta cell function. The most serious side effect is hypoglycemia, particularly with chlorpropamide (Diabinese), which has a 60-hr duration and an average half-life of 36 hr. Hypoglycemia involving the oral hypoglycemics can be severe and persistent. Nursing monitoring must be diligent. Oral hypoglycemics should be omitted several days before planned surgery. Any condition, situation, or medication that enhances the hypoglycemic effects of these drugs requires close monitoring of blood glucose when

T A B L E 5 - 2 Sulfonylurea and Biguanide Hypoglycemic Agents

Generic name (trade name)	Usual dose (mg)/ administration	Maximum dose (mg)	Duration of action (hr)
Sulfonylureas			
Acetohexamide (Dymelor)	250-1500/single or divided	1500	12-24
Chlorpropamide (Diabinese)	100-500/single	750	60
Glipizide (Glucotrol)	5-25/single or divided	40	10-24
Glipizide (Glucotrol XL)	20-30/single	30	24
Glimepiride (Amaryl)	1-8/single	8	24
Glyburide (Micronase, Glynase, DiaBeta)	1.25-10/single or divided	20	12-24
Tolazamide (Tolinase)	100-750/single or divided	1000	12-24
Tolbutamide (Orinase)	500-2000/single or divided	3000	12-24
Biguanide			
Metformin (Glucophage)	1000-2500/divided	2550	7-12

symptoms of hypoglycemia arise. Common factors in the development of hypoglycemia are fasting for diagnostic purposes, skipping meals, malnourishment related to illness or nausea and vomiting, and other medication therapy (any of which adds to the hypoglycemic action of the oral hypoglycemics). **Oral α-glucosidase inhibitors:** Acarbose is a mild antihyperglycemic that delays the digestion of carbohydrates and thus leads to a smaller rise in blood glucose in type 2 DM.

Thiazolidinediones (troglitazone [Resulin]): Thiazolidinediones are a new class of agents that act to resensitize the body to insulin by stimulating a gene to produce more insulin-controlled proteins to compensate for the gradual loss of natural insulin's ability to work. They have both hypoglycemic and hypolipidemic effects.

Insulin: Examples of short- , intermediate- , and long-acting insulins are shown in Table 5-3.

- A split-dose (twice daily) regimen of insulin administration may be preferred because it allows a higher level of blood glucose control. Daily insulin therapy usually consists of administering two thirds of the total daily intermediate-acting insulin dose in the morning, with the remaining dose given in the evening. A rapid-acting insulin might be added to either or both doses, or a mixed insulin may be used. This regimen precludes the use of the longer-acting insulins, which are rarely used in a single dose because of the risk of nocturnal hypoglycemia.

- Multiple daily injections (MDI) (2-4 injections daily) permit better control of blood glucose for some individuals. Alteration in the quantity of food and timing of meals is a benefit to the patient who values flexibility. For the self-motivated individual who has control difficulties in spite of multidose therapy, a portable insulin pump can be helpful.

- The degree to which bovine and porcine sources of insulin deviate from the protein structure of human insulin affects the extent of their antigenic properties. Biosynthetic human insulins are less likely to produce allergic responses in susceptible individuals and are used most frequently. Beef, pork, and biosynthetic human insulin should not be combined or given to the same

TABLE 5 - 3   Types of Insulin and Insulin Analogs*

Insulin type	Examples	Onset of action per SC injection	Peak action (hr)	Duration (hr)	Mixture compatibilities
Rapid acting					
Lispro (Humalog)	Humalog; insulin analog	5 min	0.5-1	2-3	None
Regular	Crystalline zinc insulin injection	0.5-1 hr	2-4	4-8	All
Semilente	Prompt insulin zinc suspension	1.0-1.5 hr	5-10	12-16	Lente
Intermediate acting					
NPH	Isophane insulin suspension	1.0-1.5 hr	4-12	20-24	Regular
Lente	Insulin zinc suspension	1.0-2.5 hr	7-16	20-24	Regular, Semilente
Long acting					
Ultralente	Extended insulin zinc suspension	4.0-8.0 hr	14-24	>36	Regular, Semilente
Intermediate/rapid					
70% NPH/30% regular	Isophane insulin suspension, insulin injection	0.5-1.0 hr	4-8	20-24	Premixed; do not mix

SC, Subcutaneous.
*Source may be beef or pork, pancreatic extracts, or biosynthetic human insulin preparations.

patient. The patient should receive only all pork, all beef, or all human biosynthetic insulin.

- Lispro (Humalog) is a new insulin analog used in the treatment of both type 1 and type 2 DM. This agent has been demonstrated to provide more consistency in low blood glucose levels and to result in fewer fluctuations. May also supplement therapy with sulfonylureas in type 2 DM and can be used in continuous infusion insulin pumps for type 1 DM.

Insulin delivery systems

Continuous subcutaneous insulin infusion (CSII)/portable insulin pumps: Devices that deliver a constant basal rate of insulin throughout the day and night with the capability of delivering a patient-programmed bolus of insulin at mealtime. The needle, which attaches to a pump via a long strip of plastic tubing, remains indwelling in the SC tissue of the abdomen. Patients program their own pumps to deliver the optimal amount of insulin, based on self-monitoring of blood glucose. Patient should be alert to soreness and erythema at the insertion site, indicators of abscess or staphylococcal infection. Current literature reports a rare incidence of a toxic shock-like syndrome with these devices. Clinical trials are investigating a variety of pump technologies, including implantable pumps. Some implantable pumps are commercially available in European countries.

Injection ports: Subcutaneous access ports inserted into the subcutaneous fat by the patient. These ports may remain in place for up to 3 days. They are constructed similarly to peripheral IV catheters, with introducer needles that are removed when the catheter is appropriately positioned. The device is secured by taping, and patients may use the port for dosage rather than puncturing the skin.

Jet injectors: Deliver insulin in a fine, pressurized stream through the skin without use of a needle for injection. Absorption, peak, and insulin levels may be altered by the injector, necessitating caution for the patient. Typically, onset and peak action occur earlier using these devices. Thorough training must be provided before allowing patients to use these devices independently.

Insulin pens: Small, prefilled insulin cartridges that are inserted into a penlike holder. After the attachment of a specially designed, shorter, and finer disposable needle, the insulin is injected by selecting a dose or depressing a button either once for each 1- to 2-U increment desired for the dosage (older device) or once for the entire selected dosage (newer device). Although patients must use needles for injection, there is no need for insulin to be drawn up from multidose vials, adding to the convenience and accuracy of administration. Patients electing to use these agents should plan on frequent blood glucose testing until use of the new device demonstrates stable glucose control.

Patient teaching about drugs that potentiate hyperglycemia: These include estrogens, corticosteroids, thyroid preparations, diuretics, phenytoin, glucagon, and medications that contain sugar, such as cough syrup.

Patient teaching about drugs that potentiate hypoglycemia: These include salicylates, sulfonamides, tetracyclines, methyldopa, anabolic steroids, acetaminophen, MAO inhibitors, ethanol, haloperidol, and marijuana. Propranolol and other β-adrenergic blocking agents mask the signs of and inhibit recovery from hypoglycemia.

Exercise: Exercise is as important as diet and insulin in treating DM. It lowers blood glucose levels, helps maintain normal cholesterol levels, and increases circulation. These effects increase the body's ability to metabolize glucose and help reduce the therapeutic dose of insulin for most patients. The exercise program must be consistent and individualized (especially for individuals with type 1 DM). Patients should be given a complete physical examination and encouraged to incorporate acceptable activities as part of their daily routine. **Note:** If blood glucose level is >250 mg/dl, exercise acts as a stressor, causing blood glucose to increase rather than decrease. Patients should monitor blood glucose levels with a monitoring device before beginning an exercise program.

Transplantation: Complete or partial pancreatic transplants have been performed on a small number of patients, usually in conjunction with kidney transplantation. Candidates must thoroughly evaluate the risks associated with antirejection medications vs. the benefits of pancreatic transplantation. Immune suppression caused by the medications may promote development of opportunistic infections. Transplantation of only beta cells is being investigated as an alternative to other methods.

NURSING DIAGNOSES AND INTERVENTIONS

Altered peripheral, cardiopulmonary, renal, cerebral, and GI tissue perfusion (or risk for same) related to interrupted blood flow secondary to development and progression of macroangiopathy and microangiopathy

Desired outcome: Optimally, patient has adequate tissue perfusion as evidenced by warmth, sensation, brisk capillary refill time (<2 sec), and peripheral pulses >2+ on a 0-4+ scale in the extremities; BP within his or her optimal range; urinary output ≥30 ml/hr; baseline vision; good appetite; and absence of nausea and vomiting.

- Compliance with the therapeutic regimen is essential for promoting optimal tissue perfusion. Check blood glucose before meals and at bedtime. Encourage patient to perform regular home blood glucose monitoring. Urine testing is less reliable and should not be used by patients with reduced renal function.
- Hypertension is a common complication of diabetes. Careful control of BP is critical in preventing or limiting the development of heart disease, retinopathy, or nephropathy. Check BP q4hr. Alert health care provider about values outside the patient's normal range. Administer antihypertensive agents as prescribed, and document the response.
- Patients may experience decreased sensation in the extremities because of peripheral neuropathy. In addition to sensation, assess capillary refill, temperature, peripheral pulses, and color. Protect patients with impaired peripheral perfusion from injury with sharp objects or heat (e.g., avoid use of heating pads). Teach patient to prevent venous stasis by avoiding pressure at the back of the knees (e.g., by not crossing the legs or "gatching" the bed under the knees) and avoiding constricting garments on the extremities and lower body. For additional information see **Impaired tissue integrity,** p. 382.
- Provide a safe environment for patients with diminished eyesight caused by diabetic retinopathy. Orient patient to the location of such items as water, tissues, glasses, and call light.
- Approximately half of all persons with type 1 DM develop chronic renal failure (CRF) and end-stage renal disease. Monitor patients for changes in renal function (e.g., increases in BUN [>20 mg/dl] and creatinine [>1.5 mg/dl] and altered urine output). Proteinuria (protein >8 mg/dl in a random sample of urine) is an early indicator of developing CRF. Individuals with DM and with reduced renal function are at significant risk for dehydration or developing acute renal failure (ARF) after exposure to contrast medium. Observe these patients for indicators of ARF. (See "Acute Renal Failure," p. 144, and "Chronic Renal Failure," p. 150, for more information.) Insulin doses will decrease as renal function decreases.
- Be alert to indicators of hypoglycemia (e.g., changes in mentation, apprehension, erratic behavior, trembling, slurred speech, staggering gait, seizure activity). Treat hypoglycemia as prescribed (see discussion in "Collaborative Management," p. 397).

In addition
- Individuals with DM may experience multiple problems resulting from autonomic neuropathy, such as the following:
  —*Orthostatic hypotension:* assist patients when getting up suddenly or after prolonged recumbency. Check BP while patient is lying down, sitting, and

TABLE 5-4 Infectious Processes Necessitating Medical Intervention	
Upper respiratory infection:	Fever, chills, cough productive of sputum, crackles (rales), rhonchi, dyspnea, inflamed pharynx, sore throat
Urinary tract infection:	Burning or pain with urination, cloudy or malodorous urine, fever, chills, tachycardia, diaphoresis, nausea, vomiting, abdominal pain
Systemic sepsis:	Fever, chills, tachycardia, diaphoresis, nausea, vomiting, hypothermia, flushed skin, hypotension
Localized (IV sites):	Erythema, swelling, purulent drainage, warmth

IV, Intravenous.

then standing to document presence of orthostatic hypotension. Alert health care provider to significant findings.

—*Impaired gastric emptying with nausea, vomiting, and diarrhea:* administer metoclopramide before meals if prescribed. Keep a record of all stools. Nausea, vomiting, and anorexia can signal developing uremia in patients with progressive renal failure.

—*Neurogenic bladder:* encourage patients to void q3-4hr during the day. Intermittent catheterization may be necessary in severe cases. Avoid use of indwelling urinary catheters because of the risk of infection. For additional information see "Neurogenic Bladder," p. 188.

NIC: Circulatory Care; Diarrhea Management; Environmental Management: Safety; Fall Prevention; Hyperglycemia Management; Hypoglycemia Management; Neurologic Monitoring; Peripheral Sensation Management

Risk for infection with risk factors related to chronic disease process (e.g., hyperglycemia, neurogenic bladder, poor circulation)
Desired outcome: Patient is asymptomatic for infection as evidenced by normothermia, negative cultures, and WBC ≤11,000/mm^3.

Note: Infection is the most common cause of DKA.

- Monitor temperature q4hr. Alert health care provider to elevations.
- Maintain meticulous sterile technique when changing dressings, performing invasive procedures, or manipulating indwelling catheters.
- Monitor for indicators of infection (Table 5-4).
- Consult health care provider about obtaining culture specimens for blood, sputum, and urine during temperature spikes or for wounds that produce purulent drainage.

NIC: Infection Protection; Risk Identification; Surveillance; Temperature Regulation; Vital Signs Monitoring

Impaired tissue integrity (or risk for same) related to altered circulation and sensation secondary to peripheral neuropathy and vascular pathology
Desired outcomes: Patient's lower extremity skin remains intact. Within the 24-hr period before hospital discharge, patient verbalizes and demonstrates knowledge of proper foot care.

- Assess integrity of the skin and evaluate reflexes of the lower extremities by checking knee and ankle deep tendon reflexes, proprioceptive sensations, two-point discrimination, and vibration sensation (using a tuning fork on the medial malleolus). If sensations are impaired, anticipate patient's inability to respond appropriately to harmful stimuli. Monitor peripheral pulses, comparing the quality bilaterally. Be alert to pulses ≤2+ on a 0-4+ scale.

- Use foot cradle on bed, space boots for ulcerated heels, elbow protectors, and pressure-relief mattress to prevent pressure points and promote patient comfort.
- To alleviate acute discomfort yet prevent hemostasis, minimize patient activities and incorporate progressive passive and active exercises into daily routine. Discourage extended rest periods in the same position.
- Teach patient the following steps for foot care:
  —Wash feet daily with mild soap and warm water; check water temperature with water thermometer or elbow.
  —Inspect feet daily for the presence of erythema or trauma, using mirrors as necessary for adequate visualization.
  —Alternate between at least two pairs of properly fitted shoes to avoid potential for pressure points that can occur by wearing one pair only.
  —Prevent infection from moisture or dirt by changing socks or stockings daily and wearing cotton or wool blends.
  —Use gentle moisturizers to soften dry skin, avoiding areas between the toes.
  —Prevent ingrown toenails by cutting toenails straight across after softening them during bath. File nails with an emery board.
  —Do not self-treat corns or calluses; visit podiatrist regularly.
  —Attend to any foot injury immediately, and seek medical attention to avoid any potential complication.
  —Do not go barefoot indoors or outdoors.

NIC: Foot Care; Incision Site Care; Peripheral Sensation Management; Pressure Ulcer Prevention; Wound Care

Knowledge deficit: Proper insulin administration and dietary precautions for promoting normoglycemia
Desired outcome: Within the 24-hr period before hospital discharge, patient verbalizes and demonstrates knowledge of proper insulin administration and the prescribed dietary regimen.

- Teach patient to check expiration date on insulin vial and to avoid using it if outdated. Also teach patient proper storage of insulin and the importance of avoiding temperature extremes.
- Explain that intermediate- and long-acting insulins require mixing (contraindicated for the intermediate/rapid). Demonstrate rolling the insulin vial between the palms to mix the contents. Caution patient that vigorous shaking produces air bubbles that can interfere with accurate dose measurement.
- Explain that insulin should be injected 30 min before mealtime; newer insulin analogs need to be injected immediately before eating.
- Explain that either making a change in insulin type or withholding a dose of insulin may be required for the following: when fasting for studies or surgery, when not eating because of nausea/vomiting, or when hypoglycemic. Remind patient that stress from illness or infection can increase insulin requirements (or necessitate insulin therapy for one who is normally controlled with oral hypoglycemics) and that increased exercise will necessitate additional food intake to prevent hypoglycemia when no change is made in insulin dose. Adjustments are always individually based and require clarification with patient's health care provider.
- Provide patient with a chart that depicts rotation of the injection sites. Explain that injection sites should be at least 1 inch apart.
- Explain the importance of inserting the needle perpendicular to the skin rather than at an angle to ensure deep SC administration of insulin. Very thin persons may need to use a 45-degree angle.
- Ensure that the patient understands and demonstrates the technique and timing for home monitoring of blood glucose using a commercial kit, which

provides ongoing data reflecting the degree of control and may identify necessary changes in diet and medication before severe metabolic changes occur. This test also allows for patient's self-control and psychologic security.
- Caution patient about the importance of following a diet that is low in fat and high in fiber as an effective means of controlling blood fats, especially cholesterol and triglycerides. Stress that diet is the sole method of control for many individuals with type 2 DM. Adequate nutrition and controlled calories are essential to maintaining normoglycemia in these persons.
- For patients who experience low blood glucose at night, inform the patient about commercially available long-acting carbohydrate sources.

NIC: Exercise Promotion; Health Education; Medication Management; Nutritional Counseling; Teaching: Disease Process; Teaching: Prescribed Diet; Teaching: Prescribed Medication

---

See Also: As appropriate, "Atherosclerotic Arterial Occlusive Disease," p. 118; Chapter 8, "Amputation," p. 602; Appendix One, "Caring for Patients With Cancer and Other Life-disrupting Illnesses," p. 791, for psychosocial nursing diagnoses and interventions.

PATIENT-FAMILY TEACHING AND DISCHARGE PLANNING

When providing patient-family teaching, focus on sensory information; avoid giving excessive information; and initiate a visiting nurse referral for necessary follow-up teaching. Consider including verbal and written information about the following:
- Importance of carrying a diabetic identification card and wearing Medic-Alert bracelet or necklace and identification card outlining diagnosis and emergency treatment. Contact the following organization:

  Medic Alert
  2323 Colorado Ave.
  Turlock, CA 95382   (209) 668-3333

- Recognizing warning signs of both hyperglycemia and hypoglycemia, treatment, and factors that contribute to both conditions. Remind patient that stress from illness or infection can increase insulin requirements (or necessitate insulin therapy for one who is normally controlled with oral hypoglycemics) and that increased exercise will necessitate additional food intake to prevent hypoglycemia when no change is made in insulin dosage under normoglycemic conditions. Blood glucose at a level >250 mg/dl at the beginning of exercise will make the exercise a stressor that elevates the glucose level rather than decreasing it.
- Drugs that potentiate **hyperglycemia:** estrogens, corticosteroids, thyroid preparations, diuretics, phenytoin, glucagon, and drugs containing sugar (e.g., cough syrup). Drugs that potentiate **hypoglycemia:** salicylates, sulfonamides, tetracyclines, methyldopa, anabolic steroids, acetaminophen, MAO inhibitors, ethanol, haloperidol, and marijuana. Propranolol and other β-adrenergic agents may mask the signs of and inhibit recovery from hypoglycemia.
- Home monitoring of blood glucose using commercial kits and possibly daily urine testing for glucose and ketones, which provide ongoing data reflecting the degree of control and may identify necessary changes in diet and medication before severe metabolic changes occur. These tests also provide a means for patient's self-control and psychologic security. In addition, kits for monitoring glycohemoglobin (HbAIC) are available for home use and may assist patients in determining the overall effectiveness of their diabetes management regimen. New, smaller lancets allow more frequent blood

glucose testing by decreasing pain from fingersticks. Stress the need for careful control of blood glucose as a means of decreasing the risk of or minimizing long-term complications of DM.

- Importance of daily exercise, maintenance of normal body weight, and yearly medical evaluation. Explain that exercise is as important as diet in treating DM. It lowers blood glucose, helps maintain normal cholesterol levels, and increases circulation. These effects increase the body's ability to metabolize glucose and help reduce the therapeutic dose of insulin for most patients. Stress that each exercise program must be individualized (especially for persons with type 1 DM) and implemented consistently. The patient should have a complete physical examination and then be encouraged to incorporate acceptable exercise activities into his or her daily routine.
- Diet that is low in fat and high in fiber as an effective means of controlling blood fats, especially cholesterol and triglycerides. Stress that diet is the sole method of control for many individuals with type 2. Adequate nutrition and controlled calories are essential to maintaining normoglycemia in these individuals.
- Necessity for individuals with type 1 to use ^{100}U syringes with ^{100}U insulin. Various *types/sources* of insulin (beef, pork, biosynthetic) should not be mixed. When mixing various *acting* insulins, draw up the regular first, followed by the intermediate- or long-acting insulin. Insulin analogs (Lispro) should not be mixed with other insulin preparations.
- Availability of syringe magnifiers that can be used for patients with poor visual acuity. Other products that permit safe and accurate filling of syringes are also available.
- Necessity of rotating injection sites and injecting insulin at room temperature. Provide a chart showing possible injection sites, and describe the system for rotating the sites. Complications related to insulin injections, including lipodystrophy, insulin resistance, and allergic reactions, should be discussed thoroughly.
- Importance of meticulous skin, wound, and foot care.
- Importance of annual eye examinations for early detection and treatment of retinopathy.
- Importance of regular dental checkups because periodontal disease poses a major problem for individuals with DM. The mouth often is the primary site of origination for low-grade infections.
- Importance of inserting the needle perpendicular to the skin rather than at an angle to ensure deep SC administration of insulin. Individuals who are very thin may need to use a 45-degree angle.
- Name, purpose, dosage, schedule, precautions, drug/drug and food/drug interactions, and potential side effects for any supplemental medications used.
- Review of appropriate sections of Tables 5-2 and 5-3 with the patient and significant other.
- Identification of available resources for ongoing assistance and information, including nurses, dietitian, patient's health care provider, and other individuals with DM in the patient care unit. Other resources include the local chapter of the American Diabetes Association (ADA) and the local library for free access to current materials on diabetes. The following is a list of resources available to patients:

American Diabetes Association
1660 Duke St.
Alexandria, VA 22314   (800) 232-3472
WWW address: *http://www.diabetes.org*

Canadian Diabetes Association
15 Toronto St., Suite 1001
Toronto, Ontario M5C2F3   (416) 363-3373
WWW address: *http://www.diabetes.ca*

Juvenile Diabetes Foundation
120 Wall St.
New York, NY 10005   (800) JDF-CURE
WWW address: *http://www.jdfcure.com*

Joslin Diabetes Center
Director, Joslin Clinic
1 Joslin Place
Boston, MA 02215   (617) 732-2501

National Diabetes Information Clearinghouse   (301) 468-2162
WWW address: *http://www.niddk.nih.gov/BROCHURES/NDIC.htm*

American Heart Association   (800) 242-8721
WWW address: *http://www.amhrt.org/*

Can-Am-Care   (800) 461-7448
(diabetes care store brand availability guide)

- The following is a list of journals available for patients:

    Diabetes 95, American Diabetes Association Subscription Department,
    1660 Duke Street, Alexandria, VA 22314

    Diabetes Forecast, American Diabetes Association Membership Center,
    Box 2055, Harlan, IA 51593-0238

    Diabetes in the News, Ames Center for Diabetes Education, Miles Inc.,
    Box 3105, Elkhart, IN 46515

    Diabetes Self-Management, Box 51125, Boulder, CO 80321-1125

    Health-O-Gram, SugarFree Center, 13725 Burbank Blvd., Van Nuys, CA
    91401

    Living Well with Diabetes, Diabetes Center, 13911 Ridgedale Drive,
    Suite 250, Minnetonka, MN 55343

    Diabetes Interview, 3715 Balboa Street, San Francisco, CA 94121

- The following Internet resources provide links to additional diabetes-related
  resources:

    http://castleweb.com/diabetes/d—07—000.htm

    http://castleweb.com/diabetes/index.html

Diabetic ketoacidosis

Diabetic ketoacidosis (DKA) is a life-threatening condition caused by severe
lack of effective insulin, resulting in abnormal carbohydrate, fat, and protein
metabolism. The intracellular environment is unable to receive necessary
glucose for oxidation and energy production without insulin to facilitate the
transport of glucose from the bloodstream across the cell membrane. The
impairment of glucose uptake results in hyperglycemia, while the intracellular
environment continues to lack necessary nutrients. Glucagon secretion increases, causing available body stores of food substances to be broken down in
an attempt to provide nourishment for the cells. Impaired amino acid transport,
protein synthesis, and protein degradation facilitate protein catabolism with a
resultant increase in serum amino acids, while the breakdown of fats results in
elevated free fatty acids (FFA) and glycerol. The liver converts the newly
available amino acids, fatty acids, and glycerol into glucose (gluconeogenesis)

in an attempt to provide nourishment for the cells, but instead the hyperglycemia worsens because of the lack of insulin to transport glucose into the cells. The liver also produces ketone bodies from available FFA, causing mild to severe acidosis. As ketone bodies increase in the extracellular fluid, the hydrogen ions within the ketones are exchanged with K^+ ions from within the cells. Thus intracellular K^+ ions are released into the extracellular fluid and therefore to circulating fluid, where they are excreted by the kidneys into the urine. Hyperglycemia acts as an osmotic diuretic, causing severe fluid and electrolyte losses, leading to hypovolemic shock if untreated. Individuals with severe DKA may lose nearly 500 mEq of Na^+, Cl^-, and K^+, along with approximately 7 L of water in 24 hr.

ASSESSMENT
See Table 5-5.

DIAGNOSTIC TESTS
See Table 5-5.

COLLABORATIVE MANAGEMENT
Fluid replacement: Usually, normal saline or 0.45% saline is administered until plasma glucose falls to 200-300 mg/dl. After that, dextrose-containing solutions usually are given to prevent rebound hypoglycemia. Initially, IV fluids are administered rapidly (i.e., 2000 ml infused during the first 2 hr of treatment and 200-300 ml/hr thereafter).

Rapid-acting insulin: Usually given IV for rapid action and because poor tissue perfusion caused by dehydration makes SC route less effective. The initial dose may vary from 10-25 U, or about 0.3 U/kg. Then the patient is maintained on 5-10 U/hr, or 0.1 U/kg/hr as a continuous infusion administered through a separate IV tubing and controlled with an infusion control device. Dosage is adjusted based on serial glucose levels and resolution of ketosis. When initiating the insulin administration, flush 50 ml of the IV insulin solution through the tubing to saturate adsorption sites in the walls of the plastic tubing, where the initial insulin molecules may adhere rather than be delivered to the patient. Insulin analogs (i.e., Lispro) may be used in place of regular insulin to lower blood glucose levels.

Restoration of electrolyte balance: Na^+ and Cl^- are replaced with IV normal saline. K^+ must be monitored and corrected carefully. Before treatment there is a risk of hyperkalemia from excess transport of intracellular K^+ to extracellular spaces. After the initiation of treatment, K^+ returns to the intracellular compartment through accelerated transport into cells via insulin and following correction of acidosis, and therefore the patient is at risk for becoming hypokalemic. Use of phosphorus replacement is controversial, but if phosphorus levels remain low, potassium phosphate solutions can be used to assist with K^+ and phosphate replacement. Studies suggest that there is no difference in the outcome of patients who receive phosphorus replacement and those who do not.

IV bicarbonate: For pH <7.10. Its use is limited because acidosis will be corrected by insulin therapy. Excessive use of sodium bicarbonate can produce alkalosis, hyperosmolality, and respiratory depression.

Insertion of gastric tube: Prevents aspiration of gastric contents, particularly in comatose patients.

Treatment of underlying cause: For example, infection is treated with appropriate antibiotics, and medications are evaluated along with diet and patient's habits.

Treatment/prevention of complications: For example, arterial thrombosis, cerebrovascular accident, renal failure, adult respiratory distress syndrome, multiple organ failure, heart failure, cerebral edema, malignant dysrhythmias, death from irreversible hypovolemic shock.

TABLE 5-5 Comparison of Diabetic Ketoacidosis (DKA), Hyperosmolar Hyperglycemic Nonketotic Syndrome (HHNK), and Hypoglycemia

	DKA	HHNK	Hypoglycemia
Type of diabetes	Usually type I (IDDM)	Usually type II (NIDDM)	
Signs, symptoms/physical assessment	Note: symptoms are a result mainly of hyperglycemia, intracellular hypoglycemia, hypotension or impending hypovolemic shock, and possible acid-base imbalance	Note: symptoms are a result mainly of hyperglycemia, intracellular hypoglycemia, and fluid-electrolyte imbalance with possible acid-base imbalance	Note: symptoms result from intracellular hypoglycemia and hypotension/impending "insulin" shock (vasogenic)
Neurologic	Altered LOC (confusion, lethargy, irritability, coma); strokelike symptoms (unilateral/bilateral weakness, paralysis, numbness, paresthesia); fatigue	Same as DKA; also possible seizures and tremors	Tremors, trembling, shaking, confusion, apprehension, erratic behavior; may be same as DKA
Respiratory	Deep, rapid Kussmaul's respirations	Shallow, rapid (tachypneic) breathing	Usually rapid (tachypneic) breathing
Cardiovascular	Tachycardia, hypotension, ECG changes	Same as DKA	Same as DKA, possibly with diaphoresis
Metabolic/GI/endocrine	Polyuria, polyphagia, polydipsia, fruity "acetone" breath, abdominal pain, weight loss, fatigue, generalized weakness, nausea, vomiting	Polyuria, polyphagia, polydipsia, fatigue, generalized weakness, nausea, vomiting	Hunger, nausea, eructation
Integumentary	Dry, flushed skin; poor turgor; dry mucous membranes	Same as DKA	Cool, clammy, pale skin
VS monitoring	BP: low (>20% below normal) HR: >100 bpm CVP: <2 mm Hg (<5 cm H_2O) Temperature: normal	BP: low (>20% below normal) HR: >100 bpm CVP: <2 mm Hg (<5 cm H_2O) Temperature: possibly elevated	BP: normal to low HR: >100 bpm CVP: usually unchanged
Diagnostic tests/laboratory values	Values reflect dehydration/metabolic acidosis (ketosis) secondary to hyperglycemia, abnormal lipolysis, and osmotic diuresis; fluid loss ≥6.5 L	Values reflect dehydration secondary to hyperglycemia, osmotic diuresis, and possible lactic acidosis from hypoperfusion; fluid loss ≥9 L	Values reflect hypoglycemia, possibly with vasodilation owing to insulin shock

Hgb/Hct	Elevated	Same as DKA	Unchanged to slightly decreased
Serum BUN/creatinine	Elevated	Same as DKA	Normal
Serum electrolytes	Initially elevated, then decreased	Same as DKA	Usually unchanged
Serum glucose	250-800 mg/dl (+ ketones)	800-2000 mg/dl (– ketones)	15-50 mg/dl
ABGs	pH 6.8-7.3; HCO_3^- 12-20 mEq/L; CO_2 15-25 mEq/L	pH 7.3-7.5; HCO_3^- 20-26 mEq/L; CO_2 30-40 mEq/L	pH 7.3-7.5; HCO_3^- 20-26 mEq/L; CO_2 30-40 mEq/L
Serum osmolality	300-350 mOsm/L	>350 mOsm/L	<280 mOsm/L
Urine glucose/acetone	Positive/positive	Positive/negative	Negative/negative
Onset	Hours to days	Same as DKA	Minutes to hours
History/risk factors for development of crisis	Undiagnosed DM, infections, acute pancreatitis, uremia, insulin resistance	Undiagnosed DM; infections, especially gram negative; acromegaly; Cushing's syndrome; thyrotoxicosis, acute pancreatitis, hyperalimentation; pancreatic carcinoma; cranial trauma/subdural hematoma; uremia, hemodialysis, peritoneal dialysis; burns, heat stroke; pneumonia, MI, CVA	Excessive dose of insulin; excessive dose of sulfonylureas/oral hypoglycemic agents; skipping meals; too much exercise with controlled blood glucose without extra food intake
	Medications: digitalis intoxication; omission/reduction of insulin dosage; failure to increase insulin to compensate for stress of infections, injury, emotional problems, or surgery	*Medications:* loop and thiazide diuretics (i.e., hydrochlorothiazide, chlorthalidone, furosemide); diazoxide; glucocorticoids (i.e., hydrocortisone, dexamethasone); propranolol (Inderal); phenytoin (Dilantin); sodium bicarbonate	*Medications:* insulin, sulfonylureas (see Tables 5-2 and 5-3)
Mortality	≤10%	10%-25%	<0.1%

IDDM, Insulin-dependent diabetes mellitus; *NIDDM,* non-insulin-dependent diabetes mellitus; *LOC,* level of consciousness; *ECG,* electrocardiogram; *VS,* vital signs; *BP,* blood pressure; *HR,* heart rate; *CVP,* central venous pressure; *Hgb,* hemoglobin; *Hct,* hematocrit; *BUN,* blood urea nitrogen; *ABGs,* arterial blood gases; *MI,* myocardial infarction; *CVA,* cerebrovascular accident; *DM,* diabetes mellitus.

NURSING DIAGNOSES AND INTERVENTIONS

Fluid volume deficit related to failure of regulatory mechanisms or decreased circulating volume secondary to hyperglycemia with osmotic diuresis

Desired outcome: Patient becomes normovolemic within 10 hr of treatment, as evidenced by BP ≥90/60 mm Hg (or within patient's normal range), HR 60-100 bpm, CVP 2-6 mm Hg (5-12 cm H_2O), good skin turgor, moist and pink mucous membranes, specific gravity <1.020, balanced I&O, and urinary output ≥30 ml/hr.

- Monitor VS q15min until stable for 1 hr. Notify health care provider promptly of the following: HR >120 bpm, BP <90/60 or decreased ≥20 mm Hg from baseline, and CVP <2 mm Hg (or <5 cm H_2O).
- Monitor patient for physical indicators of dehydration, such as poor skin turgor, dry mucous membranes, sunken and soft eyeballs, tachycardia, and orthostatic hypotension.
- Weigh patient daily, and measure I&O accurately. Monitor urinary specific gravity and report findings >1.020 in the presence of other indicators of dehydration. Decreasing urinary output may signal diminishing intravascular fluid volume or impending renal failure. Report to health care provider urine output <30 ml/hr for 2 consecutive hours.
- Administer IV fluids as prescribed to ensure adequate rehydration. Be alert to indicators of fluid overload, which can occur with rapid infusion of fluids: jugular vein distention, dyspnea, crackles (rales), CVP >6 mm Hg (>12 cm H_2O).
- Administer insulin as prescribed to correct or stabilize the existing hyperglycemia. Be aware that insulin, when added to IV solutions, may be absorbed by the container and plastic tubing. Before initiating treatment, flush the tubing with 50 ml of the insulin-containing IV solution to ensure that maximum adsorption of the insulin by the container and tubing has occurred before patient use.
- Monitor laboratory results for abnormalities. Serum K^+ should decline until it reaches normal levels. Promptly report to the health care provider serum K^+ levels <3.5 mEq/L. Serum Na^+ levels will increase gradually with appropriate IV saline replacement.
- Observe for clinical manifestations of the electrolyte, glucose, and acid-base imbalances associated with DKA as follows:
  - —*Hyperkalemia:* lethargy, nausea, hyperactive bowel sounds with diarrhea, numbness or tingling in extremities, muscle weakness.
  - —*Hypokalemia:* muscle weakness, hypotension, anorexia, drowsiness, hypoactive bowel sounds.
  - —*Hyponatremia:* headache, malaise, muscle weakness, abdominal cramps, nausea, seizures, coma.
  - —*Hypophosphatemia:* muscle weakness, progressive encephalopathy possibly leading to coma.
  - —*Hypomagnesemia:* anorexia, nausea, vomiting, lethargy, weakness, personality changes, tetany, tremor or muscle fasciculations, seizures, confusion progressing to coma.
  - —*Hypochloremia:* hypertonicity of muscles, tetany, depressed respirations.
  - —*Hypoglycemia:* headache, impaired mentation, agitation, dizziness, nausea, pallor, tremors, tachycardia, diaphoresis.
  - —*Metabolic acidosis:* lassitude, nausea, vomiting, Kussmaul's respirations, lethargy progressing to coma.

NIC: Acid-Base Monitoring; Electrolyte Management: Hyperkalemia; Electrolyte Management: Hypokalemia; Electrolyte Management: Hypomagnesemia; Electrolyte Management: Hyponatremia; Electrolyte Management: Hypophosphatemia; Fluid/Electrolyte Management; Hyperglycemia Management; Hypovolemia Management; Shock Management: Volume

Risk for infection with risk factors related to inadequate secondary defenses (suppressed inflammatory response) secondary to protein depletion
Desired outcome: Patient is free of infection as evidenced by normothermia, HR ≤100 bpm, BP within patient's normal range, WBC count ≤11,000/mm^3, and negative culture results.

- Monitor patient for evidence of infection (see Table 5-4). Monitor laboratory results for increased WBC count, and culture purulent drainage as prescribed.
- Ensure good hand-washing technique when caring for patient. Because patient is at increased risk of bacterial infection, use of invasive lines should be limited. Peripheral IV sites should be rotated q48-72hr, depending on agency policy. Central lines should be discontinued as soon as feasible and when in place should be handled carefully. Schedule dressing changes according to agency policy, and inspect the site(s) for signs of local infection, including erythema, swelling, or purulent drainage. Document the presence of any of these indicators, and notify health care provider.
- Provide good skin care to maintain skin integrity. Use pressure-relief mattress on the bed to help prevent skin breakdown. Air circulation beds are recommended for severe skin breakdown.
- Use meticulous sterile technique when caring for or inserting indwelling catheters to minimize the risk of bacterial entry via these sites. **Note:** Because of the increased risk of infection, limit use of indwelling urethral catheters to patients who are unable to void in a bedpan or when continuous assessment of urine output is essential.
- To help prevent pulmonary infection, provide incentive spirometry and encourage its use, along with deep-breathing and coughing exercises, hourly while patient is awake.

NIC: Bathing; Cough Enhancement; Infection Protection; Perineal Care; Pressure Management; Respiratory Monitoring; Tube Care: Urinary

Risk for injury with risk factors related to altered cerebral function secondary to dehydration or cerebral edema associated with DKA
Desired outcomes: Patient verbalizes orientation to person, place, and time and does not demonstrate significant change in mental status; normal breath sounds are auscultated over the patient's airway; and patient's oral cavity and musculoskeletal system remain intact and free of injury.

- Monitor patient's mental status, orientation, LOC, and respiratory status, especially airway patency, at frequent intervals. Keep an appropriate-size oral airway, manual resuscitator and mask, and supplemental oxygen at the bedside.
- Reduce the likelihood of injury from falls by maintaining bed in lowest position, keeping side rails up at all times, and using soft restraints as necessary.
- Insert gastric tube in comatose patients, as prescribed, to decrease the likelihood of aspiration. Attach gastric tube to low, intermittent suction, and assess patency q4hr.
- Elevate HOB to 45 degrees to minimize the risk of aspiration.
- Initiate seizure precautions. For details, see "Seizure Disorders," p. 324.

NIC: Environmental Management: Safety; Fall Prevention; Gastrointestinal Intubation; Neurologic Monitoring; Reality Orientation; Respiratory Monitoring; Seizure Precautions

Altered peripheral tissue perfusion (or risk for same) related to interrupted venous or arterial flow secondary to increased blood viscosity, increased platelet aggregation and adhesiveness, and patient immobility

Desired outcomes: Optimally, patient has adequate peripheral perfusion as evidenced by peripheral pulses >2+ on a 0-4+ scale; warm skin; brisk capillary refill (<2 sec); and absence of swelling, bluish discoloration, erythema, and discomfort in the calves and thighs. Alternatively, if signs of altered peripheral tissue perfusion occur, they are detected and reported promptly.

- Monitor hematocrit (Hct) results. Normal values are 40%-54% (male) or 37%-47% (female). With proper fluid replacement, results should return to normal within 24-48 hr. Assess for a falling BUN value as an indicator of improved tissue perfusion and renal function. Normal BUN is 6-20 mg/dl.
- Assess peripheral pulses q2-4hr. Report immediately any decrease in amplitude or absence of pulse(s) to health care provider.
- Be alert to indicators of deep vein thrombosis (DVT), such as erythema, pain, tenderness, warmth, and swelling over the area of thrombus and bluish discoloration, paleness, coolness, and dilation of superficial veins in the distal extremities, especially the lower extremities. Arterial thrombosis may produce pain, paresthesia (especially loss of sensation of light touch and two-point discrimination), cyanosis with delayed capillary refill, mottling, and coolness of the extremity. Report significant findings to health care provider immediately.
- Encourage active exercises to all extremities q2hr to increase blood flow to the tissues. Calf pumping and ankle circles should be encouraged q1hr in patients susceptible to DVT.
- Unless contraindicated, encourage fluid intake to >2500 ml/day to decrease potential for hemoconcentration.
- Apply antiembolic hose, Ace wraps, pneumatic alternating pressure stockings, or pneumatic foot pumps as prescribed to aid in the prevention of thrombosis.

NIC: Circulatory Precautions; Embolus Precautions; Exercise Promotion; Fluid Monitoring; Peripheral Sensation Management; Surveillance

Knowledge deficit: Cause, prevention, and treatment of DKA
Desired outcome: Within the 24-hr period before hospital discharge, patient verbalizes understanding of the cause, prevention, and treatment of DKA.

- Determine patient's knowledge about DKA and its treatment. As needed, explain the disease process of diabetes mellitus (DM) and DKA and the common early symptoms of worsening hyperglycemia, including polyuria, polydipsia, polyphagia, dry and flushed skin, and increased irritability (see also Table 5-5).
- Stress the importance of maintaining a regular diet, exercise, and insulin regimen for optimal control of serum glucose levels and prevention of adverse physical effects of DM, such as peripheral neuropathies and increased atherosclerosis.
- Explain the importance of testing urine ketone and blood glucose levels consistently and increasing the frequency of assessment during episodes of illness, injury, and stress. Blood glucose >200 mg/dl and the appearance of large amounts of urine ketones should be reported to the health care provider so that insulin dose can be increased. As indicated, review testing procedure with patient. Caution patient that DKA necessitates professional medical management and cannot be self-treated.
- Teach patient that insulin or insulin analog must be taken every day and that lifetime insulin therapy is necessary to achieve control of blood glucose. Explain that insulin is administered 1-4 times per day as prescribed and that it may require adjustment during periods of illness or stress.
- Remind patient of the importance of maintaining an adequate oral fluid intake during illness. Anorexia or nausea may limit food intake, but patient should make every effort to continue fluid intake.

- Teach patient the indicators of *insulin or insulin analog excess (hypoglycemia),* such as dizziness, impaired mentation, irritability, pallor, and tremors; and *insulin deficiency (hyperglycemia),* such as increased polyuria and polydipsia and dry and flushed skin. Teach patient the importance of receiving prompt treatment if any of these indicators occurs.
- Explain the importance of dietary changes as prescribed by the health care provider. Typically the patient is put on a fixed-calorie American Diabetes Association (ADA) diet composed of 60% carbohydrates, 20%-30% fats, and 12%-20% proteins. Explain that the fats should be polyunsaturated and the proteins chosen from low-fat sources. Teach patient the importance of eating three meals per day at regularly scheduled times and a bedtime snack.
- Explain the causes for adjustments in insulin dose: (1) increased or decreased food intake; (2) any physical (e.g., exercise) or emotional stress. Teach patient that exercise and emotional stress increase release of glucose from the liver, which may increase insulin demand. Instruct patient to monitor blood glucose and urine ketone levels closely during periods of increased emotional stress and periods of increased or decreased exercise and to adjust insulin dose accordingly.
- Explain that persons with diabetes are susceptible to infection and that preventive measures, such as good hygiene and meticulous daily foot care, are necessary to prevent infection. Stress the importance of avoiding exposure to communicable diseases, and explain that the following indicators of infection necessitate prompt medical treatment: fever, chills, increased HR, diaphoresis, nausea, and vomiting. In addition, teach patient and significant other to be alert to wounds or cuts that do not heal, burning or pain with urination, and a productive cough.
- Instruct patient to implement the following therapy when ill for any reason:
  —Do not alter insulin, insulin analog (Lispro), biguanide, sulfonylurea, or other antihyperglycemic medication dosage unless health care provider has prescribed a supplemental regimen to be implemented by individuals with type 1 DM for hyperglycemia secondary to illness.
  —Perform blood glucose monitoring and urine ketone checks q3hr, and promptly report glucose >300 mg/dl and positive ketones to the health care provider.
  —Implement small, frequent meals of soft, easily digestible, nourishing foods if regular meals are not tolerated.
  —Maintain adequate hydration, particularly if diarrhea, vomiting, or fever is persistent.
  —Use a balance of regular sodas or juices and water to ensure adequate calories yet prevent hyperosmolality caused by sugars in the beverages.
  —Report any of the above conditions to the health care provider to gain further insight into treatment modalities/prevention of dehydration.
- Provide the following address of the ADA for acquisition of pamphlets and magazines related to the disease, its complications, and appropriate treatment:

American Diabetes Association, Inc.
18 East 48th Street
New York, NY 10017   (800) 232-3472

NIC: Exercise Promotion; Health Education; Infection Protection; Nutritional Counseling; Self-Modification Assistance; Self-Responsibility Facilitation; Support Group; Weight Management

See Also: Appendix One, "Caring for Patients With Cancer and Other Life-disrupting Illnesses," p. 791, for psychosocial nursing diagnoses and interventions.

PATIENT-FAMILY TEACHING AND DISCHARGE PLANNING
See **Knowledge deficit:** Cause, prevention, and treatment of DKA, p. 392.

Hyperosmolar hyperglycemic nonketotic syndrome

Hyperosmolar hyperglycemic nonketotic (HHNK) syndrome, also known as *hyperosmolar coma, nonketotic hyperosmolar coma, hyperosmolar nonketotic syndrome, hyperosmolar hyperglycemic nonketotic coma,* and *nonketotic hyperglycemic hyperosmolar coma,* is a life-threatening emergency resulting from a lack of effective insulin, which causes severe hyperglycemia. Usually patients are elderly, with undiagnosed or inadequately treated type 2 diabetes mellitus (DM). Often HHNK is precipitated by a stressor, such as trauma or infection, that increases insulin demand. It is believed that enough insulin is present to prevent lipolysis and the formation of ketone bodies, thereby preventing acidosis, but not enough to prevent hyperglycemia. Without adequate insulin to facilitate transport into cells, glucose molecules accumulate in the bloodstream, causing serum hyperosmolality with resultant osmotic diuresis and simultaneous loss of electrolytes, most notably K^+, Na^+, and phosphate. Patients may lose up to 25% of their total body water. Fluids are pulled from individual body cells by increasing serum hyperosmolality and extracellular fluid loss, causing intracellular dehydration and body cell shrinkage. Neurologic deficits (i.e., slowed mentation, confusion, seizures, strokelike symptoms, coma) can occur as a result. Loss of extracellular fluid stimulates aldosterone release, which facilitates Na^+ retention and prevents further loss of K^+. However, the aldosterone cannot halt severe dehydration. As extracellular volume decreases, blood viscosity increases, causing slowing of blood flow. Thromboemboli are common because of increased blood viscosity, enhanced platelet aggregation and adhesiveness, and possibly patient immobility. Cardiac workload is increased and may lead to myocardial infarction (MI). Renal blood flow is decreased, potentially resulting in renal impairment or failure. Cerebrovascular accident (CVA) may result from thromboemboli or decreased cerebral perfusion. These severe complications, in addition to the initial precipitating disorder, contribute to a mortality of 10%-25%.

Unlike diabetic ketoacidosis (DKA), in which acidosis produces severe symptoms requiring fairly prompt hospitalization, symptoms of HHNK develop more slowly and frequently are nonspecific. The cardinal symptoms of polyuria and polydipsia are noted first but may be ignored by older persons or their families. Neurologic deficits may be mistaken for signs of impending CVA or senility. The similarity of these symptoms to those of other disease processes common to this age-group may delay differential diagnosis and treatment, allowing progression of pathophysiologic processes with resultant hypovolemic shock and multiple organ failure.

ASSESSMENT
See Table 5-5.

Note: Patients with HHNK usually are >50 yr of age and may have preexisting cardiac or pulmonary disorders. Assessment results often cannot be evaluated based on accepted normal values. Evaluate results based on what is normal or optimal for the individual patient. CVP, HR, and BP should be evaluated in terms of deviations from the patient's baseline and concurrent clinical status.

DIAGNOSTIC TESTS

Serum electrolytes: Serum values change as osmotic diuresis progresses. At the late stages, the patient may reflect the following electrolyte values/losses:

- Na^+: 125-160 mEq/L. Although the patient has lost large quantities of Na^+, osmotic diuresis causes abnormally high blood concentration. The Na^+ value may appear high despite probable Na^+ deficits.
- K^+: <3.5 mEq/L.
- Cl^-: <95 mEq/L.
- Phosphorus: <1.7 mEq/L.
- Magnesium: <1.5 mEq/L.

Serum osmolality: Will be >350 mOsm/L. A quick bedside calculation of serum osmolality can be obtained by using the following formula:

$$2 (Na^+ + K^+) + \frac{BUN\ (mg/dl)}{2.8} + \frac{Glucose\ (mg/dl)}{18} = mOsm/L$$

For example: $Na^+ = 140$; $K^+ = 4.5$; BUN = 20; glucose = 120

$$2 (140 + 4.5) + \frac{20}{2.8} + \frac{120}{18} = 2 (144.5) + 7 + 6.7$$
$$289 + 7 + 6.7 = 302.7\ mOsm/L$$

- See Table 5-5 for a discussion of other diagnostic tests.

COMPLICATIONS

Complications of HHNK include arterial thrombosis, CVA, renal failure, heart failure, multiple organ failure, cerebral edema, malignant dysrhythmias, and gram-negative sepsis (from infection that may have caused the problem to ensue).

COLLABORATIVE MANAGEMENT

Fluid replacement: Usually 0.9% normal saline or 0.45% saline is administered at 200-300 ml/hr until the plasma glucose is 200-300 mg/dl. For the first 2 hr of fluid infusion, >1000 ml/hr may be initiated to correct the hypovolemia and hypotension; 6-20 L may be given in the first 24 hr. Dextrose solutions (i.e., D_5/½NS or D_5/NS) are administered when blood glucose reaches 200-300 mg/dl. CVP measurements, coupled with thorough cardiovascular and pulmonary physical assessments, can be used to guide therapy and assess tolerance to the rapid fluid infusion.

Rapid-acting insulin: Initial dose of 10-25 U (0.3 U/kg) followed by continuous infusion of 5-10 U/hr (0.1 U/kg/hr) of regular insulin until blood glucose level is lowered to 200-250 mg/dl, at which time the infusion should be decreased to 2-3 U/hr. SC administration is less predictable if the patient is hypotensive, because tissue perfusion is decreased throughout the body, sometimes profoundly to the skin. Dosage is adjusted based on serial glucose levels and resolution of ketosis. When initiating insulin by continuous solution, 50 ml of the insulin IV solution should be flushed through the tubing to saturate adsorption sites, where the initial insulin molecules may adhere rather than be delivered to the patient. If the insulin is ineffective in reducing blood glucose, consider a possible insulin resistance. Insulin analogs (Lispro) may also be used to lower blood glucose levels.

Restoration of electrolyte balance: Na^+ and Cl^- are replaced with IV normal saline, and K^+ is replaced with 10-40 mEq of KCl or potassium phosphate if the patient also needs phosphorus replacement. All electrolytes are replaced carefully because fluids and electrolytes will be shifting between fluid compartments as the fluids are replaced and insulin is administered.

Supportive care: Protective measures are instituted for those who are neurologically impaired or in a coma. These measures include seizure precautions, endotracheal intubation, placement of indwelling urinary catheter, insertion of a gastric tube, pressure-relieving mattress, specialty bed, and possibly restraints for patients who are confused or agitated.

NURSING DIAGNOSES AND INTERVENTIONS

Knowledge deficit: Causes, prevention, and treatment of HHNK

Desired outcome: Within the 24-hr period before hospital discharge, patient and significant other verbalize understanding of the causes, prevention, and treatment of HHNK.

- Determine patient's understanding of HHNK and its treatment. Enable patient to verbalize fears and feelings about the diagnosis; correct any misconceptions. As needed, explain the disease process of DM and HHNK and the common early symptoms of worsening diabetes, including polyuria, polydipsia, polyphagia, dry and flushed skin, and increased irritability. Review Table 5-5.
- Teach the importance of testing urine acetone and blood glucose levels qid or as prescribed before meals and at bedtime. Explain that blood glucose >200 mg/dl should be reported to the health care provider so that insulin dose can be increased. As indicated, review testing procedure with patient.
- Stress the importance of dietary changes as prescribed by the health care provider. Typically, the person with type 2 DM is obese and will be on a reduced-calorie diet with fixed amounts of carbohydrate, fat, and protein. Explain that the fats should be polyunsaturated and the proteins chosen from low-fat sources. Teach patient the importance of eating three meals per day at regularly scheduled times and a bedtime snack. Explain that increased or decreased food intake will necessitate an adjustment in insulin dosage. Provide a referral to a dietitian as needed.
- Caution patient about the importance of taking oral hypoglycemic agents as prescribed. In addition, explain that exogenous insulin or insulin analogs may be required during periods of physical and emotional stress and that blood glucose levels should be monitored closely during these times.
- For patients with type 2 DM, explain the benefits of regular exercise for maintaining blood glucose levels. Exercise increases insulin effectiveness and reduces serum triglyceride and cholesterol levels, thus also decreasing the risk of atherosclerosis. Aerobic exercises, such as walking or swimming, are most effective in lowering blood glucose levels. Caution patient always to monitor blood glucose level before exercise. A level >250 mg/dl is indicative of abnormal metabolism. In this case exercise would be a stressor, resulting in further elevation of blood glucose.
- Explain the need for measures to prevent infection, such as good hygiene and meticulous daily foot care. Stress the importance of avoiding exposure to communicable diseases. Explain that the following indicators of infection necessitate prompt medical treatment: fever, chills, tachycardia, diaphoresis, and nausea and vomiting. In addition, teach patient and significant other to be alert to wounds or cuts that do not heal, burning or pain with urination, and cough that is productive of sputum.
- Provide booklets or pamphlets from the American Diabetes Association or pharmaceutical companies about diabetes and appropriate treatment.

See Also: "Seizure Disorders" for **Risk for trauma** related to musculoskeletal, oral, and airway vulnerability secondary to seizure activity, p. 324; "Diabetic Ketoacidosis" for **Fluid volume deficit,** p. 390; **Risk for infection,** p. 391; **Altered peripheral tissue perfusion,** p. 391; Appendix One, "Caring for Patients With Cancer and Other Life-disrupting Illnesses," p. 791, for psychosocial nursing diagnoses and interventions.

NIC: Exercise Promotion; Health Education; Infection Protection; Nutritional Counseling; Self-Modification Assistance; Self-Responsibility Facilitation; Support Group; Weight Management

PATIENT-FAMILY TEACHING AND DISCHARGE PLANNING

See **Knowledge deficit:** Causes, prevention, and treatment of HHNK, p. 396.

Hypoglycemia

Hypoglycemia is a lowering of blood glucose caused by an excessive dose of insulin or oral hypoglycemic agents, skipping meals, or too much exercise without a concomitant increase in food intake. Unlike diabetic ketoacidosis and hyperosmolar hyperglycemic nonketotic syndrome, hypoglycemia can have a sudden onset, and its course is precipitous if it is left untreated. Typically, hypoglycemia occurs during the time of the peak action of the insulin/hypoglycemic agent, particularly at night when the patient is asleep and has not eaten an adequate bedtime snack.

The patient usually becomes symptomatic when blood glucose is <50 mg/dl or a relatively significant drop in blood glucose occurs (e.g., when an older person's blood glucose drops to 90 mg/dl from 180-200 mg/dl). Alcohol consumption also can cause hypoglycemia because it depletes glycogen stores, resulting in increased insulin levels.

Caution: Mentation changes caused by severe hypoglycemia can be indistinguishable from those caused by alcoholic stupor. If hypoglycemic symptoms are misdiagnosed as alcoholic stupor and an individual with hypoglycemic is left to "sleep it off," death can ensue.

ASSESSMENT

See Table 5-5.

COLLABORATIVE MANAGEMENT

Administration of rapid-acting sugar: 10-15 g of a fast-acting sugar (e.g., 4-6 oz fruit juice or nondiet soda, 2-3 tsp honey or table sugar, 5-10 Lifesavers or small hard candies, or 2-4 commercially manufactured glucose tablets) is given by mouth. If symptoms persist for >15 min, the treatment is repeated. After resolution of the event, the patient should continue to consume a protein/complex carbohydrate snack, such as cheese or peanut butter on crackers/whole grain bread, or milk with crackers/bread.

Glucagon: For patients unable to swallow, 1 mg glucagon is injected SC or IM. Glucagon stimulates the liver to break down stored glycogen into glucose and usually results in the patient regaining consciousness in 15-30 min, at which time the patient should be given a fast-acting sugar followed by the snack just described. Patients and their significant other are instructed in glucagon administration as a part of their diabetes education. Glucagon is used rarely in the hospital setting.

50% Dextrose: Hospitalized patients may receive an IV injection of 25-50 ml of 50% dextrose (D_{50}), which usually revives the unconscious individual in

<10 min. Patients may experience hyperglycemia and headache after D_{50}, particularly if given 50 ml. These individuals may benefit from a protein or complex carbohydrate snack once consciousness is regained unless blood glucose has been elevated to >200 mg/dl. If the patient has frequent episodes of hypoglycemia, an alteration in dietary composition or insulin administration should be evaluated.

NURSING DIAGNOSES AND INTERVENTIONS

Altered protection related to potential for brain damage or death secondary to hypoglycemia
Desired outcome: Within 10-30 min of intervention, patient is alert with no significant change from his or her usual mental status and verbalizes orientation to person, place, and time.

> Caution: Hypoglycemia requires immediate intervention because, if severe, it can lead to brain damage and death. When the cause of coma in a person with diabetes mellitus (DM) is unknown, immediately draw a blood sample for evaluation of glucose and prepare to administer IV D_{50}.

- Administer a fast-acting carbohydrate: 2-3 tsp sugar, 4-6 oz fruit juice or nondiet soda, 6-10 Lifesavers, or 2-4 commercially manufactured glucose tablets. Notify health care provider if patient is incoherent, unresponsive, or incapable of taking carbohydrates by mouth. If any of these indicators occur, an IV access is required and you should prepare to administer prescribed 50-ml D_{50} by IV push. Consciousness should be restored within 10 min.
- Continue to monitor blood glucose levels q30-60min to identify recurrence of hypoglycemia.
- Once the patient is alert, question him or her about the most recent food intake. Any situation preventing food intake, such as nausea, vomiting, dislike of hospital food related to cultural preferences, or fasting for a scheduled test, should be determined and addressed immediately.
- If food intake has been adequate, consult health care provider about a reduction in patient's daily dose of antihyperglycemic medication.
- Consider use of a commercially available long-acting carbohydrate at bedtime to help prevent nocturnal hypoglycemia.

> Note: Sometimes hypoglycemia leads to rebound hyperglycemia (Somogyi phenomenon). If hypoglycemia goes undetected, the rebound hyperglycemia may be inappropriately treated with increased insulin. Suspect the Somogyi phenomenon if wide fluctuations in blood glucose occur over several hours. Notify the health care provider if these changes are observed or if the patient is experiencing nocturnal hypoglycemia.

NIC: Hypoglycemia Management; Neurologic Monitoring; Nutrition Management; Risk Identification; Teaching: Individual

Altered protection related to neurosensory alterations with risk of seizures secondary to hypoglycemia
Desired outcome: Within 4 hr of the event, patient verbalizes orientation to person, place, and time and is free of signs of trauma caused by seizures or altered LOC. Alternatively, if patient experiences a seizure, it is detected, reported, and treated promptly.
- Monitor LOC at frequent intervals. Anticipate seizure potential in presence of severe hypoglycemia, and have airway, protective padding, and suction equipment at bedside. Keep all side rails raised.

- Notify health care provider of any seizure activity; do not leave patient unattended if a seizure occurs.
- Place call light within patient's reach, and have patient demonstrate its proper use every shift. The patient's inability to use the call light properly necessitates assessments at least q30min. If necessary, consider moving patient to a room next to the nurses' station for close monitoring.
- Keep all potentially harmful objects, such as knives, forks, and hot beverages, out of patient's reach.
- If necessary to prevent patient from wandering and causing self-injury, obtain a prescription for soft restraints. Explain these safety precautions to patient and significant other.
- For other information, see "Seizure Disorders," p. 324.

NIC: Airway Insertion and Stabilization; Airway Management; Environmental Management: Safety; Fall Prevention; Hypoglycemia Management; Seizure Management; Self-Care Assistance

Knowledge deficit: Disease process, diagnostic testing, indicators of hypoglycemia, and therapeutic regimen
Desired outcome: Within the 24-hr period before hospital discharge, patient verbalizes knowledge about DM, including testing and management, indicators of hypoglycemia, and therapeutic regimen.
- Assess patient's knowledge about DM, including diagnostic testing and management. Provide information or clarify as appropriate.
- Review the indicators and immediate interventions for hypoglycemia with the patient.
- Evaluate current diet for adequate nutritional requirements, caloric content, and patient satisfaction. Assist patient in making acceptable and realistic changes. Consider patient's activity level and need for changes to achieve normoglycemia. Refer patient and significant other to dietitian as needed.
- Review with patient the onset, peak action, and duration of the hypoglycemic medication. Advise patient to avoid drugs that contribute to hypoglycemia (salicylates, sulfonamides, methyldopa, anabolic steroids, acetaminophen, ethanol, haloperidol, marijuana).
- Stress the importance of testing blood glucose at the time symptoms of hypoglycemia occur.
- Explain that injection of insulin into a site that is about to be exercised heavily (e.g., a jogger's thigh) will result in quicker absorption of the insulin and possible hypoglycemia.
- Inform patient that a change in the type of medication may require a change in dose to prevent hypoglycemia. Caution patient about the need to follow prescription directions precisely.

NIC: Exercise Promotion; Health Education; Hypoglycemia Management; Nutritional Counseling; Teaching: Individual; Teaching: Prescribed Diet; Teaching: Prescribed Medication

See Also: "General Discussion," p. 381.

PATIENT-FAMILY TEACHING AND DISCHARGE PLANNING

See **Knowledge deficit:** Disease process, diagnostic testing, indicators of hypoglycemia, and therapeutic regimen, above. See also "General Discussion," p. 384, for general care of patients with DM.

Selected Bibliography

American Diabetes Association: Consensus statement: the pharmacologic treatment of hyperglycemia in NIDDM, *Diabetes Care* 19(suppl 1):S54-S61, 1996.

American Diabetes Association: Position statement: diabetes mellitus and exercise, *Diabetes Care* 19(suppl 1):S30, 1996.

American Diabetes Association: Position statement: nutritional recommendations and principles for people with diabetes mellitus, *Diabetes Care* 19(suppl 1):S16-S19, 1996.

American Diabetes Association: Position statement: standards of medical care for patients with diabetes mellitus, *Diabetes Care* 19(suppl 1):S8-S15, 1996.

Bode BW et al: Reduction in severe hypoglycemia with long-term continuous subcutaneous insulin infusion in type I diabetes, *Diabetes Care* 19:324-327, 1996.

Childs BP et al: Clinical decision making: incorporating new diabetes oral agents into clinical practice, *Diabetes Spectrum* 9(4):266-268, 1996.

DDCT Research Group: The effects of intensive treatment of diabetes on the development and progression on long-term complications in insulin-dependent diabetes, *N Engl J Med* 329:977-986, 1993.

DCCT Research Group: Implementation of treatment protocols in the diabetes control and complications trial, *Diabetes Care* 18:361-376, 1995.

DCCT Research Group: Effects of intensive diabetes therapy on neuropsychological function in adults in the diabetes control and complications trial, *Ann Intern Med* 124:379-388, 1996.

Diabetes Interview, issues 52, 53, November/December 1996.

Farkas-Hirsch R: The process of establishing and maintaining nursing staff competence in education patients being placed on insulin pump therapy, *Diabetes Spectrum* 9(4):237-238, 1996.

Fitzgerald PA: Endocrinology. In Tierney LM et al, editors: *Current medical diagnosis and treatment,* ed 36, Stamford, Conn, 1997, Appleton & Lange.

Hermann W: *The prevention and treatment of complications of diabetes mellitus: a guide for primary care practitioners, US Department of Health and Human Services, Public Health Service, Centers for Disease Control, National Center for Chronic Disease Prevention and Health Promotion, Division of Diabetes Translation,* Washington, DC, 1992, US Government Printing Office.

Hirsch IB: Technological advances in diabetes care: where are we going? *Diabetes Spectrum* 9(4):225-226, 1996.

Interqual: *The ISD-A review system with adult ISD criteria,* Northhampton, NH, and Marlboro, Mass, August 1992, Interqual.

Kim MJ et al: *Pocket guide to nursing diagnoses,* ed 7, St Louis, 1997, Mosby.

Klein R et al: The medical management of hyperglycemia over a 10 year period in people with diabetes, *Diabetes Care* 19:744-750, 1996.

Korytowski M: Something old, something new, *Diabetes Spectrum* 9(4):211-212, 1996 (editorial).

Lyon R, Vinci DM: Nutritional management of insulin-dependent diabetes mellitus in adults, *Am Diabetes Assoc* 93(3):309-317, 1993.

Maryniuk MD: Nutrition FYI: measuring outcomes in diabetes care and education, *Diabetes Spectrum* 9(4):260-266, 1996.

McCloskey JC, Bulechek GM, editors: *Nursing interventions classification (NIC),* ed 2, St Louis, 1996, Mosby.

Nathan DM: Inferences and implications: do results from the diabetes control and complications trial apply in NIDDM? *Diabetes Care* 18:251-257, 1995.

Papadakis MA: Fluid & electrolyte disorders. In Tierney LM et al, editors: *Current medical diagnosis and treatment,* ed 36, Stamford, Conn, 1997, Appleton & Lange.

Savinetti-Rose B, Bolmer L: Understanding continuous subcutaneous insulin infusion therapy, *Am J Nurs* 97(3):42-48, 1997.

Vinicor F: Analysis of direct cost of standard compared with intensive insulin treatment of insulin-dependent diabetes mellitus and cost of complications, *Diabetes Spectrum* 9(4):246-248, 1996.

White JR, Jr: The pharmacologic management of patients with type II diabetes mellitus in the era of new oral agents and insulin analogs, *Diabetes Spectrum* 9(4):227-235, 1996.

White NH: Reduction in severe hypoglycemia with long-term continuous subcutaneous insulin infusion in type I diabetes, *Diabetes Spectrum* 9(4):235-237, 1996.

6 GASTROINTESTINAL DISORDERS

Section One: Disorders of the Mouth and Esophagus

Stomatitis

Inflammatory and infectious diseases of the mouth are commonly overlooked in the debilitated hospitalized patient. Typically, they occur secondary to systemic disease and infection, nutritional and fluid deficiencies, poorly fitting dentures, neglect of oral hygiene, side effects of drugs, or exposure to oral irritants such as alcohol, smoking, or smokeless tobacco. Patients with leukemia or neoplastic disease of the head and neck are at increased risk for stomatitis. Stomatitis (inflammation of the mouth and mucous membrane) is the term generally applied to a variety of mouth disorders characterized by mucosal cell destruction and disruption of the mucosal lining. It is one of the major side effects of radiation therapy and cancer chemotherapy, occurring in more than 30% of this population. It also is seen frequently in patients older than 65 years, patients in ICU, and individuals with human immunodeficiency virus (HIV).

ASSESSMENT

Signs and symptoms: Oral pain; sensitivity to hot, spicy foods; foul taste; oral bleeding or drainage; fever; xerostomia (dry mouth); burning sensation in the lips; difficulty chewing or swallowing; poorly fitting dentures.

Physical assessment: The oral mucosa appears swollen, red, and ulcerated; the lymph glands may be swollen; and the breath is often foul smelling. The lips may have cracks, fissures, blisters, ulcers, and lesions; the tongue may appear dry and cracked and contain masses, lesions, or exudate.

DIAGNOSTIC TESTS

In most incidences, diagnosis of the offending organism is made by physical examination. However, the following tests may be used in selected patients.

Culture: May be taken of the lesion or drainage to identify the offending organism. The most common organism is *Candida albicans,* followed by herpes simplex virus 1.

Platelet count: Done if any bleeding is present.

COLLABORATIVE MANAGEMENT

The treatment varies, depending on the type of impairment and its cause.

Identification and attempt to control or remove causative factor(s):   If appropriate (e.g., if poor nutrition is the cause of stomatitis, the goal is to improve nutrition and follow through with other treatments that may be necessary, such as antibiotics).

Oral hygiene/mouth irrigations: Teeth should be brushed with a fluoride-containing dentifrice, using a soft-bristle toothbrush. The tongue also should be lightly brushed. The mouth should be rinsed with sterile normal saline solution after brushing. Mouthwashes may be used to loosen debris, but use of commercial mouthwashes, especially those containing alcohol, should be avoided The accepted mouthwash, in particular for immunosuppressed patients with stomatitis, is sodium bicarbonate with normal saline. A typical solution is made with 500 ml of normal saline and 15 ml of sodium bicarbonate. Oral hygiene should be repeated 4-5 times per day or even more frequently, depending on the degree of oral mucosal impairment.

Pharmacotherapy
Local/systemic analgesics and local anesthetics: For relief of pain.
Topical/systemic steroids: To reduce inflammation and promote healing in severe conditions.
Antibiotic, antifungal, and antiviral agents: To combat infection.
Vitamins: To correct deficiencies (e.g., vitamin C to strengthen connective tissue in the gums; niacin and riboflavin to promote efficient cellular growth).
Dietary management: Typically, a diet high in protein to promote wound healing, high in calories for protein sparing, and high in vitamins to correct the specific deficiency. Usually, hot and spicy foods are restricted, and the consistency of the food ranges from liquid to regular, as tolerated. Fluids are encouraged.
Cauterization of ulcerations: If required.
Dental restoration and repair: If needed.
Adequate rest: For optimal tissue repair.

NURSING DIAGNOSES AND INTERVENTIONS

Altered oral mucous membrane (stomatitis) related to ineffective oral hygiene, dehydration, irritants, or pathologic condition
Desired outcomes: Patient demonstrates oral hygiene interventions and complies with the therapeutic regimen within 12-24 hr of instruction. Patient's oral mucosal condition improves, as evidenced by intact mucous membrane, moist and intact tongue and lips, and absence of pain and lesions.

- Inspect the mouth 3 times per day for inflammation, lesions, and bleeding. Record observations, and report significant findings to health care provider.
- Administer analgesics; corticosteroids; anesthetics, such as Xylocaine jelly, diphenhydramine (Benadryl), and Maalox (or other antacid); and mouthwashes (described below) as prescribed. Avoid commercial mouthwashes, which are high in alcohol. For mild stomatitis, provide mouth care after every meal and before bedtime. For moderate stomatitis, provide mouth care q4hr; for severe stomatitis, provide mouth care q2hr and twice at night or even hourly if indicated.
- Prepare a solution containing 15 ml of sodium bicarbonate and 500 ml of normal saline. Instruct patient to rinse the mouth with the solution (as often as indicated by assessments described above) to provide local relief and promote healing. Warm saline solution may be used to apply heat and aid in cleansing mucous membranes. Avoid solutions containing hydrogen peroxide.
- Instruct patient to brush teeth after meals and at bedtime, using a soft-bristle toothbrush and nonabrasive toothpaste. Patients with severe stomatitis who have dentures should remove them until the oral mucosa has healed. Dietary alterations may be necessary (e.g., changing to a full liquid or pureed diet). A dietary or nutritional consultation may be necessary.
- Use disposable foam swabs to stimulate gums and clean the oral cavity. Avoid use of lemon and glycerin swabs (glycerin is hydrophilic and will cause excessive drying of oral membranes). If platelet levels are >50,000/mm^3, encourage *gentle* flossing of teeth twice daily, using unwaxed floss.

- Advise patient to keep the lips moist with emollients, such as lanolin or any nonpetroleum surgical lubrication.
- Advise patient to avoid irritants, including alcohol, tobacco products, and foods that are hot, spicy, and rough in texture.
- Offer ice or popsicles to help anesthetize the mouth.

You may also wish to refer to the following interventions from the Nursing Interventions Classification (NIC):

NIC: Diet Staging; Medication Management; Nutrition Management; Oral Health Maintenance; Oral Health Promotion; Pain Management

Self-care deficit: Oral hygiene, related to sensorimotor deficit or decreased LOC
Desired outcome: Patient or significant other demonstrates ability to perform patient's oral care by the day of hospital discharge.

- Assess patient's ability to perform mouth care. Identify performance barriers, such as sensorimotor or cognitive deficits. Encourage patient to provide oral hygiene within the confines of the patient's self-care limitations.
- If the patient has decreased LOC or is at risk for aspiration, remove dentures and store them in a water-filled denture cup.
- If the patient cannot perform mouth care, cleanse the teeth, tongue, and mouth at least 2 times daily with a soft-bristle toothbrush and nonabrasive toothpaste. If the patient is unconscious or at risk for aspiration, turn the patient to a side-lying position. Swab the mouth and teeth with a sponge-tipped applicator or gauze pad moistened with the mouthwash solution described earlier, and irrigate the mouth with a syringe. If the patient cannot manage the secretions, use only a small amount of liquid at a time, using a suction catheter or tonsil suction catheter to remove the secretions. This regimen should be performed at least q4hr. As appropriate, teach the procedure to significant other.
- For patients with physical disabilities, the following toothbrush adaptations can be made:
  —*For patients with limited hand mobility:* enlarge the toothbrush handle by covering it with a sponge hair roller or aluminum foil, attaching with an elastic band; or by attaching a bicycle handle grip with plaster of paris.
  —*For patients with limited elbow or shoulder mobility:* extend the toothbrush handle by overlapping another handle or rod over it and taping them together.

NIC: Mutual Goal Setting; Oral Health Maintenance; Patient Contracting; Self-Care Assistance: Bathing/Hygiene; Self-Responsibility Facilitation

Knowledge deficit: Disease process, treatment, and factors that potentiate oral bleeding
Desired outcome: Within the 24-hr period before hospital discharge, patient verbalizes knowledge about the cause, preventive measures, and treatment of stomatitis and the factors that potentiate oral bleeding.

- Describe the causes of patient's stomatitis, and remind patient that the best treatment is prevention.
- Explain the importance of meticulous, frequent oral hygiene and periodic dental examinations.
- Advise patient to avoid irritating foods and substances (e.g., alcohol; tobacco; hot, spicy, and rough foods).
- Teach the importance of discontinuing flossing when the platelet count drops below 50,000/mm^3, or as suggested by health care provider, and discontinuing brushing when the count drops below 30,000/mm^3, or per health care provider's instructions, to avoid possible bleeding. Instead, instruct patient to perform oral hygiene using the mouth irrigation technique described in **Altered oral mucous membrane,** gently swabbing the mouth, teeth, and lips

with a sponge-tipped applicator moistened in a sodium bicarbonate and normal saline solution.

NIC: Discharge Planning; Teaching: Disease Process; Teaching: Prescribed Diet; Teaching: Prescribed Medication; Teaching: Procedure/Treatment

Altered nutrition: Less than body requirements related to inability to ingest food secondary to discomfort with chewing and swallowing

Desired outcome: At least 24 hr before hospital discharge, patient exhibits adequate progress toward optimal nutrition as evidenced by stable weight, serum protein 6-8 g/dl, serum albumin 3.5-5.5 g/dl, and a balanced or positive nitrogen (N) state.

- Assess the patient's ability to chew and swallow.
- Monitor I&O. Unless contraindicated, ensure that patient has optimal hydration (at least 2-3 L/day) and a diet that is high in protein, calories, and essential vitamins and minerals. Alert health care provider if the need for IV or nasogastric (NG) tube feedings becomes apparent.
- Provide any special equipment to facilitate ingestion, such as straws, nipples, or syringes.
- If the patient's mouth is very painful, encourage intake of soft foods (e.g., cooked cereals, soups, gelatin, ice cream). Drinks that are high in calories and protein are especially helpful. Consider adding Polycose to beverages, and powdered milk or protein powder to food preparations.
- Encourage mouth care after every meal or more frequently to minimize the risk of infection caused by the nonintact oral mucosa.

NIC: Nutrition Management; Teaching: Disease Process; Teaching: Prescribed Diet

PATIENT-FAMILY TEACHING AND DISCHARGE PLANNING

When providing patient-family teaching, focus on sensory information; avoid giving excessive information; and initiate a visiting nurse referral for necessary follow-up teaching. Consider including verbal and written information about the following:

- Essentials of diet, medications, and oral hygiene; adaptations that may be required at home; and the importance of monitoring for changes of LOC, which will necessitate precautions to prevent aspiration during oral hygiene (see **Self-care deficit,** p. 338).
- Importance of notifying health care provider if any of the following recurs or worsens: oral pain, fever, drainage, continuous bleeding, or inability to eat or drink.
- Necessity of follow-up care; reconfirm date and time of next medical appointment.
- Importance of visiting the dentist at least twice per year.

Hiatal hernia and reflux esophagitis

Hiatal hernia is defined as a herniation of a portion of the stomach into the chest through the esophageal hiatus of the diaphragm. Hernias are classified as (1) rolling, or esophageal, and (2) sliding, or direct. When intraabdominal pressure increases, a portion of the lower esophagus and stomach may rise up into the chest. Causative factors include degenerative changes (aging), trauma, kyphoscoliosis (a curvature of the spine), and surgery. Increased intraabdominal pressure can occur with coughing, straining, bending, vomiting, obesity, pregnancy, trauma, constricting clothing, ascites, and severe physical exertion. Complications of hiatal hernia include aspiration of reflux contents, ulceration, hemorrhage, stricture, gastritis, and in severe cases, strangulation of the hernia.

The diagnosis of diaphragmatic hernia is often suspected on the basis of reflux symptoms. However, gastroesophageal reflux disease is not caused by any one abnormality. The multiple factors that determine whether reflux esophagitis is present include (1) efficacy of the antireflux mechanism, (2) volume of gastric contents (in the stomach), (3) potency of refluxed material, (4) efficiency of esophageal clearance, and (5) resistance of the esophageal tissue to injury and the ability for tissue repair. By definition, however, the patient must have several episodes of reflux for reflux disease to be present. Reflux esophagitis is the result of an incompetent lower esophageal sphincter that allows regurgitation of acidic gastric contents into the esophagus.

The most common type of hiatal hernia is the sliding hernia, which accounts for 90% of adult hiatal hernias. It is characterized by the upper portion of the stomach and esophageal junction sliding up into the chest when the individual assumes a supine position and sliding back into the abdominal cavity when sitting or standing. The incidence of hiatal hernia increases with age. Women and obese individuals are more often affected.

ASSESSMENT

Many individuals are asymptomatic unless esophageal reflux is present.
Signs and symptoms: Reflux esophagitis often occurs 1-4 hr after eating and while sleeping or reclining, with stress, and with increased intraabdominal pressure. Heartburn (often worse with recumbency), belching, regurgitation, vomiting, retrosternal or substernal chest pain (dull, full, heavy), hiccups, mild or occult bleeding in vomitus or stools, and mild anemia also may occur. Dysphagia can occur and is associated with advanced disease and greater potential for complications. The older adult often presents with symptoms of pneumonitis caused by aspiration of reflux contents into the pulmonary system. Peptic stricture of the esophagus is a serious sequela of aggressive reflux esophagitis.
Physical assessment: Auscultation of peristaltic sounds in the chest, presence of palpitations, abdominal distention. **Note:** These findings are not diagnostic, nor are they usually helpful in making the diagnosis.

DIAGNOSTIC TESTS

For most patients with reflux, obtaining a complete history is sufficient for starting therapy without the necessity of comprehensive diagnostic tests.
Barium swallow: The most specific diagnostic test for revealing hernias and gastroesophageal and diaphragmatic abnormalities. With fluoroscopy, a hiatal hernia will appear as a barium-containing outpouching at the lower end of the esophagus. It may be necessary for the patient to be in Trendelenburg position for the hernia to appear on x-ray. Although gastric barium will move into the esophagus with reflux, the degree of esophagitis is not easily demonstrated radiographically. Scintigraphic techniques using a technetium 99m–labeled solid meal have been used to quantify the degree of esophageal reflux.
Chest x-ray: Reveals large hernias that look like air bubbles in the chest; infiltrates will be seen in the lower lobes of the lungs if aspiration has occurred.
Upper endoscopy and biopsy: Aid in differentiating between hiatal hernia and gastroesophageal lesion; exclude the possibility of neoplasm; or assess the type and severity of esophagitis.
Esophageal motility studies: Identify primary and secondary motor dysfunction before surgical repair of the hernia is performed. Included are manometry, which graphically records resting pressures and peristaltic wave pressures; pH probe, which will be low (acidic) in the presence of gastroesophageal reflux.
Gastric analysis: Assesses bleeding, which can occur if ulceration is present.
CBC: May reveal an anemic condition if bleeding ulcers are present.
Stool occult blood test: Is positive if bleeding has occurred.
ECG: Rules out cardiac origin of pain.

COLLABORATIVE MANAGEMENT

Conservative medical management, which is successful in 90% of the cases, is preferred over surgical intervention. The goals are to prevent or reduce gastric reflux caused by increased intraabdominal pressure and increased gastric acid production.

Restriction or limitation of irritating agents: For example, caffeine, nicotine, and NSAIDS.

Dietary management: Small, frequent meals; bland foods; weight reduction for obese individuals; food restriction 2-3 hr before reclining; refraining from fatty foods, acidic foods, chocolate, and alcohol. Meals low in fat and high in protein increase lower esophageal sphincter tone and decrease reflux.

Elevation of HOB: Using 4- to 6-inch blocks to prevent postural reflux at night, depending on the severity of the reflux; the more severe, the higher the blocks.

Restriction of tight, waist-constricting clothing

Pharmacotherapy

Gastric acid pump inhibitor: Omeprazole or lanisoprazole provides significant remission of symptoms in many patients.

Histamine H_2-receptor blockers: For example, cimetidine, ranitidine, famotidine, and nizatidine to suppress acid secretion.

Antacids: Do not add to the effectiveness of the H_2- receptor blockers but may be useful when side effects of the H_2 blockers preclude their use.

Prokinetic agents: For example, cisapride and metaclopromide, to augment peristalsis of the esophagus and stomach and increase lower esophageal sphincter (LES) pressure.

Antiemetics, cough suppressants, and stool softeners: To prevent increased intraabdominal pressure from vomiting, coughing, and straining with bowel movements.

Surgery: Indicated in approximately 15% of these patients to restore gastroesophageal integrity and prevent reflux if symptoms do not resolve and complications (obstruction, bleeding, aspiration) occur. The most common procedure is a fundoplication, in which a portion of the upper stomach is wrapped around the distal esophagus and sutured to itself to prevent reflux from recurring. Typically, an abdominal rather than a thoracic approach is used. Laparascopic approaches are being used with increasing frequency.

Postsurgical management: Includes chest physiotherapy to prevent respiratory complications, administration of IV fluids and electrolytes until bowel sounds are present, a gradual increase in diet as tolerated after the return of peristalsis, and in some cases, gastric tubes for decompression and feeding.

NURSING DIAGNOSES AND INTERVENTIONS

Knowledge deficit: Disease process and treatment for hiatal hernia and reflux esophagitis

Desired outcome: Within the 24-hr period before hospital discharge, patient verbalizes knowledge about the cause and therapeutic regimen for hiatal hernia and reflux esophagitis.

Note: The cornerstone for many patients with reflux is a change in life-style (e.g., smoking cessation, weight loss, decreased or omitted alcohol consumption, avoidance of irritating agents).

- Assess patient's knowledge about the disorder, its treatment, and the methods used to prevent symptoms and their complications. Provide instructions as appropriate.
- Explain the following methods of dietary management: eating a low-fat, high-protein diet; eating small, frequent meals; eating slowly; chewing well to avoid reflux; avoiding extremely hot or cold foods; limiting stimulants of

gastric acid, such as alcohol, caffeine, chocolate, spices, fruit juices, and nicotine; and losing weight if appropriate.
- Advise the patient to drink water after eating to cleanse the esophagus of residual food, which can irritate the esophageal lining.
- Explain the following alterations in body positions and activities: avoiding the supine position 2-3 hr after eating; sleeping on the right side with the HOB elevated on 4- to 6- inch blocks to promote gastric emptying; for 2-3 hr after eating, avoiding bending, coughing, lifting heavy objects, straining with bowel movements, strenuous exercise, and clothing that is too tight around the waist.
- Stress the importance of following prescribed pharmacologic regimen: omeprazole, histamine H_2-receptor blockers, gastric acid pump inhibitors, antacids, sucralfate, or prokinetic agents, even if symptoms no longer are persistent.

NIC: Discharge Planning; Nutritional Counseling; Smoking Cessation Assistance; Teaching: Prescribed Diet; Teaching: Prescribed Medication; Teaching: Procedure/Treatment

Pain, nausea, or feeling of fullness related to gastroesophageal reflux and increased intraabdominal pressure
Desired outcomes: Patient's subjective perception of discomfort decreases within 1 hr of intervention, as documented by a pain scale. Nonverbal indicators, such as grimacing, are absent or diminished.
- Assess and document the amount and character of the discomfort. Devise a pain scale with patient, rating discomfort from 0 (no pain) to 10 (worst pain).
- Administer medications as prescribed. Document their effectiveness using the pain scale.
- Encourage the patient to follow dietary and activity restrictions.
- If prescribed, insert an NG tube and connect it to suction to reduce pressure on the diaphragm and relieve vomiting.
- Determine whether a position change improves symptoms (e.g., raise the HOB or have the patient turn from side to side).
- For additional information, see **Pain,** p. 719, in Appendix One.

NIC: Analgesic Administration; Distraction; Pain Management; Progressive Muscle Relaxation; Simple Guided Imagery; Sleep Enhancement

For patients with a fundoplication
Ineffective breathing pattern related to guarding secondary to pain of thoracic incision or chest tube insertion
Desired outcome: Patient's RR is 12-20 breaths/min with normal depth and pattern (eupnea) within 1 hr after pain-relieving intervention.
- If a thoracic rather than an abdominal approach was used, chest tubes may be present. Assess the insertion site and suction apparatus for integrity, patency, function, and character of drainage. Tape all chest tube insertion sites.

> **Caution:**   Be alert to the following indications of a pneumothorax: dyspnea, cyanosis, sharp chest pain. (See "Pneumothorax/Hemothorax," p. 24, for care of the patient with a chest tube.)

- Encourage and assist patient with coughing, deep breathing, incentive spirometry, and turning q2-4hr, and note quality of breath sounds, cough, and sputum.
- Facilitate coughing and deep breathing by teaching patient how to splint incision with hands, a folded blanket, or pillow.

- To enhance compliance with the postoperative routine, medicate patient about ½ hr before major moves such as ambulation and turning. If patient-controlled analgesia (PCA) is available, advise its use accordingly. Be aware that opioid analgesics will depress respirations.
- Reassure patient that sutures will not break and tubes will not fall out with coughing and deep breathing.

◎ NIC: Chest Physiotherapy; Cough Enhancement; Fluid Monitoring; Oxygen Therapy; Respiratory Monitoring; Tube Care: Chest

PATIENT-FAMILY TEACHING AND DISCHARGE PLANNING

When providing patient-family teaching, focus on sensory information; avoid giving excessive information; and initiate a visiting nurse referral for necessary follow-up teaching. Consider including verbal and written information about the following:

- Importance of dietary management and activity (see **Knowledge deficit,** p. 407).
- Community resources for weight reduction and smoking cessation. As appropriate, refer patient to a "stop smoking" program as appropriate. The following free brochures outline ways to help patients stop smoking:

  How to Help Your Patients Stop Using Tobacco: A National Cancer Institute Manual for the Oral Health Team, from the Smoking and Tobacco Control Program of the National Cancer Institute; call 1-800-4-CANCER.

  Clinical Practice Guideline: A Quick Reference Guide for Smoking Cessation Specialists, from the Agency for Health Care Policy and Research (AHCPR); call 1-800-358-9295.

- Medications, including drug name, dosage, schedule, purpose, precautions, drug/drug and food/drug interactions, and potential side effects.
- Indicators that signal recurrence of hernia or reflux (which happens only rarely after surgery): dysphagia, hematemesis, increased pain.
- Importance of follow-up care; reconfirm date and time of next medical appointment.
- Care of incision, including dressing changes. Ensure that the patient can verbalize indicators of infection (e.g., increasing pain, local warmth, fever, purulent drainage, swelling, foul odor).
- Procedure for enteral feedings and care of tubes if appropriate.

Section Two: Disorders of the Stomach and Intestines

Peptic ulcers

Peptic ulcers are erosions of the upper GI tract mucosa. They may occur anywhere the mucosa is exposed to the erosive action of gastric acid and pepsin. Commonly, ulcers are gastric or duodenal, but the esophagus, surgically created stomas, and other areas of the upper GI tract may be affected. Autodigestion of mucosal tissue and ulceration are associated with an increase in acidity of the stomach juices or an increased sensitivity of the mucosal surfaces to erosion. Erosions can penetrate deeply into the mucosal layers and become a chronic problem; or they can be more superficial and manifest as an acute problem resulting from severe physiologic or psychologic trauma, infection, or shock (stress ulceration of the stomach or duodenum). Both duodenal and gastric ulcers can occur in association with high-stress life-style, smoking, use of irritating drugs, and presence of *Helicobacter pylori*, as well as secondary to other diseases. Ulceration may occur as a part of Zollinger-Ellison syndrome, in which gastrinomas (gastrin-secreting tumors) of the pancreas or other organs develop. Gastric acid hypersecretion and ulceration subsequently occur.

H. pylori, a gram-negative, spiral-shaped bacterium with four to six flagella on one pole, was first isolated from gastric biopsies in 1983. *H. pylori* can reside below the stomach's mucosa because it produces the enzyme *urease*, which hydrolyses urea to ammonia and carbon dioxide, providing a buffering alkaline halo. Infection can go undetected for years because there may be no symptoms until gastric or duodenal ulceration or gastritis occurs. Transmission of *H. pylori* has not been established, but the fecal-oral route of transmission is suspected.

Serious and disabling complications, such as hemorrhage, GI obstruction, perforation, peritonitis, or intractable ulcer pain, are common. With treatment, ulcer healing usually occurs within 4-6 weeks (gastric ulcers can take as long as 12-16 weeks to heal), but there is potential for recurrence in the same or another site.

ASSESSMENT

Signs and symptoms: Burning, gnawing, dull pain typically 1-3 hr after eating. Discomfort occurs more frequently between meals and at night. With duodenal ulcer, eating usually alleviates discomfort; with gastric ulcer, pain often worsens after meals. Hematemesis, melena, dizziness, and syncope are associated with an actively bleeding ulcer. Sudden, severe epigastric pain, often radiating to the right shoulder, suggests perforation of an ulcer. Pain described as piercing through to the back suggests penetration of the ulcer into adjacent posterior structures in the abdomen.

Physical assessment: Tenderness over the involved area of the abdomen. With perforation, there will be severe pain (see "Peritonitis" for more information) and rebound tenderness. With penetration the pain is usually altered by changes in back position (extension or flexion).

History of: Chronic or acute stress; smoking; use of irritating agents such as caffeine, alcohol, corticosteroids, salicylates, reserpine, indomethacin, or phenylbutazone; disorders of the endocrine glands, pancreas, or liver; and hypersecretory conditions, such as Zollinger-Ellison syndrome. Use of NSAIDs is associated with gastric ulceration.

DIAGNOSTIC TESTS

Barium swallow: Uses contrast agent (e.g., barium) to detect abnormalities. Patient should maintain NPO status and not smoke for at least 8 hr before the test. Postprocedure care involves administration of prescribed laxatives and enemas to facilitate passage of the barium and prevent constipation and fecal impaction.

Endoscopy: Allows visualization of the stomach (gastroscopy), duodenum (duodenoscopy), or both stomach and duodenum (gastroduodenoscopy), or the esophagus, stomach, and duodenum (esophagogastroduodenoscopy) via passage of a lighted, flexible tube. Patient is NPO for 8-12 hr before the procedure, and written consent is required. Before the test a sedative is administered to relax the patient, an opioid analgesic is given to prevent pain, and atropine is administered to decrease GI secretions and prevent aspiration. Local anesthetic may be sprayed into the posterior pharynx to ease passage of the tube. A biopsy may be performed as part of the endoscopy procedure. Biopsied tissue may be sent for histologic examination and for culture and sensitivity to identify *Helicobacter pylori* infection. Postprocedure care involves maintaining NPO status for 2-4 hr, ensuring return of the gag reflex before allowing the patient to eat (if local anesthetic was used), administering throat lozenges or analgesics as prescribed, and monitoring for complications, such as bleeding or perforation (e.g., hematemesis, pain, dyspnea, tachycardia, hypotension).

Gastric secretion analysis: Is helpful in differentiating gastric ulcer from gastric cancer. An NG tube is passed, and the stomach contents are aspirated and analyzed for the presence of blood and free hydrochloric acid. Achlorhydria (absence of free hydrochloric acid) suggests gastric cancer, whereas mildly elevated levels suggest gastric ulcer. Excessive elevation of free hydrochloric acid occurs with Zollinger-Ellison syndrome. A tubeless gastric analysis involves administration of a gastric stimulant followed by a resin dye. A urine specimen is obtained 2 hr later and analyzed for the presence of dye. Absence of dye indicates achlorhydria. The patient is NPO for at least 8 hr before either test.

CBC: Reveals a decrease in hemoglobin (Hgb), hematocrit (Hct), and RBCs when acute or chronic blood loss accompanies ulceration.

Helicobactor pylori **testing:** Serum antigen testing identifies exposure to *H. pylori* bacteria; this is the least expensive means of identifying *H. pylori* infection. A breath test is available to identify *H. pylori* infection by detecting carbon dioxide and ammonia as by-products of the action of the bacterium's urease in the patient's expired air.

Stool for occult blood: Is positive if bleeding is present.

COLLABORATIVE MANAGEMENT

Conservative management is preferred over surgical intervention, with the therapy aimed at decreasing hyperacidity, healing the ulcer, relieving symptoms, and preventing complications.

Activity as tolerated with adequate rest: So that tissue repair can occur. The patient who is anemic from bleeding ulcers requires activity limitations and more assistance with ADL because of fatigue.

Dietary management: Well-balanced diet with avoidance of foods that are not tolerated. Three meals per day are recommended, with elimination of bedtime snacks. Consumption of caffeine and alcohol should be reduced or eliminated. For acute episodes of upper GI hemorrhage, the patient is NPO and is given IV fluid and electrolyte replacement, with foods and fluids introduced orally after bleeding subsides.

Pharmacotherapy (generally short term and given in combination) (Table 6-1)

Histamine H₂-receptor blockers (e.g., cimetidine [Tagamet], ranitidine [Zantac], nizatidine [Axid], famotidine [Pepcid]): Administered PO or IV to suppress secretion of gastric acid and facilitate ulcer healing. They also can be used prophylactically for limited periods of time, especially in patients susceptible to stress ulceration. These medications should be administered with meals at least 1 hr apart from antacids, since antacids can reduce their absorption.

Sucralfate (Carafate): An antiulcer agent that coats the ulcer with a protective barrier so that healing can occur. This drug must be taken before meals and at bedtime. It should not be taken within 30 min of antacids, since acid facilitates adherence of sucralfate to the ulcer.

Antacids: Administered orally or through an NG tube to provide symptomatic relief, facilitate ulcer healing, and prevent further ulceration; can be administered prophylactically in patients who are especially susceptible to ulceration. They are administered after meals and at bedtime or are given periodically via NG tube for patients who are intubated.

Omeprazole (Prilosec): Deactivates the enzyme system that pumps hydrogen ions (H⁺) from the parietal cells, thus inhibiting gastric acid secretion; used for short-term treatment of active duodenal and gastric ulcers and for long-term treatment of hypersecretory conditions.

Misoprostol (Cytotec): Synthetic prostaglandin E₁ analog that enhances the body's normal mucosal protective mechanisms and decreases acid secretion. The drug is used in the healing and prevention of NSAID-induced ulcers.

T A B L E 6 - 1   Acid Suppression Therapies

	Anticholinergics (e.g., atropine, propantheline)	Antacids (e.g., Maalox, Mylanta, Riopan)	Sucralfate (Carafate)	H₂-blockers (e.g., cimetidine, ranitidine, famotidine, nizatidine)	Misoprostol (Cytotec)	Omeprazole (Prilosec)
Mechanism of action	Block secretion of acid	Neutralize acid	Coats mucosa	Block secretion of acid	Enhances mucosal protection; reduces acid secretion	Inhibits proton pump
Relative efficacy	+	++	++	++	++	+++
Drug interactions	Few	Many	Some	Many with cimetidine; some with others	Few	Some
Comments	Many side effects; not first-line therapy; not for gastric ulcers	Inconvenient; magnesium-containing type causes diarrhea; aluminum-containing type causes constipation; usually given prn for pain	Give 30 min before meal or at hs	Single daily dose often given at hs; cimetidine may cause drug interactions and other undesired effects	Used for NSAID-induced ulcers; causes diarrhea; may cause abortion; do not give to pregnant patients	Very potent; may completely inhibit secretion of gastric acid; not for long-term use

NSAID, Nonsteroidal antiinflammatory drug.

***Helicobacter pylori* eradication therapy:**   Indicated for patients in whom *H. pylori* is cultured. Triple antibiotic therapy regimen consists of amoxicillin, tetracycline, and metronidazole along with bismuth subsalicylate (Pepto-Bismol). This combination antibiotic therapy is thought to reduce the potential for antimicrobial resistance. Another regimen (clarithromycin [Biaxin] and omeprazole [Prilosec]) has been shown to be no more effective than triple antibiotic therapy but more expensive.

NG tube with gastric lavage: For acute, severe GI bleeding, to clear blood from the stomach before endoscopy and to prevent accumulation of clotted blood. For this procedure the patient should be in semi-Fowler's position or higher. A large-bore NG tube or an Ewald tube is inserted. Gastric contents are aspirated, followed by the instillation of 100-250 ml of room-temperature normal saline or tap water, as prescribed, and aspiration of the contents. The process is repeated until returns are clear or light pink and clot free. Vasopressin may be administered intravenously to diminish uncontrolled bleeding before surgery.

Surgical interventions: Indicated for hemorrhage, intractable ulcers, GI obstruction, and perforation. Common surgical procedures include the following, singly or in combination.

Pyloroplasty: Remodeling of the pyloric valve between the stomach and duodenum. This may involve enlargement to relieve obstruction and facilitate gastric emptying or tightening to reduce duodenal reflux into the stomach.

Vagotomy: Severing of the branches of the vagus nerve to inhibit gastric acid secretion. This may be done at the following three levels.

TRUNCAL VAGOTOMY: Severs the vagus nerves at the gastroesophageal junction, reducing gastric acid production and gastric mobility. This has fallen from usage recently.

SELECTIVE VAGOTOMY: Severs branches of the vagus nerve that innervate the distal two thirds of the stomach, reducing gastric acid production but maintaining antral function and thus having little impact on gastric motility.

PARIETAL CELL, OR SUPRASELECTIVE, VAGOTOMY: Severs only branches of the vagus nerve that innervate the parietal cells responsible for gastric acid production.

Subtotal gastrectomy: Removal of distal part of the stomach with anastomosis to the duodenum in a gastroduodenostomy (Billroth I for gastric ulcer) or removal of part of the stomach and the duodenum with anastomosis to the jejunum in a gastrojejunostomy (Billroth II for duodenal ulcer). Vagotomy may accompany subtotal gastrectomy.

Total gastrectomy: Removal of the entire stomach (rarely performed for ulcer disease but may be used for gastric cancer).

Postsurgical care: Involves temporary GI decompression with NG tube; analgesics for pain; IV fluid and electrolyte replacement; symptomatic relief of dumping syndrome (rapid gastric emptying characterized by abdominal fullness, weakness, diaphoresis, fatigue, tachycardia, palpitations, dizziness) with a low-carbohydrate, high-fat, high-protein diet, small meals without liquids, and supine position after meals; treatment of pernicious anemia (decreased production of intrinsic factor secondary to removal of that part of the stomach that contains the parietal cells) with vitamin B_{12} injections; and treatment with iron supplements for iron-deficiency anemia (which might occur secondary to loss of blood or iron-absorbing surface in the GI tract). Prevention of hypoventilation and subsequent atelectasis and hypoxemia is especially important in patients who have had abdominal surgery. Deep-breathing exercises are imperative (see "Atelectasis," p. 2).

Life-style alterations: Such as smoking cessation, decreased consumption of alcohol, avoidance of irritating drugs, and stress reduction therapies.

> **See Also:** "Obstructive Processes" (p. 420) for treatment of GI obstruction secondary to inflammatory edema or scar tissue formation with ulcer healing; "Peritonitis" (p. 424) for care of the patient with peritonitis caused by perforation.

NURSING DIAGNOSES AND INTERVENTIONS

Altered protection related to potential for bleeding, obstruction, and perforation secondary to ulcerative process

Desired outcome: Patient is free of signs and symptoms of bleeding, obstruction, perforation, and peritonitis as evidenced by negative results for occult blood testing, passage of stool and flatus, soft and nondistended abdomen, good appetite, and normothermia.

- Assess for indicators of bleeding, including hematemesis and melena. Check all NG aspirate, emesis, and stools for occult blood. Report positive findings.
- Monitor results of CBC and coagulation studies. Be alert for Hct <40% (male) or <37% (female) and Hgb <14 g/dl (male) or <12 g/dl (female); PTT >70 sec or PT >12.5 sec.
- If indicated, insert gastric tube to evacuate blood from the stomach, monitor for bleeding, and perform gastric lavage as prescribed. Do not use gastric tubes in patients who have or are suspected of having esophageal varices.
- If patient is actively bleeding or if the Hct is low, administer O_2. Monitor O_2 saturation via oximetry to evaluate systemic oxygenation status (report O_2 saturation <92%).
- Monitor and note indicators of obstruction, including abdominal pain, abnormal (increased peristalsis, "rushes," or "tinkles") or absent bowel sounds, distention, anorexia, nausea, vomiting, and the inability to pass stool or flatus. For more information, see "Obstructive Processes" (p. 420).
- Be alert to indicators of perforation and peritonitis, such as sudden or severe abdominal pain, distention and abdominal rigidity, fever, nausea, and vomiting. Notify health care provider immediately of significant findings. See "Peritonitis" for more information (p. 424).
- Teach patient the signs and symptoms of GI complications and the importance of reporting them promptly to the staff or health care provider if they occur.

NIC: Bedside Laboratory Testing; Oxygen Therapy; Surveillance; Teaching: Individual; Vital Signs Monitoring

Impaired tissue integrity related to exposure to chemical irritants (gastric acid, pepsin)

Desired outcomes: Patient verbalizes knowledge of the necessary life-style alterations within the 24-hr period before hospital discharge and demonstrates compliance with medical recommendations for peptic ulcer throughout the hospital stay. Gastric and duodenal mucosal tissues heal and remain intact as evidenced by reduced or absent pain and absence of bleeding.

- Encourage patient to avoid foods that seem to cause pain or increase acid secretion; this response is highly individual.
- Advise patient to avoid foods and drugs that are associated with increased acidity and GI erosions: coffee, caffeine, alcohol, aspirin, and ibuprofen and other NSAIDs.
- If applicable, recommend strategies for smoking cessation.
- Administer *Helicobacter pylori* eradication therapy (e.g., amoxicillin, tetracycline, metronidazole, bismuth subsalicylate) for *H. pylori*–associated ulceration.
- Administer acid suppression therapy (see Table 6-1) for acute episodes of ulceration.

- Stress the importance of taking medications at the prescribed intervals, not just for symptomatic relief of pain.
- Refer patient to community resources and support groups for assistance in smoking cessation or abstinence from drinking (p. 409).

NIC: Medication Management; Teaching: Prescribed Diet; Teaching: Prescribed Medication; Smoking Cessation Assistance

---

See Also: "Crohn's Disease" for **Pain,** abdominal cramping, and nausea: intestinal inflammatory process, p. 455; related discussion in "Obstructive Processes," p. 422, if the patient has a gastric obstruction; Appendix One, "Caring for Preoperative and Postoperative Patients," p. 717, for nursing diagnoses and interventions.

PATIENT-FAMILY TEACHING AND DISCHARGE PLANNING

When providing patient-family teaching, focus on sensory information; avoid giving excessive information; and initiate a visiting nurse referral for necessary follow-up teaching. Consider including verbal and written information about the following:

- Importance of following the prescribed diet to facilitate ulcer healing, prevent exacerbation or recurrence, or control postsurgical dumping syndrome. If appropriate, arrange a consultation with a dietitian.
- Medications, including drug name, rationale, dosage, schedule, precautions, drug/drug and food/drug interactions, and potential side effects (see Table 6-1).
- Signs and symptoms of exacerbation and recurrence, as well as potential complications.
- Care of the incision line and dressing change technique, as necessary.
- Signs of wound infection, including persistent redness, swelling, purulent drainage, local warmth, fever, and foul odor.
- Role of life-style alterations in preventing exacerbation or recurrence of ulcer, including smoking cessation, stress reduction (see **Health-seeking behavior:** Relaxation technique effective for stress reduction, p. 59), decreasing or eliminating consumption of alcohol, and avoidance of irritating foods and drugs. In addition, the histamine H_2-receptor blockers are more effective in individuals who are nonsmokers.
- Referral to a health care specialist for assistance with stress reduction as necessary.
- Referrals to community support groups, such as Alcoholics Anonymous.

Malabsorption/Maldigestion

Malabsorption or maldigestion refers to a condition in which a specific nutrient or a variety of nutrients are inadequately digested or absorbed from the GI tract. The causes of malabsorption are varied and can include the following.

Postgastrectomy malabsorption: This is frequently seen in individuals after subtotal gastrectomy, because of rapid gastric emptying and decreased intestinal transit time.

Inadequate presence of digestive substances in the GI tract: Examples are lactase enzyme deficiency, which is characterized by an inability to digest and absorb lactose, a disaccharide found in milk and dairy products; bile deficiency secondary to liver and gallbladder disease and biliary tract obstruction, which is characterized by inability to digest and absorb fats and fat-soluble vitamins; and pancreatic secretion deficiency secondary to pancreatic insufficiency or obstruction to the flow of pancreatic secretions, as seen with pancreatic disorders or cystic fibrosis.

Inadequate absorptive space in the GI tract: This occurs secondary to GI surgery (especially ileal resection) and is characterized by general nutrient malabsorption (short bowel syndrome).

Mucosal lesions that impair absorption: Mucosal changes occur secondary to intestinal invasion of microorganisms endemic to tropical islands (tropical sprue) or ingestion of gluten in the diet (celiac disease, nontropical sprue, gluten-induced enteropathy). Gluten-containing foods include malt, rye, barley, oats, and wheat. With Whipple's disease, which is a rare disorder, a small bowel lipodystrophy occurs, resulting in impaired absorption.

Inflammatory conditions of the GI tract: For example, ulcerative colitis (see p. 440) and Crohn's disease (see p. 450) involve significant diarrhea with malabsorption and deficiencies of various nutrients. Inflammation and mucosal ulceration secondary to chemotherapy also can impair digestion and absorption.

Use of drugs that alter intestinal fluids or mucosa (and subsequently affect absorption of specific nutrients):   These include antacids, mineral oil, broad-spectrum antibiotics, hypocholesterolemic agents, antiinflammatory agents, oral hypoglycemics, and oral potassium chloride (KCl).

Overgrowth of microbes in the GI tract: Overgrowth is secondary to diverticula (outpouchings) of the small intestine, inadequate gastric acid secretion (e.g., secondary to total or partial gastrectomy or aggressive antisecretory therapy), immunologic defects, gastroenteritis, blind loop syndrome, and intestinal obstruction.

Excessive use of enemas or cathartics: Nutrients pass too rapidly through the intestinal tract to be absorbed. Complications can include specific or generalized malnutrition, fluid and electrolyte imbalances, and acid-base imbalances, any of which may necessitate hospitalization.

ASSESSMENT

Signs and symptoms: Will vary depending on the specific nutrients that are not absorbed. Patient may have unexplained weight loss with muscle atrophy, despite normal or increased appetite; diarrhea; steatorrhea (greasy, pale, foul-smelling stools); bloating; excessive flatus; abdominal cramping; and indicators of specific nutrient deficiencies (e.g., anemia with iron or vitamin B_{12} deficiency; tetany and paresthesias with calcium deficiency; bleeding or easy bruising with vitamin K deficiency).

History of: GI surgery; excessive use of enemas or cathartics; diseases that cause diarrhea; immunologic defects; diverticulosis; liver, pancreatic, or gallbladder disease; inflammatory/infectious disorders of the intestinal tract; medications that increase GI motility and cause diarrhea; chemotherapy.

DIAGNOSTIC TESTS

72-Hr fecal fat test: Increased when steatorrhea characterizes malabsorption.

Stool culture: May be diagnostic of pathogens or bacterial overgrowth.

Schilling's test: Analysis of a 24-hr urine specimen collected after ingestion of radioactive vitamin B_{12} followed by an IM injection of nonradioactive vitamin B_{12} will reveal below-normal levels of B_{12}. Further testing, during which intrinsic factor is administered, will facilitate diagnosis of pernicious anemia from malabsorption or renal disease.

D-Xylose tolerance test: Will show inadequate presence of xylose (an easily absorbed monosaccharide) in a 5-hr collection of urine after oral administration.

Serum tests: Will show depressed levels of carotene, calcium, magnesium, and other electrolytes and minerals, depending on specific malabsorption problem. In addition, serum albumin, total iron-binding capacity, and transferrin may be decreased because of protein depletion.

Lactose tolerance test: Will show failure of fasting blood glucose levels to rise and the presence of abdominal symptoms after ingestion of lactose. These signs are diagnostic of lactase deficiency (lactose intolerance).

Hydrogen breath test: Will show an increase in hydrogen after ingestion of lactose. Because unabsorbed lactose is converted to hydrogen, this test is diagnostic of lactase deficiency.

Lactulose breath test: Assesses for presence of bacterial overgrowth. Nonabsorbent lactulose is administered, and the breath is tested for hydrogen. With the abnormal presence of bacteria in the proximal intestine, lactulose is hydrolyzed earlier than normal.

Barium swallow: Facilitates diagnosis of the specific cause of malabsorption (e.g., diverticula of the small intestine). (For a description, see "Peptic Ulcers," p. 410.) Small bowel follow-through is accomplished by serial x-rays as the barium progresses through the small intestines.

Abdominal x-ray: Facilitates diagnosis of the specific cause of malabsorption (e.g., pancreatic calcifications may be noted, which are suggestive of a pancreatic source).

CT scan of the abdomen: Facilitates diagnosis, especially for pancreatic involvement. Patients are NPO 3-4 hr before the procedure. To minimize flatus, a low-residue diet may be prescribed for 48 hr before the test. If contrast will be used, patients should be assessed in advance for allergy to iodine. Patients may be required to hold several deep breaths during scanning. Oral or IV fluids should be adequate to ensure elimination of the dye via the kidneys after the procedure.

Endoscopy with or without biopsy: Visualization of the small (duodenoscopy) or large (colonoscopy) bowel through a lighted, flexible tube (endoscope) that is inserted through the mouth (duodenoscopy) or anus (colonoscopy). The patient is NPO before the procedure. Written consent is required. Sedation is prescribed to relax the patient; atropine may be administered to decrease GI secretions; and glucagon may be administered to facilitate passage of the tube through the pylorus. Tissue samples may be taken for examination, including culture and cytologic evaluation. Hemorrhage and perforation are potential complications, and VS should be monitored closely for 4-8 hr after the procedure.

Endoscopic retrograde cholangiopancreatography (ERCP): Involves passage of an endoscope into the duodenum to the ampulla of Vater (distal end of the pancreatic and common bile duct drainage system) for visualization. A contrast medium is injected through the scope into the pancreatic ducts or biliary ducts (common bile duct, cystic duct, hepatic ducts), and x-rays are taken. This test is diagnostic for pancreatic disease and common bile duct pathology (stricture, obstruction, choledocholithiasis). Patient is NPO for 8-12 hr before the test and must be assessed for allergies to iodine (and/or to shellfish) before undergoing the test. Written consent is required. Oral or IV fluid should be adequate to ensure elimination of dye via the kidneys after the procedure. A rare but potentially fatal complication of ERCP is acute pancreatitis; monitor for increasing abdominal pain, tachycardia, hypotension, abdominal distention, nausea, and vomiting.

Hormonal stimulation test: Checks for pancreatic insufficiency. A collecting tube is passed into the duodenum of the patient who is NPO. IV secretin and/or cholecystokinin is given, and the duodenal secretions are collected and analyzed for bicarbonate and trypsin levels, which are decreased with pancreatic insufficiency. Written consent is required.

COLLABORATIVE MANAGEMENT

Management will vary, depending on the specific cause of malabsorption and the nutrient deficiencies that are exhibited.

Activity as tolerated: Patient may be fatigued and require limited activity as a consequence of diarrhea, malnutrition, and associated anemia.

TABLE 6-2   Guidelines for Low-residue, High-residue, and Gluten-free Diets

Low-residue diet	High-residue diet
Encourage intake of enriched/refined breads and cereals; rice and pasta dishes	Encourage intake of fruits, vegetables, large amounts of fluid, whole-grain breads and cereals
Avoid fruits, vegetables, whole wheat products (cereals and breads)	Avoid highly refined cereals and pasta (e.g., white rice, white bread, spaghetti noodles, ice cream)

Gluten-free diet

Avoid cereals and bakery goods made from wheat, malt, barley, rye, and oats. Also avoid the following if they contain any of the above grain products: coffee substitutes, sauces, commercially prepared luncheon meats, gravies, noodles, macaroni, spaghetti, flour tortillas, crackers, cakes, cookies, pastries, puddings, commercial ice cream, and alcoholic beverages	Use the following (if allowed): rice, corn, eggs, potatoes; breads made from rice flours, cornmeal, soybean flour, gluten-free wheat starch, and potato starch; cereals made from corn or rice (grits, cornmeal mush, cooked cream of rice, puffed rice, rice flakes); pasta made from rice or corn flour; homemade ice cream; tapioca pudding

Dietary management: Will vary, depending on the specific disorder that is precipitating the malabsorption. A *low-residue diet* may be useful for controlling diarrhea. For lactase deficiency a *low-lactose diet* (avoidance of milk and milk products) is prescribed, and for nontropical sprue, a *gluten-free diet* is prescribed (Table 6-2). Until specific problems (e.g., liver or gallbladder disorders) are corrected, dietary intake of fats is avoided. Any specific nutrient deficiencies are corrected. For the seriously malnourished patient, parenteral nutrition may be necessary (see "Providing Nutritional Therapy," p. 687).

Pharmacotherapy: Will vary, depending on the specific disorder that has precipitated malabsorption and the specific nutrient deficiencies.

Mineral, vitamin, and electrolyte supplements: To correct specific deficiencies.

Antibiotics: For treatment of bacterial overgrowth or pathogenic infection (e.g., *Clostridium difficile*).

Cholestyramine (an antihyperlipidemic agent):   May be given to control diarrhea when it is associated with ileal resection.

IV fluids and electrolytes: As necessary to rehydrate and correct electrolyte imbalances.

Surgical intervention: May be necessary to correct specific disorders that precipitate malabsorption, such as biliary tract obstruction or stricture of the sphincter of Oddi.

NURSING DIAGNOSES AND INTERVENTIONS

Diarrhea, bloating, excessive flatus, and abdominal cramping related to malabsorption in the bowel

Desired outcome: Patient is free of discomfort from diarrhea and other symptoms of malabsorption at least 24 hr before hospital discharge, as evidenced by passage of normal stools (soft, semiformed) and absence of excessive flatus and cramping.

- Assess and document presence of GI discomfort and symptoms, including the onset and duration of symptoms and the precipitating and palliative factors. Instruct patient to avoid foods associated with symptoms.

- Teach patient the importance of dietary compliance in the treatment for some malabsorptive disorders (e.g., dietary restriction, such as a low-lactose diet with lactase intolerance or a gluten-free diet with nontropical sprue, may be necessary to prevent symptoms). Have patient plan a 3-day menu that includes and excludes foods from the lists in Table 6-2 as appropriate.
- If an infectious source of diarrhea is suspected (e.g., *Clostridium difficile*), collect a stool specimen for culture and sensitivity.

NIC: Learning Readiness Enhancement; Teaching: Prescribed Diet

Risk for fluid volume deficit related to excessive loss with diarrhea
Desired outcome: Patient is normovolemic as evidenced by good skin turgor, moist mucous membranes, urinary output ≥30 ml/hr, HR ≤100 bpm, absence of orthostatic systolic BP changes, and absence of thirst.

- Assess patient for evidence of fluid volume deficit: weight loss, tachycardia, hypotension, poor skin turgor, dry skin and mucous membranes, thirst, and decreased urinary output. Consult health care provider for hypotension or urinary output ≤30 mm/hr for 2 consecutive hours.
- Ensure precise maintenance and documentation of fluid I&O records and daily weights.
- Administer IV fluids and parenteral nutrients appropriately and at prescribed rate.
- As appropriate, encourage intake of water and/or noncaffeinated clear liquids.
- Encourage prescribed dietary compliance for relief of symptomatic diarrhea.
- Administer medications, and teach patient self-administration of medications, to control diarrhea or treat underlying condition.

NIC: Diarrhea Management; Fluid/Electrolyte Management; Learning Readiness Enhancement; Perineal Care; Teaching: Prescribed Diet

> **Note:** For assessment of nutrient deficiencies, see "Providing Nutritional Support," p. 687.

PATIENT-FAMILY TEACHING AND DISCHARGE PLANNING

When providing patient-family teaching, focus on sensory information; avoid giving excessive information; and initiate a visiting nurse referral for necessary follow-up teaching. Consider including verbal and written information about the following:

- Use of medications (vitamins, antibiotics), including drug name, purpose, dosage, schedule, precautions, drug/drug and food/drug interactions, and potential side effects.
- Prescribed dietary replacement of deficiency nutrients and dietary management of symptoms if appropriate.
- The need to ensure adequate oral fluid intake during episodes of diarrhea to avoid dehydration.
- Problems that necessitate medical attention: nutrient deficiencies, fluid volume deficit, and acid-base imbalances.
- Phone numbers to call should questions or concerns arise about therapy or disease after discharge. Additional general information can be obtained by contacting the following organizations:

National Digestive Diseases Information Clearinghouse, National Institute of Diabetes and Digestive and Kidney Diseases
Project Officer
2 Information Way
Bethesda, MD 220892-3570   (301) 654-3810
WWW address: *http://www.aerie.com/nihdb/ddbase.htm*

Gluten Intolerance Group of North America
P.O. Box 23053
Seattle, WA 98102-3053   (206) 325-6980

- Additional resource (WWW address):

  http://www.demon.co.uk/webguides/nutrition/diets/glutenfree/index.html

Obstructive processes

Obstruction of the GI tract is a condition in which the normal peristaltic transport of GI contents does not take place. Therefore the digestion and absorption of foods and fluids and the elimination of wastes are impaired or totally blocked. Further, GI fluids become hypertonic, precipitating osmotic fluid loss from the body into the GI lumen. Subsequently, nutritional status and fluid and electrolyte status are compromised and distention occurs. Increased pressure in the GI tract also can result in perforation and peritonitis or necrosis of the GI mucosa. Obstruction can occur anywhere along the GI tract, but most commonly it occurs at the pyloric area of the stomach or in the small bowel because of adhesions in the ileum. Obstruction can occur as a result of the inflammation and edema that accompany GI disease (peptic ulcers, diverticulitis, colitis, gastroenteritis, trauma); GI surgery with subsequent edema and possibly adhesions (gastrectomy, appendectomy, colon resection); growths (polyps, tumors); adynamic (paralytic) ileus secondary to peritoneal insult, such as surgery or peritonitis; diminished GI motility because of hypokalemia, uremia, diabetes mellitus (DM), or use of opioids, diuretics, or anticholinergic drugs; volvulus; or incarcerated hernia. If obstruction is prolonged or infarction of intestinal tissue occurs, sepsis is likely.

ASSESSMENT

Signs and symptoms: Severe and crampy pain, vomiting, back pain, restlessness, hiccoughs, belching, and inability to pass stool or flatus (accompanied by a feeling of fullness). Symptoms vary, depending on the type and site of obstruction (Table 6-3).

Physical assessment: Abdominal distention, abdominal tenderness, high-pitched ("tinkles") and intermittent bowel sounds above the point of obstruction. Bowel sounds are absent or diminished with paralytic ileus.

TABLE 6-3   Assessment of Patients With Obstructive Processes

	Small bowel obstruction	Large bowel obstruction	Paralytic ileus
Pain*	Severe, episodic	Moderate, more continuous	Not prominent
Vomiting	Occurs early; may be projectile	Occurs late; feculent (if duodenal valve is incompetent)	Not prominent
Abdominal distention	Occurs late	Pronounced	Present
Passage of stool/flatus	Minimal to none with partial obstruction of large bowel; "pencil" stools or fecal smearing may be present		

*With obstruction associated with intestinal strangulation, pain always is severe, vomiting is present, and abdomen is distended, rigid, and tender.

Patients may have decreased urinary output, poor skin turgor, and dry skin and mucous membranes associated with intravascular volume depletion. Bleeding may be noted on rectal examination if strangulation or tumor is present.

History of: Abdominal hernia, recent or past abdominal surgery, GI inflammation or perforation secondary to various disease processes, DM, chronic renal failure, or use of opioids, diuretics, or anticholinergics.

DIAGNOSTIC TESTS

CBC count: WBCs usually elevated secondary to inflammation. Marked leukocytosis is usually present with intestinal strangulation. Hct and Hgb may be elevated because of hemoconcentration.

X-ray of abdomen: Will reveal distention of bowel loops with air and fluid proximal to the obstruction. The presence of free air under the diaphragm suggests intestinal perforation.

Contrast studies: Facilitate quick assessment to determine presence and location of obstruction. Barium or meglumine diatrizoate (Gastrografin) is commonly used as the contrast agent. Barium enema (to exclude colon obstruction) should precede barium swallow. Barium will not advance past the site of obstruction. For more information, see "Peptic Ulcers," p. 410.

Aspiration of fecal matter from NG/intestinal tube: Fecal matter, which is identified by its characteristic foul odor, is an indication of obstruction.

Endoscopy (sigmoidoscopy, colonoscopy): Identifies tumor, stricture, inflammation, or other sources of colonic obstruction.

COLLABORATIVE MANAGEMENT

The specific cause of the obstruction must be identified quickly so that the appropriate treatment can be instituted and complications prevented. In the interim, management is supportive and aimed at maintaining nutritional and fluid and electrolyte balance and promoting comfort.

Activity as tolerated: With paralytic ileus, patient encouraged to ambulate to enhance return of peristalsis. With other forms of obstruction, activity may be limited because of pain or complications.

Dietary management: Patient NPO until obstruction is resolved (or bowel sounds return in paralytic ileus).

GI decompression: Accomplished via gastric or intestinal tube connected to low, intermittent suction (Table 6-4).

IV fluid and electrolyte support: Lactated Ringer's or isotonic saline solutions (or isotonic dextrose/saline combinations) are commonly prescribed. Volume of IV fluid required often depends on the amount of gastric or intestinal tube drainage (replacement fluids often prescribed ml for ml). K^+ is added to IV fluids to correct or prevent hypokalemia. Total parenteral nutrition (TPN) may be indicated to meet nutritional needs if obstruction or recovery is prolonged.

Urinary catheterization: Allows close monitoring of urinary output.

Pharmacotherapy: May include the following.

Antibiotics: To prevent or treat infection.

Analgesics: For pain relief. However, they can mask symptoms and interfere with diagnosis. Opioids, such as morphine, can decrease intestinal motility and increase nausea and vomiting.

Antiemetic agents (e.g., hydroxyzine, ondansetron, prochlorperazine, promethazine): For relief of nausea and vomiting.

GI stimulants (e.g., metoclopramide [Reglan], dexpanthenol [Ilopan]): Used perioperatively to minimize paralytic ileus. Used cautiously because stimulant action may cause perforation in ischemic bowel. Metoclopramide is used in the management of diabetic gastric stasis.

Surgical intervention: Indicated for obstruction that does not resolve. In some cases, inflammatory processes subside and obstruction resolves without surgery. Paralytic ileus generally resolves in 2-3 days without any treatment. In most other cases, surgery is indicated to identify and relieve the source of

TABLE 6-4   **Gastric/Intestinal Tubes Used in Obstructive Processes**

Tube	Obstructive process	Purpose
Gastric tube*	Pyloric obstruction, small bowel obstruction, paralytic ileus	Decompresses gastrointestinal (GI) tract of retained fluids, alleviates abdominal distention, relieves edema in intestinal wall, prevents vomiting, and promotes comfort
Intestinal tube*† (e.g., single-lumen Cantor or Harris tube or double-lumen Miller-Abbott tube)	Small or large bowel obstruction, paralytic ileus	See gastric tube above; presence of tube may promote return of peristalsis in paralytic ileus; tube may relieve edema sufficiently to relieve obstruction, thereby avoiding need for surgery

*In some cases, gastric and intestinal tubes are used together.
†Long intestinal tubes are indicated primarily when obstruction is partial.

obstruction. Exploratory laparotomy is performed when diagnosis is uncertain. When diagnosis is known, the indicated surgery is performed (e.g., pyloroplasty for pyloric obstruction or bowel resection with or without colostomy for removal of tumor or adhesions).

NURSING DIAGNOSES AND INTERVENTIONS

Pain, nausea, and distention related to obstructive process or malfunction of gastric or intestinal drainage tube

Desired outcomes: Patient's subjective perception of discomfort decreases within 8 hr of admission and is absent by hospital discharge, as documented by a pain scale. Nonverbal indicators, such as grimacing, are absent or diminished.

- Assess the degree of the patient's discomfort. Investigate characteristics of the pain such as severity, character, location, duration, precipitating/ alleviating factors, and nonverbal indicators. Devise a pain scale with patient, rating discomfort from 0 (no discomfort) to 10 (worst discomfort). Be alert to characteristics of pain, vomiting, and distention, depending on the type of obstructive process (see Table 6-3).
- Instruct the patient in nonpharmacologic methods to provide pain relief: distraction, back rubs, conversation, relaxation therapy. See **Health-seeking behaviors:** Relaxation technique effective for stress reduction, p. 59.
- Administer prescribed analgesics and antiemetic agents as indicated. **Note:** Do not administer opioid analgesics until surgical evaluation has been completed. Instruct the patient to request analgesia before the pain becomes severe. Assess and document the degree of relief obtained using the pain scale. Be aware that opioid analgesics contribute to intestinal hypomotility.
- Maintain patency and proper functioning of the gastric or intestinal tube.
  —Maintain connection to low, intermittent suction or as prescribed.
  —Irrigate tube with 30 ml of normal saline prn or as prescribed.
  —Keep gastric tube properly positioned in stomach by securing it with tape or other adhesive.
  —Avoid occlusion of the vent side of sump suction tubes because this may result in vacuum occlusion of the tube and excessive suction and injury to gastric mucosa.

—Advance intestinal tube slowly, 2-3 inches at a time or as prescribed, until it reaches the desired location. Positioning patient in various positions (right side-lying, supine, left side-lying) may facilitate passage of the tube. Do not tape the tube to the patient's skin until it reaches the desired location.
* Keep HOB elevated 30-45 degrees as permitted, to promote comfort and facilitate ventilation. A slightly Trendelenburg, right side-lying position may reduce gas pains in patients with paralytic ileus.
* Encourage turning in bed and activity as permitted to promote peristalsis.
* Provide oral care at frequent intervals. Frequent brushing of teeth and rinsing of mouth will alleviate dryness. Provide lubricant for lips.
* Provide mouth rinses at frequent intervals to alleviate pharyngeal discomfort from tube. Apply water-soluble lubricant to naris to alleviate discomfort. Apply viscous lidocaine solution to naris or back of throat, as prescribed, to alleviate discomfort from the tube.

NIC: Analgesic Administration; Distraction; Gastrointestinal Intubation; Pain Management; Simple Relaxation Therapy; Tube Care: Gastrointestinal

Risk for fluid volume deficit with risks related to *excessive loss* secondary to obstructive process and subsequent vomiting or gastric decompression of large volumes of GI fluids; and *decreased intake* secondary to fluid restrictions
Desired outcome: Patient is normovolemic as evidenced by good skin turgor, moist mucous membranes, urinary output ≥30 ml/hr, urinary specific gravity 1.010-1.025, stable weight, HR ≤100 bpm, absence of orthostatic systolic BP changes, and absence of thirst.
* Ensure precise measurement and documentation of fluid I&O. Weigh patient daily.
* Take special note of the amount and character of GI aspirate. Check GI aspirate for electrolyte loss or pH as prescribed.
* Administer appropriate IV fluids at the prescribed rate. Replace volume of GI fluids aspirated by suction if prescribed. Weigh patient daily.
* Take careful note of the character and amount of GI aspirate. Check GI aspirate for electrolyte loss (collect specimen for laboratory analysis) or pH as prescribed.
* For other interventions, see **Risk for fluid volume deficit**, p. 730, in Appendix One.

NIC: Fluid/Electrolyte Management; Intravenous (IV) Therapy; Tube Care: Gastrointestinal; Tube Care: Urinary

See Also: Appendix One, "Caring for Preoperative and Postoperative Patients," p. 717, if surgery was performed.

PATIENT-FAMILY TEACHING AND DISCHARGE PLANNING
When providing patient-family teaching, focus on sensory information; avoid giving excessive information; and initiate a visiting nurse referral for necessary follow-up teaching. Consider including verbal and written information about the following:
* Specific disease process that precipitated the obstruction and methods to prevent recurrence, such as compliance with prescribed therapies.
* Symptoms of recurring obstruction to report to health care provider.
* Medications, including drug name, purpose, dosage, schedule, precautions, drug/drug and food/drug interactions, and potential side effects.

Peritonitis

Peritonitis is the inflammatory response of the peritoneum to offending chemical and bacterial agents invading the peritoneal cavity. The inflammatory process can be local or generalized and acute or chronic, depending on the pathogenesis of the inflammation. Common causes include abdominal trauma; postoperative leakage of GI content or blood into the peritoneal cavity; intestinal ischemia; ruptured or inflamed abdominal organs; poor sterile techniques (e.g., with peritoneal dialysis); and direct contamination of the bloodstream. The peritoneum responds to invasive agents by attempting to localize the infection with a shift of the omentum (the "guardian of the abdominal cavity") to wall off the inflamed area. Inflammation of the peritoneum results in tissue edema, the development of fibrinous exudate, and hypermotility of the intestinal tract. As the disease progresses, paralytic ileus occurs, and intestinal fluid, which then cannot be reabsorbed, leaks into the peritoneal cavity. As a result of the fluid shift, cardiac output and tissue perfusion are reduced, leading to impaired cardiac and renal function. If infection or inflammation continues, respiratory failure and shock can ensue. Peritonitis frequently is progressive and can be fatal. It is the most common cause of death following abdominal surgery.

ASSESSMENT

Signs and symptoms: Early findings: acute abdominal pain with movement, anorexia, nausea, vomiting, chills, fever, rigor, malaise, weakness, hiccoughs, diaphoresis, and abdominal distention and rigidity (often described as *boardlike*). Later findings may include those of dehydration (e.g., thirst, dry mucous membranes, oliguria, concentrated urine, poor skin turgor).

Physical assessment: Presence of tachycardia, hypotension, and shallow and rapid respirations caused by abdominal distention and discomfort. Often the patient assumes a supine position with the knees flexed or side-lying with the knees drawn up toward the chest. Palpation usually reveals peritoneal irritation as shown by distention, abdominal rigidity with general or localized tenderness, guarding, and rebound or cough tenderness. However, as many as one fourth of these patients will have minimal or no indications of peritoneal irritation. Auscultation findings include hyperactive bowel sounds during the gradual development of peritonitis and an absence of bowel sounds or infrequent high-pitched sounds ("tinkling" or "squeaky") during later stages if paralytic ileus occurs. Mild ascites may be present as demonstrated by shifting areas of dullness on percussion.

History of: Abdominal surgery, peptic ulcer disease, cholecystitis, acute necrotizing pancreatitis, GI disorders, acute salpingitis, ruptured appendix or diverticulum, trauma, peritoneal dialysis.

DIAGNOSTIC TESTS

Serum tests: May reveal the presence of leukocytosis (usually with a shift to the left), hemoconcentration, elevated BUN, and electrolyte imbalance, particularly hypokalemia. Hypoalbuminemia and prolonged prothrombin time, in combination with leukocytosis, are especially characteristic.

ABG values: May reveal hypoxemia (Pao_2 <80 mm Hg) or acidosis (pH <7.40).

Urinalysis: Often performed to rule out genitourinary involvement (e.g., pyelonephritis).

Occult fecal blood test: Should be routinely done on all patients and may reflect possible mucosal lesions that may have resulted in intestinal perforation.

Paracentesis for peritoneal aspiration with culture and sensitivity: May be performed to determine the presence of blood, bacteria, bile, pus, and amylase content and identify the causative organism. Gram stain of ascitic fluid is positive in only about 25% of these patients. Ascitic fluid with a WBC count

>500/mm^3 with more than 25% polymorphonuclear leukocytes is especially characteristic. Blood-ascitic fluid albumin gradient >1.1 g/dl, reduced pH of ascitic fluid (<7.31), and serum lactic acid elevation >33 mg/dl aid in confirmation of the diagnosis.

Abdominal x-rays: May be performed to determine the presence of distended loops of bowel and abnormal levels of fluid and gas, which usually collect in the large and small bowel in the presence of a perforation or obstruction. "Free air" under the diaphragm also may be visualized, which indicates a perforated viscus.

Chest x-ray: Abdominal distention may elevate the diaphragm. Pain from peritonitis may limit respiratory excursion and lead to associated infiltrates in the lower lobes. In later stages, changes in serum osmolality allow for pleural effusions to occur.

Contrast x-rays: May be used to identify specific intestinal pathologic conditions. Water-soluble contrast (e.g., meglumine diatrizoate [Gastrografin]) may be used to evaluate suspected upper GI perforation.

CT scan and ultrasound: May be used to evaluate abdominal pain and more clearly delineate nondistinct areas found by plain abdominal x-rays. MRI has not been an effective adjunct in abdominal surveys because of motion artifacts.

Radionuclide scans: Such as gallium, hepato-iminodiacetic acid (lidofenin, HIDA), and liver-spleen scans, may be used to identify intraabdominal abscess.

COLLABORATIVE MANAGEMENT

Bedrest: With patient in semi-Fowler's or high Fowler's position to promote fluid shift to the lower abdomen, which will reduce pressure on the diaphragm and allow deeper and easier respirations. Raising the knees will lower stress on the abdominal wall.

NG or intestinal tube: Inserted to reduce or prevent GI distention, nausea, and vomiting (Table 6-4).

IV fluids, electrolyte therapy, and parenteral feedings: To correct fluid, electrolyte, and nutritional disorders. Daily measurements of serum electrolytes and calculations of fluid volume are performed to determine the necessary types of fluid and electrolyte replacement. A urinary catheter is inserted to facilitate careful intake and output measurement. Crystalloids, colloids (albumin, Plasmanate), blood, and blood products may be administered to correct hypovolemia, hypoproteinemia, and anemia. Patient is NPO during the acute phase, and oral fluids are not resumed until the patient has passed flatus and the gastric tube has been removed. Total parenteral nutrition (TPN) usually is initiated in the early stages to promote nutrition and protein replacement.

Cardiovascular monitoring: A CVP catheter may be inserted in the critically ill patient. CVP values should be maintained at 2-6 mm Hg (5-12 cm H$_2$O). A pulmonary artery (i.e., Swan-Ganz) catheter may be inserted if the patient is unstable or develops hypovolemic shock.

Pharmacotherapy

Antibiotic therapy: Combination broad-spectrum antibiotic therapy is rapidly begun to cover gram-negative bacilli and anaerobic bacteria. Common agents include cephalosporins (cefotaxime, cefepime), aminoglycosides (gentamicin), ampicillin, floxacin (Floxin), and metronidazole. Antibiotics are commonly administered intravenously and may also be directly instilled into the peritoneal cavity via surgically placed catheters.

O$_2$: Often prescribed to support increased metabolic needs or treat hypoxia.

Analgesics and sedatives: To relieve severe pain and discomfort once the diagnosis has been confirmed. Because potent analgesics can mask diagnostic symptoms, opioids should not be administered until surgical evaluation has been completed.

Surgical intervention: May be required to repair perforations, remove the source of infection, drain the abscess or accumulated fluids, and prevent recurrent infection. This can include the removal of an organ, such as the appendix or gallbladder. Drains usually are inserted to allow continued removal of purulent drainage and excessive fluids. Intestinal decompression may be employed to decrease massive abdominal distention. Intraoperative and postoperative irrigation, with or without antibiotic solutions, may be indicated if bowel contents have grossly contaminated the peritoneal cavity.

Peritoneal lavage: May be used if the patient does not respond to the interventions just mentioned or is a surgical risk. Rapid dialysis exchanges may be performed along with antibiotic lavages.

NURSING DIAGNOSES AND INTERVENTIONS

Pain, abdominal distention, and nausea related to inflammatory process, fever, and tissue damage

Desired outcomes: Patient's subjective perception of pain decreases within 1 hr of intervention, as documented by a pain scale. Nonverbal indicators, such as grimacing and abdominal guarding, are absent or diminished.

- Assess and document the character and severity of the discomfort q1-2hr. Devise a pain scale with the patient, rating discomfort on a scale of 0 (no pain) to 10 (worst pain).
- After the diagnosis has been made, administer opioids, other analgesics, and sedatives as prescribed to promote comfort and rest. Encourage patient to request analgesic *before* pain becomes severe. Document the relief obtained, using the pain scale.
- Keep patient on bedrest to minimize pain, which can be aggravated by activity.
- Instruct the patient in methods to splint the abdomen to reduce pain on movement, coughing, and deep breathing.
- Provide a restful and quiet environment.
- Keep patient in a position of comfort, usually semi-Fowler's position with the knees bent.
- Explain all procedures to patient to help minimize anxiety, which can exacerbate discomfort.
- Offer mouth care and lip moisturizers at frequent intervals to help relieve discomfort/nausea from continuous or intermittent suction, dehydration, and NPO status.
- Administer antiemetics (e.g., hydroxyzine, ondansetron, prochlorperazine, promethazine) as prescribed to combat nausea and vomiting; instruct patient to request medication *before* the nausea becomes severe.
- See "Stomatitis," p. 403, for mouth care interventions.

NIC: Analgesic Administration; Distraction; Environmental Management; Pain Management; Positioning; Simple Relaxation Therapy; Sleep Enhancement

Impaired gas exchange related to alveolar hypoventilation and decreased depth of respirations secondary to guarding with abdominal pain or distention

Desired outcomes: Patient has an effective breathing pattern as evidenced by Pao_2 ≥80 mm Hg, oxygen saturation ≥92%, BP ≥90/60 mm Hg (or within patient's baseline range), HR ≤100 bpm, and orientation to person, place, and time. Eupnea occurs within 1 hr after pain-relieving intervention.

- Monitor ABG and oximetry results, and be alert to indicators of hypoxemia, including Pao_2 <80 mm Hg and low oxygen saturation (<92%), and to the following clinical signs: hypotension, tachycardia, tachypnea, restlessness, confusion or altered mental status, central nervous system (CNS) depression, and possibly cyanosis.
- Auscultate lung fields to assess ventilation and detect pulmonary complications. Note and document the presence of adventitious breath sounds.
- Keep patient in semi-Fowler's or high Fowler's position to aid respiratory effort; encourage deep breathing to enhance oxygenation and coughing to

clear pulmonary secretions. Instruct the patient in splinting the abdomen to facilitate respiratory hygiene.
- Administer oxygen as prescribed.

NIC: Chest Physiotherapy; Cough Enhancement; Fluid Monitoring; Infection Protection; Oxygen Therapy; Respiratory Monitoring

Altered protection related to potential for worsening/recurring peritonitis or development of septic shock secondary to inflammatory process
Desired outcome: Patient is free of symptoms of worsening/recurring peritonitis or septic shock as evidenced by normothermia, BP ≥90/60 mm Hg (or within patient's normal range), HR ≤100 bpm, absence of chills, presence of eupnea, urinary output ≥30 ml/hr, CVP 2-6 mm Hg (5-12 cm H_2O), decreasing abdominal girth measurements, and minimal tenderness to palpation.
- Assess the abdomen q1-2hr during the acute phase and q4hr once the patient is stabilized. Monitor for increasing distention by measuring abdominal girth; use a permanent marker to identify the placement of the tape measure to ensure consistent measurement by caregivers. Auscultate bowel sounds to assess motility. Bowel sounds often are frequent during the beginning phase of peritonitis but are absent in the presence of paralytic ileus. *Lightly* palpate the abdomen for evidence of increasing rigidity or tenderness, which indicates disease progression. If the patient experiences increased pain on removal of your hand, rebound tenderness is present. Notify health care provider of significant findings.
- If prescribed, insert gastric tube and connect it to suction to prevent or decrease distention. If an intestinal tube is placed, note orders for allowing tube advancement or fixed placement. If prescribed to allow intestinal tube advancement, do *not* attach the tube to suction; allow enough laxity in the tube to facilitate its movement, but stabilize it on the bed to decrease inadvertent removal. Carefully note and document tube length at least q8hr until advancement ceases. Carefully monitor drainage from gastric or intestinal tubes; examine suspicious drainage for occult blood.
- Monitor VS at least q2hr and more frequently if the patient's condition is unstable. Be alert to signs of septic shock: increased temperature, hypotension, tachycardia, shallow and rapid respirations, urine output <30 ml/hr, and CVP <2 mm Hg (<5 cm H_2O). In the early (warm) stage of shock, the skin usually is warm, pink, and dry secondary to peripheral venous pooling, and the BP and CVP begin to drop. In the late (cold) stage of shock, the extremities become pale and cool because of the decreasing tissue perfusion.
- Administer antibiotics as prescribed; ensure close adherence to schedules for maintenance of bacteriocidal serum levels. Collect peak and trough antibiotic determinations as prescribed.
- Monitor CBC count for the presence of leukocytosis, which signals infection, and hemoconcentration (increased Hct and Hgb), which occurs with a decrease in plasma volume. Normal values are as follows: WBC: 4,500-11,000/mm^3; Hgb: 14-18 g/dl (male) or 12-16 g/dl (female); and Hct: 40%-54% (male) or 37%-47% (female). With peritonitis, WBC count usually is >20,000/mm^3. Notify health care provider of significant findings.
- Maintain sterile technique with dressing changes and all invasive procedures.
- Teach patient the signs and symptoms of recurring peritonitis and the importance of reporting them promptly if they occur: fever, chills, abdominal pain, vomiting, and abdominal distention.

NIC: Gastrointestinal Intubation; Infection Protection; Teaching: Prescribed Activity/Exercise; Tube Care: Gastrointestinal; Tube Care: Urinary; Wound Care

Altered nutrition: Less than body requirements related to vomiting and intestinal suctioning

Desired outcome: By at least 24 hr before hospital discharge, patient demonstrates optimal progress toward adequate nutritional status as evidenced by stable weight, balanced or positive nitrogen (N) state, serum protein 6-8 g/dl, and serum albumin 3.5-5.5 g/dl.

- Keep patient NPO as prescribed during acute phase of the disorder. If the patient has an ileus, an NG tube will be inserted to decompress the abdomen. Reintroduce oral fluids gradually once motility has returned, as evidenced by presence of bowel sounds, decreased distention, and passage of flatus.
- Maintain intestinal tubes as prescribed; closely monitor the amount and consistency of the drainage.
- Support patient with peripheral parenteral nutrition (PPN) or TPN, as prescribed, depending on the duration of the acute phase (usually by day 3).
- Administer replacement fluids, electrolytes, and vitamins as prescribed.
- Instruct patient in the rationale for tube placement and NPO status, underlying pathologic condition (as appropriate), the need for close monitoring of fluid intake and output, and, eventually, diet advancement.

See Also: "Providing Nutritional Support," p. 687, for the care of patients receiving enteral or parenteral feedings; "Obstructive Processes," p. 420, if paralytic ileus occurs; Appendix One, "Caring for Preoperative and Postoperative Patients," p. 717, for nursing diagnoses and interventions; Appendix One, "Caring for Patients on Prolonged Bedrest" for **Risk for activity intolerance,** p. 738; **Risk for disuse syndrome,** p. 740.

NIC: Diet Staging; Fluid/Electrolyte Management; Gastrointestinal Intubation; Nutrition Management; Teaching: Procedure/Treatment

PATIENT-FAMILY TEACHING AND DISCHARGE PLANNING

When providing patient-family teaching, focus on sensory information; avoid giving excessive information; and initiate a visiting nurse referral for necessary follow-up teaching. Consider including verbal and written information about the following:

- Medications, including drug name, dosage, schedule, purpose, precautions, drug/drug and food/drug interactions, and potential side effects.
- Activity alterations as prescribed by health care provider, such as avoiding heavy lifting (>10 lb), resting after periods of fatigue, getting maximum amounts of rest, and gradually increasing activities to tolerance.
- Notifying health care provider of the following indicators of recurrence: fever, chills, abdominal pain, vomiting, abdominal distention.
- If patient has undergone surgery, indicators of wound infection: fever, pain, chills, incisional swelling, persistent erythema, purulent drainage.
- Importance of follow-up medical care; confirm date and time of next medical appointment.

Appendicitis

Appendicitis is the most frequently occurring inflammatory lesion of the bowel and one of the most common reasons for abdominal surgery. Appendicitis occurs most often in adolescents and young adults, especially males. Approximately 200,000 appendectomies for acute appendicitis are performed yearly in the United States. The appendix is a blind, narrow tube that extends from the inferior portion of the cecum and does not serve any known useful function. Appendicitis is usually caused by obstruction of the appendiceal lumen by a fecalith (hardened bit of fecal material), inflammation, a foreign body, or a neoplasm. Obstruction prevents drainage of secretions that are produced by epithelial cells in the lumen, thereby increasing intraluminal pressure and compressing mucosal blood vessels. This tension eventually impairs local blood flow, which can lead to necrosis and perforation. Inflammation and infection result from normal bacteria invading the devitalized wall. Mild cases of appendicitis can heal spontaneously, but severe inflammation can lead to a ruptured appendix, which can cause local or generalized peritonitis.

ASSESSMENT

Signs and symptoms vary because of differences in anatomy, size, and age.
Early stage: The onset of abdominal pain usually occurs in either epigastric or umbilical area and may be vague and diffuse or associated with mild cramping. Abdominal discomfort is accompanied by fever, nausea, and vomiting.
Intermediate (acute) stage: Over a period of a few hours, pain that shifts from the midabdomen or epigastrium to the right lower quadrant (RLQ) at McBurney's point (approximately 2 inches from the anterior superior iliac spine on a line drawn from the umbilicus) and is aggravated by walking, coughing, and movement. The pain may be accompanied by a sensation of constipation (gas-stoppage sensation). Anorexia, malaise, occasionally diarrhea, and diminished peristalsis also can occur.

On *physical assessment* the patient experiences pain in the RLQ elicited by *light* palpation of the abdomen; presence of rebound tenderness; RLQ guarding, rigidity, and muscle spasms; tachycardia; low-grade fever; absent or diminished bowel sounds; and pain elicited with rectal examination. A palpable, tender mass may be felt in the peritoneal pouch if the appendix lies within the pelvis.
Acute appendicitis with perforation: Increasing, generalized pain; recurrence of vomiting.

On *physical assessment* the patient usually exhibits temperature increases >38.5° C (101.4° F) and generalized abdominal rigidity. Typically, the patient remains rigid with flexed knees. Presence of abscess can result in a tender, palpable mass. The abdomen may be distended.

DIAGNOSTIC TESTS

WBC with differential: Reveals presence of leukocytosis and an increase in neutrophils. A shift to the left with more than 75% neutrophils is found in about 90% of cases or more.
Urinalysis: To rule out genitourinary conditions mimicking appendicitis; may reveal microscopic hematuria and pyuria.
Abdominal x-ray: May reveal presence of a fecalith. About half of these patients may have x-ray findings of localized air-fluid levels, increased soft tissue density in the RLQ, and indications of localized ileus. If perforation has occurred, the presence of free air is noted. Barium enemas do not aid in diagnosis.
Intravenous pyelogram: May be performed to rule out ureteral stone or pyelitis.
Abdominal ultrasound: May be done to rule out appendicitis or conditions that mimic it, such as Crohn's disease, diverticulitis, or gastroenteritis.
Abdominal CT scan: May reveal an appendiceal abscess or acute appendicitis.

COLLABORATIVE MANAGEMENT

Preoperative care
Bedrest: For observation.
NPO status: Parenteral fluids begun if surgery is imminent.
Pharmacotherapy: Opioids avoided until diagnosis is certain because they mask clinical signs and symptoms.
Antibiotics: To prevent systemic infection.

Tranquilizing agents: For sedation.
Gastric tube: Inserted for gastric suction and lavage, if needed.

> Note: Cathartics and enemas are contraindicated because they increase peristalsis and can cause perforation.

Surgery
Appendectomy: Performed as soon as the diagnosis is confirmed and fluid imbalance and systemic reactions have been controlled. The appendix is removed through an incision made over McBurney's point or through a right paramedian incision. In the presence of abscess, rupture, or peritonitis, an incisional drain is inserted.

Laparoscopic appendectomy incidental to gynecologic procedures (e.g., endometriosis involving the appendix) or for acute or chronic appendicitis (in the absence of rupture or signs of peritonitis) is gaining popularity and is performed using from one umbilical portal to three or four abdominal portals. Advantages to this technique over traditional surgery include earlier ambulation and hospital discharge, decreased risk of wound infection, improved cosmesis, and less pain. Direct costs of laparoscopic appendectomy are greater than with open appendectomy, but there may be economic benefits from more rapid recovery.

Postoperative care
Activities: Ambulation on the day of surgery. The patient may be hospitalized for 1-3 days. Normal activities are resumed 2-3 wk after surgery.
Diet: Advances from clear liquids to soft solids during the second through fifth postoperative day; parenteral fluids are continued if required.
Pharmacotherapy
Antibiotics: May be used prophylactically or provided in the presence of infection.
Mild laxatives: Given if necessary, but enemas continue to be contraindicated during the first few postoperative weeks until adequate healing has occurred and bowel function has been restored.
Analgesics: For postoperative pain.

NURSING DIAGNOSES AND INTERVENTIONS

Risk for infection with risk factors related to inadequate primary defenses (danger of rupture, peritonitis, abscess formation) secondary to inflammatory process
Desired outcomes: Patient is free of infection as evidenced by normothermia, HR ≤100 bpm, BP ≥90/60 mm Hg, RR 12-20 breaths/min with normal depth and pattern (eupnea), absence of chills, soft and nondistended abdomen, and bowel sounds 5-34/min in each abdominal quadrant. Following instruction, patient verbalizes the rationale for not administering enemas or laxatives preoperatively and enemas postoperatively and demonstrates compliance with the therapeutic regimen.
- Assess and document quality, location, and duration of pain. Be alert to pain that becomes accentuated and generalized or to the presence of recurrent vomiting, and note whether patient assumes side-lying or supine position with flexed knees. Any of these signs can signal worsening appendicitis, which can lead to rupture. Be alert to pain that worsens and then disappears—a signal that rupture may have occurred.
- Monitor for ambulation with a limp or pain with extension of the hip. Retrocecal abscess may irritate the psoas muscle as it traverses the area of the posterior RLQ of the abdomen and result in pain with hip extension.
- Monitor VS for elevated temperature, increased pulse rate, hypotension, and shallow/rapid respirations; and assess the abdomen for presence of rigidity,

distention, and decreased or absent bowel sounds, any of which can occur with rupture. Report significant findings to health care provider.

- Caution patient about the danger of preoperative self-treatment with enemas and laxatives because they increase peristalsis, which increases the risk of perforation. If constipation occurs postoperatively, health care provider may prescribe laxatives/stool softeners at bedtime after the third day. Remind patient that enemas should be avoided until approved by health care provider (usually several weeks after surgery). Instruct the patient in an anticonstipation diet with added roughage and fluid intake.
- Teach patient about postoperative incisional care, as well as care of drains if patient is to be discharged with them.
- Provide instructions about prescribed antibiotics if patient is to be discharged with them.
- See "Peritonitis" for more information (p. 424).

NIC: Bowel Management; Diet Staging; Infection Protection; Postanesthesia Care; Surgical Preparation; Teaching: Procedure/Treatment; Tube Care; Wound Care

Pain and nausea related to the inflammatory process

Desired outcomes: Within 1-2 hr of pain-relieving intervention, patient's subjective perception of pain decreases, as documented by a pain scale. Objective indicators, such as grimacing, are absent or diminished.

- Assess and document quality, location, and duration of pain. Devise a pain scale with patient, rating discomfort from 0 (no pain) to 10 (worst pain). Be aware of the characteristics of discomfort during the following stages of appendicitis:
  - —*Early stage:* abdominal pain (either epigastric or umbilical) that may be vague and diffuse; nausea and vomiting; fever; and sensitivity over the appendix area.
  - —*Intermediate (acute) stage:* pain that shifts from the epigastrium to the RLQ at McBurney's point (approximately 2 inches from the anterior superior iliac spine on a line drawn from the umbilicus) and is aggravated by walking or coughing. The pain may be accompanied by a sensation of constipation (gas-stoppage sensation). Anorexia, malaise, occasional diarrhea, and diminished peristalsis also can occur.
  - —*Acute appendicitis with perforation:* increasing, generalized pain; recurrence of vomiting; increasing abdominal rigidity.
- Medicate patient with antiemetics, sedatives, and analgesics as prescribed; evaluate and document patient's response, using the pain scale. Encourage the patient to request medication *before* symptoms become severe.
- Keep patient NPO before surgery; after surgery, nausea and vomiting usually disappear. If prescribed, insert gastric tube for decompression.
- Teach technique for slow, diaphragmatic breathing to reduce stress and help relax tense muscles.
- Help position patient for optimal comfort. Many patients find comfort from a side-lying position with the knees bent, whereas others find relief when supine with pillows under the knees. Avoid pressure on the popliteal area.

See Also: Appendix One, "Caring for Preoperative and Postoperative Patients," p. 717, for nursing diagnoses and interventions.

NIC: Analgesic Administration; Anxiety Reduction; Coping Enhancement; Pain Management; Progressive Muscle Relaxation; Simple Guided Imagery; Simple Relaxation Therapy; Sleep Enhancement

PATIENT-FAMILY TEACHING AND DISCHARGE PLANNING

When providing patient-family teaching, focus on sensory information; avoid giving excessive information; and initiate a visiting nurse referral for necessary follow-up teaching. Consider including verbal and written information about the following:

- Medications, including drug name, dosage, purpose, schedule, precautions, drug/drug and food/drug interactions, and potential side effects.
- Care of incision, including dressing changes and bathing restrictions if appropriate.
- Indicators of infection: fever, chills, incisional pain, redness, swelling, and purulent drainage.
- Postsurgical activity precautions: avoid lifting heavy objects (>10 lb) for the first 6 wk or as directed, be alert to and rest after symptoms of fatigue, get maximum rest, gradually increase activities to tolerance.
- Importance of avoiding enemas for the first few postoperative weeks. Caution patient about the need to check with health care provider before having an enema.

Section Three: Intestinal Neoplasms and Inflammatory Processes

Diverticulosis and diverticulitis

Diverticulosis is acquired small pouches or sacs (diverticula) in the colon formed by the herniation of mucosal and submucosal linings through the muscular layers of the intestine. Although diverticula can be found anywhere in the colon, they are seen most frequently in the sigmoid colon because it is the narrowest part of the colon, harbors the firmest stool, and, as a result, must generate higher intraluminal pressures than the rest of the colon. It is theorized that diverticula develop secondary to a low-residue diet and increased intracolonic pressure, such as that created with straining to have a bowel movement. It has been estimated that 50% of people in Western countries develop diverticula, with cultural factors, especially diet, playing a significant role in this development.

Diverticulitis is a complication of diverticulosis. It is an inflammatory process that is theorized to begin with a single diverticulum, usually in the sigmoid colon, and to be caused by the irritating presence of trapped fecal material within the diverticulum. When the obstructing fecal plug (called a *fecalith*) remains and bacteria proliferate, the inflammation can spread from the thin wall at the apex of the diverticulum to peridiverticular tissue. The resulting inflammation creates edema that may compromise blood flow to the diverticulum, resulting in tissue ischemia. If unrelieved, tissue ischemia may eventually allow perforation of the diverticulum. The resulting infection can be localized (diverticular abscess) or more extensive (peritonitis) and life threatening.

ASSESSMENT

Diverticulosis: Lower GI bleeding that may be minute or may present as a massive hemorrhage (hematochezia) that can be life threatening. Such hemorrhage is usually self-limiting. Other findings include symptoms of irritable bowel syndrome, such as steady or crampy abdominal pain in the LLQ associated with alternating constipation or diarrhea and increased flatulence. The patient may be asymptomatic.

Diverticulitis: See the indicators just mentioned. Pain may be mild to severe, cramping or aching, or described as similar to that of appendicitis, only occurring in the LLQ. Cecal diverticulitis presents with findings similar to appendicitis. Passing flatus or stool may reduce pain. In addition, fever, nausea, vomiting, and obstipation can be present if obstruction or peritonitis occurs. Fistulas to the bladder, vagina, or skin and gas or stool elimination from the involved site also may be present.

Physical assessment: Presence of tender, palpable mass, usually in the LLQ; rebound tenderness secondary to infection or abscess formation; abdominal distention; hypoactive or hyperactive bowel sounds; and possibly, absence of stool felt on rectal examination. Often the patient assumes a side-lying position with the knees flexed to relieve pain. Tachycardia, hypotension, and shallow respirations can be present if there is severe abdominal discomfort. **Note:** With massive hemorrhage, patients may present with findings of hypovolemic shock.

DIAGNOSTIC TESTS

Diverticulosis

Barium enema: To determine presence and number of diverticula.

CBC: To determine if anemia is present.

Rigid sigmoidoscopy or colonoscopy: To reveal presence of diverticula, thickening of bowel wall, diverticular openings, and stricture (decrease in intraluminal size from scarring following repeated attacks). **Caution:** Sigmoidoscopy and colonoscopy are contraindicated during acute attacks.

Diverticulitis

Abdominal x-rays: To determine presence of abnormal gas and fluid levels, which collect in the intestine above the affected area of the colon, indicating the presence and degree of bowel obstruction or ileus; and to reveal the presence of free air in the peritoneal cavity, signaling noncontainment of diverticular perforation. These films also may show the presence of air in the urinary bladder if a colovesical fistula is present.

CBC with differential: Usually reveals leukocytosis with a shift to the left and an increase in neutrophils, indicating presence of infection.

Blood culture: May reveal presence of bacteremia in severely ill patients.

Urinalysis: To rule out bladder involvement; may show red and white cells in the presence of colovesical fistula.

Barium enema: To support the diagnosis of diverticulitis by demonstrating the presence of barium outside the lumen of the colon or outside a diverticulum, a fistula or fistulas leading from the colon, an intramural abscess, or a pericolic mass. This examination should be deferred during the acute phase of illness if perforation is suspected. Water-soluble agents can be used if risk of perforation is great or fistula formation is suspected.

CT scan: To demonstrate diverticula, changes in the wall of the colon that indicate diverticulitis (effacement of pericolonic fat), and related abscesses and fistulas. Oral or IV contrast may be used to enhance imaging. Because this examination is noninvasive, it can be used in acutely ill or septic individuals for whom barium enema studies can be hazardous.

Radionuclide "bleeding" scan (technetium 99m-sulfur colloid, technetium 99m-labeled red blood cells): To identify active bleeding sites during lower GI hemorrhage.

MRI and ultrasound: May aid in clarifying abnormal findings.

COLLABORATIVE MANAGEMENT

Diverticulosis

The goal of medical therapy for uncomplicated disease is to relieve symptoms and prevent or postpone complications.

High-residue diet: Including fruits and vegetables and the use of wheat bran in the form of 100% bran cereal or 2 tbsp/day (10-25 g/day) of unprocessed bran to increase moisture content of the stool, thus softening it to promote elimination and reduce intracolonic pressure (see Table 6-2). Fluid intake should also be encouraged (2500-3000 ml/day).

Pharmacotherapy: Commercial *bulk laxative,* such as psyllium (Metamucil), 1-2 tsp PO bid, which can replace bran in the diet.

Diverticulitis

The goal of medical therapy is to rest the bowel, resolve infection and inflammation, and prevent or decrease the severity of complications.

Bed rest and NPO status: To promote physical, emotional, and bowel rest.

Gastric suction: To relieve nausea, vomiting, or abdominal distention if present.

Parenteral replacement of fluids, electrolytes, and blood products: As indicated by laboratory test results to maintain intravascular volumes, electrolyte and acid-base balance, urinary output, and caloric intake.

Pharmacotherapy

Parenteral antibiotics: To limit secondary infection.

Analgesics: To relieve pain. Meperidine (Demerol) is the agent of choice. In addition to producing analgesia, it decreases GI motility and spasm. In analgesic doses, pentazocine (Talwin) also reduces sigmoid activity. It should be used with caution in older persons since it may cause confusion, disorientation, and hallucinations. The use of morphine and other opiates is contraindicated since they increase intraluminal pressure in the sigmoid colon, thus potentially increasing the risk of perforation.

Emergency diverting colostomy: In severely unstable patients (i.e., advanced peritonitis) a transverse colostomy for stool diversion can be created using local anesthesic. This creates a double-barreled colostomy; the proximal barrel empties stool from the GI tract whereas the distal barrel (or mucous fistula) allows rest of the distal diseased colon. After the patient stabilizes, more definitive surgery may be performed. Hartmann's procedure involves removal of the inflamed bowel, creation of a temporary colostomy, and temporary closure of the distal colon. After 3-6 mo, the patient returns for take-down of the temporary colostomy and reanastomosis to the distal colon.

NURSING DIAGNOSES AND INTERVENTIONS

For *diverticulitis* treated by emergency surgical intervention with diverting temporary colostomy, see "Fecal Diversions" for **Bowel incontinence,** p. 460; **Body image disturbance,** p. 461; **Impaired peristomal skin integrity** (or risk for same), p. 459; Appendix One, "Caring for Preoperative and Postoperative Patients," p. 717; "Caring for Patients With Cancer and Other Life-disrupting Illnesses," p. 791, for nursing diagnoses and interventions.

PATIENT-FAMILY TEACHING AND DISCHARGE PLANNING

When providing patient-family teaching, focus on sensory information; avoid giving excessive information; and initiate a visiting nurse referral for necessary follow-up teaching. Consider including verbal and written information about the following:

- Medications, including drug name, rationale, dosage, schedule, precautions, drug/drug and food/drug interactions, and potential side effects.
- Signs and symptoms that necessitate medical attention, including fever; nausea or vomiting; cloudy or malodorous urine; diarrhea or constipation; change in stoma color from the normal bright and shiny red; peristomal skin irritation; and incisional pain, increased local skin temperature, drainage, swelling, or redness.
- Importance of a normal diet that includes all four food groups (meat, eggs, and fish; fruits and vegetables; milk and cheese; cereal and breads) and drinking adequate fluids (at least 2500-3000 ml/day). Also teach the patient to add fiber to the diet in the form of uncooked fruits and vegetables, and whole-grain cereals with the addition of bran in the form of 100% bran cereal

or 2 tbsp/day of coarse, unprocessed bran that can be taken with milk or juice or sprinkled over cereal. Because bran initially may cause abdominal distention and excessive flatus, instruct the patient to begin with 1 tbsp/day and increase gradually. Caution patient to avoid nuts and berries and foods with seeds.

- Gradual resumption of ADL, excluding heavy lifting (>10 lb), pushing, or pulling for 6 wk to prevent development of incisional herniation.
- Care of incision, dressing changes, and permission to take baths or showers once sutures and drains are removed.
- Care of stoma and peristomal skin; use of ostomy skin barriers, pouches, and accessory equipment; and method for obtaining supplies.
- Referral to community resources, including enterostomal therapy (ET) nurse, home health care agency, and the United Ostomy Association:

  United Ostomy Association
  19722 MacArthur Blvd.
  Irvine, CA 92612-2405   (800) 826-0826
  WWW address: *http://www.uoa.org/*

- Importance of follow-up care with health care provider or ET nurse; confirm date and time of next appointment.

Colorectal cancer

Colorectal cancer is second only to lung cancer and nonmelanoma skin cancer in the annual number of newly diagnosed cancer cases. It is estimated that 150,000-160,000 new cases of colorectal cancer are reported each year in the United States. More than 90% of colorectal cancers are adenocarcinomas, of which 50% are located in the rectum, 20% in the sigmoid colon, 6% in the descending colon, 8% in the transverse colon, and 16% in the cecum and ascending colon. Many arise from malignant degeneration of benign adenomatous polyps. Metastatic disease occurs through lymph nodes, direct extension to adjacent tissues, and the bloodstream (via the portal venous system to the liver or the lumbar or vertebral veins to the lungs). Right colon (ascending colon) cancer occurs more frequently in women, whereas carcinoma of the rectum is more common in men.

The cause of colorectal cancer is unknown, but risk factors include a high-fat, low-fiber diet, age >40 years, a personal history of colorectal polyps or colorectal carcinoma, a family history of polyposis syndromes (i.e., familial polyposis coli, Gardner's syndrome, Turcot's syndrome, Muir's syndrome, Peutz-Jeghers syndrome, familial juvenile polyposis from adenomas), first-degree relatives with colorectal cancer, and a personal history of inflammatory bowel disease (i.e., chronic ulcerative colitis, Crohn's colitis).

ASSESSMENT

Right colon cancer: Vague, dull abdominal pain; often postprandial and attributed to gallbladder or ulcer disease. Because stool in the ascending colon is still comparatively liquid, enlarging tumors do not create demonstrable changes in stool or noticeable symptoms (i.e., the patient is commonly asymptomatic). Gradual blood loss (occult melena) may create symptoms of anemia (e.g., weakness, fatigue).

Physical assessment: Possible presence of a palpable mass in the RLQ (in 10%) and presence of abdominal distention. Stools may appear black or dark red, or they may appear normal but be positive for occult blood. The patient also may appear anemic with a microcytic, hypochromic anemia.

Left colon cancer: Increasing abdominal cramping ("gas pains"), change in bowel elimination patterns (constipation and increased frequency of stools, but not typical watery stools), decrease in caliber of stools (pencil- or ribbon-shaped), vomiting, obstipation, and acute large bowel obstruction causing progressive increase in abdominal pain. Patient may be asymptomatic.

Physical assessment: Possible absence of stool felt on rectal examination, presence of bright red blood intermixed with or coating the surface of the stool, and abdominal distention.

Rectal cancer: Sensation of incomplete evacuation, tenesmus, perineal or sacral pain caused by local invasion of surrounding nerves, bladder, or vaginal wall. Pain is a late manifestation. The patient may be asymptomatic.

Physical assessment: Potential presence of palpable mass on digital rectal examination; bright red blood coating surface of the stool.

History of (for all types of colorectal cancer): Blood on or in stools, change in stool elimination pattern, vague abdominal discomfort or pain.

DIAGNOSTIC TESTS

Occult blood test of three serial stool specimens: To detect presence of blood associated with tumor mass bleeding.

Proctosigmoidoscopy or colonoscopy: To examine intraluminal areas of intestine visually. Because rectal and sigmoid lesions sometimes are difficult to diagnose radiologically, proctosigmoidoscopy should be used to complement air contrast barium enemas (ACBaE). If a neoplasm is detected radiographically or on sigmoidoscopy or if the patient is at high risk because of personal or family history, a full colonoscopic examination should be performed.

Biopsy: To confirm diagnosis.

CBC: To detect presence of anemia.

ACBaE: To detect colon irregularities suspicious of tumor. ACBaE examinations are more accurate than single contrast barium enemas in diagnosing cancers and detecting small neoplastic lesions. Typically, right-sided tumors appear as an intraluminal mass or constriction; left-sided tumors have a typical "apple-core" appearance of an annular growth 2-6 cm in length.

CT scan and MRI: To identify metastatic colon cancer by imaging tissue outside the rectal wall and distant metastases. However, because these techniques cannot discriminate the individual layers of the rectal wall, they are not conclusive for early-stage disease.

Endorectal ultrasound: To identify lesions confined to the layers of the bowel wall and to distinguish involved lymph nodes. This technique is useful in early-stage disease.

Carcinoembryonic antigen (CEA): Serum elevation can be indicative of intestinal tumor. CEA is not useful as a screening test because of its lack of sensitivity in detecting early colorectal cancer. However, CEA may be useful in preoperative staging and postoperative follow-up to identify early recurrence. Other serologic tumor markers are being examined for sensitivity for early detection and diagnosis of colorectal cancer; their effectiveness for screening is still undetermined.

COLLABORATIVE MANAGEMENT

Surgery: Resection of tumor mass and lymph nodes that drain the area, with reanastomosis of colon. If bowel ends cannot be reanastomosed, a colostomy is created. The exact extent of the colonic resection is determined by the distribution of regional lymph nodes and by the blood supply. The margins of the resection should be at least 2-5 cm from either side of the tumor. Surgical treatment includes right hemicolectomy for lesions located in the right colon; left hemicolectomy for lesions located in the left colon; a subtotal or total colectomy for synchronous right- and left-sided lesions; low anterior resection for lesions in the rectosigmoid and upper rectum; and abdominoperineal resection (APR) with colostomy for lesions in the mid-rectum and low rectum. With the development of end-to-end stapling devices, APR is being replaced by low anterior resection with reanastomosis for lesions of the mid-rectum and even for low rectal lesions if a distal margin of at least 2 cm of normal bowel can be resected below the lesion. At present, there appears to be no significant difference in survival and recurrence rates with low anterior resection compared with APR as long as a 2- to 5-cm distal margin is preserved. Alternatives to radical operations are being investigated for lesions confined to a local site. These methods used to ablate tumors locally include local excision, electrofulguration with tumor destruction by burning via electrocautery, cryotherapy with liquid nitrogen probes, thermal destruction by laser, and endocavitary irradiation (delivering a large dose of radiation [i.e., 9,000-15,000 cGy] to a limited field).

Radiation therapy: To eliminate cancer cells, reduce tumor mass, or decrease pain from advanced disease. As a method of treatment of colorectal cancer, radiation therapy generally is ineffective. It may provide palliation of pelvic pain or rectal or vaginal bleeding secondary to tumor invasion in advanced rectal disease. It is used mainly as adjuvant therapy to surgery. Preoperatively it is used to reduce tumor mass, converting unresectable large tumors and tumors fixed to pelvic organs to resectable lesions. It also is used preoperatively or postoperatively to decrease local recurrence in patients at high risk (penetration of bowel wall and positive lymph nodes) or in a combined preoperative-postoperative "sandwich" technique.

Chemotherapy: For advanced disease, usually fluorouracil (5-FU) alone or in combination with other agents, such as levamisole, to eliminate cancer cells and provide relief from pain with advanced disease. Generally it is used as adjuvant therapy, combined with surgery or with both surgery and radiation therapy. For more information, see Appendix One, "Caring for Patients With Cancer and Other Life-disrupting Illnesses," p. 747.

Nutritional management: May include elemental fluid supplements and/or parenteral nutrition if oral intake is inadequate. For further details, see "Providing Nutritional Support," p. 687.

NURSING DIAGNOSES AND INTERVENTIONS

Altered health maintenance related to recommendations for increased dietary fiber and increased fluid intake

Desired outcome: Before hospital discharge, patient verbalizes understanding of recommendations and rationale for increased dietary fiber and fluid intake and sources of dietary insoluble fiber.

- Instruct patients that the National Research Council advises increasing fiber intake by consuming five or more servings of fresh fruits and vegetables and six or more servings of legumes, whole-grain breads, and cereals per day. The National Cancer Institute recommends 25-30 g of fiber daily.
- Explain to patients that increased insoluble fiber is speculated to reduce exposure of the bowel mucosa to potential carcinogens by reducing intestinal transit time and diluting carcinogens in bulky stools.
- Instruct patients on the sources of insoluble dietary fiber (e.g., wheat bran; navy, kidney, pinto, and lima beans; skins of fruits and vegetables; raspberries and strawberries; sesame and poppy seeds).
- Instruct patients that inadequate fluid intake in the presence of a high bulk diet may lead to constipation. Emphasize the importance of maintaining a fluid intake of 2500-3000 ml/day to provide adequate fluids.

NIC: Fluid Monitoring; Nutritional Counseling; Risk Identification; Teaching: Disease Process; Teaching: Prescribed Diet

Health-seeking behaviors: Recommendations for follow-up diagnostic care after colon resection or polypectomy for malignant polyps

Desired outcome: Before hospital discharge, patient and/or significant other verbalizes accurate information about recommendations for follow-up diagnostic care.

For patients who have had colorectal cancer resections
- Teach patient that colonoscopy is recommended 6-12 mo after surgery, followed by yearly colonoscopy for 2 consecutive yr; if the aforementioned are negative, colonoscopy or ACBaE plus proctosigmoidoscopy is performed every 3 years.
- Explain that fecal occult blood testing is performed every year.
- Remind patient that serum CEA levels are measured at regular intervals (three times at 6-mo intervals, then annually for 5 yr).

For postpolypectomy patients with malignant polyps
- Teach patient that a colonoscopy is performed within 6 mo of polypectomy; if this second examination is negative, colonoscopy is performed every 2 years. However, if the second examination is positive, colonoscopy is performed at yearly intervals until negative, and then colonoscopy is done at 2-yr intervals.
- Explain that fecal occult blood testing is performed between colonoscopies.

NIC: Health Education; Health Screening; Risk Identification; Teaching: Disease Process; Teaching: Procedure/Treatment

---

See Also: "Fecal Diversions" for **Bowel incontinence,** p. 460; **Body image disturbance,** p. 461; **Risk for impaired peristomal skin integrity** and **Impaired stomal tissue integrity,** p. 459; **Knowledge deficit:** Colostomy irrigation procedure, p. 462; Appendix One, "Caring for Preoperative and Postoperative Patients," p. 717; "Caring for Patients With Cancer and Other Life-disrupting Illnesses," p. 747, for nursing diagnoses and interventions.

PATIENT-FAMILY TEACHING AND DISCHARGE PLANNING

When providing patient-family teaching, focus on sensory information; avoid giving excessive information; and initiate a visiting nurse referral for necessary follow-up teaching. Consider including verbal and written information about the following:
- Medications, including drug name, rationale, dosage, schedule, precautions, drug/drug and food/drug interactions, and potential side effects.
- Signs and symptoms that necessitate medical attention, including fever, nausea and vomiting, diarrhea, or constipation.
- If an intestinal stoma is present, the importance of reporting change in stoma color from the normal bright and shiny red; presence of peristomal skin irritation; and incisional pain, local increased temperature, drainage, swelling, or redness.
- Importance of a diet based on the Food Guide Pyramid for daily food choices:
  —Bread, cereal, rice, and pasta group: 6-11 servings
  —Vegetable group: 3-5 servings
  —Fruit group: 2-4 servings
  —Milk, yogurt, and cheese group: 2-3 servings
  —Meat, poultry, fish, dry beans, eggs, and nuts group: 2-3 servings
  —Fats, oils, and sweets: use sparingly
- Recommendations for increasing dietary fiber intake: see **Altered health maintenace,** p. 437.
- Importance of drinking adequate fluids (at least 2500-3000 ml/day).
- Enteral or parenteral feeding instructions if patient is to supplement diet or is NPO.
- Gradual resumption of ADL, excluding heavy lifting (>10 lb), pushing, or pulling for 6 wk to prevent incisional herniation.

- Care of incision and perianal wounds, including dressing changes, and bathing once sutures and drains are removed. Sitz baths may be recommended for perianal wound.
- If stoma is present, care of stoma and peristomal skin; use of ostomy skin barriers, pouches, and accessory equipment; and method for obtaining supplies.
- Referral to community resources, including home health care agency, American Cancer Society, and, if appropriate, ET nurse and United Ostomy Association:

    United Ostomy Association
    19722 MacArthur Blvd.
    Irvine, CA 92612-2405   (800) 826-0826
    WWW address: *http://www.uoa.org/*

- Importance of follow-up care with health care provider (or ET nurse if appropriate); confirm date and time of next appointment.
- Recommendations for follow-up diagnostic care after colon resection or polypectomy: see **Health-seeking behaviors,** p. 435.

Polyps/Familial adenomatous polyposis

Of the single, multiple, sessile, and pedunculated polypoid colon tumors, the adenomatous polyp is the most common. The practical significance of these polyps is their tendency to become malignant (see "Colorectal Cancer"). *Familial adenomatous polyposis (FAP)* is characterized by, but distinct from, frequent colon polyp formation. FAP is also known as *multiple familial adenomatosis, adenomatosis coli,* and *hereditary multiple polyposis.* In this disorder the glandular epithelia of the colon and rectum undergo excessive proliferation throughout the mucous membranes, which leads to the formation of sessile or pedunculated polyps. These are soft and red or purplish red in color, vary in size from a few millimeters to several centimeters, and range in number from a few to several thousand. They can be found anywhere along the entire length of the colon, but the rectum is almost always involved. Every individual with untreated familial polyposis will develop cancer because at some point in time one or more of these polyps will undergo malignant degeneration. This is a hereditary disease passed from generation to generation as an autosomal dominant trait, and it appears most often during late childhood through the early 30s. The incidence of FAP is estimated at approximately 1 in 8300 births.

ASSESSMENT

FAP: Mild, early symptoms, such as diarrhea or melena, although many patients remain asymptomatic for years. Once malignant degeneration has begun, these symptoms become more pronounced and there can be intermittent or constant colicky pain. Tenesmus and a frequent urge to defecate also can be present. If blood loss is significant, anemia, weight loss, loss of appetite, and fatigue can occur.

Physical assessment: In the presence of a well-developed malignant growth, a mass can be palpated on abdominal examination. Digital rectal examination may detect presence of polyps.

History of: FAP, mild colicky abdominal discomfort with or without diarrhea, presence of blood in stools.

DIAGNOSTIC TESTS

Proctosigmoidoscopy or colonoscopy: To visualize polyposis.

Biopsy: To confirm diagnosis. Histopathologic criteria for malignant potential are polyp size, histologic type, and degree of dysplasia.

X-ray examination with barium enema and air contrast: To determine extent of the disease.

CBC: To detect presence of anemia.

COLLABORATIVE MANAGEMENT

Because colorectal cancer is inevitable, appearing approximately 10-15 years after the onset of the polyposis if the colon is not removed, surgical resection is the treatment of choice for FAP. Once the diagnosis has been made, it is not advisable to delay surgery.

Proctocolectomy: Surgical cure via removal of colon and rectum with continent (Kock) ileostomy, conventional (Brooke) ileostomy, or ileoanal reservoir for fecal diversion (see "Fecal Diversions," p. 457).

Colectomy with preservation of rectum and ileorectal anastomosis: After this procedure, follow-up proctoscopies are necessary at frequent intervals to assess the rectum for further evidence of the disease or malignant changes.

Radiation or chemotherapy: May be indicated as adjuvant therapy or for advanced malignant disease.

NURSING DIAGNOSES AND INTERVENTIONS

See "Colorectal Cancer" for **Health-seeking behaviors:** Recommendations for follow-up diagnostic care following colon resection or polypectomy for malignant polyps, p. 435; "Fecal Diversions" for **Bowel incontinence,** p. 460; **Body image disturbance,** p. 461; **Risk for impaired peristomal skin integrity** and **impaired stomal tissue integrity,** p. 459; Appendix One, "Caring for Preoperative and Postoperative Patients," p. 717; "Caring for Patients With Cancer and Other Life-disrupting Illnesses," p. 747, for nursing diagnoses and interventions.

PATIENT-FAMILY TEACHING AND DISCHARGE PLANNING

When providing patient-family teaching, focus on sensory information; avoid giving excessive information; and initiate a visiting nurse referral for necessary follow-up teaching. Consider including verbal and written information about the following:

- Importance of informing all close family members that because familial polyposis is inherited, periodic examinations of the rectum and colon are essential.
- For other guidelines, see teaching and discharge planning in "Colorectal Cancer," p. 438.

Ulcerative colitis

Ulcerative colitis is a nonspecific, chronic inflammatory disease of the mucosa and submucosa of the colon. Generally the disease begins in the rectum and sigmoid colon, but it can extend proximally and uninterrupted as far as the cecum. In some instances, a few centimeters of distal ileum are affected. This is sometimes referred to as *backwash ileitis*, and it occurs in only about 10% of patients with ulcerative colitis involving the entire colon. Ulcerative colitis initially affects the mucosal layer. Eventually small mucosal layer abscesses form that ultimately penetrate the submucosa, spread horizontally, and allow sloughing of the mucosa, creating ulcerative lesions. The muscular layer (muscularis) generally is not affected, but the serosal layer may have congested and dilated blood vessels.

The cause of ulcerative colitis is unknown, but theories posit an interaction of external agents, host responses, and genetic immunologic factors creating the pathogenic responses. Factors that have been associated with ulcerative colitis include infection, allergy, immunologic abnormalities, psychosomatic factors, and heredity. Individuals with ulcerative colitis develop colonic adenocarcinomas at 10 times the rate of the general population. This process is found more commonly in Western countries, and females are affected slightly more often than males.

ASSESSMENT

Signs and symptoms: Bloody diarrhea (the cardinal symptom). The clinical picture can vary from acute episodes with frequent discharge of watery stools mixed with blood, pus, and mucus, accompanied by fever, abdominal pain, rectal urgency, and tenesmus, to loose or frequent stools, to formed stools coated with a little blood. However, nearly two thirds of patients have cramping abdominal pain and varying degrees of fever, vomiting, anorexia, weight loss, and dehydration. Remissions and exacerbations are common. Extracolonic manifestations also can occur, including polyarthritis, skin lesions (erythema nodosum, pyoderma gangrenosum), liver impairment, and ophthalmic complications (iritis, uveitis) (Tables 6-5 and 6-6).

Physical assessment: With severe disease, the abdomen will be tender, especially in the LLQ; distention and a tender, spastic anus also may be present. With rectal examination, the mucosa may feel gritty and the examining gloved finger may be covered with blood, mucus, or pus.

Risk factors: Duration of active disease >10 yr, pancolitis, and family history of colonic cancer.

DIAGNOSTIC TESTS

Stool examination: Reveals the presence of frank or occult blood. Stool cultures and smears rule out bacterial and parasitic disorders. **Note:** Collect specimens *before* barium enema is performed.

Sigmoidoscopy: Reveals red, granular, hyperemic, and extremely friable mucosa; strips of inflamed mucosa undermined by surrounding ulcerations, which form pseudopolyps; and thick exudate composed of blood, pus, and mucus. **Note:** Enemas should not be given before the examination because they can produce hyperemia and edema and may cause exacerbation of the disease.

Colonoscopy: Will help determine the extent of the disease and differentiate ulcerative colitis from Crohn's disease through both endoscopic appearance and histologic examination of biopsy tissues. Serial colonoscopy is also done to

T A B L E   6 - 5   Comparison of Gross Pathologic Features of Ulcerative Colitis and Crohn's Disease

Pathologic feature	Ulcerative colitis	Crohn's disease
Thickened mesentery	Rare	Common
Enlarged mesenteric lymph nodes	Rare	Common
Shortening of colon	Frequent	Rare
Small bowel involvement	Never	May occur
Serositis	Not present	Common
Thickening of intestinal wall	Rare	Common
Segmental disease	Never	Frequent
Strictures	Never	Frequent
Abdominal wall and internal fistulas	None	Frequent
Cobblestoning of mucosa	Rare	Common
Mucosal ulcerations	Diffuse	Normal mucosa between ulcers
Pseudopolyps	Frequent	Rare

From Broadwell DC, Jackson BS: *Principles of ostomy care,* St Louis, 1982, Mosby.

TABLE 6-6 Comparison of Clinical Features of Inflammatory Bowel Disease

Clinical feature	Ulcerative colitis (mucosal)	Crohn's disease (transmural)
Age	Young to middle age	Young
Gender distribution	Equal	Equal
Diarrhea	Remission	More constant
Tenesmus	Constant	Occurs
Fever (intermittent)	Occurs	Common
Weight loss	Common	Severe
Abdominal cramping pains	Occurs	Severe
Gross bleeding	Common	Infrequent
Fistulas	Rare	Common
Perforation	Common	Rare
Abdominal mass	Rare	Occurs
Anal lesions	Occurs	Common
Toxic megacolon	Common	Occurs
Carcinoma	Common	Occurs
Proctoscopic findings	Rectum involved in most cases	Rectum may be spared
Extracolonic complications: arthralgia, ocular (uveitis), skin disorders (erythema nodosum, pyoderma gangrenosum)	Frequent	Common

From Broadwell DC, Jackson BS: *Principles of ostomy care,* St Louis, 1982, Mosby.

monitor patients with chronic ulcerative colitis at risk for colon carcinoma. **Note:** This test may be contraindicated in patients with acute disease because of the risk of perforation or hemorrhage.

Rectal biopsy: Aids in differentiating ulcerative colitis from carcinoma and other inflammatory processes.

Barium enema: Reveals mucosal irregularity from fine serrations to ragged ulcerations, narrowing and shortening of the colon, presence of pseudopolyps, loss of haustral markings, and the presence of spasms and irritability. Double-contrast technique may facilitate detection of superficial mucosal lesions. With a double-contrast technique, barium is instilled into the colon as with a conventional barium enema, but most of the barium is then withdrawn and the colon is inflated with air, which causes a thin coating of barium to line the intestinal wall. The double-contrast technique has become the "gold standard" for evaluating patients for colitis. **Note:** Irritant cathartics and enemas should not be given before the examination, since they produce hyperemia and edema and may cause exacerbation of the disease.

Abdominal plain films (flat plate): An important tool for screening severely ill patients when colonoscopy and barium enema are contraindicated. An abdominal flat plate may reveal fecal residue, the appearance of mucosal margins, widening or thickening of visible haustra, and the diameter of the colonic wall. In patients with suspected ileus, obstruction, or perforation, the flat plate film reveals abnormal gas and fluid levels or the presence of free air in the peritoneal cavity.

CT: Used to identify suspected complications of ulcerative colitis (i.e., toxic megacolon, pneumatosis coli).

Radionuclide imaging:　To identify the extent of disease activity, especially when colonoscopy and barium enema are contraindicated. Injections of indium-111–labeled autologous leukocytes are used to identify areas of active inflammation.

Blood tests:　Anemia, with hypochromic microcytic red blood indices in severe disease, usually is present because of blood loss, iron deficiency, and bone marrow depression. WBC count may be normal to markedly elevated in severe disease. Sedimentation rate is usually increased according to the severity of illness. Hypoalbuminemia and negative nitrogen (N) state occur in moderately severe to severe disease and result from decreased protein intake, decreased albumin synthesis in the debilitated condition, and increased metabolic needs. Electrolyte imbalance is common; hypokalemia is often present because of colonic losses (diarrhea) and renal losses in patients taking high doses of corticosteroids. Bicarbonate may be decreased because of colonic losses and may signal metabolic acidosis.

COLLABORATIVE MANAGEMENT

Medical therapy is symptomatic. The goals are to terminate the acute attack, reduce symptoms, and prevent recurrences.

Parenteral replacement of fluids, electrolytes, and blood products:　To maintain acutely ill patient, as indicated by laboratory test results.

Physical and emotional rest:　Including bedrest and limitation of visitors.

Pharmacotherapy

Sedatives and tranquilizers:　To promote rest and reduce anxiety.

Hydrophilic colloids (e.g., kaolin and pectin mixture) and anticholinergic and antidiarrheal preparations (e.g., tinctures of belladonna and opium, diphenoxylate hydrochloride, loperamide, codeine phosphate):　To relieve cramping and diarrhea. **Note:** Opiates and anticholinergics should be administered with extreme caution since they contribute to the development of toxic megacolon.

Antiinflammatory agents:　Corticosteroids to reduce mucosal inflammation. Dosage and routes of administration vary with the severity and extent of the disease. In patients with mild disease limited to the rectum and sigmoid colon, rectal instillation of steroids (enema or suppository) may induce or maintain remission. In patients with more extensive (pancolonic) more active disease, oral corticosteroid therapy with prednisone or prednisolone usually is initiated. In severely ill patients, IV corticosteroids are given. Once clinical remission is achieved, IV and oral corticosteroids are tapered until discontinuation since these medications have not been shown to prolong remission or prevent future exacerbations. Budesonide, a new steroidal agent, shows promise for providing the benefits of traditional therapy without the side effects; budesonide is undergoing clinical trials in North America and Europe.

Sulfasalazine:　To help maintain remissions. This drug generally is effective in the treatment of mild to moderate attacks of ulcerative colitis and appears to decrease the frequency of subsequent relapse. Sulfasalazine is considered inferior to corticosteroids in the treatment of severe attacks of disease; once remission has been attained by use of corticosteroid therapy, sulfasalazine appears to be superior to systemic corticosteroids in the maintenance of remission.

　　When administered orally, sulfasalazine is broken down by colonic bacteria into its two constituents: 5-aminosalicylic acid (5-ASA), which is considered the active therapeutic component, and sulfapyridine, which is the carrier and responsible for the side effects experienced by more than one third of the individuals treated with this therapy. To avoid side effects of sulfapyridine, several agents have been developed using a variety of delivery mechanisms that allow release of the active agent in the colon or ileum. These agents include the 5-ASA derivatives: mesalamine (in enteric-coated and time-release forms), olsalazine, and balsalazide. These three agents are useful alternatives to patients unable to tolerate sulfapyridine; however, these agents have their own side effects.

Topical therapy with 5-ASA via retention enemas for patients with proctosigmoiditis (involvement to 40 cm) and suppositories for patients with proctitis have provided encouraging results. If relapses occur after cessation of interim topical therapy, maintenance therapy may be accomplished with 5-ASA enemas or suppositories every 2-3 nights. Although the therapeutic benefit of 5-ASA enemas is the same as that achieved with hydrocortisone enemas, the 5-ASA therapy is preferred because of the systemic side effects found with corticosteroids.

Immunosuppressive therapy: To reduce inflammation in patients not responding to steroids and sulfasalazine; in patients unwilling or unable to undergo colectomy; or as an alternative to steroid dependency. Azathioprine and 6-mercaptopurine have been used alone and in combination with steroids. These agents may have steroid-sparing and steroid-enhancing effects and are used with the goal of gradually withdrawing, or substantially reducing the dosage of, corticosteroids. Immunosuppressive therapy has been used to maintain remission in patients with frequent relapses. From 3-6 mo may be required to achieve therapeutic response, and patients need to be closely monitored for hematologic toxicity.

IV cyclosporine has been used in severe, intractable ulcerative colitis. If there is no response within 4-7 days, cyclosporine is unlikely to be effective. Cyclosporine is toxic and associated with many side effects and thus is used with caution.

Antibiotics: To limit secondary infection. Antibiotics are not indicated in the management of mild to moderate disease since infectious agents generally are not thought to be responsible for ulcerative colitis. In the patient with acute pancolitis or toxic megacolon, broad-spectrum IV antibiotic therapy is recommended since secondary bacterial infection of deeply inflamed colonic mucosa is likely (Table 6-7).

Nutritional management: Varies with patient's condition. In severely ill patients, total parenteral nutrition (TPN) along with NPO status is prescribed to replace nutritional deficits while allowing complete bowel rest and improving patient's nutritional status before surgery. For less severely ill patients, a low-residue elemental diet provides good nutrition with low fecal volume to allow bowel rest. A bland, high-protein, high-calorie, low-residue diet with vitamin and mineral supplements and excluding raw fruits and vegetables provides good nutrition and decreases diarrhea. Milk and wheat products are restricted to reduce cramping and diarrhea in patients with lactose and gluten intolerance (see Table 6-2).

Referral to mental health practitioner: As indicated for supportive psychotherapy for patient who has difficulty dealing with any type of chronic or disabling illness.

Surgical interventions: Indicated only when the disease is intractable to medical management or when the patient develops a disabling complication. *Total proctocolectomy* cures ulcerative colitis and results in construction of a permanent fecal diversion, such as Brooke ileostomy, continent (Kock pouch) ileostomy, or ileoanal reservoir. See "Fecal Diversions," p. 458, for additional details.

Postoperative management: Includes routine chest physiotherapy to prevent respiratory complications; IV fluid and electrolyte replacement or TPN as the patient's condition warrants; NG tube for decompression until bowel sounds are present and the patient is eliminating flatus or stool; gradual resumption of diet as tolerated following NG tube removal and return of bowel function; aseptic incisional care to prevent infection; and fecal diversion care and teaching.

NURSING DIAGNOSES AND INTERVENTIONS

Fluid volume deficit related to active loss secondary to diarrhea and gastrointestinal bleeding/hemorrhage

Desired outcome: Patient is normovolemic within 24 hr of admission as evidenced by balanced I&O, urine output ≥30 ml/hr, urine specific gravity <1.030, good skin turgor, moist mucous membranes, stable weight, BP ≥90/60 mm Hg (or within patient's normal range), and RR 12-20 breaths/min.

- Monitor I&O and urine specific gravity; weigh patient daily; and monitor laboratory values to evaluate fluid, electrolyte, and hematologic status. Optimal values are serum K^+ ≥3.5 mEq/L, Hct 40%-54% (male) and 37%-47% (female), Hgb 14-18 g/dl (male) and 12-16 g/dl (female), and RBCs 4.5-6.0 million/mm^3 (male) and 4.0-5.5 million/mm^3 (female).
- Monitor frequency and consistency of stool. For frequent bowel movements keep a stool count; measure liquid stools. Assess and record presence of blood, mucus, fat, and undigested food.
- Monitor patient for indicators of dehydration: thirst, poor skin turgor (may not be a reliable indicator of hydration in the older adult), dryness of mucous membranes, fever, and concentrated (specific gravity >1.030) and decreased urinary output.
- Monitor patient for signs of hemorrhage: hypotension, increased HR and RR, pallor, diaphoresis, and restlessness. Assess stool for quality (e.g., is it grossly bloody and liquid?) and quantity (e.g., is it mostly blood or mostly stool?). Report significant findings to health care provider.
- Maintain parenteral replacement of fluids, electrolytes, and vitamins as prescribed.
- Administer blood products and iron as prescribed to correct existing anemia and losses caused by hemorrhage.
- Provide bland, high-protein, high-calorie, low-residue diet, as prescribed when patient is taking food by mouth. Assess tolerance to diet by determining incidence of cramping, diarrhea, and flatulence.

NIC: Bleeding Precautions: Gastrointestinal; Blood Products Administration; Fluid/Electrolyte Management; Hypovolemia Management; Intravenous (IV) Therapy; Nutrition Management

Altered protection related to risk of perforation secondary to deeply inflamed colonic mucosa

Desired outcome: Patient is free of signs of perforation as evidenced by normothermia; HR 60-100 bpm; RR 12-20 breaths/min with normal depth and pattern (eupnea); normal bowel sounds; absence of abdominal distention, tympany, or rebound tenderness; negative culture results; no mental status changes and orientation to person, place, and time.

Note: Patients with severe ulcerative colitis can have markedly elevated WBC counts: >20,000/mm^3 and occasionally as high as 50,000/mm^3.

- Monitor patient for fever, chills, increased respiratory and heart rates, diaphoresis, and increased abdominal discomfort, which can occur with perforation of the colon and potentially result in localized abscess or generalized fecal peritonitis and septicemia. **Note:** Systemic therapy with corticosteroids and antibiotics can mask the development of this complication.
- Report any evidence of sudden abdominal distention associated with the preceding symptoms because they can signal toxic megacolon. Factors contributing to the development of this complication include hypokalemia, barium enema examinations, and use of opiates and anticholinergics.

TABLE 6-7   Drug Therapy for Ulcerative Colitis and Crohn's Disease

Drug	Ulcerative colitis	Crohn's disease
Sulfasalazine	Used in treating mild to moderate disease and in maintaining remission	Used in treating acute disease; most effective in disease limited to colon; does not prevent recurrence
5-Aminosalicylic acid (5-ASA) derivatives		
Oral		
Mesalamine (Asacol, Pentasa) Olsalazine (Dipentum)	Used in patients unable to tolerate sulfasalazine; Asacol and Dipentum used for colonic disease	Used in patients unable to tolerate sulfasalazine; slow-release Pentasa and delayed-release Asacol used for ileocolonic and ileal disease and are being studied for maintenance therapy
Topical		
Mesalamine (Rowasa)	Suppository or foam used for proctitis and retention enema used for proctosigmoiditis; used for maintenance therapy	Same as for ulcerative colitis
Corticosteroids		
Oral	Used in treating acute, active pancolonic disease; not beneficial in maintaining remission	Used in treating acute, active disease and in controlling exacerbations in chronic disease; most effective for disease limited to small intestine
Topical	Suppository, foam, or enema used in inducing or maintaining remission for mild to moderate active disease limited to rectum or rectosigmoid colon	Same as for ulcerative colitis
Parenteral	Used in treating severe, fulminant disease	Used in treating disease with severe, inflammatory activity

Antibiotics	Used in preventing secondary bacterial infection for acute pancolitis or toxic megacolon	Used in treating mild to moderate ileocolonic or colonic disease and perianal fistulas; used as adjunct in treating suppurative complications and bacterial overgrowth
Immunosuppressive agents		
Axathioprine; 6-mercaptopurine	Used in maintaining remission in patients with frequent relapses and in reducing or eliminating need for corticosteroids in steroid-dependent patients	Same as for ulcerative colitis; also used in treating perianal fistulas
Cyclosporine	Used intravenously in treating severe or intractable disease	Used intravenously in treating refractory disease and resistant fistulas
Methotrexate	Under study for use in chronically active disease and for use in reducing or eliminating steroid dosage	Same as for ulcerative colitis

- If patient has a sudden temperature elevation, culture blood and other sites as prescribed. Monitor culture reports, notifying health care provider promptly of any positive cultures.
- Administer antibiotics as prescribed and in a timely fashion.
- Evaluate patient's mental status, orientation, and LOC q2-4hr.

NIC: Surveillance; Vital Signs Monitoring

Pain, abdominal cramping, and nausea related to intestinal inflammatory process
Desired outcomes: Within 4 hr of intervention, patient's subjective perception of discomfort decreases as documented by a pain scale. Objective indicators, such as grimacing, are absent or diminished.

- Monitor and document characteristics of discomfort, and assess whether it is associated with ingestion of certain foods or medications or with emotional stress. Devise a pain scale with patient, rating discomfort from 0 (no pain) to 10 (worst pain). Eliminate foods that cause cramping and discomfort.
- As prescribed, maintain patient on NPO or TPN to provide bowel rest.
- Provide nasal and oral care at frequent intervals to lessen discomfort from NPO status or presence of NG tube.
- Keep patient's environment quiet. Facilitate coordination of health care providers to provide rest periods between care activities. Allow 90 min for undisturbed rest.
- Administer sedatives and tranquilizers as prescribed to promote rest and reduce anxiety.
- Administer hydrophilic colloids, anticholinergics, and antidiarrheal medications as prescribed to relieve cramping and diarrhea. Instruct the patient to request medication before discomfort becomes severe.
- Document the degree of relief obtained, rating it according to the pain scale.
- Observe for intensification of symptoms, which can indicate the presence of complications. Notify health care provider of significant findings.

NIC: Anxiety Reduction; Environmental Management: Comfort; Gastrointestinal Intubation; Medication Administration; Pain Management; Simple Relaxation Therapy; Tube Care: Gastrointestinal

Diarrhea related to inflammatory process of the intestines
Desired outcome: Patient's stools become normal in consistency, and frequency is lessened within 3 days of admission.

- Monitor and record amount, frequency, and character of patient's stools. When possible, measure liquid stools.
- Provide covered bedpan, commode, or bathroom that is easily accessible and ready to use at all times.
- Empty bedpan and commode to control odor and decrease patient's anxiety and self-consciousness.
- Administer hydrophilic colloids, anticholinergics, and antidiarrheal medications as prescribed to decrease fluidity and number of stools.
- Administer topical corticosteroid preparations and antibiotics via retention enema, as prescribed, to relieve local inflammation. If patient has difficulty retaining the enema for the prescribed amount of time, consult health care provider about the use of corticosteroid foam, which is easier to retain and administer.
- Monitor serum electrolytes, particularly K^+, for abnormalities. Alert health care provider to K^+ <3.5 mEq/L.

NIC: Diarrhea Management; Electrolyte Management: Hypokalemia; Fluid/ Electrolyte Management; Medication Administration; Perineal Care

Risk for impaired perineal/perianal skin integrity related to risk of persistent diarrhea

Desired outcome: Patient's perineal/perianal skin remains intact with no erythema.
- Provide materials or assist patient with cleansing and drying perineal area after each bowel movement. Use a nonirritating cleansing agent.
- Apply protective skin care products (skin preparations, gels, or barrier films) to prevent irritation from frequent liquid stools.
- Administer hydrophilic colloids, anticholinergics, and antidiarrheal medications as prescribed to decrease fluidity and number of stools.

NIC: Bathing; Perineal Care; Skin Care: Topical Treatments; Surveillance

> **See Also:** "Fecal Diversions" for **Bowel incontinence,** p. 460; **Body image disturbance,** p. 461; **Risk for impaired peristomal skin integrity** and **impaired stomal tissue integrity,** p. 459; Appendix One, "Caring for Preoperative and Postoperative Patients" for nursing diagnoses and interventions, p. 717, if surgery is performed; "Caring for Patients With Cancer and Other Life-disrupting Illnesses," p. 747.

PATIENT-FAMILY TEACHING AND DISCHARGE PLANNING

When providing patient-family teaching, focus on sensory information; avoid giving excessive information; and initiate a visiting nurse referral for necessary follow-up teaching. Consider including verbal and written information about the following:
- Medications, including drug name, rationale, dosage, schedule, route of administration, precautions, drug/drug and food/drug interactions, and potential side effects. **Note:** Caution patients receiving high-dose steroid therapy about abrupt discontinuation of steroids to prevent precipitation of adrenal crisis. Withdrawal symptoms include weakness, lethargy, restlessness, anorexia, nausea, and muscle tenderness. Instruct patient to notify health care provider if these symptoms occur.
- Signs and symptoms that necessitate medical attention, including fever, nausea and vomiting, diarrhea or constipation, and any significant change in appearance and frequency of stools, any of which can signal exacerbation of the disease.
- Dietary management to promote nutritional and fluid maintenance and prevent abdominal cramping, discomfort, and diarrhea.
- Importance of perineal care after bowel movements.
- Enteral or parenteral feeding instructions if patient is to supplement diet or is NPO.
- Referral to community resources, including the following organization:

  Crohn's and Colitis Foundation of America
  386 Park Ave. South, 17th Floor
  New York, NY 10016-8804 (800) 932-2423
  WWW address: *http://www.cefa.org/*

- Importance of follow-up medical care, particularly for patients with long-standing disease, since so many of them develop colonic adenocarcinoma.
- Referral to a mental health specialist if recommended by the health care provider.

In addition, if patient has a fecal diversion
- Care of incision, dressing changes, and permission to take baths or showers once sutures and drains are removed.
- Care of stoma, peristomal/perianal skin, or perineal wound; use of ostomy equipment; and method for obtaining supplies. Sitz baths may be indicated for perineal wound.

- Medications that are contraindicated (e.g., laxatives) or that may not be well tolerated or absorbed (e.g., antibiotics, enteric-coated tablets, long-acting tablets).
- Gradual resumption of ADL, excluding heavy lifting (>10 lb), pushing, or pulling for 6-8 wk to prevent incisional herniation.
- Referral to community resources, including home health care agency, enterostomal (ET) nurse, and the local chapter of the United Ostomy Association:

  United Ostomy Association
  19722 MacArthur Blvd.
  Irvine, CA 92612-2405   (800) 826-0826
  WWW address: *http://www.uoa.org/*

- Importance of reporting signs and symptoms that require medical attention, such as change in stoma color from the normal bright and shiny red; peristomal or perianal skin irritation; diarrhea; incisional pain, local increased temperature, drainage, swelling, or redness; signs and symptoms of fluid and electrolyte imbalance; and signs and symptoms of mechanical or functional obstruction.

Crohn's disease

Crohn's disease, also known as *regional enteritis*, *granulomatous colitis*, or *transmural colitis*, is a chronic inflammatory disease that can involve any part of the GI tract from the mouth to the anus. Usually the disease occurs segmentally, demonstrating discontinuous areas of disease with segments of healthy bowel in between. The terminal ileum is the most frequent site of involvement, followed by the colon. The disease affects all layers of the bowel: the mucosa, submucosa, circular and longitudinal muscles, and serosa. A family history of this disease or ulcerative colitis occurs in 15%-20% of affected patients. The cause is unknown, but theories include infection, immunologic factors, environmental factors, and genetic predisposition.

During the past 20 years, the incidence of Crohn's disease has increased dramatically, whereas that of ulcerative colitis has not changed. This rise may reflect increased diagnostic awareness rather than a real change in frequency in Crohn's disease.

ASSESSMENT

Signs and symptoms: Clinical presentation varies as a direct reflection of the location of the inflammatory process, its extent, severity, and relationship to contiguous structures. Sometimes the onset is abrupt, and the patient can appear to have appendicitis, ulcerative colitis, intestinal obstruction, or a fever of obscure origin. Acute symptoms include RLQ pain, tenderness, spasm, flatulence, nausea, fever, and diarrhea. A more typical picture is insidious onset with more persistent but less severe symptoms, such as vague abdominal pain, unexplained anemia, and fever. Diarrhea—liquid, soft, or mushy stools—is the most common symptom. The presence of gross blood is rare. Abdominal pain is a frequent symptom, and it may be colicky or crampy, initiated by meals, centered in the lower abdomen, and relieved by defecation because of the chronic partial obstruction of the small intestine, colon, or both. As the disease progresses, anorexia, malnutrition, weight loss, anemia, lassitude, malaise, and fever can occur in addition to fluid, electrolyte, and metabolic disturbances. See Tables 6-5 and 6-6 for comparisons of ulcerative colitis and Crohn's disease. **Physical assessment:**   In the early stages the examination is often normal but may demonstrate mild tenderness in the abdomen over the affected bowel. In more advanced disease, a palpable mass may be present, especially in the RLQ with terminal ileum involvement. Persistent rectal fissure, large ulcers, perirectal abscess, or rectal fistula is the first indication of disease in 15%-25% of patients with small bowel involvement and in 50%-75% of patients with colonic involvement. Rectovaginal, abdominal, and enterovesical fistulas also can occur. Extraintestinal manifestations characteristic of ulcerative colitis do occur, but less frequently (10%-20%).

DIAGNOSTIC TESTS

Stool examination: Usually reveals occult blood; frank blood may be noted in stools of patients with colonic involvement or with ulcerations and fistulas of the rectum. A few patients present with bloody diarrhea. Stool cultures and smears rule out bacterial and parasitic disorders. Specimens are also examined for fecal fat.

Sigmoidoscopy: Evaluates possible colonic involvement and obtains rectal biopsy. The finding of granulomas on mucosal biopsy argues strongly for the diagnosis of Crohn's disease. However, because granulomas are more numerous in the submucosa, suction biopsy of the rectum provides deeper, larger, and less traumatized specimens for a better diagnostic yield than mucosal biopsy obtained through an endoscope.

Colonoscopy: May help differentiate Crohn's disease from ulcerative colitis. Characteristic patchy inflammation (skip lesions) rules out ulcerative colitis. However, colonoscopy usually does not add useful diagnostic information in the presence of positive findings from sigmoidoscopy or radiologic examination. When the diagnosis is unclear and there is a question of malignancy, colonoscopy provides the means of directly visualizing mucosal changes and obtaining biopsies, brushings, and washings for cytologic examination. Colonoscopy also may assist in planning for surgery by documenting the extent of colonic disease. **Note:** This procedure may be contraindicated in patients with acute phases of Crohn's colitis or when deep ulcerations or fistulas are known to be present because of the risk of perforation.

Endoscopic ultrasonography: Aids in the diagnosis of perirectal fistula and abscesses and in detecting the transmural depth of inflammation in the bowel or esophagus, using an endoscopically placed ultrasound probe.

Small bowel enteroscopy: Permits visualization of the upper GI tract to identify areas of inflammation and bleeding to the level of the midjejunum.

Barium enema and upper GI series with small bowel follow-through: Contribute to the diagnosis of Crohn's disease. Involvement of only the terminal ileum or segmental involvement of the colon or small intestine almost always indicates Crohn's disease. Thickened bowel wall with stricture (string sign) separated by segments of normal bowel, cobblestone appearance, and presence of fistulas and skip lesions are common findings. A double-contrast barium enema technique may increase sensitivity in detecting early or subtle changes. **Note:** Barium enema may be contraindicated in patients with acute phases of Crohn's colitis because of the risk of perforation. Upper GI barium series is contraindicated in patients in whom intestinal obstruction is suspected.

CT scan: Complements information gathered via endoscopy and conventional radiography. In advanced disease, CT scanning clearly delineates extraluminal complications (e.g., abscess, phlegmon, bowel wall thickening, mesenteric inflammation). CT has been used also to percutaneously drain fistulas (colovesicular, enterovesicular, colovaginal, enterocolonic) and to evaluate perirectal disease, enterocutaneous fistula, and sinus tracts.

Radionuclide imaging: Intravenous indium-111 labeled leukocytes migrate to areas of active inflammation and are then identified by scans done after 4 and 24 hr. This procedure aids in differentiating Crohn's disease from ulcerative colitis and evaluating abscess and fistula formation.

Blood tests: Are nonspecific for the diagnosis of Crohn's disease but help determine whether the inflammatory process is active and evaluate the patient's overall condition. Anemia may be present and may be (1) microcytic because of iron deficiency from chronic blood loss and bone marrow depression secondary to chronic inflammatory process or (2) megaloblastic because of folic acid or vitamin B_{12} deficiency (usually seen only in patients with extensive ileitis causing malabsorption). Increased WBC count and sedimentation rate reflect disease activity and inflammation. Hypoalbuminemia corresponds with the disease activity and results from decreased protein intake, extensive malabsorption, and significant enteric loss of protein. Hypokalemia is seen in patients with chronic diarrhea; hypophosphatemia and hypocalcemia are seen in patients with significant malabsorption. Liver function studies may be abnormal secondary to pericholangitis.

Urinalysis and urine culture: May reveal urinary tract infection secondary to enterovesicular fistula.

Tests for malabsorption: Because patients with active, extensive disease (especially when it involves the small intestine) may develop malabsorption and malnutrition, the following tests are clinically significant: D-xylose tolerance test (for upper jejunal involvement); Schilling's test (for ileal involvement); serum albumin, carotene, calcium, and phosphorus levels; and fecal fat (steatorrhea).

COLLABORATIVE MANAGEMENT

The initial treatment is nonoperative, and it is individualized and based on symptomatic relief. Medical treatment is more likely to be successful early in the course of the disease before permanent structural changes have occurred.

Parenteral replacement of fluids, electrolytes, and blood products: Maintenance therapy for acute exacerbation as indicated by laboratory test results.

Physical and emotional rest: Complete bedrest and assistance with ADL during acute phases.

Pharmacotherapy: It has not been proven that drugs, singly or in combination, can prolong remission and prevent relapse of Crohn's disease.

Sedatives and tranquilizers: To promote rest and reduce anxiety.

Antidiarrheal medications: To decrease diarrhea and cramping. Codeine or loperamide often reduces diarrhea with a concomitant decrease in abdominal cramping. Anticholinergics are not recommended because they may mask obstructive symptoms and precipitate toxic megacolon. For these reasons, antidiarrheal medications should be administered with caution. If a patient does not respond appropriately to standard antidiarrheal medications and mild sedation, the presence of obstruction, bowel perforation, or abscess formation is suspected.

Sulfasalazine: To treat acute exacerbations of colonic and ileocolonic disease. It appears to be more effective in patients with mild to moderate disease limited to the colon than in those with disease limited to the small bowel. Sulfasalazine has not been shown to prevent recurrence of Crohn's disease, but patients who respond tend to benefit from long-term therapy and tend to relapse when the agent is discontinued. **Note:** Because sulfasalazine impairs folate absorption, patients receive folic acid supplements during treatment.

5-Aminosalicylic acid (5-ASA) preparations: Slow-release mesalamine (Pentasa) and enteric-coated mesalamine (Asacol) have demonstrated effectiveness in maintenance therapy for preventing recurrence of Crohn's disease. These agents are undergoing clinical trials to determine their effectiveness in preventing recurrence in patients after surgical resection.

Corticosteroids: To reduce the active inflammatory response, decrease edema in moderate to severe forms, and control exacerbations. Prednisone is effective in diminishing activity of the disease process but is more beneficial in patients with small bowel involvement than it is in those with disease limited to the colon. As active disease subsides, prednisone is tapered with the goal of eliminating the drug. However, many patients with Crohn's disease become steroid dependent, meaning they are symptomatic with low-dose therapy (5-15 mg/day) or with total discontinuation of the drug. In some cases of chronic disease, continuous corticosteroid therapy may be necessary. A new steroidal agent (budesonide) shows promise for providing the benefits of traditional therapy without the side effects; budesonide is undergoing clinical trials in the United States to determine its effectiveness in controlling active Crohn's disease and in maintaining remission. Topical therapy with hydrocortisone has controlled inflammation via retention enemas for patients with proctosigmoiditis (involvement to 40 cm), and suppositories have been used for patients with Crohn's proctitis.

Immunosuppressive agents: To allow dosage reduction or withdrawal of corticosteroids in steroid-dependent patients, for maintenance therapy with a lower relapse rate, and to aid in healing and reduce drainage of perianal fistulas. Oral immunosuppressive agents include azathioprine and 6-mercaptopurine (6-MP).

IV cyclosporine has been used to treat refractory Crohn's disease and treatment-resistant fistulas. Oral cyclosporine has not proven effective for maintenance therapy because relapse occurs when dosage is reduced or stopped. Because of the frequency and severity of toxicity and side effects, short-term IV administration has proven to be the best method for cyclosporine.

Parenteral (IM, SC) methotrexate provides both immunosuppressive and antiinflammatory effects and allows for reduction or cessation of steroid therapy in some patients with chronically active Crohn's disease. However, long-term efficacy, incidence of side effects, and toxicity need to be determined.

Antibiotics: To control suppurative complications (e.g., bacterial overgrowth) and perianal fistulas in patients with mild to moderate colonic or ileocolonic Crohn's disease (see Table 6-7). In patients who are allergic, intolerant, or unresponsive to sulfasalazine, metronidazole (Flagyl) appears to be effective in colonic disease and in promoting healing of perianal disease. Long-term use of metronidazole is limited because of potential for peripheral neuropathy and other side effects. Patients with bacterial overgrowth in the small intestine may be treated with broad-spectrum antibiotics. Ciprofloxacin (Cipro) may be useful in treating patients who are intolerant or unresponsive to metronidazole therapy.

New pharmacotherapies: The following agents are undergoing development or clinical trials but have shown potential for treating Crohn's disease.

MONOCLONAL ANTIBODIES (E.G., ANTI-TNF [TUMOR NECROSING FACTOR]): Shows promise in combating the effect of cytokine, an agent that incites inflammation.

INTERLEUKIN 10 (IL-10): To suppress inflammation in patients unresponsive to steroids.

EICOSAPENTAENOIC ACID (EPA): To augment steroid therapy to allow lower steroid dosages in patients with chronic inflammatory disease. This agent is found in fish oil, and new slow-release preparations are being developed.

ANTICOAGULANT THERAPY (HEPARIN): To combat thrombus formation in blood vessels of the intestines. Some investigators have linked thrombus formation to increased inflammation in some patients with Crohn's disease.

Nutritional management: A major adjunct to standard medical therapy. During acute exacerbations, total parenteral nutrition (TPN) and NPO status can be used to replace nutritional deficits and allow complete bowel rest. Elemental diets that are free of bulk and residue, low in fat, and digested in the upper jejunum provide good nutrition with low fecal volume to allow bowel rest in selected patients. Use of elemental diets is being investigated for effectiveness as primary therapy, as an alternative to steroids and bowel rest, in treating patients with acute Crohn's disease. Bland diets low in residue, roughage, and fat but high in protein, calories, carbohydrates, and vitamins provide good nutrition and reduce excessive stimulation of the bowel. A diet free of milk, milk products, gas-forming foods, alcohol, and iced beverages reduces cramping and diarrhea. When remission occurs, a less restricted diet can be tailored to the individual patient, excluding foods known to precipitate symptoms. Personal exclusion diets have been associated with a decrease in the number of relapses, but further research is needed to substantiate these findings. Patients with involvement of the small intestine frequently require supplementation of vitamins and minerals, especially calcium, iron, folate, and magnesium, secondary to malabsorption or to compensate for foods excluded from the diet. Patients with extensive ileal disease or resection frequently require vitamin B_{12} replacement, and if bile salt deficiency exists, cholestyramine and medium-chain triglycerides may be needed to control diarrhea and reduce fat malabsorption and steatorrhea. Vitamin D deficiency is common in these patients and may require replacement with cholecalciferol.

Referral to mental health practitioner for supportive psychotherapy: If indicated, because of the chronic and progressive nature of Crohn's disease.

Surgical management: Because surgery is not a cure for Crohn's disease, it is reserved for complications rather than used as a primary form of therapy. Common indications for surgery include bowel obstruction, internal and enterocutaneous fistulas, intraabdominal abscesses, and perianal disease. Conservative resection of the affected bowel segments with restoration of bowel continuity, preserving as much of the intestine as possible, is the preferred surgical approach. If fecal diversion using an ostomy is required, the type of diversion used will depend on the location and amount of intestinal segment(s) to be resected. (For details, see"Fecal Diversions," p. 457.)

NURSING DIAGNOSES AND INTERVENTIONS

Fluid volume deficit related to active loss secondary to diarrhea or presence of GI fistula

Desired outcomes: Patient is normovolemic within 24 hr of admission as evidenced by balanced I&O, urinary output ≥30 ml/hr, specific gravity 1.010-1.030, BP ≥90/60 mm Hg (or within patient's normal range), RR 12-20 breaths/min, stable weight, good skin turgor, and moist mucous membranes. Patient reports that diarrhea is controlled.

- Monitor I&O and urinary specific gravity, weigh patient daily, and monitor laboratory values to evaluate fluid and electrolyte status. Optimal values are serum K^+ 3.5-5.0 mEq/L, serum Na^+ 137-147 mEq/L, and serum Cl^- 95-108 mEq/L.
- Monitor frequency and consistency of stools. Keep a stool count, and measure the volume of liquid stools. Assess and record presence of blood, mucus, fat, or undigested food.
- Monitor patient for indicators of dehydration: thirst, poor skin turgor, dryness of mucous membranes, fever, and concentrated (specific gravity >1.030) and decreased urinary output.
- Maintain patient on parenteral replacement of fluids, electrolytes, and vitamins as prescribed to promote anabolism and healing.
- When the patient is taking food by mouth, provide bland, high-protein, high-calorie, low-fat, low-residue diet, as prescribed. Assess tolerance to diet by determining incidence of cramping, diarrhea, and flatulence. Modify diet plan accordingly.

NIC: Diarrhea Management; Fluid/Electrolyte Management; Hypovolemia Management; Intravenous (IV) Therapy; Total Parenteral Nutrition (TPN) Administration

Risk for infection/altered protection with risks related to potential complications caused by intestinal inflammatory disorder

Desired outcome: Patient is free from indicators of infection and intraabdominal injury as evidenced by normothermia; HR 60-100 bpm; RR 12-20 breaths/min; normal bowel sounds; absence of abdominal distention, rigidity, or localized pain and tenderness; absence of nausea and vomiting; negative culture results; and no significant change in mental status and orientation to person, place, and time.

- Monitor patient for indicators of intestinal obstruction, including abdominal distention, abdominal rigidity, and increased episodes of nausea and vomiting. **Note:** Contributing factors to the development of intestinal

obstruction include use of opiates and the prolonged use of antidiarrheal medication.
- Monitor patient for fever, increased RR and HR, chills, diaphoresis, and increased abdominal discomfort, which can occur with intestinal perforation, abscess or fistula formation, or generalized fecal peritonitis and septicemia. **Note:** Systemic therapy with corticosteroids and antibiotics can mask development of the preceding complications.
- Evaluate patient's mental status, orientation, and LOC q2-4hr.
- Obtain cultures of blood, urine, fistulas, or other possible sources of infection, as prescribed if the patient has a sudden temperature elevation. Abscesses or fistulas to the abdominal wall, bladder, or vagina are common in Crohn's disease, as well as abscesses or fistulas to other loops of small bowel and colon. Monitor culture reports, and notify health care provider promptly of any positive results.
- If draining fistulas or abscesses are present, change dressings and pouching system or irrigate tubes or drains as prescribed. Note color, character, and odor of all drainage. Report the presence of foul-smelling or abnormal drainage or the loss of tube/drain patency.
- Administer antibiotics as prescribed and on the prescribed schedule to maintain a therapeutic serum level.
- Prevent the transmission of potentially infectious organisms by good hand-washing technique before and after caring for the patient and by disposing of dressings and drainage using Standard Precautions (see p. 817).

NIC: Infection Control; Surveillance; Tube Care; Vital Signs Monitoring; Wound Care: Closed Drainage

Pain, abdominal cramping, and nausea related to intestinal inflammatory process
Desired outcomes: Patient's subjective perception of discomfort decreases within 4 hr of intervention, as documented by a pain scale. Objective indicators, such as grimacing, are absent or diminished.
- Monitor and document characteristics of discomfort, and assess whether it is associated with ingestion of certain foods or with emotional stress. Devise a pain scale with patient, rating discomfort from 0 (no discomfort) to 10 (worst discomfort). Eliminate foods that cause cramping and discomfort.
- As prescribed, keep patient NPO and provide parenteral nutrition to allow bowel rest.
- Administer antidiarrheal medications and analgesics as prescribed to reduce abdominal discomfort. Instruct the patient to request analgesic before pain becomes severe.
- Provide nasal and oral care at frequent intervals to lessen discomfort from NPO status and presence of nasogastric tube.
- Administer antiemetic medications before meals to enhance appetite when nausea is a problem.
- Document relief obtained, using the pain scale.
- For additional information, see **Pain,** p. 719, in Appendix One.

NIC: Anxiety Reduction; Environmental Management: Comfort; Gastrointestinal Intubation; Medication Administration; Pain Management; Simple Relaxation Therapy; Tube Care: Gastrointestinal

Diarrhea related to intestinal inflammatory process
Desired outcome: Patient reports a reduction in frequency of stools and a return to more normal stool consistency within 3 days of hospital admission.
- If the patient is experiencing frequent and urgent passage of loose stools, provide covered bedpan or commode or be sure the bathroom is easily accessible and ready to use at all times.
- Empty the bedpan or commode promptly to control odor and decrease patient's anxiety and self-consciousness.

- Administer antidiarrheal medication as prescribed to decrease fluidity and number of stools.
- If bile salt deficiency (because of ileal disease or resection) is contributing to diarrhea, administer cholestyramine as prescribed to control diarrhea.
- Eliminate or decrease fat content in the diet because it can increase diarrhea in individuals with malabsorption syndromes. Also, restrict foods and beverages that can precipitate diarrhea and cramping, such as raw vegetables and fruits, whole-grain cereals, condiments, gas-forming foods, alcohol, iced and carbonated beverages, and, in lactose-intolerant patients, milk and milk products.

NIC: Diarrhea Management; Medication Management; Nutritional Counseling; Perineal Care

Activity intolerance related to generalized weakness secondary to intestinal inflammatory process
Desired outcome: Patient adheres to prescribed rest regimen and sets appropriate goals for self-care as the condition improves (optimally within 3-7 days of admission).
- Keep patient's environment quiet to facilitate rest.
- Because adequate rest is necessary to sustain remission, assist patient with ADL and plan nursing care to provide maximum rest periods. Keep patient's environment quiet. Facilitate coordination of health care providers to allow rest periods between care activities. Allow 90 min for undisturbed rest.
- As prescribed, administer sedatives and tranquilizers to promote rest and reduce anxiety.
- As the patient's physical condition improves, encourage self-care to the greatest extent possible and assist patient with setting realistic, attainable goals.
- For additional information, see **Risk for activity intolerance,** p. 738, in Appendix One.

NIC: Activity Therapy; Energy Management; Mutual Goal Setting; Self-Care Assistance; Teaching: Individual

---

See Also: *If surgery is performed:* "Fecal Diversions" for **Bowel incontinence,** p. 460; **Body image disturbance,** p. 461; **Risk for impaired peristomal skin integrity** and **impaired stomal tissue integrity,** p. 459; Appendix One, "Caring for Preoperative and Postoperative Patients," p. 717; "Caring for Patients With Cancer and Other Life-disrupting Illnesses," p. 747, for nursing diagnoses and interventions.

PATIENT-FAMILY TEACHING AND DISCHARGE PLANNING

When providing patient-family teaching, focus on sensory information; avoid giving excessive information; and initiate a visiting nurse referral for necessary follow-up teaching. Consider including verbal and written information about the following:
- Medications, including drug name, rationale, dosage, schedule, route of administration, precautions, drug/drug and food/drug interactions, and potential side effects.
- Signs and symptoms that necessitate medical attention, including fever, nausea and vomiting, abdominal discomfort, any significant change in appearance and frequency of stools, or passage of stool through the vagina or stool mixed with urine, any of which can signal recurrence or complications of Crohn's disease.
- Importance of dietary management to promote nutritional and fluid maintenance and prevent abdominal cramping, discomfort, and diarrhea.
- Importance of perineal/perianal skin care after bowel movements.

- Importance of balancing activities with rest periods, even during remission, because adequate rest is necessary to sustain remission.
- Referral to community resources, including the following organization:

  Crohn's and Colitis Foundation of America
  386 Park Ave. South, 17th Floor
  New York, NY 10016-8804   (800) 932-2423
  WWW address: *http://www.cefa.org/*

- Importance of follow-up medical care, including supportive psychotherapy, because of the chronic and progressive nature of Crohn's disease.

In addition, if the patient has a fecal diversion
- Care of incision, dressing changes, and bathing.
- Care of stoma and peristomal skin, use of ostomy equipment, and method for obtaining supplies.
- Gradual resumption of ADL, excluding heavy lifting (>10 lb), pushing, or pulling for 6-8 weeks to prevent incisional herniation.
- Referral to community resources, including home health care agency, ET nurse, and local chapter of the United Ostomy Association:

  United Ostomy Association
  19722 MacArthur Blvd.
  Irvine, CA 92612-2405   (800) 826-0826
  WWW address: *http://www.uoa.org/*

- Importance of reporting signs and symptoms that require medical attention, such as change in stoma color from the normal bright and shiny red; lesions of stomal mucosa that may indicate recurrence of the disease; peristomal skin irritation; diarrhea or constipation, fever, chills, abdominal pain, distention, nausea, and vomiting; and incisional pain, local increased temperature, drainage, swelling, or redness.

Fecal diversions

For a discussion of diverticulitis, see p. 432; colorectal cancer, p. 435; polyps/familial adenomatous polyposis, p. 439; ulcerative colitis, p. 440; Crohn's disease, p. 450.

SURGICAL INTERVENTIONS

It is sometimes necessary to interrupt the continuity of the bowel because of intestinal disease or its complications. A fecal diversion may be necessary to divert stool around a diseased portion or, more commonly, out of the body. A fecal diversion can be located anywhere along the bowel, depending on the location of the diseased or injured portion; and it can be permanent or temporary. The most common sites for fecal diversion are the colon and ileum.
Colostomy: Created when the surgeon brings a portion of the colon to the surface of the abdomen. An opening in the exteriorized colon permits elimination of flatus and stool through the stoma. Any part of the colon may be diverted into a colostomy.
Transverse colostomy: Most frequently created stoma to divert the feces on a temporary basis. Surgical indications include relief of bowel obstruction before definitive surgery for tumors, inflammation, or diverticulitis and colon perforation secondary to trauma. Stool can be liquid to pastelike or soft and unformed, and bowel elimination is unpredictable. A temporary colostomy may be double barreled, with a proximal stoma through which stool is eliminated and a distal stoma adjacent to the proximal stoma called a *mucous fistula*. More commonly, a loop colostomy is created with a supporting rod placed beneath it until the exteriorized loop of colon heals to the skin.

Descending or sigmoid colostomy: Usually a permanent fecal diversion. Cancer of the rectum is the most common cause for surgical intervention. Stool is usually formed, and some individuals may have stool elimination at predictable times. In a permanent colostomy, the surgeon brings the severed end of the colon to the abdominal skin surface. The diseased or injured portion of the colon and/or rectum is resected and removed. To create the stoma, the colon above the skin surface is rolled back on itself to expose the mucosal surface of the intestine. The end of the cuff is sutured to the subcutaneous tissues with absorbable sutures to hold it in place as it heals.

Temporary colostomy: Typically created when there is significant inflammation in the diseased portion of the bowel (e.g., perforated diverticulum or ulcerative colitis). When a temporary colostomy is created, the severed end of the colon is brought through the abdominal wall as for a permanent colostomy. The diseased or injured portion of the colon is resected and removed. The remaining rectum or rectosigmoid is oversewn, left in the peritoneal cavity, and is referred to as Hartmann's pouch. After the inflammatory process has resolved (e.g., 3-6 mo), the colostomy is taken down and reattached to the bowel of Hartmann's pouch, thus reconstructing continuity of the bowel and normal bowel elimination.

Cecostomy or ascending colostomy: Not a commonly seen procedure. A temporary diverting colostomy is most commonly used to bypass an unresectable tumor. The stool from an ascending colostomy is soft, unformed, pastelike, semiliquid, or liquid, and bowel elimination is unpredictable. Surgical procedure is similar to that with transverse colostomies.

Ileostomy

Conventional (Brooke) ileostomy: Created by bringing a distal portion of the resected ileum through the abdominal wall. A permanent ileostomy is created by the same procedure discussed with a permanent colostomy. Surgical indications include ulcerative colitis, Crohn's disease, and familial adenomatous polyposis (FAP) requiring excision of the entire colon and rectum. For any ileostomy, the output is usually liquid (or more rarely, pastelike) and is eliminated continually. The more proximal the ileostomy, the more active are digestive enzymes within the effluent (stool) and the greater their potential for irritation to exposed skin around the stoma. A collection pouch is worn over the stoma on the abdomen to collect gas and fecal discharge.

Temporary ileostomy: Usually a loop stoma with or without a supporting rod in place beneath the loop of the ileum until the exteriorized loop of ileum heals to the skin. The purpose is to divert the fecal stream away from a more distal anastomotic site or fistula repair until healing has occurred.

Continent (Kock pouch) ileostomy: An intraabdominal pouch constructed from approximately 30 cm of distal ileum. Intussusception of a 10-cm portion of ileum is done to form an outlet nipple valve from the pouch to the skin of the abdomen, where a stoma is constructed flush with the skin. The intraabdominal pouch is continent for gas and fecal discharge and is emptied approximately qid by inserting a catheter through the stoma. No external pouch is needed, and a Band-Aid or small dressing is worn over the stoma to collect mucus. Surgical indications include ulcerative colitis and FAP requiring removal of the colon and rectum. Crohn's disease is generally a contraindication for this procedure because the disease can recur in the pouch, necessitating its removal.

Ileoanal reservoir (or restorative protocolectomy):   A two-stage surgical procedure developed to preserve fecal continence and prevent the need for a permanent ileostomy. During the first stage after total colectomy and removal of the rectal mucosa, an ileal reservoir is constructed and lowered into position in the pelvis just above the rectal cuff. Then the ileal outlet from the reservoir is brought down through the cuff of the rectal muscle and anastomosed to the anal canal. The anal sphincter is preserved, and the resulting ileal reservoir provides a storage place for feces. A temporary diverting ileostomy is required for 2-3 mo to allow healing of the anastomosis. The second stage occurs when the diverting ileostomy is taken down and fecal continuity is restored. Initially, the patient experiences fecal incontinence and 10 or more bowel movements per day. After 3-6 mo, the patient experiences a decrease in urgency and frequency with 4-8 bowel movements per day. This procedure is an option for patients requiring colectomy for ulcerative colitis or FAP. It is contraindicated in patients with Crohn's disease and incontinence problems.

NURSING DIAGNOSES AND INTERVENTIONS

Risk for impaired peristomal skin integrity related to risk factors from exposure to effluent or sensitivity to appliance material; *and*
Impaired stomal tissue integrity (or risk for same) related to improperly fitted appliance resulting in impaired circulation
Desired outcome: Patient's stomal and peristomal skin and tissue remain nonerythemic and intact.

After colostomy or conventional ileostomy (permanent or temporary)
- Apply a pectin, gelatin, methylcellulose-based, or synthetic, solid-form skin barrier around the stoma to protect the peristomal skin from irritation caused by contact with stool.
  —Cut an opening in the skin barrier the exact circumference of the stoma or as recommended by the manufacturer. Remove the release paper, and apply the sticky surface directly to the peristomal skin. For some pouching systems, the skin barrier may be a separate barrier to be used with an adhesive-backed pouch, part of a two-piece system, or an integral part of a one-piece pouch system. Pectin-based paste may also be used to "caulk" around the barrier and compensate for irregular surfaces on the peristomal skin. A pectin-based paste may prevent undermining of the barrier with effluent and protect skin immediately adjacent to the stoma.
  —Remove the skin barrier and inspect the skin q3-4days. Monitor peristomal skin for changes (e.g., erythema, erosion, serous drainage, bleeding, induration) that may signal the presence of infection, irritation, or sensitivity to materials placed on the skin. Carefully document abnormal findings, and report them to the health care provider. Discontinue use of irritating materials, and substitute other materials. Patch-test the patient's abdominal skin to determine sensitivity to suspected materials.
  —Recalibrate the skin barrier opening to the size of the stoma with each change. Stomas become less edematous over a period of weeks after surgery, necessitating changes in the size of the skin barrier opening. The skin barrier opening should be the exact circumference of the stoma to prevent contact of stool with the skin. Commercial templates are available to aid in estimating the size of opening needed for the skin barrier.
- Apply a two-piece pouch system or a pouch with access cap so that the stoma can be inspected for viability q12-24hr in the immediate postoperative period. A mature stoma will be red in color with overlying mucus. A nonmature stoma will be red and moist where the mucous membrane is exposed but can be a darker, mottled, grayish red with a transparent or translucent film of serosa elsewhere.
- Cleanse the patient's skin with warm water when removing the skin barrier and pouch for routine care. Dry peristomal skin completely so the skin retains its normal integrity and the skin barrier and pouch materials adhere well.
- Empty the pouch when it is one-third to one-half full of stool or gas to maintain a secure pouch seal.

After continent ileostomy (Kock pouch)
- Avoid stress on the ileostomy catheter and its securing suture. As prescribed, maintain catheter on low, continuous suction or gravity drainage. The catheter was inserted through the stoma into the continent ileostomy pouch during surgery to prevent stress on the nipple valve and maintain pouch

decompression so that suture lines are allowed to heal without stress or tension.
- Monitor the site for erythema, induration, drainage, or erosion around the stoma. Report significant findings to health care provider.
- Check the catheter q2hr for patency, and irrigate with sterile saline (30 ml) to prevent obstruction. Notify health care provider if solution cannot be instilled, if there are no returns from the catheter, or if leakage of irrigating solution or pouch contents appears around the catheter.
- Change 4×4 dressing around the stoma q2hr or as often as it becomes wet to prevent peristomal skin irritation. The drainage will be serosanguineous at first and mixed with mucus. Report presence of frank bleeding to health care provider.
- Assess stoma for viability with each dressing change. It should be red in color and moist and shiny with mucus. A stoma that is pale or dark purple to black or dull in appearance may indicate circulatory impairment and should be reported to health care provider immediately and documented.

After ileoanal reservoir
- Perform routine care for diverting ileostomy (see earlier discussion).
- After the first stage of the operation, the patient may have incontinence of mucus. Maintain perineal/perianal skin integrity by irrigating the mucus out of the reservoir daily with 60 ml of water or gently cleansing the area with water and cotton balls or soft tissues. (**Note:** Pouch irrigation to remove mucus rarely is indicated now because of new reservoir configurations that allow spontaneous emptying of the reservoir.) Avoid soap, which can cause itching or irritation. Use an absorbent pad at night to absorb oozing mucus.
- After the second stage of operation (when the ileostomy is taken down), expect the patient to experience frequency and urgency of defecation.
- Wash perineal/perianal area with warm water or commercial perianal/perineal cleansing solution, using a squeeze bottle, cotton balls, or soft tissues. Do not use toilet paper, because it can cause irritation. If desired, dry the area with a hair dryer on a cool setting.
- Provide sitz baths to promote comfort and help clean the perineal/perianal area.
- Apply protective skin sealants or ointments. Skin sealants should not be used on irritated or eroded skin because of the high alcohol content, which would cause a painful burning sensation.

NIC: Bathing; Heat/Cold Application; Ostomy Care; Skin Care: Topical Treatments; Surveillance; Teaching: Psychomotor Skill

Bowel incontinence related to disruption of normal function with fecal diversion
Desired outcomes: Within 2-4 days after surgery, patient has bowel sounds and eliminates gas and stool via the fecal diversion. Within 3 days after teaching has been initiated, patient verbalizes understanding of measures that will maintain normal elimination pattern and demonstrates care techniques specific to the fecal diversion.

After colostomy and conventional ileostomy (permanent and temporary)
- Empty stool from the bottom opening of the pouch, and assess the quality and quantity of stool to document return of normal bowel function. Record volume of liquid stool and its color and consistency.
- If the colostomy is not eliminating stool after 3-4 days and bowel sounds have returned, gently insert a gloved, lubricated finger into the stoma to determine presence of stricture at the skin or fascial levels and note presence of any stool within reach of the examining finger. To stimulate elimination of gas and stool, health care provider may prescribe colostomy irrigation. (For procedure, see **Knowledge deficit:** Colostomy irrigation procedure, p. 462.)

After continent ileostomy (Kock pouch)

- Monitor I&O, and record amount, color, and consistency of output.
- Expect aspiration of bright red blood or serosanguineous liquid drainage from the Kock pouch during the early postoperative period.
- As GI function returns after 3-4 days, expect the drainage to change in color from blood-tinged to greenish brown liquid. When ileal output appears, suction (if used) is discontinued and the pouch catheter is placed to gravity drainage.
- As the patient's diet progresses from clear liquids to solid food, the ileal output thickens. Check and irrigate the catheter q2hr and as needed to maintain patency. If the patient reports abdominal fullness in the area of the pouch along with decreased fecal output, check placement and patency of the catheter.
- When the patient is alert and taking food by mouth, teach catheter irrigation procedure, which should be performed q2hr; demonstrate how to empty the pouch contents through the catheter into the toilet.
- Before hospital discharge, teach patient how to remove and reinsert the catheter.

After ileoanal reservoir

- Monitor I&O, observing quantity, quality, and consistency of output from diverting ileostomy and reservoir. Monitor patient for elevation of temperature accompanied by perianal pain and discharge of purulent, bloody mucus from drains and anal orifice. Report significant findings to health care provider.
- If drains are present, irrigate them as prescribed to maintain patency, decrease stress on suture lines, and decrease incidence of infection.
- After the first stage of the operation, patient may experience oozing of mucus. Advise patient to wear small pad to avoid soiling outer garments.
- After the second stage of the operation (when the ileostomy is taken down), expect incontinence and 15-20 bowel movements per day with urgency when patient is on a clear-liquid diet. Assist patient with perianal care, and apply protective skin care products. If nocturnal incontinence is especially troublesome, the catheter can be placed in the reservoir and connected to gravity drainage bag overnight.
- Expect the number of bowel movements to decrease to 6-12/day and the consistency to thicken when the patient is eating solid foods.
- Administer hydrophilic colloids and antidiarrheal medications as prescribed to decrease frequency and fluidity of stools.
- Provide diet consultation so that patient can avoid foods that cause liquid stools (spinach, raw fruits, highly seasoned foods, green beans, broccoli, prune and grape juices, alcohol) and increase intake of foods that cause thick stools (cheese, ripe bananas, applesauce, creamy peanut butter, gelatin, pasta).
- Reassure patient that frequency and urgency are temporary and that as the reservoir expands and absorbs fluid, bowel movements should become thicker and less frequent.

NIC: Diet Staging; Nutritional Counseling; Ostomy Care; Perineal Care; Self-Care Assistance: Toileting; Teaching: Prescribed Diet; Teaching: Procedure/Treatment

Body image disturbance related to presence of fecal diversion
Desired outcome: Within 5-7 days after surgery, patient demonstrates actions that reflect beginning acceptance of the fecal diversion and incorporates changes into self-concept as evidenced by acknowledging body changes, viewing the stoma, and participating in the care of the fecal diversion.

- Expect the following fears, which may be expressed by patients experiencing a fecal diversion: physical, social, and work activities will be curtailed significantly; rejection, isolation, and feelings of uncleanliness will occur; everyone will know about the altered pattern of fecal elimination; and loss of voluntary control may occur (many patients view incontinence as a return to infancy).

- Encourage patient to discuss feelings and fears; clarify any misconceptions. Involve family members in the discussions because they too may have anxieties and misconceptions.
- Provide a calm and quiet environment for patient and significant other to discuss the surgery. Initiate an open, honest discussion. Monitor carefully for and listen closely to expressed or nonverbalized needs because each patient will react differently to the surgical procedure.
- Encourage acceptance of fecal diversion by having patient participate in care. Assure patient that education offers a means of control.
- Assure patient that physical, social, and work activities will not be affected by the presence of a fecal diversion.
- Expect the patient to have fears about sexual acceptance, although these fears usually are not expressed overtly. Concerns center on change in body image; fears about odor and the ostomy appliance interfering with intercourse; conception, pregnancy, and discomfort from perineal wound and scar in women; and impotence and failure to ejaculate in men, especially after more radical dissection of the pelvis in the patient with cancer. If you are uncomfortable talking about sexuality with patients, be aware of these potential concerns and arrange for a consultation with someone who can speak openly and honestly about these problems.
- Consult patient's health care provider about a visit by another person with an ostomy. Patients gain reassurance and build positive attitudes by seeing a healthy, active person who has undergone the same type of surgery.

NIC: Active Listening; Anxiety Reduction; Body Image Enhancement; Emotional Support; Environmental Management; Learning Facilitation; Ostomy Care; Sexual Counseling

Knowledge deficit: Colostomy irrigation procedure
Desired outcome: Within 3 days after initiation of teaching, patient demonstrates proficiency with the procedure for colostomy irrigation.

> **Note:** Teach prescribed colostomy irrigation to patient with permanent descending or sigmoid colostomy. Colostomy irrigation is performed daily or every other day so that wearing a pouch becomes unnecessary. An appropriate candidate is a patient who has 1 or 2 formed stools each day at predictable times (same as normal stool elimination pattern before illness). In addition, the patient must be able to manipulate the equipment, remember the technique, and be willing to spend approximately 1 hr/day performing the procedure. It may take 4-6 weeks for the patient to have stool elimination regulated with irrigation.

Instruct patient about the following steps
- Position an irrigating sleeve over the colostomy, centering the stoma in the opening. Secure the sleeve in place with the adhesive disk on the sleeve or with a sleeve belt.
- Fill an enema/irrigation container with 500-1000 ml (1-2 pints) warm water. With the patient in a sitting position on the toilet or on a chair facing the toilet, position the sleeve so that it empties into the toilet. Hang the enema/irrigation container so that the bottom surface is at the patient's shoulder level.
- Open the slide or roller clamp and flush the tubing with the water to remove air from the tubing; reclamp the tubing.

- Gently dilate the stoma with a gloved finger lubricated with water-soluble lubricant; this allows the patient to identify the direction of the intestinal lumen. Lubricate the cone and catheter, and slowly insert them into the stoma. (**Note:** If a cone and catheter are used, insert the catheter no more than 3 inches.) Hold the cone gently, but firmly, in place against the stoma to prevent backflow of irrigant.
- Allow the water to slowly enter the stoma from the container through tubing; it should take 15 min for fluid to slowly enter the colon. **Note:** If cramping occurs while the water is flowing, stop the flow and leave the cone in place until the cramping passes; then the flow of water may be resumed. If cramping does not resolve, the colon is probably ready to evacuate and should be allowed to do so.
- After water has entered the colon, advise the patient to hold the cone in place for a few seconds and then to gently remove it. The sleeve should be left in place for 30-40 min to allow the water and stool to be eliminated.
- When elimination is complete, remove the irrigation sleeve and cleanse and dry the peristomal area.
- Apply a small dressing or security pouch over the colostomy between irrigations.

NIC: Learning Readiness Enhancement; Learning Facilitation; Teaching: Individual; Teaching: Psychomotor Skill

---

See Also: Appendix One, "Caring for Preoperative and Postoperative Patients," p. 717; "Caring for Patients With Cancer and Other Life-disrupting Illnesses," p. 747, for nursing diagnoses and interventions.

PATIENT-FAMILY TEACHING AND DISCHARGE PLANNING

When providing patient-family teaching, focus on sensory information; avoid giving excessive information; and initiate a visiting nurse referral for necessary follow-up teaching. Consider including verbal and written information about the following:

- Medications, including drug name, rationale, dosage, schedule, route of administration, precautions, drug/drug and food/drug interactions, and potential side effects.
- Importance of dietary management to promote nutritional and fluid maintenance.
- Care of incision, dressing changes, and permission to take baths or showers once sutures and drains are removed.
- Care of stoma, peristomal, and perianal skin; use of ostomy equipment; and method for obtaining supplies.
- Gradual resumption of ADL, excluding heavy lifting (>10 lb), pushing, or pulling for 6-8 weeks to prevent development of incisional herniation.
- Referral to community resources including home health care agency, ET nurse, and local chapter of the United Ostomy Association:

    United Ostomy Association
    19722 MacArthur Blvd.
    Irvine, CA 92612-2405   (800) 826-0826
    WWW address: *http://www.uoa.org/*

- Importance of follow-up care with health care provider and ET nurse; confirm date and time of next appointment.
- Importance of reporting signs and symptoms that require medical attention, such as change in stoma color from the normal bright and shiny red; peristomal or perianal skin irritation; any significant changes in appearance, frequency, and consistency of stools; fever, chills, abdominal pain, or

distention; and incisional pain, increased local warmth, drainage, swelling, or redness.

Section Four: Abdominal Trauma

Injury to abdominal contents is related to the nature of the force applied and the consistency of the affected structures. Forces involved are classified as blunt (e.g., those caused by falls, physical assault, motor vehicle collisions, crush injury) or penetrating (e.g., stab, gunshot wounds). Organs are categorized as solid (e.g., liver, spleen, pancreas) or hollow (e.g., stomach, intestine, urinary bladder). Blunt abdominal trauma typically results in injury to solid viscera because hollow viscera tend to be more compressible. However, hollow organs may rupture, especially when full, if there is a sudden increase in intraluminal pressure. Usually injury inflicted by stab wounds follows a more predictable pattern and involves less tissue destruction than injury from gunshot wounds, although stab wounds to major vascular structures and organs can be fatal. Removing penetrating objects can result in additional injury, so attempts at removal are made only in a controlled surgical environment. High-velocity weapons (e.g., rifles) cause injury not only to tissue in the direct path of the missile but also to adjacent organs because of energy shock waves that surround the missile path. Tissue destruction is not as great with low-velocity pistols. The rate of complications and death increases greatly if injury to multiple abdominal organs is sustained.

Abdominal trauma results in direct injury to organs, blood vessels, and supporting structures. Other pathophysiologic changes associated with abdominal trauma include (1) fluid shifts related to tissue damage, blood loss, and shock; (2) metabolic changes mediated by the CNS and macroendocrine/microendocrine systems; (3) coagulation problems associated with massive hemorrhage and multiple transfusions; (4) inflammation, infection, and abscess formation caused by release of GI secretions and bacteria into the peritoneum; and (5) nutritional and electrolyte alterations that develop as a consequence of disruption of GI tract integrity. The following is a brief overview of common injuries.

Spleen: The spleen is the organ most frequently injured following blunt trauma. Massive hemorrhage from splenic rupture is common. All efforts are made to repair the spleen, since total splenectomy increases the long-term risk of sepsis, especially in children and young adults.

Liver: Because of its size and location, it is the organ most frequently involved in penetrating trauma and often is affected by blunt injury as well. Control of bleeding and bile drainage from liver lacerations are major concerns with hepatic injury.

Lower esophagus and stomach: Occasionally the lower esophagus is involved in penetrating trauma. Because the stomach is flexible and readily displaced, it usually is not injured with blunt trauma but may be injured by direct penetration. Any serious injury to the lower esophagus and stomach results in the escape of irritating gastric fluids and the release of free air below the level of the diaphragm.

Pancreas and duodenum: Although traumatic pancreatic or duodenal injury occurs relatively infrequently, it is associated with high morbidity and mortality because of the difficulty of detecting these injuries and the likelihood of massive injury to nearby organs. These organs are retroperitoneal, and clinical indicators of injury often are not obvious for several hours.

Small intestine and mesentery: These injuries are common and may be caused by penetrating or nonpenetrating forces. Compromised intestinal blood flow with eventual infarction is the consequence of undetected mesenteric damage. Perforations or contusions can result in release of bacteria and intestinal contents into the abdominal cavity, causing serious infection.

Colon: Injury is most frequently caused by penetrating forces, although lap safety belts, direct blows, and other blunt forces cause a small percentage of colonic injuries. Because of the high bacterial content, infection is always a serious concern. Many patients with colon injury require a temporary colostomy (see "Fecal Diversions," p. 457).

Major vessels: Injuries to the abdominal aorta and inferior vena cava are most often caused by penetrating trauma but also occur with deceleration injury. Hepatic vein injuries frequently are associated with juxtahepatic vena caval injury and result in rapid hemorrhage. Blood loss after major vascular injury is massive, and survival depends on rapid prehospital transport and immediate surgical intervention.

Retroperitoneal vessels: Tears in retroperitoneal vessels associated with pelvic fractures or damage to retroperitoneal organs (pancreas, duodenum, kidney) can cause bleeding into the retroperitoneum. Even though the retroperitoneal space can accommodate up to 4 L of blood, clinical detection of retroperitoneal hematomas is difficult, and CT scanning is commonly required.

ASSESSMENT

Signs and symptoms: A wide variation can occur. Mild tenderness to severe abdominal pain may be present, with the pain either localized to the site of injury or diffuse. Blood or fluid collection within the peritoneum causes irritation, resulting in involuntary guarding, distention, rigidity, and rebound tenderness. Fluid or air under the diaphragm may cause referred shoulder pain. Kehr's sign (left shoulder pain caused by splenic bleeding) also may be noted, especially when the patient is recumbent. Nausea and vomiting may be present, and the conscious patient who has sustained blood loss often complains of thirst, an early sign of hemorrhagic shock. Symptoms of abdominal injury may be minimal or absent in the patient who is intoxicated or has sustained head or spinal cord injury. **Note:** The absence of signs and symptoms does not exclude the presence of major abdominal injury.

Physical assessment: Abdominal assessment is highly subjective, and serial evaluations by the same examiner are strongly recommended to detect subtle changes.

Inspection: Abrasions and ecchymoses are suggestive of underlying injury (e.g., ecchymosis over LUQ suggests splenic rupture; ecchymotic areas on the flank are suggestive of retroperitoneal bleeding; erythema and ecchymosis across the lower abdomen suggest intestinal injury caused by lap belts). Ecchymoses may take hours to days to develop, depending on the rate of blood loss.

Auscultation: It is important to auscultate before palpation and percussion because these maneuvers can stimulate the bowel and confound assessment findings. Bowel sounds are likely to be decreased or absent with abdominal organ injury, intraperitoneal bleeding, or recent surgery. However, the presence of bowel sounds does not exclude significant abdominal injury. Bowel sounds should be auscultated frequently, especially in the first 24-48 hr after injury. Absence of bowel sounds is expected immediately after surgery. Inability to auscultate bowel sounds within 24-48 hr after surgery is suggestive of ileus or other complications, such as bleeding, peritonitis, or bowel infarction.

Palpation: Tenderness or pain to palpation strongly suggests abdominal injury. Blood or fluid in the abdomen can result in signs and symptoms of peritoneal irritation (Table 6-8).

Percussion: Tympany suggests the presence of gas. Percussion may reveal unusually large areas of dullness over ruptured blood-filled organs (e.g., a fixed area of dullness in the LUQ suggests a ruptured spleen).

Vital signs and hemodynamic measurements: Ventilatory excursion often is diminished because of pain, thoracic injury, or limited diaphragmatic

---

T A B L E 6 - 8   Signs and Symptoms Suggestive of Peritoneal Irritation

Generalized abdominal pain or tenderness
Involuntary guarding of abdomen
Abdominal wall rigidity
Rebound tenderness
Abdominal pain with movement or coughing
Decreased or absent bowel sounds

---

movement caused by abdominal distention. Initial compensatory tachycardia and vasoconstriction secondary to blood loss usually maintain a normal BP until blood loss becomes major. At that point, BP rapidly deteriorates.

History: Details regarding circumstances of the accident and mechanism of injury are invaluable in detecting the possibility of specific injuries. In addition, ascertain time of patient's last meal, previous abdominal surgeries, and use of safety restraints (if appropriate). If possible, determine current medications and allergies, particularly to contrast material, antibiotics, and tetanus toxoid. The history may be difficult to obtain because of alcohol or drug intoxication, head injury, breathing difficulties, or impaired cerebral perfusion. In such cases, family members may be valuable sources of information.

DIAGNOSTIC TESTS

Hct: Serial levels reflect the amount of blood lost. If drawn immediately after the injury, Hct may be normal, but serial levels will reveal dramatic decreases during resuscitation and as extravascular fluid mobilizes during the recovery phase.

WBC count: Leukocytosis is expected immediately after injury. Splenic injuries, in particular, result in rapid development of a moderate to high WBC count. A later increase in WBCs or a shift to the left reflects an increase in the number of neutrophils, which signals an inflammatory response and possible intraabdominal infection. In the patient with abdominal trauma, ruptured abdominal viscera must be considered as a potential source of infection.

Platelet count: Mild thrombocytosis is seen immediately after traumatic injury. After massive hemorrhage, thrombocytopenia may be noted. Platelet transfusion usually is not required unless spontaneous bleeding is present.

Glucose: Glucose is initially elevated because of catecholamine release and insulin resistance associated with major trauma. Glucose metabolism is abnormal after major hepatic resection, and patients should be monitored to prevent hypoglycemic episodes.

Amylase: Elevated serum levels are associated with pancreatic or upper small bowel injury, but values may be normal even with severe injury to these organs.

Serum glutamic-oxaloacetic transaminase (SGOT; aspartate aminotransferase [AST]), serum glutamic-pyruvic transaminase (SGPT; alanine aminotransferase [ALT]), lactic dehydrogenase (LDH): Elevations of these enzymes reflect hepatic dysfunction caused by liver ischemia during prolonged hypotensive episodes or direct traumatic damage. Fluctuations in these enzymes during the postoperative period can be used to detect evidence of liver necrosis.

X-rays: Initially, flat and upright chest x-rays exclude chest injuries (frequently associated with abdominal trauma) and establish a baseline. Subsequent chest x-rays aid in detecting complications, such as atelectasis and pneumonia. In addition, chest, abdominal, and pelvic x-rays may reveal fractures, missiles, foreign bodies, free intraperitoneal air, hematoma, or hemorrhage.

Occult blood: Gastric contents, urine, and stool should be tested for blood in the initial and recovery periods because bleeding can occur as a result of both direct injury and later complications.

Diagnostic peritoneal lavage (DPL): DPL involves insertion of a peritoneal dialysis catheter into the peritoneum to check for intraabdominal bleeding. It is indicated for confirmed or suspected blunt abdominal trauma for the following patients: (1) those in whom signs and symptoms of abdominal injury are obscured by intoxication, head or spinal cord trauma, opioids, or unconsciousness; (2) those about to undergo general anesthesia for repair of other injuries (e.g., orthopedic, facial); and (3) any patient with equivocal assessment findings. DPL is unnecessary for patients who have obvious intraabdominal bleeding or other indications for immediate laparotomy (see "Surgical Considerations," p. 468).

CT scan: CT can detect intraperitoneal and retroperitoneal bleeding and free air (associated with rupture of hollow viscera). It is most useful in assessing injury to solid abdominal organs. This procedure also is helpful in detecting abscesses and other complications. **Caution:** Because of the risk of rapid deterioration, patients with recent injuries (24-48 hr) or in unstable condition should be accompanied by a nurse during the CT scan. Appropriate monitoring and resuscitation equipment must be readily available.

Angiography: Angiography is performed selectively with blunt trauma to evaluate injury to spleen, liver, pancreas, duodenum, and retroperitoneal vessels when other diagnostic findings are equivocal. **Caution:** Because of the large amount of contrast material used during this procedure, ensure adequate hydration and monitor urine output closely for 24-48 hours, especially in older patients or patients with preexisting cardiovascular or renal disease. Decreased urinary output and increased BUN and creatinine may indicate contrast-associated acute tubal necrosis.

● ● ●

Abdominal injuries often are associated with multisystem trauma. See also diagnostic test discussions under "Pneumothorax/Hemothorax," p. 27; "Spinal Cord Injury," p. 259; "Head Injury," p. 276.

COLLABORATIVE MANAGEMENT

Oxygen: Individuals sustaining abdominal trauma are likely to be tachypneic, with the potential for poor ventilatory effort. Supplemental O_2 is delivered until patient's ABG or oximetry values while breathing room air are acceptable.

Fluid management: Massive blood loss is frequently associated with abdominal injuries. Restoration and maintenance of adequate volume are essential. Initially, Ringer's lactate or similar balanced salt solution is given. Colloid solutions, such as albumin, are helpful in the postoperative period if the patient has hypoalbuminemia. Typed and cross-matched fresh blood is the optimal fluid for replacement of large blood losses. However, because fresh whole blood is rarely available, a combination of packed cells and fresh frozen plasma most often is used. For the hemodynamically stable patient, balanced crystalloid solutions with additional K^+ are used until the patient can tolerate enteral or oral feedings.

Gastric intubation: A gastric tube permits gastric decompression, aids in removal of gastric contents, and prevents accumulation of gas or air in the GI tract. Aspirated contents can be checked for blood to aid in the diagnosis of lower esophageal, gastric, or duodenal injury. The tube usually remains in place until bowel function returns.

Urinary drainage: An indwelling catheter is inserted soon after admission to obtain a specimen for urinalysis, monitor hourly urine output, and aid in the diagnosis of genitourinary trauma. Monitoring urine specific gravity may provide an indirect measure of the patient's hydration status.

TABLE 6-9 Tetanus Prophylaxis in Routine Wound Management—United States

History of adsorbed tetanus toxoid (doses)	Clean, minor wounds		All other wounds*	
	Td†	TIG	Td†	TIG
Unknown or <3	Yes	No	Yes	Yes
≥3‡	No§	No	No‖	No

Modified from Centers for Disease Control: *Morbid Mortal Weekly Rep* 34(27):422, 1985.

Td, Adult tetanus toxoid (full dose) and diphtheria toxoid (reduced dose) for adult use; *TIG,* tetanus immune globulin; *DPT,* diphtheria-pertussis-tetanus (vaccine); *DT,* diphtheria and tetanus toxoids, pediatric type.

*Such as, but not limited to, wounds resulting from missiles, crushing, burns, and frostbite.

†For children <7 yr old; *DPT (DT,* if pertussis vaccine is contraindicated) is preferred to tetanus toxoid alone. For persons 7 yr old and older, Td is preferred to tetanus toxoid alone.

‡If only 3 doses of *fluid* toxoid have been received, a fourth dose of toxoid, preferably an adsorbed toxoid, should be given.

§Yes, if >10 yr since last dose.

‖Yes, if >5 yr since last dose. (More frequent boosters are not needed and can accentuate side effects.)

Pharmacotherapy

Antibiotics: Abdominal trauma is associated with a high incidence of intraabdominal abscess, sepsis, and wound infection, particularly injury to the terminal ileum and colon. Individuals with suspected intestinal injury are given parenteral antibiotic therapy immediately. Broad-spectrum antibiotics are continued postoperatively and stopped after several days unless there is evidence of infection.

Analgesics: Because opioid analgesics alter the sensorium, making evaluation of the patient's condition difficult, they are used cautiously in the early stages of trauma. Small doses of IV analgesics are preferred because absorption from IM sites may be prolonged and erratic. Narcotic analgesics are used in the immediate postoperative period to relieve pain and promote ventilatory excursion. They may be delivered intermittently by the nurse or via patient-controlled pumps. As the severity of pain lessens, alternate analgesics such as NSAIDs (e.g., ketorolac, ibuprofen) may be prescribed. The risk of excessive bleeding and gastric stress ulcers must be weighed against the potential benefit of NSAIDs.

Tetanus prophylaxis: Tetanus immune globulin and tetanus toxoid are considered, based on Centers for Disease Control and Prevention recommendations (Table 6-9).

Nutrition: Patients with abdominal trauma have complex nutritional needs because of the hypermetabolic state associated with major trauma and traumatic or surgical disruption of normal GI function. Often infection and sepsis contribute to negative nitrogen (N) state and increased metabolic needs. Prompt initiation of parenteral feedings in patients unable to accept enteric feedings and the administration of supplemental calories, proteins, vitamins, and minerals are essential for healing.

Surgical considerations for penetrating abdominal injuries: The issue of mandatory surgical exploration vs. observation and selective surgery, especially with stab wounds, remains controversial. Patients without obvious injury or peritoneal signs generally are observed for positive peritoneal signs and stability of VS. Indications for laparotomy include one or more of the following: (1) penetrating injury suspected of invading the peritoneum; (2) positive peritoneal signs (see Table 6-8); (3) shock; (4) GI hemorrhage; (5) free air in the peritoneal cavity as seen on x-ray; (6) evisceration;

(7) massive hematuria; or (8) positive DPL. **Note:** Recently injured patients should be evaluated for peritoneal signs at hourly intervals by the same professional. Notify the health care provider immediately if the patient develops peritoneal signs, evidence of shock, gastric or rectal bleeding, or gross hematuria.

Surgical considerations for nonpenetrating abdominal injuries: Physical examination usually is reliable in determining the necessity for surgery in alert, cooperative, unintoxicated patients. Additional diagnostic tests such as DPL or CT scan are necessary to evaluate the need for surgery in the patient who is intoxicated, is unconscious, or has sustained head or spinal cord trauma. Immediate laparotomy for blunt abdominal trauma is indicated under the following circumstances: (1) clear signs of peritoneal irritation (see Table 6-8); (2) free air in the peritoneum; (3) hypotension caused by suspected abdominal injury or persistent and unexplained hypotension; (4) positive DPL; (5) GI aspirate or rectal smear positive for blood; or (6) other positive diagnostic tests, such as CT scan or arteriogram. Carefully evaluated stable patients with blunt abdominal trauma may be admitted to critical care for observation. These patients should be evaluated in the same manner as that just described for penetrating abdominal injuries. It is important to note that damage to retroperitoneal organs, such as the pancreas and duodenum, may not cause significant signs and symptoms for 6-12 hr or longer. Relatively slow bleeding from abdominal viscera may not be clinically apparent for 12 hr or longer after the initial injury. In addition, the nurse should be aware that complications, such as bowel obstruction, may develop days or weeks after the traumatic event. The need for vigilant assessment in the care of these patients cannot be overemphasized.

NURSING DIAGNOSES AND INTERVENTIONS

Fluid volume deficit related to active loss secondary to bleeding/hemorrhage
Desired outcomes: Within 4 hr of admission or on definitive repair (e.g., surgery), patient is normovolemic as evidenced by systolic BP ≥90 mm Hg (or within patient's baseline range), HR 60-100 bpm, CVP 2-6 mm Hg (5-12 cm H_2O), urinary output ≥30 ml/hr, warm extremities, brisk capillary refill (<2 sec), distal pulses >2+ on a 0-4+ scale, and absence of orthostasis.

- In *recently injured patients,* monitor BP hourly or more frequently in the presence of obvious bleeding or unstable VS. Be alert to increasing diastolic BP and decreasing systolic BP. Even a small but sudden decrease in systolic BP signals the need to notify health care provider, especially with the trauma patient in whom the extent of injury is unknown. Most trauma patients are young, and excellent neurovascular compensation results in a near normal BP until there is a large intravascular volume depletion. In the *stable postoperative patient,* perform routine VS assessment.
- Be alert to the clinical indicators of fluid volume deficit (Table 6-10), and report them accordingly.
- Monitor HR and cardiovascular status hourly until the patient's condition is stable. Note and report sudden increases or decreases in HR, especially if associated with indicators of fluid volume deficit, as noted above.
- Monitor for physical indicators of fluid volume deficit, including diaphoresis, cool extremities, delayed capillary refill ≥2 sec, and absent or decreased strength of distal pulses.
- In the patient with evidence of volume depletion or active blood loss, administer prescribed fluids rapidly through one or more large-caliber (16-gauge or larger) IV catheters. **Caution:** Evaluate patency of IV catheters frequently during rapid volume resuscitation. Monitor patient closely to avoid fluid volume overload and complications such as heart failure (see p. 68) and pulmonary edema (see p. 103).

T A B L E　6 - 1 0　Indicators of Fluid Volume Deficit

Increasing diastolic BP (early)
Decreasing systolic BP (later)
Tachycardia (>100 bpm)
Tachypnea (>20 breaths/min)
Anxiety (early)
Confusion, lethargy, coma (later)
Delayed capillary refill (≥2 sec)
Cool, pale skin
Low or decreasing CVP
Low urinary output (<30 ml/hr)

BP, Blood pressure; *CVP,* central venous pressure.

- Measure CVP q1-4hr if indicated. Be alert to low or decreasing values. Report sudden decreases in CVP, especially if associated with other indicators of fluid volume deficit, as just noted.
- Measure urinary output q4hr (or when patient voids). Be alert to decreasing urinary output and to infrequent voidings. Low urine output usually reflects inadequate intravascular volume in the abdominal trauma patient. Before administering diuretics, evaluate patient for evidence of fluid volume deficit, as just noted.
- Estimate ongoing blood loss. Measure all bloody drainage from drainage tubes or catheters, noting drainage color (e.g., coffee ground, burgundy, bright red). Monitor for, and measure when possible, bloody stools. Note the frequency of dressing changes because of saturation with blood to estimate amount of blood lost via wound site. Note and report significant increases in the amount of drainage, especially if it is bloody.

NIC: Bleeding Precautions; Fluid/Electrolyte Management; Hemorrhage Control; Hypovolemia Management; Intravenous (IV) Therapy; Shock Management: Volume; Tube Care

Pain related to irritation caused by intraperitoneal blood or secretions, actual trauma or surgical incision, and manipulation of organs during surgery
Desired outcomes:　Within 4 hr of admission, patient's subjective perception of pain decreases, as documented by a pain scale. Nonverbal indicators, such as grimacing, are absent or diminished.
- Evaluate patient for presence of preoperative and postoperative pain. Devise a pain scale with patient, rating discomfort from 0 (no pain) to 10 (worst pain). Preoperative pain is anticipated and is a vital diagnostic aid. The location and character of postoperative pain also can be important. Incisional and some visceral pain can be anticipated, but intense or prolonged pain, especially when accompanied by other peritoneal signs (see Table 6-8), can signal bleeding, bowel infarction, infection, or other complications. Recognize that the autonomic nervous system (ANS) response to pain can complicate assessment of abdominal injury and hypovolemia. For details, see **Pain,** p. 719, in Appendix One.
- Administer analgesics as prescribed. Avoid administering analgesics preoperatively until the patient has been evaluated thoroughly by a trauma surgeon. Administer postoperatively prescribed analgesics on a continual or regular schedule promptly with additional analgesia as needed, or provide patient with patient-controlled analgesia (PCA). Analgesics are helpful in relieving pain as well as aiding the recovery process by promoting greater ventilatory excursion. Encourage the patient to request analgesic before pain becomes severe.

- Be aware that intoxication often is involved in traumatic events; therefore victims may be drug or alcohol users, with a higher-than-average tolerance for opioids, requiring adjusted dosage. These same individuals may suffer symptoms of alcohol withdrawal (tremors, weakness, tachycardia, elevated BP, delusions, agitation, hallucinations) or narcotic withdrawal (lacrimation, rhinorrhea, anxiety, tremors, muscle twitching, mydriasis, nausea, abdominal cramps, vomiting) that need recognition and treatment. In addition, recognize that narcotic analgesics can decrease GI motility and may delay return to normal bowel function. Document the degree of relief obtained, using the pain scale.
- Monitor PCA, if prescribed, and document effectiveness, using the pain scale.
- Supplement analgesics with nonpharmacologic maneuvers (e.g., positioning, back rubs, distraction) to aid in pain reduction. Provide these instructions to the patient and family members.

NIC: Analgesic Administration; Environmental Management: Comfort; Medication Management; Pain Management; Patient-Controlled Analgesia (PCA) Assistance; Surveillance

Risk for infection with risk factors related to inadequate primary defenses secondary to disruption of the GI tract (particularly of the terminal ileum and colon) and traumatically inflicted open wound; multiple indwelling catheters and drainage tubes; and compromised immune state caused by blood loss and metabolic response to trauma

Desired outcome: Patient is free of infection as evidenced by core or rectal temperature <37.7° C (100° F); HR ≤100 bpm; no significant changes in mental status and orientation to person, place, and time; and absence of unusual erythema, edema, tenderness, warmth, or drainage at surgical incisions or wound sites.

- Monitor VS for evidence of infection, noting temperature increases and associated increases in heart and respiratory rates. Notify health care provider of sudden temperature elevations.
- Evaluate mental status, orientation, and LOC q8hr. Note mental status changes, confusion, or deterioration from baseline LOC.
- Ensure patency of all surgically placed tubes or drains. Irrigate or attach to low-pressure suction as prescribed. Maintain continuity of closed drainage systems; use sterile technique when emptying drainage and recharging suction containers. Promptly report unrelieved loss of tube patency.
- Evaluate incisions and wound sites for evidence of infection: unusual erythema, warmth, tenderness, edema, delayed healing, and purulent or unusual drainage.
- Note amount, color, character, and odor of all drainage (Table 6-11). Report the presence of foul-smelling or abnormal drainage. Test drainage for pH and the presence of blood; compare with expected characteristics.
- Administer antibiotics in a timely fashion. Reschedule parenteral antibiotics if a dose is delayed more than 1 hr. Recognize that failure to administer antibiotics on schedule may result in inadequate blood levels and treatment failure.
- As prescribed, administer pneumococcal vaccine to patients with total splenectomy to minimize the risk of postsplenectomy sepsis.
- Administer tetanus immune globulin and tetanus toxoid as prescribed (see Table 6-9).
- Change dressings as prescribed, using sterile technique. Prevent cross contamination from various wounds by changing one dressing at a time.
- Use drains, closed drainage systems, or drainage bags to remove and collect GI secretions and avoid contamination of the surgical incision site.
- If patient has or develops evisceration, do not reinsert tissue or organs. Place a sterile, saline-soaked gauze over the evisceration, and cover with a sterile

TABLE 6-11 Characteristics of Gastrointestinal Drainage

Source	Composition and usual character
Mouth and oropharynx	Saliva; thin, clear, watery; pH 7.0
Stomach	Hydrochloric, gastrin, pepsin, mucus; thin, brownish to greenish; acidic
Pancreas	Enzymes and bicarbonate; thin, watery, yellowish brown; alkaline; usually abundant after surgery
Biliary tract	Bile, including bile salts and electrolytes; bright yellow to brownish green
Duodenum	Digestive enzymes, mucus, products of digestion; thin, bright yellow to light brown, may be greenish; alkaline
Jejunum	Enzymes, mucus, products of digestion; brown, watery with particles
Ileum	Enzymes, mucus, digestive products, greater amounts of bacteria; brown, liquid feculent
Colon	Digestive products, mucus, large amounts of bacteria; brown to dark brown, semiformed to firm stool
Postoperative (GI surgery)	Initial drainage expected to contain fresh blood; later drainage mixed with old blood and then approaches normal composition
Infection present	Drainage cloudy, may be thicker than usual; strong or unusual odor; drain site often erythematous and warm

GI, Gastrointestinal.

towel until the evisceration can be evaluated by the surgeon. Keep the patient on bedrest with the bed in semi-Fowler's position with the knees bent. Maintain NPO status for patient, and anticipate the need for emergency surgery.

NIC: Infection Control; Infection Protection; Neurologic Monitoring; Surveillance; Tube Care; Vital Signs Monitoring; Wound Care; Wound Care: Closed Drainage

Ineffective breathing pattern related to pain from injury or surgical incision; chemical irritation of blood or bile on pleural tissue; and diaphragmatic elevation caused by abdominal distention
Desired outcome: Within 24 hr of admission or surgery, patient is eupneic with RR 12-20 breaths/min and clear breath sounds.
- Administer supplemental oxygen as prescribed. Monitor and document effectiveness.
- Administer analgesics at dose and frequency that relieves pain and associated impaired chest excursion.
- Encourage and assist patient with coughing, deep breathing, incentive spirometry, and turning q2-4hr, and note quality of breath sounds, cough, and sputum.
- Instruct patient in methods to splint the abdomen to reduce pain on movement, coughing, and deep breathing.
- Monitor oximetry readings q2-4hr, and report O_2 saturation <92%.
- For additional interventions, see **Ineffective breathing pattern,** p. 729, in Appendix One, "Caring for Preoperative and Postoperative Patients."

NIC: Bedside Laboratory Testing; Respiratory Monitoring; Teaching: Individual

Altered gastrointestinal tissue perfusion (or risk for same) related to interrupted blood flow to abdominal viscera secondary to vascular disruption or occlusion or related to moderate to severe hypovolemia caused by hemorrhage
Desired outcomes: Patient has adequate GI tissue perfusion as evidenced by normoactive bowel sounds; soft, nondistended abdomen; and return of bowel elimination. Gastric secretions, drainage, and excretions are negative for occult blood.

- Auscultate for bowel sounds hourly in recently injured patients and q8hr during the recovery phase. Report prolonged or sudden absence of bowel sounds because these signs may signal bowel ischemia or infarction. Anticipate absent or diminished bowel sounds for up to 72 hr after surgery.
- Evaluate patient for peritoneal signs (see Table 6-8), which may occur acutely secondary to injury or may not develop until days or weeks later if complications caused by slow bleeding or other mechanisms occur.
- Ensure adequate intravascular volume (see discussion in **Fluid volume deficit,** p. 469).
- Evaluate laboratory data for evidence of bleeding (e.g., serial Hct) or organ ischemia (e.g., SGPT, SGOT, LDH). Optimal values are Hct >30%; SGOT (AST) 5-40 IU/L; SGPT (ALT) 5-35 IU/L; and LDH 90-200 IU/ml.
- Document amount and character of GI secretions, drainage, and excretions. Note changes suggestive of bleeding (presence of frank or occult blood), infection (e.g., increased or purulent drainage), or obstruction (e.g., failure to eliminate flatus or stool within 72 hr after surgery).

NIC: Bowel Management; Intravenous (IV) Therapy; Laboratory Data Interpretation; Vital Signs Monitoring

Risk for impaired skin integrity related to risk of exposure to irritating GI drainage; *and*
Impaired tissue integrity (or risk for same) related to direct trauma and surgery, catabolic posttraumatic state, and altered circulation
Desired outcome: Patient exhibits wound healing by time of hospital discharge, and the skin remains nonerythemic and unbroken.

- Promptly change all dressings that become soiled with drainage or blood.
- Protect the skin surrounding tubes, drains, or fistulas, keeping the areas clean and free from drainage. Gastric and intestinal secretions and drainage are irritating and can lead to skin excoriation. If necessary, apply ointments, skin barriers, or drainage bags to protect the surrounding skin. Apply reusable dressing supports such as Montgomery straps or Surginet gauze to prevent excessive injury to the surrounding skin. Consult ET nurse for complex or involved cases.
- Inspect wounds, fistulas, and drain sites for signs of irritation, infection, and ischemia.
- Identify infected and devitalized tissue. Aid in their removal by irrigation, wound packing, or preparing patient for surgical debridement.
- Ensure adequate protein and calorie intake for tissue healing (see **Altered nutrition** below).
- For more information, see "Managing Wound Care," p. 704.

NIC: NIC: Diet Staging; Incision Site Care; Ostomy Care; Skin Care: Topical Treatments; Skin Surveillance; Wound Care; Wound Irrigation

Altered nutrition: Less than body requirements related to decreased intake secondary to disruption of GI tract integrity (traumatic or surgical) and increased need secondary to hypermetabolic posttrauma state
Desired outcome: By at least 24 hr before hospital discharge, patient has adequate nutrition as evidenced by maintenance of baseline body weight and positive or balanced nitrogen (N) state.

- Collaborate with health care provider, dietitian, and pharmacist to estimate patient's metabolic needs, based on type of injury, activity level, and nutritional status before injury.
- Consider patient's specific injuries when planning nutrition (e.g., expect patients with hepatic or pancreatic injury to have difficulty with blood sugar regulation; patients with trauma to the upper GI tract may be fed enterally, but feeding tube must be placed distal to the injury; disruption of the GI tract may require feeding gastrostomy or jejunostomy; patients with major hepatic trauma may have difficulty with protein tolerance).
- Ensure patency of gastric or intestinal tubes to maintain decompression and encourage healing and return of bowel function. Avoid occlusion of the vent side of sump suction tubes because this may result in vacuum occlusion of the tube and excessive suction to gastric mucosa. Use caution and consult surgeon before irrigating NG or other tubes that have been placed in or near recently sutured organs.
- Confirm placement of feeding tube before each tube feeding. After initial insertion, check x-ray for position of feeding tube. Insufflation with air and aspiration of stomach contents do not always confirm placement of small-bore feeding tubes. Mark to determine tube migration, secure tubing in place, and reassess q4hr and before each feeding. Assess aspirate for pH <5 for gastric tube placement.
- Do not start enteral feeding until bowel function returns (i.e., bowel sounds are present, patient experiences hunger).
- Recognize that opioid analgesics decrease GI motility and may contribute to nausea, vomiting, abdominal distention, and ileus. Consider administration of prescribed nonnarcotic analgesics (e.g., ketorolac).
- For more information, see "Providing Nutritional Support," p. 687.

NIC: Diet Staging; Enteral Tube Feeding; Gastrointestinal Intubation; Nutrition Management; Total Parenteral Nutrition (TPN) Administration

Posttrauma response related to life-threatening accident or event resulting in trauma

Desired outcomes: By at least 24 hr before hospital discharge, patient verbalizes that the psychosocial impact of the event has abated, and he or she does not exhibit signs of severe stress reaction, such as display of inconsistent affect, suicidal or homicidal behavior, or extreme agitation or depression. Patient cooperates with treatment plan.

> **Note:** Many victims of major abdominal trauma sustain life-threatening injury. The patient is often aware of the situation and fears death. Even after the physical condition stabilizes, the patient may have a prolonged or severe reaction triggered by recollection of the trauma.

- Evaluate mental status at regular intervals. Be alert to indicators of severe stress reaction, such as display of affect inconsistent with statements or behavior, suicidal or homicidal statements or actions, extreme agitation or depression, and failure to cooperate with instructions related to care.
- Consult specialists such as psychologist, psychiatric nurse clinician, or pastoral counselor if patient displays signs of severe stress reaction described previously.
- Consider organic causes that may contribute to posttraumatic response (e.g., severe pain, alcohol intoxication or withdrawal, electrolyte imbalance, metabolic encephalopathy, impaired cerebral perfusion).
- For other psychosocial interventions, see Appendix One, "Caring for Patients With Cancer and Other Life-disrupting Illnesses," p. 791.

NIC: Anxiety Reduction; Coping Enhancement; Crisis Intervention; Emotional Support; Security Enhancement; Suicide Prevention

See Also: "Fecal Diversions," p. 457; Appendix One, "Caring for Preoperative and Postoperative Patients," p. 717; "Caring for Patients on Prolonged Bedrest," p. 738; "Caring for Patients With Cancer and Other Life-disrupting Illnesses," p. 747, for nursing diagnoses and interventions.

PATIENT-FAMILY TEACHING AND DISCHARGE PLANNING

Anticipate extended physical and emotional rehabilitation for the patient and significant other. When providing patient-family teaching, focus on sensory information; avoid giving excessive information; and initiate a visiting nurse referral for necessary follow-up teaching. Consider including verbal and written information about the following:

- Probable need for emotional care, even for patients who have not required extensive physical rehabilitation. Provide referrals to support groups for trauma patients and family members.
- Availability of rehabilitation programs, extended care facilities, and home health agencies for patients unable to accomplish self-care on hospital discharge.
- Availability of rehabilitation programs for substance abuse, as indicated. Immediately after the traumatic event, the patient and family members are very impressionable, making this period an ideal time for the substance abuser to begin to resolve the problem.
- Medications, including drug name, purpose, dosage, schedule, precautions, drug/drug and food/drug interactions, and potential side effects. Encourage patients taking antibiotics to take the medications for the prescribed length of time, even though they may be asymptomatic. If patient received tetanus immunization, ensure that he or she receives a wallet-size card documenting the immunization.
- Wound and catheter care. Have patient or caregiver describe and demonstrate proper technique before hospital discharge.
- Importance of seeking medical attention if indicators of infection or bowel obstruction occur (e.g., fever, severe or unusual abdominal pain, nausea and vomiting, unusual drainage from wounds or incisions, a change in bowel habits).
- Injury prevention. Immediately after a traumatic injury, the patient and family members are especially likely to respond to injury prevention education. Provide instructions on proper seat-belt applications (across the pelvic girdle rather than across soft tissue of the lower abdomen), safety for infants and children, and other factors suitable for the individuals involved.

Section Five: Hepatic and Biliary Disorders

The liver lies directly beneath the diaphragm and occupies most of the RUQ of the abdomen. It has many functions, among them the storage of vitamins, synthesis of blood proteins (including albumen and many clotting factors), conjugation of the sex hormones, destruction of worn-out red blood cells, removal of toxic substances from the body, and management of the formation and secretion of bile.

The gallbladder, which lies directly beneath the right lobe of the liver, and the hepatic, cystic, and common bile ducts make up the biliary system. The biliary duct system transports bile from the liver to the gallbladder. Bile is concentrated and stored in the gallbladder and released to the small intestine (duodenum), where it facilitates the breakdown of fats, fat-soluble vitamins, and certain minerals and also activates the release of pancreatic enzymes. If an obstructive lesion is present in the biliary ducts, the flow of bile is blocked, eventually resulting in its backup into the bloodstream in the form of bilirubin. When this occurs, a variety of clinical manifestations can surface, including jaundice, dark-amber urine, and clay-colored stools. Pruritus occurs because the bile salts begin to be excreted through the skin. Steatorrhea and bleeding tendencies result from the inability of the duodenum to absorb fats and fat-soluble vitamins A, D, E, and K. Vitamin K is necessary for adequate clotting of the blood.

Hepatitis

Viral hepatitis may be caused by one of five viruses that are capable of infecting the liver: A (HAV), B (HBV), C (HCV), D (HDV), or E (HEV). Although symptomatology is similar, immunologic and epidemiologic characteristics are different (Table 6-12). When hepatocytes are damaged, necrosis and autolysis can occur, which in turn lead to abnormal liver functioning. Generally these changes are completely reversible after the acute phase. In some cases, however, massive necrosis can lead to acute liver failure and death.

Chronic hepatitis is inflammation of the liver for more than 6 mo. The term is used to describe a spectrum of inflammatory liver diseases ranging from mild chronic persistent hepatitis to severe chronic active hepatitis. Forms of chronic hepatitis are associated with infection from HBV, HCV, or HDV; viral infections such as cytomegalovirus (CMV); excessive alcohol consumption; inflammatory bowel disease; and autoimmunity (chronic active lupoid hepatitis). *Alcoholic hepatitis* occurs as a result of tissue necrosis caused by alcohol abuse. Generally it is a precursor to cirrhosis (see p. 484), but it may occur simultaneous with cirrhosis.

Jaundice is discoloration of body tissues from increased serum levels of bilirubin (total serum bilirubin >2.5 mg/dl). Jaundice may be seen in any patient with impaired hepatic function and occurs as the bilirubin begins to be excreted through the skin. There is also an increased excretion of urobilinogen and bilirubin by the kidneys, resulting in darker, almost brownish, urine. Jaundice is classified as follows.

Prehepatic (hemolytic):   Caused by increased production of bilirubin following erythrocyte destruction. Prehepatic jaundice is implicated when the indirect (unconjugated) serum bilirubin is >0.8 mg/dl.

Hepatic (hepatocellular):   Caused by the dysfunction of the liver cells (hepatocytes), which reduces their ability to remove bilirubin from the blood and form it into bile. Hepatic jaundice is also implicated with indirect serum bilirubin and is associated with hepatitis.

Posthepatic (obstructive):   Caused by an obstruction of the flow of bile out of the liver and resulting in backed-up bile through the hepatocytes to the blood. Posthepatic jaundice is implicated when the direct serum bilirubin is >0.3 mg/dl.

ASSESSMENT

Signs and symptoms: Nausea, vomiting, malaise, anorexia, muscle or joint aches, fatigue, irritability, slight to moderate temperature increases, epigastric discomfort, dark urine, clay-colored stools, pruritus, aversion to smoking.

Acute hepatic failure: Nausea, vomiting, and abdominal pain tend to be more severe. Jaundice is likely to appear earlier and deepen more rapidly. Mental status changes (possibly progressing to encephalopathy), coma, seizures, ascites, sharp rise in temperature, significant leukocytosis, coffee-ground emesis, GI hemorrhage, purpura, shock, oliguria, and azotemia all may be present.

Physical assessment: Presence of jaundice; palpation of lymph nodes and abdomen may reveal lymphadenopathy, hepatomegaly, and splenomegaly. Liver size usually is small with acute hepatic failure.

TABLE 6-12 Types and Characteristics of Viral Hepatitis

	Hepatitis A virus (HAV)	Hepatitis B virus (HBV)	Hepatitis C virus (HCV)	Hepatitis D virus (HDV)	Hepatitis E virus (HEV)
Likely modes of transmission	Fecal-oral; food-borne most common; parenteral transmission rare; most infectious 2 wk before symptoms appear	Contact with blood or serum; sexual contact; perinatal transmission; often transmitted by chronic carriers; most infectious before symptoms appear and for 4-6 mo after acute infection	Contact with blood or serum; perinatal transmission rare unless mother is HIV infected; often transmitted by chronic carriers; most infectious 1-2 wk before symptoms appear and throughout acute infection	Similar to HBV; can cause infection only if individual already has HBV; blood infectious throughout HDV infection	Fecal-oral; foodborne; waterborne

Continued

From Keen JH: Gastrointestinal disorders. In Swearingen PL, editor: *Pocket guide to medical-surgical nursing*, ed 2, St Louis, 1996, Mosby. *HIV*, Human immunodeficiency virus; *IgG*, immunoglobulin G; *HBsAg*, hepatitis B surface antigen; *HBeAg*, hepatitis B early antigen; *IgM*, immunoglobulin M; *HBcAg*, hepatitis B core antigen; *HBIG*, hepatitis B immune globulin; *CDC*, Centers for Disease Control and Prevention.

TABLE 6-12 Types and Characteristics of Viral Hepatitis—cont'd

	Hepatitis A virus (HAV)	Hepatitis B virus (HBV)	Hepatitis C virus (HCV)	Hepatitis D virus (HDV)	Hepatitis E virus (HEV)
Population most often affected	Children; individuals living in or traveling to areas with poor sanitation	Injecting drug users; health care and public safety workers exposed to blood; patients and staff of institutions for the developmentally disabled; homosexual men; men and women with multiple heterosexual partners; young children of infected mothers; recipients of certain blood products; hemodialysis patients	Injecting drug users; individuals who received blood products before 1991; potential risk to health care and public safety workers exposed to blood	Injecting drug users; hemophiliacs; recipients of multiple blood transfusions (infects only individuals who already have HBV)	People living in or traveling to parts of Asia, Africa, or Mexico where sanitation is poor
Incubation	2-6 wk	6 wk–6 mo	18-180 days	Varies; not well established	

Serum markers of acute infection	Antibody to HAV (anti-HAV); IgG-class antibody to HAV (IgG anti-HAV) indicates immunity	HBsAg; HBeAG; IgM-class antibody to HBcAg (IgM anti-HBc)	Only test available is antibody to HCV (anti-HCV), which detects chronic but not acute cases	Antibody to HDV (anti-HDV)
Measures for reducing exposure	Hand washing; good personal hygiene; sanitation; appropriate infection control measures (see Appendix Two)	Hand washing; good personal hygiene; appropriate infection control measures (see Appendix Two), autoclaving of all nondisposable items; careful handling of needles and sharps; ensuring that needles are not reused and are discarded carefully in special containers	Same as for HBV	Same as for HBV
				Same as for HAV

Continued

T A B L E   6 - 1 2   Types and Characteristics of Viral Hepatitis—cont'd

	Hepatitis A virus (HAV)	Hepatitis B virus (HBV)	Hepatitis C virus (HCV)	Hepatitis D virus (HDV)	Hepatitis E virus (HEV)
Prophylaxis	Sanitation measures; immunization; immunoglobulin within 1-2 wk after exposure	Screening of donated blood; protective devices for providers and immunization for all health care workers who come in contact with blood, as well as for risk groups noted above; use of condoms; HBIG for known exposure to HBsAg-contaminated material; also, CDC recommends routine immunization of all children	Screening of donated blood; protective devices for health care providers; no vaccine exists for HCV	Immunization against HBV	Effectiveness of immunoglobulin manufactured in the United States is not known
Comments	Symptoms usually mild; rarely causes fulminant hepatic failure	HBsAg persists in carrier state; chronic hepatitis may develop; fulminant hepatic failure may result	Carrier state and chronic hepatitis may develop; fulminant hepatic failure may result	Increased risk of serious complications (including fulminant hepatic failure) and death; carrier state and chronic hepatitis may develop	Disease is not endemic in United States or western Europe

From Keen JH: Gastrointestinal disorders. In Swearingen PL, editor: *Pocket guide to medical-surgical nursing*, ed 2, St Louis, 1996, Mosby.
HIV, Human immunodeficiency virus; *IgG,* immunoglobulin G; *HBsAg,* hepatitis B surface antigen; *HBeAg,* hepatitis B early antigen; *IgM,* immunoglobulin M; *HBcAg,* hepatitis B core antigen; *HBIG,* hepatitis B immune globulin; *CDC,* Centers for Disease Control and Prevention.

History of: Clotting disorders, multiple blood transfusions, excessive alcohol ingestion, parenteral drug use, exposure to hepatotoxic chemicals or medications, travel to developing countries.

DIAGNOSTIC TESTS

Hematologic tests: Anti-HAV immunoglobulin M (IgM) is present with HAV, as is hepatitis B surface antigen (HBsAg) with HAV. Anti-HCV is present approximately 15 wk after infection with HCV. Serum glutamic-oxaloacetic transaminase (SGOT; aspartate aminotransferase [AST]) and serum glutamic-pyruvic transaminase (SGPT; alanine aminotransferase [ALT]) are elevated initially and then drop. Total bilirubin is elevated, and prothrombin time (PT) is prolonged. Differential WBC count reveals leukocytosis, monocytosis, and atypical lymphocytes; γ-globulin levels are increased.

Urine tests: Reveal elevation of urobilinogen, mild proteinuria, and mild bilirubinuria.

Liver biopsy: Performed percutaneously or via laparoscopy to collect a specimen for histologic examination to confirm differential diagnosis.

COLLABORATIVE MANAGEMENT

Monitoring of activity level: Bedrest may be indicated when symptoms are severe, with a gradual return to normal activity as symptoms subside.

Diet: In general, dietary management consists of giving palatable meals as tolerated without overfeeding. If oral intake is substantially decreased, parenteral or enteral nutrition may be initiated. Na^+ restrictions may be indicated in the presence of fluid retention. Protein is moderately restricted, or eliminated, depending on the degree of mental status changes (i.e., encephalopathy). If no mental status changes are noted, normal amounts of high biologic value protein are indicated to facilitate tissue healing. All alcoholic beverages are strictly forbidden. Vitamins usually are given, and folic acid may be indicated in alcoholic hepatitis.

Management of pruritus: Alkaline soaps are restricted; emollients and lipid creams (i.e., Eucerin) are prescribed. Antihistamines and tranquilizers, if used, are administered with caution and in low doses because they are metabolized by the liver. See Table 6-13 for a list of hepatotoxic drugs.

Pharmacotherapy

Parenteral vitamin K: For patients with prolonged PT. **Note:** Patients with severe hepatic failure may not respond to vitamin K and require transfusions of fresh frozen plasma.

Antihistamines (e.g., diphenhydramine): For symptomatic relief of pruritus. However, they may cause excessive sedation.

Antiemetics (e.g., hydroxyzine, ondansetron): For patients with nausea. Avoid phenothiazines, such as prochlorperazine (Compazine), because they cause excessive sedation.

Immune globulin (IG): Given routinely to all close personal contacts of patients with HAV.

Hepatitis B immune globulin (HBIG): Recommended for individuals exposed to HBsAg-contaminated material.

HAV vaccine: Recommended for people with potential for exposure to HAV (i.e., persons who travel to areas where it is endemic, such as eastern Asia).

HBV vaccines: Developed for prevention of hepatitis, they reduce the incidence of HBV by approximately 92%. Immunization is recommended for all health care workers and others with risk of exposure to blood and body secretions. Health departments in some states have begun to recommend childhood immunizations with HBV vaccine.

Corticosteroids: Used in some patients to control symptomatology and reduce abnormal liver function.

Recombinant interferon: An antiviral agent that inhibits viral replication.

Restriction of hepatotoxic drugs: See Table 6-13.

TABLE 6-13   Drugs That Can Cause Hepatotoxicity

Prescription drugs
  Allopurinol
  Amiodarone
  Androgenic steroids
  Carbamazepine
  Carmustine (BCNU)
  Chlorpromazine (CPZ)
  Cyclosporine
  Dantrolene
  Diazepam
  Erythromycin
  Glucocorticoids
  Haloperidol
  Halothane (and related anesthetics)
  Isoniazid (INH)
  Ketoconazole
  Mercaptopurine (6-MP)
  Methotrexate (MTX)
  Methyldopa
  Mitomycin
  Monoamine oxidase (MAO) inhibitors
  Oral contraceptives
  Oxacillin
  Phenindione
  Phenylbutazone
  Phenytoin sodium
  Rifampin
  Sulfonamides
Nonprescription drugs
  Acetaminophen
  Alcohol
  Aspirin and other salicylates
  NSAIDs
  Vitamin A

NSAIDs, Nonsteroidal antiinflammatory drugs.

NURSING DIAGNOSES AND INTERVENTIONS

Fatigue related to decreased metabolic energy production secondary to liver dysfunction, which causes faulty absorption, metabolism, and storage of nutrients
Desired outcome: By at least 24 hr before hospital discharge, patient relates decreasing fatigue and increasing energy.
- Take a diet history to determine food preferences. Encourage significant other to bring in desirable foods if permitted.
- Monitor and record intake.
- Encourage small, frequent feedings, and provide emotional support during meals. Consult dietitian regarding increased intake of carbohydrates or other high-energy food sources within prescribed dietary limitations.
- Obtain prescription for vitamin and mineral supplements if appropriate.

- Provide rest periods of at least 90 min before and after activities and treatments. Avoid activity immediately after meals.
- Keep frequently used objects within easy reach.
- Promote rest and sleep by decreasing environmental stimuli, providing back massage and relaxation tapes, and speaking with patient in short, simple terms.
- Administer acid suppression therapy (see Table 6-1), antiemetics, antidiarrheal medications, and cathartics as prescribed to minimize gastric distress and promote absorption of nutrients.

NIC: Environmental Management: Comfort; Medication Management; Nutrition Therapy; Simple Relaxation Therapy; Sleep Enhancement

Knowledge deficit: Causes of hepatitis and modes of transmission
Desired outcome: Within the 24-hr period before hospital discharge, patient verbalizes knowledge about the causes of hepatitis and measures that help prevent transmission.

- Assess patient's knowledge about the disease process, and educate as necessary (see Table 6-12). Make sure patient knows you are not making moral judgments about alcohol/drug use or sexual behavior.
- Teach patient and significant other the importance of good handwashing and of wearing gloves if contact with feces is possible.
- If appropriate, advise patients with HAV that crowded living conditions with poor sanitation should be avoided to prevent recurrence.
- Remind patients with HBV and HCV that they should modify sexual behavior as directed by health care provider. Explain that blood donation is no longer possible.
- Advise patients with HBV that their sexual partners should receive HBV vaccine.
- Refer patient to drug treatment programs as necessary.

NIC: Health Education; Learning Readiness Enhancement; Teaching: Disease Process; Teaching: Prescribed Medication; Teaching: Safe Sex

Risk for impaired skin integrity with risk factors related to pruritus secondary to hepatic dysfunction
Desired outcome: Patient's skin remains intact.

- Keep patient's skin moist by using tepid water or emollient baths, avoiding alkaline soap, and applying emollient lotions at frequent intervals.
- Encourage patient not to scratch skin and to keep nails short and smooth. Suggest use of the knuckles if patient must scratch. Wrap or place gloves on patient's hands (especially comatose patients).
- To prevent infection, treat any skin lesion promptly.
- Administer antihistamines as prescribed; observe closely for excessive sedation.
- Encourage patient to wear loose, soft clothing; provide soft linens (cotton is best).
- Keep the environment cool.
- Change soiled linen as soon as possible.

NIC: Bathing; Environmental Management; Skin Care: Topical Treatments; Skin Surveillance

Altered protection related to increased risk of bleeding secondary to decreased vitamin K absorption, thrombocytopenia
Desired outcome: Patient is free of bleeding as evidenced by negative tests for occult blood in the feces and urine, absence of ecchymotic areas, and absence of bleeding at the gums and injection sites.

- Monitor PT levels daily for increases; optimal range is 10.5-13.5 sec.
- Monitor platelet count daily for thrombocytopenia; optimal range is 150,000-400,000/mm^3.

- Monitor Hct and Hgb daily for decreases that may indicate occult bleeding; optimal ranges are Hct 40%-54% (male) and 37%-47% (female), Hgb 14-18 g/dl (male) and 12-16 g/dl (female).
- Handle patient gently (e.g., when turning or transferring).
- Minimize IM injections. Rotate sites, and use small-gauge needles. Apply moderate pressure after an injection, but do not massage the site. Administer medications orally or intravenously when possible.
- Observe for ecchymotic areas. Inspect the gums, and test the urine and feces for bleeding. Report significant findings to health care provider.
- Teach patient to use electric razor and soft-bristle toothbrush.
- Administer vitamin K as prescribed.

NIC: Bleeding Precautions; Laboratory Data Interpretation; Medication Administration

---

See Also: "Cirrhosis" for **Altered protection,** p. 492, if the patient develops encephalopathy.

PATIENT-FAMILY TEACHING AND DISCHARGE PLANNING

When providing patient-family teaching, focus on sensory information; avoid giving excessive information; and initiate a visiting nurse referral for necessary follow-up teaching. Consider including verbal and written information about the following:

- Importance of rest and getting adequate nutrition. When appropriate, provide a list of high biologic value protein food sources or protein foods to avoid and sample menus to demonstrate how these foods may be incorporated into or excluded from the diet. Instruct patient to eat frequent, small meals, to eat slowly, and to chew all food thoroughly. Teach the patient to rest for 30-60 min after meals.
- Importance of avoiding hepatotoxic agents, including OTC drugs (see Table 6-13).
- Prescribed medications (e.g., multivitamins), including drug name, purpose, dosage, schedule, drug/drug and food/drug interactions, potential side effects, and precautions.
- Importance of informing health care providers, dentists, and other health care workers of hepatitis diagnosis.
- Potential complications, including delayed healing, skin injury, and bleeding tendencies.
- Importance of avoiding alcohol during recovery.
- Referral to alcohol/drug treatment programs as appropriate.

Cirrhosis

Cirrhosis is a chronic, serious disease in which normal configuration of the liver is changed, resulting in cell death. When new cells are formed, the resulting scarring causes disruption of blood and lymph flow. Although pathologic changes do not occur for many years, structural changes gradually lead to total liver dysfunction. Manifestations of cirrhosis are related to hepatocellular necrosis and portal hypertension. Complications caused by cellular failure are similar to those of acute hepatitis and include inability to metabolize bilirubin and resultant jaundice; difficulty producing serum proteins, including albumin and certain clotting factors; hyperdynamic circulation and decreased vasomotor tone; pulmonary changes (ventilation-perfusion [V/Q] mismatch) and sometimes cyanosis; changes in nitrogen (N) metabolism (e.g., inability to convert ammonia to urea); and difficulty metabolizing some hormones (especially the sex hormones). Complications related to portal hypertension include development of ascites, bleeding esophageal and gastric varices, portal-systemic collaterals, encephalopathy, and splenomegaly.

Alcoholic (Laennec's) cirrhosis: Associated with long-term alcohol abuse; accounts for 50% of all cases. Changes in liver structure caused by cirrhosis are irreversible, but compensation of liver function can be achieved if the liver is protected from further damage by alcohol cessation and proper nutrition. The histologic definition of this form of cirrhosis is micronodular cirrhosis.

Postnecrotic cirrhosis: Associated with history of viral hepatitis or hepatic damage from drugs or toxins; accounts for 20% of all cases. This type appears to predispose the patient to the development of a hepatoma. The histologic definition of this form of cirrhosis is macronodular cirrhosis.

Biliary cirrhosis: Associated with chronic retention of bile and inflammation of bile ducts; accounts for 15% of all cases. The histologic definition of this form of cirrhosis is mixed nodular cirrhosis; it may be further classified as follows:

Primary biliary cirrhosis (nonsuppurative destructive cholangitis):   Results from cholestasis from an unknown cause. This progressive disease has other findings, including steatorrhea, xanthomatous (yellow tumors) neuropathy, osteomalacia, and portal hypertension.

Secondary biliary cirrhosis: Results from chronic obstruction to bile flow, usually from an obstruction outside the liver, such as calculi, neoplasms, or biliary atresia.

ASSESSMENT

Signs and symptoms: Weakness, fatigability, weight loss, fever, anorexia, nausea, occasional vomiting, abdominal pain, diarrhea, menstrual abnormalities, sterility, impotence, loss of libido, hematemesis. Urine may be dark (brownish) because of the presence of urobilinogen, and stools may be pale and clay colored because of the absence of bilirubin.

Physical assessment: Jaundice, hepatomegaly, ascites, peripheral edema, pleural effusion, and fetor hepaticus (a musty, sweetish odor on the breath). There may be slight changes in personality and behavior, which can progress to coma (a result of hepatic encephalopathy); spider angiomas, testicular atrophy, gynecomastia, pectoral and axillary alopecia (a result of hormonal changes); splenomegaly; hemorrhoids (a result of portal hypertension complications); spider nevi; purpuric lesions; and palmar erythema. Asterixis may be present in advanced cirrhosis, that is, jerking movements of the hands and wrists when the wrists are dorsiflexed with the fingers extended.

History of: Excessive alcohol ingestion; hepatitis B, C, or D infection; exposure to hepatotoxic drugs (see Table 6-13) or chemicals; biliary or metabolic disease; poor nutrition.

DIAGNOSTIC TESTS

Hematologic: RBCs are decreased in hypersplenism and decreased with hemorrhage. WBCs are decreased with hypersplenism and increased with infection. Platelet counts are less than normal.

Serum biochemical tests

Bilirubin levels: Elevated because of failure in hepatocyte metabolism and obstruction in some instances. Very high or persistently elevated levels are considered a poor prognostic sign.

Alkaline phosphatase levels: Normal to mildly elevated.

Serum glutamic-oxaloacetic transaminase (SGOT; aspartate aminotransferase [AST]) and serum glutamic-pyruvic transaminase (SGPT; alanine aminotransferase [ALT]) levels: Usually elevated >300 U with acute failure. Normal or mildly elevated with chronic failure. SGPT (ALT) is more specific for hepatocellular damage.

Albumin levels: Reduced, especially with ascites. Persistently low levels suggest a poor prognosis.

Na$^+$ levels: Normal to low. Na$^+$ is retained but is associated with water retention, which results in normal serum Na$^+$ levels or even a dilutional hyponatremia. Often severe hyponatremia is present in the terminal stage and is associated with tense ascites and hepatorenal syndrome.

K$^+$ levels: Slightly reduced unless patient has renal insufficiency, which would result in hyperkalemia. Chronic hypokalemic acidosis is common in patients with chronic alcoholic liver disease.

Glucose levels: Hypoglycemia possible because of impaired gluconeogenesis and glycogen depletion in patients with severe or terminal liver disease.

BUN levels: May be slightly decreased because of failure of Krebs cycle enzymes in the liver or elevated because of bleeding or renal insufficiency.

Ammonia levels: Elevation expected because of inability of the failing liver to convert ammonia to urea and shunting of intestinal blood via collateral vessels. GI hemorrhage or an increase in intestinal protein from dietary intake increases ammonia levels. **Note:** Keep patient NPO except for water for 8 hr before drawing the ammonia level. Notify laboratory of all antibiotics taken by patient because they may lower the ammonia level.

Coagulation: Prothrombin time (PT) is prolonged and, in severe liver disease, unresponsive to vitamin K therapy. Coagulation abnormalities usually include factor V, but also factors II, VII, IX, and X.

Urine tests: Urine bilirubin is increased; urobilinogen is normal or increased. There may be proteinuria.

Liver biopsy: Obtains a specimen of liver for microscopic analysis and diagnosis of cirrhosis, hepatitis, or other liver disease. After local anesthetic is administered and the patient's skin is prepared, a large needle is inserted into the eighth or ninth intercostal space in the midaxillary line. It is critical that patients hold their breath at the end of expiration to elevate the liver maximally. Patient movement or failure to sustain expiration can result in puncture through the lung rather than liver. Type and cross-matching sometimes are performed before the procedure in anticipation of hemorrhagic complications. Percutaneous liver biopsy is contraindicated in patients with markedly prolonged PT or very low platelet counts because of the risk of hemorrhage. In these patients a transvenous biopsy via the jugular and hepatic vein may be attempted instead (see Table 6-14 for care of patients undergoing liver biopsy). Open liver biopsy, or minilaparotomy, may also be done for liver biopsy.

Barium swallow: Used in nonemergency situations (i.e., for patients without active bleeding) to verify the presence of gastroesophageal varices. **Note:** The patient should be NPO from midnight until completion of the test. Because of the constipating effects of barium, enemas should be given upon the patient's return from the procedure.

Radiologic studies: Ultrasound differentiates hemolytic and hepatocellular jaundice from obstructive jaundice and shows hepatomegaly and intrahepatic tumors. CT scan of the liver/spleen is done to evaluate size and location of tumors and to rule out gallbladder disease. Percutaneous transhepatic cholangiography reveals the extent of obstruction via contrast dye. Endoscopic retrograde cholangiopancreatography (ERCP) is a fiberoptic technique used to show obstructions of the common bile and pancreatic ducts as potential causes of jaundice. Liver scans enable visualization of the spleen and liver via injection of radioisotopes. **Note:** After injection of the dye, the patient may experience nausea, vomiting, and transient elevated temperature.

Angiographic studies: Establish patency of the portal vein and visualize the portosystemic collateral vessels to determine cause and effective treatment for variceal bleeding. Portal venous anatomy must be established before such operations as portal systemic shunt or hepatic transplantation. In patients with previously constructed surgical shunts, loss of patency may be confirmed as a

T A B L E 6 - 1 4 Nursing Care of the Patient Undergoing Liver Biopsy

Prebiopsy

Explain procedure to patient and significant other

Intrabiopsy

Assist patient with remaining motionless.

Coach patient in sustaining exhalation during puncture (or manually ventilate intubated patient to prevent lung inflation during puncture) to prevent pneumothorax.

Postbiopsy

Auscultate breath sounds immediately after procedure and at 1- to 2-hr intervals for 6-8 hr after procedure to detect pneumothorax or hemothorax (unlikely but serious complications). Diminished sounds on the right side and tachypnea suggest pneumothorax or hemothorax.

Position patient on the right side for several hours after biopsy to tamponade puncture site.

Enforce bedrest for 8-12 hr after biopsy to minimize risk of hemorrhage from puncture site.

Administer analgesics as prescribed. Avoid NSAIDs (see Table 8-1, p. 555), which may affect clotting, and hepatotoxins (see Table 6-13).

Monitor patient for indicators of peritonitis or intraperitoneal bleeding, which can occur as a result of puncture of blood vessels or major bile duct: severe abdominal pain, abdominal distention and rigidity, rebound tenderness, nausea, vomiting, tachycardia, tachypnea, pallor, decreased BP, and rising temperature.

NSAIDs, Nonsteroidal antiinflammatory drugs; *BP,* blood pressure.

factor leading to the present bleeding episode. See Table 6-15 for nursing implications of angiographic studies.

- The most common procedure is portal venography by indirect angiography. The femoral artery is catheterized, and contrast material is injected into the splenic artery. Contrast material flows through the spleen into the splenic and portal veins.
- Hepatic vein wedge pressure is measured by introducing a balloon catheter into the femoral vein and threading it into a hepatic vein branch.
- Direct access to the portal vein may be achieved through transhepatic portography. During this procedure, varices may be obliterated by injection of thrombin or gel foam into veins that supply the varices. **Note:** Transhepatic portography involves a direct puncture through the liver and has many of the same risks as liver biopsy. Patients returning from this procedure should be positioned on their right side and monitored closely.

Esophagoscopy: Visualizes the esophagus and stomach directly via a fiberoptic esophagoscope. Varices in the esophagus and upper portion of the stomach are identified, and attempts are made to identify the exact source of bleeding. Variceal bleeding may be treated by sclerotherapy, electrocautery, laser, vasoconstrictive agents, or other methods during the endoscopic procedure (see "Collaborative Management" below). See Table 6-16 for nursing implications of esophagoscopy.

Peritoneoscopy or laparoscopy: Visualizes the liver (to identify characteristic "hobnailed" appearance in cirrhosis) and allows for biopsy.

EEG: Traces the electrical impulses of the brain to detect or confirm encephalopathy. EEG changes occur very early, usually before behavioral or biochemical alterations.

TABLE 6-15   Nursing Care for the Patient Undergoing Angiographic Studies

Preprocedure

Explain procedure to patient and significant other.

Maintain NPO status for 8 hr before procedure.

Verify patency of IV catheter.

Note allergies to seafood, iodine, and contrast material.

Administer sedatives as prescribed. Be aware that dosage usually is reduced if cirrhosis or hepatitis is diagnosed.

Intraprocedure

Assist radiology personnel with positioning and draping patient.

Monitor VS q15min or more often for evidence of anaphylaxis or hemorrhagic shock.

Postprocedure

Check VS q15min initially and q1-2hr once patient's condition has stablized.

Maintain patient in supine position.

Keep pressure dressing and sandbag over puncture site for 6-8 hr.

Evaluate distal pulses and perfusion in affected extremity q1-2hr for 8 hr. Arterial thrombosis and large hematomas that compromise femoral blood flow may develop as a result of manipulation of the artery and clotting abnormalities associated with liver disease.

Promote adequate hydration via PO intake or IV fluids as indicated.

Monitor urine output q1-2hr, and report volume <30 ml/hr.

TABLE 6-16   Nursing Care for the Patient Undergoing Esophagoscopy

Preprocedure

Explain procedure to patient and significant other.

Maintain NPO status for 8 hr before procedure.

Clear stomach of blood and gastric contents immediately before endoscope is passed.

Verify patency of two large-bore IV catheters, which are used for rapid administration of fluids and medications.

Administer sedatives as prescribed. Be aware that dosage usually is reduced if cirrhosis or hepatitis is diagnosed.

Intraprocedure

Maintain patient in side-lying position to reduce likelihood of aspiration.

Have pharyngeal and tracheal suction readily available.

Monitor LOC, VS, and oxygenation status during procedure.

Postprocedure

Maintain side-lying position until patient is fully alert.

Note evidence of change in rate of hemorrhage.

Be alert for immediate complications, such as aspiration pneumonia (evidenced by difficulty breathing, diminished breath sounds, coarse crackles, rhonchi) and perforation (rare—evidenced by severe retrosternal pain and bleeding).

LOC, Level of consciousness; *VS,* vital signs.

Psychometric testing: Evaluates for hepatic encephalopathy. A common test is the Reitan number connection (trail-making) test. The patient's speed and accuracy at connecting a series of numbered circles are evaluated at intervals. A daily handwriting test is an easy check of intellectual deterioration or improvement.

COLLABORATIVE MANAGEMENT

Treatment of underlying causes: For example, exposure to hepatotoxins, use of alcohol, biliary obstruction.

Pharmacotherapy

Diuretics: To reduce edema. Potassium (K^+)-sparing diuretics (e.g., spirono-lactone) often are used. If indicated, teach patient to avoid excessive ingestion of K^+-rich foods (see Table 3-4, p. 146) or salt substitutes.

Neomycin: To control intestinal flora that aggravate encephalopathy.

Lactulose: To neutralize intraluminal ammonia in the intestine in an attempt to control encephalopathy.

Propranolol: To reduce portal blood pressure to aid in controlling bleeding esophageal or gastric varices.

Vasopressin: Used with acute variceal bleeding to vasoconstrict mesenteric blood vessels and reduce portal blood flow. Nitroglycerin also is commonly administered to counteract the potential for myocardial ischemia or other serious cardiovascular side effects.

Hematinics (iron preparations such as ferrous sulfate):   To control anemia. They are used to replace iron after abnormal blood loss.

Blood coagulants: To control bleeding.

Laxatives and stool softeners: To prevent straining and rupture of varices.

Antihistamines (e.g., diphenhydramine):   For pruritus.

Topical anesthetics: For hemorrhoids.

Supplemental vitamins and minerals: Such as folic acid for macrocytic anemia and vitamin K for prolonged PT.

Note: Opioids and sedatives, which are metabolized by the liver, are contraindicated. Small doses of benzodiazepines with a short half-life, such as oxazepam (Serax), may be administered if absolutely necessary. See Table 6-13 for a list of hepatotoxic drugs.

Dietary management: With fluid retention and ascites, Na^+ and fluids are restricted. Usually half the calories are supplied as carbohydrates. Protein is restricted in hepatic coma or precoma because the action of intestinal bacteria on protein increases blood ammonia levels, which causes or worsens the coma state. Parenteral or enteral nutrition is administered in the presence of bleeding or coma.

Bedrest: In the presence of fever, infection.

Treatment of complications

GI hemorrhage: Upper GI hemorrhage is common in patients with chronic liver disease and can result from esophageal varices, portal hypertensive gastropathy, duodenal or gastric ulcers, or Mallory-Weiss tear (mucosal laceration at the juncture of the distal esophagus and proximal stomach). Early diagnosis is essential to allow appropriate intervention.

ESOPHAGEAL VARICES: The therapeutic goal is to reduce portal hypertension and blood flow.

- Pharmacotherapy includes β-blockers, vasopressin, and somatostatin.
- Gastroesophageal balloon tamponade (via Minnesota, Linton, or Sengstaken-Blakemore tubes) applies direct pressure on acutely bleeding varices until definitive therapy is possible. Complications can include airway obstruction, pulmonary aspiration, gastroesophageal mucosal pressure necrosis, and esophageal rupture.

TABLE 6-17   Side Effects and Complications of Esophageal
             Sclerotherapy

Anticipated mild side effects
   Mild retrosternal pain
   Transient fever
   Diminished breath sounds
   Transient dysphagia
   Local ulcerations

Serious side effects/complications
   Bleeding from remaining varices or ulcers
   Stricture formation evidenced by prolonged dysphagia
   Perforation evidenced by bleeding, severe pain, or fever
   Pulmonary problems, including aspiration pneumonia, pleural effusion, ARDS,
      mediastinitis
   Bacteremia evidenced by fever, tachycardia, positive blood culture results

---

ARDS, Adult respiratory distress syndrome.

- Endoscopic therapies include variceal sclerosis (Table 6-17) (using sodium morrhuate or sodium tetradecyl sulfate, electrocautery, laser cautery, topical vasoconstrictive agents, or variceal band ligation.
- Portosystemic shunt procedures are used to divert portal blood flow away from the liver. Transjugular intrahepatic portosystemic shunting (TIPS) is a nonoperative procedure that achieves portal decompression by transvenous placement of a stent between the hepatic and portal veins. Surgical shunts, such as portocaval or distal splenorenal shunts, may be performed if medical therapies are unsuccessful. Operative mortality is much higher for emergent vs. elective procedures.

PORTAL HYPERTENSIVE GASTROPATHY: Results in bleeding from the gastric mucosa from severe portal hypertension. Treatment focuses on reducing portal blood pressure with propranolol or a portosystemic shunt.

Ascites: Dietary management may include Na^+ and fluid restrictions. Diuretics, usually aldosterone antagonists, are often given to minimize fluid collection. If indicated, surgical management includes a peritoneovenous (LeVeen or Denver) shunt, which provides a route for reinfusion of ascitic fluid into the venous system. Monitor for these potential complications: cardiac or renal overload (see "Heart Failure," p. 68; "Pulmonary Hypertension," p. 73; "Pulmonary Edema," p. 103), shunt occlusion, disseminated intravascular coagulation (DIC, see p. 535), hemorrhage, infection, and extravasation of ascitic fluid from the incisions. Paracentesis is usually not indicated unless there is severe respiratory distress or discomfort or unless it is essential for diagnosis of a tumor or other source of peritonitis.

Hepatic encephalopathy (hepatic coma):   Dietary management includes restriction of protein from the diet to decrease blood ammonia levels, giving sweetened fruit juices to provide the necessary carbohydrates for energy, and administering parenteral/enteral nutrition if the patient is comatose. Pharmacologic management includes neomycin to inhibit intestinal bacteria and magnesium sulfate or enemas to cleanse the intestines after GI bleeding. Lactulose is administered to neutralize ammonia and aid in evacuating stool to improve mentation. The following drugs are contraindicated: barbiturates and opioids (because of the liver's inability to detoxify them), K^+-depleting diuretics (aldosterone antagonists are the first-line choice since edema is related to inadequate detoxification of aldosterone), and ammonia-containing medications or food, which would cause or worsen hepatic coma.

Spontaneous bacterial peritonitis: Occurs in cirrhotic patients with ascites. Abdominal pain, worsening ascites, fever, and progressive encephalopathy suggest peritonitis. Mortality is high. See "Peritonitis," p. 425, for treatment.
Irreversible end-stage liver disease: Individuals with irreversible liver failure caused by chronic active hepatitis, primary biliary cirrhosis, sclerosing cholangitis, alcoholic cirrhosis, metabolic liver disease, acute fulminant hepatic necrosis, and other conditions may be considered for transplantation. Severe failure is manifested by serum bilirubin >10 mg/dl, albumin <2.5 g/dl, and prothrombin time >5 sec beyond the control. The patient must be refractory to all medical and other surgical treatments and have no absolute contraindications to transplantation (e.g., active substance abuse, metastatic disease). Patients are referred to specialized medical centers where they receive extensive preoperative evaluation and preparation. Posttransplant survival rates at 1 and 5 years are 70% and 60%, respectively.

NURSING DIAGNOSES AND INTERVENTIONS

Altered nutrition: Less than body requirements related to anorexia, nausea, or malabsorption
Desired outcome: By at least 24 hr before hospital discharge, patient demonstrates adequate progress toward adequate nutritional status as evidenced by stable weight, balanced or positive N state, serum protein 6-8 g/dl, and serum albumin 3.5-5.5 g/dl.

- Explain dietary restrictions; remember that sodium and fluids are restricted (see Table 3-2, p. 133, for a list of foods high in sodium). Encourage the patient to eat foods that are permitted within dietary restrictions. If the ammonia level rises (normal levels are whole blood 70-200 μg/dl and plasma 56-150 μg/dl), protein and foods high in ammonia also will be restricted.
- Monitor I&O; weigh patient daily.
- Encourage small, frequent meals to ensure adequate nutrition.
- Encourage significant other to bring desirable foods as permitted.
- Have nourishing foods available to patient at night.
- Administer vitamin and mineral supplements as prescribed.
- Administer the following prescribed medications to decrease gastric distress: acid suppression agents, antiemetics, and cathartics.
- Implement prescribed measures to relieve/mobilize ascites and decrease pressure on intraabdominal structures.
- Promote bedrest to reduce metabolic demands on the liver.
- Provide soft diet if patient has esophageal varices that are not bleeding. Patients with bleeding esophageal varices are NPO.
- Discuss need for feeding supplements and enteral or parenteral nutrition (see "Providing Nutritional Support," p. 687) with health care provider if appropriate.

NIC: Diet Staging; Enteral Tube Feeding; Gastrointestinal Intubation; Nutrition Management; Total Parenteral Nutrition (TPN) Administration

Impaired gas exchange related to alveolar hypoventilation secondary to shallow breathing occurring with ascites or pleural effusion; altered oxygen-carrying capacity of the blood secondary to erythrocytopenia; and possible ventilation/perfusion mismatching
Desired outcome: Within 24 hr of admission, patient has adequate gas exchange as evidenced by $Paco_2$ ≤45 mm Hg, Pao_2 ≥80 mm Hg, O_2 saturation ≥92%, and RR 12-20 breaths/min with normal depth and pattern (eupnea).

- During complaints of dyspnea or orthopnea, assist patient into semi-Fowler's or high Fowler's position to promote gas exchange.
- Administer oxygen as prescribed.
- Monitor ABG values and pulse oximetry; notify health care provider of Pao_2 <80 mm Hg or O_2 saturation <92%.

- Encourage patient to change positions and deep-breathe at frequent intervals to promote gas exchange. If secretions are present, ensure that the patient coughs frequently.
- Notify health care provider of indicators of respiratory infection, such as spiking temperatures, chills, diaphoresis, and adventitious breath sounds.
- Position patient in a side-lying position during episodes of vomiting to prevent aspiration.
- Obtain baseline abdominal girth measurement, and measure girth either daily or every shift. Measure around the same circumferential area each time; mark the site with indelible ink. Report significant findings to health care provider.

NIC: Bedside Laboratory Testing; Oxygen Therapy; Positioning; Respiratory Monitoring

Altered protection related to increased risk of esophageal bleeding secondary to portal hypertension and altered clotting factors
Desired outcomes: Patient is free of esophageal bleeding as evidenced by BP ≥90/60 mm Hg; HR ≤100 bpm; warm extremities; distal pulses >2+ on a 0-4+ scale; brisk capillary refill (<2 sec); and orientation to person, place, and time.

- Monitor VS q4hr (or more frequently if VS are outside of patient's baseline values). Be alert to hypotension and increased HR, as well as to physical indicators of hypovolemia and hemorrhage, including cool extremities, delayed capillary refill, decreased amplitude of distal pulses, mental status changes, and decreasing LOC.
- Teach patient to avoid swallowing foods that are chemically or mechanically irritating (e.g., rough or spicy foods, hot foods, hot liquids, alcohol) and therefore injurious to the esophagus.
- Instruct patient to avoid actions that increase intraabdominothoracic pressure, such as coughing, sneezing, lifting, or vomiting.
- Administer stool softeners as prescribed to help prevent straining with defecation.
- Inspect stools for presence of blood, which would signal bleeding within the GI tract; perform stool occult blood test as indicated.
- Monitor PT for abnormality (normal range is 10.5-13.5 sec), and assess patient for signs of bleeding such as altered VS, irritability, air hunger, pallor, weakness, melena, and hematemesis.
- As appropriate, encourage intake of foods rich in vitamin K (e.g., spinach, cabbage, cauliflower, liver) to help decrease the PT.
- As often as possible, avoid invasive procedures such as giving injections and taking rectal temperatures.
- Monitor the patient undergoing injection sclerotherapy for evidence of perforation, including increased HR, decreased BP, pallor, weakness, and air hunger. If signs of perforation occur, notify health care provider immediately, keep the patient NPO, and prepare for gastric suction. For more information see Table 6-17. Administer antibiotics as prescribed to prevent infection.

NIC: Bleeding Precautions; Teaching: Disease Process; Teaching: Individual; Vital Signs Monitoring

Sensory/perceptual alterations (all) related to increased risk of neurosensory changes secondary to hepatic coma occurring with cerebral accumulation of ammonia or GI bleeding
Desired outcome: Patient verbalizes orientation to person, place, and time; exhibits intact signature; and is free of symptoms of injury caused by neurosensory changes.

- Perform a baseline assessment of patient's personality characteristics, LOC, and orientation. Enlist the aid of significant other to help determine slight changes in personality or behavior.
- Have patient demonstrate his or her signature daily. If the writing deteriorates, ammonia levels may be increasing. Be alert to generalized

muscle twitching and asterixis (flapping tremor induced by dorsiflexion of wrist and extension of fingers). Report significant findings to health care provider.

- Remind patient to avoid protein and foods high in ammonia, such as gelatin, onions, and strong cheeses. The diseased liver cannot convert ammonia to urea, and the build-up of ammonia adds to the progression of hepatic encephalopathy.
- Monitor for indicators of GI bleeding, including melena or hematemesis. GI bleeding can precipitate hepatic coma. Report bleeding promptly to health care provider, and obtain prescription for cleansing enemas if indicated.
- Protect patient against injury that can be precipitated by confused state (e.g., keep the side rails up and the bed in its lowest position, and assist patient with ambulation when need is determined).
- Use caution when administering sedatives, antihistamines, and other agents affecting the central nervous system. Avoid opiate analgesics and phenothiazines.

NIC: Neurologic Monitoring; Surveillance: Safety

Fluid volume excess related to compromised regulatory mechanism with sequestration of fluids secondary to portal hypertension and hepatocellular failure

Desired outcome: By at least 24 hr before hospital discharge, patient is normovolemic as evidenced by stable or decreasing abdominal girth, RR 12-20 breaths/min with normal depth and pattern (eupnea), HR ≤100 bpm, edema ≤1+ on a 0-4+ scale, and absence of crackles (rales).

- Obtain baseline abdominal girth measurement. Place patient in the supine position, and mark abdomen with indelible ink to ensure serial measurements from the same circumferential site. Measure girth daily or every shift as appropriate.
- Monitor weight and I&O. Output should be equal to or exceed intake. Weight loss should not exceed 0.23 kg/day (½ lb). Assess the degree of edema, from 1+ (barely detectable) to 4+ (deep, persistent pitting), and document accordingly.
- Be alert to clinical indicators of pulmonary edema, including dyspnea, basilar crackles that do not clear with coughing, orthopnea, and tachypnea.
- Give frequent mouth care, and provide ice chips to help minimize thirst.
- Monitor serum Na^+ and K^+ values and report abnormalities to health care provider. Optimal values are serum Na^+ 137-147 mEq/L and serum K^+ 3.5-5.0 mEq/L. Restrict Na^+ and replace K^+ as prescribed.
- Remind patient to avoid food (see Table 3-2, p. 133) and nonfood items that contain Na^+, such as antacids, baking soda, and some mouthwashes.
- Elevate extremities to decrease peripheral edema. Apply antiembolism hose (AEH) support stockings, sequential compression devices, or pneumatic foot compression devices as prescribed.
- Remember that rapid increases in intravascular volume can precipitate variceal hemorrhage in susceptible patients. Monitor for hemorrhage accordingly (see **Altered protection,** p. 492).
- Teach the patient to inhale against resistance, using a blow bottle to facilitate the flow of ascitic fluid through the shunt (if a LeVeen peritoneovenous or Denver shunt is in place). Inhaling against resistance raises intraperitoneal pressure sufficiently to enable ascitic fluid to flow through the shunt. In addition, provide instructions about the following: importance of life-style changes such as low-Na^+ diet (see Table 3-2, p. 133), abstinence from alcohol, practicing breathing exercises, obtaining daily weight and abdominal girth measurements, and monitoring I&O and edema.

NIC: Fluid/Electrolyte Management; Respiratory Monitoring; Teaching: Disease Process; Teaching: Individual

See Also: "Hepatitis" for **Knowledge deficit:** Causes of hepatitis and modes of transmission, p. 483.

PATIENT-FAMILY TEACHING AND DISCHARGE PLANNING

When providing patient-family teaching, focus on sensory information; avoid giving excessive information; and initiate a visiting nurse referral for necessary follow-up teaching. Consider including verbal and written information about the following:

- Medications, including drug name, purpose, dosage, schedule, precautions, drug/drug and food/drug interactions, and potential side effects.
- Dietary restrictions, in particular that of Na^+ (see Table 3-2, p. 133), protein, and ammonia.
- Potential need for life-style changes, including avoiding alcoholic beverages. Stress that alcohol cessation is a major factor in survival of this disease. Include appropriate referrals (e.g., to Alcoholics Anonymous, Al-Anon, and Al-Ateen). As appropriate, provide referrals to community nursing support agencies.
- Awareness of hepatotoxic agents (see Table 6-13), especially OTC drugs, including acetaminophen and aspirin.
- Importance of breathing exercises (see p. 491) when ascites is present.
- Indicators of variceal bleeding/hemorrhage (i.e., vomiting blood, change in LOC) and the need to inform health care provider should they occur.
- Phone numbers to call should questions or concerns arise about therapy or disease after discharge. Additional general information can be obtained by contacting the following organization:

    National Digestive Diseases Information Clearinghouse, National Institute of Diabetes and Digestive and Kidney Diseases
    Project Officer
    2 Information Way
    Bethesda, MD 220892-3570   (301) 654-3810
    WWW address: *http://www.aerie.com/nihdb/ddbase.htm*

- For patients awaiting transplantation, provide the following information as appropriate:

    The United Network for Organ Sharing
    UNOS Communication Department
    P.O. Box 13770
    Richmond, VA 23225   (804) 330-8561 or (800) 243-6667 (voice mail)
    WWW address: *http://www.unos.org*

- As an additional information source, refer patients to the following organization:

    American Liver Foundation
    1425 Pompton Ave.
    Cedar Grove, NJ 07009   (800) 223-0179
    WWW address: *http://sadieo.ucsf.edu/alf/alffinal/homepagealf.html*

Cholelithiasis and cholecystitis

Cholelithiasis is characterized by the presence of stones in the gallbladder. Gallstones may cause pain or other symptoms or remain asymptomatic for years. *Choledocholithiasis* is the term used to describe gallstones in the common bile duct. Gallstones are classified as cholesterol or pigment stones.

Cholesterol stones are more common in the United States. Black-pigment stones are composed mainly of calcium bilirubinate and are associated with cirrhosis and chronic hemolysis. Brown-pigment stones are the predominant type found in native Asians and may be associated with bacterial infection of the bile. Precipitating factors for stone formation include disturbances in metabolism, biliary stasis, obstruction, and infection. Gallstones are especially prevalent in women who are multiparous, are taking estrogen therapy, or use oral contraceptives. Other risk factors include obesity, dietary intake of fats, sedentary life-style, and familial tendencies. The incidence increases with age, and it is estimated that one of every three persons who reach age 75 has gallstones. Cholelithiasis is frequently seen in disease states such as diabetes mellitus, regional enteritis, and certain blood dyscrasias. Usually cholelithiasis is asymptomatic until a stone becomes lodged in the cystic tract. If the obstruction is unrelieved, biliary colic (intermittent painful episodes) and cholecystitis can ensue.

Cholecystitis is most commonly associated with cystic duct obstructions caused by impacted gallstones; however, it may result also from stasis, bacterial infection, or ischemia of the gallbladder. Cholecystitis involves acute inflammation of the gallbladder and is associated with pain, tenderness, and fever. With obstruction, structural changes can occur, such as swelling and thickening of the gallbladder walls. If the edema is prolonged, the walls become scarred and fibrosed and the constant pressure of bile can lead to mucosal irritation. As a complication of the impaired circulation and edema, pressure ischemia and necrosis can develop, resulting in gangrene or perforation. With chronic cholecystitis, stones almost always are present and the gallbladder walls are thickened and fibrosed.

ASSESSMENT

Cholelithiasis: History of intolerance to fats and occasional discomfort after eating. As the stone moves through the duct or becomes lodged, a sudden onset of mild, aching pain occurs in the mid-epigastrium after eating (especially after a high-fat meal) and increases in intensity during a colic attack, potentially radiating to the RUQ and right subscapular region. Nausea, vomiting, tachycardia, and diaphoresis also can occur. Many individuals with gallstones are entirely asymptomatic.

Cholecystitis: History of intolerance to fats and discomfort after eating, including regurgitation, flatulence, belching, epigastric heaviness, indigestion, heartburn, chronic upper abdominal pain, and nausea. Amber-colored urine, clay-colored stools, pruritus, jaundice, steatorrhea, and bleeding tendencies can be present if there is bile obstruction. Symptoms may be vague. An acute attack may last 7-10 days, but it usually resolves in several hours.

Physical assessment

Cholelithiasis: Palpation of RUQ reveals a tender abdomen during colic attack. Otherwise, between attacks, the examination is usually normal.

Cholecystitis: Palpation elicits tenderness localized behind the inferior margin of the liver. With progressive symptoms, a tender, globular mass may be palpated behind the lower border of the liver. Rebound tenderness and guarding may also be present. With the patient taking a deep breath, palpation over the RUQ elicits Murphy's sign (pain and inability to inspire when the examiner's hand comes in contact with the gallbladder).

DIAGNOSTIC TESTS

Ultrasonography: Preferred test for confirming the presence of gallstones, as well as their number and size. Ultrasonography of the gallbladder and biliary tract may be used to determine the location of gallstones and detect tumors.

Radiologic studies: For example, oral cholangiogram, IV cholangiogram, nuclear scans, and percutaneous transhepatic cholangiogram; may be performed to determine the patency of the biliary or cystic ducts and help rule out other conditions that mimic cholelithiasis or cholecystitis. Chest, abdominal, upper GI, and barium enema x-rays often are used to rule out pulmonary or other GI disorders.

Hepato-iminodiacetic acid (lidofenin) (HIDA) scan: Radioisotopic scan that is highly sensitive for diagnosis of acute cholecystitis.

Oral cholecystogram: Measures gallbladder function and demonstrates the number and size of gallstones. This test requires ingestion of iodine-based tablets (i.e., Telepaque) for 2 consecutive nights, with x-ray films taken the following morning. Failure to visualize the gallbladder indicates a nonfunctioning gallbladder, usually because of complete obstruction of the cystic duct or chronic irritation of the gallbladder wall. Diarrhea may be caused by the iodine tablets and sometimes results in nonvisualization of the gallbladder.

CT scan: To detect dilated bile ducts and the presence of gallbladder cysts or tumors.

Endoscopic retrograde cholangiopancreatography (ERCP): Visualization and evaluation of the biliary tree or pancreatic duct.

ECG: To rule out cardiac disease.

CBC with differential: To assess for presence of infection or blood loss.

Prothrombin time: To assess for a prolonged clotting time secondary to faulty vitamin K absorption.

Bilirubin tests (serum and urine) and urobilinogen tests (urine and fecal): To differentiate between hemolytic disorders, hepatocellular disease, and obstructive disease. Usually there is an increase of bilirubin in the plasma and urine with biliary disease.

Serum liver enzyme test: Usually normal in cholecystitis but often becomes abnormal in the presence of prolonged cholecystitis or common duct stones.

COLLABORATIVE MANAGEMENT

Pharmacologic therapy

Analgesics: NSAIDs or opioid analgesics may be indicated, depending on the severity of the pain. For the postoperative patient, epidural, continuous IV, and patient-controlled infusions of opioid analgesics are used with increasing frequency and superior efficacy (see Appendix One, "Caring for Preoperative and Postoperative Patients" for **Pain,** p. 719, for more information). Recently, IV ketorolac (Toradol) q6hr for 4-8 doses has shown benefit in controlling postoperative pain with these patients, reducing the need for opioid analgesics.

Acid suppression therapy: To neutralize gastric hyperacidity and reduce associated pain.

Antibiotics: For infection.

Antiemetics (e.g., hydroxyzine, ondansetron, prochlorperazine, promethazine): For nausea and vomiting.

Bile sequestrant therapy: Cholestyramine (Questran) and colestipol (Colestid) bind with bile salts in the intestine to facilitate their excretion and may be given to provide relief from pruritus caused by prolonged obstructive jaundice.

Gallstone-solubilizing agents: Indicated for patients in whom open or laparoscopic cholecystectomy is contraindicated. Ursodeoxycholic acid (UDCA; ursodiol [Actigall]) or, rarely, chenodeoxycholic acid (CDCA; chenodiol [Chenix]) may be used in selected patients with relatively small, uncalcified (cholesterol) stones to reduce size and eventually dissolve them. Treatment duration ranges from months to years with variable results. Patients should be advised of the many potential drug interactions, serious side effects, and need for careful follow-up treatment.

Chemical dissolution of cholesterol gallstones with a solvent: May be used in patients with a functioning gallbladder and an unobstructed biliary tract. The solvent is infused via a T-tube or endoscopically placed catheter. Agents such as monoctanoin are used in carefully selected patients. Oral solubilizing agents (see above) are administered after chemical dissolution to prevent recurrence of stones.

Dietary management: Varies according to the patient's condition. During an acute attack, NPO status with IV fluids may be instituted. With severe nausea and vomiting, a gastric tube is inserted and attached to low, intermittent suction. Diet advances to patient's tolerance, and small, frequent feedings of a low-fat diet are recommended for both the acute and chronic conditions.

ERCP: The common bile duct may be cannulated, and if a stone is present, an endoscopic sphincterotomy (a technique that cuts the opening of the bile duct) can be performed with stone extraction via a snare or balloon catheter.

Nonoperative biliary stone removal: One method of stone extraction, which is performed using fluoroscopy in the radiology department. The stone is removed with a basket that is inserted via a catheter or T-tube through a surgically created sinus tract into the common duct. If this technique is unsuccessful, forceps are used to manipulate the stone. A cholangiogram is done before and after the procedure. If the x-ray is normal after the procedure, the T-tube is removed; if stones are still present, a new T-tube or catheter is inserted and the patient returns the following day for the same procedure. This technique may be ideal for an individual who is not a good surgical candidate.

Lithotripsy: Gallstones, like kidney stones, can be fragmented by exposure to extracorporeal shock waves. The stones are broken up into small granules that can be passed through the intestine or dissolved with ursodiol. Patients are carefully selected and evaluated before therapy. During the approximately 1-hr procedure the patient is mildly sedated and may feel some RUQ tenderness immediately after the procedure.

Surgical interventions: Usually required for relief of long-term symptoms of cholelithiasis and acute cholecystitis. Surgery is the best treatment choice for patients with frequent or severe episodes of biliary pain, cholecystitis, diabetes, or suspected gallbladder cancer. The type of surgery depends on the severity and length of illness, site of obstruction, and condition of the patient. The following procedures may be performed.

Laparoscopic cholecystectomy (removal of the gallbladder): Three to four small incisions are made in the abdominal wall. A laparoscope and specialized, long-handled instruments are used to resect the gallbladder with electrocautery or laser cautery. Although laparoscopic cholecystectomy is more costly, surgical complications are fewer and postoperative recovery is more rapid than with conventional cholecystectomy.

Cholecystectomy: If laparascopic cholecystectomy is unsuccessful (or contraindicated), a traditional open cholecystectomy is done via a right subcostal incision. The gallbladder is excised, and the cystic duct, vein, and artery are ligated. A closed drainage system may be needed for drainage of blood, serum, and bile from the gallbladder bed. The drain is brought out through a separate stab wound away from the incision. An intraoperative cholangiogram is done if stones are suspected in the common bile duct; that is, a small catheter is threaded through the amputated cystic duct, and radiopaque dye is injected. If stones are identified, a common duct exploration (CDE) is done to remove the stones, using either gallbladder scoops or embolectomy catheters. Because of edema after the CDE, a T-tube may be inserted to drain bile until the edema resolves and patency of the common bile duct returns.

Cholecystostomy: Opening and draining the gallbladder in grossly septic or unstable patients. This is a palliative surgery and is generally followed by more definitive cholecystectomy once the patient is stable.

Choledochotomy: Opening the common bile duct to remove stones.

Choledochoduodenostomy or choledochojejunostomy: Anastomosis of the common bile duct to the duodenum or jejunum; done for neoplasms involving the duodenum or common bile duct.

NURSING DIAGNOSES AND INTERVENTIONS

Pain, spasms, nausea, and itching related to obstructive or inflammatory process

Desired outcomes: Patient's subjective perception of discomfort decreases within 1 hr of intervention, as documented by a pain scale. Nonverbal indicators, such as grimacing, are absent or diminished.

- Monitor patient for the presence of pain or other discomfort. Devise a pain scale with patient, rating discomfort on a scale of 0 (no pain) to 10 (worst pain).
- Explain to patient that a low-Fowler's position will minimize pressure in the RUQ.
- Teach patient to avoid fatty and rough or fibrous foods to prevent nausea and spasms.
- Administer bile salt binding agent (e.g., cholestyramine) as prescribed for itching.
- Help control itching by providing cool Alpha Keri baths and cold water or ice for topical application and using soft linens on the bed.
- For additional interventions, see **Pain**, p. 719, in Appendix One.

NIC: Nutritional Counseling; Pain Management; Teaching: Prescribed Medication

Altered protection related to recurrence of biliary obstruction
Desired outcomes: Patient is free of symptoms of postsurgical perforation as evidenced by graduallly diminishing dark brown drainage of <1000 ml/day and the presence of a soft and nondistended abdomen. Patient is free of symptoms of recurring biliary obstruction as evidenced by normal skin color, brown-colored stools, and straw-colored urine.

- Monitor the color of the skin, sclera, urine, and stool. If obstruction recurs and bile is forced back into the bloodstream, jaundice will be present, the urine will be amber, and the stools will be clay colored (clay color is normal if bile is drained via a T-tube). The brown color should return to the stools once bile begins to drain normally into the duodenum.
- Note and record the color, amount, odor, and consistency of drainage from the T-tube or wound drain q2hr on the day of surgery and at least every shift thereafter. Initially the drainage will be dark brown with small amounts of blood and can amount to 500-1000 ml/day. Report greater amounts of blood or drainage to health care provider. The amount should subside gradually as the swelling diminishes in the common duct and drainage into the duodenum normalizes.
- Ensure that drainage collection devices are positioned lower than the level of the common bile duct to prevent reflux of drainage when ambulating patients.
- Be alert to abdominal distention, rigidity, and complaints of diaphragmatic irritation along with a cessation or significant decrease in the amount of drainage. If these occur, notify health care provider immediately and anticipate tube replacement with a 14 Fr catheter.

NIC: Surveillance; Tube Care

See Also: "Hepatitis" for **Risk for impaired skin integrity** related to pruritus, p. 483; Appendix One, "Caring for Preoperative and Postoperative Patients," p. 717, for nursing diagnoses and interventions.

PATIENT-FAMILY TEACHING AND DISCHARGE PLANNING

When providing patient-family teaching, focus on sensory information; avoid giving excessive information; and initiate a visiting nurse referral for necessary follow-up teaching. Consider including verbal and written information about the following:

- Notifying health care provider if the following indicators of recurrent biliary obstruction occur: dark urine, pruritus, jaundice, clay-colored stools. Inform

patient that loose stools may occur for several months as the body adjusts to the continuous flow of bile.
- Medications, including drug name, dosage, schedule, purpose, precautions, drug/drug and food/drug interactions, and potential side effects.
- Care of dressings and tubes if patient is discharged with them, and monitoring the incision and drain sites for signs of infection (e.g., fever, persistent redness, pain, purulent discharge, swelling, increased local warmth).
- Importance of maintaining a diet low in fat and eating frequent, small meals for medically managed patients.
- Importance of follow-up appointments with health care provider; reconfirm time and date of next appointment.
- Avoiding alcoholic beverages during the first 2 postoperative mo to minimize the risk of pancreatic involvement.
- Necessity of postsurgical activity precautions: avoid lifting heavy objects (>10 lb) for the first 4-6 wk or as directed, rest after periods of fatigue, get maximum amounts of rest, and gradually increase activities to tolerance.
- Postsurgical patients may experience fatty food intolerance (e.g., flatulence, cramps, diarrhea) for several months postoperatively until the body acclimates to loss of the gallbladder.
- For more information contact the following organization:

  National Digestive Diseases Information Clearinghouse,
  National Institute of Diabetes and Digestive and Kidney Diseases
  Project Officer
  2 Information Way
  Bethesda, MD 20892   (302) 468-6344
  WWW address: *http://www.aerie.com/nihdb/ddbase.htm*

Section Six: Pancreatic Disorders

The pancreas serves both endocrine (hormonal) and exocrine (nonhormonal) functions. Pancreatic endocrine function is discussed in Chapter 5 (see p. 374). The exocrine portion comprises 98% of the tissue mass of the pancreas. Its function is the secretion of potent enzymes that act to reduce proteins, fats, and carbohydrates into simpler chemical substances. Pancreatic lipase acts on fats to produce glycerides, fatty acids, and glycerol; pancreatic amylase acts on starch to produce disaccharides. Pancreatic proteases (trypsin, chymotrypsin, carboxypeptidases A and B, elastase, phospholipase A) aid in the digestion of proteins. The pancreas also secretes sodium bicarbonate to neutralize the strongly acidic gastric contents as they enter the duodenum. The resultant mixture of acids and bases provides an optimal pH for the activation of pancreatic enzymes.

Pancreatitis

Acute pancreatitis occurs when pancreatic ductal flow becomes obstructed and digestive enzymes escape from the pancreatic duct into surrounding tissue. Self-destruction of the pancreas produces edema, hemorrhage, and necrosis of pancreatic and surrounding tissue. Biochemical abnormalities and disruption of cardiopulmonary, renal, metabolic, and GI function are likely. Pancreatitis has been associated with cholelithiasis, choledocholithiasis, alcoholism, surgical manipulation, abdominal trauma, abdominal vascular disease, heavy metal poisoning, infectious agents (viral, bacterial, mycoplasma, parasitic), and some allergic reactions.

Chronic pancreatitis is characterized by varying degrees of pancreatic insufficiency, which results in decreased production of enzymes and bicarbonate and malabsorption of fats and proteins. The digestion of fat is affected most severely. As a result, a high-fat content in the bowel stimulates water and electrolyte secretion, which produces diarrhea. The action of bacteria on fecal fat produces flatus, fatty stools (steatorrhea), and abdominal cramps. Often diabetes mellitus occurs as a result of chronic pancreatitis because of damage to the insulin-producing beta cells and resultant deficient insulin production. Complications of acute pancreatitis include pancreatic abscess, hemorrhage, pancreatic pseudocyst, fistula formation, and transient hypoglycemia. Acute, life-threatening complications include renal failure, hemorrhagic pancreatitis, septicemia, adult respiratory distress syndrome (ARDS), shock, and disseminated intravascular coagulation (DIC). Chronic pancreatitis is associated with complications of diabetes mellitus, chronic pain, and maldigestion.

ASSESSMENT

Acute pancreatitis: Sudden onset of constant, severe epigastric pain, often after a large meal or alcohol intake. The pain frequently radiates to the back or left shoulder and is somewhat relieved by a sitting position. Nausea and vomiting, sometimes with persistent retching, usually occur. Jaundice suggests biliary tree obstruction. Extreme malaise, restlessness, respiratory distress, and diminished urinary output may be present. Hypovolemic shock may be present with hemorrhagic events, or distributive shock may occur secondary to systemic inflammatory response syndrome.

Physical assessment: Diminished or absent bowel sounds, suggesting presence of ileus; mild to moderate ascites; generalized abdominal tenderness; tachypnea, crackles (rales) at the lung bases related to atelectasis, and interstitial fluid accumulation; diminished ventilatory excursion related to splinting and guarding with pain; low-grade fever (37.7°-38.8° C [100°-102° F]) or pronounced fever with abscess or sepsis; and agitation, confusion, and altered mental status may occur because of electrolyte/metabolic abnormalities or acute alcohol withdrawal. Gray-blue discoloration of the flank (Grey Turner's sign) or around the umbilicus (Cullen's sign) sometimes is present with pancreatic hemorrhage.

Chronic pancreatitis: Constant, dull epigastric pain; steatorrhea resulting from malabsorption of fats and protein; severe weight loss; and onset of symptoms of diabetes mellitus: polydipsia, polyuria, polyphagia. In addition, chemical addiction is often seen because of the chronic pain.

History of: Biliary tract disease, chronic excessive alcohol consumption, physical trauma to the abdomen (especially in young people), peptic ulcer disease, viral infection, endoscopic retrograde cholangiopancreatography (ERCP), cystic fibrosis, neoplasms, shock, and use of certain medications, such as estrogen-containing oral contraceptives, glucocorticoids, sulfonamides, chlorothiazides, and azathioprine.

DIAGNOSTIC TESTS

Serum amylase: When significantly elevated (>500 U/dl), rules out acute abdomen conditions, such as cholecystitis, appendicitis, bowel infarction/obstruction, and perforated peptic ulcer, and confirms presence of pancreatitis. These levels return to normal 48-72 hr after the onset of acute symptoms, even though clinical indicators may continue.

Serum lipase: Rises more slowly than serum amylase and persists longer. Both lipase and amylase levels reflect the degree of necrotic pancreatic tissue.

Hyperglycemia: Occurs because of interference with beta cell function. It is transient with acute pancreatitis but common with chronic pancreatitis, during which diabetes mellitus is likely to develop.

Serum calcium and magnesium: May be lower than normal. On ECG, hypocalcemia is evidenced by prolonged QT segment with a normal T wave.

CBC: Elevated WBCs caused by inflammatory process. Polymorphonuclear bodies may increase if bacterial peritonitis is present secondary to duodenal rupture.

BUN and serum creatinine: To evaluate renal function.

Urinalysis: May show presence of glycosuria, which can signal the onset of diabetes mellitus. Elevated urine amylase levels are useful diagnostically when serum levels have dropped off. An elevated specific gravity reflects the presence of dehydration.

Abdominal x-rays: May show dilation of the small or large bowel and presence of pancreatic calcification in chronic pancreatitis.

Ultrasound, MRI, or CT scan: May reveal an enlarged and edematous pancreatic head, or abscess, pseudocyst, or calcification.

ERCP: A combined endoscopic-radiographic tool that is used to study the degree of pancreatic disease via assessment of biliary-pancreatic ductal systems. It allows direct visualization of the ampulla of Vater, diagnoses biliary stones and duct stenosis, and distinguishes cancer of the pancreas from pancreatic calculi. ERCP is not performed until the acute episode has subsided.

Secretin stimulation test: To diagnosis chronic pancreatitis.

COLLABORATIVE MANAGEMENT

Medical goals are to reduce stimuli for pancreatic secretion to permit healing and rehydrate with fluids.

For acute pancreatitis

Fluid and electrolyte replacement/monitoring: To maintain adequate circulating blood volume (e.g., parenteral solutions that do not stimulate the pancreas, such as glucose or free amino acids, and blood volume expanders, such as albumin and plasma protein fraction). Close monitoring of urinary output is accomplished to assess for renal complications.

NPO status and NG suction: Initiated early in the course of illness to decrease stimulus for pancreatic secretions and reduce stress in the GI tract. After acute pain and ileus have resolved, the patient is given clear liquids and diet is advanced as tolerated.

Bedrest: To reduce metabolic demands on the body and thereby minimize need for pancreatic activity.

Pharmacotherapy

Meperidine, morphine: For pain. **Note:** Both morphine and meperidine may cause spasms at the sphincter of Oddi, although meperidine may be less likely to do so. Response varies with the individual. Pentazocine may be used as an alternative analgesic.

Broad-spectrum antibiotics: For infection or abscess if present or suspected.

Steroids: To reduce inflammation in certain types of pancreatitis when infection is not a problem.

Histamine H₂-receptor blockers: To reduce gastric acid secretion, which stimulates pancreatic enzymes (Table 6-18).

Antiemetics (e.g., hydroxyzine, ondansetron, prochlorperazine, promethazine): For nausea and vomiting.

Antacids: To neutralize gastric acid and reduce associated pain.

Other pharmacotherapies: Atropine (to reduce sphincter of Oddi spasm), glucagon, somatostatin, aprotinin, and indomethacin.

Ruling out underlying factors (e.g., hyperparathyroidism, hyperlipoproteinemia): These factors can contribute to the development of pancreatitis.

Peritoneal lavage: Removes toxic factors present in peritoneal exudate and can result in immediate clinical improvement. The procedure is similar to peritoneal dialysis. A soft lavage catheter is positioned in the peritoneum, and continual lavage is instituted for 2-7 days, depending on the patient's clinical course.

TABLE 6-18   **Histamine H$_2$-Receptor Blockers**

Generic name	Trade name	Usual dosage	Comments
Cimetidine	Tagamet	800-1200mg/day*	Reduces hepatic blood flow; inhibits metabolism of some drugs in the liver
Ranitidine	Zantac	150-300mg/day*	5-12 times more potent than cimetidine; fewer drug interactions than with cimetidine
Famotidine	Pepcid	40-120mg/day*	30-100 times more potent than cimetidine
Nizatidine	Axid	150-300mg/day†	

From Keen JH. In Swearingen PL, Keen JH: *Manual of critical care,* ed 3, St Louis, 1995, Mosby.
*PO, IM, or IV administration or continuous IV infusion titrated to gastric pH value.
†Available in oral form only.

Surgery: In general, nonsurgical management of acute pancreatitis is preferred. Surgical interventions may not improve the patient's condition, and the risk of respiratory and other complications is great. Because symptoms of acute pancreatitis are easily confused with those of other acute abdominal emergencies that require urgent surgery, exploratory laparotomy is necessary for some patients. For unstable patients with severe acute pancreatitis, prompt surgical debridement sometimes is necessary to limit vessel erosion and bleeding or to drain pseudocysts and abscesses. Surgery in these patients carries a high mortality rate, and complications are numerous.

For chronic pancreatitis
For exacerbations: See treatment for acute pancreatitis.
Alcohol rehabilitation: If alcoholism is the cause of pancreatitis.
Long-term pain management: With lowest effective dose of analgesic. Acetaminophen is used for initial pain control, but pain may require oral opioids using the lowest effective dose. Referral to a pain management team is recommended for these patients. Nerve blocks that interfere with transmission of pain sensations along visceral nerve fibers are effective in the relief of pancreatic pain. Bilateral splanchnic nerve or left celiac ganglion blocks may be performed.
Oral enzyme supplements (e.g., pancreatin, pancrelipase):   To treat maldigestion.
Histamine H$_2$-receptor blockers: Used as with acute pancreatitis.
Diet: High in carbohydrates and protein and low in fat; avoidance of spicy foods, caffeine, and nicotine.
Insulin therapy: May be required to ensure adequate carbohydrate metabolism if endocrine function is impaired. Laboratory values of fasting blood sugar and bedside monitoring of blood glucose will reveal abnormalities in blood glucose levels and direct the appropriate insulin therapy (see "Diabetes Mellitus," p. 378, for more information).
Surgical interventions: Indicated when pancreatitis is caused by an obstructive process, such as gallstone formation or cancer. When gallstones are the cause of the pancreatitis, surgical removal of the stone(s) and usually the gallbladder is performed (see "Cholelithiasis and Cholecystitis," p. 497). The surgery is performed when the acute symptoms of pancreatitis have abated. A common bile duct exploration may be done at the time of surgery to uncover and retrieve all stones. (See "Pancreatic Tumors," p. 508, for a discussion of

total pancreatectomy and other surgical procedures performed if cancer of the pancreatic head is present.)

NURSING DIAGNOSES AND INTERVENTIONS

Fluid volume deficit related to active loss secondary to NG suctioning, vomiting, diaphoresis, or pooling of fluids in the abdomen and retroperitoneum
Desired outcome: Patient is normovolemic within 8 hr of admission as evidenced by HR 60-100 bpm, CVP 2-6 mm Hg (5-12 cm H_2O), brisk capillary refill (<2 sec), peripheral pulse amplitude >2+ on a 0-4+ scale, urinary output ≥30 ml/hr, and stable weight and abdominal girth measurements.

- Monitor VS q2-4hr, and be alert to falling BP and increasing HR, which can occur with moderate to severe fluid loss.
- Measure I&O and CVP, if available, q2-4hr. Because fluid loss requires immediate replacement to prevent shock and acute renal failure, be alert to and report I&O imbalances. CVP <2 mm Hg can occur with volume-related hypotension. Measure orthostatic VS initially and q8hr. Be alert to decreasing BP and increasing HR on standing, which suggests the need for crystalloid and/or colloid volume expansion. Weigh daily, and note trends. Correlate weights with I&O ratios.
- Administer plasma volume expanders as prescribed. Monitor closely for fluid overload and pulmonary edema.
- Administer electrolytes (K^+, calcium [Ca^{++}]) as prescribed to prevent cardiac dysrhythmias and tetany.
- Be alert to indicators of hypocalcemia, such as positive Chvostek's sign (facial muscle spasm) and Trousseau's sign (carpopedal spasm), muscle twitching, tetany, or irritability, which can occur with electrolyte loss.
- Monitor values of the following for irregularities: Hct, Hgb, Ca^{++}, glucose, BUN, creatinine, and K^+. Normal values are as follows: Hct 40%-54% (male) and 37%-47% (female); Hgb 14-18 g/dl (male) and 12-16 g/dl (female); Ca^{++} 8.5-10.5 mg/dl (4.3-5.3 mEq/L); glucose <145 mg/dl (2-hr postprandial) and 65-110 mg/dl (fasting); BUN 6-20 mg/dl; and K^+ 3.5-5.0 mEq/L.

NIC: Fluid/Electrolyte Management; Gastrointestinal Intubation; Intravenous (IV) Therapy; Surveillance; Vital Signs Monitoring

Pain related to inflammatory process of the pancreas
Desired outcomes: Within 6 hr of intervention, patient's subjective perception of discomfort decreases, and it is controlled within 24 hr, as documented by a pain scale. Nonverbal indicators, such as splinting of abdominal muscles, are absent or diminished.

- Assess for and document the degree and character of the patient's discomfort. Devise a pain scale with the patient, rating the discomfort on a scale of 0 (no pain) to 10 (worst pain).
- Assess patient's previous responses to pain and previously effective pain relief measures. Consider possible cultural and spiritual influences.
- To minimize pancreatic secretions and pain and to maximize needed rest, ensure that patient maintains limited activity or bedrest.
- Maintain NPO status to minimize stimulation of pancreatic secretions. Monitor NG tube function, and maintain patency.
- Administer analgesics, histamine H_2-receptor blockers (see Table 6-18), antiemetics, and other medications as prescribed; be alert to patient's response to medications, using the pain scale. Instruct the patient to request analgesic before pain becomes severe. If analgesic is ineffective, notify health care provider because patient may require a nerve block or other intervention. Optimally, analgesics are administered via patient-controlled pumps. Transdermal analgesic or small, frequent doses of IV opiates usually are more effective than IM injections. Avoid IM injections in individuals with clotting or bleeding complications.

- Assist patient in attaining a position of comfort. A sitting or supine position with knees flexed often helps to relax abdominal muscles.
- Emphasize nonpharmacologic pain interventions (e.g., relaxation techniques, distraction, guided imagery, massage). These interventions are especially important for patients who develop chronic pancreatitis and are prone to chemical dependence. (See **Health-seeking behaviors:** Relaxation technique effective for stress reduction, p. 59.)
- Pancreatitis can be very painful. Prepare significant other for personality changes and behavioral alterations associated with extreme pain and opioid analgesic. Family members sometimes misinterpret patient's lethargic or unpleasant disposition and may even blame themselves. Reassure them that these are normal responses.
- Monitor patient's respiratory pattern and LOC closely because both may be depressed by the large amount of opioids usually required to control pain. Continuous pulse oximetry identifies decreasing oxygen saturation associated with hypoventilation (report O_2 saturation <92%). **Note:** Opioid analgesics decrease intestinal motility and delay return to normal bowel function.
- Consider referral to a pain management team.
- For additonal pain interventions, see **Pain**, p. 719, in Appendix One.

NIC: Analgesic Administration; Distraction; Environmental Management: Comfort; Pain Management; Simple Relaxation Therapy; Tube Care: Gastrointestinal

Impaired gas exchange (or risk for same) related to ventilation-perfusion mismatching secondary to atelectasis or accumulating pulmonary fluid
Desired outcome: Patient has adequate gas exchange as evidenced by RR 12-20 breaths/min with normal depth and pattern (eupnea); oxygen saturation ≥92%; no significant changes in mental status and orientation to person, place, and time; and breath sounds that are clear and audible throughout the lung fields.

- Monitor and document RR q2-4hr as indicated by patient's condition. Note pattern, degree of excursion, and whether patient uses accessory muscles of respiration. Report significant deviations from baseline to the health care provider.
- Auscultate both lung fields q4-8hr. Note presence of abnormal (crackles [rales], rhonchi, wheezes) or diminished breath sounds.
- Monitor sputum production, and promptly report to the health care provider any respiratory secretions indicating respiratory tract infection or pulmonary edema.
- Be alert to early signs of hypoxia, such as changes in mental status, restlessness, agitation, and alterations in mentation.
- Monitor pulse oximetry q8hr or as indicated (report oxygen saturation <92%). Monitor ABG results as available (report Pao_2 <80 mm Hg).
- Administer oxygen as prescribed. Monitor the oxygen delivery system at regular intervals.
- Maintain body position that optimizes ventilation and oxygenation. Elevate HOB 30 degrees or higher, depending on patient comfort. If pleural effusion or other defect is present on one side, position patient with the unaffected lung dependent to maximize the ventilation-perfusion relationship.
- Avoid overaggressive fluid resuscitation.
- Explain to the patient and significant other that pancreatitis results in decreased production of surfactant and pain limits adequate respiratory excursion, increasing the potential for hypostatic pneumonia.
- Instruct patient in the use of hyperinflation device (e.g., incentive spirometer). Instruct the patient that the emphasis of this therapy is on inhalation to expand the lungs maximally. Ensure that patient inhales slowly and deeply 2× normal tidal volume and holds the breath at least 5 sec at the end of inspiration. Ten breaths/hr is recommended to maintain adequate alveolar

inflation. Deep breathing expands the alveoli and aids in mobilizing secretions to the airways, whereas coughing further mobilizes and clears the secretions. Monitor patient's progress, and document in nurses' notes.
- When appropriate, instruct the patient in methods of splinting wounds or the upper abdomen to enable cough.
- Instruct patients who cannot cough effectively in cascade cough, that is, a succession of more short and forceful exhalations.
- Encourage activity as prescribed to help mobilize secretions and promote effective airway clearance.

NIC: Airway Management; Analgesic Administration; Cough Enhancement; Respiratory Monitoring

Risk for infection related to risk of tissue destruction with resulting necrosis secondary to release of pancreatic enzymes
Desired outcome: Patient remains free of infection as evidenced by body temperature <37.7° C (<100° F); negative culture results; HR 60-100 bpm; RR 12-20 breaths/min; BP within patient's normal range; and orientation to person, place, and time.
- Check patient's temperature q4hr for increases. Be aware that hypothermia may precede hyperthermia in some individuals.
- If there is a sudden elevation in temperature, obtain specimens for culture of blood, sputum, urine, wound, drains, and other sites as indicated. Monitor culture reports, and report findings promptly to the health care provider.
- Evaluate patient's mental status, orientation and LOC q4-8hr. Document and report significant deviations from baseline.
- Monitor BP, HR, and RR q4hr. Be alert to increases in HR and RR associated with temperature elevations.
- Administer parenteral antibiotics in a timely fashion to maintain bacteriocidal serum levels. Reschedule antibiotics if a dose is delayed for >1 hr. Recognize that failure to administer antibiotics on schedule can result in inadequate blood levels and treatment failure.
- Observe all secretions and drainage for changes in appearance or odor that may signal infection.
- Prevent transmission of potentially infectious agents by using good hand-washing technique before and after caring for the patient and by disposing of dressings and drainage carefully.

NIC: Infection Protection; Medication Administration; Surveillance; Teaching: Disease Process; Vital Signs Monitoring; Wound Care

Altered nutrition: Less than body requirements related to anorexia, dietary restrictions, and digestive dysfunction
Desired outcomes: Patient maintains baseline body weight and exhibits a positive or balanced nitrogen (N) state on N studies by 24 hr before hospital discharge.
- Initiate parenteral nutrition and adjust insulin amounts according to capillary blood glucose levels, as prescribed.
- Provide oral hygiene at frequent intervals to enhance appetite and minimize nausea.
- Monitor capillary blood sugar levels for presence of hyperglycemia, and be alert to dysphagia, polydipsia, and polyuria, which occur with a hyperglycemic state. These indicators reflect the need for health care provider evaluation and intervention to ensure proper metabolism of carbohydrates.
- When the gastric tube is removed, provide diet as prescribed (e.g., small, high-carbohydrate, low-fat meals at frequent intervals [6/day] with protein added according to patient's tolerance). Instruct patient to avoid stimulants that increase pancreatic enzyme secretion, such as coffee, tea, alcohol, and nicotine or other gastric irritants.

- Weigh patient daily to assess gain or loss. Progressive weight loss may signal the need to change the diet or provide enzyme replacement therapy.
- Note amount and degree of steatorrhea (foamy, foul-smelling stools high in fat content) as an indicator of fat intolerance. As prescribed, administer pancreatic enzyme supplements, which are given before introducing fat into the diet.
- If prescribed, administer other dietary supplements that support nutrition and caloric intake. These may include products that consist of medium-chain triglycerides (MCTs), such as Isocal or MCT oil. These supplements do not require pancreatic enzymes for absorption.
- Avoid administering pancreatin with hot foods or drinks, which will deactivate enzyme activity.
- To help alleviate the bloating, nausea, and cramps experienced by some patients, provide meals in small feedings throughout the day.

NIC: Diet Staging; Enteral Tube Feeding; Gastrointestinal Intubation; Nutrition Management; Teaching: Prescribed Diet; Total Parenteral Nutrition (TPN) Administration

> **See Also:** Appendix One, "Caring for Preoperative and Postoperative Patients," p. 717, for nursing diagnoses and interventions.

PATIENT-FAMILY TEACHING AND DISCHARGE PLANNING

When providing patient-family teaching, focus on sensory information; avoid giving excessive information; and initiate a visiting nurse referral for necessary follow-up teaching. Consider including verbal and written information about the following:

- Cause for current episode of pancreatitis, if known, so that recurrence may be avoided.
- Alcohol consumption, which can cause or exacerbate chronic pancreatitis.
- Availability of chemical dependency programs to prevent/treat drug dependence, which is a common occurrence with chronic pancreatitis; or to treat alcoholism. Availability of community support groups, such as the following:

  Alcoholics Anonymous
  WWW address: *http://www.alcoholics-anonymous.org/*

  Narcotics Anonymous
  WWW address: *http://www/netwizrds.net/recovery/na*

- Diet: frequent, small meals that are high in carbohydrates and protein. Food should be bland until gradual return to normal diet is prescribed. Remind patient to avoid enzyme stimulants, such as coffee, tea, nicotine, and alcohol.
- Medications, including drug name, purpose, dosage, schedule, precautions, drug/drug and food/drug interactions, and potential side effects.
- Signs and symptoms of diabetes mellitus, including fatigue, weight loss, polydipsia, polyuria, and polyphagia.
- Necessity of medical follow-up; confirm time and date of next medical appointment.
- Potential for recurrence of steatorrhea as evidenced by foamy, foul-smelling stools that are high in fat content. Steatorrhea can indicate recurrence of disease process or ineffectiveness of drug therapy and should be reported to health care provider.
- Weighing daily at home; importance of reporting weight loss to health care provider.

- If surgery was performed, the indicators of wound infection: redness, swelling, discharge, fever, pain, or increased local warmth.
- For more information contact the following organization:

National Digestive Diseases Information Clearinghouse, National Institute of Diabetes and Digestive and Kidney Diseases Project Officer
2 Information Way
Bethesda, MD 20892   (302) 468-6344
WWW address: *http://www.aerie.com/nihdb/ddbase.htm*

Pancreatic tumors

Pancreatic tumors, either benign (adenoma) or malignant (carcinoma), can develop anywhere within the pancreas. The most frequent site for pancreatic tumors is the pancreatic head, particularly in the region around the ampulla of Vater. These are malignant tumors (adenocarcinomas), whose detection is difficult and for which the prognosis is poor. Because of vague, ill-defined symptoms that appear early in the disease process with pancreatic cancer, metastasis often occurs before a diagnosis can be made. Tumors that develop at beta cells of the islet cells of Langerhans are called insulinomas. These tumors are characterized by hypersecretion of insulin, which leads to significant hypoglycemia. Usually they are treated surgically with a subtotal pancreatectomy.

ASSESSMENT

Signs and symptoms: Progressive, unexplained, rapid weight loss; upper or midabdominal pain that radiates to the back, can be aggravated by eating, and is not related to posture or activity. The patient also may have clay-colored stools, dark urine, pruritus, anorexia, nausea, vomiting, steatorrhea caused by fat and protein malabsorption, bleeding tendencies, malnutrition, and electrolyte disturbances. In addition, diabetes mellitus (DM) symptoms often appear as early indicators of the disorder (see "Diabetes Mellitus," p. 374).

Insulinomas: Characterized by signs and symptoms of associated hypoglycemia. These symptoms appear irregularly and are associated with fasting or exercise. Hypoglycemia results in irritability, confusion, delirium, palpitations, tachycardia, angina, tremors that may progress to seizures and coma.

Physical assessment: Jaundice caused by obstruction of the flow of bile from the liver, mild ascites, abdominal tenderness, hepatomegaly, muscle wasting, generalized bruising and ecchymosis, generalized weakness, and poor skin turgor.

DIAGNOSTIC TESTS

Serum alkaline phosphatase: Elevated with obstructive bile duct disease.
Serum bilirubin: Elevated if the pancreatic tumor obstructs the flow of bile from the liver. Levels >3 mg/dl will result in jaundice; levels >25 mg/dl are common with pancreatic adenocarcinoma.
Prothrombin time (PT):   Prolonged because of vitamin K deficiency. Vitamin K is required for synthesis of prothrombin in the liver, and it is absorbed poorly in the presence of pancreatic insufficiency because it is a fat-soluble vitamin.
Hct and Hgb   Often decreased. Stools for occult blood may reveal blood with involvement of the head of the pancreas.
GI x-rays: May show displacement of visceral organs by the enlarged pancreatic tumor.
CT or MRI scan of pancreas: To delineate pancreatic mass.
Endoscopic retrograde cholangiopancreatography (ERCP):   Permits direct visualization of the ampulla of Vater via injection of a radiopaque dye into

the pancreatic and biliary ducts. Biopsy, collection of pancreatic secretions, and collection of cytology specimens may be accomplished.

Percutaneous transhepatic cholangiogram (PTHC): To determine the level of biliary obstruction and confirm the presence of cholelithiasis. There is a risk of postprocedure bleeding (see "Liver Biopsy," p. 487), and it is contraindicated for patients with bleeding tendencies.

5-Hr glucose tolerance test: Helps confirm diagnosis of insulinoma.

Cytologic examination of duodenal contents: Reveals malignant cells if present.

Fine-needle aspiration biopsy: To confirm diagnosis. It may be guided by CT scan.

Laparoscopy: Allows direct visualization of the pancreas and collection of biopsies.

COLLABORATIVE MANAGEMENT

Pancreatic cancer frequently results from metastasis; and even when the pancreas is the primary site, diagnosis and interventions are thwarted by the vague symptomatology and insidious onset of this disease. The medical and surgical approaches vary depending on the status of the tumor found with the initial exploratory surgery (exploratory laparotomy).

Preoperative/postoperative pain control: Pain may be severe and require significant amounts of opioid analgesics. Regularly scheduled, transcutaneous patches, or PCA may be used to provide analgesia. **Note:** Opioids may result in spasm of the sphincter of Oddi and an increase in pain. If increasing pain is noted, notify the health care provider and request a pain management team consultation to investigate alternative opioid or other pain management strategies.

Whipple's procedure (pancreatoduodenectomy): A surgical attempt to cure cancer of the pancreatic head when the tumor is judged to be resectable (e.g., it has not metastasized and is not interfering with major blood vessels). This extensive surgery involves resection of the head of the pancreas and duodenum and three anastomoses of the following: common bile duct to the jejunum (choledochojejunostomy); the remainder of the pancreas to the jejunum (pancreaticojejunostomy); and the stomach to the jejunum (gastrojejunostomy).

Total pancreatectomy: May be performed for patients with cancer of the pancreatic head. The location of the surgical incision varies with the extent of the surgery; however, whether it is vertical or oblique, the incision usually extends high into the abdomen. The patient has one or two drains, depending on the extent of the surgery. Closed wound drainage system are commonly used to drain the pancreatic bed. For patients who have undergone a total pancreatectomy, the resultant pancreatic endocrine and exocrine deficiency requires treatment with insulin, pancreatic enzymes, and a low-fat diabetic diet.

Partial (subtotal) pancreatectomy: Removes the distal pancreas (tail of the pancreas) to control insulinomas.

Palliative measures: Initiated when the tumor is not resectable (90% of the cases).

Choledochoduodenostomy: The unresectable tumor is left intact, and the common bile duct is anastomosed to the duodenum to permit bile from the liver to bypass the tumor and flow directly into the duodenum.

Percutaneous biliary drain: Used for inoperable liver, pancreatic, or bile duct carcinoma. A tube or catheter, which is perforated with holes at the distal end, is inserted percutaneously through the liver, past the obstructed common bile and pancreatic ducts, and into the duodenum. The catheter collects fluid from the surrounding tissues and permits their passage into the duodenum for excretion. It is a palliative measure to prolong life and minimize discomfort.

The catheter must be changed q6-8wk and flushed qod with small amounts of saline to maintain patency.

Postoperative chemotherapy: Multiple drug protocols are used but commonly are delayed until the patient has recovered from surgery.

NURSING DIAGNOSES AND INTERVENTIONS

Risk for fluid volume deficit with risks of postsurgical hemorrhage (caused by vascularity of surgical site or multiple anastomosis sites) or fluid shift to third-space (interstitial) compartments

Desired outcome: Patient is normovolemic as evidenced by BP ≥90/60 mm Hg (or within patient's baseline range), HR ≤100 bpm, RR ≤20 breaths/min with normal depth and pattern (eupnea), good skin turgor, brisk capillary refill (<2 sec), balanced I&O, urinary output ≥30 ml/hr, stable weight, and moist mucous membranes.

- Monitor BP, HR, and RR, and check capillary refill in nail beds at frequent intervals. Tachycardia, hypotension, increased respirations, and slow capillary refill can signal the presence of dehydration and hypovolemia, which can lead to shock. Also be alert to cool, clammy skin, which can occur with hemorrhage, and to a low urinary output (<30-40 ml/hr for 2 consecutive hr). Report significant findings to health care provider.
- Administer crystalloids and colloids (e.g., albumin) as prescribed. Large amounts of fluid may be necessary because of fluid sequestration, surgical loss, and loss from incisions or drains. Fluid often is prescribed as a baseline amount with additional amounts according to previous 8-hr output, including drainage from surgical sites and drains.
- Prevent increased pressure on suture lines by keeping all drainage tubes patent and free of kinks. Keep gravity drains dependent to the wound site, and secure all connections with tape.
- Prevent abdominal distention by maintaining function of the NG drainage system. *Gently* irrigate NG tube with air or saline q2-4hr or as needed.
- Note and document the amount and character of drainage from the tubes. Drainage from the surgical incision or drains may be profuse. Increasing amounts of fluid from the surgical incision or drains can suggest infection or fistula formation. Note the amount, consistency, color, and odor, and inform the health care provider accordingly. Persistent, bloody drainage in steady or increasing amounts signals active bleeding. Foul-smelling, cloudy, creamy, thick drainage suggests infection. Report significant findings to health care provider.
- Monitor blood study results, including PT, for clotting factor and Hct and Hgb, which can fall with blood loss. Optimal values are as follows: PT 11-15 sec, Hct 40%-54% (male) and 37%-47% (female), and Hgb 14-18 g/dl (male) and 12-16 g/dl (female).
- Monitor serum protein levels (normal range for random specimen is 2-8 mg/dl), and be alert to weight gain, which may signal interstitial spacing of fluids. Monitor I&O; note if intake exceeds output. Preoperatively, most of these patients are protein deficient. Low serum protein alters serum colloid osmotic pressure, resulting in fluid shift from intravascular to interstitial compartments (third spacing of body fluids). Supplemental colloids, such as albumin, plasma protein fraction (PPF), or Plasmanate may be required. **Note:** Intravascular fluid loss can occur despite adequate fluid replacement.
- Monitor laboratory study results for evidence of electrolyte imbalances, especially K^+ and Na^+. Normal K^+ range is 3.5-5.0 mEq/L, and normal Na^+ range is 137-147 mEq/L.

NIC: Fluid/Electrolyte Management; Surveillance; Tube Care; Tube Care: Gastrointestinal; Wound Care

Risk for impaired skin integrity with risk factors related to wound drainage, pressure on incision, or pruritus

Desired outcome: Patient's skin remains nonerythemic and intact, with evidence of good wound healing.

- Promote adequate drainage from drainage tubes to prevent pressure from fluid collection around wound site. Evaluate proper functioning of the wall suction and drains. Do not occlude the air port of the sump drainage devices, which could result in excessive suction. Be certain to protect surrounding skin by using Karaya or other nonirritating adhesive disks and stoma pouches over the drain or wound sites. Consult ET nurse or wound specialist as indicated.

- Assess and document condition of incision and quality and quantity of wound drainage. Fistula formation is a major complication of Whipple's procedure, so it is important to monitor periincisional skin carefully for signs of irritation. If irritation occurs or a fistula does form, cover the irritated area with a pectin wafer skin barrier and use stoma pouch to collect drainage from the fistula.

- Keep patient in semi-Fowler's position to minimize pressure on the incision. Use pressure-relief mattress to minimize potential for skin breakdown.

- When regular diet is resumed after surgery, provide small, frequent meals that are high in protein, vitamins, and calories and low in fat. Administer pancreatic enzyme replacements and insulin, as prescribed, for patient who has had a total pancreatectomy. These interventions help ensure optimal tissue repair by improving digestion.

- For patients with jaundice or increased serum bilirubin levels, administer diphenhydramine, phenothiazines, or cholestyramine to aid in relieving pruritus.

- For more information, see "Managing Wound Care," p. 704.

NIC: Incision Site Care; Ostomy Care; Pressure Management; Skin Care: Topical Treatments; Skin Surveillance; Wound Care

---

See Also: "Hepatitis" for **Risk for impaired skin integrity** related to pruritus, p. 483; **Altered protection** related to increased risk of bleeding secondary to decreased vitamin K absorption, p. 483; "Diabetes Mellitus," p. 376, for interventions relating to blood glucose control; Appendix One, "Caring for Preoperative and Postoperative Patients," for **Pain** or **Chronic Pain** related to disease process, injury, or surgical procedure and other nursing diagnoses and interventions, p. 719; "Caring for Patients With Cancer and Other Life-disrupting Illnesses," p. 747.

PATIENT-FAMILY TEACHING AND DISCHARGE PLANNING

When providing patient-family teaching, focus on sensory information; avoid giving excessive information; and initiate a visiting nurse referral for necessary follow-up teaching. Consider including verbal and written information about the following:

- For patients with DM, a review of insulin action, dosage, and administration; diabetic diet; and signs and symptoms of hyperglycemia and hypoglycemia. See "Diabetes Mellitus," p. 376, for more information.

- Wound care, such as cleansing, dressing changes, and care of drains if patient is discharged with them; indicators of wound infection, such as drainage, warmth along incision line, persistent incisional redness, swelling, fever, and pain.

- Medications, including drug name, purpose, dosage, schedule, precautions, drug/drug and food/drug interactions, and potential side effects.

- Arrangements for hospice services; contact the following organization:

  National Hospice Association
  1901 North Moore St., Suite 901
  Arlington, VA 22209   (703) 243-5900;   (703) 525-5762 FAX
  WWW address: *http://www.nho.org/*

- For additional information, refer patients to the following organization:

  National Cancer Institute
  Department of Health and Human Services
  Office of Cancer Communications
  9000 Rockville Pike
  Bethesda, MD 20892   (301) 496-5583
  WWW address: *http://www.icic.nic.nigh.gov/*

  The American Cancer Society
  1599 Clifton Road NE
  Atlanta, GA 30329   (800) ACS-2345
  WWW address: *http://www.cancer.org*

Selected Bibliography

Ambrose M, Dreher H: Pancreatitis, *Nurs 96* 26(4):33-39, 1996.

Apelgren KN: Laparoscopic appendectomy and the management of gyneco-logic pathologic conditions found at laparoscopy for presumed appendicitis, *Surg Clin North Am* 76(3):469-482, 1996.

Armstrong T: Stomatitis in the bone marrow transplant patient: an overview and proposed oral care protocol, *Cancer Nurs* 17(5):403-410, 1994.

Bauley G et al: Transjugular intrahepatic portosystemic shunt: an alternative, *Crit Care Nurs* 16(1):23-29, 1996.

Boey JH: The acute abdomen, In Way LW, editor: *Current surgical diagnosis & treatment,* ed 10, Norwalk, Conn, 1994, Appleton & Lange.

Butler RW: Managing the complications of cirrhosis, *Am J Nurs* 94(3):46-49, 1994.

Caroline DF, Friedman AC: The radiology of inflammatory bowel disease, *Med Clin North Am* 78(6):1353-1385, 1994.

Cohen S, Parkman H: Treatment of achalasia—from whalebone to botulinum toxin, *N Engl J Med* 332(12):815-816, 1995.

Deglin JH, Vallerand AH: *Davis's drug guide for nurses,* ed 5, Philadelphia, 1997, Davis.

Dose AM: The symptom experience of mucositis, stomatitis and xerostomia, *Semin Oncol Nurs* 11(4):248-255, 1995.

Gore RM, Ghahremani GG: Radiologic investigation of acute inflammatory and infectious bowel disease, *Gastroenterol Clin North Am* 24(2):353-384, 1995.

Hampton BG, Bryant PA: *Ostomies and continent diversions,* St Louis, 1992, Mosby.

Hanauer SB, Baert F: Medical therapy of inflammatory bowel disease, *Med Clin North Am* 78(6):1413-1426, 1994.

Handerhan B: Investigating peritoneal irritation, *Am J Nurs* 94(4):71-73, 1994.

Heslin JM: Peptic ulcer disease: making a case against the prime suspect, *Nurs 97* 27(1):34-39, 1997.

Hirschfeld S, Clearfield HR: Pharmacologic therapy for inflammatory bowel disease, *Am Fam Physician* 51(8):1971-1975, 1995.

Interqual: *ISD-A review system with adult ISD criteria,* Northhampton, NH, and Marlboro, Mass, August 1992, Interqual.

Jackson MM, Rymer TE: Viral hepatitis: anatomy of a diagnosis, *Am J Nurs* 94(1):43-48, 1994.

Kahng KU, Roslyn JJ: Surgical treatment of inflammatory bowel disease, *Med Clin North Am* 78(6):1427-1441, 1994.

Keen J: Abdominal trauma. In Keen J, Swearingen P, editors: *Mosby's critical care consultant,* St Louis, 1997, Mosby.

Kim MJ et al: *Pocket guide to nursing diagnoses,* ed 7, St Louis, 1997, Mosby.

Krumberger J: Acute pancreatitis, *Crit Care Nurs Clin North Am* 5(1):185-201, 1993.

Lewis JD, Fisher RL: Nutrition support in inflammatory bowel disease, *Med Clin North Am* 78(6):1443-1456, 1994.

MacRae HM et al: Comparison of hemorrhoidal treatment modalities: a meta-analysis, *Dis Colon Rectum* 38(7):687-694, 1995.

Mazier WP: Hemorrhoids, fissures, and pruritus ani, *Surg Clin North Am* 74(6):1277-1291, 1994.

McCloskey JC, Bulechek GM, editors: *Nursing interventions classification,* ed 2, St Louis, 1996, Mosby.

McDonald M et al: Severe liver disease. In Ayers S et al, editors: *Textbook of critical care*, Philadelphia, 1995, Saunders.

Mercer L: Pancreatic cancer, exocrine. In Dambro M: *Griffith's 5 minute clinical consult*, Baltimore, 1995, Williams & Wilkins.

Moyer LA, Mast EE: Hepatitis B: virology, epidemiology, disease, and prevention, and an overview of viral hepatitis, *Immunization in Medical Education, Am J Prev Med* 10(suppl):45-55, 1994.

Nathens AB, Rothstein OD: Therapeutic options in peritonitis, *Surg Clin North Am* 76(3):451-457, 1996.

NIH Consensus Development Conference: *Helicobacter pylori* in peptic ulcer disease, *JAMA* 272:65-69, 1994.

Oddsdottir M: Laparoscopic management of achalasia, *Surg Clin North Am* 76(3):451-457, 1996.

Pasricha PJ et al: Intrasphincteric botulinum toxin for the treatment of achalasia, *N Engl J Med* 332(12):774-778, 1995.

Pelligrini CA, Way LW: Esophagus & diaphragm. In Way LW, editor: *Current surgical diagnosis & treatment*, ed 10, Norwalk, Conn, 1994, Appleton & Lange.

Quinn PG et al: The role of endoscopy in inflammatory bowel disease, *Med Clin North Am* 78(6):1331-1352, 1994.

Rosenstein B: New drugs on the horizon, *Foundation Focus* 11:17, 1996.

Rueden KT, Dunham CM: Sequelae of massive fluid resuscitation in trauma patients, *Crit Care Nurs Clin North Am* 6(3):463-472, 1994.

Russell TR: Anorectum. In Way LW, editor: *Current surgical diagnosis & treatment*, ed 10, Norwalk, Conn, 1994, Appleton & Lange.

Schrock TR: Large intestine. In Way LW, editor: *Current surgical diagnosis & treatment*, ed 10, Norwalk, Conn, 1994, Appleton & Lange.

Schrock TR: Small intestine. In Way LW, editor: *Current surgical diagnosis & treatment*, ed 10, Norwalk, Conn, 1994, Appleton & Lange.

Seifrit B: *Helicobacter pylori*, *AORN J* 65(3):614-620, 1997.

Sherlock S: *Diseases of the liver and biliary system*, ed 9, Oxford, England, 1992, Blackwell.

Spiro HM: Hiatus hernia and reflux esophagitis, *Hosp Pract* 29(1):51, 1994.

Stamatos CS et al: Meeting the challenge of the older trauma patient, *Am J Nurs* 96(5):40-48, 1996.

Steinberg W, Tanner S: Acute pancreatitis, *N Engl J Med* 330(17):1198-1210, 1994.

Sugarbaker DJ et al: Esophageal physiology and pathophysiology, *Surg Clin North Am* 73(6):1101-1115, 1993.

Swearingen PL, Howard C: *Addison-Wesley's photo-atlas of nursing procedures,* ed 3, Redwood City, Calif, 1996, Addison-Wesley.

US Department of Health and Human Services: *Acute pain management: operative or medical procedures and trauma,* AHCPR 92-0032, Rockville, Md, 1992, Public Health Service, Agency for Health Care Policy and Research.

Way LW: Appendix. In Way LW, editor: *Current surgical diagnosis & treatment,* ed 10, Norwalk, Conn, 1994, Appleton & Lange.

Zurita VF et al: Nutritional support in inflammatory bowel disease, *Dig Dis* 13(2):92-107, 1995.

7 HEMATOLOGIC DISORDERS

Section One: Disorders of the Red Blood Cells

The erythrocyte, or RBC, is the transport mechanism for hemoglobin (Hgb), which carries O_2 from the heart and lungs to the tissues, exchanges it for CO_2, and then returns it to the heart and lungs. RBCs are very flexible and capable of bending, elongating, and squeezing through tiny capillaries. Normal RBCs can travel under high pressure and speed, are extremely active metabolically, and have an average life span of 120 days. The bone marrow produces and replaces RBCs every day and can respond to an increased need for RBCs by increasing production. However, with increased production, immature RBCs (reticulocytes) often are released into the circulation; a high or abnormally low level of reticulocytes often aids in the diagnosis of RBC disorders.

Anemia is a common hematopoietic disorder, defined as a reduced RBC volume (hematocrit [Hct]) or a reduced concentration of Hgb. Consideration of the patient's intravascular volume (i.e., hydration status) is essential for proper interpretation of the Hct and Hgb. The general effects of anemia result from a deficiency in the O_2-carrying mechanism, although some effects are related to varied pathogeneses. Three basic types of anemias are discussed in this section: erythropoietin deficiency, hemolytic, and hypoplastic (aplastic).

Erythropoietin deficiency anemia

Erythropoietin (EPO) is a naturally occurring protein hormone produced and released by the kidney (90%) and liver (10%). EPO stimulates stem cells in the bone marrow to develop and produce RBCs. The kidney is stimulated to release EPO in response to low blood oxygenation. Patients with decreased renal function (e.g., chronic renal failure) often become anemic because their kidneys cannot produce EPO. Development of recombinant human erythropoietin (epoetin alpha) has provided dramatic benefits for patients with chronic renal failure, patients receiving chemotherapy for cancer, and patients receiving AZT for treatment of HIV infection.

ASSESSMENT

Chronic indicators: The patient may be asymptomatic or have brittle hair and nails. In the presence of severe and chronic disease, dysphagia, stomatitis, and inflammation of the tongue may be present. History of chronic renal disease, dialysis therapy, cancer chemotherapy, or AZT therapy for HIV infection may also be present.

Acute indicators: Fatigue, decreased ability to concentrate, cold sensitivity, menstrual irregularities, and loss of libido.

Physical assessment: Tachycardia, palpitations, tachypnea, exertional dyspnea, pale mucous membranes, pale nail beds, vertigo.

DIAGNOSTIC TESTS

Blood count: Usually RBCs and Hgb are decreased; Hct usually is low because the percentage of RBCs in the total blood volume is decreased.
Peripheral blood smear to examine RBC indices: Morphology may be normal, or there may be microcytosis or hypochromia.
Total iron-binding capacity: Decreased.
Reticulocyte count: Normal to slightly elevated.
Serum iron levels: Decreased.

COLLABORATIVE MANAGEMENT

Correction of the underlying cause: For example, kidney transplant.
Erythropoietin replacement: Recombinant EPO (epoetin-α), 150 U/kg intravenously 3 times each week or 600 U/kg subcutaneously each week. Although side effects are few, deep vein thrombosis may occur and patients with renal insufficiency must be observed for hypertension and iron deficiency.
Iron replacement: To provide concurrent iron replacement therapy.

NURSING DIAGNOSES AND INTERVENTIONS

See "Lymphomas" for **Activity intolerance** related to imbalance between oxygen-carrying capacity of the blood caused by anema.

PATIENT-FAMILY TEACHING AND DISCHARGE PLANNING

When providing patient-family teaching, focus on sensory information; avoid giving excessive information; and initiate a visiting nurse referral for necessary follow-up teaching. Consider including verbal and written information about the following:

- Importance of a well-balanced diet, especially iron intake, which is found in foods such as red meat, dark green vegetables, legumes, and certain fruits (apricots, figs, raisins).
- Special instructions for taking iron, depending on type prescribed. Therapy may need to be continued for 4-6 mo to adequately replace iron stores.
- EPO replacement therapy will need to be continued for life, unless the underlying condition (e.g., cancer chemotherapy) is corrected.
- When self-administering EPO, patients should understand the need to *avoid* shaking medication vial before administration. Shaking the vial may denature glycoprotein in the solution and render it biologically inactive. Any discolored solution or solution with particulate matter should not be used.

Hemolytic anemia

Hemolytic anemia is characterized by abnormal or premature destruction of RBCs. Hemolysis can be intrinsic or result from such conditions as infection or radiation. *Sickle cell anemia* is a form of chronic hemolytic anemia characterized by abnormal, crescent-shaped, rigid, and elongated erythrocytes. Because of their abnormal shape and rigidity, these "sickled" RBCs interfere with circulation because they cannot get through the microcirculation and are destroyed in the process. Sickle cell anemia can affect almost every body system through decreased O_2 delivery, decreased circulation caused by occlusion of the vessels by RBCs, and inflammatory process. This disorder occurs when the gene is inherited from both parents (homozygous); a carrier state for the sickle cell trait exists when it is inherited from one parent (heterozygous). Sickle cell anemia is seen predominantly in African-Americans and with less frequency in hereditary descendants of Greece and southern Italy.

Acquired hemolytic anemia is usually the result of an abnormal immune response that causes premature destruction of RBCs. Hemolysis can occur because of a foreign antigen, as from a transfusion reaction, or an autoimmune reaction in which the hemolytic agent is intrinsic to the patient's body. Other possible causes include exposure to radiation and ingestion of some drugs (e.g., sulfisoxazole [Gantrisin], phenacetin, methyldopa [Aldomet]).

Hemolytic crisis: Individuals with chronic hemolytic anemia may do relatively well for a time, but many factors can precipitate a hemolytic crisis or acute hemolysis (i.e., an individual with mild hemolytic anemia can become severely anemic with an acute infectious process or with any other physiologic or emotional stressor, including surgery, trauma, or emotional upset). Widespread hemolysis causes an acute decrease in O_2-carrying capacity of the blood, resulting in decreased O_2 delivery to the tissues. Organ congestion from the hemolyzed blood cells occurs, and this affects organ function and precipitates a shock state.

Although medical therapy has improved the general prognosis of these patients, there is still an overall decrease in life expectancy.

ASSESSMENT

Chronic indicators: Pallor (e.g., conjunctival), fatigue, dyspnea on exertion, and intermittent dizziness, all of which depend on the severity of the anemia. With chronic hemolytic anemia, the individual sometimes will exhibit jaundice, arthritis, renal failure, and skin ulcers because of hemolysis and chronic organ damage. In children and adolescents, sickle cell disease impairs and distorts skeletal growth and increases the potential for hematogenic osteomyelitis.

Acute indicators: Fever; headache, visual blurring, temporary blindness; severe abdominal pain, vomiting, splenomegaly, hepatomegaly; back, lower leg, and joint pain; palpitations; shortness of breath (SOB); chills; lymphadenopathy; and decreased urinary output (signs and symptoms of hemolytic crisis). Peripheral nerve damage can result in paralysis or paresthesias. Occasionally a low-grade fever may occur 1-2 days after a crisis event. Attacks last a few hours to a few days, resolving spontaneously.

DIAGNOSTIC TESTS

Sickle cell test (Sickledex): Screens for sickle cell anemia or the trait.

Hgb electrophoresis: Discriminates between Hgb AS, the sickle cell trait, and Hgb SS, sickle cell anemia.

Cold agglutinin titer: Markedly elevated (>1:1000).

Hgb and Hct: Decreased because of RBC destruction.

Serum tests: Lactate dehydrogenase (LDH) elevated because of the release of this enzyme when the RBC is destroyed. Bilirubin is elevated because the liver cannot process the excess that occurs from rapid RBC destruction.

Urine and fecal urobilinogen: Levels increased. These are more sensitive indicators of RBC destruction than serum bilirubin levels.

Bone marrow aspiration: Reveals erythroid hyperplasia, especially with chronic hemolytic anemia.

Reticulocyte count: Elevated because of the rapid destruction of RBCs.

Serum haptoglobin: Decreased because the Hgb released from hemolyzed RBCs is bound to haptoglobin.

Chorionic biopsy: Determines presence of sickle cell disease in the first 6-8 wk of pregnancy.

COLLABORATIVE MANAGEMENT

Elimination or discontinuation of causative factor: If possible (e.g., chemical, drug, incompatible blood).

Volume replacement: Adequate hydration important to prevent complications from decreased organ perfusion secondary to hemolysis.

O_2 therapy: Routine pulse oximetry to determine need for oxygen therapy for patients who are hypoxemic (e.g., O_2 saturation <92%).

Supportive therapy for shock state: If it occurs.

Transfusion: If circulatory failure or severe anemic anoxia occurs; especially at risk are older persons or others with limited cardiopulmonary reserve.

Erythrocytapheresis (RBC exchange):   A relatively new procedure that removes abnormal RBCs and infuses healthy RBCs to correct the anemia.

Patient assessment during erythrocytapheresis
- Monitor for symptom relief following one RBC exchange.
- Monitor arterial Pao$_2$ for evidence of improvement, optimally ≥80 mm Hg.
- Monitor Hct. Values ≥30% are necessary to prevent bone marrow stimulation.

Corticosteroids: To help stabilize cell membranes and decrease the inflammatory response. Usually prednisone, 50-100 mg, is given with antacids.

Folic acid: To help prevent hemolytic crisis by increasing the production of RBCs in individuals with chronic hemolytic anemias.

Splenectomy: To provide symptomatic relief, depending on the cause of the anemia. May also be done prophylactically to reduce potential for rupture and massive blood loss. The spleen is the site of RBC destruction.

NURSING DIAGNOSES AND INTERVENTIONS

Risk for impaired skin integrity *or* **impaired tissue integrity** with risk factors related to altered circulation (occlusion of the vessels), resulting in impaired oxygen transport to the tissues and skin

Desired outcome: Patient's skin and tissue remain nonerythematous and intact.

- Assess the patient's skin, especially over bony prominences and extremities. Document changes in integrity, such as erythema, increased warmth, and blisters.
- Use a bed cradle to keep pressure of bed linens and blankets off patient's tissue and skin.
- Keep extremities warm to promote circulation.
- Encourage moderate exercises or ROM to promote circulation q1hr while awake. **Caution:** Avoid any activity or exercise if signs and symptoms of hemolytic crisis are present (see "Patient-Family Teaching and Discharge Planning," p. 518).
- Caution patient about the importance of avoiding trauma or injury to the skin and tissues.
- Apply dry, sterile dressings or transparent or hydrocolloidal dressing materials such as Duoderm, Comfeel, Op-Site, or Tegaderm to areas of tissue breakdown. Use sterile technique to help prevent infection. See "Managing Wound Care," p. 704, for more information.

You may also wish to refer to the following interventions from the Nursing Interventions Classification (NIC):

NIC: Circulatory Precautions; Exercise Promotion; Pressure Management; Pressure Ulcer Care; Skin Surveillance; Teaching: Prescribed Activity/Exercise

Altered peripheral and cardiopulmonary tissue perfusion related to interrupted blood flow secondary to inflammatory process and occlusion of blood vessels with RBCs

Desired outcome: Following treatment, patient has adequate peripheral and cardiopulmonary perfusion as evidenced by systolic BP ≤10 mm Hg lower than baseline systolic BP, peripheral pulses >2+ on a 0-4+ scale, HR ≤100 bpm, RR 12-20 breaths/min with normal depth and pattern (eupnea), and normal skin color.

- Assess BP at frequent intervals, and report significant drops (>10 mm Hg from baseline systolic readings).
- Assess amplitude of peripheral pulses as an indicator of peripheral perfusion. Be alert to pulses ≤2+ (on a 0-4+ scale) in amplitude.

- Be alert to signs of cardiac depression, including decreased BP, increased HR, decreased pulse amplitude, dyspnea, and decreased urine output.
- Assess for and report indicators of hypoxia or respiratory dysfunction, such as increased RR, dyspnea, SOB, and cyanosis.
- Administer oxygen as prescribed if hypoxemia is present.
- Assist patient with ROM exercises and positioning to enhance tissue perfusion as well as to maintain and increase joint mobility. **Caution:** Exercise should be avoided if any early signs of hemolytic crisis appear (see "Patient-Family Teaching and Discharge Planning" below) because exercise can aggravate hemolysis.
- Report significant findings to patient's health care provider.

NIC: Circulatory Care; Exercise Therapy: Joint Mobility; Fluid Management; Positioning; Vital Signs Monitoring

Pain related to joint hemolysis secondary to hemolytic crisis
Desired outcomes: Within 1 hr of intervention, patient's subjective perception of discomfort decreases, as documented by a pain scale. Objective indicators, such as grimacing, are absent or diminished. Life-style behaviors are not compromised because of discomfort.

- Monitor for the presence of pain. Devise a pain scale with the patient, rating the discomfort on a scale of 0 (no pain) to 10 (worst pain). Administer pain medications as prescribed, and document effectiveness using the pain scale.
- Instruct patient to request analgesic before the pain becomes too intense.
- Reassure patient that pain will subside when acute hemolytic episode is over.
- Elevate extremities to promote comfort.
- Apply moist heat packs to the joints to increase circulation and decrease pain. Use heat cautiously, especially for patients with decreased peripheral sensations.
- Apply elastic stockings or wraps, if prescribed, to protect skin, support joints, and promote circulation.

NIC: Analgesic Administration; Heat/Cold Application; Pain Management

PATIENT-FAMILY TEACHING AND DISCHARGE PLANNING

When providing patient-family teaching, focus on sensory information; avoid giving excessive information; and initiate a visiting nurse referral for necessary follow-up teaching. Consider including verbal and written information about the following:

- If patient is discharged taking corticosteroids, the side effects of steroids, including weight gain, headache, capillary fragility, hypertension, moon facies, thinning of arms and legs, mood changes, acne, buffalo hump, edema formation, risk of gastrointestinal hemorrhage and delayed wound healing, and increased appetite. Review need to take the medication with food, to immediately take missed doses, and to avoid precipitously discontinuing medication.
- Provide information on phone numbers and contact person for local and/or national support groups available for sickle cell anemia and thalassemia, such as the following organization:

  Sickle Cell Disease Association of America
  200 Corporate Point
  Suite 495
  Culver City, CA 90230-7633   (800) 421-8453; FAX (310) 215-3722
  WWW address: *http://www.stepstn.com/nord/org_sum/280.htm*

- Indicators of hemolytic crisis, including jaundice, dyspnea, SOB, joint or abdominal pain, decreasing BP, and increased HR; and factors that precipitate

hemolytic crisis, such as emotional stress, physical stress, infection, trauma, chemicals, and toxic drug reactions (e.g., to penicillin, methyldopa, sulfonamides, quinine).
- Importance of maintaining a calm environment for the patient. Teach patient stress reduction techniques, such as meditation and relaxation exercises. See **Health-seeking behaviors:** Relaxation technique effective for stress reduction, p. 59.
- Importance of avoiding infectious processes, such as upper respiratory infections, and getting prompt medical attention if infection occurs.
- Medications, including drug name, purpose, schedule, dosage, precautions, drug/drug and food/drug interactions, and potential side effects.
- Caution against taking any over-the-counter (OTC) drugs before consulting primary health care provider.
- Refer for genetic counseling as indicated.
- Importance of medical follow-up.
- Importance of obtaining a Medic-Alert bracelet and identification card outlining diagnosis and emergency treatment. Contact the following organization:

Medic Alert
2323 Colorado Ave.
Turlock, CA 95382   (209) 668-3333

Hypoplastic (aplastic) anemia

Hypoplastic anemia results from inability of erythrocyte-producing organs, specifically the bone marrow, to produce erythrocytes. The causes of hypoplastic anemia are varied but can include use of antineoplastic or antimicrobial agents, an infectious process, pregnancy, hepatitis, and radiation. Approximately half the patients with hypoplastic anemia have had exposure to drugs or chemical agents, whereas the remaining half have had immunologic disorders. Hypoplastic anemia most often involves pancytopenia, the depression of production of all three bone marrow elements: erythrocytes, platelets, and granulocytes. Usually the onset of hypoplastic anemia is insidious, but it can evolve quickly in some cases. Prognosis usually is poor for these individuals.

ASSESSMENT

Chronic indicators: Weakness, fatigue, pallor, dysphagia, and numbness and tingling of the extremities.
Acute indicators: Fever and infection (because of decreased neutrophils); bleeding (because of thrombocytopenia), dizziness, dyspnea on exertion, progressive weakness, and oral ulcerations.
History of: Exposure to chemical toxins or radiation; use of antibiotics, such as chloramphenicol; viral infections, such as hepatitis C; antineoplastic therapy.

DIAGNOSTIC TESTS

CBC with differential: Low levels of Hgb, WBCs, and RBCs; however, RBCs usually appear to be normal morphologically.
Platelet count: Low.
Bleeding time: Prolonged.
Bone marrow aspiration: Reveals hypocellular or hypoplastic tissue with a fatty and fibrous appearance and depression of erythroid elements.
Reticulocyte count: This test, which is a determinant of bone marrow function, shows a marked decrease because of the bone marrow's inability to respond.

Peripheral blood smear: Shows nucleated RBCs as well as immature granulocytes.
Cultures: If infection is suspected.

COLLABORATIVE MANAGEMENT

Determination of the cause of anemia
Transfusion with packed RBCs or frozen plasma: See Table 7-1. **Note:** Because of the potential for antibody formation, patients considered candidates for bone marrow transplants should be given leukocyte-poor and cytomegalovirus (CMV)–negative blood products.
Transfusion with concentrated platelets: To keep platelet count >20,000/mm^3. Hemorrhage occurs less frequently when platelet count is above this level (see Table 7-1).
Bone marrow transplantation (BMT):   In this procedure, 500-700 ml of bone marrow is aspirated from the pelvic bones of the donor and then filtered and infused into the patient. Optimally, the donated marrow is antigen compatible (using human leukocyte antigen [HLA] tissue typing), and for that the donor should be an identical twin or sibling. However, only about one third of potential BMT recipients have an HLA-matched sibling donor. The use of unrelated donors is an area of research and potential benefit. **Note:** This procedure is costly (approximately $100,000) and associated with significant risk (5% morbidity and mortality) and carries the requirement for permanent life-style changes.
Treatment with antilymphocyte globulin: To cause immunosuppression before BMT.
Antibiotic therapy: If infection is found.
Steroid therapy: To stimulate granulocyte production, although results with adults are not always successful.
O$_2$:   If anemia is severe.
Granulocyte transfusion: See Table 7-1. Although rarely used today, the following are indications for use: documented infection, fever unresponsive to antibiotics, WBC <500/mm^3, and expectations for bone marrow regeneration.
Androgen therapy: An attempt to stimulate bone marrow activity.

NURSING DIAGNOSES AND INTERVENTIONS

Risk for infection with risk factors related to inadequate secondary defenses secondary to leukopenia with granulocytopenia
Desired outcome: Patient is free of infection as evidenced by normothermia; full, but not bounding, HR ≤100 bpm; RR 12-20 breaths/min with normal depth and pattern (eupnea); urine that is straw colored, clear, and of characteristic odor; absence of adventitious breath sounds; absence of diaphoresis or chills; and absence of unusual erythema, swelling, local warmth, tenderness, or drainage at any wound sites.
- Perform meticulous handwashing before patient contact.
- If appropriate, maintain protective/reverse isolation, using gloves, gown, and mask; make sure that visitors follow the same protocol. Discourage delivery of plants and flowers to the room. Thoroughly wash all fresh fruits and vegetables.
- Screen and restrict the number of visitors to reduce infection via communicable disease.
- Instruct patient or significant other in the assessment of infections and the need to report these quickly to the care provider.
- Report any signs of systemic infection (e.g., fever); obtain prescription for blood, wound, and urine cultures as indicated. Administer antibiotics as prescribed.
- Monitor for and report any signs of local infection, such as sore throat or erythematous or draining wounds. **Note:** With decreased or absent granulo-

TABLE 7-1 Commonly Used Blood Products*†

Product	Approximate volume	Indications	Precautions/comments
Whole blood	500-510 ml (450 ml of WB; 50-60 ml of anticoagulants)	Acute, severe blood loss; hypovolemic shock. Increases both red cell mass and plasma. WB transfusion is used rarely today, and the patient with hematologic disorders is not usually considered an autologous donor. The specific blood components are in lieu of WB.	Must be ABO and Rh compatible. Do not mix with dextrose solutions; always prime tubing with normal saline. Observe for dyspnea, orthopnea, cyanosis, and anxiety as signs of circulatory overload; monitor VS. Administer as rapidly as indicated but not to exceed 4 hr.
Packed RBCs	250 ml	Increase RBC mass and O_2-carrying capacity of blood	Must be ABO and Rh compatible. Leukocyte-depleted RBCs may be used to reduce risk of antibody formation and nonhemolytic reactions. Irradiated RBCs may be used to prevent graft vs. host disease in patients who are immunocompromised. Packed RBCs have less volume than WB, thus reducing risk of fluid overload. Administer over 1.5-2 hrs
Fresh frozen plasma	250 ml	Treatment of choice for combined coagulation factor deficiencies and factor V and XI deficiencies; alternate treatment for factor VII, VIII, IX, and X deficiencies when concentrates are not available	Must be ABO compatible. Supplies clotting factors. Usual dose is 10-15 mg/kg body weight. Transfuse within 24 hr of thawing. Do not use if patient needs volume expansion.

Continued

WB, Whole blood; *VS*, vital signs; *RBC*, red blood cell.

*NOTE: DNA recombinant technology may decrease complications from factor concentrates.

†NOTE: When administering blood products, it is important to recognize that most blood products have risk associated with delivery. Risks include transmission of human immunodeficiency virus, hepatitis B, hepatitis C, cytomegalovirus, and human T-cell leukemia/lymphoma virus (HTLV-I).

‡These products carry no risk of disease transmission.

TABLE 7-1   Commonly Used Blood Products*†—cont'd

Product	Approximate volume	Indications	Precautions/comments
Random-donor platelet concentrate	50 ml (usual adult dose is 5-6 U)	Treatment of choice for thrombocytopenia. Also used for leukemia and hypoplastic anemia.	Usual dose is 0.1 U/kg body weight to increase platelet count to 25,000/mm^3. Administer as rapidly as tolerated. ABO compatibility is preferable. Effectiveness is decreased by fever, sepsis, and splenomegaly. Febrile reactions are common. Use special platelet tubing and filter. Special filters are available for removing leukocytes and thus decreasing the risk of alloimmunization to HLA. Platelets must be infused within 4 hr of initiation.
Platelet concentrate by platelet pheresis (single-donor platelets)	200 ml but may vary	Treatment for thrombocytopenic patients who are refractory to random-donor platelets	Involves removing donor's venous blood, removing platelets by differential centrifuge, and returning blood to donor. Approximately 3-4 L of WB is processed to obtain a therapeutic dose of platelets. May use special donors who are HLA matched to the patient.
Cyroprecipitate (factor VIII)	10-25 ml	Routine treatment for hemophilia (factor VIII deficiency) and fibrinogen deficiency (factor XIII deficiency). Occasionally used to control bleeding in anemic patients.	Made from fresh frozen plasma. Infuse immediately on thawing, 1-2 ml/min in 8-12 hr to achieve desired effect.

AHG (factor VIII) concentrates	20 ml	Alternate treatment for hemophilia A	Allergic and febrile reactions occur frequently. Administer by syringe or component drip set. Can store at refrigerator temperature, making it convenient for persons with hemophilia during travel.
Factor II, VII, IX, X concentrate	20 ml	Treatment of choice for hemophilia B and factor IX deficiencies	Can precipitate clotting. Allergic and febrile reactions occur occasionally. Contraindicated in liver disease.
Albumin‡	50 or 250 ml	Hypovolemic shock, hypoalbuminemia, protein replacement for burn patients	Osmotically equal to 5× its volume of plasma. Used as a volume expander in conjunction with crystalloids. Also used in hypoalbuminemic states. Commercially available.
Plasma protein fraction‡	250 ml (83% albumin with some alpha and beta globulins)	Volume expansion	Commercially available; expensive. Certain lots reported to have hypotension, possibly related to vasoactive amines used in preparation.
Granulocyte transfusion (collected from a single donor)	200 ml but may vary	Leukemia with granulocytopenia related to treatment	Not a common treatment. Febrile and allergic symptoms are frequent. Must be ABO compatible.

WB, Whole blood; *HLA*, human leukocyte antigen; *AHG*, antihemophilic globulin.

*NOTE: DNA recombinant technology may decrease complications from factor concentrates.

†NOTE: When administering blood products, it is important to recognize that most blood products have risk associated with delivery. Risks include transmission of human immunodeficiency virus, hepatitis B, hepatitis C, cytomegalovirus, and human T-cell leukemia/lymphoma virus (HTLV-I).

‡These products carry no risk of disease transmission.

cytes, pus may not form; therefore it is important to look for other signs of infection.

- Provide oral care at frequent intervals to prevent oral lesions, which may result in bleeding and infection.
- Provide and encourage adequate perianal hygiene to prevent rectal abscess. Avoid giving medications or taking temperature rectally.
- Avoid invasive procedures if possible.
- Encourage ambulation, deep breathing, turning, and coughing to prevent problems of immobility, which can result in pneumonia and skin breakdown.
- Arrange for patient to have a private room when possible to permit optimal environmental control.
- Institute reverse isolation if granulocyte count is <200/mm^3. Discuss with patient granulocyte transfusion and BMT if appropriate.
- Teach patient and significant other signs and symptoms of infection and the importance of notifying staff or health care provider promptly if they are noted.

NIC: Infection Protection; Respiratory Monitoring; Surveillance; Teaching: Disease Process; Wound Care

Knowledge deficit: Potential for bleeding (caused by low platelet count) and measures that can help prevent it
Desired outcome: After patient teaching, patient or significant other verbalizes knowledge about the potential for bleeding and measures that can prevent it.
- Teach patient about the potential for bleeding and the importance of monitoring for hematuria, melena, frank bleeding from the mouth, epistaxis, coughing up blood (hemoptysis), or excessive vaginal bleeding (menometrorrhagia) and notifying staff promptly if they occur.
- Teach patient to use an electric razor and soft-bristle toothbrush.
- Explain the importance of maintaining regularity with bowel movements to prevent straining and potential bleeding. Monitor fluid (should be >2.5 L/day) and dietary fiber intake; administer stool softeners as indicated.
- Teach patient to avoid potentially traumatic procedures (e.g., enemas, rectal temperatures) and high-risk recreational life-style.
- Caution patient to avoid using aspirin, aspirin products, or nonsteroidal antiinflammatory drugs (NSAIDs), which decrease platelet aggregation and further increase the potential for bleeding.
- Discourage smoking and excessive alcohol consumption.
- Explain that concentrated platelets usually are transfused to keep the platelet count >20,000/mm^3. Hemorrhage occurs less frequently when the platelet count is maintained above this level.

NIC: Bleeding Precautions; Health Education; Surveillance; Teaching: Disease Process; Teaching: Procedure/Treatment

Altered protection related to neurosensory and musculoskeletal alterations secondary to tissue hypoxia occurring with decreased production of erythrocytes
Desired outcome: Patient verbalizes orientation to person, place, and time and is free of mental status changes or symptoms of injury caused by neurosensory alterations.
- Perform neurologic checks and assess mental status as indicators of cerebral perfusion. If signs of decreasing cerebral perfusion occur, establish precautionary measures (e.g., keeping side rails up and the bed in the lowest position) to protect patient from injury. Request restraints and pad side rails if indicated.
- Request one-on-one supervision by family or staff member if patient becomes confused or restless.

- Assess sensorimotor status to help evaluate nervous system oxygenation. Be alert to paresthesias, decreased muscle strength, and altered gait.
- Prevent injury from heat or cold applications for patients with paresthesias.
- Do not allow patient to ambulate unassisted if muscle or gait alterations are present. Carefully assess the patient's reliability in complying with assisted ambulation.
- As indicated, monitor oximetry; report O_2 saturation <92%. Administer oxygen as prescribed.
- Teach patient and then encourage deep breathing to augment oxygen delivery to the tissues. Cue patient q1-2 hr while awake.
- Report indicators of a worsening condition promptly to patient's health care provider.

NIC: Neurologic Monitoring; Oxygen Therapy; Peripheral Sensation Management; Respiratory Monitoring; Surveillance: Safety

---

See Also: Appendix One, "Caring for Patients on Prolonged Bedrest" for **Risk for activity intolerance** related to deconditioned status, p. 738.

PATIENT-FAMILY TEACHING AND DISCHARGE PLANNING

When providing patient-family teaching, focus on sensory information; avoid giving excessive information; and initiate a visiting nurse referral for necessary follow-up teaching. Consider including verbal and written information about the following:

- Medications, including drug name, purpose, dosage, schedule, precautions, drug/drug and food/drug interactions, and potential side effects.
- Indicators of systemic infection, including fever, malaise, fatigue, as well as signs and symptoms of upper respiratory infection, urinary tract infection, and wound infection (see pp. 162, 704).
- Importance of avoiding exposure to individuals known to have acute infections; preventing trauma, abrasions, and breakdown of the skin; and maintaining good nutritional intake to enhance resistance to infections.
- Signs of bleeding/hemorrhage that necessitate medical attention: melena, hematuria, epistaxis, hemoptysis (coughing up blood), excessive vaginal bleeding (menometrorrhagia), ecchymosis, and bleeding gums.
- Measures to prevent hemorrhage, such as using electric razor and soft-bristle toothbrush and avoiding activities that can traumatize tissues.
- Importance of reporting general symptoms of anemia, including fatigue, weakness, paresthesias, palpitations, or exertional dyspnea.
- Importance of avoiding aspirin, aspirin products, or NSAIDs in the presence of a bleeding disorder.
- Phone numbers to call if questions or concerns arise about therapy or disease after discharge. In addition, some cities have local support groups for patients who may require BMT. Information for these patients can be obtained by contacting the following organization:

    Bone Marrow Transplant Family Support Network
    P.O. Box 845
    Avon, CT 06001   (800) 826-9376
    WWW address: *http://www.ai.mit.edu/people/laurel/Bmt-talk/bmt-talk.html*

Polycythemia

Polycythemia is a chronic disorder characterized by excessive production of RBCs, platelets, and myelocytes. As these increase, blood volume, blood viscosity, and Hgb concentration increase, causing excessive workload for the heart and congestion of some organ systems (e.g., liver, kidney).

Secondary polycythemia results from an abnormal increase in erythropoietin production (e.g., because of hypoxia that occurs with chronic lung disease or prolonged living in altitudes >10,000 ft) or with renal tumors. *Polycythemia vera* is a primary disorder of unknown cause affecting men of Jewish descent, with onset in late mid-life. Polycythemia vera results in increased RBC mass, leukocytosis, and slight thrombocytosis. Because of increased viscosity and decreased microcirculation, mortality is high if the condition is left untreated. In addition, there is a potential for this disorder to evolve into other hematopoietic disorders, such as acute leukemia.

ASSESSMENT

Signs and symptoms: Headache, dizziness, paresthesias, visual disturbances, dyspnea, thrombophlebitis, joint pain, pruritus, night sweats, fatigue, chest pain, and a feeling of "fullness," especially in the head.

Physical assessment: Hypertension, engorgement of retinal blood veins, crackles (rales), weight loss, cyanosis, ruddy complexion (especially palmar aspects of hands and plantar surfaces of feet), hepatosplenomegaly.

DIAGNOSTIC TESTS

CBC: Increased RBC mass (8-12 million/mm^3), Hgb (18-25 g/dl), Hct (>54% in men and >49% in women), and leukocytes; overproduction of thrombocytes.

Platelet count: Elevated as a result of increased production.

Bone marrow aspiration: Reveals RBC proliferation.

Uric acid levels: May be increased because of increased nucleoprotein, an end product of RBC breakdown.

Erythropoietin levels: Elevated in secondary polycythemia and decreased in polycythemia vera.

O$_2$ saturation: Normal ($\geq$92%).

COLLABORATIVE MANAGEMENT

Phlebotomy: Blood withdrawn from the vein to decrease blood volume (and decrease Hct to 45%). Usually 500 ml is removed every 2-3 days until the Hct is 40%-45%. For the older adult, 250-300 ml is removed.

Myelosuppressive therapy: Via alkylating and nonalkylating agents to inhibit bone marrow function, for example, hydroxyurea (preferred), busulfan, chlorambucil, and/or radioactive phosphorus (especially for older persons and those refractive to other agents).

Histamine antagonists: To provide symptomatic relief of pruritus.

Investigational drug therapy: Recombinant interferon alfa has demonstrated promising results in controlling RBC production.

NURSING DIAGNOSES AND INTERVENTIONS

Pain related to headache, angina, and abdominal and joint discomfort secondary to altered circulation because of hyperviscosity of the blood

Desired outcomes: Within 1 hr of intervention, patient's subjective perception of discomfort decreases, as documented by a pain scale. Objective indicators, such as grimacing, are absent or diminished. Life-style behaviors are not compromised because of discomfort.

- Assess patient for the presence of headache, angina, abdominal pain, and joint pain. Devise a pain scale with the patient, rating discomfort from 0 (no pain) to 10 (worst pain).
- In the presence of joint pain, rest the joint and elevate the extremity; apply moist heat or ice to ease discomfort.

- Administer analgesics as prescribed. **Note:** Avoid analgesics containing aspirin or NSAIDs, which may exacerbate bleeding associated with thrombocytosis.
- Instruct patient to request analgesic before the pain becomes too intense.
- Encourage use of nonpharmacologic pain control, such as relaxation and distraction.
- Document the degree of pain relief using the pain scale.
- Be alert to indicators of peripheral thrombosis, such as calf pain and tenderness.
- Report significant findings to patient's health care provider.

NIC: Analgesic Administration; Embolus Precautions; Heat/Cold Application; Pain Management

Altered renal, peripheral, and cerebral tissue perfusion related to interrupted blood flow secondary to hyperviscosity of the blood
Desired outcome: Following treatment, patient has adequate renal, peripheral, and cerebral perfusion as evidenced by urinary output ≥30 ml/hr, peripheral pulses >2+ on a scale of 0-4+, distal extremity warmth, adequate (baseline) muscle strength, no mental status changes, and orientation to person, place, and time.
- Monitor I&O; report urine output <30 ml/hr in the presence of adequate intake, which can signal congestion and decreased perfusion.
- In the absence of signs of cardiac and renal failure, encourage fluid intake to decrease viscosity.
- Monitor peripheral perfusion by palpating peripheral pulses. Be alert to amplitude ≤2+ on a scale of 0-4+ and coolness in the distal extremities.
- Encourage patient to change position q1hr when in bed or to exercise and ambulate to tolerance to enhance circulation.
- Instruct patient to avoid tight or restrictive clothing.
- Monitor patient for indicators of impending neurologic damage, such as muscle weakness and decreases in sensation and LOC. If these indicators are present, protect patient by assisting with ambulation or raising side rails on the bed, depending on the degree of deficit.
- Administer myelosuppressive agents, as prescribed, to inhibit proliferation of RBCs.
- If the patient smokes, encourage enrollment in a smoking cessation program because smoking significantly increases the potential of a thromboembolic event.
- Report significant findings to patient's health care provider.

NIC: Activity Therapy; Embolus Precautions; Exercise Promotion; Fluid Management; Neurologic Monitoring; Teaching: Disease Process

Altered nutrition: Less than body requirements related to anorexia secondary to feelings of fullness occurring with organ system congestion
Desired outcome: By at least 24 hr before hospital discharge, patient exhibits adequate nutrition as evidenced by maintenance of or return to baseline body weight or a 1- to 2-lb weight gain.
- Weigh patient daily to identify trend.
- Monitor fluid volume intake, and encourage intake if necessary.
- Encourage patient to eat small, frequent meals. Document intake.
- Request that significant other bring in patient's favorite foods if they are unavailable in the hospital.
- Advise patient to avoid spicy foods and to eat mild foods, which are better tolerated.
- Teach patient to avoid intake of iron to help minimize abnormal RBC proliferation.

- As indicated, obtain a dietary consultation.
- Teach patient or significant other how to record and maintain a fluid and food intake diary.

◎ NIC: Discharge Planning; Nutritional Counseling; Teaching: Disease Process; Teaching: Individual; Teaching: Prescribed Diet

Altered cerebral and cardiopulmonary tissue perfusion (or risk for same) related to hypovolemia secondary to phlebotomy
Desired outcome: Patient has adequate cerebral and cardiopulmonary perfusion as evidenced by no mental status changes and orientation to person, place, and time; HR ≤100 bpm; BP ≥90/60 mm Hg (or within patient's baseline range); absence of chest pain; and RR ≤20 breaths/min.

- During procedure, keep patient recumbent to prevent dizziness or hypotension.
- Assess for tachycardia, hypotension, chest pain, or dizziness during procedure; notify patient's health care provider of significant findings.
- After the procedure, assist patient with sitting position for 5-10 min before ambulation to prevent orthostatic hypotension. For more information about orthostatic hypotension, see Appendix One, "Caring for Patients on Prolonged Bedrest" for **Altered cerebral tissue perfusion,** p. 743.
- Teach patients, especially older persons and chronically ill persons, about the potential for orthostatic hypotension and the need for caution when standing for at least 2-3 days after the phlebotomy.

◎ NIC: Activity Therapy; Positioning; Teaching: Individual

PATIENT-FAMILY TEACHING AND DISCHARGE PLANNING

When providing patient-family teaching, focus on sensory information; avoid giving excessive information; and initiate a visiting nurse referral for necessary follow-up teaching. Consider including verbal and written information about the following:

- Need for continued medical follow-up, including potential for phlebotomy every 1-3 mo.
- Medications, including drug name, purpose, dosage, schedule, precautions, drug/drug and food/drug interactions, and potential side effects.
- Importance of augmenting fluid intake (e.g., >2.5 L/day) to decrease blood viscosity.
- Signs and symptoms that necessitate medical attention: angina, muscle weakness, numbness and tingling of extremities, decreased tolerance to activity, mental status changes, and joint pain.
- Nutrition: importance of maintaining a balanced diet to increase resistance to infection, and limiting dietary or supplemental intake of iron to help minimize abnormal RBC proliferation.

Section Two: Disorders of Coagulation

The formation of a visible fibrin clot is the conclusion of a complex series of reactions involving different clotting factors in the blood that are identified by Roman numerals I through XIII. All are plasma proteins except factor III (thromboplastin) and factor IV (calcium ion). When a vessel injury occurs, these factors interact to form the end product, a clot. The clots that are formed are eventually dissolved by the fibrinolytic system.

Platelets play a role in coagulation by releasing substances that activate the clotting factors. At the time of vascular injury, platelets migrate to the site and adhere to collagen fibrils in vascular subendothelium and subsequently to each other to form a temporary plug to stop the bleeding.

Thrombocytopenia

Thrombocytopenia is a common coagulation disorder that results from a decreased number of platelets. It can be congenital or acquired, and it is classified according to cause. Common causes include deficient formation of thrombocytes, as occurs with bone marrow disease or destruction; accelerated platelet destruction, loss, or increased use, as in hemolytic anemia, diffuse intravascular coagulation, or damage by prosthetic heart valves; and abnormal platelet distribution, as in hypersplenism and hypothermia. Potential triggers include autoimmune disorder, severe vascular injury, and spleen malfunction. In addition, thrombocytopenia can occur as a side effect of certain drugs. Regardless of the cause or trigger, the disorder affects coagulation and hemostasis. With chemical-induced thrombocytopenia, prognosis is good after withdrawal of the offending drug. Prognosis for other types depends on the form of thrombocytopenia and the individual's baseline health status and response to treatment.

> **Note:** Thrombocytopenia may be the first sign of systemic lupus erythematosus (SLE) or HIV infection.

Thrombotic thrombocytopenic purpura (TTP) is an acute, often fatal disorder. The cause is presumed to be the absence of a factor in the plasma or the presence of a platelet-stimulating factor. Platelets become sensitized and clump in blood vessels, occluding them. *Idiopathic thrombocytopenic purpura (ITP)* is believed to be an immune disorder specifically involving antiplatelet immunoglobulin G (IgG), which destroys platelets. The acute form is most often seen in children (2-6 yr of age) and may be related to a previous viral infection. The chronic form is seen more often in adults (18-50 yr of age) and is of unknown origin.

ASSESSMENT

Chronic indicators: Long history of mild bleeding or hemorrhagic episodes from the mouth, nose, gastrointestinal (GI) tract, or genitourinary (GU) tract. Increased bruising (ecchymosis) and petechiae also have been noted.

Acute indicators: Fever, splenomegaly, acute and severe bleeding episodes, weakness, lethargy, malaise, hemorrhage into mucous membranes, gum bleeding, and GU or GI bleeding. Prolonged bleeding can lead to a shock state with tachycardia, SOB, and decreased LOC. Optic fundal hemorrhage decreases vision and may preclude potentially fatal intracranial hemorrhage.

Note: With TTP the individual may exhibit signs associated with platelet thrombus formation and ischemic organs, such as decreased renal function or neurologic changes.

History of: Recent infection; recent vaccination; binge alcohol consumption; positive family history of thrombocytopenia; or use of chlorothiazide, digitalis, quinidine, rifampin, sulfisoxazole, chloramphenicol, phenytoin, or heparin.

DIAGNOSTIC TESTS

Platelet count: Can vary from only slightly decreased to nearly absent. Less than $100,000/mm^3$ is significantly decreased; $<20,000/mm^3$ results in a serious risk of hemorrhage.

Peripheral blood smear: Reveals megathrombocytes (large platelets), which are present during premature destruction of platelets.

CBC: Low Hgb and Hct levels because of blood loss; WBC count usually is within normal range.

Coagulation studies

Bleeding time: Increased because of decreased platelets.

Partial thromboplastin time (PTT):   Increased.

Prothrombin time (PT):   Increased.

International normalized ratio (INR):   Increased.

International sensitivity index (ISI):   Increased.

Bone marrow aspiration: Reveals increased number of megakaryocytes (platelet precursors) in the presence of ITP but may be decreased with certain causes of thrombocytopenia.

Platelet antibody screen: May be positive because of the presence of IgG antibodies.

COLLABORATIVE MANAGEMENT

Treatment of underlying cause or removal of precipitating agent

Platelet transfusion: Unless platelet destruction is the cause of the disorder (see Table 7-1). Provides only temporary relief because the half-life of platelets is only 3-4 days; may be even shorter with ITP (i.e., minutes to hours).[1]

Corticosteroids: To enhance vascular integrity or diminish platelet destruction.

Intravenous immunoglobulin (IVIgG):   To raise platelet count; dosage is 1 g/kg.[2]

Splenectomy: Removal of the organ responsible for platelet destruction. This is considered viable treatment unless patient has acute bleeding, a severe deficiency of platelets, or a cardiac disorder that contraindicates surgery.

Inoculation: In anticipation of splenectomy, vaccination for pneumococcal, meningococcal, and *Haemophilus influenzae* infection should be accomplished.[3]

Plasma exchange via apheresis: Removes the antibody or immune complex; used for short-term therapy.

NURSING DIAGNOSES AND INTERVENTIONS

Altered protection related to increased risk of bleeding secondary to decreased platelet count

Desired outcome: Patient is free of the signs of bleeding as evidenced by secretions and excretions negative for blood, BP ≥90/60 mm Hg or within patient's baseline range, HR ≤100 bpm, RR 12-20 breaths/min with normal depth and pattern (eupnea), and absence of bruising or active bleeding.

• Monitor patient for hematuria, melena, epistaxis, hematemesis, hemoptysis, menometrorrhagia, bleeding gums, or severe ecchymosis. Teach patient to be alert to and report these indicators promptly.

• When appropriate, protect patient from injury by padding and keeping up side rails.

• When possible, avoid venipuncture. If performed, apply pressure on site for 5-10 min or until bleeding stops.

• Avoid IM injections. If injections are necessary, preferably use SC routine and with small-gauge needle when possible.

• Monitor platelet count daily. Optimal range is 150,000-400,000/mm³.

• Advise patient to avoid straining at stool and coughing, which increase intracranial pressure and can result in intracranial hemorrhage. Obtain

---

[1] Edwards C: *Davidson's principles and practice of medicine*, ed 17, Edinburgh, 1995, Churchill Livingstone, p. 831.

[2] Ibid.

[3] Ibid.

prescription for stool softeners, if indicated, to prevent constipation. Teach patient anticonstipation routine as described in Appendix One, "Caring for Patients on Prolonged Bedrest" for **Constipation,** p. 743.
- Administer corticosteroids as prescribed to help minimize platelet destruction.
- Teach patient to use electric razor and soft-bristle toothbrush.
- Instruct patient about the association of alcohol consumption, smoking, and use of aspirin or NSAIDs with increased risk of bleeding.
- Administer platelets as prescribed. Double-check type and crossmatching with a colleague, and monitor for and report signs of transfusion reaction, including chills, back pain, dyspnea, hives, and wheezing.
- Alert patient's health care provider to significant findings.

NIC: Blood Products Administration; Bleeding Precautions; Bowel Management; Medication Administration; Teaching: Individual

Altered cerebral, peripheral, and renal tissue perfusion (or risk for same) related to interrupted blood flow secondary to presence of thrombotic component, which results in sensitization and clumping of platelets in the blood vessels
Desired outcome: Patient's cerebral, peripheral, and renal perfusion is adequate as evidenced by no mental status changes and orientation to person, place, and time; normoreactive pupillary responses; absence of headaches, dizziness, and visual disturbances; peripheral pulses >2+ on a 0-4+ scale; and urine output ≥30 ml/hr.
- Assess patient for changes in mental status, LOC, and pupillary response.
- Monitor for headaches, dizziness, or visual disturbances.
- Palpate peripheral pulses on all extremities. Be alert to pulses ≤2+ on a 0-4+ scale. Compare distal extremities for color, warmth, and character of pulses.
- Assess urine output. Adequate perfusion is reflected by urine output ≥30 ml/hr for 2 consecutive hr.
- Monitor I&O. The patient should be well hydrated (2-3 L/day) to increase perfusion of the small vessels.

NIC: Circulatory Care; Fluid Management; Neurologic Monitoring

Pain related to joint discomfort secondary to hemorrhagic episodes or blood extravasation into the tissues
Desired outcomes: Within 1 hr of intervention, patient's subjective perception of discomfort decreases, as documented by a pain scale. Objective indicators, such as grimacing, are absent or diminished.
- Monitor patient for the presence of fatigue, malaise, and joint pain. Devise a pain scale with patient, rating discomfort on a scale of 0 (no pain) to 10 (worst pain).
- Maintain a calm, restful environment.
- Facilitate coordination of care providers to provide rest periods as needed between care activities, allowing time for periods of undisturbed rest.
- Elevate legs to minimize joint discomfort in the lower extremities. Support legs with pillows. Avoid gatching the bed at the knee.
- Choose chairs with, or provide, padding on seats of chairs to prevent occluding the popliteal vessels.
- Use a bed cradle to decrease pressure on the tissues of the lower extremities; socks may be needed for warmth.
- Administer analgesics as prescribed. Document relief obtained, using the pain scale. **Caution:** Aspirin and other NSAIDs are contraindicated because of their antiplatelet action.
- Instruct patient to request analgesic before pain becomes severe.

NIC: Analgesic Administration; Pain Management; Teaching: Individual

---

See Also: Appendix One, "Caring for Preoperative and Postoperative Patients" for **Risk for fluid volume deficit** related to postoperative bleeding/hemorrhage, p. 729.

PATIENT-FAMILY TEACHING AND DISCHARGE PLANNING

When providing patient-family teaching, focus on sensory information; avoid giving excessive information; and initiate a visiting nurse referral for necessary follow-up teaching. Consider including verbal and written information about the following:

- Importance of preventing trauma, which can cause bleeding.
- Seeking medical attention for *any* signs of bleeding or infection. Review the signs and symptoms of common infections, such as upper respiratory, urinary tract, and wound infections. Signs and symptoms of common infections are described in "Care of the Renal Transplant Recipient," **Risk for infection,** p. 162. Also teach patient to assess for hematuria, melena, hematemesis, hemoptysis, menometrorrhagia, oozing from mucous membranes, and petechiae.
- Importance of regular medical follow-up for platelet counts.
- If patient is discharged taking corticosteroids, the side effects of steroids, including weight gain, headache, capillary fragility, hypertension, moon facies, thinning of arms and legs, mood changes, acne, buffalo hump, edema formation, risk of GI hemorrhage, delayed wound healing, and increased appetite. Review need to take the medication with food, to immediately take missed doses, and not to precipitously discontinue medication.
- Other medications, including drug name, dosage, purpose, schedule, precautions, drug/drug and food/drug interactions, and potential side effects.
- Importance of obtaining a Medic-Alert bracelet and identification card outlining diagnosis and emergency treatment. Contact the following organization:

  Medic Alert
  2323 Colorado Ave.
  Turlock, CA 95382   (209) 668-3333

Hemophilia

Hemophilia is a hereditary bleeding disorder characterized by a deficiency of one or more clotting factors. Classic hemophilia is caused by deficiency of factors VIII (hemophilia A) and IX (hemophilia B). Estimated incidence of hemophilia A is 1:20,000, and of hemophilia B is 1:100,000. Both may be classified as mild, moderate, or severe.

Both types of hemophilia are sex-linked inherited disorders. Individuals affected are usually males, whereas their mothers and sisters are asymptomatic carriers. This disorder also can occur in females if it is inherited from an affected male and a female carrier or if it is caused by X chromosome inactivation during embryologic development. Hemarthroses (bleeding in a joint), particularly of the knee, elbow, ankle, and hip, affect 75% of adults with hemophilia. Hemorrhage may also occur in the kidneys and CNS; intracranial hemorrhage is the most common cause of death.

ASSESSMENT

Chronic indicators: Bruising after minimal trauma, joint pain.
Acute indicators: Acute bleeding episodes after minimal trauma. Hemarthrosis is the most common and debilitating symptom, causing painful and swollen joints. Large ecchymoses can occur, as well as bleeding from the gums, tongue, GI tract, urinary tract, or cuts in the skin. Shock can result from severe bleeding.

DIAGNOSTIC TESTS

Partial thromboplastin time (PTT):   Prolonged.
Bleeding time: Prolonged.
Fibrinogen level: Normal.
Prothrombin time (PT):   Normal.
Thrombin time: Normal.
Platelet count: Usually normal.
Activated clotting time: Prolonged.
Assays of factors VIII and IX: Reveal low activity.
Prenatal fetal serum: For DNA analysis.

COLLABORATIVE MANAGEMENT

Factor transfusion: For hemophilia B (see Table 7-1).
Transfusion of fresh frozen plasma: See Table 7-1.
Cryoprecipitate: For infusion of factor VIII with classic hemophilia A (see Table 7-1). **Note:** Commercially prepared, heat-treated factor VIII is also being used to decrease the risk of disease and contamination. A product called monoclonal antibody-derived factor VIII has no risk of disease transmission. However, its use is limited by cost and availability.
Agents such as desmopressin (DDAVP) and aminocaproic acid (Amicar): To enhance intrinsic coagulation mechanisms and decrease the need for factor replacement.
Gene transfer therapy: Experimental research being conducted to correct the basic genetic defect responsible for the disorder (not presently available).

NURSING DIAGNOSES AND INTERVENTIONS

Risk for impaired skin integrity *and* **impaired tissue integrity** with risk factors related to altered blood circulation to the tissues secondary to bleeding
Desired outcome: Patient's skin and tissue remain intact with absence of bruising and swelling.
- Inspect patient's skin at least q4hr, being alert to bruising, pressure areas, and swelling.
- Apply ice or pressure over sites of intradermal or subcutaneous bleeding to promote vasoconstriction. If appropriate, rest and elevate the area to reduce blood flow.
- Handle patient gently to minimize the risk of tissue trauma.
- To maintain joint mobility and pliability of the periarticular tissues, assist patient with gentle, passive, or active-assistive ROM exercises daily. However, avoid exercise for 48 hr after bleeding to prevent recurrence.
- Assist patient with ambulation as tolerated.

NIC: Activity Therapy; Exercise Promotion; Exercise Therapy: Joint Mobility; Heat/Cold Application; Skin Surveillance

Pain related to swollen joints (hemarthrosis)
Desired outcomes: Within 1 hr of intervention, patient's subjective perception of discomfort decreases, as documented by a pain scale. Objective indicators, such as grimacing, are absent or diminished.

- Monitor patient for joint discomfort. Devise a pain scale with the patient, rating discomfort on a scale of 0 (no pain) to 10 (worst pain).
- Apply splints or other supportive devices to joints. Immobilize joints in slight flexion or neutral position; avoid extremes of flexion, extension, or rotation. Some health care providers advocate use of elastic wraps around involved joints to control hemorrhage.
- Elevate or position pillows under affected joints to promote comfort.
- Administer analgesics as prescribed; avoid aspirin or NSAIDs because of their anticoagulant action. Document pain relief achieved, using the pain scale.
- Assist patient with ambulation as needed.
- As needed, use ice for its topical analgesia and ability to constrict the vessels, which will decrease swelling. **Caution:** Avoid use of warm thermotherapy for these patients because it will increase bleeding and/or edema formation. (See also "Ligamentous Injuries" for **Knowledge deficit**: Need for elevation of the involved extremity, use of thermotherapy, and prescribed exercise, p. 566.)
- Discuss with patient the importance of frequent assessment of joint function to enable rapid identification and treatment of hemophilic arthritis.

NIC: Exercise Therapy: Joint Mobility; Heat/Cold Application; Pain Management; Positioning; Teaching: Procedure/Treatment

> **See Also:**   "Acute Leukemia" for **Altered protection** related to increased risk of bleeding secondary to decreased platelet count, p. 547.

PATIENT-FAMILY TEACHING AND DISCHARGE PLANNING

When providing patient-family teaching, focus on sensory information; avoid giving excessive information; and initiate a visiting nurse referral for necessary follow-up teaching. Consider including verbal and written information about the following:

- Importance of avoiding trauma, and necessity of seeking medical attention for any obvious or suspected bleeding.
- Phone numbers to call in the event of emergency.
- Procedure in case of bleeding: application of cold compresses and gentle, direct pressure; elevation and rest of affected part if possible; seeking medical attention promptly.
- Importance of notifying health care provider if dental procedures need to be done.
- Importance of lifetime medical follow-up and regular factor transfusions.
- Importance of obtaining a Medic-Alert bracelet and identification card outlining diagnosis and emergency treatment. Contact the following organization:

  Medic Alert
  2323 Colorado Ave.
  Turlock, CA 95382   (209) 668-3333

- Importance of frequent assessment of joint function to allow rapid identification and treatment of hemophilic arthritis.
- Phone number and address of local or national hemophiliac support groups, such as the following:

  National Hemophilia Foundation
  110 Greene St., Suite 303
  New York, NY 10012   (800) INFO-NHF
  WWW address: *http://www.hemophilia.org*

- If indicated, information on resources for genetic counseling.

In addition
- In patients for whom factor VIII prophylaxis is used, the patient or significant other will require instruction in the IV administration of factor VIII.

Disseminated intravascular coagulation

Disseminated intravascular coagulation (DIC) is an acute coagulation disorder characterized by paradoxic clotting and hemorrhage. The sequence usually progresses from massive clot formation, depletion of the clotting factors, and activation of diffuse fibrinolysis to hemorrhage (Figure 7-1). DIC occurs secondary to widespread coagulation factors in the bloodstream caused by extensive surgery, burns, shock, neoplastic diseases, or abruptio placentae; extensive destruction of blood vessel walls caused by eclampsia, anoxia, or heat stroke; or damage to blood cells caused by hemolysis, sickle cell disease, or transfusion reactions (Table 7-2). DIC is also associated with sepsis. Prompt assessment of the disorder can result in a good prognosis. Usually affected patients are transferred to the ICU for careful monitoring and aggressive therapy. DIC may be classified as low grade (compensated or chronic) or fulminant (acute).

ASSESSMENT

Clinical indicators: Bleeding of abrupt onset, oozing from venipuncture sites or mucosal surfaces; bleeding from surgical sites; the presence of hematuria, blood in the stool (melena or hematochezia), spontaneous ecchymosis (bruising), petechiae, purpura fulminans, pallor, or mottled skin. The patient also may bleed from the vagina (menometrorrhagia), nose (epistaxis), and mucous membranes. Joint pain and swelling may signal bleeding into the joints. Complaint of headache or mental status changes may indicate intracranial hemorrhage. Symptoms of hypoperfusion can occur, including decreased urine output and abnormal behavior.

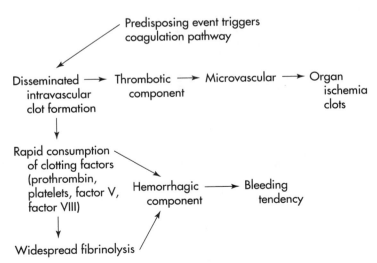

Figure 7-1:   Overview of DIC syndrome.

TABLE 7-2 Clinical Conditions That Can Activate Disseminated Intravascular Coagulation

Obstetric	GI disorders	Tissue damage	Infections	Hemolytic processes	Vascular disorders	Miscellaneous
Abruptio placentae	Cirrhosis	Surgery	Viral	Transfusion reaction	Shock	Fat or pulmonary embolism
Toxemia	Hepatic necrosis	Trauma	Bacterial	Acute hemolysis	Aneurysm	Snake bite
Amniotic fluid embolism	Pancreatitis	Burns	Rickettsial	secondary to	Giant hemangioma	Neoplastic disorders
Septic abortion	Peritoneovenous	Prolonged	Protozoal	infection or		(leukemias, solid tumors,
Retained dead fetus	shunts	extracorporeal		immunologic		or metastatic disease and
	Necrotizing	circulation		disorder		their related treatments)
	enterocolitis	Transplant rejection				Acute anoxia
		Heat stroke				

Physical assessment: Abdominal assessment may reveal signs of GI bleeding, such as guarding; distention (increasing abdominal girth measurements); hyperactive, hypoactive, or absent bowel sounds; and a rigid, boardlike abdomen. With significant hemorrhage, patients may exhibit the following: systolic BP <90 mm Hg and diastolic BP <60 mm Hg; HR >100 bpm; peripheral pulse amplitude <2+ on a 0-4+ scale; RR >22 breaths/min; SOB; urinary output <30 ml/hr; secretions and excretions positive for blood; cool, pale, clammy skin; and lack of orientation to person, place, and time or changes in mental status.

Risk factors: Infection, burns, trauma, hepatic disease, hypovolemic shock, severe hemolytic reaction, obstetric complications, and hypoxia (see Table 7-2).

DIAGNOSTIC TESTS

Serum fibrinogen: Low because of abnormal consumption of clotting factors in the formation of fibrin clots.

Platelet count: Will be <250,000/mm^3 because of platelets' role in clot formation.

Fibrin split products (FSPs), also known as *fibrin degradation products (FDPs):*   Increased, indicating widespread dissolution of clots. Fibrinolysis produces FSPs as an end product.

Prothrombin time (PT):   Increased because of depletion of clotting factors.

Partial thromboplastin time (PTT):   High because of depletion of clotting factors.

Peripheral blood smear: Shows fragmented RBCs.

Bleeding time: Prolonged because of decreased platelets.

COLLABORATIVE MANAGEMENT

Identification and treatment of primary disorder: See Table 7-2.

Hemodynamic and cardiovascular support: Fluid management, oxygen supplementation, and invasive monitoring.

Anticoagulant therapy: Although this therapy is controversial, heparin may be administered. Heparin interferes with the coagulation process and activation of the fibrinolytic system in an attempt to prevent clot formation within organs. Heparin dose is regulated and determined by the PTT. Warfarin may be used in compensated DIC.

Replacement of platelets and clotting factors: Replacement of clotting factors by administering fresh frozen plasma, packed RBCs, and platelets may counteract deficiencies. Blood replacement also supports blood volume (see Table 7-1).

Aminocaproic acid (Amicar):   Although controversial, ϵ-aminocaproic acid has been used to disrupt the fibrinolysis process and may be administered to stop bleeding.

DIC scoring system: A rigorous scoring system may be used to assess the severity of DIC to objectively evaluate the response to therapy. The DIC scoring system includes laboratory and clinical parameters that are assessed q4-8hr (Table 7-3). A definitive diagnosis is usually known within 72 hr.

NURSING DIAGNOSES AND INTERVENTIONS

Altered cardiopulmonary, peripheral, renal, and cerebral tissue perfusion related to interrupted blood flow secondary to coagulation/fibrinolysis processes
Desired outcome: Following treatment, patient has adequate cardiopulmonary, peripheral, renal, and cerebral perfusion as evidenced by BP ≥90/60 mm Hg and HR ≤100 bpm (or within patient's baseline range); peripheral pulse amplitude >2+ on a 0-4+ scale; urinary output ≥30 ml/hr; equal and normoreactive pupils; normal/baseline motor function; orientation to person, place, and time; and no mental status changes.

TABLE 7-3 Scoring System for Severity and Response to Therapy in DIC

	High score				Normal	Low score			
	Plus 4	Plus 3	Plus 2	Plus 1	0	Plus 1	Plus 2	Plus 3	Plus 4
Fibronpeptide A	>70	41-70	11-40	3-10	<3	—	—	—	—
Profragment 1.2	>10	7.5-10.0	6.0-7.4	2.7-5.9	0.2-2.7 nM	—	—	—	—
D-dimer (a neoantigen)	>3000	2001-2999	1001-2000	500-1000	<500	—	—	—	—
Fibrinogen degradation products (FDPs)	>120	81-120	41-80	10-40	<10	—	—	—	—
Antithrombin	—	—	—	—	85-125	75-85	65-74	54-64	<54
α_2-Antiplasmin	—	—	—	—	75%-120%	65%-74%	55%-64%	45%-54%	<45%
Fibrinogen	—	—	—	—	150-350	100-150	75-99	50-74	<50
Platelet count	—	—	—	—	150-450	100-149	75-99	50-74	<50
Temperature	>41	39-40.9	—	38.5-38.9	36-38.4	34-35.9	32-33.9	30-31.9	<29.9
Mean arterial pressure (MAP)	>160	130-159	110-129	—	70-109	—	50-69	—	<49
Pulse rate	>180	140-179	110-139	—	70-109	—	55-69	40-54	<39
Respiratory rate	>50	35-49	—	25-34	12-24	10-11	6-9	—	<5
Partial pressure of dissolved oxygen in arterial blood (Pao_2)	—	—	—	—	80-100	70-79	60-69	55-60	<55

Hydrogen ion concentration (pH)	>7.7	7.6-7.69	—	7.5-7.59	7.33-7.49	—	7.25-7.32	7.15-7.24	<7.15
Creatinine	>3.5	2-3.4	1.5-1.9	—	0.6-1.4	—	<0.6	—	—
Lactic dehydrogenase (LDH)	>275	251-275	226-250	194-225	<193	—	—	—	—
Albumin	—	—	—	—	3.5-5.5	3.0-3.4	2.9-2.6	2.5-2.1	<2.0
Sodium (NA⁺)	>180	160-170	155-159	150-154	130-149	—	120-129	111-119	<110
Potassium (K⁺)	>7.0	6.0-6.9	—	5.5-5.9	3.5-5.4	3.0-3.4	2.5-2.9	—	<2.5
Hematocrit	>60	—	50.0-59.9	46.0-49.9	30.0-45.9	—	20.0-29.9	—	<20.0
Total white blood cell (WBC) count	>40 K	—	20.0-39.9 K	15.0-19.9 K	3.0-14.9 K	—	1.0-2.9 K	—	<1.0 K
Column total (CT)									
DIC score (100 minus CT)									
DIC grading severity criteria	Score ≥90: DIC *unlikely*	Score 75-89: DIC is *mild*			Score 50-74: DIC is *moderate*		Score <49: DIC is *severe*		

Modified from Bick RL: *Med Clin North Am* 78(3):511-543, 1994.

DIC, Disseminated intravascular coagulation.

- Monitor VS. Be alert to and report decreased BP, increased HR, or decreased amplitude of peripheral pulses, which may signal that coagulation and thrombus formation are occurring.
- Monitor I&O; report output <30 ml/hr in the presence of adequate intake, which may indicate renal vessel thrombosis.
- Perform neurologic checks, including orientation, mental status assessments, pupillary reaction to light, and motor response, and assess mental status and LOC to evaluate cerebral perfusion. If signs of impaired cerebral perfusion occur, protect patient from injury by instituting measures such as keeping bed in the lowest position and side rails up.
- Monitor for hemorrhage from surgical wounds, GI and GU tracts, and mucous membranes, which can occur after fibrinolysis.
- Monitor laboratory work for values suggestive of DIC, including low serum fibrinogen (<200 mg/dl), low platelet count (<250,000/mm^3), increased fibrin split products (>8 μm/ml), increased PT (>11-15 sec), and increased PTT (>40-100 sec).
- Monitor O_2 saturation via pulse oximetry q4hr or as indicated; report O_2 saturation <92%.
- Report significant findings to patient's health care provider; prepare for transfer to ICU if condition worsens.

NIC: Circulatory Care; Fluid Management; Neurologic Monitoring; Oxygen Therapy; Surveillance; Vital Signs Monitoring

Altered protection related to increased risk of bleeding secondary to hemorrhagic component of DIC
Desired outcome: Patient is free of signs of bleeding as evidenced by systolic BP ≥90 mm Hg; HR ≤100 bpm (or within patient's normal range); RR 12-20 breaths/min with normal depth and pattern (eupnea); urinary output ≥30 ml/hr; secretions and excretions negative for blood; stable abdominal girth measurements; orientation to person, place, and time; and no changes in mental status.

- Monitor VS and LOC at frequent intervals; report significant changes. Be alert to hypotension, tachycardia, dyspnea, disorientation, and changes in mental status, which can signal hemorrhage. **Note:** Be cautious of the pressure used with BP cuffs. Frequent BP readings may cause bleeding under the cuff. Rotate arm use to reduce repeated trauma.
- Monitor coagulation studies, being alert to PTT >40-100 sec.
- Use a reagent screening agent to check stool, urine, emesis, and nasogastric drainage for blood.
- Monitor for internal bleeding by assessing for abdominal pain, abdominal distention, changes in bowel sounds, and a boardlike abdomen, which are signs of GI bleeding.
- Assess puncture sites regularly for oozing or bleeding. When possible, treat bleeding sites with ice, pressure, rest, and elevation. Some health care providers promote use of thrombin- soaked gauze, such as Gelfoam or topical thrombin powder, to reduce external bleeding or oozing.
- Be alert to other signs of bleeding, including joint pain and headache. Visual changes may signal retinal hemorrhage.
- Avoid giving IM injections or performing venipunctures for blood drawing.
- Administer blood products (fresh frozen plasma, packed RBCs, platelets [see Table 7-1]) and IV fluids as prescribed.
- Teach patient to use electric shaver and soft-bristle toothbrush.

NIC: Bedside Laboratory Testing; Bleeding Reduction; Medication Administration; Neurologic Monitoring; Surveillance

Risk for impaired skin integrity *or* **impaired tissue integrity** with risk factors related to altered circulation secondary to hemorrhage and thrombosis
Desired outcome: Patient's skin and tissue remain nonerythemic and intact.

- Assess patient's skin, noting erythema that does not clear after removal of pressure or changes in color, temperature, and sensation, which may signal decreased perfusion and can lead to tissue damage.
- Eliminate or minimize pressure points by ensuring that the patient turns q2hr and by using sheepskin on elbows and heels and enhanced pressure-distribution mattress padding. Do not pull on extremities when turning patient.
- Encourage active ROM of all extremities q2hr to reduce pressure and enhance circulation.
- Keep patient's extremities warm to prevent tissue hypoxia.
- Use alternatives to tape to hold dressings in place, such as gauze wraps or net gauze.
- If patient has areas of breakdown, see "Managing Wound Care," p. 704.

NIC: Circulatory Precautions; Exercise Promotion; Pressure Management; Pressure Ulcer Care; Skin Surveillance; Teaching: Prescribed Activity/ Exercise

See Also: "Pulmonary Embolus" for **Altered protection** related to increased risk of bleeding or hemorrhage secondary to anticoagulant therapy, p. 18.

PATIENT-FAMILY TEACHING AND DISCHARGE PLANNING

See patient's primary diagnosis.

Section Three: Neoplastic Disorders of the Hematopoietic System

WBCs, also called *leukocytes*, are the blood cells responsible for both immunity and the body's response to infectious organisms. WBCs are classified according to structure, specialized function, and response to dye in the laboratory. The three main classifications of WBCs are granulocytes, lymphocytes, and monocytes, all of which may undergo malignant transformations. The bone marrow has a reserve of approximately 10 times the number of circulating WBCs, and these are released into the circulation during an infectious process.

Lymphomas

Lymphomas are disorders that cause neoplastic proliferation of lymphoid cells and tissue (e.g., lymph nodes, spleen). This results in abnormal functioning of the lymph cells responsible for immunity and eventually results in system obstruction. Lymphomas are classified as Hodgkin's lymphoma and non-Hodgkin's lymphoma.

Hodgkin's lymphoma (or Hodgkin's disease [HD]) is a tumor of the lymph tissue. It is distinguished from other lymphomas by the presence of large, variable cells called *Reed-Sternberg* cells, which proliferate and invade normal lymph tissue throughout the body. Lymph tissue is found in the spleen, liver, bone marrow, lymph nodes, and lymph channels (which connect virtually all tissues). Clinical presentation depends on the degree of malignant cell growth, extent of the invasion, and the tissues affected. Hodgkin's disease frequently affects young people, and it can be treated successfully, particularly with early diagnosis and intervention. The cause of the disorder is unclear, but a hereditary component has been implicated. Although no infectious organism has been identified, infection has been suggested as a potential cause. Long-term survival (20 yr) is now possible.

Non-Hodgkin's lymphomas (NHLs) are characterized by disseminated spread, often with extranodal infiltration. They can appear in the GI tract, bone marrow, and testes. They tend to affect individuals around 50 yr of age and are more common than Hodgkin's lymphomas. NHL involves an abnormal, malignant lymphocytic invasion of the lymph nodes; Reed-Sternberg cells are not involved in this malignancy.

ASSESSMENT

Chronic indicators: Nonspecific symptoms, such as unexplained and persistent fever, night sweats, malaise, weight loss (>10% of body weight), back pain, and pruritus (termed *B symptoms* [symptomatic] for staging).

Acute indicators: Worsening of the symptoms just mentioned, in addition to unexplained pain in the lymph nodes after drinking alcohol. Also, individuals with NHL may experience GI symptoms, including nausea, vomiting, and abdominal pain.

Physical assessment: Enlarged (painless) lymph nodes that may cause symptoms associated with compression of adjacent tissues (e.g., upper airway obstruction, paresthesias, muscular weakness, ureteral obstruction). Splenomegaly or hepatomegaly may also occur.

DIAGNOSTIC TESTS

CBC: Decreased Hgb and Hct (confirming anemia); increased, decreased, or normal levels of WBCs. Neutrophilic leukocytosis may occur, and lymphocyte levels will be low.

Platelet count: May be low.

Lymph node biopsy: May reveal characteristic giant, multinuclear Reed-Sternberg cells.

Lymphangiogram: To determine extent of involvement. Cannulas are inserted into the lymph vessels, and contrast medium is injected. Before the procedure, patient should be assessed regarding allergy to contrast medium. This procedure is less useful in NHL since it does not allow visualization of mesenteric nodes, which often are involved.

Biopsy of the bone marrow, lung, liver, pleura, or bone: May be performed to determine involvement and assist in staging the degree of disease.

Serum alkaline phosphatase: If elevated, indicates liver involvement or bone involvement.

Erythrocyte sedimentation rate: Elevated.

Staging laparotomy with splenectomy and liver biopsy: To determine extent of the disease and plan of care.

Chest x-ray or abdominal CT scan: To help determine presence of nodal involvement.

Bone scan: To detect bone involvement.

COLLABORATIVE MANAGEMENT

Staging: To determine extent of the disease. A simplified description of staging follows (based on the Ann Arbor Staging Classification).

Stage I: Limited to a single lymph node region or a single extralymphatic organ.

Stage II: Involves two or more lymph node regions on the same side of the diaphragm, or there is localized involvement of an extralymphatic organ.

Stage III: Involves lymph node regions on both sides of the diaphragm, accompanied by involvement of an extralymphatic region or the spleen.

Stage IV: Diffuse involvement of one or more extralymphatic regions or tissues.

Prognosis based on staging: For HD the 5-yr survival rate varies: 85% for stages I and II and 50%-70% for stages III and IV. Prognosis for NHL varies, but without therapy the survival rate is less than 2 yr. If treated aggressively, patients may achieve a cure. Patients who are not going to respond to therapy demonstrate their lack of response rapidly.

Radiation therapy to lymph node regions: For stages I and II. Whole-body radiation may be used for individuals with lymphoma who are symptomatic.

Chemotherapy in combination with radiation: For stages III and IV. One common combination of chemotherapeutic agents includes mechlorethamine hydrochloride (nitrogen mustard), vincristine, prednisone, and procarbazine. For NHL a variety of antineoplastic drugs are being used, including cyclophosphamide (Cytoxan), vincristine, prednisone, procarbazine, doxorubicin, and bleomycin. **Note:** Adults with NHL often have central nervous system involvement, and therefore intrathecal chemotherapy may be administered. For more information, see Appendix One, "Caring for Patients With Cancer and Other Life-disrupting Illnesses," p. 747.

Interferon, monoclonal antibodies, and autologous bone marrow transplant (BMT): Research is being conducted regarding efficacy. Currently, BMT has been found to provide long-term remission for only a few patients. The cost (>$100,000) and risks inherent in this therapy need to be thoroughly explained to potential recipients before obtaining consent.

NURSING DIAGNOSES AND INTERVENTIONS

Activity intolerance related to imbalance between oxygen supply and demand secondary to decreased oxygen-carrying capacity of the blood because of anemia

Desired outcome: After treatment, the patient rates perceived exertion at ≤3 on a 0-10 scale and exhibits tolerance to activity as evidenced by RR 12-20 breaths/min with normal depth and pattern (eupnea), HR ≤100 bpm, and absence of dizziness and headaches.

- As patient performs ADL, be alert for signs of activity intolerance and decreased tissue oxygenation: dyspnea on exertion, dizziness, palpations, headaches, and verbalization of increased exertion level. Ask patient to rate perceived exertion (see Appendix One, "Caring for Patients on Prolonged Bedrest" for **Risk for activity intolerance,** p. 738).
- Facilitate coordination of care providers to provide rest periods as needed between care activities, allowing time for at least 90 min of undisturbed rest.
- As indicated, monitor oximetry; report O_2 saturation <92%. Administer oxygen as prescribed, and encourage deep breathing to augment oxygen delivery to the tissues.
- Administer blood components (usually RBCs) as prescribed. Double-check type and crossmatching with a colleague, and monitor for and report signs of transfusion reaction.
- Encourage gradually increasing activities to tolerance as patient's condition improves. Set mutually agreed on goals with patient (e.g., "Let's plan this morning's activity goals. Do you feel you could walk up and down the hall once, or twice?" or appropriate amount, depending on patient's tolerance).
- Reassure patient that symptoms are usually relieved and tolerance for activity increases with therapy.

NIC: Blood Products Administration; Cardiac Care: Rehabilitative; Energy Management; Mutual Goal Setting; Oxygen Therapy

Altered nutrition: Less than body requirements related to decreased intake secondary to fatigue, impairment of oral mucosa, or anorexia

Desired outcome: By at least 24 hr before hospital discharge, patient exhibits adequate nutrition as evidenced by maintenance of or return to baseline body weight or a 1- to 2-lb weight gain.

- Weigh patient daily to identify trend.
- Monitor fluid volume and dietary intake, and encourage intake if necessary.
- If patient is easily fatigued, encourage him or her to eat small, frequent meals. Document intake.
- Request that significant other bring patient's favorite foods if they are unavailable in the hospital and stay with patient to encourage eating.
- Monitor for oral lesions or soreness of the gums, tongue, and esophagus. If oral lesions or cracks are present, encourage soft, bland foods. Advise patient to avoid spicy foods.
- Teach patient or significant other how to record and maintain a fluid and food intake diary.
- Administer vitamins and minerals as prescribed.

◎ **NIC:**   Discharge Planning; Nutritional Counseling; Teaching: Disease Process; Teaching: Individual; Teaching: Prescribed Diet

Risk for infection with risk factors related to inadequate secondary defenses secondary to altered WBC count and patient's decreased resistance to infection because of radiation therapy or chemotherapy

Desired outcome: Patient is free of infection as evidenced by normothermia, HR ≤100 bpm, RR 12-20 breaths/min with normal depth and pattern (eupnea), and absence of erythema, warmth, and drainage at any invasive or wound sites.

- Perform meticulous handwashing before touching the patient.
- Report any signs of systemic infection (e.g., fever); obtain prescription for blood, wound, and urine cultures as indicated. Administer antibiotics as prescribed.
- Monitor for and report any signs of local infection, such as sore throat or erythematous or draining wounds.
- Provide oral care at frequent intervals to prevent oral lesions, which may result in bleeding and infection.
- Provide and encourage adequate perianal hygiene to prevent rectal abscess. Avoid giving medications or taking temperatures rectally (i.e., use a tympanic thermometer if possible).
- Avoid invasive procedures whenever possible.
- Encourage ambulation, deep breathing, coughing, and turning to prevent problems from immobility, which can result in pneumonia or skin breakdown.
- Teach patient and significant other the signs and symptoms of infection and the importance of notifying staff or health care providers promptly if they develop.

◎ **NIC:**   Activity Therapy; Health Education; Infection Control; Oral Health Maintenance; Perineal Care; Surveillance

See Also: "Disseminated Intravascular Coagulation" for **Altered protection** related to increased risk of bleeding, p. 540; Appendix One, "Caring for Preoperative and Postoperative Patients," p. 717; "Caring for Patients With Cancer and Other Life-disrupting Illnesses," p. 747.

PATIENT-FAMILY TEACHING AND DISCHARGE PLANNING

When providing patient-family teaching, focus on sensory information; avoid giving excessive information; and initiate a visiting nurse referral for necessary follow-up teaching. Consider including verbal and written information about the following:

- For patients in stage I or II, the resumption of normal life-style with minor adjustments, as prescribed.
- Continuing radiation or chemotherapy, if prescribed, which is given on an outpatient basis; confirm date and time of next appointment.
- Signs and symptoms that necessitate medical attention: persistent fever, weight loss, enlarged lymph nodes, malaise, dyspnea, and decreased exercise tolerance.
- Importance of preventing infection and avoiding exposure to individuals with infection, which is essential because of alterations in WBC count and patient's decreased resistance to infection secondary to therapy. Teach patient the indicators of common infections, such as urinary tract infection, upper respiratory infection, and wound infection. See "Care of the Renal Transplant Recipient" for **Risk for infection,** p. 162.
- Importance of maintaining good nutritional habits to increase resistance to infection.
- Referral to American Cancer Society and local support groups, including phone numbers and addresses. For information on local resources or more general information contact the following organizations:

    The American Cancer Society
    1599 Clifton Road NE
    Atlanta, GA 30329   (800) ACS-2345
    WWW address: *http://www.cancer.org*

    National Cancer Institute Information Service (CIS)
    Bldg. 31, Room 10A16
    9000 Rockville Pike
    Bethesda, MD 20892   (800) 422-6237
    WWW address: *http://wwwicic.nic.nih.gov/*

- Some cities have local support groups for patients who may require BMT. Information for these patients can be obtained by contacting the following organization:

    Bone Marrow Transplant Family Support Network
    P.O. Box 845
    Avon, CT 06001   (800) 826-9376
    WWW address: *http://www.stepstn.com/nord/org_sum/280.htm*

- Avoiding trauma, which can cause bruising, especially in the presence of thrombocytopenia, which can occur secondary to chemotherapy.
- If appropriate, measures for assisting patient with ADL or referral for home health care.
- Importance of obtaining a Medic-Alert bracelet and identification card outlining diagnosis and emergency treatment. Contact the following organization:

    Medic Alert
    2323 Colorado Ave.
    Turlock, CA 95382   (209) 668-3333

Acute leukemia

Acute leukemia is an abnormal, malignant proliferation of WBC precursors, also called *blasts*. These abnormal cells accumulate in bone marrow, body tissues, and blood vessels and eventually cause malfunction by encroachment, hemorrhage, or infection. In addition, they function inappropriately in response to infection and prevent normal WBC maturation. Moreover, the accumulation of WBCs in the bone marrow alters and decreases the production of RBCs and platelets. The two most common types of acute leukemia are *myelocytic* (arising from the myeloblast, which matures into a neutrophil) and *lymphocytic* (arising from the lymphoblast, which matures into a lymphocyte). Identification of specific genetic translocations directly reflects the prognosis. Untreated acute leukemia invariably is fatal, and even with treatment the prognosis varies. Acute lymphocytic leukemia (ALL) most often affects children younger than 15 yr, whereas acute myelocytic leukemia (AML) usually affects individuals older than 20 yr.

ASSESSMENT

Chronic indicators: Fever, pallor, chills, and weakness, which can be present for days, weeks, or months before acute crisis occurs. Gingivitis, easy bruising, and prolonged menstruation (menorrhagia) also may occur.
Acute indicators: High fever, diffuse petechiae, ecchymosis, epistaxis, anorexia, nausea, vomiting, headaches, visual disturbances, weakness, feeling of abdominal fullness, lethargy, and seizures.
Physical assessment: Sternal and bone tenderness on palpation, splenomegaly, hepatomegaly, palpable lymph nodes, pallor, papilledema, cranial nerve disorders, and diffuse bleeding of mucous membranes.

DIAGNOSTIC TESTS

CBC: Hgb is decreased; WBC count usually is high (often >50,000/mm^3) and includes many immature cells.
Bone marrow aspiration: Reveals increased numbers of myeloblasts or lymphoblasts.
Platelet count: Decreased.
Prothrombin time (PT) and partial thromboplastin time (PTT):   May be increased because of clotting deficiencies.
Uric acid: Increased secondary to rapid cell destruction.
Chromosomal study: Permits realistic estimates of prognosis and disease staging.

COLLABORATIVE MANAGEMENT

The goal is complete remission or reduction in the number of malignant cells and increased number of normal leukocytes by normal hematopoiesis. Secondary management goals are to return the erythrocyte index and thrombocyte count to normal.
Chemotherapy/pharmacotherapy: Used in combination to produce remission (less than 5% blast cells and no identifiable leukemic cells in the bone marrow). Treatment may be continued for 1½-2 yr after remission occurs. **Note:** For children with ALL, treatment may last as long as 3 yr.
For ALL: Vincristine sulfate, prednisone, and daunorubicin with or without l-asparaginase and methotrexate may be given intrathecally for central nervous system prophylaxis. Although l-asparaginase is a valuable adjunct, the incidence of hypersensitivity reactions in children ranges from 3% to 73%, rising with increasing dosage and frequency of administration.
For AML: Treated initially with intensive combination chemotherapy with an antimetabolite (e.g., thioguanine), as well as an anthracycline antineoplastic antibiotic (e.g., daunorubicin hydrochloride or cytarabine). Postremis-

sion therapy dosages are much higher than those used during standard induction therapy.

Note: For lymphocytic leukemias, therapeutic lymphocytapheresis or leukocytapheresis may be performed to decrease tumor load before and at the start of chemotherapy. Usually this is performed when the WBC count is >100,000/mm^3 and the individual has signs of decreased circulation.

Transfusion of packed RBCs: To restore erythrocytes. Leukocyte-poor packed RBCs are preferable to whole blood because febrile reactions to WBCs or platelet antibodies are prevented. Because of possible antibody formation and increased transfusion reactions over time, transfusions are given conservatively, especially in individuals for whom long-term transfusions of platelets and granulocytes are anticipated. Therefore patients may need to tolerate a certain degree of anemia (see Table 7-1).

Platelet transfusion: To restore platelet levels to >20,000/mm^3 (see Table 7-1).

Bone marrow and peripheral blood progenitor cell transplantation: Available in specialized centers. See discussion for Bone Marrow Transplantation under "Hypoplastic (Aplastic) Anemia," p. 520.

NURSING DIAGNOSES AND INTERVENTIONS

Risk for infection with risk factors related to inadequate secondary defenses secondary to myelosuppression from disease process or therapy

Desired outcome: Patient is free of infection as evidenced by normothermia, negative culture results, absence of adventitious breath sounds, HR ≤100 bpm, and the presence of well-healing wounds.

- Monitor patient's temperature frequently. In the presence of any suspected infections, obtain prescription for a culture. Report temperature >38° C (100.4° F) that lasts >24 hr and occurs concurrently with chills and/or HR >100 bpm.
- Be aware that as the neutrophil count decreases, the risk of infection increases. When the patient becomes neutropenic, perform reverse (protective) isolation using a gown, mask, and gloves.
- When appropriate, provide a private room in an air-controlled, positive-pressure room.
- Control access to the patient; restrict visitors.
- Allow no fresh fruits or vegetables in the diet; allow no contact with plants, flowers, or pets.
- Perform meticulous handwashing before caring for patient.
- Avoid all invasive procedures (e.g., catheterization) unless absolutely necessary. When such procedures are performed, use strict sterile technique.
- Assist patient with ambulation when possible. Institute turning, coughing, and deep breathing at frequent intervals to help prevent problems of immobility that can result in infection, such as skin breakdown and respiratory dysfunction.
- Provide oral hygiene and perianal care at frequent intervals.
- Monitor I&O, and maintain adequate hydration by encouraging fluid intake of 3 L/day unless contraindicated.
- Administer antibiotic therapy if prescribed.
- Administer transfusion of granulocytes if prescribed.

NIC: Blood Products Administration; Environmental Management; Fluid Management; Infection Protection; Medication Management; Oral Health Maintenance; Perineal Care; Vital Signs Monitoring

Altered protection related to increased risk of bleeding secondary to decreased platelet count

Desired outcomes: Patient is free of symptoms of bleeding as evidenced by BP ≥90/60 mm Hg, HR ≤100 bpm (or within patient's baseline range), and excretions and secretions negative for blood.

- Monitor platelet counts. Counts <50,000/mm³ dramatically increase the risk of bleeding. Monitor Hct and Hgb values for levels that suggest bleeding. Report values outside the following normal ranges: Hct 40%-54% (male) and 37%-47% (female); Hgb 14-18 g/dl (male) and 12-16 g/dl (female).
- Request that patient alert staff members to oozing of blood from the gums.
- Inspect patient's skin, mouth, nose, urine, feces, sputum, emesis, and IV sites for signs of bleeding.
- Use a reagent stick to check stool, urine, emesis, and nasogastric drainage for blood.
- Monitor VS at frequent intervals, and be alert to signs of bleeding such as hypotension, tachycardia, dyspnea, and increased RR.
- Monitor LOC at frequent intervals; report significant changes. Be alert to disorientation and changes in mental status, which can signal intracranial hemorrhage.
- Limit invasive procedures to those that are absolutely necessary.
- When injections are necessary, use small-gauge needle when possible. Maintain gentle pressure on injection site until bleeding stops.
- If bleeding occurs, elevate the affected part, if possible, and apply cold compresses and gentle pressure.
- Pad side rails to prevent trauma.
- Administer stool softeners as prescribed to minimize risk of rectal bleeding.
- Teach patient the signs and symptoms of bleeding and the importance of notifying staff promptly if they occur.
- Teach patient to use soft-bristle toothbrush or sponge-tipped applicator and electric shaver.

NIC: Bedside Laboratory Testing; Bleeding Precautions; Bleeding Reduction; Neurologic Monitoring; Surveillance

Activity intolerance related to imbalance between oxygen supply and demand secondary to decreased oxygen-carrying capacity of the blood because of erythrocyte destruction
Desired outcome: Following treatment, patient rates his or her perceived exertion at ≤3 on a 0-10 scale and exhibits tolerance to activity as evidenced by HR ≤100 bpm, RR ≤20 breaths/min, and absence of headache and dizziness.

- Monitor patient's response to activity, and ask patient to rate his or her perceived exertion. Be alert to indicators of decreased tissue oxygenation: dyspnea on exertion, dizziness, palpitations, or headaches. See Appendix One, "Caring for Patients on Prolonged Bedrest" for **Risk for activity intolerance,** p. 738.
- As indicated, monitor oximetry; report O₂ saturation <92%. Administer oxygen as prescribed, and encourage deep breathing to augment oxygen delivery to the tissues.
- If prescribed, administer packed RBCs to restore normal erythrocyte level (see Table 7-1).
- Assist patient with ADL as necessary.
- Facilitate coordination of care providers to provide rest periods as needed between care activities, allowing time for at least 90 min of undisturbed rest.
- Minimize restlessness, which increases oxygen use, by providing frequent comfort measures such as back rubs, music therapy, assisted relaxation, and cognitive and attentional distraction.

- Monitor dietary intake to ensure adequate caloric intake.
- As patient's condition improves, encourage activities to tolerance. Set mutually agreed on goals (e.g., "Can you walk the length of the hall two or three times [or appropriate number, depending on tolerance] this morning?"). Be alert to and document activity intolerance as evidenced by pallor, weakness, increase in pulse rate, headache, and dizziness. Discontinue activity and assist patient with getting back into bed if these symptoms occur.

NIC: Cardiac Care: Rehabilitative; Distraction; Energy Management; Mutual Goal Setting; Oxygen Therapy; Progressive Muscle Relaxation; Simple Massage

Altered renal tissue perfusion related to interrupted blood flow secondary to destruction of RBCs and their precipitation in the kidney tubules
Desired outcome: By at least 24 hr before hospital discharge, patient has adequate renal perfusion as evidenced by balanced I&O, urinary output ≥30 ml/hr, and stable weight.

- Monitor for and report signs of renal insufficiency, including positive fluid balance, edema formation, weight gain, and urinary output <30 ml/hr in the presence of adequate intake.
- Maintain adequate hydration of at least 2-3 L/day (unless contraindicated) to enhance urinary flow.
- Encourage ambulation or in-bed exercises to patient's tolerance to promote renal circulation.
- Alert patient's health care provider to significant findings.

NIC: Activity Therapy; Fluid Management

See Also: Appendix One, "Caring for Patients With Cancer and Other Life-disrupting Illnesses," p. 747, for nursing diagnoses and interventions.

PATIENT-FAMILY TEACHING AND DISCHARGE PLANNING

When providing patient-family teaching, focus on sensory information; avoid giving excessive information; and initiate a visiting nurse referral for necessary follow-up teaching. Consider including verbal and written information about the following:

- Importance of avoiding infections and bleeding and measures to prevent same, including the following: avoid exposure to individuals with infection, maintain good hygiene, avoid situations with high risk of trauma or injury, and report any signs of infection to patient's health care provider (e.g., fever, chills, malaise).
- Side effects of chemotherapy: constipation, alopecia, nausea and vomiting, anorexia, diarrhea, stomatitis, skin rash, nail changes, hyperpigmentation of the skin, weight gain from steroid use, ecchymosis, and cystitis. For more information, see Appendix One, "Caring for Patients With Cancer and Other Life-disrupting Illnesses," p. 747.
- Importance of good nutrition, eating small and frequent meals, consuming 2-3 L of fluids per day (unless contraindicated by cardiac or renal disorder), and using soft-bristle toothbrush and electric razor.
- Referrals to American Cancer Society, Leukemia Society of America, local support groups, and home care or hospice groups, if appropriate:

The American Cancer Society
1599 Clifton Road NE
Atlanta, GA 30329   (800) ACS-2345
WWW address: *http://www.cancer.org*

National Cancer Institute Information Service (CIS)
Bldg. 31, Room 10A16
9000 Rockville Pike
Bethesda, MD 20892   (800) 422-6237
WWW address: *http://wwwicic.nic.nih.gov/*

Leukemia Society of America
600 3rd Ave.
New York, NY 10016   (800) 955-4572
WWW address: *http://www.leukemia.org*

National Hospice Association
1901 North Moore St., Suite 901
Arlington, VA 22209   (703) 243-5900; (703) 525-5762 FAX
WWW address: *http://www.hospice.org*

Chronic leukemia

Chronic leukemias are characterized by malignant proliferation of abnormal immature WBCs. These abnormal cells eventually infiltrate body tissues and organs and prevent maturation of normal WBCs, thus preventing usual and necessary WBC function. The proliferation of abnormal WBCs in the bone marrow inhibits the formation of other bone marrow elements, including RBCs and platelets. Chronic leukemic cells are a more mature form than is seen in acute leukemias, and they accumulate much more slowly. The two most common types of chronic leukemia are *chronic myelocytic leukemia (CML;* sometimes called *granulocytic)* (involves the myelocyte, precursor of the neutrophil) and *chronic lymphocytic leukemia (CLL)* (involves the lymphocyte). Causes of chronic leukemia are unclear, although chromosomal abnormality is suspected in many cases of myelogenous leukemia. Also implicated are hereditary factors and immunologic defects.

ASSESSMENT

Chronic indicators: Fatigue, anorexia, weight loss, gingivitis, prolonged menstruation, sensation of heaviness in the spleen area, malaise, unexplained low-grade fever, and lymph node enlargement.
Acute indicators: High fever, diffuse petechiae, ecchymosis, epistaxis, anorexia, headaches, visual disturbances, weakness, sensation of abdominal fullness, and lethargy.

DIAGNOSTIC TESTS

CBC with differential: Elevated WBC; decreased Hgb and neutrophils.
Platelet count (thrombocytes):   Low.
Bone marrow aspiration: Usually identifies abnormal distribution or increased number of cells.
Chromosomal study: Permits realistic estimates of prognosis and disease staging.

COLLABORATIVE MANAGEMENT

For chronic lymphocytic leukemia
Chemotherapy: Chlorambucil or cyclophosphamide and prednisone to produce remission. Cladribine (2-CdA) is a new agent that has demonstrated a response rate up to 85%. IV immunoglobulin has been effectively used for prophylaxis, but this therapy is very expensive.
Local irradiation of spleen and lymph nodes: Performed when drug therapy has failed. This procedure is associated with decreasing peripheral leukocyte counts.

For chronic myelocytic leukemia

Bone marrow transplantation: Uses matched sibling donors and is the treatment of choice. Marrow grafting using unrelated donors is a potentially beneficial treatment.

Chemotherapy

Busulfan, hydroxyurea, interferon alfa-2a, and interferon alfa-2b: During the stable chronic phase.

Daunorubicin, cytarabine, vincristine, prednisone, and thioguanine: During the acute phase.

Splenectomy: May be necessary if the spleen is destroying platelets.

Whole-brain irradiation or leukapheresis: May be done during an acute crisis for rapid reduction of WBCs.

NURSING DIAGNOSES AND INTERVENTIONS

See "Acute Leukemia," p. 547.

> Note: Although patients survive longer and the severity of symptoms is less with chronic leukemias, the same principles and nursing interventions apply. See also Appendix One, "Caring for Preoperative and Postoperative Patients," p. 717, if splenectomy is performed; "Caring for Patients With Cancer and Other Life-disrupting Illnesses," p. 747.

PATIENT-FAMILY TEACHING AND DISCHARGE PLANNING

See this section in "Acute Leukemia," p. 549.

Selected Bibliography

Asimacopulous PJ et al: Angina pectoris caused by pernicious anemia, *Chest* 105(3):653-654, 1994.

Bick RL: DIC: objective criteria for diagnosis and management, *Med Clin North Am* 78(3):511-543, 1994.

Cahill M: Hematologic problems in pediatric patients, *Semin Oncol Nurs* 12(1):38-50, 1996.

Caudell KA: Psychoneuroimmunology and innovative behavioral interventions in patients with leukemia, *Oncol Nurs Forum* 23(3):493-501, 1996.

DeGowin RI, editor: *DeGowin & DeGowin's diagnostic examination,* ed 6, New York, 1994, McGraw-Hill.

Edwards C: *Davidson's principles and practice of medicine*, ed 17, Edinburgh, 1995, Churchill Livingstone.

Erickson JM: Anemia, *Semin Oncol Nurs* 12(1):2-14, 1996.

Horne MM, Heitz UE, Swearingen PL: *Pocket guide to fluid, electrolyte, and acid-base balance,* ed 3, St Louis, 1997, Mosby.

Isselbacher KJ et al, editors: *Harrison's principles of internal medicine,* ed 13, New York, 1994, McGraw-Hill.

Kim MJ et al: *Pocket guide to nursing diagnoses*, ed 7, St Louis, 1997, Mosby.

Knoop T: Polycythemia vera, *Semin Oncol Nurs* 12(1):70-77, 1996.

Krantz SB: Pathogenesis and treatment of anemia of chronic disease, *Am J Med Sci* 307:353-359, 1994.

Lundquist DM, Stewart FM: An update on non-Hodgkin's lymphomas, *Nurse Pract* 19(10):41-54, 1994.

Seidel HM et al, editors: *Mosby's guide to physical examination*, ed 3, St Louis, 1995, Mosby.

Shelton B: Disorders of hemostasis in sepsis, *Crit Care Nurs Clin North Am* 6(2):273-387, 1995.

Shirley KM: Platelet-associated bleeding disorders, *Semin Oncol Nurs* 12(1): 51-58, 1996.

Viele CS: Chronic myelogenous leukemia and acute promyelocytic leukemia: new bone marrow transplant options, *Oncol Nurs Forum* 23(3):488-492, 1996.

Wiycik D et al: Leukemia management strategies: the next generation, *Oncol Nurs Forum* 23(3):477-487, 1996.

8 MUSCULO-SKELETAL DISORDERS

Section One: Inflammatory Disorders

Arthritis is simply defined as inflammation of a joint. Arthritis is an expression of one of many diffuse connective tissue diseases, including osteoarthritis, gouty arthritis, rheumatoid arthritis, Reiter's syndrome, ankylosing spondylitis, systemic lupus erythematosus, and psoriatic arthritis. Osteoarthritis and rheumatoid arthritis are frequently seen in hospitalized patients and therefore are discussed in this section.

Osteoarthritis

Osteoarthritis (OA), also known as *degenerative joint disease* (*DJD*), is an extremely prevalent disorder. It is a chronic, progressive disease characterized by increasing pain, deformity, and loss of function. About 20 million Americans exhibit signs of OA. OA is the second leading cause of disability in people older than 50 yr. By 40 yr, 90% of all people show radiographic evidence of OA. Incidence increases with age, but it can be found in any age-group, usually following trauma or as a complication of congenital malformation. OA is characterized by hypertrophy of bone at articular margins and degeneration of cartilage. True joint inflammation seldom is present (except in the distal interphalangeal joints). Hereditary and mechanical factors are suspected to be the primary causes of this process. OA may be classified as idiopathic or secondary.

Idiopathic osteoarthritis may be localized or generalized and occurs in the distal interphalangeal (DIP), proximal interphalangeal (PIP), metacarpophalangeal (MCP), and carpometacarpal (CMC) joints of the thumb; hip; knee; first metatarsophalangeal (MTP) joint; cervical and lumbosacral spine; or other single joints. Generalized OA involves three or more of the previously listed joints. *Secondary osteoarthritis* can occur in any joint and usually follows some form of intraarticular injury or extraarticular change that affects joint dynamics. Examples include posttraumatic, congenital (e.g., Legg-Calvé-Perthes), or developmental (e.g., scoliosis) processes; calcium deposition disease; other bone or joint disorders (e.g., septic arthritis, osteitis deformans); and other diseases (e.g, endocrine, neuropathic arthropathy, frostbite).

ASSESSMENT

Involvement can range from incidental findings on x-ray to pervasive disease that affects the patient's independence in the performance of ADL.

Signs and symptoms: Onset is insidious, beginning with joint stiffness, especially early morning stiffness lasting <15 min. It evolves into joint pain, which worsens with activity and is relieved with rest. Signs of local inflammation usually are absent, except occasionally in the DIP, PIP, and CMC joints. There are no systemic signs or symptoms.

Physical assessment: Characteristic findings include limited joint motion, Heberden's nodes (enlargement of the DIP joint), Bouchard's nodes (enlargement of the PIP joint), varus or valgus deformity of the knee, bony enlargement of the joint, and flexion contracture of the knee. Frequently crepitation is found.

DIAGNOSTIC TESTS

No characteristic laboratory studies are associated with OA. Erythrocyte sedimentation rate and WBC counts may be assessed to rule out other arthropathic conditions (e.g., rheumatoid arthritis, infection).

X-ray studies: May reveal narrowing of the joint space, osteophytosis (bony projections) of the joint margins, bone cysts, sharpened articular margins, and dense subchondral bone.

COLLABORATIVE MANAGEMENT

Rest: Principal therapy for preventing progression. The patient is advised to avoid activities that will stress the joint further. Use of ambulatory assistive devices, splints, or orthotics may be prescribed to allow rest or decreased stress on affected joints, and the patient is instructed in methods that prevent postural strain. Regular rest periods of 30-60 min often are advised for patients likely to overwork.

Weight reduction: For patients for whom excessive weight contributes to the pathologic condition.

Local moist heat: To decrease stiffness and provide some subjective pain relief. Hydrotherapy with warm water is especially useful in aiding ROM exercises. Patients who cannot afford to purchase a device to supply moist heat may be required to use a traditional heating pad. Some patients find greater subjective relief from cold packs than from moist heat.

ROM and muscle-strengthening exercises: May be useful in selected cases to increase joint function and supplement joint strength (e.g., quadriceps exercises for OA of the knee). Exercises may include passive ROM, active ROM, active-assisted ROM, and isometric and isotonic exercises. The maxim that is followed for the appropriate amount of exercise is that pain that lasts until the next exercise period (or several hours) indicates the exercise was too strenuous.

Intraarticular steroids: Some health care practitioners recommend intermittent use of triamcinolone hexacetonide (Aristospan) for transient relief of symptoms. However, steroids do not halt the progression of the disease and run the risk of introducing refractory infections.

Pharmacotherapy: Includes the use of analgesics and antiinflammatory agents. Analgesics may be necessary to combat the pain associated with DJD. Aspirin, acetaminophen, and the nonsteroidal antiinflammatory drugs (NSAIDs; Table 8-1) usually are satisfactory, but occasionally narcotic analgesics may be required for short periods after physical therapy or surgical interventions. In addition, the NSAIDs may be used as maintenance therapy to control or reduce symptoms. Cytokinine modulation with tenidap shows promise for future use in amelioration of OA.

Surgical interventions: May be used to correct underlying congenital anomalies or defects created by trauma. Arthroplastic surgery allows damaged joint surfaces to be augmented, repaired, or replaced; whereas periarticular tissues may be repaired to improve joint strength. Joint replacement has been used to replace most joints, but the greatest success has been found with hip (see p. 611) and knee (see p. 616) implant arthroplasties. Although morbid obesity and neuropathic joints do not contraindicate joint replacement surgery, patients with these conditions have greater potential for poor surgical outcomes. In joints that are chronically infected or not amenable to standard or implant arthroplasties, an arthrodesis (joint fusion) may provide joint stability and

T A B L E 8 - 1   Nonsteroidal Antiinflammatory Drugs

Generic name	Common brand names	Usual daily dosage (mg)
Acetylsalicylic acid	Aspirin	650-1300 q4hr
Choline magnesium trisalicylate	Trilisate	1000-1250 bid
Choline salicylate	Arthropan	650 q4-6hr
Diclofenac potassium	Cataflam	75-100 qd
Diclofenac sodium	Voltaren	100-150 bid or tid
Diflunisal	Dolobid	500-1000 qd or divided q12hr
Etodolac	Lodine	600-1200 bid, tid, or qid
Fenoprofen calcium	Nalfon	300-600 qid
Flurbiprofen	Ansaid	200-300 bid, tid, or qid
Ibuprofen	Motrin, Advil, Nuprin	200-400 qid
Indomethacin	Indocin	20-50 tid
Ketoprofen	Orudis	25-75 q6-8hr
Ketorolac tromethamine	Toradol	10 q4-6hr
Magnesium salicylate	Mobidin	600-1200 tid or qid
Meclofenamate sodium	Meclomen	50 tid or qid
Mefenamic acid	Ponstel	250 qid
Nabumetone	Relafen	1000-2000 qd or divided bid
Naproxen	Naprosyn	250-375 qid
Naproxen sodium	Anaprox	275 q6-8hr
Oxaprozin	Daypro	1200-1800 qd
Oxyphenbutazone	Oxalid	100-200 tid
Piroxicam	Feldene	20 qd
Salsalate	Disalcid	500 q4hr
Sulindac	Clinoril	150-200 bid
Tolmetin sodium	Tolectin	200-400 tid

permit some function. Arthroscopy may be used to debride osteoarthritic joints of loose bodies, osteophytes, frayed cartilage, and hypertrophied synovium. Valgus osteotomy has been successful in transferring the weight-bearing stresses of the proximal tibia from the medial compartment to the usually less diseased lateral compartment. Osseous tissue transplants from contralateral joints show promise in treating isolated lesions of OA.

Splints and orthotic devices: May be used to supplement joint strength or protect the joint from excessive strain.

Assistive devices: A great variety have been developed to help patients perform ADL independently, even in cases of significant joint function loss. Examples include stocking helpers, built-up eating utensils, pickup sticks, and raised toilet seats.

NURSING DIAGNOSES AND INTERVENTIONS

Pain related to joint changes and corrective therapy

Desired outcomes: Within 1-2 hr of intervention, patient's subjective perception of pain decreases, as documented by a pain scale. Objective indicators are absent or diminished. Patient demonstrates ability to perform ADL without complaints of discomfort.

- Devise and help patient use a rating system to evaluate pain and analgesic relief on a scale of 0 (no pain) to 10 (worst pain).

- Administer analgesics and antiinflammatory agents as prescribed (or 30 min before strenuous activity), and document their effectiveness, using the pain scale. As appropriate, teach patient about the function of epidural anesthesia or patient-controlled analgesia (PCA).
- Provide maintenance antiinflammatory agents at scheduled intervals to ensure maximum effect.
- Teach patient use of nonpharmacologic methods of pain control, including guided imagery; graduated breathing (as in the Lamaze method); enhanced relaxation; massage; biofeedback; cutaneous stimulation (via a counterirritant, e.g., oil of wintergreen); a transcutaneous electrical nerve stimulation (TENS) device; warm or cool thermotherapy; music therapy; and tactile, auditory, visual, or verbal distractions.
- Use traditional nursing interventions to counteract the pain, including back rubs, repositioning, and encouraging the patient to verbalize feelings.
- Incorporate rest, local warmth or cold, and elevation of the affected joints, when possible, to help control discomfort.
- Advise patient to coordinate the time of peak effectiveness of the antiinflammatory agent with periods of exercise or mandatory use of arthritic joints.
- Instruct patient in the use of moist heat and hydrotherapy, which will help reduce long-term discomfort.
- For additional interventions, see **Pain** related to joint changes and corrective therapy, p. 719, in Appendix One, "Caring for Preoperative and Postoperative Patients"; and **Pain** related to surgical repair and rehabilitation therapy, p. 573, in "Torn anterior cruciate ligament."

You may also wish to refer to the following interventions from the Nursing Interventions Classification (NIC):

NIC: Acupressure; Analgesic Administration; Cutaneous Stimulation; Distraction; Heat/Cold Application; Meditation; Music Therapy; Pain Management; Progressive Muscle Relaxation; Simple Guided Imagery; Simple Massage; Simple Relaxation Therapy

Knowledge deficit: Use of a heating device
Desired outcome: Within 24 hr of instruction, patient verbalizes and demonstrates proper use of the heating device.
- Assess patient's baseline knowledge in the use of a heating device.
- As appropriate, provide patient with instructions for the proper use of moist or dry heat. Because older individuals, especially persons with diabetes, may have decreased peripheral neurologic function and skin that is more easily traumatized, instruct them in the use of a thermometer (with adequate-size numbers for reading) or a controlled warming device.
- Caution patients about the potential for increasing their tolerance to heat. This can occur when heat has been used for long periods and may cause the patient to feel the need for a higher degree of heat than that which is safe.

NIC: Heat/Cold Application; Teaching: Individual; Teaching: Prescribed Activity/Exercise; Teaching: Procedure/Treatment

Impaired physical mobility related to musculoskeletal impairment and adjustment to a new walking gait with an assistive device
Desired outcomes: By hospital discharge, patient demonstrates adequate upper body strength for use of an assistive device. Patient demonstrates appropriate use of the assistive device on flat and uneven surfaces.
- Before ambulation, ensure the necessary strength of the patient's upper extremities for using the assistive device by incorporating the interventions listed in Appendix One, "Caring for Preoperative and Postoperative Patients" for **Risk for disuse syndrome,** p. 740. Triceps muscle strength is especially

important for ambulation with crutches or a walker. Having patients push down on the bed as they extend their arms to lift their buttocks off the bed will strengthen the triceps muscles.

- Provide a thorough discussion with a demonstration to teach the patient how the assistive device is used.
- When fitting crutches, ensure that the patient is wearing flat-heel, properly fitting, supportive shoes. With the patient standing and with his or her elbows slightly flexed at 10-30 degrees, be sure that the crutch tops rest 1-1.5 inches (or the width of two fingers) below the axillae. Be aware that complaints of upper extremity paresthesia may indicate improperly fitted crutches. Ensure that the crutches have rubber tips to prevent slipping; cleat tips are also available to reduce slipping on ice. Rubber axillary pads should be placed to reduce pressure at the axillae.
- Once the assistive device is in position, repeat the instructions and then supervise the ambulation. Ambulation should begin in small increments on level ground and eventually progress to all surfaces the patient is expected to encounter after hospital discharge.
- Ensure that before discharge, the patient is able to demonstrate independence in ambulation with the assistive device on level surfaces and stairs and with getting in and out of a car.

NIC: Activity Therapy; Exercise Therapy: Ambulation; Exercise Therapy: Joint Mobility; Fall Prevention; Mutual Goal Setting; Teaching: Prescribed Activity/Exercise

---

See Also: "Ligamentous Injuries" for **Knowledge deficit:** Potential for joint weakness, and the techniques for applying external supports and assessing neurovascular status, p. 568; "Fractures" for **Knowledge deficit:** Potential for infection, p. 592; Appendix One, "Caring for Patients on Prolonged Bedrest," p. 738; "Caring for Preoperative and Postoperative Patients" (if surgery is performed), p. 717, for nursing diagnoses and interventions.

PATIENT-FAMILY TEACHING AND DISCHARGE PLANNING

When providing patient-family teaching, focus on sensory information; avoid giving excessive information; and initiate a visiting nurse referral for necessary follow-up teaching. Consider including verbal and written information about the following:

- Medications, including drug name, dosage, purpose, schedule, precautions, drug/drug and food/drug interactions, and potential side effects.
- Importance of systemic rest as well as rest of the affected joints.
- Weight reduction, if it is appropriate for the patient.
- Proper use of moist heat.
- Necessity of ROM and muscle-strengthening exercises.
- Use of splints or orthotics, including care and cleansing and where to get replacements.
- Use, care, and replacement of assistive devices.
- If surgery was performed, the precautions related to the procedure, wound care (see "Wounds Closed by Primary Intention," p. 704), indicators of wound infection (i.e., persistent redness, swelling, increasing pain, wound drainage, local warmth, fever), or complications of surgery.
- Importance of follow-up care and the date of the next appointment; a phone number to call if any questions arise.
- Phone numbers to call if questions or concerns arise about therapy or disease after discharge. In addition, many cities have local arthritis support groups.

Information for these patients can be obtained by writing to the following organization:

Arthritis Foundation
1330 West Peachtree St.
Atlanta, GA 30309   (800) 283-7800
WWW address: *http://www.arthritis.org*

- Additional information on arthritis is available through the following organization:

National Arthritis and Musculoskeletal and Skin Diseases Information Clearinghouse, National Institute of Arthritis and Musculoskeletal and Skin Diseases
Information Specialist
1 AMS Circle
Bethesda, MD 20892-3675   (301) 495-4484; (301) 587-4352 FAX
WWW address:
http://www.social.com/health/nhic/data/hr0000/hr0036.html

Rheumatoid arthritis

Rheumatoid arthritis (RA) is associated with severe morbidity, functional decline, and shortened longevity. It has a prevalence of 1%-2% in the general population, with females outnumbering males 3:1. It is an immune system disease characterized by remissions and exacerbations of inflammation of the connective tissue throughout the body. Although many connective tissues have potential for involvement (heart, blood vessels, lungs, spleen, eyes, kidney) and generalized systemic effects may be noted, this discussion centers on the arthritic aspects of this process (see Table 8-2 for a list of the extraarticular effects of RA). RA most commonly affects the synovial joints, but the effects of this disease are highly variable. Recent research into the pathogenesis of RA indicates that the chronic inflammatory reaction in the rheumatoid synovial membrane is the result of active immune response. Susceptibility to RA is determined genetically. The originating stimulus of this response is still unknown, but it has been speculated to be food allergies; hereditary deficit; or infection by parvovirus, Epstein-Barr virus, or rubella. The disease onset and progression can be rapid and fulminating or slow and chronic.

The inflammatory process results in chronic synovitis with the formation of pannus, an inflammatory exudate that accumulates over the surface of the synovial membrane. Continued inflammation eventually erodes cartilage and subchondral bone, creating dynamic joint changes that contribute to ligamentous and tendinous weakening. Involvement of periarticular tissues results in loss of support structures and leads to characteristic joint changes that further contribute to the pathologic condition.

ASSESSMENT

Specific criteria have been developed by the American Rheumatism Association (ARA) to enable a more accurate diagnosis of this process. A diagnosis of RA is made by documenting at least four of the following seven criteria:

1. Morning stiffness in and around the joints lasting ≥1 hr before maximal improvement
2. Polyarthritis of ≥3 joints simultaneously with soft tissue swelling observed by a health care provider involving the following joints: proximal interphalangeal (PIP), metacarpophalangeal (MCP), wrist, elbow, knee, ankle, and metatarsophalangeal (MTP)
3. At least one of the preceding joints should be the wrist, MCP, or PIP
4. Simultaneous involvement of symmetric joints (bilateral involvement)

T A B L E 8 - 2   Extraarticular Effects of Rheumatoid Arthritis

Location	Effects
General	Weakness
	Fatigue
	Morning stiffness
	Weight loss
Organ/system	
Skin	Rheumatoid nodules
	Superficial vasculitis (brown spots, ulcerations)
Mucous membranes	Sjogren's or sicca syndrome (dry mucous membranes)
Heart	Pericarditis
Eyes	Sjogren's syndrome ("dry eye")
	Scleromalacia (thinned sclera)
	Episcleritis (inflamed conjunctival membrane)
Nervous	Carpal/tarsal tunnel syndromes
	Cervical cord compression (cervical vertebra subluxation)
	Peripheral neuropathy
Pulmonary	Lung nodules
	Pleuritis (causing pleural effusions)
	Caplan's syndrome (pneumoconiosis, e.g., dense infiltrates)
	Interstitial pneumonitis (diffuse infiltrates)
	Bronchiolitis obliterans (emphysema-like)
Vascular	Rheumatoid vasculitis
Hematologic	Leukopenia (Felty's syndrome, e.g., severe neutropenia)
	Anemia
Other	Amyloidosis (deposition of protein in kidney, intestine, heart)
	Osteoporosis

5. Subcutaneous nodules found over bony prominences, extensor surfaces, or juxtaarticular areas
6. Abnormal amounts of the serum rheumatoid factor by any method found positive in <5% of control subjects
7. Radiographic changes characteristic of RA (bone erosion or decalcification) adjacent to involved joints

Acute indicators: Morning stiffness lasting >60 min, symmetric joint involvement, joint effusion, periarticular edema, pain, local warmth, tenderness, and limited motion. Joint stiffness usually is worsened by stress placed on the joint, and it can follow periods of inactivity as well. Especially characteristic of RA is polyarthritis, that is, involvement of ≥3 of the following joints: PIP and MCP joints, wrists, knees, ankles, and/or toes. Prodromal signs and symptoms may include malaise, weight loss, vague periarticular pain, low-grade fever, and vasomotor disturbances resulting in paresthesia and Raynaud's phenomenon. Sometimes an acute exacerbation is related to stress, such as infection, surgery, trauma, emotional strain, or the postpartum period.

Chronic indicators: Progressive thickening of the periarticular tissues; subluxation; fibrous ankylosis; atrophy of skin and muscle; severe limitation of ROM with progressive loss of function; joint and muscle contractures; juxtaarticular and generalized osteoporosis; synovial cysts (ganglion on the dorsum of the wrist or Baker's cyst in the popliteal space); tendon rupture; nerve entrapment (carpal or tarsal tunnel syndrome); dryness of the eyes and mucous membranes; subluxation of the cervical vertebrae; swan neck, boutonnière deformity of the fingers; ulnar deviation of the wrist and joints of the hands and fingers; and subcutaneous nodules. Some patients develop splenomegaly and enlarged lymph nodes.

DIAGNOSTIC TESTS

Serologic studies: Many performed to detect certain macroglobulins.

Rheumatoid factor (an IgM antibody directed against other globulins): Positive in 75% of the individuals with RA. Higher titers are associated with more severe clinical disease. Because false-positive results are common, a definite diagnosis cannot be made on this test alone.

Antinuclear antibodies: May appear in 20% of cases, but titers are lower in RA than in systemic lupus erythematosus.

Erythrocyte sedimentation rate (ESR):   An indicator of inflammation if elevated; especially useful in monitoring disease activity in RA.

γ-Globulins, especially IgM and IgG: If elevated, strongly suggest an autoimmune process as the cause of RA.

Normocytic hypochromic anemia: Usually present secondary to long-standing inflammation.

WBC count: Usually normal or slightly elevated, but leukopenia can be present, especially in the presence of splenomegaly.

Joint fluid aspiration from the involved joint: May reveal synovial fluid greater in volume than normal, opaque and cloudy yellow in appearance, glucose level lower than serum level, and elevated WBC and polymorphonuclear leukocytes in the presence of RA.

X-ray studies of the involved joints: In the early phases will illustrate soft tissue swelling, erosion of joint surfaces normally covered by articular cartilage, and osteoporosis of adjacent bone. Diagnosis of RA using ARA criteria (see p. 558 requires radiographic evidence of bony erosion and/or unequivocal evidence of bony decalcification (osteopenia) via hand and wrist radiographs. In long-standing disease, the joint will show instability, subluxation, joint space narrowing, bone cyst formation, and concurrent osteoarthritic changes. Special attention is paid to upper cervical vertebrae, where subluxation of C1 or C2 can result in life-threatening neurologic complications.

Radionuclide joint scanning: To identify inflamed synovium in patients with appropriate symptoms.

MRI: Shows promise as a sensitive measure of inflammation and cartilage loss; may also enhance identification of soft tissue nodules and spinal cord compression with cervical subluxation.

COLLABORATIVE MANAGEMENT

Systemic rest: Mandatory throughout all phases of this disease. In exacerbations, bedrest may be required until significant clinical joint findings have decreased for 2 wk. During this period, proper joint positioning is essential to prevent contractures. Concurrent physical therapy is prescribed to put joints through passive ROM at least once daily. During remissions, the patient should receive 8 hr of sleep each night and 1-2 hr of rest at midday. Any increase in symptoms necessitates increasing the amount of rest.

Emotional support: To lessen stress and help patients deal with fear, feelings of helplessness, disability, and the many losses they will incur. Patients need to be introduced to the concept of chronic disease control through multiple methods that will change in response to the disease progression. Coping strategies have been shown to reduce pain for RA patients and include relaxation techniques, distraction, and prayer. Self-efficacy (the belief that one is able to perform specific actions in specific circumstances) has been shown to effectively decrease disability and increase coping behaviors in patients with RA.

Rest of inflamed joints: Imperative. Unstable joints should be splinted or braced to provide support and put through passive ROM 2-3 times daily while inflamed. Reduction of inflammation in affected joints is aided by articular rest. Relaxing hip and knee muscles to prevent contractures is best performed by prone positioning for at least 15 min tid. Because sitting is not an effective method of joint rest, sitting should be limited to short periods (e.g., <1 hr). **Joint exercise:** Essential to maintain joint function and muscle strength, with the amount of exercise increasing as inflammation decreases. A graded exercise program should include the following: passive ROM, active-assisted ROM, active ROM, and resistive ROM with gradually increasing levels of resistance. ROM should be accomplished 2-3 times daily in active disease (e.g., arthritic flare-up) and up to 10 times daily when inflammation is quiescent. Isometric exercise is used to maintain muscle strength during active joint inflammation. During active disease, the patient should be taught to perform one 6-sec isometric contraction of each involved muscle group at least once daily. As active joint inflammation decreases, isotonic exercise may begin (e.g., movement of a limb against constant load through the ROM). Isotonic exercise may be accomplished through graded weight lifting, walking, stationary bicycling, or pool exercise. Once arthritis is quiescent, muscle and periarticular tissue strength may be rebuilt via carefully adjusted isokinetic exercise (e.g., control of limb movement and speed to maximally exercise the limb). Any signs of increasing joint inflammation are cause for regression to a less stressful exercise until joint inflammation has again decreased. Inflamed weight-bearing joints should be protected from stress by orthotics and ambulatory adjuncts (cane, crutches, walker, or a wheelchair if imperative).

Nutritional therapy: Current evidence suggests that, other than a healthy and balanced diet, no nutritional program is beneficial for RA. Fish oils containing polyunsaturated fatty acids may be important in modulating joint inflammation, but this finding needs further substantiation in research.

Thermotherapy: To relax muscles and reduce pain. Cold therapy is used during inflammatory stages to reduce pain. Moist heat (especially warm tub baths) is useful for exercising stiffened joints because the heat and buoyancy aid motion. When submersion is not possible, use of moist, warm cloths before exercise decreases the patient's discomfort. Caution must be employed to avoid thermal injury to atrophied skin over affected joints. Paraffin baths may be used to provide heat to involved small joints (e.g., in the hands and feet).

Assistive devices: For example, stocking helpers, raised toilet seats, pickup sticks.

Antiinflammatory agents: See Table 8-1. NSAIDS have been effective in reducing pain and inflammation but have not effectively altered the disease process in RA. No one NSAID is more effective than another; therefore the choice of NSAID commonly has been based on expense, individual response to each NSAID, and profile of common side effects. Aspirin (ASA) has been the mainstay of pharmacotherapy in RA. Dosage is determined by the ability to provide adequate symptom relief without toxic reactions. Adult doses may reach 4-6 g per day, producing serum levels of 20-30 mg/dl. Tinnitus and GI upset are prodromal signs of ASA toxicity, indicating a need to reduce dosages until these symptoms clear. Other NSAIDs commonly are associated with GI, hepatic, renal, and CNS toxicity. Significant morbidity and mortality are associated with NSAID-related gastric mucosal injury. GI upset may be decreased by taking NSAIDs with food or antacids or using enteric-coated forms. Renal toxicity related to NSAIDs is shown by fluid retention, edema, hyperkalemia, and worsening kidney function. Baseline and q6mo serum creatinine, BUN, and serum electrolyte determinations should be done.

More potent antiinflammatory agents also used in the treatment of RA include the slow-acting antirheumatic drugs (SAARDs), also known as disease-modifying antirheumatic drugs (DMARD). The DMARDs are now being introduced earlier in the course of RA in an attempt to slow the progression of disease. However, the DMARDs are associated with significant, possibly life-threatening, side effects. DMARDs include the following drugs.

Methotrexate: Has become the DMARD of choice for active RA. Initial therapy usually begins with bolus dosages of 5-7.5 mg/wk. Most patients respond with clinical improvement within 4-6 wk, but improvement generally plateaus in 12-16 wk. GI side effects are usually self-limiting, lasting 3-4 days. Mucosal ulceration may limit the usefulness of this therapy. Cytopenia and anemia may also occur. Because of the potential for blood, liver, and renal toxicity, baseline CBCs, liver function studies (aspartate aminotransferase [AST], alanine aminotransferase [ALT], albumin) and renal function (BUN and creatinine) should be done at the beginning of therapy (baseline level) and every 4-8 wk during therapy. Abnormal liver function studies may require liver biopsy before continuing therapy. Because of its effect on bone repair, methotrexate therapy may be discontinued during preparation for joint replacement procedures or following fractures.

Antimalarials (chloroquine phosphate, 250 mg/day, or hydroxychloroquine sulfate, 200 mg/day): Effective in the long-term control of disease in roughly half of patients with RA. Clinical improvement may take several months. Side effects include nausea, keratitis, and retinitis. Ophthalmologic examinations should be performed q6mo in the first year of therapy and then annually.

Chrysotherapy (use of medicinal gold salts): One of the traditional second-line therapies in the treatment of RA. Although up to 60% of patients who begin gold therapy have a clinical response, the long-term outcome has not been satisfactory. Most patients end up discontinuing gold therapy either because of side effects or lack of efficacy. Contraindications include severe drug allergies, previous gold toxicity, hepatotoxicity, renal toxicity, or hematologic pathologic findings. Chrysotherapy is administered by weekly injections of increasing dosage (up to 50 mg/wk) until clinical results are noted or toxic reactions encountered. Usual dosage of auranofin (an oral agent) is 3 mg bid. A significant antiinflammatory effect often takes several months of therapy. Oral forms of gold have not been shown to be as clinically effective as injectable forms but have also been associated with less serious side effects. Potential toxic reactions include exfoliative dermatitis, thrombocytopenia, bone marrow depression, stomatitis, and nephritis. Before each injection and periodically for oral forms, the patient should have a urinalysis (for proteinuria and microscopic hematuria) and CBC with differential for hemoglobin (Hgb), platelet levels, and WBC count. The patient also should be assessed for skin or mucous membrane lesions. Periodic hepatic function tests should be done. The patient should be advised to use sunscreen and avoid direct sunlight to avoid dermatoses.

Corticosteroids: The benefits of continued low-dose steroids are believed to outweigh their risks while slowing the progress of RA. The main risk of long-term low-dose steroids is osteoporosis, which may be countered with supplemental calcium and vitamin D. Deflazacort, a corticosteroid with bone-sparing properties, shows some promise for long-term therapy. Corticosteroids may be used systemically or injected intraarticularly during arthritis flare or as a "bridge" therapy until second-line agents begin to work. Low-dose oral steroids are given in ≤10 mg doses daily or every other day. Side effects of systemic steroids include hypertension, carbohydrate intolerance, myopathy, steroid psychosis, cataracts, osteoporosis, avascular necrosis, masked infection, and GI bleeding. Intraarticular injections are provided for acute inflammation in one or a few joints. Intraarticular injections have been associated with tendon rupture, postinjection flare (temporary worsening of symptoms), skin atrophy, and nerve injury.

Penicillamine: Once a popular treatment for RA, penicillamine recently has been found to be less effective than was once thought. Penicillamine is effective for a short term, but efficacy usually plateaus and then declines. Side effects are dose related and include stomatitis, pruritus, rash, nephrosis, and bone marrow suppression. Immune-mediated toxicities are also associated with penicillamine, including myasthenia gravis and systemic lupus erythematosus. During therapy a CBC and urinalysis should be done q2-6wk to monitor for toxicity. Doses need to be taken between meals to aid absorption.

Less conventional therapies for RA

Sulfasalazine: Has been effectively used to treat RA in Europe. Side effects include nausea, anorexia, headache, and gastrointestinal distress. Because of renal and liver toxicity and potential blood dyscrasia, CBC and liver functions studies should be monitored throughout therapy.

Azathioprine: An immunosuppressant showing response for some patients with RA. Side effects include blood dyscrasia, hypersensitivity, GI upset, and liver toxicity. Monitoring CBC and liver functions studies should be done throughout therapy.

Surgical interventions

Synovectomy: To remove the inflamed synovium and prevent pannus formation. This may be performed by either surgical excision or instillation of a radioactive solution to "burn" the synovium.

Arthroplasty: To correct periarticular weakness, which in turn will correct subluxation and external stressors on the diseased joint.

Osteotomy: To correct disruptive force vectors placed on the joint surfaces or to correct bony malalignments.

Carpal tunnel release, tarsal tunnel release, ganglionectomy, tendon repair, and removal of Baker's cyst: Surgeries performed to correct concurrent connective tissue defects associated with RA.

Implant arthroplasty: Significantly increases functional capabilities for selected RA patients. Used for many joints, but greatest success has been seen with the hip and knee. The rate of success depends on the joint, patient's general condition, stage of disease, and rate of compliance with therapy.

Arthroscopy: May be used for diagnosis or treatment. Loose bodies may be excised, plica (redundant tissue) incised, and cartilage abraded (or "shaved") through an arthroscope.

Arthrodesis: Although less often used since the advent of implant arthroplasty, joint fusion allows for a stable, painless joint in severely affected joints with very weakened periarticular tissues and muscle atrophy.

Experimental therapies under trial in the United States: Include additional NSAIDs, an anthelmintic agent (levamisole), cyclophosphamide, azathioprine, sulfasalazine (for preceding two therapies, see discussion above), chlorambucil, chondroprotective agents (e.g., rumalon, a bovine bone marrow and cartilage extract that affects the growth and metabolism of articular cartilage), plasmapheresis, leukapheresis, lymphocytapheresis, and irradiation of the lymph nodes. Recent research in antirheumatic drugs focuses on the modulation of cytokines and adhesion molecules. Three such agents are (1) tenidap (which inhibits cyclooxygenase and production of interleukin-1 [IL-1], interleukin-6 [IL-6], and tumor necrosis factor-α [TNF-α]), (2) intercellular adhesion molecule 1 (ICAM-1), and (3) TNF-α antibodies. Experimental surgeries include various new implant designs and joint transplantation.

NURSING DIAGNOSES AND INTERVENTIONS

Fatigue related to state of discomfort, psychoemotional demands, and the effects of prolonged immobility

Desired outcome: Within 24 hr of admission, patient verbalizes a reduction in fatigue.

- Assess the time the fatigue occurs, its relationship to required activities, and activities that relieve or aggravate the symptoms.
- Investigate the patient's sleep pattern and intervene as appropriate to ensure adequate rest (see Appendix One, "Caring for Preoperative and Postoperative Patients" for **Sleep pattern disturbance**, p. 734).
- Assess for dietary and physiologic sources of fatigue, and intervene to correct as needed.

- Determine whether patient's pain is adequately controlled, and intervene with pharmacologic and nonpharmacologic treatments as indicated.
- Assess patient for stress or psychoemotional distress; intervene as necessary or seek assistance from an appropriate clinical specialist in psychiatric nursing.
- Discuss the rationale for a graded exercise regimen to increase endurance and strength (see Appendix One, "Caring for Preoperative and Postoperative Patients" for **Risk for activity intolerance,** p. 738; **Risk for disuse syndrome,** p. 740). Encourage patient to set realistic goals, and post these goals to facilitate participation of associated health care professionals.
- Pace activities, and intersperse rest periods of at least 90 min in duration.
- Teach patient use of adjunctive and assistive devices.

NIC: Body Mechanics Promotion; Energy Management; Exercise Therapy: Ambulation; Exercise Therapy: Joint Mobility; Teaching: Prescribed Activity/Exercise

---

See Also: "Intervertebral Disk Disease" for **Health-seeking behavior:** Pain control measures, p. 251; "Osteoarthritis" for **Pain,** p. 555; **Knowledge deficit:** Use of heating device, p. 556; **Impaired physical mobility** related to musculoskeletal impairment and adjustment to new walking gait, p. 556; "Ligamentous Injuries" for **Knowledge deficit:** Need for elevation of the involved extremity, use of thermotherapy, and prescribed exercise, p. 566; **Knowledge deficit:** Care and assessment of the casted extremity, p. 567; **Knowledge deficit:** Potential for joint weakness, and the techniques for applying external supports and assessing neurovascular status, p. 568; "Torn Anterior Cruciate Ligament" for **Pain** related to surgical repair and rehabilitation therapy, p. 573; **Knowledge deficit:** Use of postoperative cryotherapy with a commercial iced knee cuff and automatic ice slush circulator, p. 574; "Fractures" for **Self-care deficit,** p. 590; "Total Hip Arthroplasty" for **Knowledge deficit:** Potential for infection caused by foreign body reaction to the endoprosthesis, p. 614; "Total Knee Arthroplasty" for **Risk for fluid volume deficit** related to postsurgical hemorrhage or hematoma formation, p. 617; Appendix One, "Caring for Preoperative and Postoperative Patients," p. 717; "Caring for Patients on Prolonged Bedrest," p. 738, for nursing diagnoses and interventions; Appendix One, "Caring for Patients With Cancer and Other Life-disrupting Illnesses," p. 791, for psychosocial nursing interventions.

PATIENT-FAMILY TEACHING AND DISCHARGE PLANNING

When providing patient-family teaching, focus on sensory information; avoid giving excessive information; and initiate a visiting nurse referral for necessary follow-up teaching. Consider including verbal and written information about the following:

- Treatment regimen, including physical therapy, systemic rest, rest of inflamed joints, exercise, and thermotherapy. For more information, see "Ligamentous Injuries" for **Knowledge deficit:** Need for elevation of the involved extremity, use of thermotherapy, and prescribed exercise, p. 566; "Torn Anterior Cruciate Ligament" for **Knowledge deficit:** Use of postoperative cryotherapy with a commercial iced knee cuff and automatic ice slush circulator, p. 574.
- Monitoring therapy (blood and urine testing) needed while patient is taking selected medications.
- Medications, including drug name, dosage, schedule, precautions, drug/drug and food/drug interactions, and potential side effects.

- Potential complications of the disease and therapy and the need to recognize and seek medical attention promptly if they occur.
- Potential concurrent pathologic conditions, such as pericarditis (see p. 77) and ocular lesions, and the need to report them promptly to health care professional.
- Use and care of splints and orthotics, including return demonstration.
- Use of adjunctive aids as appropriate, such as pickup sticks, long-handled shoehorn, elastic shoelaces, Velcro fasteners, crutches, walker, and cane, including return demonstration.
- As necessary, referral to visiting or public health nurses for ongoing care after discharge.
- Phone numbers to call if questions or concerns arise about therapy or disease after discharge. In addition, many cities have local arthritis support groups. Information for these patients can be obtained by writing to the following organizations:

  Arthritis Foundation
  1330 West Peachtree St.
  Atlanta, GA 30309   (800) 283-7800
  WWW address: *http://www.arthritis.org*

  Juvenile Rheumatoid Arthritis Research
  3333 Burnet Ave.
  Cincinnati, OH 45229-3039   (800) 559-7011
  WWW address: *http://www.jraregistry.org*

- Additional information on arthritis is available through the following organization:

  National Arthritis and Musculoskeletal and Skin Diseases Information Clearinghouse, National Institute of Arthritis and Musculoskeletal and Skin Diseases
  Information Specialist
  1 AMS Circle
  Bethesda, MD 20892-3675   (301) 495-4484; (301) 587-4352 FAX
  WWW address: *http://www.social.com/health/nhic/data/hr0000/ hr0036.html*

Section Two: Muscular and Connective Tissue Disorders

Ligamentous injuries

Ligaments are collections of fascial tissues that connect bone to bone, thereby supplementing joint strength. Ligaments reinforce stress applied to the joint in a specific direction; that is, most joints have several ligaments supporting different planes of joint motion. Ligamentous trauma occurs when the ligament is stressed in a direction other than the one evolved to accept the stress or when stress exceeds inherent structural strength. Ligament tears usually result from direct trauma or transmission of a force to the joint (i.e., twisting the distal arm may injure shoulder ligaments). The degree of trauma incurred will vary with the strength of the involved ligament, the force applied (e.g., strong ligaments will require more force before tearing than will ligaments weakened by previous injury or disease), and the direction in which the force is applied. Tears can be longitudinal, transverse, tangential, complete, or partial and can involve avulsion fractures of their origin or insertion.

ASSESSMENT

Signs and symptoms: Patients may state that they felt a tearing or heard a "pop" when the trauma occurred. Localized ecchymosis, edema, tenderness, weakness, pain, joint effusion, limited ROM, joint instability, or inability to use the joint for ambulation or ADL. Tenderness on palpation is characteristic over the area of the injury. A diagnosis is based primarily on consideration of the patient's complaints, the mechanism of the injury, and the physical assessment.

Ankle sprains may be graded for severity, from grade 1, least severe, to grade 3, most severe. Grading is based on edema/hemorrhage, point tenderness, decreased function, decreased ligament strength, anterior drawer test (anterior joint instability), and talar tilt test (mediolateral joint instability).

DIAGNOSTIC TESTS

X-ray studies: Stressing the weakened joint during x-ray examination may reveal an enlarged joint space.

Arthrogram (instillation of a radiopaque dye or radiolucent gas into the joint): To identify torn or weakened ligaments.

Arthroscopy: To rule out concurrent intraarticular pathologic conditions or trauma.

COLLABORATIVE MANAGEMENT

Treatment for uncomplicated ligamentous injuries: RICE is a useful acronym for treatment of ligamentous injuries: **R**est, **I**ce, **C**ompression, and **E**levation. Rest is accomplished by avoiding active use of the joint and/or splinting, casting, or bracing. Splinting may be accomplished with plaster of paris splints, pre-prepared splints, and air or gel splints. Cryotherapy is well established as a means of controlling inflammation from trauma. Compression via elastic wraps prevents swelling and supports joints. Elevation decreases further edema formation while aiding resolution of existing edema. NSAIDS are used for analgesic and antiinflammatory effects.

Surgical repair: For injuries resulting in grossly unstable joints. The surgery involves removal of the nonviable ligament and suture repair or reefing of the stretched ligament, using strong, absorbable suture material. An avulsion injury (tearing away of a bony insertion) without fracture may be reinserted onto its bony insertion site by using bone staples or passing a suture through holes drilled into the area of the bony insertion site. Additional procedures may involve use of prosthetic devices to stent, temporarily replace, or augment ligament repairs.

ROM and muscle-strengthening exercises: Begun after an appropriate period of immobilization of the injured area (several days to 3 wk).

NURSING DIAGNOSES AND INTERVENTIONS

Knowledge deficit: Need for elevation of the involved extremity, use of thermotherapy, and prescribed exercise

Desired outcome: Within 8 hr of instruction, patient verbalizes understanding about the rationale for treatment and returns a demonstration of the exercise regimen and the use of elevation and thermotherapy.

- Teach patient the pathophysiology of the injury and the concomitant inflammatory response. Provide the patient with instructions in the need for a graded muscle-strengthening and joint ROM exercise regimen to allow return of normal joint function.
- Instruct patient to keep the injured extremity elevated until edema no longer is a problem (usually 3-7 days). Explain that the involved extremity should be kept above the level of the heart, with each successively distal joint elevated above the level of the preceding joint.
- Explain that ice usually is applied for the first 48-72 hr to prevent excessive edema. **Note:** Ice is contraindicated for patients with suspected compartment

syndrome or those with peripheral vascular disease, decreased local sensation, coagulation disorders, or a similar pathologic condition that increases the potential for thermal injury. Advise the patient to apply thermotherapy with at least two thicknesses of terry cloth to protect the skin from injury.

- Explain each prescribed exercise in detail, including the rationale. The optimal method is to teach it to the patient, demonstrate it, and then have the patient return the demonstration. Provide written instructions that describe the exercises, and list the frequency and number of repetitions for each. Include a phone number in case the patient has questions after hospital discharge.

NIC: Exercise Promotion; Exercise Therapy: Muscle Control; Heat/Cold Application; Pain Management; Positioning; Teaching: Prescribed Activity/ Exercise

Knowledge deficit: Care and assessment of the casted extremity

Desired outcome: Within 12 hr of instruction, patient verbalizes understanding about the care of the casted extremity and knowledge of self-assessment of neurovascular status and returns a demonstration of the use of ambulatory aids, exercise, and general cast care.

- Explain the function of the patient's cast.
- Instruct patient in the rationale and procedure for neurovascular checks of the casted extremity. Explain that they should be performed q2-4hr for the first 2 days, and then 4 times daily until the cast is removed. Advise patient to be alert to and promptly report increasing pain, changes in sensation (especially loss of two-point discrimination), pain that increases with passive or active movement of distal digits, pallor, cyanosis, coolness, decreased pulse or capillary refill, and muscle weakness or paralysis of the distal portion of the casted limb.
- Ensure that patient demonstrates independence in ADL and ambulation before discharge. If ambulatory aids (crutches, walker, cane) are used, be sure patient demonstrates independent use on all surfaces likely to be encountered (especially stairs) and that patient understands and verbalizes precautions. Be sure patient will have adequate assistance or is independent in self-care before discharge. If necessary, initiate a referral for home care.
- Instruct patient to exercise the parts of the extremity that are not immobilized by the cast (e.g., wiggling the toes or fingers and putting the most proximal joints through complete ROM) unless doing so is contraindicated by the injury or the health care practitioner. Isometric exercises for muscles beneath the cast will be prescribed for some patients. When prescribed, provide patient with the rationale and instructions for these exercises, including written instructions that review the information and list the frequency and number of repetitions of each exercise.
- Provide patient with a phone number for the appropriate person to call if problems or questions arise after hospital discharge.
- Instruct patient in the following basic components of cast care.

With plaster of paris cast
- Use plastic bags while showering or in the rain to avoid getting cast wet. Damp cloths can be used to clean soiled cast surfaces, but saturation must be avoided.
- White shoe polish may be used *sparingly* to cover stains.
- Petal the cast edges with tape if they are rough or if cast crumbs are falling into the cast. If the edges continue to irritate the skin, they can be padded with moleskin, sheepskin, or foam rubber. Notify the health care practitioner if irritation continues.
- Avoid putting anything beneath the cast because skin under the cast is more susceptible to injury.

- Report any pain, burning, changes in sensation, increased warmth, drainage on the cast, or foul odor because they can signal the presence of pressure necrosis.

With synthetic cast material

- Immersion in water may be permitted by health care practitioner, depending on the materials used, the type of injury, and whether surgery was performed. If immersion is permitted, it is necessary to dry the cast thoroughly (using a hair dryer on a cool setting) to prevent skin maceration.
- If permitted, dirt or sand can be rinsed from the cast.
- Avoid overexercising the casted extremity; perform exercises within the prescribed range.
- Avoid putting anything under the cast because skin under the cast is more susceptible to injury.
- Report any pain, burning, changes in sensation, increased warmth, drainage on the cast, or foul odor because they can indicate the presence of pressure necrosis.

NIC: Cast Care: Maintenance; Cast Care: Wet; Exercise Promotion; Pain Management; Teaching: Prescribed Activity/Exercise; Traction/Immobilization Care

Knowledge deficit: Potential for joint weakness, and the techniques for applying external supports and assessing neurovascular status
Desired outcome: Within 8 hr of the instruction, patient verbalizes understanding about the potential for joint weakness and returns a demonstration of applying external supports and self-checking neurovascular status.

- Advise patient about the potential for joint weakness and the need for limiting or omitting activities that aggravate the condition.
- If the health care practitioner has prescribed elastic wraps, elastic supports, or orthotic devices to supplement joint strength until exercise has compensated for the joint laxity, explain and demonstrate their use and application. Show the patient how to apply elastic wraps diagonally from the distal to proximal areas with an overlap of two-thirds to one-half the width of the wrap for each successive layer.
- Teach patient how to self-check neurovascular status 15 min after application and to rewrap the joint if a deficit is found. For details, see **Knowledge deficit:** Care and assessment of the casted extremity, above.
- Ensure that the patient receives two wraps, supports, or orthotic devices to allow for cleaning. These devices typically are washed with mild soap and water and allowed to air dry without stretching (or see manufacturer's recommendations).

NIC: Circulatory Care; Exercise Therapy: Joint Mobility; Teaching: Disease Process; Teaching: Procedure/Treatment; Traction/Immobilization Care

---

See Also: "Total Knee Arthroplasty" for **Risk for fluid volume deficit** with risks related to postsurgical hemorrhage or hematoma formation, p. 617, if surgery was performed; "Torn Anterior Cruciate Ligament" for **Pain** related to surgical repair and rehabilitation therapy, p. 573, if surgery was performed; Appendix One, "Caring for Preoperative and Postoperative Patients," p. 717, for nursing diagnoses and interventions.

PATIENT-FAMILY TEACHING AND DISCHARGE PLANNING

When providing patient-family teaching, focus on sensory information; avoid giving excessive information; and initiate a visiting nurse referral for necessary

follow-up teaching. Consider including verbal and written information about the following:

- Prescribed therapies, such as rest, ice, compression, elevation, cast care, exercise, and external supports.
- Potential complications, including subluxation/dislocation (see below), wound infection (i.e., local warmth, persistent redness, swelling, wound drainage, foul odor from within the cast, sensation of burning from within the cast, drainage from the cast, fever), and neurovascular deficit (see p. 568), all of which necessitate immediate medical attention.
- ADL and ambulation. Ensure that patient demonstrates independence before hospital discharge.
- Medications, including drug name, rationale, dosage, schedule, precautions, drug/drug and food/drug interactions, and side effects.

Dislocation/Subluxation

A dislocation occurs when the joint surfaces are completely out of contact. A subluxation is an incomplete dislocation in that some of the joint surfaces remain in contact. Most dislocations and subluxations are the result of trauma and can involve significant periarticular damage, including fractures. Some subluxations are associated with pronounced connective tissue disease, such as ulnar deviation of the phalanges and metacarpals, which is seen with severe rheumatoid arthritis.

ASSESSMENT

Signs and symptoms: Vary with the joint involved. Although any joint can dislocate, some joints are more susceptible than others. One finding common to most forms of dislocation is limb shortening. Usually there is significant pain, ecchymosis, loss of normal bony contour, edema, and loss or limitation of joint ROM. Complications include recurrent dislocation, joint contracture, neurovascular injury, and eventual traumatic arthritis.

DIAGNOSTIC TESTS

X-rays: Both anteroposterior (AP) and lateral views commonly used. Occasionally an oblique view or other special approach is required. Because muscle spasms frequently force the dislocated bones back into normal alignment, it is sometimes necessary to stress the joint to permit visualization of the injury (called a *stress film*). CT scans or MRI may be necessary to aid in diagnosis.

Bone scans: May demonstrate nondisplaced avulsion fractures, areas of recent excessive stress, or bony insertions of joint ligaments following dislocation.

Arthrocentesis: May show blood from trauma or excessive fluid from joint effusion. Free fat globules in joint aspirate are indicative of fracture involving joint surfaces.

Arthrogram: Use of radiopaque dye or radiolucent gas for outlining the joint cavity to visualize injured ligaments, capsule, or intraarticular structures, such as the menisci or cruciate ligaments.

Arthroscopy: May be used to rule out injury to joint surfaces or intraarticular structures.

COLLABORATIVE MANAGEMENT

Interventions vary with the degree of subluxation or dislocation and the joint involved. Many patients are discharged from the hospital with instructions for the use of temporary immobilization of the part, thermotherapy, elevation, and pain medication.

Dislocation of the sternoclavicular joint: Usually reduced manually using local anesthetic. After reduction, the joint is immobilized with a clavicular strap (figure-of-8 bandage) for 2-6 wk. Occasionally, an open reduction with internal fixation (ORIF) using screws, pins, or wire is necessary to maintain reduction.

Uncomplicated subluxation or dislocation of the acromioclavicular (AC) joint: May be classified as type I (least severe) to type III (most severe). The AC joint may be immobilized with a sling, clavicular strap, brace, or harness, or it might require ORIF. After satisfactory joint stability has been achieved, the patient begins a regimen of progressively more rigorous exercise to regain muscle strength and ROM.

Dislocation of the shoulder: Careful assessment necessary for complications of nerve and blood vessel injury, fractures, and rotator cuff tears. This dislocation is reduced with the patient under anesthesia or strong sedation and then immobilized in a Velpeau bandage, sling and swathe binder, shoulder immobilizer, or spica cast of the shoulder, all of which support the arm while immobilizing the shoulder. Immobilization usually is continued for 3-6 wk, followed by progressive exercises to regain muscle strength and ROM. Surgical procedures usually include reefing (taking up redundant ligament with sutures) of the articular capsule and transferring or shortening the subcapsular muscle to tighten the periarticular tissues. (See also "Repair of Recurrent Shoulder Dislocation," p. 609.)

Dislocation of the elbow: Frequently associated with fractures of the humerus, ulna, or radius. The elbow and associated fractures are carefully reduced, usually with the patient under general anesthesia, and the area is immobilized in a posterior splint at approximately 90-degree flexion for 2-4 wk. ORIF may be required. Because of the area of the injury, these patients are at risk for nerve injury and Volkmann's ischemic contracture (acute compartment syndrome), and therefore the extremity must be monitored carefully for evidence of neurovascular deficit (see "Acute Compartment Syndrome," p. 575). Progressive exercises are used to regain muscle strength and ROM.

Dislocation of the radioulnar or radiocarpal joints: Frequently involves fractures. This dislocation is usually reduced using regional anesthesia and then immobilized in a posterior splint or long arm cast for 2-6 wk. However, an ORIF may be performed. Progressive exercise is used to regain muscle strength and ROM.

Dislocation of the finger: Usually reduced using regional or digital block anesthesia. The finger may be immobilized with a metal splint or taped to an adjacent finger, followed by progressive mobilization. Surgery may be performed to reef the stretched periarticular tissues, followed by transfixion of the joint with a Kirschner wire (K-wire) during the healing period—usually 10-14 days.

Dislocation of the metacarpophalangeal joint of the thumb: Surgery usually indicated because of the importance of this joint for hand grip strength and function. Surgical repair includes suturing torn ligaments, repair of avulsion injuries, and transfixion of the joint with a K-wire to maintain joint stability in slight (15-degree) flexion. A thumb spica cast immobilizes the joint for 4 wk, followed by an Orthoplast splint, which is used intermittently for an additional 4 wk, during which ROM exercises are instituted gradually.

Dislocation of the hip: Usually requires general anesthesia with significant muscle relaxation with paralytic agents (e.g., succinylcholine chloride) for reduction. Immobilization may be accomplished via balanced suspension traction or a hip-knee-ankle (HKA) orthosis for 3-6 wk, followed by progressive ambulation, mobilization of the joint, and muscle-strengthening exercises. Open reduction with surgical repair of the torn capsule and ligaments might be required for severe or recurrent dislocations or for patients who cannot tolerate prolonged immobility. Dislocation of the hip may precipitate avascular necrosis of the femoral head, necessitating hemiarthroplasty. A fractured acetabulum may require internal fixation or replacement via total hip arthroplasty.

Dislocation of the patella: Often self-limiting, in that the patella usually reduces itself. Immobilization may be accomplished with a knee immobilizer, posterior splint, cylinder cast, or long leg cast for 10-21 days, followed by progressive mobilization and quadriceps setting exercises. Surgery may be required to reef the periarticular tissues or reattach the insertion of the patellar tendon to overcorrect distorted joint vectors that cause recurrent dislocation.

Dislocation of the ankle: Commonly associated with malleolar fractures. This dislocation is usually reduced with the patient under regional or general anesthesia. The joint is immobilized in a long leg plaster cast for 6-12 wk. Surgery may be necessary to reef stretched periarticular tissues and/or to internally fix malleolar fractures. Progressive mobilization and exercises are used to regain motion and strength.

Dislocation of the toe: Usually reduced using regional anesthesia. Often the toe is immobilized for 3-5 days, using an adjacent toe as a splint (strapping or taping the toes together).

NURSING DIAGNOSES AND INTERVENTIONS

See "Osteoarthritis" for **Pain,** p. 555; **Impaired physical mobility** related to musculoskeletal impairment and adjustment to a new walking gait, p. 556; "Ligamentous Injury" for **Knowledge deficit:** Need for elevation of the involved extremity, use of thermotherapy, and prescribed exercise, p. 566; "Torn Anterior Cruciate Ligament" for **Knowledge deficit**: Use of postoperative cryotherapy with a commercial iced knee cuff and automatic ice slush circulator, p. 574; **Knowledge deficit:** Care and assessment of the casted extremity, p. 567; "Fractures" for **Self-care deficit,** p. 590; "Total Knee Arthroplasty" for **Risk for fluid volume deficit** related to postsurgical hemorrhage or hematoma formation, p. 617, if surgery was performed; "Torn Anterior Cruciate Ligament" for **Pain** related to surgical repair and rehabilitation therapy, p. 573, if surgery was performed; Appendix One, "Caring for Preoperative and Postoperative Patients," p. 717; "Caring for Patients on Prolonged Bedrest," p. 738, for nursing diagnoses and interventions.

PATIENT-FAMILY TEACHING AND DISCHARGE PLANNING

When providing patient-family teaching, focus on sensory information; avoid giving excessive information; and initiate a visiting nurse referral for necessary follow-up teaching. Consider including verbal and written information about the following:

- Therapy that will be used at home, including thermotherapy, elevation, and exercises (see "Ligamentous Injuries," p. 564; "Torn Anterior Cruciate Ligament" for **Knowledge deficit**: Use of postoperative cryotherapy with a commercial iced knee cuff and automatic ice slush circulator, p. 574); use of immobilization devices (p. 568); cast care (see p. 567); and medications.
- Potential complications that should be observed for at home, such as recurrent dislocations, neurovascular deficit (see "Ligamentous Injuries," p. 568), or wound infection (i.e., persistent redness, swelling, fever, local warmth, increasing pain, wound discharge, foul odor from within the cast, burning sensation from within the cast, drainage from the cast).
- Precautions that should be taken at home, including activity limitations (as directed by health care practitioner), monitoring for changes in neurovascular status qid, and following the guidelines described for cast, splint, or orthotic care.
- Medications, including drug name, rationale, dosage, schedule, precautions, drug/drug and food/drug interactions, and potential side effects.

Torn anterior cruciate ligament

The anterior cruciate ligament (ACL) prevents excessive forward motion and internal rotation of the tibia. Injury to this ligament can result in strain, with microtears, partial tears, complete tears, or avulsion of the tibial or femoral attachments. Stresses that can result in tears include forceful contraction of the quadriceps muscles combined with restricted extension, "clipping" injuries incurred in football, forced pivoting on the knee, or excessive forward motion of the tibia, which can occur when stopping quickly while running and skiing.

ASSESSMENT

Acute indicators: Sensation of the knee giving way, joint effusion, restricted ROM, joint instability and pain.
Chronic indicators: Untreated tears of the ACL result in gross instability, which eventually can cause osteoarthritis (see assessment for osteoarthritis, p. 553).

DIAGNOSTIC TESTS

Lachman test: Positive if the ACL is torn. The patient's knee is partially flexed at 15-20 degrees, and the foot is planted flat on the examining table. The examiner then pulls the tibia forward while holding the femur stable. Excessive forward movement of the tibia is evidenced by a convex curve of the patellar tendon, and this indicates an ACL tear.
Drawer test: Performed with the knee flexed at 60-90 degrees and the foot planted flat on the table. The tibia is pulled forward as the femur is stabilized. Excessive forward movement (≥6 mm) indicates a tear. The test is then repeated with the foot externally rotated 15 degrees to assess concurrent injury of medial joint structures (meniscus or periarticular ligaments). Finally, the test is repeated with the foot internally rotated 30 degrees to assess concurrent lateral joint injury.
Pivot shift maneuver (jerk test):   Provides evidence of anterolateral instability of the knee. The tibia is internally rotated with one hand while the other hand is used to apply valgus stress on the knee. The knee is then flexed 20-30 degrees. The test is positive when the tibia subluxates anteriorly as evidenced by a palpable clunk on the lateral aspect of the knee.
Arthrometry: Measures AP displacement of the tibial tuberosity as related to the patella. A ≥3-mm difference compared with the contralateral knee measurement indicates ACL compromise.
Arthrocentesis: Done immediately after ACL injury occurs; will reveal hemarthrosis.
Arthrography: Outlines tears via injection of radiopaque dye and radiolucent gas.
Radiography of the knee (including AP, lateral, patellar [tunnel], and intercondylar notch [skyline] views, with and without stress on the joint): Evaluates for the presence of abnormal joint contours.
MRI: Allows identification of ACL tears and other soft tissue injuries not visible on radiographs.
Arthroscopy: Allows direct visualization of the ACL injury to determine degree of injury and assess need for surgery.

COLLABORATIVE MANAGEMENT

The type of therapy is determined by the type of injury, length of time since the original injury, concurrent joint pathologic findings, and the patient's age and functional goals.
Bracing: To provide primary support for an incompletely torn ACL or to supplement adjunctive joint support structures (posterior oblique ligament, collateral ligaments, lateral capsular ligament, menisci). Functional braces provide support and immobilization following reconstruction and allow control

of ROM in rehabilitation. Any of several commercial braces can be used to provide AP, lateral, and rotational stability of the joint. Concurrent physiotherapy is provided to strengthen periarticular structures and muscles.

Primary ACL repair: Involves direct suturing of the torn ligament via an arthrotomy or arthroscopy. The suture is heavy and nonabsorbable and is used in repairing incomplete tears that are less than 6 wk old.

ACL reconstruction: Involves use of either anatomic grafts (autograft or allograft) or prosthetics. Autografts are taken from the patellar tendon, semitendinosus tendon, or hamstring tendon. Allograft patellar tendon has also been used for repair. Regardless of the type of reconstructive procedure used, an open arthrotomy ACL repair requires prolonged knee immobilization (6-12 wk in partial flexion in a long leg cast and/or a splint), followed by extensive physical therapy (PT) and bracing. PT is continued until the knee is functionally normal. In addition, some patients return from surgery with a closed wound drainage system consisting of a wound drain, tubing, and a reservoir. Most surgeons bring the drainage tubing out through the area using a separate stab wound. Arthroscopy allows endoscopic ACL repair or reconstruction, permitting dramatically less joint trauma, earlier hospital discharge (1-3 days), more rapid initiation of PT (1-3 days), and excellent long-term results.

NURSING DIAGNOSES AND INTERVENTIONS

Pain related to surgical repair and rehabilitation therapy

Desired outcomes: Within 1-2 hr of intervention, patient's subjective perception of pain decreases, as documented by a pain scale. Objective indicators are absent or diminished. Patient demonstrates ability to perform ADL without complaints of discomfort.

- Devise and help patient use a rating system to evaluate pain and analgesic relief on a scale of 0 (no pain) to 10 (worst pain).
- If intraarticular bupivacaine or morphine is used, instruct the patient that the lack of pain in the immediate 2-6 hr after surgery should *not* be mistaken as a license to move the joint excessively.
- Instruct the patient in the use of patient-controlled analgesia (PCA). Monitor for the effectiveness of pain control while observing for excessive sedation, respiratory depression, and decreased level of consciousness (ensure that the appropriate reversal medication is available— most commonly naloxone). Ensure that the PCA pump has the prescribed medication and concentration with settings for each dose and a 4-hr maximum dosage.
- If appropriate, teach patient about the function of epidural anesthesia.
- Administer antiinflammatory agents as prescribed (most commonly in divided dosages around the clock), and document their effectiveness, using the pain scale. IM or IV ketorolac is commonly prescribed for 1-2 days postoperatively to reduce inflammation and therefore pain. Because of the potential for hemorrhage following ketorolac administration, closely observe for hemorrhage at the incision site and through drains.
- Provide maintenance antiinflammatory agents at scheduled intervals to ensure maximum affect.
- Teach patient use of nonpharmacologic methods of pain control, including guided imagery; graduated breathing (as in the Lamaze method); enhanced relaxation; massage; biofeedback; cutaneous stimulation (via a counterirritant, e.g., oil of wintergreen); acupressure; a transcutaneous electrical nerve stimulation (TENS) device; warm or cool thermotherapy; music therapy; and tactile, auditory, visual, or verbal distractions.
- Use traditional nursing interventions to counteract the pain, including back rubs, repositioning, and encouraging the patient to verbalize feelings.
- Advise patient to coordinate the time of peak effectiveness of the antiinflammatory agent with periods of exercise or ambulation.
- For additional interventions, see **Pain**, p. 719, in Appendix One, "Caring for Preoperative and Postoperative Patients."

NIC: Analgesic Administration; Distraction; Environmental Management; Heat/Cold Application; Pain Management; Progressive Muscle Relaxation

Knowledge deficit: Use of postoperative cryotherapy with a commercial iced knee cuff and automatic ice slush circulator
Desired outcomes: Within 8 hr of intervention, patient verbalizes understanding of the use of cryotherapy to control postoperative swelling and pain. Patient demonstrates ability to perform cryotherapy safely.
- Instruct patient in the use of cold to reduce edema formation and postoperative pain.
- Ensure that a layer of cloth is placed between the knee cuff and patient's skin (e.g., Stockinette).
- Instruct patient in the placement of the knee cuff to ensure that all surgical incisions are included in the therapy and that the cuff is not applied too tightly (patient should be able to comfortably fit one finger freely beneath the filled knee cuff).
- Instruct patient in how to fill the ice reservoir with ice and water to provide a slush solution and the need to check for refilling q4hr.
- Instruct patient in filling the knee cuff to prevent overfilling and possible excessive pressure on underlying skin.
- Instruct patient to inspect skin underneath the knee cuff at least q4hr for erythema that is not relieved after removal of the cuff. If erythema persists, patient should call the health care provider for advice.
- If appropriate (i.e., patient will be discharged with the device), instruct patient in how to connect the Autocirculator and precautions in its use.
- Allow patient adequate guided repetitions to ensure that he or she understands the instructions and can properly use the device.

NIC: Heat/Cold Application; Incision Site Care; Positioning; Pressure Management; Skin Surveillance; Teaching: Procedure/Treatment

> **See Also:** "Osteoarthritis" for **Impaired physical mobility** related to musculoskeletal impairment and adjustment to new walking gait, p. 556; "Ligamentous Injury" for **Knowledge deficit:** Need for elevation of the involved extremity, use of thermotherapy, and prescribed exercise, p. 566; **Knowledge deficit:** Potential for joint weakness, and the techniques for applying external supports and assessing neurovascular status, p. 568; "Fractures" for **Self-care deficit,** p. 590; Appendix One, "Caring for Preoperative and Postoperative Patients," p. 717, for nursing diagnoses and interventions.

PATIENT-FAMILY TEACHING AND DISCHARGE PLANNING

When providing patient-family teaching, focus on sensory information; avoid giving excessive information; and initiate a visiting nurse referral for necessary follow-up teaching. Consider including verbal and written information about the following:
- Phone number of appropriate person for patient's questions after hospital discharge.
- Use of external support devices (elastic wraps, knee immobilizer, orthosis), including care of the device, care of the skin beneath the device, and monitoring for areas of irritation and neurovascular deficit (see "Ligamentous Injuries," p. 568).
- Prescribed exercise regimen, including rationale, how it is performed, number of repetitions, and frequency.
- Prescribed medications, including drug name, rationale, dosage, schedule, precautions, drug/drug and food/drug interactions, and potential side effects.

- Indicators of wound infection that necessitate medical attention: erythema, edema, joint effusion, purulent discharge, local warmth, pain, and fever.
- Ambulation with assistive device, including patient's demonstration of independence on level and uneven ground and stairs (see "Osteoarthritis," p. 556).

Acute compartment syndrome

Acute compartment syndrome results from an interruption in local blood flow to muscles within an anatomic myofascial compartment. This is a progressive disorder associated with changes in compartmental tissue pressures from internal sources (e.g., edema, hemorrhage), external forces (e.g., tight casts/dressings, circumferential eschar formation), or alterations in local blood flow (venostasis, vasospasm). Volkmann's ischemic contracture of the forearm and march gangrene (anterior tibial compartment syndrome) are sequelae that may follow this process. Edema within a myofascial compartment can eventually lead to ischemia that damages the capillary endothelium and leads to leakage of fluid into the interstitial space (i.e., further edema formation in a self-perpetuating cycle). Similarly, impaired venous return from a compartment can lead to distention of the compartment that can eventually lead to disruption of the capillary bed fluid dynamics and to ischemia. Arterial injury, from fracture fragments or the mechanism of injury, with resultant reflex vasospasm, also has been implicated as a potential cause of this process. Elevation and application of ice may aggravate the process by contributing to decreased blood supply.

An iatrogenic compartment syndrome can result from any circumferential cast or dressing that adversely affects the circulation of tissues. This syndrome is most commonly seen in trauma or surgery involving the elbow, wrist, knee, or ankle or fractures of the humerus, radius, ulna, tibia, and/or fibula. Additional causes include bleeding disorders (hemophilia), major vascular surgery, thermal injuries (especially circumferential burns or frostbite), snake bite, and infiltration of IV infusions into deep tissues. Systemic hypotension increases the risk of compartment syndrome because it will further aggravate decreases in local blood flow. Because muscle tissue requires large amounts of blood to meet the muscle's demands, necrosis will occur rapidly if the blood supply is inadequate. Irreversible injury to muscle and nerve may occur after 5-6 hr of ischemia. If not corrected quickly, ischemic myositis can lead to myonecrosis and result in a severely contracted, functionally useless, and disfiguring limb distal to the area of injury. Complications of acute compartment syndrome include infection, renal failure from excessive release of myoglobin (myoglobinemia), hyperkalemia because of K^+ loss from injured muscle cells, and metabolic acidosis caused by loss of built-up lactic acid in injured muscle.

ASSESSMENT

Signs and symptoms: The hallmark indicator of compartment syndrome is pain more than normally expected for the injury or the need for increasing amounts of narcotic analgesic. Pain increases with passive movement of distal digits (causing a stretching of muscle within the compartment) or when pressure is applied over the involved compartment. The most reliable physical findings are sensory deficits, especially loss of two-point discrimination, decreased sensation to light touch, decreased sensation of pinprick, and decreased proprioception. The involved compartment may be palpably tense, and the overlying skin may be tense and shiny. The distal extremity may be pale, cool, and edematous. Distal circulation through the compartment may be impaired as shown by slowed capillary refill and impaired venous return. Weakness of involved muscle groups generally precedes frank paralysis. Paralysis may actually represent pseudoparalysis because of the patient's avoidance of movements that stress the involved compartment, or it may be frank paralysis of muscle that is innervated by injured nerves in the involved compartment. Pulselessness and true paralysis are late findings.

DIAGNOSTIC TESTS

Compartment pressure: Can be measured via a variety of devices (e.g., slit, wick, or large-bore catheter) that are introduced into the compartment and attached to a saline-primed manometer or transducer. Normal tissue pressures are <15 mm Hg; sustained pressures >30 mm Hg are considered significantly elevated above normal. Continuous monitoring of high-risk patients may be necessary to warn of impending acute compartment syndrome. Patients with low blood pressure are at increased risk and may develop compartment syndrome with lower tissue pressures. In such patients, the delta pressure should be determined. Delta pressure equals the mean arterial pressure minus the compartment tissue pressure. Delta pressure ≤30 mm Hg for 6 hr or 40 mm Hg for 8 hr should be reported promptly to the health care practitioner.
Arteriogram and venogram: To rule out vasospasm, thrombus, embolus, or arterial trauma, which can result in acute compartment syndrome, especially in patients with supracondylar fracture of the humerus. Angiography is not useful in identifying compartment syndrome. **Note:** Pulse oximetry has not been demonstrated as reliable in identifying vascular compromise in distal extremities.
Doppler ultrasound: May be used to assess peripheral circulation.
Electromyography (EMG) and nerve conduction tests: May be done to rule out intrinsic muscle or nerve pathologic conditions.
MRI: May show muscle ischemia.

COLLABORATIVE MANAGEMENT

Conservative measures: Used initially when acute compartment syndrome is suspected. The constriction limiting the swelling (e.g., cast, splint, circumferential dressing) is loosened down to skin level, ideally via bivalving (splitting both sides) the cast. However, if a fracture is involved, adequate immobilization should be maintained by a splint or immobilizer that allows uninhibited swelling. After a fracture, the limb is elevated to enhance venous return and ice is applied to cause vasoconstriction in the area of the injury and inhibit further edema formation. However, if compartment syndrome is suspected, **ice and elevation are contraindicated** because they may contribute to decreased vascular supply. Often, larger-than-normal levels of narcotics with potentiation, such as aspirin, acetaminophen, promethazine (Phenergan), or hydroxyzine (Vistaril), are required for pain control.
Fasciotomy: Necessary if conservative measures fail to control the progressive symptoms. Fasciotomy is the surgical incision of the fascia for the entire length of the involved compartment to decompress tissues and remove any restriction to swelling. In the lower leg all compartments are incised (e.g., anterior, lateral, and superficial and deep posterior compartments). (Some authors include a fifth compartment, the posterior tibial compartment.) After several days the fasciotomy is debrided and closed primarily or the area is grafted with skin.
Surgical repair of a lacerated artery: Performed if the cause is arterial injury. If vasospasm is the suspected cause, some surgeons will expose the involved artery and apply topical papaverine to control the problem; if unsuccessful, resection of the involved artery with reanastomosis frequently is necessary.

NURSING DIAGNOSES AND INTERVENTIONS

For patients at risk for acute compartment syndrome
Risk for peripheral neurovascular dysfunction with risk factors related to interruption of capillary blood flow secondary to increased pressure within the myofascial compartment

Desired outcomes: Patient has adequate peripheral neurovascular function in the involved limb as evidenced by absence of paresthesia, normal muscle tone, brisk (<2 sec) capillary refill (or capillary refill consistent with the contralateral extremity), normal skin color and temperature, peripheral pulse amplitude >2+ on a 0-4+ scale, normal tissue pressures (<15 mm Hg), and absence of edema or tautness. Patient verbalizes understanding about the importance of reporting symptoms indicative of impaired neurovascular status.

- Monitor neurovascular status of injured extremity with each VS check (at least q2hr). Monitor for loss of two-point discrimination, decreased sensation of light touch or pinprick, decreased proprioception, pain on passive movement of distal digits or with pressure applied to involved compartment(s), sluggish capillary refill, impaired venous return, increasing limb edema, coolness, tense shiny skin, and tautness over individual compartments. Also assess for muscle weakness, paralysis, or pseudoparalysis. To assess for pseudoparalysis use distraction to facilitate examination.
- Report deficits in neurovascular status promptly. Apply ice when appropriate (see p. 576), and loosen all circumferential dressings down to the skin unless contraindicated. **Caution:** When compartment syndrome is suspected, ice and elevation are contraindicated because they may compromise vascular supply further.
- Teach patient the symptoms that necessitate prompt reporting: increasing pain, paresthesia (diminished sensation, hyperesthesia, anesthesia), paralysis, and coolness.
- Monitor tissue pressures on a continuous basis if an intracompartmental pressure device is present. Alert health care practitioner to pressures higher than normal. Be aware that pressures >30 mm Hg may be significantly elevated above normal.
- Ensure that fluid resuscitation is accomplished as necessary to ensure adequate systemic circulation to the involved compartments. Fluid resuscitation also aids in flushing myoglobin from the circulation to reduce the potential for acute tubular necrosis and renal failure.
- In patients with lowered systemic BP, monitor delta pressure (mean arterial pressure minus compartment tissue pressure). Report delta pressure ≤30 mm Hg for 6 hr or ≤40 mm Hg for 8 hr.

NIC: Cast Care: Maintenance; Circulatory Precautions; Exercise Therapy: Joint Mobility; Heat/Cold Application; Peripheral Sensation Management; Shock Management; Skin Surveillance; Teaching: Disease Process

For patients experiencing acute compartment syndrome

Pain related to tissue ischemia secondary to compartment syndrome

Desired outcomes: Within 8 hr of treatment, patient's subjective perception of discomfort decreases as documented by a pain scale. Nonverbal indicators of discomfort are absent or diminished. Patient verbalizes understanding of the need to report uncontrolled or increasing pain.

- Assess the patient's complaints of pain for onset, duration, progression, and intensity. Devise a pain scale with patient, rating discomfort from 0 (no pain) to 10 (worst pain).
- Determine if passive stretching of digits and pressure over limb compartments increase the pain, because both are likely to occur with compartment syndrome.
- Adjust the medication regimen to the patient's needs; document medication effectiveness.
- Prevent pressure on involved compartment and neurovascular structures. When not contraindicated by evidence of impaired circulation, apply ice if it has been prescribed.
- If patient has had a fasciotomy, be aware that if the pain does not subside after this procedure, it could signal an incomplete fasciotomy. Pain that increases several days after a fasciotomy may signal compartmental infection.

- Continue to monitor neurovascular function with each VS check to assess for recurring compartment syndrome or infection.

NIC: Analgesic Administration; Anxiety Reduction; Coping Enhancement; Pain Management; Progressive Muscle Relaxation; Simple Guided Imagery

Risk for infection with risk factors related to inadequate primary defenses secondary to necrotic tissue, wide compartmental fasciotomy, and open wound
Desired outcome: Patient is free of infection as evidenced by normothermia, WBC count ≤11,000/mm^3, erythrocyte sedimentation rate (ESR) ≤20 mm/hr (female) or ≤15 mm/hr (male), and absence of wound erythema and other clinical indicators of infection.

- Monitor patient for fever, increasing pain, and laboratory data indicative of infection (e.g., increased WBC count, increased ESR).
- Assess exposed wounds and dressings for erythema, increasing wound drainage, purulent wound drainage, increasing wound circumference, edema, and localized tenderness.
- Monitor distal neurovascular status for deficit, which may indicate infection or pressure on these structures caused by nearby deep infection.
- After primary closure or grafting of wound, continue to assess wound for signs of infection (see above).
- Be aware of and assess for chronic infection and osteomyelitis as potential complications after compartment syndrome. Teach patient about the increased potential for infection with this type of wound and that chronic infection and osteomyelitis are late complications after compartment syndrome has occurred.
- Use sterile technique when changing dressings and providing wound care. As indicated, teach sterile technique to patient before hospital discharge.
- Notify health care practitioner promptly of significant findings.

NIC: Environmental Management; Infection Protection; Medication Management; Surveillance; Vital Signs Monitoring; Wound Care; Wound Care: Closed Drainage

---

See Also: "Osteoarthritis" for **Pain,** p. 555; "Ligamentous Injuries" for **Knowledge deficit:** Need for elevation of the involved extremity, use of thermotherapy, and prescribed exercise, p. 566; **Pain** related to surgical repair and rehabilitation therapy, p. 573; Appendix One, "Caring for Preoperative and Postoperative Patients," p. 717, for nursing diagnoses and interventions if surgery was performed.

PATIENT-FAMILY TEACHING AND DISCHARGE PLANNING

When providing patient-family teaching, focus on sensory information; avoid giving excessive information; and initiate a visiting nurse referral for necessary follow-up teaching. Consider including verbal and written information about the following:

- Phone number of appropriate person to call for questions after hospital discharge.
- Instructions regarding the process of acute compartment syndrome, use of elevation and ice, and loosening of restrictive dressings.
- Discharge instructions for patients with fractures (see "Fractures," p. 593).
- Importance of seeking medical attention promptly if signs and symptoms of wound infection occur.
- Importance of monitoring for vascular changes in patients who have undergone vascular surgery (exploration or resection). Teach patient to be alert to color changes (pallor, cyanosis, duskiness), coolness, pulselessness, and decreased or absent capillary refill. Caution patient about the importance of reporting these findings promptly.

Section Three: Skeletal Disorders

Osteomyelitis

Osteomyelitis is an acute or a chronic infection involving a bone. Patients at risk for osteomyelitis include those who are undernourished, older persons, and individuals with DM and COPD. *Primary osteomyelitis* is a direct implantation of microorganisms into bone via open (compound) fractures, penetrating wounds, diagnostic bone marrow aspiration, or surgery. *Secondary* or *acute hematogenic osteomyelitis* is an infection of bone that occurs through vascular seeding following bacteremia or by infection from contiguous soft tissues (especially ischemic, diabetic, or neurotrophic ulcers), IV drug users, or joints involved with septic arthritis. Although osteomyelitis often remains localized, it can spread through the marrow, cortex, and periosteum. Conditions favoring the development of osteomyelitis include recent bone trauma or bone with low O_2 tension, such as that found in sickle cell anemia. Acute hematogenic osteomyelitis is most frequently caused by *Staphylococcus aureus* (90%-95%), but it also can result from *Escherichia coli, Pseudomonas* species, *Klebsiella, Enterobacter, Proteus, Salmonella, Streptococcus* (groups A, B, and G), and *Haemophilus influenzae.* As many as 25% of the cases of osteomyelitis involve multiple infectious agents. The incidence of tuberculosis of the musculoskeletal system is on the rise in the United States and should be considered, especially with spinal column symptoms. Chronic osteomyelitis is comparatively rare and is characterized by persistent, multiple, draining sinus tracts.

ASSESSMENT

Acute osteomyelitis: Pain, warmth, and swelling in the involved area; fever; malaise; limited motion. Pseudoparalysis is especially indicative of osteomyelitis in children who refuse to move an adjacent joint because of pain.

Chronic osteomyelitis: Bone infection that persists intermittently for years, usually flaring up after minor trauma to the area or lowered systemic resistance. Edema and erythema over the involved bone, weakness, irritability, and generalized signs of sepsis can occur. Sometimes the only symptom is persistent purulent drainage from an old pocket or sinus tract. With implant arthroplasty osteomyelitis, the symptoms involve aseptic loosening (demonstrated radiologically) and pain 3-5 mo postoperatively. Tuberculosis of the spine (Pott's disease) presents with back pain and possible radiculopathy.

History of: Total joint replacement, open (compound) fracture, penetrating trauma, use of external fixator, vascular insufficiency (e.g., with DM, sickle cell disease, COPD), recurrent urinary tract infections, bone marrow aspiration, advanced age, malnutrition, or IV drug use.

DIAGNOSTIC TESTS

CBC: Reveals leukocytosis and anemia in the presence of osteomyelitis.

Erythrocyte sedimentation rate: Elevated in the presence of osteomyelitis.

C-reactive protein: Elevated within 6-8 hr of onset of the assessments of osteomyelitis and septic arthritis (especially higher levels with the latter).

Bone biopsy: Will provide infectious material for accurate culture and sensitivity studies. This study is limited to large bones because of the risk of fracture in small bones. Bone biopsy is the "gold standard" for diagnosis of osteomyelitis and is considered positive when there is evidence of necrosis, acute or chronic inflammatory cells (including polymorphonuclear leukocytes), and aggregates of lymphocytes and/or plasma cells. Biopsy may also provide infectious material for the most accurate culture and sensitivity studies. Bone biopsy is especially important to establish musculoskeletal tuberculosis.

Blood or sequestrum cultures: To identify the causative organism via Gram stain and culture and sensitivity. Sequestrum is a piece of necrotic bone that is separated from surrounding bone as a result of osteomyelitis.

X-rays: May reveal subtle areas of radiolucency (osteonecrosis) and new bone formation. No x-ray changes will be evident until the disease has been active at least 5 days in infants, 8-10 days in children, and 2-3 wk in adults.

Radioisotope scanning: Methods include bone scans with technetium-99 or gallium-67 and leukocyte scans with indium-111. These scans may reveal areas of increased vascularity (called *hot spots*), which may be indicative of osteomyelitis >80% of the time. False-positive results can occur with contiguous soft tissue infection, and they are used cautiously for this reason. Negative bone scan results do not guarantee that osteomyelitis is not present.

CT and MRI scans: CT scans may demonstrate bone damage and soft tissue inflammation. MRI will not reveal bone changes, but it is an excellent means for identifying pockets of purulence, especially intramedullary infections, osteitis, and diskitis with Pott's disease.

COLLABORATIVE MANAGEMENT

IV antimicrobial therapy: When agent-specific antibiosis is possible, may be given for 2 wk, followed by 2-4 wk of oral antibiotic therapy. When the infective agent is not specifically identified, broad-spectrum antibiotic IV therapy may be required for 4-6 wk. Therapy frequently requires agents such as vancomycin, ticarcillin (Timentin), aminoglycosides, third-generation cephalosporins, clindamycin, fluoroquinolones, or combinations of these.

Bedrest

Immobilization of affected extremity: With splint, cast, or traction to relieve pain and decrease the potential for pathologic fracture.

Blood transfusions: To correct any accompanying anemia.

Removal of internal fixation device or endoprosthesis, if present: To help control the infection. Total joint replacements may need to be removed to allow adequate treatment of osteomyelitis. Removal of the prosthesis will result in a flail joint until revision replacement is possible.

Surgical decompression of infected bone: May be followed by primary closure when small areas are involved. For large areas of involvement, myocutaneous flaps may be needed to cover denuded bone. Sometimes the area is left open to drain and heal by secondary intention or with secondary closure. Radical débridement, bone grafting, and antituberculosis chemotherapy are used to prevent kyphotic deformity in Pott's disease.

Drains: May be inserted into the affected bone to drain the site or act as ingress-egress tubes to funnel topical antibiotics directly into the area of infection. This system may incorporate suction to aid drainage.

Topical antibiotics: May be used via continuous or intermittent infusion into the wound and are continued until three successive drain cultures have been negative. As an alternative, antibiotic-impregnated polymethylmethacrylate (PMMA) beads may be packed into affected sites for 2-4 wk, after which the wound is reopened, the beads are removed, and bone graft is packed in the deficit. Intramedullary or intraarticular antibiotic solutions also may be used.

Long-term antibiotic therapy: May be continued for 3-6 mo.

Hyperbaric O_2:   Has shown promise in treating refractory osteomyelitis associated with adjacent pressure necrosis. Routine therapy lasts 90 min at 2-3 atmospheres (atm) pressure.

Amputation: Although rarely performed, may be required for extremities in which persistent infection severely limits function.

NURSING DIAGNOSES AND INTERVENTIONS

Risk for infection *(for others)* related to risk of cross-contamination; *(for patient)* related to disease chronicity

Desired outcomes: At the time of patient's hospital discharge, patient is free of symptoms of infection as evidenced by normothermia and WBC count ≤11,000/mm^3. Within 24 hr of instruction, patient verbalizes knowledge of the potential chronicity of the disease and the importance of strict adherence to the prescribed antibiotic therapy.

- When appropriate for the infecting organism, isolate the patient from other patients, especially immunocompromised patients.
- Use Transmission-based Precautions: Contact, for patients known to be or suspected of being infected or colonized with epidemiologically important microorganisms (e.g., methicillin-resistant *Staphylococcus aureus* [MRSA], vancomycin-resistant *Enterococcus* [VRE]) that can be transmitted by direct contact.
- In addition to Standard Precautions, wear gloves when providing direct care or having hand contact with potentially contaminated surfaces or items in the patient's environment.
- When possible, dedicate use of noncritical patient care equipment to the patient with osteomyelitis to avoid sharing between patients.
- Ensure that the patient's drainage system is properly handled, using Standard Precautions, and that careful hand washing is observed between patients by all staff members to prevent cross-contamination.
- Teach patient about the disease and potential for chronic infection. Stress the importance of adherence to the prescribed antibiotic therapy.
- Follow Standard Precautions (i.e., use of gloves, goggles, and an impervious gown) when performing irrigations, changing dressings, or handling contaminated dressings (see Appendix Two, p. 817). Wash hands well between patients.
- Monitor for fever, increasing pain, and laboratory data indicative of infection (e.g., increased WBC, increased ESR).
- Assess exposed wounds and dressings for erythema, increasing wound drainage, purulent wound drainage, increasing wound circumference, edema, warmth, and localized tenderness.
- Assess neurovascular structures for deficit, which can signal infection or pressure from inflamed tissues.
- After primary closure or grafting of wound, continue to assess for indications of infection.
- Observe for superimposed infections, especially fungal, by assessing for fever, black and furry tongue, complaint of sore mouth or tongue, nausea, diarrhea, oral monilial growth, or vaginal monilial growth. If a venous access device (VAD) is used for antibiotic administration, monitor infusion site closely for irritation that does not respond to usual treatments with topical antibiotics. As indicated, obtain cultures of suspicious inflammation.

NIC: Environmental Management; Home Maintenance Assistance; Infection Control; Medication Management; Wound Care; Wound Care: Closed Drainage

Knowledge deficit: Side effects from prolonged use of potent antibiotics
Desired outcome: Within 24 hr of instruction, patient verbalizes knowledge about potential side effects of antibiotic therapy and precautions that must be taken.

AMINOGLYCOSIDE ANTIBACTERIALS: Gentamicin sulfate, kanamycin sulfate, neomycin, streptomycin, and tobramycin are used to combat gram-negative organisms. Potential toxic reactions include ototoxicity (exhibited by dizziness, vertigo, tinnitus, and decreased auditory acuity); nephrotoxicity (evidenced by rising BUN and serum creatinine levels from progressive renal tubular necrosis, which can progress to renal failure if untreated); and superimposed infections, which occur because of loss of normal body flora protection against bacterial overgrowth. Peak and trough serum levels are monitored during therapy to ensure an adequate bacteriocidal level is obtained and maintained with the lowest possible dosage and schedule.

- Teach patient about the potential complications and the need to report symptoms as early as possible.
- Advise patient that with long-term therapy, a baseline audiogram with frequent audiograms should be performed to identify potential hearing deficit; serum creatinine and BUN should be drawn weekly while patient is taking aminoglycosides; and weight should be checked daily to help assess for fluid retention (patients should report weight gain ≥2 lb/day). Monitor I&O during patient's hospitalization to help assess renal function.
- Advise patient to observe for superimposed infections, especially fungal infections, by assessing for fever, black or furry tongue, nausea, diarrhea, oral candidiasis, or vaginal candidiasis. If a VAD is used for antibiotic administration, the infusion site should be closely monitored for indicators of irritation that do not respond to usual treatments with topical antibiotics. During hospitalization, consult health care practitioner about culturing suspicious areas of inflammation.

PENICILLINS: Ampicillin, carbenicillin, cyclacillin, methicillin, mezlocillin, oxacillin, and piperacillin are used to combat organisms that demonstrate sensitivity to them. Potential toxic reactions include anemia, hypersensitivity reactions, and overgrowth of nonsusceptible organisms.

- Teach patient about the potential complications and the need to report symptoms promptly.
- Use penicillin cautiously in patients with allergies or allergic pathologic conditions, such as asthma, hay fever, or dermatitis. Erythematous, maculopapular rash; urticaria; and anaphylaxis can occur. Caution patient about these potential reactions.
- Instruct patient to seek medical attention if rash, fever, chills, or signs of infection/inflammation develop (e.g., erythema, edema, local tenderness, local warmth)

CEPHALOSPORINS: Cefadroxil, cefamandole, cefazolin, cefepime, cefoperazone, cefotetan, cefoxitin, ceftazidime, ceftriaxone, cefuroxime, cephalothin, cephapirin, cephradine, and tazicef are used in the treatment of susceptible organisms. Potential toxic reactions include overgrowth of nonsusceptible organisms, photosensitivity, increased BUN, hepatotoxicity, and pseudomembranous colitis.

- Advise patient about the potential complications, which necessitate prompt medical attention.
- Explain that patients with suspected renal or hepatic disease should have baseline and serial (weekly) serum liver enzymes (lactate hydrogenase [LDH], serum glutamic-oxaloacetic transaminase [SGOT; aspartate aminotransferase {AST}], serum glutamic-pyruvic transaminase [SGPT; alanine aminotransferase {ALT}]), BUN, and serum creatinine evaluations. I&O should be monitored along with daily weight to determine hydration status. Scleral and skin icterus, as well as darkening of the urine (from increased urobilinogen), should be noted. Persistent diarrhea (>3 liquid stools or liquid stools for >2 days) should be reported promptly to the health care provider.
- Advise patient to avoid direct sunlight or ultraviolet light sources. Suggest the use of sunscreen agents to help prevent photosensitivity reactions.
- When oral medications are used, instruct patient to avoid concurrent intake with dairy or iron products because they can inhibit absorption from the gut.

SULFONAMIDES: Sulfadiazine, sulfamethoxazole, sulfapyridine, and sulfisoxazole can cause toxic reactions, including disruption of intestinal flora, which results in decreased production of metabolically active vitamin K and hemorrhagic tendencies; agranulocytosis; nephrotoxicity; and crystalluria.

- Teach patient about the potential complications and the importance of seeking prompt medical attention if they occur.
- Advise patients taking long-term sulfonamide therapy of the need to have baseline BUN and serum creatinine level determinations along with weekly

levels to rule out nephrotoxicity. Baseline and serial (weekly) granulocyte determinations also should be performed. Agranulocytosis can manifest as lesions of the throat, mucous membranes, GI tract, and skin. Daily weight and I&O should be evaluated to help assess hydration status.

- Teach patient how to monitor for bleeding, especially epistaxis, bleeding gums, hemoptysis, hematemesis, melena, hematuria, prolonged bleeding from wounds, and ecchymosis. During patient's hospitalization, perform a Hematest on suspicious secretions or send them to the laboratory if prescribed, to determine if blood is present. Teach patient to control bleeding with ice, pressure, or elevation and to seek medical assistance promptly if unable to control hemorrhage.

- Advise patient to consume at least 2-3 L of fluids daily (unless contraindicated by cardiac or renal disease) to prevent crystalluria. Teach the indicators of urinary calculi and the importance of getting medical attention if they occur: hematuria, pyuria, retention, frequency, urgency, and pain in the flank, lower back, perineum, thighs, groin, labia, or scrotum.

NIC: Health Education; Teaching: Prescribed Activity/Exercise; Teaching: Preoperative; Teaching: Prescribed Diet; Teaching: Procedure/Treatment

Knowledge deficit: Potential for infection and air embolus related to use of Hickman catheter, peripherally inserted central catheters (PICC lines), or other VAD for long-term intermittent antibiotic therapy

Desired outcome: By at least 24 hr before hospital discharge, patient demonstrates care of the catheter and verbalizes knowledge about the indicators of infection and air embolus.

- Teach patient how to care for the catheter and monitor the entry site for indicators of infection or inflammation if therapy is to be continued at home. Use sterile technique for dressing changes, following hospital protocol for the procedure, which usually includes initial preparation of the skin with alcohol, applying povidone-iodine, and covering the site with an air-occlusive dressing. Have patient or significant other return the demonstration before hospital discharge. If appropriate, arrange for a visit by a home health care nurse.

- If appropriate, caution patient about the importance of keeping the tubing clamped unless he or she is aspirating or injecting solutions into the catheter. Some VAD catheters are designed to omit the need for clamping (e.g., Groshong catheters). Teach patient and significant other to be alert to indicators of air embolism: labored breathing, cyanosis, cough, chest pain, syncope. Explain that if air embolism is suspected, the patient should be rolled immediately to the left side and placed in Trendelenburg position while reclamping the catheter, and medical assistance should be obtained as rapidly as possible.

- Teach patient the importance of preventing inadvertent puncture or breakage of the tubing and checking for kinks or cracks daily. Explain the necessity of taping all tube junctures to prevent accidental separation and positioning the clamp over tape tabs to minimize stress on the tubing.

NIC: Embolus Precautions; Teaching: Preoperative; Teaching: Prescribed Activity/Exercise; Teaching: Procedure/Treatment; Teaching: Psychomotor Skill

Impaired physical mobility related to musculoskeletal immobilization devices and pain

Desired outcomes: By at least 24 hr before hospital discharge, patient maintains appropriate body alignment, with external fixation devices in place, or demonstrates setup and use of home traction device. Patient verbalizes understanding of use of analgesics and adjunctive methods to decrease pain when performing prescribed exercises or activity.

- Instruct patient in proper body alignment, most commonly with joints in neutral position. If orthotic devices are used to maintain position, provide instruction in the application of the device, assessments of areas of excess pressure beneath the device (increasing the risk of pressure necrosis), and exercises and ROM to do when the device is removed.
- Instruct patient and/or significant other in active and/or passive ROM of adjacent joints q8hr as appropriate.
- When appropriate, instruct patient and significant other in the setup and maintenance of home traction, including appropriate indicators of untoward effects (e.g., pressure necrosis, impaired neurovascular function).
- Instruct patient and significant other in the care of an extremity in an external fixator (i.e., pin site care), knowing how to identify problems associated with fixator, performing prescribed exercises, monitoring neurovascular status of the limb, and monitoring pin sites for indicators of infection.
- Instruct patient and significant other in the care of a casted extremity, that is, caring for the cast, monitoring neurovascular status of the distal extremity, watching for evidence of pressure necrosis beneath the cast, performing prescribed exercises, preventing skin maceration, and preventing disuse osteoporosis (see also **Knowledge deficit**: Care and assessment of the casted extremity, p. 567).
- Instruct patient and significant other in use of analgesics and other methods to control pain (see "Intervertebral Disk Disease" for **Health-seeking behavior:** Pain control measures, p. 251).

NIC: Bathing; Cast Care: Maintenance; Environmental Management; Health Education; Medication Management; Teaching: Prescribed Activity/Exercise

See Also: "Intervertebral Disk Disease" for **Health-seeking behavior:** Pain control measures, p. 251; "Osteoarthritis" for **Pain,** p. 555; "Fractures" for **Self-care deficit,** p. 590; Appendix One, "Caring for Preoperative and Postoperative Patients," p. 717; "Caring for Patients on Prolonged Bedrest," p. 738, for nursing diagnoses and interventions.

PATIENT-FAMILY TEACHING AND DISCHARGE PLANNING

When providing patient-family teaching, focus on sensory information; avoid giving excessive information; and initiate a visiting nurse referral for necessary follow-up teaching. Consider including verbal and written information about the following:

- Necessary patient care after hospital discharge (e.g., analgesia, dressing changes, warm soaks, ROM exercises, activity limitations, use of ambulatory aids). Involve significant other in patient care during hospitalized period to familiarize him or her with care activities after discharge.
- When parenteral antibiotic therapy is to be given at home (usually via a Hickman catheter, Portacath, or similar long-term VAD), the method of administering medications and care of the device used.
- Medications, including drug name, route, dosage, purpose, schedule, precautions, drug/drug and food/drug interactions, and potential side effects.
- For complex drug therapy regimen, including graphic illustration of dosage and frequency to facilitate adherence to therapy.
- Involving a public health nurse, visiting nurse, or similar home health care service professional to ensure adequate follow-up at home.
- Indicators of potential complications, such as recurring infection, pathologic fracture, joint contracture, pressure necrosis, and medication reactions or toxic effects, and a phone number to call if untoward effects occur.

Fractures

A fracture is a break in the continuity of a bone. It occurs when stress is placed on the bone that exceeds the bone's biologic loading capacity. Most commonly the stress is the result of trauma. *Pathologic fractures* are the result of decreased biologic loading capacity so that even normal stress can result in a break.

ASSESSMENT

Chronic indicators: These are rare. Osteoporotic fractures of the vertebral column may be found incidental to an x-ray in an asymptomatic patient or in a patient who complains of back discomfort. Delayed union is a failure of the bone to unite within the normally accepted time frame for that bone's healing, and a chronic fracture may result. Nonunion is demonstrated by nonalignment and lost function secondary to lost bony rigidity. Pseudoarthrosis is a state in which the fracture fails to heal and a false joint forms at the fracture site. Avascular necrosis occurs when the fracture interrupts the blood supply to a segment of bone, which then eventually necroses. Reflex sympathetic dystrophy is an incompletely understood process that appears to be a "short circuiting" of neurotransmission, resulting in pain, reduced function, joint stiffness, and trophic changes in soft tissues and skin following fracture. Symptoms of reflex sympathetic dystrophy include severe pain in the involved extremity, edema, muscle spasm and atrophy, stiffness, decreased mobility, vasospasm, loss of bone mass, and contractions. Myositis ossificans is heterotrophic (abnormal, out of the normal area) bone formation, most commonly in the arms, thighs, and hips. Other fracture complications can include altered sensation, limb length discrepancies, and chronic lymphatic or venous stasis.

Acute indicators: Insidious and progressive or sudden onset of severe pain, which usually is associated with trauma or physical stress, such as jogging, strenuous exercise, or a fall. In pathologic fractures, the patient may describe signs and symptoms associated with the underlying pathologic condition (see "Benign Neoplasms," p. 594; "Malignant Neoplasms," p. 596).

Physical assessment: Loss of normal bony or limb contours, edema, ecchymosis, limb shortening, decreased ROM of adjacent joints, false motion (movement that occurs outside a joint), and crepitus, which should not be elicited purposely because of the risk of injury to surrounding soft tissues. Complicated and complex fractures can present with signs and symptoms of perforated viscus (internal organ), neurovascular deficit, joint effusion, or excessive joint laxity. Open (or compound) fractures involve a break in the skin and will demonstrate a wound in the area of suspected fracture, or bone may be exposed in the wound (Table 8-3).

> **Note:**   Any patient with a suspected fracture should be treated as though a fracture is present until it is ruled out. Interventions should include immobilization and elevation of the involved area, application of ice, and careful monitoring of the neurovascular status distal to the injury. Any restrictions to swelling (e.g., rings, wristwatches, bracelets) should be removed before they impair neurovascular function.

DIAGNOSTIC TESTS

Most fractures are identified easily with standard AP and lateral x-rays. MRI may be useful in evaluating complicated fractures; its usefulness in identifying different bone densities is limited. Occasionally it is necessary to involve

T A B L E 8 - 3   Wound Classification of Open Fractures

Type	Description
I	Wound ≤1 cm
	Minimal contamination
	Simple transverse or oblique with presumed wound resulting from bone spike
	Minimal soft tissue trauma
II	Wound >1 cm
	Moderate contamination
	Moderately involved comminuted fractures with crush injuries
	Moderate soft tissue injuries (e.g., skin flaps or avulsion)
III	Significant contamination
	Severe fractures with comminution and gross instability
	Extensive soft tissue injury involving skin, muscle, and neurovascular structures
	Traumatic amputations
IIIA	Adequate soft tissue coverage of fractures
	Segmental or severely comminuted fractures
IIIB	Extensive soft tissue loss or injury
	Massive tissue contamination
	Severely comminuted fractures
IIIC	Any open fracture with arterial injury, regardless of the amount of soft tissue injury

From Snyder PE: In Maher AB et al, editors: *Orthopaedic nursing,* ed 2, Philadelphia, 1998, Saunders.

special techniques, such as the mortise view with bimalleolar ankle fractures (showing the joint spaces between the fibula, tibia, and talus) or x-rays through the open mouth to identify fractures of the odontoid process. Bone scans, tomograms, CT scans, stereoscopic films, and arthrograms also can be used. Intraarticular fractures sometimes may be diagnosed with arthroscopy.

COLLABORATIVE MANAGEMENT

The choice of treatment varies with the complexity of the fracture and with the patient's age, concurrent health problems, and functional goals. The goal of treatment is to provide immobilization of the bone until healing occurs. The length of time for immobilization varies with the type of fracture. The following is a brief overview of common examples of treatment interventions.

Bedrest: May be all that is required to maintain reduction for simple, uncomplicated fractures, such as those of the posterior elements of the vertebrae and some pelvic fractures.

Traction

Cervical fractures: Skeletal traction via Turner, Cone, Vinke, or Crutchfield tongs, which are inserted into the outer plate of the cranial vault. An alternative is the halo vest, which allows the insertion of four pins into the outer plate of the cranium. The pins are attached to a halo device that is connected to four metal posts encompassed within a body jacket, cast, or orthosis. This "four-posted" jacket allows exposure of the head and neck yet maintains immobilization of the fracture. Cervical collars and a wide variety of orthotics can be used to provide support for some simple fractures or to maintain stability of more complex fractures following therapy with traction or ORIF.

Humeral fractures: Dunlop's side arm or overhead or side arm 90/90 traction. Skeletal traction may be applied with a Kirschner wire through the proximal ulna.

Pelvic fractures: Balanced suspension, pelvic sling, or pelvic belt may be used for nondisplaced fractures, but skeletal traction with pins in the ilium or femur may be required for displaced fractures.

Femoral fractures: Skin traction (Buck's extension; Bohler-Braun, Russell's, or balanced suspension traction) may be applied until skeletal traction can be used or the fracture is internally or externally fixated. Skeletal traction may involve a Steinmann pin or Kirschner wire positioned through the distal femur or proximal tibia. When skeletal traction is used, it is provided in combination with balanced suspension or Russell's traction and is used for 1-4 mo.

Tibial fractures: Temporary traction can be accomplished with Buck's extension or for longer periods of time with a pin placed through the distal tibia or calcaneus, augmented with balanced suspension, Bohler-Braun, or Russell's traction.

Immobilization devices

Uncomplicated, simple fractures of cervical vertebrae: A variety of orthotics, soft or hard cervical collars, or a Minerva jacket cast for less stable fractures.

Dorsal and lumbar vertebral fractures: Plaster of paris body cast or a variety of orthotic devices.

Clavicular fractures: Figure-of-8 dressing, modified Velpeau dressing (a wrap that holds the arm against the thorax with the elbow flexed at 90 or 45 degrees), sling and swathe shoulder immobilizer, clavicular straps.

Humeral fractures: Velpeau cast, shoulder spica cast (which abducts or extends the upper arm), or Caldwell's hanging plaster cast, which is a long arm cast with additional layers of plaster of Paris that provide weight to distract fracture fragments and aid in alignment. Patients in Caldwell's casts should be instructed to maintain the cast in dependent position, which will help ensure adequate fracture distraction. A coaptation splint may be used to immobilize midshaft humeral fractures. The coaptation splint consists of a long plaster splint applied over a thick layer of padding, beginning at the medial aspect of the upper arm in the axilla and extending around the elbow and up the outside of the upper arm. An elastic wrap secures the splint. Posterior splints may immobilize distal shaft fractures temporarily. Posterior or coaptation splints accommodate progressive edema, reducing the potential for acute compartment syndrome. Undisplaced, stable fractures may require immobilization only, with a sling and swathe shoulder immobilizer or functional bracing. Prefabricated polypropylene sleeves have been used successfully to immobilize fractures of the lower half of the humerus.

Ulnar or radial fractures: Long arm casts for proximal fractures or short arm casts for distal fractures. In the presence of significant edema, a sugar tong splint may be used to provide immobilization while accommodating progressive edema. A sugar tong splint is applied over heavy padding and consists of one long plaster splint that extends from the back of the wrist, bends around the elbow, covers the underside of the forearm to the wrist, and is held in place with an elastic wrap. Some fractures are immobilized in a posterior splint for 3-7 days before casting to allow the edema to subside. Fractures involving both the radius and ulna usually are immobilized in a long arm cast.

Hand fractures: Short arm posterior splints until edema subsides, and then a short arm cast can be applied. Some fractures of the hand may be immobilized safely in splints or orthoses. A thumb spica cast may be used for various fractures involving the thumb.

Pelvic fractures: Corsets, orthoses, or external fixators.

Femoral fractures: Spica cast that extends from the thorax and completely encompasses the affected leg and opposite leg to the midthigh, or a long leg cast may be applied. After sufficient callus has formed, it may be possible to use a cast brace to allow motion of the knee and weight-bearing stress, which can facilitate bony union in fractures that involve the articular surface of the femoral condyles.

Patellar fractures: Cylinder cast for nondisplaced fractures. After knee surgery, the leg may be immobilized in a Jones dressing, which includes AP and lateral splints over bulky padding and is held in place with an elastic wrap. Once swelling subsides, a cylinder or long leg cast is applied. A commercial knee immobilizer or orthotic may provide sufficient immobilization for some stable patellar fractures.

Tibial fractures: Cylinder or long leg cast; short leg cast for easily stabilized fractures. Some casts will be converted to walking casts at a later time. For fractures involving the articular surface of the tibial plateau, a long leg cast may be initially applied that is later converted to a cast brace to allow motion of the knee and weight-bearing stress, which can facilitate bony union.

Fibular shaft fractures: Although some fibular fractures may not require casting, a short leg walking cast is often applied if adequate support is not provided by the tibia.

Malleolar fractures: Short leg cast that is converted to a walking cast after callus has formed; long leg cast for nondisplaced bimalleolar fractures. Trimalleolar fractures require ORIF to ensure joint integrity.

Avulsion fractures of the insertion of the Achilles tendon from the calcaneus: Often require a long leg cast with the knee flexed at 30 degrees and the ankle slightly plantar flexed to reduce stress on the Achilles tendon.

Tarsal and metatarsal fractures: For unstable fractures, a short leg cast may be initially applied and later converted to a walking cast. For stable fractures a stiff-sole shoe or slipper cast may be used.

Phalangeal fractures: Splints made of plaster, metal, or plastic, or the phalanx can be immobilized by taping it to an adjacent phalanx.

Closed reduction: Allows for manipulation of displaced fragments to their normal anatomic alignment. It can be done with the patient under general, regional, local, or hematoma-block anesthesia (where local anesthetic is injected into the area of the fracture hematoma).

ORIF: Indicated for fractures that are grossly unstable or for patients who cannot tolerate prolonged bedrest or traction. Internal fixation may be accomplished with screws, pins, cannulated screws or nails, staples, wires, plates, bone grafts (either allograft or autograft), methylmethacrylate, or rods. **Note:** For specific information on allograft bone tissue, see *http://quality.red-cross.org/tissue.* In some fractures in which avascular necrosis is likely or the fracture is severely comminuted, placement of an endoprosthesis may be necessary. Endoprostheses most commonly are used to replace the head of the humerus or femur. Open (compound) fractures need definitive treatment within 6-8 hr to prevent limb compromise. Fibrin sealant may be used to aid in the internal fixation of some small fractures, avulsion fractures, and osteochondral fractures, as well as to aid in the internal fixation of bone grafts. Bioelectric stimulators, autogenous bone graft substitutes, osteoconductors, and osteoinductors are being used experimentally to compensate for bone loss or stimulate fracture healing via pulsed electromagnetic fields (PEMFs).

External fixation: Consists of skeletal pins (similar to Kirschner wires or Steinmann pins) that penetrate the fracture fragments and are attached to universal joints, which in turn are attached to rods to provide stabilization. These rods form a frame around the fractured limb for immobilization. Biaxial frames with transfixing pins or uniaxial frames with bicortical half pins may be used. The external fixator is left in place until sufficient soft tissue repair or bony callous formation allows either application of a cast or complete removal of any form of immobilization. Sometimes the skeletal pins are left in place (after removing the external fixation rods) and incorporated into a cast that immobilizes the limb until the fracture has healed. The external fixator can be used to treat massive open comminuted fractures with extensive soft tissue injury or neurovascular injury in which there is increased risk of infection. It is also the treatment of choice for infected nonunion, segmental bone loss, limb-lengthening procedures, arthrodesis (joint fusion), and multiple trauma with injuries involving other body systems.

Ilizarov procedure: Use of a ring-shaped external fixator that can be arranged in more than 600 configurations to enable maintenance of limb position for a myriad of orthopedic conditions. As with other external fixators, the connection between the device and bone is accomplished with Kirschner wires or Steinmann pins.

Progressive ROM and muscle-strengthening exercises: Begun after the designated period of immobilization to help the patient regain joint function.

Continuous passive movement (CPM): A motor-driven device developed to place a joint through repeated extension and flexion. It is used as an adjunctive treatment for femoral condyle, tibial plateau, humeral head, and other fractures and after total joint arthroplasty.

Electrical bone stimulation: Has been shown to enhance fracture healing in situations in which the healing has been delayed. Electrical stimulation devices may be incorporated into overlying casts with electrodes either surgically placed in the area of the fracture or incorporated into the overlying cast. The electrical stimulation device may also be completely implanted in the area of the fracture and utilizes PEMFs to stimulate bone growth.

NURSING DIAGNOSES AND INTERVENTIONS

See "Intervertebral Disk Disease" for **Health-seeking behavior:** Pain control measures, p. 251; "Osteoarthritis" for **Pain,** p. 555; **Pain** related to surgical repair and rehabilitation therapy, p. 573; **Impaired physical mobility** related to musculoskeletal impairment and adjustment to new walking gait, p. 556 (useful for any patient with spinal or lower extremity injuries); "Rheumatoid Arthritis" for **Fatigue,** p. 563; "Ligamentous Injuries" for **Knowledge deficit:** Need for elevation of the extremity, use of thermotherapy, and prescribed exercise, p. 566; "Torn Anterior Cruciate Ligament" for **Knowledge deficit**: Use of postoperative cryotherapy with a commercial iced knee cuff and automatic ice slush circulator, p. 574 (useful for patients discharged after a recent fracture or surgery); **Knowledge deficit:** Care and assessment of the casted extremity, p. 567 (applies to any patient in a cast); "Repair of Recurrent Shoulder Dislocation" for **Risk for impaired skin integrity** related to trapping of moisture on the axillary skin, p. 610 (useful for any patient with moist areas trapped by a therapeutic device that is necessary to treat a fracture); "Total Hip Arthroplasty" for **Knowledge deficit:** Potential for and mechanism of total hip arthroplasty (THA) dislocation, p. 613 (for patients undergoing hemiarthroplasty for replacement of the femoral head); **Knowledge deficit:** Potential for infection caused by foreign body reaction to an endoprosthesis, p. 614 (useful for any patient with an internal fixation device, especially large devices); **Risk for peripheral neurovascular dysfunction,** p. 614 (can be adapted for any patient in traction); "Total Knee Arthroplasty" for **Risk for fluid volume deficit** related to postsurgical hemorrhage or hematoma formation, p. 617 (for patients with ORIF); Appendix One, "Caring for Preoperative and Postoperative Patients," p. 717; "Caring for Patients on Prolonged Bedrest," p. 738, for nursing diagnoses and interventions.

Specific nursing diagnoses for patients with casts, traction, ORIF, and external fixators

Fatigue related to the state of discomfort, reactive depression, psychoemotional demands, and effects of prolonged immobility

Desired outcome: Within 24 hr of admission, patient verbalizes reduction in fatigue.

• Assess when fatigue occurs, any relationship to required activities, and activities that aggravate or improve symptoms.

- Investigate patient's sleep pattern and intervene as appropriate to ensure adequate rest (see Appendix One, "Caring for Preoperative and Postoperative Patients" for **Sleep pattern disturbance**, p. 734). Discuss the need to avoid excess naps since these disrupt nighttime sleeping patterns. Encourage rest and naps for fatigue but discourage naps from boredom.
- Assess for dietary and physiologic (e.g., low Hgb and Hct) sources of fatigue, and correct as needed. Request a prescription for multivitamin and/or iron supplementation as indicated.
- Assess the patient's pain control, and intervene with pharmacologic and nonpharmacologic treatments as indicated to obtain adequate control and thus permit increasing activity.
- Assess for psychoemotional distress, and intervene as necessary or seek assistance from an appropriate clinical specialist in psychiatric nursing.
- Discuss the reason for a graded exercise regimen to increase endurance and strength (see Appendix One, "Caring for Preoperative and Postoperative Patients" for **Risk for activity intolerance**, p. 738; **Risk for disuse syndrome**, p. 740). Encourage the patient to set realistic goals, and post these goals to facilitate participation of associated health care providers.
- Pace activities, and intersperse rest periods of at least 90 min. Fatigue that lasts to the next exercise/activity period probably indicates excessive exercise/activity in the preceding period.
- Teach patient how to use adjunctive and assistive devices to minimize energy consumption.

NIC: Energy Management; Exercise Promotion; Mutual Goal Setting; Nutrition Management; Self-Care Assistance; Sleep Enhancement; Support System Enhancement; Teaching: Prescribed Activity/Exercise

Self-care deficit: bathing/hygiene, dressing/grooming, feeding, or toileting related to physical limitations secondary to cast or surgical procedure (applies to patients with casts, ORIF, external fixators, immobilizers, or orthotic devices) *Desired outcome:*   Within 48 hr of the surgical procedure or immobilizing device's application, patient demonstrates independence with ADL.
- For patients with insufficient strength to manipulate immobilized extremities to allow independence in self-care, incorporate a structured exercise regimen that will increase strength and endurance. Direct the regimen toward development of those muscle groups necessary for the patient's activity deficit. See the guidelines described in "Amputation" for **Risk for disuse syndrome,** p. 603; Appendix One, "Caring for Patients on Prolonged Bedrest" for **Risk for disuse syndrome** related to inactivity secondary to prolonged bedrest, p. 740.
- Use assistive devices liberally. These include stocking helpers, Velcro fasteners, enlarged handles on eating utensils, pickup sticks, raised toilet seats, and similar self-help devices.
- As appropriate, ask social services department of hospital for assistance with funding for purchasing assistive equipment or for home help.
- Because pain control is an essential element in enhancing self-care activities, ensure that the patient is as comfortable as possible (see "Osteoarthritis" for **Pain** related to joint changes and corrective therapy, p. 555; "Intervertebral Disk Disease" for **Health-seeking behavior:** Pain control measures, p. 251; "Torn Anterior Cruciate Ligament" for **Pain** related to surgical repair and rehabilitation therapy, p. 573).
- When needed, teach significant other how to assist patient with self-care.
- As appropriate, use adaptive clothing (e.g., garments with Velcro fasteners for easy removal and application) that is designed to accommodate the cast.

NIC: Bathing; Behavior Modification; Environmental Management; Fall Prevention; Mutual Goal Setting; Patient Contracting; Self-Care Assistance; Self-Responsibility Facilitation

Risk for impaired skin integrity and/or **impaired tissue integrity** with risk factors related to irritation and pressure secondary to the presence of a cast (applies to patients with casts, ORIF, immobilization devices, or CPM)
Desired outcomes: Patient relates the absence of discomfort under the cast or immobilization device and exhibits intact skin once the cast or immobilization device is removed. Within 8 hr of cast or immobilization device application, patient verbalizes knowledge about the indicators of pressure necrosis.

- When assisting with cast or immobilization device application, ensure that adequate padding is put on bony prominences of the affected extremity.
- While a cast is curing (drying), handle it only with the palms of the hands to avoid pressure points caused by finger indentations. Ensure that the cast surface is exposed to facilitate drying.
- Petal the edges of plaster casts with tape or moleskin to prevent cast crumbs from falling into the cast and causing pressure necrosis. Pad surfaces of immobilization devices or CPM machines that cause excessive pressure on underlying skin, that is, areas of erythema that do not clear within 5 min of removal of pressure.
- Instruct patient never to insert anything between the cast or immobilization device and skin. In the presence of severe itching, advise patient to notify health care practitioner, who may prescribe a medication (hydroxyzine) to relieve itching.
- Teach patient the indicators of pressure necrosis under the cast or immobilization device or areas in contact with the CPM device: pain, burning sensation, foul odor from cast opening, or drainage on the cast.

NIC: Cast Care: Maintenance; Circulatory Precautions; Incision Site Care; Perineal Care; Pressure Ulcer Prevention; Skin Surveillance; Splinting

Altered cerebral or cardiopulmonary tissue perfusion (or risk of same) related to interrupted arterial flow secondary to fat embolization (applies to patients with multiple trauma, multiple long bone or pelvic fractures, or surgical repair of these fractures)
Desired outcome: Patient has adequate cerebral and cardiopulmonary perfusion as evidenced by oximetry oxygen saturation $\geq 92\%$; Pao_2 ≥ 80 mm Hg, HR ≤ 100 bpm, RR ≤ 20 breaths/min, normothermia, normal skin color, absence of adventitious breath sounds over the tracheobronchial tree, absence of petechial rash, absence of inappropriate verbalizations indicating confusion, and orientation to time, place, and person.

- Ensure strict maintenance of fracture immobilization to help prevent embolization.
- Carefully monitor patient for the initial 72 hr after injury or surgery for indicators of fat embolism: tachycardia, tachypnea, profuse tracheobronchial secretions, pulmonary edema, chest pain, cyanosis, fever, petechial rash (involving the conjunctivae, trunk, neck, proximal arms, and axillae), anxiety, apprehension, progressive mental dysfunction (confusion, disorientation), and the presence of fat globules in the sputum or retina of the eye. The Hct may drop, serum lipase may rise, and fat may be noted on urinalysis. Frequent specimens for ABG levels should be drawn from patients at risk for fat embolus for the first 48 hr after injury because early hypoxemia that is indicative of fat embolism is apparent on laboratory measurement only. In addition, a platelet count indicative of thrombocytopenia ($<150,000/mm^3$) is diagnostic of fat embolism.
- Because fat embolism is a life-threatening emergency, notify health care practitioner immediately if any of the preceding occurs. Inform patient and significant other of these potential indicators so that they can notify the staff if they occur.
- As prescribed, perform respiratory support measures with oxygen and rigorous pulmonary hygiene. Intubation with ventilation using positive end expiratory pressure (PEEP) may be necessary. In general, all patients with

significant trauma and fractures should receive oxygen at 40% concentration via mask or 2-8 L/min via nasal prongs until the threat of fat embolism has been ruled out. Oximetry monitoring should be accomplished to ensure oxygen saturation ≥92%.

- Cardiovascular support may be provided through fluid resuscitation to correct hypovolemic shock while carefully monitoring for indications of pulmonary compromise. Decreased cardiac and urinary output may be combated with dopamine.
- Administer IV steroids, diuretics, and dextran as prescribed.

NIC: Cerebral Perfusion Promotion; Embolus Precautions; Fluid/Electrolyte Management; Neurologic Monitoring; Respiratory Monitoring; Temperature Regulation

Knowledge deficit: Potential for infection because of an open fracture or orthopedic procedure or presence of the internal or external device (appropriate for patients with open fractures, ORIF, or external fixators)
Desired outcome: Within 24 hr of instruction, patient verbalizes knowledge about the potential for infection, lists the indicators that may occur, and relates the significance of reporting them promptly.

- Advise patient about the potential for infection, which can occur as a result of the surgical procedure.
- Teach patient the following indicators of infection and the importance of reporting them to a health care professional promptly if they occur: persistent redness, swelling, increasing pain, wound drainage, local warmth, foul odor from within the cast, sensation of burning within the cast, drainage into the cast material or from the cast, and fever.
- Alert patients with internal fixation devices to the potential for infection for as long as the implant is present. Instruct them to report any of the preceding indicators promptly.

NIC: Infection Protection; Medication Management; Surveillance; Teaching: Disease Process; Wound Care: Closed Drainage

Knowledge deficit: Function of external fixation, pin care, and signs and symptoms of pin site infection
Desired outcomes: By at least 24 hr before hospital discharge, patient verbalizes knowledge about the rationale for the external fixator and demonstrates ways to adapt life-style to the fixator. Patient demonstrates knowledge of pin care and verbalizes knowledge of the indicators of infection at the pin sites.

- Teach patient the rationale for use of the fixator with type of fracture or injury, emphasizing benefits for the patient.
- Discuss ways in which the patient can adapt his or her life-style to accommodate the fixator (e.g., by wearing adaptive clothing that fits the device).
- Instruct patient and significant other in pin care as prescribed by health care practitioner. Some health care practitioners prescribe daily pin site care with hydrogen peroxide or skin preparation solutions, such as povidone-iodine. Some health care practitioners request that buildup of crusts from serous drainage be removed when cleansing pin sites, whereas others request that the crust be left intact to minimize the risk of infection. If prescribed, teach the patient how to apply antibacterial ointments and small dressings to the pin site. Some health care practitioners require that external fixator pins be cleansed with alcohol daily. **Note:** Literature supplied with some external fixators cautions against the use of iodine-based mixtures, which may cause corrosion of the device.
- Instruct patient and significant other to *avoid* using the external fixator as a handle or support for the extremity. Repeated use of the external fixator as a "handle" may lead to loosening of the skeletal pins. Teach them to support

the extremity with pillows, two hands, slings, and other devices as necessary to prevent excessive stress on the skeletal pins.

- Teach patient how to monitor the pin sites for indicators of infection, including persistent redness, swelling, drainage, increasing pain, temperature >38.3° C (101° F), and local warmth, and to be alert to pin migration or "tenting" of the skin on the pin, which can signal movement of the pin or infection. Instruct patient to report significant findings promptly to health care practitioner.
- If orthotics are added to the external fixator to prevent wristdrop, footdrop, or similar joint contractures, ensure that patient and/or significant other is aware of the purpose of the orthotic, knows to check for areas of excessive pressure, and knows the schedule for adjunctive and ROM exercises.
- Advise patient of the need for follow-up care to ensure that the device is functioning properly and for maintaining adequate immobilization of the fracture(s).

NIC: Infection Protection; Medication Management; Surveillance; Teaching: Procedure/Treatment; Wound Care

PATIENT-FAMILY TEACHING AND DISCHARGE PLANNING

When providing patient-family teaching, focus on sensory information; avoid giving excessive information; and initiate a visiting nurse referral for necessary follow-up teaching. Consider including verbal and written information about the following:

- Medications, including drug name, dosage, purpose, schedule, precautions, drug/drug and food/drug interactions, and potential side effects.
- Importance of elevation, use of thermotherapy, and prescribed exercise (see "Ligamentous Injuries," p. 566; "Torn Anterior Cruciate Ligament" for **Knowledge deficit:** Use of postoperative cryotherapy with a commercial iced knee cuff and automatic ice slush circulator, p. 574).
- Rationale for the individual's therapy after discharge and how that therapy will be accomplished (e.g., casting, external fixation, internal fixation).
- Precautions of therapy:
  —*Casts:* caring for the cast, monitoring neurovascular status of the distal extremity, watching for evidence of pressure necrosis beneath the cast, performing prescribed exercises, preventing skin maceration, and preventing disuse osteoporosis (see also **Knowledge deficit:** Care and assessment of the casted extremity, p. 567).
  —*Internal fixation devices:* caring for the wound, noting signs of wound infection, preventing refracture of the limb, performing prescribed exercises, and monitoring for delayed infection.
  —*External fixator:* demonstrating understanding of pin care, knowing when to notify health care practitioner of problems with the fixator, performing prescribed exercises, use of accompanying orthotics, monitoring neurovascular status of the limb, and monitoring pin site for indicators of infection.
- Ways in which patient can control discomfort (see "Intervertebral Disk Disease" for **Health-seeking behavior:** Pain control measures, p. 251).
- Use of assistive devices and ambulatory aids. Ensure that the patient can perform a return demonstration and is independent with devices and aids before hospital discharge (see "Osteoarthritis," p. 556). If needed, initiate a referral for a home visit early after discharge to ensure patient safety.
- Materials that are necessary for care at home and agencies that can supply materials.
- For patients who require home help, a collaborative effort between hospital nurses and community care agencies should be made to ensure continuity of care. The appropriate agency should see patient before hospital discharge.

- For patients who receive allograft bone for bone graft and who have questions about these grafts, resources for information include the following organizations:

  American Red Cross
  Tissue Services   (800) 847-7838
  WWW address: *http://quality.redcross.org/tissue*

  AlloSource
  8085 E. Harvard Ave.
  Denver, CO 80231   (800) 557-3587
  WWW address: *http://www.allosource.org*

Benign neoplasms

The three most common benign bone tumors are osteochondromas, enchondromas, and giant cell tumors. *Osteochondromas* (bony exostoses) are the most common, representing 45% of all benign tumors. Usually they are found in the metaphysis (wider portion of the shaft) of the long bones, typically the distal femur or proximal humerus, although they also can occur in a rib or vertebra. Individuals younger than 20 yr are most commonly affected. Some osteochondromas are the result of an inheritable autosomal dominant trait that causes concurrent growth retardation and bowing of the long bones. *Enchondromas* (chondromas) are most commonly found in the hand (metacarpals or phalanges) or the proximal humerus. They represent approximately 10% of all diagnosed benign tumors. Although they occur most commonly in people in their 30s, they may be seen at any time. *Giant cell tumors* are found most often around the proximal humerus, distal radius, sacrum, or the knee (most common) in the area of the fused epiphyseal growth plate in individuals 30-40 yr old. Giant cell tumors occur with a female/male ratio of 3:2. About 2% of these tumors degenerate into malignancy with a potential for metastasis. Giant cell tumors recur 40% of the time.

ASSESSMENT

Osteochondromas: Indicators arise from mechanical irritation of surrounding musculotendinous structures and include pain upon specific movements of the involved areas or from irritation.
Enchondromas: Local pain is often the presenting symptom. Unless the growth is in an area with little soft tissue, the growth usually is not palpable.
Giant cell tumors: Pain occurs before the mass becomes palpable.

DIAGNOSTIC TESTS

AP and lateral x-rays are most commonly used for preliminary diagnosis. Osteochondromas appear on x-ray as a bony stalk with a cartilaginous cap that arises from the metaphyseal area. Radiographic evidence of enchondroma includes a cystic, slightly expansive lesion of the shaft of a long bone with scalloping defect of the cortex but no evidence of new bone formation. Within the cystic lesion the x-ray appears speckled with calcified areas and shadows. Radiographic appearance is that of a cystic expansion of bone with an area of destruction that appears like a soap bubble with small amounts of reactive bone formation at the margins. CT scans, tomograms, contrast radiography, bone scans, and angiograms can be used to clarify the extent of the tumor. MRI may be useful in determining precise areas for surgical resection.

SURGICAL INTERVENTION

All three types of tumors are best treated with surgical removal. Resection can require allografting, prosthetic replacement, or use of methylmethacrylate to replace resected bone. When removal is impossible, curettage (scraping) of the lesion usually is done.

NURSING DIAGNOSES AND INTERVENTIONS

See "Osteoarthritis" for **Pain,** p. 555; "Fractures," p. 584, for nursing diagnoses as appropriate; Appendix One, "Caring for Preoperative and Postoperative Patients," p. 717, for nursing diagnoses and interventions.

PATIENT-FAMILY TEACHING AND DISCHARGE PLANNING

When providing patient-family teaching, focus on sensory information; avoid giving excessive information; and initiate a visiting nurse referral for necessary follow-up teaching. Consider including verbal and written information about the following:

- Description of the disease process.
- For patients having surgery, the indicators of wound infection (swelling, persistent redness, wound drainage, pain, local warmth, and fever) and the necessity of reporting these indicators promptly to health care practitioner.
- For patients with casts and orthotics, care of the extremity and immobilization device. For more information about casts, see **Knowledge deficit:** Care and assessment of the casted extremity, p. 567.
- Medications, including drug name, dosage, purpose, schedule, precautions, drug/drug and food/drug interactions, and potential side effects.
- Posthospitalization therapy and the importance of follow-up.
- For patients who receive allograft bone for bone graft and who have questions about these grafts, resources for information include the following organizations:

> American Red Cross
> Tissue Services   (800) 847-7838
> WWW address: *http://quality.redcross.org/tissue*

> AlloSource
> 8085 E. Harvard Ave.
> Denver, CO 80231   (800) 557-3587
> WWW address: *http://www.allosource.org*

Malignant neoplasms

The most common malignant tumors affecting bones are osteogenic sarcoma, primary chondrosarcoma, and myeloma. *Osteogenic sarcoma* is the most common true tumor originating from bone tissue, occurring most frequently in adolescents. It is found (in order of prevalence) in the distal femoral metaphysis, proximal tibial metaphysis, proximal humeral metaphysis, pelvis, and proximal femur. Most osteosarcomas become apparent during the time of a skeletal growth spurt, and these tumors occur more often in males than females (3:2). This tumor is associated with early metastasis to the lung, lymph involvement, and rapid death unless rigorous treatment is begun early in the disease process. The current survival rate following resection and adjunctive chemotherapy is 60%. Children treated with radiation or alkylating agents for other cancers have a greatly increased risk of developing osteosarcoma. *Chondrosarcomas* occur half as frequently as osteogenic sarcomas and usually are seen at ages 50-60 yr with twice as many males affected as females. Most of these tumors originate in the pelvic girdle, ribs, or shoulder girdle. Resection of all of the tumor results in an excellent 5-yr cure rate; however, inadequate resection frequently results in recurrence and late metastasis to the lung. *Myelomas* arise from bone marrow and thus are not truly bone tumors, but they are the most common malignant tumor that affects bones. The peak time of onset is the 60s and 70s age-groups. Myelomas can occur in any bone, although they are seen less frequently in smaller bones. Average survival after diagnosis is 1-2 yr.

ASSESSMENT

Osteogenic sarcomas: Pain, tenderness, limited ROM, and swelling near a joint. Night pain usually is more severe. A history of trauma is frequently noted.
Chondrosarcomas: Localized pain, rarely with a demonstrable mass.
Myelomas: Pain is the usual presenting symptom. Also, anemia, weight loss, tenderness, backache, or pathologic and spontaneous fracture may be present.

DIAGNOSTIC TESTS

Standard x-rays, CT scans, MRI, tomograms, and radioisotope (gallium) uptake tests: To delineate extent of the disease. X-ray evidence of osteogenic sarcoma usually involves a destructive bone lesion with a sunburstlike area of calcification and a periphery of periosteal new bone formation. Low-grade chondrosarcomas appear on x-ray as an expanded area of radiolucency with a central area of flocculent calcific density. High-grade chondrosarcomas may have an x-ray appearance similar to osteosarcomas. Myelomas present with radiologic evidence of areas of osteolysis with little or no reactive bone formation. MRI is useful in delineating the extent of cortical involvement and degree of medullary spread and may prove useful in identifying metastasis.

For myelomas
Standard blood and electrolyte tests: May reveal moderate normocytic anemia and a markedly elevated sedimentation rate. Serum calcium level and alkaline phosphatase usually are elevated, indicating bone turnover.
Bence Jones protein: Urine will be positive in 40% of patients with myeloma.
Bone marrow aspiration: May reveal plasma cells with large nuclei and nucleoli typical of myeloma.
Electrophoresis: Immunoelectrophoresis will show an abnormal amount of either immunoglobulin G (IgG) or immunoglobulin A (IgA) produced by the tumor cells. Serum protein electrophoresis will show a paraprotein, a hallmark of myeloma.

COLLABORATIVE MANAGEMENT

Osteogenic sarcoma: Treated with resection of the tumor, most commonly by amputation. Less radical resections (en bloc tumor resection with limb salvage procedures), including therapy with chemotherapeutic agents (especially methotrexate, leucovorin [Citrovorum], cyclophosphamide, vincristine, and adriamycin in various combinations), have resulted in longer survival rates.
Chondrosarcoma: Usually treated with resection; the degree of resection depends on the stage of tumor development. Radiotherapy and chemotherapy have not proven to be effective in treating this disease.
Multiple myeloma: Requires extensive therapy with radiation and chemotherapy. Radiation is used to control localized bone pain and treat areas with pathologic fractures. Chemotherapy with melphalan, prednisone, and vincristine has been shown to be helpful. Vincristine, doxorubicin, and dexamethasone may be useful in treating refractory cases of myeloma, which occur in as many as 50% of patients. Occasionally hypercalcemia requires additional therapy with increased volumes of IV fluids, furosemide, prednisone, or mithramycin. Laminectomy may be required for spinal cord compression caused by vertebral lesions. Pathologic fractures frequently require ORIF. Blood transfusions and

potent analgesics are usually required. Bone marrow transplantation has been used experimentally.

NURSING DIAGNOSES AND INTERVENTIONS

See "Intervertebral Disk Disease" for **Health-seeking behavior:** Pain control measures, p. 251; "Osteoarthritis" for **Pain,** p. 555; **Impaired physical mobility** related to musculoskeletal impairment and adjustment to new walking gait, p. 556; "Total Knee Arthroplasty" for **Risk for fluid volume deficit** related to postsurgical hemorrhage or hematoma formation, p. 617.

> Note: When postoperative casts, orthotics, exercises, or similar therapies are prescribed, refer to appropriate nursing diagnoses throughout this chapter. See "Amputation," p. 603, if the patient undergoes amputation; Appendix One, "Caring for Preoperative and Postoperative Patients," p. 717; "Caring for Patients on Prolonged Bedrest," p. 738; "Caring for Patients With Cancer and Other Life-disrupting Illnesses," p. 747, for nursing diagnoses and interventions.

PATIENT-FAMILY TEACHING AND DISCHARGE PLANNING

When providing patient-family teaching, focus on sensory information; avoid giving excessive information; and initiate a visiting nurse referral for necessary follow-up teaching. Consider including verbal and written information about the following:

- Medications, including drug name, rationale, dosage, schedule, precautions, drug/drug and food/drug interactions, and potential side effects.
- Phone numbers to call if questions or concerns arise about therapy or disease after discharge. In addition, many cities have local support groups. Information for these patients can be obtained by contacting the following organizations:

American Cancer Society
1599 Clifton Road NE
Atlanta, GA 30329   (800) ACS-2345
WWW address: *http://www.cancer.org*

National Cancer Institute Information Service (CIS)
Bldg. 31, Room 10A16
9000 Rockville Pike
Bethesda, MD 20892   (800) 422-6237
WWW address: *http://wwwicic.nic.nih.gov/*

- For surgical patients the following indicators of wound infection and the importance of notifying health care practitioner if they occur: persistent redness, swelling, local warmth, fever, discharge from the wound, or pain. As appropriate, see also "Ligamentous Injuries" for **Knowledge deficit:** Need for elevation of the involved extremity, use of thermotherapy, and prescribed exercise, p. 566; "Torn Anterior Cruciate Ligament" for **Knowledge deficit**: Use of postoperative cryotherapy with a commercial iced knee cuff and automatic ice slush circulator, p. 574.
- For patients with casts, orthotics, prosthetics, ambulatory aids, assistive devices, or similar therapies, instructions for their use, including a return demonstration by patient and a phone number to call if any questions arise after hospital discharge. See **Impaired physical mobility** related to adjustment to a new walking gait, p. 556; "Ligamentous Injuries" for **Knowledge deficit:** Care and assessment of the casted extremity, p. 567.
- Referral to hospice or agency that provides home help. This should occur before discharge planning begins to ensure continuity of care between the hospital and home or hospice.

- Phone numbers to call if questions or concerns arise about hospice after discharge. Information for these patients can be obtained by contacting the following organization:

  National Hospice Association
  1901 North Moore St., Suite 901
  Arlington, VA 22209   (703) 243-5900; (703) 525-5762 FAX
  WWW address: *http://www.hospice.org*

Osteoporosis

Osteoporosis is a condition in which the amount of bony mass/density decreases while the size of the bone remains constant, making bone more brittle and more susceptible to fractures. It is a major health problem in the United States, potentially affecting as many as 15-20 million Americans and causing more than 1 million fractures per year in people older than 45 yr. The risk of osteoporosis increases with age and is higher in females than in males. It is estimated that >50% of females in the United States older than 50 yr will experience an osteoporotic fracture.

ASSESSMENT

Signs and symptoms: Documented loss of bone density, most commonly found in conjunction with pathologic fractures secondary to osteoporosis. Most fractures occur in the dorsal (thoracic) and lumbar vertebral bodies (usually D8 through L2), the neck and intertrochanteric regions of the femur, and the distal radius. Vertebral compression fractures can develop gradually, resulting in loss of height, kyphosis (dowager's hump), back discomfort, and constipation. Severe chronic flexion of the vertebral column (kyphosis) may inhibit function of multiple organ systems. Fractures of the hip result in significant morbidity and mortality.

History and risk factors: Loss of ovarian function (surgical or physiologic menopause), race (non-African-American, especially white or Asiatic), family history, nulliparity, preexisting skeletal disease, underweight, inadequate childhood nutrition (lifelong low-calcium intake), high caffeine intake, sedentary life-style, high alcohol intake, increased protein intake, slender figure, and cigarette smoking. Secondary causes include some metastatic cancers, drugs (heparin, phosphate-binding antacids, corticosteroids, phenytoin, isoniazid), subtotal gastrectomy, hyperparathyroidism, immobilization, hypercortisolism, chronic renal disease, hyperthyroidism, hypogonadism, and connective tissue disease.

DIAGNOSTIC TESTS

Standard AP and lateral x-rays of the spine: Provide a diagnosis for osteoporotic fractures. Bone density loss is not easily demonstrated by standard radiographs, since 20%-30% of bone density must be lost before it can be noted on x-ray.

Radiogrammetry, photodensitometry, single- and dual-photon absorptiometry, neutron activation, quantitative digital radiography, and single- and dual-energy T-scan: These are some of the sophisticated noninvasive tests that can be used to determine bone density. However, the availability of these tests varies, and their usefulness in predicting fracture has been questioned. Bone mass/density measurement is indicated in individuals who are at risk.

Posture measurement: Measuring posture at the time of diagnosis will allow monitoring progress in therapy. A flexible ruler (e.g., the Flexicurve found in art supply stores) can be used to measure four parameters of posture: thoracic width and length and lumbar width and length. These parameters reflect relative kyphosis and lordosis and allow quantitative measurement of improvement following initiation of therapy.

COLLABORATIVE MANAGEMENT

Hormonal replacement: Estrogen doses as low as 0.625 mg or 2 mg of estradiol valerate have been shown to be effective in preventing osteoporosis in postmenopausal women. Estrogen may be given orally or by dermal patch, topical gel, implanted subcutaneous pellets, or vaginal pessary or creams. Once begun, estrogen replacement therapy must be used continually to provide protection. Use of cyclic estrogen/progesterone also may reduce the risk of endometrial cancer. Osteoporotic men may require testosterone replacement.

Calcium intake: Dietary intake should exceed 1000-1500 mg/day for women approaching menopause. Each 8-oz glass of milk provides 275-300 mg of calcium, indicating that an intake of 4-6 glasses/day is ideal. Vegetable calcium sources (e.g., dark green, leafy vegetables; sesame seeds) are also good. For lactose-intolerant patients or those unable to consume dietary calcium, calcium supplementation is prescribed. Some antacids (e.g., Tums) contain calcium and may serve as a calcium supplement. Calcium supplementation is associated with constipation and abdominal distention. In individuals prone to osteoporosis, lifelong intake of adequate amounts of calcium should be stressed. Adequate (1200 mg/day) calcium intake in adolescents is especially important to meet pubertal growth spurt. **Note:** Supplemental calcium in doses more than 1250 mg is suspected to bind dietary iron and result in iron deficiency anemia. Because smoking and a high-sugar, high-meat diet affect the phosphorus/calcium ratio, and therefore calcium utilization, individuals who do not smoke or eat red meat or sugar have a lower calcium requirement.

Vitamin D: Necessary to allow adequate intestinal absorption and usage of calcium. Adequate dietary vitamin D usually is supplied in vitamin-enriched cereals and milk products. When necessary, the recommended daily intake of this vitamin is 600-800 U twice daily. Because excessive vitamin D is associated with significant toxicity, higher intake is discouraged without clear documentation of need. Patients with liver or renal disease may require synthetic, biologically active vitamin D (ergocalciferol). Vitamin D requires activation in the skin by sunlight to be effective.

Moderate weight-bearing exercise: To stress bones and activate osteoblastic bone formation, because inactivity has been shown to result in disuse osteoporosis. Williams' back extension exercises, pectoral stretching, isometric abdominal exercises, and walking often are recommended. For older individuals, swimming appears to be the best all-around exercise, but this "no-load" exercise does little to stimulate bone growth. **Note:** Back flexion exercises are associated with increased risk of vertebral compression fractures and should be avoided. Women athletes who become hypogonadal lose bone despite high-intensity exercise.

Antiresorptive and other agents: To reduce further bone mass loss. Calcitonin acts directly on osteoclasts to reduce bone resorption. Dosage is 50-100 IU subcutaneously or intramuscularly every other day. A recently released nasal spray shows promise for use but has been associated with nasal membrane irritation. Anabolic steroids positively affect bone density, but masculinizing side effects are usually prohibitive. Diphosphonate etidronate (Didronel) to suppress osteoclastic function cycled with calcium and vitamin D supplementation may inhibit bone loss and foster increased bone density. Alendronate (Fosamax), a biphosphonate, is a new antiresorptive agent that shows promise in reducing bone loss. Fluoride is the only therapeutic agent known to stimulate osteoblastic activity. However, fluoride has not demonstrated the ability to restore the normal architecture of osteoporotic bone. Fluoride therapy must have accompanying calcium supplementation to prevent impaired bone mineralization. Thiazide diuretics reduce urinary calcium excretion and may reduce bone loss in patients with hypercalciuria.

NURSING DIAGNOSES AND INTERVENTIONS

Health-seeking behaviors: Prevention of osteoporosis, its treatment, and the importance of choosing and using calcium supplements effectively

Desired outcome: Within 48 hr of instruction, patient verbalizes knowledge about the disease process and understanding of the most effective calcium supplements and the way in which they are used.

> **Note:** It is important to begin instructing all individuals at risk for osteoporosis as early in their lives as possible because of the prolonged period of time involved in developing, and thus preventing, this process. Individuals at risk for osteoporosis include those with loss of ovarian function (surgical or physiologic menopause, women athletes), family history, nulliparity, preexisting skeletal disease, underweight, inadequate childhood nutrition (lifelong low-calcium intake), high caffeine intake, increased protein intake, sedentary life-style, slender figure, high alcohol intake, and cigarette smoking; whites; and Asians. The risk of osteoporosis increases with age and is higher in females than in males. Secondary causes include metastatic disease, drugs (heparin, alcohol, phosphate-binding antacids, corticosteroids, phenytoin, isoniazid), hyperparathyroidism, chronic renal disease, subtotal gastrectomy, immobilization, hypercortisolism, hyperthyroidism, hypogonadism, and connective tissue disease.

- Ensure that the health care practitioner has recommended or approves use of calcium supplements for the patient. Increased calcium can result in nephrolithiasis in susceptible individuals.
- Be sure patient is aware of the silent nature of this disorder and realizes that by the time symptoms arise, it is too late for effective treatment.
- Teach patient that calcium supplements come in many varieties. The most effective form is calcium carbonate, which delivers about 40% calcium. Bone meal and dolomite should be avoided because they may contain high amounts of lead or other toxic substances.
- Teach patient to look for the amount of elemental calcium available when evaluating supplement labels, rather than the weight of the total compound, and to avoid supplements with added vitamin D because hypervitaminosis of this vitamin is possible. Remind patients of the need for sunlight, 15 min/day, to allow activation of vitamin D.
- Teach patient not to take calcium and iron supplements simultaneously, because iron absorption will be impaired. Calcium also may reduce the absorption of some medications. Similarly, some foods inhibit absorption of calcium (e.g., red meats, spinach, colas, bran, bread, whole-grain cereals). Therefore calcium should be taken 2 hr before or after other medications or meals. Calcium is best absorbed at night and should be taken at hs.
- Caution patient to avoid taking more than 500-600 mg of calcium at one time and to spread doses over the entire day. Remind patient to drink a full glass of water with each supplement to minimize the risk of developing renal calculi.

NIC: Activity Therapy; Exercise Promotion; Nutrition Management; Risk Identification; Smoking Cessation Assistance; Teaching: Individual; Weight Management

Altered nutrition: Less than body requirements for calcium and vitamin D
Desired outcome: Patient demonstrates adequate intake of calcium and
vitamin D within the 24-hr period before hospital discharge and plans a 3-day
menu that provides sufficient intake of both.

- Ensure that the patient demonstrates understanding of foods high in calcium,
  including cheese, milk, dark green leafy vegetables, eggs, peanuts, sesame
  seeds, and oysters. Provide patient with a list of these foods, including the
  relative amounts of calcium in each.
- Teach patient how to plan menus that provide sufficient daily intake of
  calcium and vitamin D-fortified foods, such as eggs, halibut, herring, fortified
  dairy products, liver, mackerel, oysters, salmon, and sardines.
- Provide patient with sample menus that include adequate daily amounts of
  calcium and vitamin D. Have patient plan a 3-day menu that incorporates
  these foods.
- Provide patient with phone numbers to call if questions arise after hospital
  discharge.

NIC: Teaching: Disease Process; Teaching: Individual; Teaching: Prescribed Diet

PATIENT-FAMILY TEACHING AND DISCHARGE PLANNING

When providing patient-family teaching, focus on sensory information; avoid
giving excessive information; and initiate a visiting nurse referral for necessary
follow-up teaching. Consider including verbal and written information about
the following:

- Medications, including drug name, dosage, purpose, schedule, precautions,
  drug/drug and food/drug interactions, and potential side effects.
- Instructions for the prescribed dietary regimen, including the rationale for the
  diet and foods to include and avoid, if appropriate.
- Prescribed exercise regimen, including how to perform the exercise, number
  of repetitions of each, and frequency of exercise periods (see **Knowledge
  deficit:** Postsurgical exercise regimen, p. 566).
- Importance of establishing measures for preventing falls in the home (e.g.,
  placing a handrail in the bathtub, installing night lights, avoiding use of throw
  rugs). Arrange for a home visit for fall prevention as necessary.
- Importance of reporting to health care provider indicators of pathologic
  fracture (i.e., deformity, pain, edema, ecchymosis, limb shortening, false
  motion, decreased ROM, or crepitus). Stress promptly reporting indicators of
  vertebral fractures resulting in spinal cord or nerve compression (e.g.,
  paresthesias, weakness, paralysis, or loss of bowel or bladder function).
- Phone numbers to call if questions or concerns arise about therapy or disease
  after discharge. In addition, many cities have local osteoporosis support
  groups. Information for these patients can be obtained by contacting the
  following organizations:

National Osteoporosis Foundation, Chicago Office
c/o AMA
515 North State St.
Chicago, IL 60610   (312) 464-5110; (312) 464-5863 FAX
WWW address: *http://www.nof.org*

Osteoporosis and Related Bone Disease National Resource Center
National Institute of Arthritis & Musculoskeletal and Skin Diseases
1150 17th Street, NW
Suite 500
Washington, DC 20036   (202) 223-0344/2237; (800) 624-BONE
(Voice/FAX)
WWW address: *http://www.osteo.org*

Section Four: Musculoskeletal Surgical Procedures

Amputation

Today amputation is less frequently required as an orthopedic surgical intervention than it was before the advent of antibiotics and microsurgery techniques. However, amputation is still required for certain disorders, such as atherosclerotic arterial occlusive disease, complications of diabetes mellitus, osteomyelitis, severe trauma, malignant tumors, or congenital anomalies. In the United States, most amputations are performed for advanced atherosclerotic arterial occlusive disease, especially in individuals older than 60 yr with diabetes mellitus who have pronounced peripheral vascular disease, as evidenced by gangrene. When it is possible to increase a person's function with a prosthesis, amputation is sometimes offered as an optional treatment. The majority of amputations are of the lower extremity.

ASSESSMENT

Signs and symptoms: Patients with advanced atherosclerotic arterial occlusive disease may have gangrene, a chronic stasis ulcer, or an infected wound that fails to heal. The patient usually complains of pain, and there can be rubor (a dark red color) when the limb is dependent, as well as atrophy of the skin and subcutaneous tissues.

> **See Also:**   "Atherosclerotic Arterial Occlusive Disease," p. 116; "Osteomyelitis," p. 579; "Malignant Neoplasms," p. 595, as appropriate.

DIAGNOSTIC TESTS

Angiography: Confirms inadequacy of circulation to determine the appropriate level for amputation.
CT scan: Determines the degree of neoplastic or osteomyelitic involvement.
Biopsy: May be used to confirm presence of osteomyelitis or neoplasm.
Extensive evaluations by occupational therapist for fine motor function and by physical therapist for gross motor function: Document functional loss and potential for compensation.
Noninvasive vascular testing: Documents lack of perfusion of blood vessels using a Doppler ultrasound device and pneumatic cuffs. Doppler ultrasound is used to examine blood vessel waveforms. Plethysmography may be used to assess differing systolic pressures of the affected extremity to determine arterial flow. Thermography examines temperatures in the extremity to determine areas of decreased vascularity.
Xenon-133 studies: Skin clearance of this agent after intradermal injection is determined using a gamma camera and computer. Skin clearance reflects skin blood flow as a measure of the appropriate level of amputation.
Skin fluorescence: Measured with a fluorometer after IV injection of a fluorescein dye; useful in determining blood supply.
Oximetry: Transcutaneous determination of Pao_2 aids in determining levels of tissue perfusion. Levels >40 mm Hg usually support tissue healing.
Laboratory tests: Serum albumin <3.5 g/ml and a total lymphocyte count <1500 cells/mm^3 portend significant problems with healing.

COLLABORATIVE MANAGEMENT

Amputation: The procedure used for amputation depends on the area of the limb involved. Generally the surgical goals are to remove the least amount of tissue possible, provide adequate tissue for a viable myocutaneous flap to create a residual limb, and ensure adequate provision for a prosthetic device. Large blood vessels are individually identified and suture-ligated. Nerves are stretched and then suture-ligated to allow them to retract back into the residual limb (stump) to prevent trauma when the residual limb is used. Usually bone ends are beveled to prevent trauma from sharp edges. Infected limbs are closed loosely to allow adequate drainage until infected tissues have been treated adequately.

Persons with an amputation expend more energy in ambulation than persons without an amputation: 40% more energy in ambulation with a below-knee amputation (BKA) and 60% more energy with an above-knee amputation (AKA). Levels of lower extremity amputation include the following: ray (phalanges and metatarsal), transmetatarsal, hindfoot, ankle (Syme), below-knee, knee disarticulation and above-knee, hemipelvectomy, and translumbar (hemicorporectomy). En bloc resections for osteosarcoma allow for extensive procedures that replace the knee, such as the reversed ankle (rotationplasty), which allows for greater postoperative function. Upper extremity amputations include the following: ray (phalanges and metacarpal), transmetacarpal, below elbow (transradial), above elbow, and shoulder disarticulation.

Postoperative period: Immediately after surgery, an immediate postoperative prosthesis (IPOP) may be used to promote wound healing, minimize residual limb edema, decrease the length of rehabilitation, and prevent postsurgical complications of immobility. A cast is applied over the postoperative dressing, which incorporates a device that allows subsequent attachment of a pylon prosthesis to enable ambulation while the first prosthesis is being made. Plain casts or air splints may be applied to postoperative dressings to reduce edema. Patient-controlled analgesia facilitates early ambulation. Early ambulation prevents flexion contractures, allows earlier gait training, improves psychologic state, prevents loss of muscle strength, and increases local circulation to improve wound healing, which subsequently decreases edema and pain. Complications associated with amputations include infection and thromboembolism in the early postoperative period, increased mortality (fewer than 50% of all persons with lower extremity amputations survive 5 yr), fractures in the residual limb following falls, and residual limb ischemia.

NURSING DIAGNOSES AND INTERVENTIONS

Risk for disuse syndrome with risk factors related to severe pain and immobility secondary to amputation

Desired outcomes: Within 24 hr of instruction, patient verbalizes understanding about the exercise regimen and performs the exercises independently. Patient is free of symptoms of contracture formation as evidenced by complete ROM of the joints and maintenance of muscle mass.

- Control patient's pain to ensure appropriate movement.
- After providing elevation for the first 2 days postoperatively, intersperse elevation with periods of ROM to the remaining joints of the involved extremity. **Caution:** Both elevation and ROM are performed only if prescribed by health care practitioner. A residual limb with marginal vascular supply must not be elevated.
- Prevent flexion contractures of the knee and hip by assisting the patient with lying prone for 1 hr three times daily.
- Another method for preventing flexion contractures is to teach the patient to perform exercises that increase the strength of the muscle extensors. Consult health care practitioner about prescriptions for the following exercises:
  - *AKA:* have patient attempt to straighten the hip from a flexed position against resistance or perform gluteal setting exercises.
  - *BKA:* have patient attempt to straighten the knee against resistance or perform quadriceps-setting exercises. These patients also should perform the exercises just described for AKA.
    - For other interventions, see **Risk for disuse syndrome,** p. 740, in Appendix One.

◎ NIC: Analgesic Administration; Coping Enhancement; Pain Management; Teaching: Prescribed Activity/Exercise; Teaching: Procedure/Treatment; Teaching: Psychomotor Skill

Knowledge deficit: Care of the residual limb and prosthesis; signs and symptoms of skin irritation or pressure necrosis
Desired outcomes: Within the 24-hr period before hospital discharge, patient verbalizes knowledge about the care of the residual limb and prosthesis and independently returns demonstration of wrapping the residual limb. Patient verbalizes knowledge about the indicators of pressure necrosis and irritation from the wrapping device or prosthesis.

> Note: A residual limb that is inappropriately treated will become edematous and more prone to injury, which will delay proper fitting of the permanent prosthesis.

- For the first 24-48 hr the residual limb is elevated to reduce edema formation (for cautions to observe with elevation, see also **Risk for disuse syndrome**, p. 603). After this period, lower limbs are usually not elevated to prevent hip flexion contractures. When the patient is up in a chair, it is usually advisable to elevate lower residual limbs to reduce dependent edema.
- If molding of the residual limb for eventual prosthetic fitting is prescribed, instruct the patient in the technique for application of an elastic sleeve or wrap: application of the elastic wrap is begun with a recurrent turn over the distal end of the residual limb, and then diagonal circumferential turns are made, overlapping one-half to two-thirds the width of the wrap. Traction applied to the wrap should ensure more pressure on the distal portion of the residual limb. The elastic device should be snug but not excessively so, because a tight wrap can impede circulation and healing. Rewrapping should be performed q4hr, combined with careful inspection of the residual limb. Areas prone to pressure, such as bony prominences or prominent tendons, should be assessed for evidence of excess pressure. Ensure that all tissue is contained by the elastic device. If any tissue is allowed to bulge, proper fitting of the prosthesis will be difficult.
- Teach patient to monitor the residual limb for indicators of skin irritation or pressure necrosis caused by the elastic device or prosthesis, including blebs, abrasions, and erythemic or tender areas. Explain that if erythema persists after massage, the patient should seek the help of the public health nurse or visiting nurse or notify the health care practitioner.
- For areas that are susceptible to pressure, provide extra padding with sheet wadding, moleskin, or lamb's wool to prevent irritation.
- The day after the sutures have been removed (and assuming the incision is dry and intact), instruct the patient to cleanse the residual limb daily with mild soap and water. Caution against the use of emollients, which can create skin maceration beneath the prosthesis.
- Advise patient that when molding is no longer necessary (after 1-6 mo), he or she will be fitted with a residual limb sock that will allow air to circulate around the residual limb.
- Ensure that the patient receives complete instructions in care of the prosthesis by the certified prosthetist-orthotist or knowledgeable nurse.

◎ NIC: Circulatory Care; Exercise Therapy: Joint Mobility; Pain Management; Pressure Ulcer Prevention; Teaching: Prescribed Activity/Exercise; Teaching: Procedure/Treatment

Pain related to phantom limb sensation
Desired outcomes: Within 24 hr of intervention (s), patient relates a reduction in phantom limb sensations as documented by a pain scale. Objective indicators are absent or diminished.

- Explain to patient that continued sensations often arise from the amputated part and they can be painful, irritating, or simply disconcerting. As appropriate, devise a pain scale with patient, rating discomfort on a scale of 0 (no pain) to 10 (worst pain).
- Instruct patient in the basis for pharmacologic interventions. β-Blockers may be used to control dull, constant aching by increasing central and peripheral nervous system serotonin level. Anticonvulsant agents may be used to treat severe lancinating (sharply cutting or tearing) pain by decreasing neuronal excitability. Tricyclic antidepressants may be used to elevate the mood of the person with an amputation. Local anesthetics may be used in trigger zones on the contralateral limb. β-Blockers and sodium channel blockers have also been used to treat phantom limb pain.
- Manage these painful sensations with the interventions discussed in "Osteoarthritis" for **Pain,** p. 555. For this type of pain, counterirritation is especially useful. Other phantom limb sensations may respond to similar tactics, such as distraction, guided imagery, relaxation, biofeedback, psychotherapy, behavior modification, hypnosis, whirlpool, ultrasound, reciprocal motion (cycling), or use of cutaneous stimulation via oil of wintergreen, heat, acupressure, or massage. Transcutaneous electrical nerve stimulation (TENS) has been found to be especially effective in managing phantom limb sensation.
- Some health care practitioners advocate vigorous stimulation of the end of the residual limb to alter the feedback loop of the resected nerve. Advise patient that this can be accomplished by hitting the end of a *well-healed* residual limb with a rolled towel.
- Chronic phantom limb sensation may require exploration of the residual limb to resect a neuroma at the site of the nerve resection. Inform patient that this may be a possibility if phantom limb sensation continues for more than 6 mo. Use of epidural anesthesia in the perioperative period shows promise in reducing phantom limb pain.
- For additional interventions, see **Pain,** p. 719, in Appendix One, "Caring for Preoperative and Postoperative Patients."

NIC: Analgesic Administration; Biofeedback; Cutaneous Stimulation; Distraction; Heat/Cold Application; Meditation; Music Therapy; Simple Guided Imagery; Simple Massage; Sleep Enhancement

Body image disturbance *and/or* **altered role performance** related to loss of limb
Desired outcome: Within 72 hr of surgery, patient begins to show adaptation toward loss of the limb and demonstrates role-related responsibilities.

- Be aware that use of a prosthesis immediately after surgery allows patients to continue to perceive themselves as ambulatory (and thus "whole") individuals.
- Gently encourage patient to look at and touch the residual limb and verbalize feelings about the amputation. The nurse and other caregivers must show an accepting attitude, as well as encourage significant other to accept the patient as he or she now appears. Provide privacy for the patient and significant other to express their grief.
- Assist patient with adapting to the loss of the limb while maintaining a sense of what is perceived as the normal self. This may be accomplished by introducing patient to others who have successfully adapted to a similar amputation. In addition, teaching aids, such as audiovisuals, books, pamphlets, and videotapes, can be used to demonstrate how others have adapted to the amputation.
- For patients who continue to have difficulty adapting to the amputation, provide a referral to an appropriate resource person, such as a psychologist or psychiatric nurse.

- For additional interventions, see **Body image disturbance,** p. 799, in Appendix One, "Caring for Preoperative and Postoperative Patients."

NIC: Active Listening; Amputation Care; Anticipatory Guidance; Body Image Enhancement; Coping Enhancement; Counseling; Grief Work Facilitation

> **See Also:** Appendix One, "Caring for Preoperative and Postoperative Patients" for **Risk for fluid volume deficit:** Postoperative bleeding/hemorrhage, p. 721; "Intervertebral Disk Disease" for **Health-seeking behavior:** Pain control measures, p. 251; "Osteoarthritis" for **Pain,** p. 555; "Fractures" for **Knowledge deficit:** Potential for infection, p. 592; Appendix One, "Caring for Preoperative and Postoperative Patients," p. 717; "Caring for Patients With Cancer and Other Life-disrupting Illnesses," p. 747, for nursing diagnoses and interventions.

PATIENT-FAMILY TEACHING AND DISCHARGE PLANNING

When providing patient-family teaching, focus on sensory information; avoid giving excessive information; and initiate a visiting nurse referral for necessary follow-up teaching. Consider including verbal and written information about the following:

- How and where to purchase necessary supplies and equipment for self-care.
- Care of the residual limb and prosthesis.
- Indicators of wound infection that necessitate medical attention: swelling, persistent redness, discharge, local warmth, systemic fever, and pain. Suggest the use of a small hand mirror, if necessary, to examine the incision and residual limb.
- Medications, including drug name, rationale, dosage, schedule, precautions, drug/drug and food/drug interactions, and potential side effects.
- Phone numbers to call if questions or concerns arise about therapy or adaptation after discharge. In addition, many cities have local support groups. Information for these patients can be obtained by contacting the following organization:

  National Amputation Foundation
  73 Church St.
  Malverne, NY 11565   (518) 887-3600; (516) 887-3667 FAX
  WWW address: *http://www.social.com/health/nhic/data/hr0300/hr0359*

- Prescribed exercise regimen, including rationale for each exercise, number of repetitions for each, and frequency of the exercise periods. Be sure patient independently demonstrates understanding of the exercises and gives a return demonstration before hospital discharge.
- Referral to appropriate resource person if grieving or body image disturbance continues.
- Ambulation with assistive device and prosthesis on level and uneven surfaces and on stairs. Patient should demonstrate independence before hospital discharge. For patients with an upper extremity amputation, independence with ADL should be demonstrated before discharge. If necessary, arrange for a follow-up home visit.

Tendon transfer

A tendon transfer involves the transference of the insertion site of a functioning musculotendinous unit to a new position to change the action of that unit. This enables compensation for a deficit created by a congenital defect or paralyzed or severed muscle. Because there is considerable overlap in function, in that multiple muscles can serve one purpose, tendon transfer may allow the patient to regain function.

DIAGNOSTIC TESTS

Electromyography: Can be used to ensure adequate muscle function of the units proposed for transfer.

Dynmography: Grip or pinch strength may be assessed preoperatively or postoperatively.

COLLABORATIVE MANAGEMENT

Surgical procedure: Involves transection of the tendon at an appropriate level, transfer to the new position, and fixation to the appropriate insertion site with permanent sutures, staples, screws, or wire. It also is possible to attach "new" tendon to the resected tendon above the insertion site, using tendon repair suture techniques. Examples of disorders in which tendon transfer procedures are performed include radial nerve paralysis, congenital talipes equinovarus (a form of clubfoot), thumb carpometacarpal joint osteoarthritis, and extensive injury to the extensor pollicis longus that limits thumb extension.

Postsurgical immobilization: Immobilization of the operant area in a cast, splint, or orthosis until there has been sufficient healing of the tendon repair (2-6 wk) or stabilization of the bony insertion (4-12 wk).

Physical therapy (PT) regimen: After immobilization, the patient begins an intense, progressive PT regimen to regain strength in the transferred tendon, retrain new muscle function, and compensate for decreased strength at the site of the transfer. Various orthotics, dynamic splints, and special exercise rigs can be constructed to aid the patient in regaining function.

NURSING DIAGNOSES AND INTERVENTIONS

See "Osteoarthritis" for **Pain,** p. 555; **Impaired physical mobility** related to musculoskeletal impairment and adjustment to new walking gait, p. 556; "Ligamentous Injuries" for **Knowledge deficit:** Care and assessment of the casted extremity, p. 567; "Total Knee Arthroplasty" for **Risk for fluid volume deficit** related to postsurgical hemorrhage or hematoma formation, p. 617; "Fractures" for **Self-care deficit,** p. 590; Appendix One, "Caring for Preoperative and Postoperative Patients," p. 717; "Caring for the Patient on Prolonged Bedrest," p. 738, for nursing diagnoses and interventions.

PATIENT-FAMILY TEACHING AND DISCHARGE PLANNING

When providing patient-family teaching, focus on sensory information; avoid giving excessive information; and initiate a visiting nurse referral for necessary follow-up teaching. Consider including verbal and written information about the following:

- Use of therapies such as thermotherapy and elevation (see "Ligamentous Injuries," p. 566; "Torn Anterior Cruciate Ligament" for **Knowledge deficit**: Use of postoperative cryotherapy with a commercial iced knee cuff and automatic ice slush circulator, p. 574).
- Use of external support devices, such as elastic wraps, splints, orthotics, or similar items (see "Ligamentous Injuries," p. 568). This should include care of the device, care of the skin beneath the device, monitoring the area for presence of irritation, and monitoring for neurovascular deficit.
- Cast care instructions if patient is discharged with a cast (see "Ligamentous Injuries," p. 567).
- Prescribed exercise regimen, including rationale for each exercise, method of performing the exercise, number of repetitions for each, and frequency of the exercise periods (see "Ligamentous Injuries," p. 566). Be sure the patient can return the demonstration independently before hospital discharge.

- Medications, including drug name, rationale, dosage, schedule, precautions, drug/drug and food/drug interactions, and potential side effects.
- Indicators of wound infection that necessitate medical attention: persistent redness, swelling, wound discharge, local warmth, and increase in pain.
- Use of ambulatory aid if patient is discharged with one (see "Osteoarthritis," p. 556). This should include return demonstration of independence with ambulation on level and uneven surfaces and stairs before discharge.
- Phone number of resource person if questions arise after patient has been discharged.

Bone grafting

A bone graft procedure refers to the transfer of cancellous and cortical bone from one site to another. The bone can be from the patient (autogenic), another human (homogenic), or another species (heterogenic or xenogeneic). Currently, the most successful results are achieved with autogenic grafts, but homogenic grafting (using donated cadaver bone) is showing increasing promise as a therapeutic resource. Bone grafts can be required to create bony fusion of a joint (arthrodesis), compensate for lost or inadequately developed bone, or correct bony nonunion of fractures. Fibrin sealant has been used to aid in securing bone grafts and controlling bleeding, especially in patients with hemorrhagic disorders.

Current microsurgical techniques permit myocutaneous-bone or muscle-bone grafts that include bone, overlying muscle, and/or skin. These complex grafting procedures increase the potential for success of the graft in procedures used to rebuild large areas of tissue loss from trauma or necessary surgical resection. The following discussion focuses on traditional, simple autogenic bone grafting procedures.

DIAGNOSTIC TESTS

The need for bone grafts can be documented by the following: AP x-rays, gallium scans (to rule out osteomyelitis), and angiograms to evaluate blood supply when myocutaneous-bone or muscle-bone grafts are to be done.

COLLABORATIVE MANAGEMENT

Bone graft procedure: Most commonly, bone grafts are taken from the anterior or posterior iliac crest. However, bone grafts also can be harvested from the fibula, tibia, or ribs. The graft usually involves resection of a piece of cortical bone that is fashioned to replace the deficit, enhance bony fusion, or aid internal fixation. Usually cancellous bone is taken from the same site and packed in and around the cortical graft to facilitate new bone formation. The donor site frequently oozes blood, so a postoperative drain is often placed.

Postoperative regimen: Usually the recipient site requires immobilization (most often with a cast) to prevent dislodging of the graft. Some bone grafts require internal fixation to hold them in place. A closed drainage system frequently is used at the donor site.

NURSING DIAGNOSES AND INTERVENTIONS

See "Osteoarthritis" for **Pain,** p. 555; **Impaired physical mobility** related to musculoskeletal impairment and adjustment to new walking gait, p. 556; "Ligamentous Injuries" for **Knowledge deficit:** Care and assessment of the casted extremity, p. 567; "Total Knee Arthroplasty" for **Risk for fluid volume deficit** related to postsurgical hemorrhage or hematoma formation, p. 617; Appendix One, "Caring for Preoperative and Postoperative Patients," p. 717; "Caring for the Patient on Prolonged Bedrest," p. 738, for nursing diagnoses and interventions.

PATIENT-FAMILY TEACHING AND DISCHARGE PLANNING

Patients who receive allograft bone for bone graft and who have questions about these grafts should contact the following organizations:

American Red Cross
Tissue Services   (800) 847-7838
WWW address: *http://quality.redcross.org/tissue*

AlloSource
8085 E. Harvard Ave.
Denver, CO 80231   (800) 557-3587
WWW address: *http://www.allosource.org*

See Also: "Tendon Transfer," p. 607.

Repair of recurrent shoulder dislocation

The shoulder is a complex set of joints including the glenohumeral, sternoclavicular, acromioclavicular, and thoracoscapular joints, all of which act in combination to allow function. Of these joints, the glenohumeral joint is most commonly affected by dislocation. Most glenohumeral dislocations originate with trauma, usually a fall. During a fall the person instinctively lifts the arm (abducts it) and externally rotates it to protect the body. Force transmitted along the axis of the humerus pushes the humeral head out of the glenoid cavity, frequently tearing or stretching the glenoid labrum, supporting ligaments, and joint capsule to allow anterior dislocation. Anterior shoulder dislocation is the most common shoulder dislocation. Once periarticular weakness and laxity are established, the shoulder can dislocate with minimal stress during abduction, such as serving tennis balls, swimming, throwing, or gymnastic activity. Traditional therapy for initial traumatic anterior dislocation involved immobilization, supervised rehabilitation, and gradual return to full activity. However, recurrent dislocation following traditional therapy frequently occurred. Research by Arciero et al (1994) demonstrated the effectiveness of early arthroscopic repair to reduce recurrent dislocations. Otherwise, shoulder repair is indicated when the patient has significant pain and compromised function.

See Also: "Dislocation/Subluxation," p. 569, for a discussion of assessment, diagnostic tests, and collaborative management.

COLLABORATIVE MANAGEMENT

Bristow procedure: Transfers the short ends of the biceps and coracobrachialis muscular origin sites from the coracoid process to the scapular neck. The new positions allow these muscles to hold the head of the humerus in its anatomic position within the glenoid cavity.
Bankart procedure: Reattaches the anterior joint capsule to the front rim of the glenoid cavity to reduce laxity and prevent anterior dislocation.
Putti-Platt procedure: Reefs (shortens) the subscapularis tendon to prevent excessive lateral rotation, which can contribute to dislocation.
Postoperative care: Surgery may be performed arthroscopically or via traditional open methods. Arthroscopic laser surgery may facilitate resection, incisions, and cautery. Internal fixation devices may be used, including staples, screws, special sutures and suture anchors, and/or biodegradable tacks. Bupivacaine may be injected into periarticular tissues at the end of the procedure to reduce immediate postoperative pain. For some other shoulder surgeries, such as rotator cuff repair, a continuous passive movement (CPM)

device may be used to facilitate postoperative rehabilitation (for information on use of a CPM, see "Total Knee Arthroplasty" for **Risk for impaired skin integrity,** p. 618). Cryotherapy may be used in the immediate postoperative period to reduce edema formation and pain (see "Torn Anterior Cruciate Ligament" for **Knowledge deficit:** Use of postoperative cryotherapy with a commercial iced knee cuff and automatic ice slush circulator, p. 574, for information on nursing care of patients using a commercial iced knee cuff with automatic slush circulator). A shoulder immobilizer is usually used for 3-6 wk with no motion of the shoulder permitted until adequate healing has occurred. If the patient has large shoulder muscles, a postoperative drain may be required. Elbow flexion and extension, forearm pronation and supination, and hand exercises with putty or a soft ball are begun immediately after surgery. After immobilization, a regimen of progressive shoulder ROM and pendulum exercises is begun, first to regain ROM and then to increase muscle strength. Orthotics may be used to permit motion in specific planes or limit motion in multiple planes.

NURSING DIAGNOSES AND INTERVENTIONS

Risk for impaired skin integrity with risk factors related to trapping of moisture on the axillary skin secondary to shoulder immobilization
Desired outcomes: Patient's skin remains dry, nonerythematous, and intact. Before hospital discharge, patient verbalizes knowledge of the established plan of prevention and the signs and symptoms of maceration.

- Assess patient's axillary skin before surgery to evaluate the potential for breakdown, including open wounds, areas of irritation, and excessive perspiration.
- Teach patient the rationale and interventions used for preventing breakdown and the need to report indicators such as pain, burning, irritation, and foul odor.
- Cleanse the axilla well before surgery.
- Before the shoulder immobilizer is positioned, the operating room nurse will place a cotton pad in the axilla. After 2-3 days, remove the pad. Then cleanse, dry thoroughly, and inspect the axilla (as well as possible) without abducting the shoulder. Usually this can be done by holding a washcloth dampened in alcohol and sliding the washcloth back and forth through the axilla. Talc or cornstarch should be used judiciously because of buildup and creation of a reservoir for moisture. Replace the cotton pad with a new one, and document the condition of the skin. A deodorant pad may be used if the patient is not allergic.

NIC: Bathing; Incision Site Care; Skin Care: Topical Treatments; Skin Surveillance

Risk for peripheral neurovascular dysfunction with risk factors related to interrupted arterial flow to and compression of a musculocutaneous nerve secondary to pressure from the immobilization device
Desired outcomes: Patient has adequate peripheral neurovascular function in the operant arm as evidenced by the ability to contract the biceps muscle, presence of normal sensations along the radial portion of the forearm, brisk capillary refill (<2 sec or consistent with preoperative assessment), adequate pulses (>2+ on a 0-4+ scale), normal color, and warmth in the distal extremity. Within 8 hr of the instruction, patient verbalizes knowledge about the signs and symptoms of impaired neurovascular function and the importance of notifying the staff promptly if they occur.

- Unless it is contraindicated, encourage flexion and extension of the fingers and wrist to enhance perfusion to the distal tissues.
- Monitor the wrist and upper arm for evidence of pressure and irritation from the immobilizer. Be aware, however, that the device must be sufficiently tight to ensure adequate immobilization.

- With every VS assessment, evaluate upper extremity neurovascular function. Be especially alert to patient's inability to contract the biceps muscle and to absent or abnormal sensations along the radial portion of the forearm. Notify health care practitioner of significant findings.
- Instruct patient to notify the staff promptly if any alterations in sensory or motor function occur.

NIC: Circulatory Precautions; Exercise Therapy: Joint Mobility; Peripheral Sensation Management; Skin Surveillance; Teaching: Disease Process; Teaching: Prescribed Activity/Exercise

---

See Also: "Osteoarthritis" for **Pain,** p. 555; "Fractures" for **Self-care deficit,** p. 590; Appendix One, "Caring for Preoperative and Postoperative Patients," p. 717, for nursing diagnoses and interventions.

PATIENT-FAMILY TEACHING AND DISCHARGE PLANNING

When providing patient-family teaching, focus on sensory information; avoid giving excessive information; and initiate a visiting nurse referral for necessary follow-up teaching. Consider including verbal and written information about the following:

- Prescribed exercise regimen, including rationale for each exercise, method of performing the exercise, number of repetitions for each, and frequency of the exercise periods (see "Ligamentous Injuries," p. 566). Be sure the patient can return the demonstration independently before hospital discharge.
- Indicators of wound infection that necessitate medical attention: swelling, persistent redness, local warmth, fever, and pain.
- For patients discharged with brace or immobilizer, use and care of the device and care of the axilla on the operant side.
- Indicators of neurovascular deficit: decreasing sensation, paresthesias, weakness or paralysis, coolness, pallor, cyanosis, decreased pulses, delayed capillary refill, and increasing pain in the distal extremity.
- Medications, including drug name, rationale, dosage, schedule, precautions, drug/drug and food/drug interactions, and potential side effects.
- Phone number of a resource person if questions arise after hospital discharge.

Total hip arthroplasty

Total hip arthroplasty (THA) is surgery involving resection of the hip joint and its replacement with an endoprosthesis. Conditions resulting in the need for a THA include, among others, osteoarthritis, rheumatoid arthritis, ankylosing spondylosis (Marie-Strumpell disease), Legg-Calvé-Perthes disease, avascular necrosis, traumatic arthritis, benign and malignant bone tumors, and severe hip trauma. Usually, THA is restricted to older patients because the duration of the implant life is unknown. However, younger patients with severe disease also undergo this procedure. In addition, advanced age alone is not a contraindication for THA, since poor outcomes appear to be more related to co-morbidities than to advanced age alone.

The bipolar or universal endoprosthesis is an intermediary step between replacement of just the femoral head and a complete THA. For this device a polyethylene-lined metal cup fits over the femoral component. Articulation occurs between the femoral component and the inside of the metal cup and between the outside of the metal cup and the anatomic acetabulum. The advantages of this system are that it reduces wear on the acetabulum and allows ease in converting the joint to a THA later. Porous, roughened, and calcium phosphate ceramic implant surfaces have been designed to improve implantation fixation; however, long-term efficacy has not been established. Robotic procedures are undergoing clinical trials to determine their efficacy in providing more precise component manufacture and placement.

THA is performed when the joint has been severely affected by disease, resulting in significant pain and a dysfunctional femoroacetabular articulation. Because it is an irreversible procedure involving the removal of significant amounts of bone, several conditions should be met before the patient is considered a serious candidate. In addition to severe pain and loss of function, conservative therapies need to have been exhausted and the patient should have adhered to past therapeutic regimens and should be free of any concurrent infectious process. Complications of THA include aseptic loosening of the implant (most frequent), recurrent dislocations, osteolysis, disabling pain, and sepsis. Of these, infection is the most serious and eventually may necessitate removal of the prosthesis, with resultant flail joint and severe limb shortening. Risk factors for implant infection include rheumatoid arthritis, diabetes mellitus, urinary tract infection (UTI), pneumonia, tuberculosis, avascular necrosis, sickle cell disease, obesity, hematoma, seroma, acute dislocation, reoperation, and protein malnutrition.

DIAGNOSTIC TESTS

Gallium scan and erythrocyte sedimentation rate: May be indicated to rule out concurrent infection.

Scintigraphy: Can be used to document leg length discrepancy, which can be surgically compensated for by using alternative neck lengths on the femoral prosthesis.

COLLABORATIVE MANAGEMENT

Surgical procedure: Although the surgical procedure for THA can be accomplished via a variety of approaches, it is most commonly done through a posterolateral approach. Methylmethacrylate may be used as a grouting agent to hold the endoprosthesis in place, or special prosthetics coated with porous materials may be used to allow bony ingrowth to fix the device internally. Once the prosthetic acetabulum is positioned, the femoral canal is reamed to accept the femoral prosthesis. A drain is then inserted into the deeper layers of the wound.

Antibiotics: Because the potential for infection is increased with the presence of the massive endoprosthesis, the patient is given prophylactic antibiotics before, during, and for at least 3-5 days after surgery. Infection of the THA may require its temporary or permanent removal.

Blood replacement: Because of significant blood loss from THA and total knee replacement procedures and the perceived dangers of bloodborne disease transmission from the general blood pool (e.g., HIV, hepatitis, cytomegalovirus, Epstein-Barr virus, syphilis, malaria), blood transfusion has become an issue of concern. Autologous transfusion of the patient's own previously banked blood is being used with increasing frequency. Family members with appropriate blood types may also specifically donate blood. Blood salvage during and after joint replacement arthroplasty has also been used. During surgery, lost blood is salvaged by suctioning it from the sterile field to a cell saver machine. The cell saver washes and filters the blood, spins it down into packed RBCs, and allows return to the patient in 225-ml increments. Postoperative collection is accomplished via drain tubes that empty through a 40-μm filter into a 400-ml blood salvage canister. Blood collection is limited to 6 hr before reinfusion, and a citrate anticoagulant is added to each canister (a minimum of 320 ml of blood is needed to allow transfusion without risk of citrate poisoning). Present research is exploring the ability to salvage blood without citrate and allow reinfusion of smaller amounts of lost blood.

Postsurgical immobilization: The patient is commonly immobilized in balanced suspension or a similar device (A-frame, abduction pillow, or wedge abduction pillow) to prevent internal rotation, adduction, and flexion past 90 degrees, which can cause dislocation of the endoprosthesis. If methyl-methacrylate is used, the patient will be more quickly mobile (usually within 2 days) with weight bearing as tolerated because of the immediate fixation of the device. If a porous-coated device is used, it is not immediately fixed in place and the patient may require longer immobilization (several days) and restricted weight bearing. If the greater trochanter was removed to allow visualization or correct muscle weakness, it will require wiring, longer immobilization (sometimes as long as 1-3 wk in balanced suspension), and/or limited weight-bearing and abduction exercises for several weeks.

Antithrombus regimen: Because of increased risk of deep vein thrombosis (DVT), THA patients are given anticoagulant therapy (heparin, low-molecular-weight heparin, or warfarin) or antiplatelet agents (dextran), antiembolism hose, intermittent pneumatic compression device, venous foot pump compression device, calf pumping exercises and ankle circles, early ambulation, and close monitoring for assessments of DVT. (See also Appendix One, "Caring for Preoperative and Postoperative Patients" for **Altered peripheral tissue perfusion,** p. 742.)

Progressive physical therapy: To regain muscular strength and to ensure that the patient has adequate upper extremity strength to allow ambulation. The patient must be reminded to avoid internal rotation, adduction, and flexion of the hip past 90 degrees. Exercises begin with early active range of motion with assistance, transfer from bed to chair, sitting in the proper position (i.e., without violating the 90-degree hip flexion restriction), standing with the prescribed amount of weight bearing, and ambulation with assistance using a walker, crutches, and, eventually, a cane.

NURSING DIAGNOSES AND INTERVENTIONS

Knowledge deficit: Potential for and mechanism of THA dislocation, preventive measures, positional restrictions, prescribed ambulation regimen, potential for loosening, and use of assistive devices

Desired outcome: At least 24 hr before hospital discharge, patient verbalizes knowledge about the potential for, preventive measures for, and mechanism of THA dislocation and the indicators of implant loosening and demonstrates the prescribed regimen for ambulation and performance of ADL without experiencing dislocation.

Note: There is a high risk of dislocation until the periarticular tissues scar down around the endoprosthesis. Once dislocation occurs, there is increased potential for recurrence because of stretching of the periarticular tissues. Dislocation is treated with reduction with the patient under anesthesia and immobilization. Recurrent dislocation may require surgical intervention to tighten periarticular tissues or revise the THA. After 3-6 wk, the THA has significantly decreased potential for dislocation. The following discussion relates to the *posterolateral approach* for THA surgery. Other approaches require different positional restrictions.

- During the preoperative period, advise patient about the potential for dislocation.
- Show patient what the endoprosthesis looks like (using a model or similar implant) and how easily it can be dislocated when positional restrictions (e.g., flexion of the hip to 90 degrees; internal rotation or adduction of the affected leg) are not followed.
- During the preoperative period, instruct patient in the use of ambulatory aids and ADL-assistive devices that allow independence without violating positional restrictions. Explain the use of devices to maintain positional restrictions.

- After surgery, discuss positional restrictions and activities that involve these restrictions, including pivoting on the affected leg, sitting on a regular-height toilet seat, bending over to tie shoelaces, or crossing the legs.
- Advise patient about the need for long-handled shoehorn, pickup sticks, stocking helpers, elastic shoelaces, Velcro fasteners, and a raised toilet seat for use after discharge. Provide addresses of stores that sell these items.
- Be sure the patient verbalizes and demonstrates understanding of the positional restrictions and can ambulate and perform ADL independently, using assistive devices.
- Instruct patient to report hip, buttock, or thigh pain or prolonged limp as indicators of implant loosening.

NIC: Exercise Therapy: Ambulation; Exercise Therapy: Balance; Exercise Therapy: Joint Mobility; Exercise Therapy: Muscle Control; Pain Management; Teaching: Disease Process; Teaching: Prescribed Activity/Exercise

Knowledge deficit: Potential for infection caused by foreign body reaction to the endoprosthesis
Desired outcome: Within 24 hr of instruction, patient verbalizes knowledge about the ongoing potential for infection, its indicators, and the importance of seeking prompt medical care if they occur.

- Advise patient that infection potential will be a permanent situation. Because of foreign body reaction and increased blood supply resulting from associated inflammatory response, these patients are at increased risk for hematogenic (bloodborne) infection. Introduce this as a potential complication during the informed consent process, and review it during preoperative teaching.
- Before hospital discharge, ensure that the patient verbalizes understanding of the indicators of wound, urinary tract, upper respiratory, and dental infections (see "Care of the Renal Transplant Recipient" for **Risk for infection**, p. 162; Table 5-4, p. 382). Include this information on a written handout that reviews the information and lists a phone number to call if questions arise after hospital discharge.
- Advise patient to wear a Medic-Alert bracelet and always to request prophylactic antibiotics for procedures that can result in bacterial seeding of the bloodstream, such as minor or major surgery or dental extractions.
- Advise patient to call health care practitioner promptly if indicators of infection from the THA occur. These signs can include drainage, pain, fever, local warmth, swelling, restricted ROM of the joint, or feelings of pressure in the hip.

NIC: Health Education; Infection Protection; Teaching: Prescribed Activity/ Exercise; Teaching: Procedure/Treatment; Teaching: Psychomotor Skill

Risk for peripheral neurovascular dysfunction with risk factors related to interrupted arterial flow secondary to compression from traction or abduction device
Desired outcomes: Patient has adequate peripheral neurovascular function in distal tissues as evidenced by warmth, normal color, and the ability to dorsiflex the involved foot and feel sensations on testing of the peroneal nerve dermatome. Following instruction, patient verbalizes knowledge about potential neurovascular complications and the importance of reporting indicators of impairment promptly.

- Because the traction sling or abduction device can press on neurovascular structures, it is imperative that neurovascular status of the affected leg, especially peroneal nerve function, be assessed along with the VS. The peroneal nerve runs superficially by the neck of the fibula and can be assessed by testing the dermatome of the first web space between the great and second

toes and having the patient dorsiflex the foot. Loss of sensation or movement signals impaired peroneal nerve function. Promptly report significant findings to health care practitioner.
- Be sure patient is aware of the potential for neurovascular impairment and the importance of reporting alterations in sensation, muscle strength, movement, temperature, and color of the immobilized extremity.
- Encourage patient to reposition the leg within the restrictions of the sling and positional limitations.
- Encourage patient to perform prescribed exercises as a means of stimulating circulation in the area.

NIC: Circulatory Precautions; Exercise Therapy: Joint Mobility; Peripheral Sensation Management; Positioning; Skin Surveillance; Teaching: Prescribed Activity/Exercise

---

See Also: "Osteoarthritis" for **Pain,** p. 252; **Impaired physical mobility** related to musculoskeletal impairment and adjustment to new walking gait, p. 556; "Fractures" for **Self-care deficit,** p. 590; **Knowledge deficit:** Potential for infection, p. 592; "Total Knee Arthroplasty" for **Risk for fluid volume deficit** related to postsurgical hemorrhage or hematoma formation, p. 617; Appendix One, "Caring for Preoperative and Postoperative Patients," p. 717; "Caring for Patients on Prolonged Bedrest" (in particular **Altered peripheral tissue perfusion,** p. 742, which discusses deep vein thrombosis), for nursing diagnoses and interventions.

PATIENT-FAMILY TEACHING AND DISCHARGE PLANNING

When providing patient-family teaching, focus on sensory information; avoid giving excessive information; and initiate a visiting nurse referral for necessary follow-up teaching. Consider including verbal and written information about the following:
- Prescribed exercise regimen, including rationale for each exercise, number of repetitions for each, and frequency of the exercise periods. Be sure patient independently demonstrates understanding of the exercises and gives a return demonstration before hospital discharge.
- Indicators of the types of infections, including the following: wound (persistent redness, swelling, discharge, local warmth, restricted hip ROM, feelings of hip pressure, fever, pain); UTI (dysuria; pyuria; fever; malodorous urine; cloudy urine; urgency; frequency; pain in the suprapubic, flank, groin, scrotal, or labial area); URI (change in color or amount of sputum, cough, sore throat, malaise, fever); and dental (pain, swelling of the jaw, difficulty with mastication, fever). Advise patient to notify health care practitioner promptly if any of these indicators occur and to obtain prophylactic antibiotics for minor surgical procedures.
- Use of assistive devices (pickup sticks, stocking helpers, long-handled shoehorns, elastic shoelaces, Velcro fasteners, raised toilet seat). Ensure that patient demonstrates independence in their use before hospital discharge.
- Independent ambulation with crutches on level and uneven surfaces (see "Osteoarthritis," p. 556).
- Getting in a car safely without risking dislocation. The patient should be able to demonstrate this procedure before hospital discharge.
- Medications, including drug name, rationale, dosage, schedule, precautions, drug/drug and food/drug interactions, and potential side effects.
- Indications of implant loosening, including continuing hip, buttock, or thigh pain or prolonged limp.
- Phone number of a resource person if questions arise after hospital discharge.

Total knee arthroplasty

Total knee arthroplasty (TKA) is surgery that involves resection of the knee joint and its replacement with an endoprosthesis. Several pathologic conditions can result in the need for TKA, including osteoarthritis, rheumatoid arthritis, gouty arthritis, hemophilic arthritis, and severe knee trauma. Generally, TKA is restricted to older patients because the life span of the implant is unknown. However, younger patients also undergo this procedure, depending on the severity of the disease, amount of pain, and degree of functional deficit in the femorotibial or femoropatellar articulations. Because this procedure is irreversible and involves the removal of a significant amount of bone from the femur, tibia, and patella, several conditions must be met before the patient is considered a potential candidate. Conservative methods of therapy must have been exhausted, and there must be pain and significant loss of function that severely limit ambulation and ADL. In addition, the patient must have demonstrated adherence with past medical regimens and be free of any concurrent infectious process.

Complications of TKA have resulted in the need for reoperation in as many as 15% of these patients. Complications include loosening of the prosthesis, peroneal nerve palsy, delayed wound healing, and infection. Loosening is by far the most common complication, and it occurs most frequently in patients with varus deformity, obesity, overactivity, or decreased bone stock (i.e., osteoporosis).

DIAGNOSTIC TESTS

See discussion under "Total Hip Arthroplasty," p. 612. In addition, arthroscopy may be useful in confirming the extent of the pathologic condition to identify the appropriate prosthesis.

COLLABORATIVE MANAGEMENT

Surgical procedure: The approach varies with the type of prosthetic device used. During the procedure a skin flap is created around the patella. If the blood supply is compromised during surgery or from postoperative hematoma formation, the flap can necrose and jeopardize the success of the operation; therefore it requires careful monitoring. The implant is internally fixed with methylmethacrylate or bony ingrowth. The wound is sutured closed in layers, and a drain may be left in place.

Postoperative immobilization: Usually accomplished with a commercially prepared knee immobilizer or Jones dressing, which is composed of a bulky padding with anterior, posterior, and lateral plaster splints that are held in place with an elastic wrap. The Jones dressing ensures immobilization while allowing for edema formation to minimize the risk of iatrogenic compartment syndrome. A commercial iced knee cuff with automatic ice slush circulator may be used for cryotherapy to inhibit edema formation and combat pain (see "Torn Anterior Cruciate Ligament" for **Knowledge deficit**: Use of postoperative cryotherapy with a commercial iced knee cuff and automatic ice slush circulator, p. 574). Cryotherapy may be continued in the home after each exercise period to reduce edema and pain. If the implant is to be held in place with bony ingrowth, the leg may be immobilized within a cylinder cast after postoperative edema has subsided.

Ambulation: If methylmethacrylate was used to internally fix the implant, the patient may be permitted to ambulate with partial weight bearing or weight bearing as tolerated on the first postoperative day, with increasing activity and exercise over the rehabilitative period. ROM of the knee is often done the first postoperative day under supervision of a physical therapist. For implants held in place with bony ingrowth, ambulation may be restricted for several days or accomplished with non-weight bearing or toe-touch weight bearing for the first few weeks postoperatively. If there is a cast, ROM begins when the cast has been removed.

Continuous passive movement (CPM): Usually advocated for patients who undergo a TKA. The CPM device is applied to the patient's bed, and the operant extremity is positioned in two slings (one above and one below the knee) in the device. The device then moves the leg through preset limits of ROM in preset timed cycles (commonly 45 sec/cycle). The CPM initially may be set at 45-60 degrees, with daily progression during patient's hospitalization as determined by physical therapist or the health care practitioner. Use of CPM allows greater ROM with less pain. (The minimal flexion for a successful TKA is 90-110 degrees.)

NURSING DIAGNOSES AND INTERVENTIONS

Risk for fluid volume deficit with risks related to postsurgical hemorrhage or hematoma formation

Desired outcome: Within 36 hr after surgery, patient is free of symptoms of excessive bleeding or hematoma formation as evidenced by BP ≥90/60 mm Hg (or within patient's normal range); HR ≤100 bpm; RR ≤20 breaths/min; balanced I&O; output from drainage device ≤50 ml/hr; and brisk capillary refill (<2 sec or consistent with preoperative assessment), peripheral pulses >2+ on a 0-4+ scale, warmth, and normal color in the involved extremity distal to the surgical site.

Note: A hematoma is a collection of extravasated blood within the tissues after surgery (or trauma). During most orthopedic surgeries, a tourniquet is used to restrict blood flow from the operative field. Sometimes the tourniquet is left inflated until after the dressing or cast has been applied; therefore major bleeding may not be noted during surgery. Even when the tourniquet is deflated, it is possible that a significant bleeding vessel may be overlooked or that bleeding will begin later during the patient's recovery.

- When taking VS, monitor drainage from the drainage system as well as that on the dressings or cast. Report output from the drainage system that exceeds 50 ml/hr.
- Because noting the amount of drainage on the cast does not always provide an accurate assessment of drainage within the cast, carefully evaluate the patient's VS, subjective complaints, and neurovascular status.
- Be alert to and report patient complaints of warmth within the cast or beneath the dressing, things "crawling" under the cast, aching, increasing pressure or pain, or coolness distal to the area of surgery, which can occur with hemorrhage or hematoma formation.
- Monitor for and report VS indicative of shock or hemorrhage, including hypotension and increasing pulse rate.
- Monitor for pallor, decreased posterior tibial or dorsalis pedis pulses, slowed capillary refill, or coolness of the distal extremity, which can occur with hemorrhage or hematoma formation.
- If hemorrhage or hematoma formation is suspected, notify health care practitioner promptly. If the limb is in a cast, elevate it above the level of the patient's heart to slow the bleeding. If the limb is not in a cast, apply an elastic wrap for direct pressure on the site of bleeding.
- If hemorrhage or hematoma formation is suspected and the patient's VS are indicative of shock but a health care practitioner is unavailable, the surgical area should be exposed by windowing the cast or loosening the dressing to allow direct inspection of the area. Direct pressure usually will control hemorrhage; if not, apply a thigh blood pressure cuff over sheet wadding to serve as a tourniquet until the health care practitioner arrives for definitive therapy.

◎ NIC: Bleeding Precautions; Bleeding Reduction; Blood Products Administration; Hemodynamic Regulation; Shock Prevention; Wound Care

Risk for impaired skin integrity with risk factors related to irritation; *and/or*
impaired tissue integrity   (or risk of same) related to altered circulation
secondary to presence of CPM device
Desired outcomes: Skin and tissue of the affected leg remain intact and
nonerythematous. Following instruction, patient verbalizes knowledge about
the importance of reporting indicators of skin irritation promptly while
undergoing CPM.
- Preoperatively, assess the skin on the operant extremity, being alert to areas
  of irritation or redness.
- Preoperatively, introduce the patient to the use of the CPM, demonstrating
  how it will be used postoperatively. Point out areas susceptible to pressure or
  irritation from the device. Teach patient to report alterations in sensation or
  discomfort.
- Postoperatively, ensure correct positioning of the extremity within the CPM
  device (i.e., neutral position of the leg, with the knee resting over the area
  flexed by the device).
- Encourage patient to perform quadriceps sets, gluteal sets, and ankle circles
  to promote extremity circulation.
- During VS, or more often if erythema is noted, examine the medial, lateral,
  and posterior aspects of the extremity in the CPM device for areas of
  erythema. Also question patient about alterations in sensation or areas of
  discomfort.
- Pad areas of excessive pressure as noted by the presence of erythema.
  Reposition the leg within the confines of the CPM device. Report areas of
  erythema that do not resolve.

◎ NIC: Exercise Promotion; Incision Site Care; Infection Protection; Medication Administration: Topical; Perineal Care; Pressure Management; Skin
Surveillance; Traction/Immobilization Care

See Also: "Total Hip Arthroplasty," all nursing diagnoses (except
Knowledge deficit: Potential for and mechanism of THA dislocation),
p. 613.

PATIENT-FAMILY TEACHING AND DISCHARGE PLANNING
See "Total Hip Arthroplasty," p. 615.

Selected Bibliography

Arciero RA et al: Arthroscopic Bankart repair versus nonoperative treatment for
acute, initial anterior shoulder dislocations, *Am J Sports Med* 22(5):589-594,
1994.
Altizer L: Total hip arthroplasty, *Orthop Nurs* 14(4):7-18, 1995.
Blackburn WD: Management of osteoarthritis and rheumatoid arthritis:
prospects and possibilities, *Am J Med* 100(2A):24S-30S, 1996.
Bradford DS et al: Orthopedics. In Way LW, editor: *Current surgical diagnosis
and treatment,* ed 10, Norwalk, Conn, 1994, Appleton & Lange.
Brown FM, Jr: Anterior cruciate ligament reconstruction as an outpatient
procedure, *Orthop Nurs* 15(1):15-20, 1996.
Broy SB: A "whole patient" approach to managing osteoporosis, *J Musculo-
skeletal Med* 13(2):15, 1996.
Crutchfield J et al: Preoperative and postoperative pain in total knee
replacement patients, *Orthop Nurs* 15(2):65-72, 1996.
Davis S et al: Management of compartment syndrome in lower extremity,
Trauma Q 10(2):143-151, 1993.

DeGeorge P, Dunwoody C: Transfer techniques of the lower extremity with an external fixator, *Orthop Nurs* 14(6):17-21, 1995.

Dunwoody CJ: Modalities for immobilization. In Maher AB et al, editors: *Orthopaedic nursing,* ed 2, Philadelphia, 1998, Saunders.

Duong TT: Complications of fractures, *Phys Med Rehabil* 9(1):17-30, 1995.

Esquenazi A, Meier RH: Rehabilitation in limb deficiency. 4. Limb amputation, *Arch Phys Med Rehabil* 77:S-18–S-26, 1996.

Goldberg VM: Surgical treatment of osteoarthritis, *J Musculoskeletal Med* 11(12):13-24, 1994.

Gray MA: Osteoporosis medications: what's your source of information? *Orthop Nurs* 13(5):55-58, 1994.

Gray MA: Local application of antibiotics in orthopaedic infections, *Orthop Nurs* 14(5):69-70, 1995.

Halverson PB: Extraarticular manifestations of rheumatoid arthritis, *Orthop Nurs* 14(4):47-50, 1995.

Hefti D: Complications of trauma: the nurse's role in prevention, *Orthop Nurs* 14(6):9-15, 1995.

Hovis SER: Musculo-tendinous transfers of the hand and forearm, *Clin Neurol Neurosurg* 95(suppl):S92-S94, 1993.

Interqual: *The ISD-A review system with adult ISD criteria,* Northhampton, NH, and Marlboro, Mass, August 1992, Interqual.

Kim MJ et al: *Pocket guide to nursing diagnoses,* ed 7, St Louis, 1997, Mosby.

Krupski WC et al: Amputation. In Way LW, editor: *Current surgical diagnosis and treatment,* ed 10, Norwalk, Conn, 1994, Appleton & Lange.

Laughlin RT et al: Osteomyelitis, *Curr Opin Rheumatol* 7:315-321, 1995.

Long JS: Shoulder arthroscopy, *Orthop Nurs* 15(2):21-31, 1996.

Maher AB et al, editors: *Orthopaedic nursing,* Philadelphia, ed 2, 1998 Saunders.

Matkovic V et al: Primary prevention of osteoporosis, *Phys Med Rehabil Clin North Am* 6(3):595-627, 1995.

McCloskey JC, Bulechek, GM, editors: *Nursing interventions classification (NIC),* ed 2, St Louis, 1996, Mosby.

McLeod KJ, Rubin CT: Clinical use of electrical stimulation in fracture healing, *Phys Med Rehabil* 9(1):67-76, 1995.

Moehring HD, Johnson PG: The use of cannulated screws in musculoskeletal trauma: a review of surgical techniques, *Orthop Rev: Aspects Trauma* Suppl:10-21, 1994.

Naftulin S, Niergarth S: Continuous passive motion, *Phys Med Rehabil* 9(1):51-65, 1995.

NIH Consensus Development Panel on Total Hip Replacement: Total hip replacement, *JAMA* 273(24):1950-1956, 1995.

Paganna KD, Pagana TJ: *Mosby's diagnostic and laboratory test reference,* ed 3, St Louis, 1996, Mosby.

Rankin JA: Pathophysiology of the rheumatoid joint, *Orthop Nurs* 14(4):39-46, 1995.

Rosenthal AK, Ryan LM: Treatment of refractory crystal-associated arthritis, *Rheum Dis Clin North Am* 21(1):151-161, 1995.

Ross DG: Compartment syndrome. In Keen JH, Swearingen PL, editors: *Mosby's critical care nursing consultant,* St Louis, 1997, Mosby.

Schenck RC, Heckman JD: Injuries of the knee, *Clin Symp* 45(1):2-32, 1993.

Semble EL: Rheumatoid arthritis: new approaches for its evaluation and management, *Arch Phys Med Rehabil* 76(2):190-201, 1995.

Snyder PE: Fractures. In Maher AB et al, editors: *Orthopaedic nursing,* ed 2, Philadelphia, 1998, Saunders.

Spencer-Green G: Drug treatment of arthritis: update on conventional and less conventional methods, *Postgrad Med* 93(7):129-140, 1994.

Star VL: Gout: options for its therapy and prevention, *Hosp Med* 31(11):25-37, 1995.

Swenson TM, Harner CD: Knee ligament and meniscal injuries, *Sports Med* 26(3):529-546, 1995.

US Department of Health and Human Services, Public Health Service, Agency for Health Care Policy and Research: *Acute pain management: operative or medical procedures and trauma,* AHCPR 92-0032, Rockville, Md, 1992, The Department.

Westrich GH, Sculco TP: Prophylaxis against deep venous thrombosis after total knee arthroplasty, *J Bone Joint Surg Am* 78(6):826-834, 1996.

Yandrich TJ: Preventing infection in total joint replacement surgery, *Orthop Nurs* 14(2):15-19, 1995.

Yetzer EA: Helping the patient through the experience of an amputation, *Orthop Nurs* 15(6):45-49, 1996.

9 REPRODUCTIVE DISORDERS

Section One: Surgeries and Disorders of the Breast

Breast reduction

Breast reduction involves removal of breast tissue and skin to decrease breast size. The decision for surgery is made by the patient, and it is performed by a plastic surgeon or breast specialist.

ASSESSMENT

Clinical indicators: The procedure may be reconstructive or cosmetic, depending on symptoms and degree of enlargement. Complaints may include neck, shoulder, and back pain; postural alterations from attempting to mask breast size; skin irritation or maceration in the inframammary fold; deep ridges from bra straps; and withdrawal from social encounters.

Physical assessment: The breasts are large and may be pendulous or unequal in size; ptosis of the nipple may be present. Any signs of malignant (e.g., nipple discharge) or benign breast disease should be fully investigated before surgical consideration (see also "Malignant Breast Disorders," p. 627).

SURGICAL INTERVENTION

Markings using a keyhole pattern are made before surgery to determine the ultimate position of the nipple and incision lines. Scars result in the area around the areola and on the breast as vertical and horizontal dimensions are reduced. During surgery a pedicle flap may be created to carry the nipple/areola complex to its new position, or the nipple and areola may be removed and replaced as a graft after resection of the extra breast tissue and skin.

NURSING DIAGNOSES AND INTERVENTIONS

Body image disturbance related to breast size
Desired outcome: Before surgery, patient expresses positive and realistic reasons for having breast surgery.

- Discuss with patient the perceptions she holds of her breasts, including likes and dislikes (both ideal and real).
- Review patient's expectations for the outcome of surgery. The patient should not have unrealistic expectations, as evidenced by statements such as "Surgery will change my life or marriage."
- Review for informed consent the potential risks involved with breast reduction, such as impaired breastfeeding, nipple or skin necrosis, scarring, asymmetry, delayed healing, and diminished nipple sensation.
- Provide support for the patient's decision to have this surgery by encouraging her to verbalize fears and concerns.

You may also wish to refer to the following interventions from the Nursing Interventions Classification (NIC):

NIC: Active Listening; Body Image Enhancement; Counseling; Emotional Support; Self-Esteem Enhancement

Pain related to surgical procedure
Desired outcomes: Patient's subjective perception of pain decreases within 1 hr of intervention, as documented by a pain scale; objective indicators, such as grimacing, are absent or diminished. Patient is pain free 5-7 days after surgery.

- Assess and document location, quality, and duration of the pain, using a pain scale from 0 (no pain) to 10 (worst pain).
- Medicate patient with analgesics as prescribed; evaluate and document the response, based on the pain scale.
- Instruct patient to request analgesia before pain becomes severe.
- Ensure that patient has a comfortable bra that adequately supports her breasts.
- Teach patient relaxation techniques, such as slow, diaphragmatic breathing and guided imagery.
- Provide distractions, such as television or soothing music.
- Encourage activity as tolerated.
- Instruct patient to avoid exposing the breast to excessive cold, which will cause nipple/areola constriction.
- For additional interventions, see **Pain,** p. 719, in Appendix One.

NIC: Analgesic Administration; Distraction; Pain Management; Progressive Muscle Relaxation; Simple Guided Imagery

Knowledge deficit: Incisional site care and the need for monthly breast self-examination (BSE)
Desired outcome: Before hospital discharge, patient verbalizes and demonstrates knowledge about incisional site care and verbalizes the importance and knowledge of BSE and the signs of infection at the incisional site.

- Instruct patient to cleanse the incisional site after the sutures have been removed, using basic hygiene, such as soap and water. Explain that heavy lotions, medications, or creams should not be used around the incisional sites (except for transplanted nipples) unless specified by health care provider.
- As prescribed, teach patient how to apply lotions or creams to the transplanted nipple or nipples.
- In preparation for hospital discharge, instruct patient in BSE, using models of the breast, and emphasize the importance of monthly BSE when the incisions have healed.
- Teach patient the signs of infection to report to a health care professional if they occur after hospital discharge: redness, odor, pain, local warmth, swelling, discharge, fever.

NIC: Health Education; Learning Readiness Enhancement; Teaching: Disease Process; Teaching: Procedure/Treatment

Ineffective breastfeeding related to breast surgical procedure
Desired outcome: In the preoperative period, patient verbalizes knowledge that breast-feeding will be impaired as a result of the surgical procedure.

- Before surgery, explain to patient that breast reduction surgery will impair breastfeeding in future pregnancies.
- As indicated, arrange for a session with a lactation consultant if patient requires more information.

NIC: Anticipatory Guidance; Breastfeeding Assistance; Truth Telling

See Also: "Breast Reconstruction" for **Risk for fluid volume deficit** with risks related to postsurgical hemorrhage or hematoma formation, p. 625; Appendix One, "Caring for Preoperative and Postoperative Patients," p.717.

PATIENT-FAMILY TEACHING AND DISCHARGE PLANNING

When providing patient-family teaching, focus on sensory information; avoid giving excessive information; and initiate a visiting nurse referral for necessary follow-up teaching. Consider including verbal and written information about the following:

- Medications for pain relief, including drug name, purpose, dosage, schedule, precautions, drug/drug and food/drug interactions, and potential side effects.
- Indicators of wound infection that require follow-up care by health care provider: persistent redness, local warmth, fever, pain, swelling, and drainage at the incisional areas.
- Care of the incision site, including cleansing and dressing, if indicated.
- Changes in the nipple, which may include decreased sensation and loss of color. Nipple sensation may return within 2 yr.
- Importance of monthly BSE. Teach or review the technique as appropriate.
- Activity restrictions, which may include limited use of arms for 2 wk postoperatively and resumption of full activity after 3 wk.

Breast reconstruction

After a mastectomy, a woman may elect to have breast reconstruction in an attempt to create a breast "mound" in place of the lost breast. Although there is no medical indication for breast reconstruction, it offers a significant psychologic focal point for recovery. Women who elect immediate reconstruction often have less sense of "mutilation," perceive it less as a replacement, and tend to be more satisfied with the results. Breast reconstruction can be performed at the time of mastectomy, but it is more commonly delayed until the primary mastectomy wound has healed. This surgery has become more common in recent years because techniques continue to improve and patients are becoming more aware of the procedure and its benefits. Many insurance carriers (some under state legislative mandate) now reimburse expenses for this procedure as part of the general treatment for breast cancer.

ASSESSMENT

Clinical indicators: Scheduled mastectomy or absence of the breast, patient's desire for surgery, and absence of progressive disease. For postmastectomy reconstruction, chemotherapy and/or radiation therapy should have been completed.
Physical assessment: There should be no evidence of infection, and healing of the mastectomy scar should be complete if a surgical delay was indicated.

COLLABORATIVE MANAGEMENT

Analgesics (NSAIDs and opioids): To control postsurgical discomfort.
IV therapy: To treat dehydration secondary to blood loss and surgical intervention.
Physical therapy: For arm exercises to maintain or improve range of motion.
Balanced diet: As tolerated to promote tissue restoration; increased protein and vitamin C facilitate tissue healing.
Surgical procedure: Varying procedures involved, depending on the amount of tissue left at the reconstruction site.
Sufficient tissue coverage: An implant may be placed under the pectoralis and serratus muscles. Implants are generally composed of a silicone bag filled with saline, air, or a combination of the two. (**Note:** The Food and Drug

Administration has placed a moratorium on the use of silicone gel implants because of a possible association between leaked silicone gel and autoimmune disorders.) If the area of the implant is restricted, a tissue expander can be used. The tissue expander is injected with increasing increments of saline or air through a port at intervals to provide gradual enlargement of the site over a period of about 6 wk. Once the area has been expanded to at least 25% more than the needed volume, the expander is replaced with a permanent implant. *Insufficient soft tissue, muscle, and skin coverage (usually following a radical or modified radical mastectomy):* It then becomes necessary to graft tissue from other locations, such as the latissimus dorsi flap or transrectus abdominis musculocutaneous (TRAM) flap. Latissimus dorsi flap reconstruction involves the transfer of the muscle, skin, and subcutaneous tissue from the back to the mastectomy site. Commonly the latissimus dorsi flap does not provide sufficient fullness to the breast mound, requiring supplementation with an implant. Contralateral breast flaps may be used when there is sufficient tissue to allow the graft. The TRAM flap involves the transfer of one of the rectus abdominis muscles, overlying skin, subcutaneous fat (lipectomy), and artery to the mastectomy site. If a nipple is desired on the reconstructed breast, it can be created from a full-thickness skin graft from the inner thigh, buttock, labia, postauricular area, or the other nipple; tattooing may be used to provide coloring.

Closed drainage and suction: Placed in the wound to minimize the chance of hematoma formation.

Leech therapy: May be used to reduce hematoma formation under the surgically created nipple by applying the leech(es) to the areola.

NURSING DIAGNOSES AND INTERVENTIONS

Knowledge deficit: Surgical procedure, preoperative care, and postoperative regimen

Desired outcome: Before surgery, patient verbalizes knowledge about the surgical procedure and expected results, preoperative care, and postoperative regimen.

- Consult health care provider to arrange a visit by a woman who has had breast reconstruction surgery to share feelings and demonstrate the cosmetic results. Support patient's decision for the type of procedure or implant to be used. Clarify any questions that may arise.
- During the preoperative period, focus on sensory information; avoid giving excessive information; and use a variety of teaching modalities (e.g., printed materials, demonstration, computer simulations, videotapes). Initiate a teaching plan to ensure adequate follow-up on the following areas of instruction during or soon after hospitalization, as appropriate:
  —Explain that after surgery a suction apparatus that removes blood will be present to minimize the potential for hematoma formation. Usually this apparatus is removed after 48 hr or when drainage is less than 10-20 ml for a 24-hr period.
  —Explain that movement and activity may be restricted after surgery, depending on the procedure used. When an implant is placed under ample tissue, recovery is more rapid and hospitalization is usually 1-3 days; flap reconstruction is more involved, and movement and activity may be more restricted. Patients with a latissimus flap reconstruction are usually discharged after 2-5 days when the drains are removed. A rectus abdominis procedure is more extensive, and because of the lipectomy, the patient may require 5-7 days of hospitalization. Contralateral breast flap procedure may require 2-3 days of hospitalization.
- Be aware that patients who undergo immediate reconstruction frequently require follow-up surgery to provide an adequate cosmetic result.
- Teach patient to monitor the reconstructed nipple and report to staff members delayed capillary refill (≥2 sec) and duskiness. Hematoma or seroma formation beneath the graft may require leech therapy for removal. Although

painless, leech therapy may be disconcerting and requires tactful introduction and careful patient instruction. Patients who undergo nipple reconstruction usually are more satisfied with the results than those who do not; however, they may experience more anxiety during the recovery period and thus require more reassurance.

- Explain the following areas of concern that often arise after hospital discharge:
  - —Caring for the incision: explain that a gauze dressing usually covers the incision until the sutures are removed on about the seventh day. After the sutures are removed, Micropore tape strips usually are placed over the incision until healing has taken place and are replaced when they loosen. Instruct patient to notify health care provider if signs of infection, including persistent redness, pain, local warmth, swelling, or drainage, appear at the incision site.
  - —Taking showers: showers usually are permitted after the suction catheter has been removed, but they may be postponed until the sutures have been removed. If a dressing is present, it should be removed from the operative site and replaced after bathing.
  - —Restricting activity: usually for the first 4-6 wk or as directed, strenuous exercise, contact sports, excessive stretching, and heavy lifting (>10 lb) are avoided. Activity that involves movement below the waist usually can be resumed after 1 wk.
  - —Avoiding putting pressure on the chest wall for 4-6 wk: for example, patient should use superior position during coitus.
  - —Wearing a comfortable bra after removal of the drains: explain that it takes 3-6 mo for the reconstructed breast to appear natural in contour.
  - —Applying prescribed lotion to the nipple daily if a nipple transplant was performed.
  - —Performing monthly breast self-examination (BSE) of both breasts: teach or review the procedure as appropriate.
  - —Making follow-up visits if a tissue expander was used for gradual enlargement of the implant site.
  - —Massaging the breast to prevent fibrocapsular formation, depending on the placement and type of implant used. Explain that the procedure involves a gentle motion in which the breast is squeezed and flattened. This procedure usually is performed 3 times daily.

NIC: Incision Site Care; Leech Therapy; Skin Care: Topical Treatments; Teaching: Preoperative; Wound Care

Risk for fluid volume deficit with risks related to postsurgical hemorrhage or hematoma formation

Desired outcomes: Patient is normovolemic as evidenced by BP ≥90/60 mm Hg (or within patient's normal range), HR 60-100 bpm, RR ≤20 breaths/min, warm and dry skin, and urinary output ≥30 ml/hr. Drainage in suction apparatus is ≤50 ml/hr initially and <20 ml/hr within 24 hr after surgery. If patient develops a hematoma, it is detected and reported promptly.

- Monitor patient for clinical indicators of hemorrhage (e.g., drop of systolic BP 10-20 mm Hg below trend, rapid HR, cool and clammy skin, pallor, confusion, diaphoresis). Report significant findings.
- Assess for the appearance of a hematoma as evidenced by swelling, pain, and possibly a bluish discoloration of the skin. Report significant findings to health care provider.
- Assess the suction apparatus for patency, and document the amount and character of the drainage. Report drainage >50 ml/hr for 2 hr. Reestablish suction as necessary. Usually the suction apparatus is removed after 48 hr or if the total drainage is less than 10-20 ml in 24 hr.

NIC: Bleeding Precautions; Circulatory Care; Shock Management: Volume; Wound Care: Closed Drainage

Body image disturbance related to body changes before and after breast reconstruction surgery
Desired outcomes: Patient relates realistic expectations before surgery (e.g., that the breast will look normal under clothing) and demonstrates movement toward acceptance of body changes after surgery.
- Review with patient her expectations for the outcome of surgery.
- Discuss the emotional responses that women often have after breast reconstruction, such as elation during the early postoperative period followed by depression or confusion.
- Explain that some of the depression and confusion may be a result of the memory of the mastectomy and fear of cancer. Reassure patient that these feelings are normal and usually disappear after a short time.
- Provide emotional support by being with the patient when the dressing is first removed. Explain that the reconstructed breast will not look like the other breast at first but that the molding process will begin during the recovery period and continue for 3-6 mo.

NIC: Body Image Enhancement; Coping Enhancement; Crisis Intervention; Emotional Support; Self-Esteem Enhancement

If a silicone breast implant has been previously used
Anxiety related to use of silicone breast implant
Desired outcome: Within the 24-hr period before hospital discharge, patient discusses concerns related to silicone implant and identifies potential systemic and local reactions.
- Advise patient that removal of the silicone breast implant generally is not considered unless there are problems.
- Inform patient that surgical substitution can be made with saline or air implants if necessary.
- Teach patient to report symptoms of the body's reaction to silicone, such as joint swelling and pain, skin erythema and swelling, glandular swelling, unusual fatigue, or swelling of the feet or hands.
- Teach patient to report symptoms of fibrocapsular formation, such as breast hardness, which may be painful and result in a displaced breast.
- Provide patient with the name of the type of implant used and the manufacturer's applicable implant identification number.

NIC: Anxiety Reduction; Learning Readiness Enhancement; Teaching: Disease Process; Teaching: Individual

> See Also: Appendix One, "Caring for Preoperative and Postoperative Patients," p. 717; "Caring for Patients With Cancer and Other Life-disrupting Illnesses," p. 747, for nursing diagnoses and interventions.

PATIENT-FAMILY TEACHING AND DISCHARGE PLANNING

When providing patient-family teaching, focus on sensory information; avoid giving excessive information; and initiate a visiting nurse referral for necessary follow-up teaching. Consider including verbal and written information about the following:
- Care of the incision, including applying a gauze dressing until the sutures are removed on about the seventh day. After the sutures are removed, Micropore tape strips usually are placed over the incision until healing has taken place and are replaced when they loosen. Instruct patient to notify health care provider if signs of infection, including persistent redness, pain, local warmth, fever, swelling, or drainage, appear at the incision site.
- Taking showers, which usually are permitted after the suction catheter is removed. If present, the dressing should be removed from the operative site and replaced after bathing.

- Activity restriction for the first 4-6 wk or as directed, including strenuous exercise, contact sports, excessive stretching, and heavy lifting (>10 lb).
- Importance of not putting pressure on the chest wall for 4-6 wk (e.g., patient should use superior position during coitus).
- Importance of breast massage 3 times daily for at least the first year after surgery. Explain that it takes 3-6 mo for the reconstructed breast to appear natural in contour.
- Potential recommendation to avoid wearing a bra for 3 mo to allow for unrestricted movement of the implant.
- Necessity of applying prescribed lotion to the nipple daily if a nipple transplant was performed.
- Importance of monthly BSE of both breasts. Teach or review the procedure as appropriate. In addition, stress the importance of follow-up care. Successful reconstruction may give a false sense of security.
- Importance of regular mammograms once healing is complete. Reconstruction does not decrease the need for mammography for screening or diagnostic purposes. If implants have been used, the woman should consult a radiologist on availability of and experience with special techniques needed for postimplant mammography.
- Medications, including drug name, purpose, dosage, schedule, precautions, drug/drug and food/drug interactions, and potential side effects.

Malignant breast disorders

Breast cancer is one of the three most common types of breast disease, second only to fibrocystic condition in occurrence. In the United States, it is the most frequently occurring cancer in females. Breast cancer usually is diagnosed in women 40-70 yr of age, with 50-60 yr being the peak of occurrence. However, in the past few years the number of newly diagnosed cases in women in their 20s and 30s has increased.

The histopathology of breast tumors involves the progression of the tumor from a local preinvasive disease state to an invasive malignancy. The changes that occur in the breast are caused primarily by hyperplasia of the epithelium. Although carcinoma in situ is noninvasive, it can develop into invasive carcinoma. The differentiation between noninvasive and invasive cancers requires extensive examination of tissue cells obtained during biopsy.

ASSESSMENT

Signs and symptoms: In the earliest stages, an appearance of abnormalities in the ducts and microcalcifications on mammogram examination may indicate cancer. A later indicator is a palpable mass. Signs of advanced disease include nipple retraction, change in breast contour, nipple discharge, redness or heat of the breast, palpable lymph glands, dimpling of the skin of the breast, ridging, and *peau d'orange* (orange peel) appearance of the breast. Ulceration also may be a sign of advanced disease.

Physical assessment: Palpable mass, which often is located in the upper outer quadrant of the breast; the subareolar area is the second most common location. Usually the mass is painless, unilateral, irregular in shape, poorly delineated, and nonmotile. Signs of edema, venous engorgement, and abnormal contours may be present.

Risk factors: Previous breast cancer in the contralateral breast; family history of cancer and breast cancer, especially a mother or sister, particularly if bilateral and developed before menopause; patient's age >50 yr; postmenopausal weight gain; early age at menarche (11 yr or younger); late age of menopause (>52 yr); nulliparity or late age at first full-term delivery (>30 yr). In addition, it is theorized that exposure to carcinogens and a high-fat diet are other factors in the development of breast cancer. **Note:** Only one quarter of women with breast cancer have the known risk factors; therefore *all* women should be considered at risk.

DIAGNOSTIC TESTS

The most specific test for detection of breast disease is the excisional biopsy. Mammography may detect breast masses in patients who do not have a palpable mass. However, there is the risk of false-negative results. The American Cancer Society recommends a baseline mammogram for women at age 40 yr and a mammogram every 1-2 yr for women 40-50 yr of age and annually for women 50 yr and older.

COLLABORATIVE MANAGEMENT

Staging of the tumor: Provides a way to formulate the prognosis and treatment plan. The size of the tumor, the degree and extent of axillary lymph node involvement, and the presence of distant metastases determine the degree of staging (Table 9-1). Lymphoscintigraphy, with technetium-99m sulfur colloid, has been used to map axillary lymph nodes. This procedure identifies the so-called *sentinel node*—the lymph node suspected to be primarily responsible for lymphatic drainage of a portion of the breast. Histologic examination of the sentinel node that is positive for cancer cells implies possible metastasis, whereas a negative finding implies no metastasis. Although further clinical evidence is needed to verify these findings, this procedure shows significant promise for further refining the staging of breast cancer.

Radiation therapy: Excision of the tumor along with some of the adjacent tissue, followed by external radiation or radioactive implants. This procedure has the same 5-yr survival rate as modified radical mastectomy.

Modified radical mastectomy: Removal of the breast tissue, the nipple and areola, the tumor and surrounding skin, the axillary lymph nodes, and possibly the pectoralis minor muscle.

Total mastectomy: Removal of the breast tissue and the nipple/areola complex, but the lymph nodes are left intact. It is used in patients with in situ carcinoma, for prophylactic mastectomy, or for patients who develop local recurrence after partial mastectomy.

Partial mastectomy (lumpectomy, tylectomy, or segmental resection): Excision of the tumor and a small amount of the tissue surrounding it. Axillary nodal dissection is usually done.

Quadrantectomy: Removal of the entire quadrant of the breast where the tumor is located. Axillary nodal dissection is usually done.

Adjuvant treatment: Given after primary treatment to reduce the risk of recurrence and prolong general survivability. Includes chemotherapy, hormone therapy, and/or radiation therapy.

Chemotherapy: Includes either a single agent or a combination of agents. This management pattern is used either as an adjunct to surgery or, in advanced disease, when metastases have occurred. Cytotoxic drugs have been found to be more effective when used in combination and are given IV every 3-4 wk for 6-12 mo. Standard combinations for first-line therapy include cyclophosphamide, doxorubicin (or methotrexate), and fluorouracil. For patients not responding to first-line therapy, other agents, such as vinblastine, paclitaxel (Taxol), and plicamycin (Mithramycin C), have shown efficacy.

Hormonal therapy: Depends on whether the tumor is estrogen receptor positive or estrogen receptor negative; can be used as adjuvant therapy or to treat recurrent disease. These hormonal agents include antiestrogens (tamoxifen; as first-line therapy), progestins (megestrol), luteinizing hormone-releasing hormone (LHRH; leuprolide), steroid blockers (aminoglutethimide), and androgens.

T A B L E 9 - 1	Cancer Staging by the Tumor, Node, Metastasis (TNM) Classification System

Stage 0

T = carcinoma in situ: intraductal lobular carcinoma in situ, or Paget's disease of the nipple with no tumor

N = no regional lymph node metastasis

M = no distant metastasis

Stage I

T = tumor ≤2 cm in greatest dimension

N = no regional lymph node metastasis

M = no distant metastasis

Stage IIA

T = from no evidence of tumor to tumor >2 cm but <5 cm in greatest dimension

N = no regional lymph node metastasis if tumor >2 cm; or metastasis to movable ipsilateral axillary lymph node(s) if tumor <2 cm

M = no distant metastasis

Stage IIB

T = tumor >2 cm in greatest dimension

N = no regional lymph node metastasis if tumor >5 cm; or metastasis to movable ipsilateral axillary lymph node(s) if tumor <5 cm

M = no distant metastasis

Stage IIIA

T = from no evidence of tumor to tumor >5 cm in greatest dimension

N = metastasis to movable or fixed ipsilateral axillary lymph node(s) if tumor >5 cm in greatest diameter; or metastasis to ipsilateral axillary lymph node(s) fixed to one another or to other structures if tumor <5 cm

M = no distant metastasis

Stage IIIB

T = tumor of any size including direct extension to chest wall or skin and inflammatory carcinoma

N = from no node involvement to metastasis to ipsilateral internal mammary lymph node(s) if tumor extends directly to chest wall or skin; or any tumor size with metastasis to ipsilateral internal mammary lymph node(s)

M = no distant metastasis

Stage IV

T = tumor of any size

N = any lymph node involvement or none

M = distant metastasis, including metastasis to ipsilateral supraclavicular lymph node(s)

Condensed from American Joint Committee on Cancer: *Manual for staging of cancer,* ed 4, Chicago, 1992, The Committee.

NURSING DIAGNOSES AND INTERVENTIONS

Anxiety related to the possibility of cancer and its treatment

Desired outcome: Within 12 hr of hospital admission, patient expresses concerns and exhibits increasing psychologic comfort as evidenced by participation in decisions regarding her care and the statement that she is able to rest and sleep adequately.

- Assess patient's understanding of the potential diagnosis and treatment plan; clarify and explain as appropriate. Also determine what the patient may have learned about breast cancer from books, TV, or friends and relatives, and correct any misconceptions.
- Provide time for patient to express feelings and fears about the diagnosis.
- Evaluate patient's emotional status, and explore with patient what her breasts mean to her. Breasts may represent nurturing, sexuality, femininity, and desirability to her.
- Assess your own feelings about the diagnosis of cancer and the psychologic meaning of the breast. Your attitudes may be reflected in the patient's care; therefore a positive attitude is essential for optimal patient support.
- Provide a nonthreatening, relaxed atmosphere for the patient and significant other by using therapeutic communication techniques, such as open-ended questions and reflection.
- For additional interventions, see **Anxiety,** p. 791, in Appendix One.

NIC: Active Listening; Anxiety Reduction; Emotional Support; Presence; Teaching: Preoperative

Ineffective individual coping related to situational crisis (diagnosis of breast cancer)
Desired outcomes: Within the 24-hr period before hospital discharge, patient expresses her feelings and identifies positive coping patterns (e.g., using support systems, planning daily activities).
- Assist patient in identifying and developing a support system.
- Provide support to patient's significant other. Refer significant other to a support group that addresses specific concerns.
- If a mastectomy was performed, recognize the signs of grief, such as denial, anger, withdrawal, or inappropriate affect. Provide emotional support, and describe the stages of grief to the patient and significant other. Provide explanations to significant other, who may misunderstand the meaning of the patient's behavior or actions.
- Consult the surgeon regarding a visit from a woman who has had a diagnosis similar to that of the patient. Reach to Recovery volunteers from the American Cancer Society are trained to share their experiences with breast cancer patients (see "Patient-Family Teaching and Discharge Planning, p. 633). Additional support programs include "Look Good, Feel Better;" "I Can Cope;" and "Can Care."
- See "Caring for Patients With Cancer and Other Life-disrupting Illnesses," p. 791, for this and other psychosocial nursing diagnoses and interventions.

NIC: Coping Enhancement; Emotional Support; Support Group; Support System Enhancement; Teaching: Individual

Risk for disuse syndrome with risks related to upper extremity immobilization secondary to discomfort, lymphedema, or infection after mastectomy
Desired outcomes: Before surgery, patient verbalizes knowledge about the importance of and rationale for upper extremity movements and exercises. Upon recovery, patient has full ROM of the upper extremity.
- Consult surgeon before the mastectomy to determine the type of surgery anticipated. With surgeon, develop an individualized exercise plan specific to patient's needs, considering factors of wound healing, suture lines, and extent of the surgical procedure.
- Encourage finger, wrist, and elbow movement to aid circulation and help minimize edema as soon as patient returns to her room.
- Elevate the extremity as tolerated.
- Encourage progressive exercise by having patient use the affected arm for personal hygiene and ADL the morning after surgery. Other exercises (clasping the hands behind the head and "walking" the fingers up the wall) should be added as soon as patient is ready. After drains and sutures have

been removed (usually 7-10 days postoperatively), patient should begin exercises that will enhance external rotation and abduction of the shoulder. Patient should be able to achieve maximum shoulder flexion by touching her fingertips together behind her back. A Reach for Recovery volunteer can visit and provide patient with verbal instructions and written handouts for these exercises. Exercises should be continued daily for 6 mo.

- Assist patient with ambulation until her gait is normal. Encourage correct posture with the back straight and shoulders back.
- For patients who have had an axillary dissection (with lumpectomy or radical mastectomy) be aware that loss of lymph nodes increases their risk of being unable to combat infection. To minimize the risk of lymphedema and infection, avoid giving injections, measuring BP, or taking blood samples from the affected arm. Remind patient about her lowered resistance to infection and the importance of promptly treating any breaks in the skin. To help prevent infection after hospital discharge, advise patient to treat minor injuries with soap and water and to notify her health care provider if signs of infection occur.
- Advise patient to wear a Medic-Alert bracelet that cautions against injections and tests in the involved arm.
- To protect the hand and arm from injury, advise patient to wear a thimble when sewing and a protective glove when gardening or doing chores that require exposure to harsh chemicals, such as cleaning fluids. Explain that cutting cuticles should be avoided and that lotion should be used to keep the skin soft. An electric razor should be used for shaving the axilla.

NIC: Activity Therapy; Infection Protection; Positioning; Teaching: Disease Process; Teaching: Prescribed Activity/Exercise

Pain related to the surgical procedure
Desired outcomes: Patient's subjective perception of pain decreases within 1 hr of intervention, as documented by a pain scale; objective indicators, such as grimacing, are absent or diminished. Patient relates that pain is relieved with IV or IM narcotics for the first 24-48 hr after surgery and with oral medications for the following 2 wk, with pain decreasing daily.

- Assess and document the location, quality, and duration of the pain, rating it with the patient on a scale of 0 (no pain) to 10 (worst pain).
- Medicate patient with the prescribed analgesics before the pain becomes too severe, or provide instructions for individuals who are using patient-controlled analgesia. Evaluate and document the response, using the pain scale.
- Reassure patient that phantom breast sensations, numbness of the incision, and hyperesthesia or dysesthesia of the chest wall are common.
- Provide a comfortable in-bed position, and support the affected arm with pillows.
- Encourage movement of the fingers on the affected arm to reduce muscle tension in the distal arm. Inform patient that although progressive exercise will cause some discomfort, it will aid in the mobility of the affected arm and enhance recovery.
- Reassure patient that exercise movements will be adapted to her level of tolerance.
- If appropriate, instruct patient in relaxation techniques and use of guided imagery.
- Provide distraction, such as television, radio, or books.
- Use touch to help relieve tension (e.g., by giving a gentle massage).
- For additional interventions, see **Pain,** p. 719, in Appendix One.

NIC: Analgesic Administration; Distraction; Exercise Therapy: Muscle Control; Pain Management; Patient-Controlled Analgesia (PCA) Assistance; Simple Relaxation Therapy

Body image disturbance related to loss of a breast
Desired outcome: Within the 24-hr period before hospital discharge, patient demonstrates movement toward acceptance of the loss of her breast.

- Encourage patient to express her feelings and concerns. Reassure her that it is normal to grieve loss of the breast.
- Recognize that loss of a breast is perceived in different ways by different women. It is frequently more traumatic for the young or middle-age woman.
- Provide emotional support by being with the patient when the surgical dressing is removed.
- As appropriate, explain that sexual relations can be resumed as soon as the surgical pain has decreased. Assure patient that relations that were positive before surgery usually remain positive. Use of a soft pillow or temporary prosthesis for padding may decrease fear of discomfort during sexual relations.
- Recognize the need for a supportive person, such as a Reach for Recovery volunteer who has experienced the same procedure. Consult health care provider about a visit from this individual, if indicated. Support systems also should be made available to significant other.
- If reconstruction is to be delayed or if it is contraindicated or not desired, provide patient with a breast prosthesis after surgery to help her feel "normal." A temporary prosthesis, made of nylon and filled with Dacron fluff, should be worn for a few weeks until the incision heals and swelling lessens. Provide patient with information about where to get a breast prosthesis. The American Cancer Society has lists of distributors and types of prostheses available.
- Assure patient that few changes in her wardrobe will be needed, but supply resources about where to purchase swimwear and lingerie.
- Be aware that use of touch often enhances the patient's self-concept.
- Provide information and answer questions about breast reconstruction (see p. 623).
- For additional interventions, see **Body image disturbance,** p. 799, in Appendix One.

NIC: NIC: Body Image Enhancement; Coping Enhancement; Crisis Intervention; Emotional Support; Self-Esteem Enhancement; Support System Enhancement; Touch

Altered family processes related to breast malignancy and treatment with radiation therapy and/or chemotherapy
Desired outcome: Within the 24-hr period before hospital discharge, the patient of childbearing age verbalizes accurate information about pregnancy and parenthood after breast cancer and its treatment.

Note: Reproductive counseling should take into account the patient's age, stage of disease, type of cancer treatment, and pretreatment fertility status.

- Explain that childbearing should be delayed for approximately 2 yr after cancer diagnosis and treatment. This interval varies depending on the stage of the disease, use of adjuvant therapy, and other factors. Explain that use of oral contraceptives is contraindicated in a woman with a history of breast cancer.
- Explain to the patient that she can breastfeed with either breast after chemotherapy but that after radiation therapy she should use only the nonirradiated breast.
- Explore adoption as an alternative for the infertile couple.
- As indicated, discuss the importance of communicating the diagnosis and treatment implications with children in the family, based on the child's

developmental age. See psychosocial nursing diagnoses and interventions in Appendix One, "Caring for Patients With Cancer and Other Life-disrupting Illnesses," p. 791.

NIC: Counseling; Emotional Support; Family Process Maintenance; Family Support; Family Therapy; Teaching: Disease Process

---

See Also: Appendix One, "Caring for Preoperative and Postoperative Patients," p. 717; "Caring for Patients With Cancer and Other Life-disrupting Illnesses," p. 747, for nursing diagnoses and interventions.

PATIENT-FAMILY TEACHING AND DISCHARGE PLANNING

When providing patient-family teaching, focus on sensory information; avoid giving excessive information; and initiate a visiting nurse referral for necessary follow-up teaching. Consider including verbal and written information about the following:

- Medications, including drug name, purpose, dosage, schedule, precautions, drug/drug and food/drug interactions, and potential side effects.
- Type and dates of follow-up treatment.
- Resumption of sexual activity, which usually can occur as soon as pain is diminished.
- Care of the incision site, including cleansing, and drain care. Explain the components of good hygiene.
- Progressive exercise regimen, which should be continued at home. Advise patient to stop the exercise movement if a pulling sensation or pain is felt.
- Informing health care professionals to avoid measuring BP or giving injections in the affected arm.
- For the incision site and any wound of the affected arm, the indicators of infection (e.g., fever, erythema, local warmth, drainage, tenderness, swelling, skin discoloration) and the importance of reporting them to health care professional.
- Permanent breast prosthesis, including distributors and types available.
- Name and telephone number of a support person who can be called during the first postoperative year. An ideal individual is a Reach for Recovery volunteer. To contact Reach for Recovery volunteers, call your local American Cancer Society office (see below).
- Importance of performing monthly breast self-examination (BSE). In addition, as a part of the BSE, teach patient to palpate the scar, sweep down the chest wall, and palpate the axillary, supraclavicular, and subclavian lymph nodes to assess for lumps. Teach patient that skin changes, such as rashes and erythema, are suggestive of recurrence and should be reported promptly.
- Importance of follow-up care.
- Phone numbers to call if questions or concerns arise about therapy or disease after discharge. Additional general information can be obtained by contacting the following organizations:

The American Cancer Society
1599 Clifton Road NE
Atlanta, GA 30329   (800) ACS-2345
WWW address: *http://www.cancer.org*

National Cancer Institute Information Service (CIS)
Bldg. 31, Room 10A16
9000 Rockville Pike
Bethesda, MD 20892   (800) 422-6237
WWW address: *http://wwwicic.nic.nih.gov/*

The National Alliance of Breast Cancer Organizations (NABCO)
9 East 37th Street
10th Floor
New York, NY 10016   (800) 719-9154
WWW address: *http://www.nabco.org/*

Y-ME National Breast Cancer Organization
212 West Van Buren
4th Floor
Chicago, IL 60607   (312) 986-8228
WWW address: *http://www.y-me.org/*

Reach to Recovery Program
c/o American Cancer Society (see p. 633)   (404) 320-3333

- When appropriate, referral to hospice or agency that provides home help. This should occur before discharge planning begins to ensure continuity of care between the hospital and home or hospice.
- Phone numbers to call if questions or concerns arise about hospice after discharge. Information for these patients can be obtained by contacting the following organization:

National Hospice Association
1901 North Moore St., Suite 901
Arlington, VA 22209   (703) 243-5900; (703) 525-5762 FAX
WWW address: *http://www.nho.org*

Section Two: Neoplasms of the Female Pelvis

Cancers of the cervix and ovaries are frequently occurring reproductive cancers in women. Statistics published by the American Cancer Society for 1996 estimated 49,400 new cases of uterine cancer per year (14,500 cases of invasive cervical cancer and 34,900 cases of endometrial cancer) and 26,800 new cases of ovarian cancer. Women of all ages can develop cancer of these structures, although it is most often found in individuals age 40-60 yr.

Cancer of the cervix

Generally, cervical cancer is considered a sexually transmitted disease. The probable agents are human papillomaviruses (16 and 18) and herpes simplex virus, type 2. The following risk factors have been associated with this disease: early age of first coitus, multiple sexual partners (or exposure to partners who have had multiple sexual partners), exposure to sexually transmitted diseases, low socioeconomic status, cigarette smoking, and a diet low in vitamins A and C and folic acid. The two types of cervical cancer are squamous cell, which is the most common, and adenocarcinoma. *Preinvasive* describes cancerous cells that are limited to the cervix, and *invasive* refers to cancer that is present in the cervix, in other pelvic structures, and possibly in the lymphatic system as well. Treatment of preinvasive cancer has a greater success rate.

ASSESSMENT

Preinvasive: Patient asymptomatic; Pap smear abnormal (blood tinged).
Invasive: Patient asymptomatic or may have abnormal vaginal bleeding; persistent, watery vaginal discharge; postcoital pain and bleeding; abnormal Pap smear. With advanced disease patients may present with leg or flank pain, lower extremity edema, dysuria, and rectovaginal or cystovaginal fistula.

DIAGNOSTIC TESTS

Pap smear: Cells collected from the endocervix and squamocolumnar junction on the cervix with an applicator, placed on a slide, fixed, and sent to the laboratory for analysis. Pap smear results may be reported as follows:

- Normal or atypical benign.
- Cervical intraepithelial neoplasia (CIN):
  —Grade 1: mild dysplasia (one-third involvement of the epithelial thickness).
  —Grade 2: moderate to severe dysplasia (up to two-thirds involvement).
  —Grade 3: severe dysplasia and carcinoma in situ (two-thirds to full-thickness involvement).
- Invasive squamous cell carcinoma.
- Adenocarcinoma.
- Atypical cells present; repeat to rule out.
- Specimen insufficient for diagnosis.

Colposcopy: Procedure providing a microscopic view of the transformation zone of the cervix and allowing cervical staining with a 3%-6% acetic acid solution. Areas that do not absorb the stain are considered abnormal; biopsy specimens of these areas are obtained and are sent for histologic examination. Endocervical curettage (ECC) is also done to rule out disease in the endocervical canal. This procedure takes approximately 20 min.

Conization biopsy: Surgical procedure performed with the patient under general anesthesia or IV sedation: a cone-shaped area of the cervix, with the apex of the cone containing part of the external os, is excised for laboratory analysis to determine the extent of the malignancy. Cone biopsy is done if ECC is positive or inconclusive or if there is a discrepancy between the Pap smear and biopsy results.

CT scanning and MRI: Radiologic detection techniques used to determine the degree and extent of the pathologic process within the pelvis and the spread of the disease outside the pelvis.

Chest x-ray: May reveal presence of metastasis to the lungs.

Staging of the disease: The following guidelines are used, based on clinical classification by the International Federation of Gynecology and Obstetrics (FIGO):

- *Stage 0:* carcinoma in situ; preinvasive.
- *Stage I:* cancer cells in the cervix only.
  —*Stage IA:* microscopic disease measuring not more than 5 mm in depth from its base and not more than 7 mm horizontally.
  —*Stage IB:* lesions greater in size than IA, seen clinically or microscopically.
- *Stage II:* cancer involving cervix and vagina (upper two thirds only) but not the pelvic wall.
  —*Stage IIA:* no involvement of uterine tissue.
  —*Stage IIB:* involvement of uterine tissue.
- *Stage III:* involvement of the pelvic wall or lower third of the vagina.
  —*Stage IIIA:* no extension onto the pelvic wall.
  —*Stage IIIB:* extension onto pelvic wall and/or causes hydronephrosis (obstructed flow of urine to kidney, producing kidney atrophy).
- *Stage IV:* cancer in bladder, rectum, and other organs of the pelvis.
  —*Stage IVA:* metastasis to adjacent organs.
  —*Stage IVB:* metastasis to distant organs.

COLLABORATIVE MANAGEMENT

Therapies will vary depending on the type and extent of the lesion.

Preinvasive

Laser surgery: Precise destruction of small lesions without destruction of normal tissue. May be accomplished in surgeon's office.

Cryosurgery: Involves freezing the cervix with carbon dioxide or nitrous oxide. It is used only for superficial lesions that do not involve the endocervix and is contraindicated in pregnancy.

Conization: Removal of a cone-shaped wedge of the cervix around the os for microinvasive lesions up to 3 mm in depth. Conization is contraindicated in pregnancy.

Loop electrosurgical excision procedure (LEEP):   Done during colposcopy with the patient under local anesthesia. The transformation zone is excised using a low-voltage (25-50 watts) diathermy loop. Advantages include minimal side effects while allowing diagnosis and treatment at the same time.

Invasive

External radiation therapy: Used to treat all stages of cancer; performed on an outpatient basis in the radiotherapy department. Accumulative dose is 4000-6000 cGy given over a 4- to 6-wk period.

Radium implants: Used to deliver large doses directly to the tumor; may be used in combination with external radiation. While the patient is sedated, an applicator is positioned in the cervix through the vagina and its position is confirmed by x-ray. After the patient returns to her room, the radiologist inserts a radioactive isotope and leaves it in place for 1-3 days. During this time the patient is radioactive and therefore is in a private room with limited contact from visitors and caregivers.

A combination of external radiation and implants gives the best therapeutic results. While the implant is in place, the patient is kept on strict bedrest, has an indwelling catheter, is on a low-residue diet, and is given analgesics. After the implant has been removed, the patient is assisted to ambulate and a douche and sodium phosphate enema are administered.

Hysterectomy (simple to radical):   Limited to patients with stage I or II disease as a single treatment modality. It may involve removal of the uterus, ovaries, fallopian tubes, upper third of the vagina, and parametrium on each side, as well as pelvic lymph node dissection. Because ovarian metastasis is rare, the ovaries may be preserved in younger women. The extent of the procedure varies depending on the stage of disease.

Chemotherapy: Platinum-based combinations or single agents such as ifosfamide may be given simultaneously with pelvic irradiation in locally advanced disease. The role of chemotherapy in advanced disease is limited, but clinical trials are underway to investigate the most effective treatment combinations.

NURSING DIAGNOSES AND INTERVENTIONS

Pain related to surgery or radiation implant

Desired outcomes: Within 1 hr of intervention, patient's subjective perception of pain decreases, as documented by a pain scale. Objective indicators, such as grimacing, are absent or diminished.

- Provide back rubs, which are especially helpful for patients who were in the lithotomy position during surgery. Massage the shoulders and upper back of patients with radium implants, who are not allowed position changes.
- For other interventions, see **Pain,** p. 719, in Appendix One.

NIC: Analgesic Administration; Distraction; Pain Management; Simple Massage; Simple Relaxation Therapy

Risk for fluid volume deficit with risks related to operative, postoperative, or postimplant bleeding

Desired outcomes: Patient is normovolemic as evidenced by BP ≥90/60 mm Hg (or within patient's usual range), HR 60-100 bpm, urinary output ≥30 ml/hr, RR ≤20 breaths/min with normal depth and pattern (eupnea), skin dry and of normal color, and a soft and nondistended abdomen. Patient and significant other verbalize knowledge about the signs and symptoms of excessive bleeding and are aware of the need to alert staff promptly if they are noted.

- Monitor VS q2-4hr during the first 24 hr. Be alert to indicators of hemorrhage and impending shock: hypotension, increased pulse and respirations, pallor, and diaphoresis.
- Assess postoperative bleeding q2-4hr by noting amount and quality of drainage on dressings and perineal pads if abdominal approach was used or on perineal pads alone if vaginal approach was used. Normally the patient's postoperative bleeding is minimal. It should be dark in color (or serosanguineous if an abdominal hysterectomy was performed). If an implant is in place, check for vaginal bleeding, a sign that erosion is occurring.
- If a closed drainage system is used, note the amount of drainage and report >50 ml/hr for 2 hr.
- Inspect the abdomen for distention, and assess patient for presence of severe abdominal pain; both are indicators of internal bleeding.
- Review CBC values for evidence of bleeding: decreases in hemoglobin (Hgb) and hematocrit (Hct). Notify health care provider of significant findings. Optimal values are Hct ≥37% and Hgb ≥12 g/dl.
- Inform patient and significant other about the signs of excessive bleeding and the need to alert staff immediately if they occur.

NIC: Bleeding Precautions; Circulatory Care; Shock Management: Volume; Teaching: Individual; Wound Care: Closed Drainage

Risk for injury with risks related to radiation implant
Desired outcome: Implant remains in place for the duration of treatment.
- Assign patient to a private room.
- Elevate the head of the bed 30-50 degrees and maintain position restrictions, as per health care provider's directive.
- Maintain the indwelling catheter placed at the time of implantation.
- Monitor abdominal assessments q8hr.
- Assess skin integrity q2-4hr.
- Assess for vaginal discharge q8hr.
- Maintain a low-residue diet, and administer antidiarrheal medications as prescribed.

NIC: Medication Management; Positioning; Radiation Therapy Management; Skin Surveillance

Altered urinary elimination (oliguria or anuria) related to inadequate intake, obstruction of indwelling catheter, or ureteral ligation
Desired outcome: Within 24 hr of surgery, patient demonstrates a balanced I&O, with urinary output ≥30 ml/hr immediately following surgery.
- Monitor I&O, and document every shift. Notify health care provider if urinary output falls below 30 ml/hr for 2 hr in the presence of adequate intake. Along with low back pain or costovertebral angle tenderness, this sign can indicate ureteral ligation during surgery.
- Ensure patency of the indwelling catheter. **Caution:** For patients with radiation implants, bladder distention can result in radiation burns to the bladder.
- Administer oral or parenteral fluids as prescribed. Ensure totals of 2-3 L/day in nonrestricted patients.
- Assess for bladder distention by inspecting the suprapubic area and percussing or palpating the bladder.

NIC: Fluid Management; Intravenous (IV) Therapy; Tube Care: Urinary; Urinary Elimination Management; Urinary Retention Care

Grieving related to actual or perceived loss or changes in body image, body function, or role performance secondary to diagnosis of cancer

Desired outcomes: Before hospital discharge, patient and significant other express grief, explain the meaning of the loss, and communicate concerns with each other. The patient completes self-care activities as her condition improves.

- Anticipate patient's concern about loss of uterus, presence of cancer, the potential for recurrence, and "loss of womanhood." Provide emotional support and an unhurried atmosphere for patient and significant other to ask questions and express concerns, frustrations, and fears.
- Recognize the covert signs of grief that can accompany self-image disturbances: anger, withdrawal, demanding behavior, or inappropriate affect. Clarify patient's coping behaviors to significant other as necessary.
- To enhance patient's sense of control over her situation, encourage her to perform ADL and begin self-care as soon as her condition warrants.
- Provide materials by organizations such as the American Cancer Society, and arrange for a contact person from such an organization if appropriate.
- For additional interventions, see Appendix One, "Caring for Patients With Cancer and Other Life-disrupting Illnesses" for **Anticipatory grieving,** p. 796.

NIC: Emotional Support; Grief Work Facilitation; Self-Care Assistance; Support System Enhancement; Teaching: Individual

> **See Also:** Appendix One, "Caring for Preoperative and Postoperative Patients," p. 717; "Caring for Patients With Cancer and Other Life-disrupting Illnesses," p. 747, for nursing diagnoses and interventions.

PATIENT-FAMILY TEACHING AND DISCHARGE PLANNING

When providing patient-family teaching, focus on sensory information; avoid giving excessive information; and initiate a visiting nurse referral for necessary follow-up teaching. Consider including verbal and written information about the following:

- Phone numbers to call if questions or concerns arise about therapy or disease after discharge. Additional general information can be obtained by contacting the following organizations:

  The American Cancer Society
  1599 Clifton Road NE
  Atlanta, GA 30329   (800) ACS-2345
  WWW address: *http://www.cancer.org*

  National Cancer Institute Information Service (CIS)
  Bldg. 31, Room 10A16
  9000 Rockville Pike
  Bethesda, MD 20892   (800) 422-6237
  WWW address: *http://wwwicic.nic.nih.gov/*

For patients who have had radium implants

- Necessity of notifying health care provider if the following problems occur: vaginal bleeding, rectal bleeding, foul-smelling vaginal discharge, abdominal pain or distention, dysuria, urinary frequency, hematuria.
- Resumption of sexual intercourse, typically 6 wk after surgery or as directed by health care provider. Describe, as indicated, use of a vaginal dilator to prevent atrophy. It is usually inserted once daily for 5 min.
- Medications, including drug name, dosage, purpose, schedule, precautions, drug/drug and food/drug interactions, and potential side effects.
- Need for follow-up care; confirm date and time of next medical appointment if known.
- Patient is *not* radioactive once the implant has been removed.

- Side effects of radium implants: vaginal dryness, burning sensation, vaginal discharge, and dyspareunia.

For patients who have had a hysterectomy
- Necessity of notifying health care provider if the following indicators of infection occur: incisional swelling, local warmth around the incision, fever, redness, purulent drainage, vaginal bleeding, odorous vaginal discharge, incisional or abdominal pain.
- Care of the incision.
- Restriction of activities as directed, such as heavy lifting (>10 lb) and sexual intercourse. Advise patient to get maximum amounts of rest and avoid fatigue.
- Medications, including drug name, dosage, purpose, schedule, precautions, drug/drug and food/drug interactions, and potential side effects.
- Need for follow-up care; confirm date and time of next medical appointment if known.
- Phone numbers to call if questions or concerns arise following hysterectomy. Additional general information can be obtained by contacting the following organization:

Hysterectomy Educational Resources and Services (HERS) Foundation
422 Bryn Mawr Ave.
Bala Cynwyd, PA 19004   (610) 667-7757
e-mail: *74053.2441@compuserve.com*

Ovarian tumors

There are numerous types of ovarian tumors, both benign and malignant. They include solid tumors and cysts of various cell types and can occur in females of all ages. The most common enlargements arise from the normal follicular apparatus of the ovary (i.e., follicle and corpus luteum cysts) and hyperplasias, such as polycystic ovaries. The most common benign neoplasms are the cystadenomas, which make up 55% of the tumors. The most common malignant tumors are of epithelial tissue origin. *Malignant ovarian tumors* rarely are diagnosed early because the patient tends to be asymptomatic. Because their detection usually occurs during an advanced stage, survival rate is low. Therefore this is the most lethal type of gynecologic cancer. Although malignant ovarian tumors are found in women of all ages, the greatest incidence occurs between 60-64 yr. Although rare, germ cell ovarian cancer is the most common malignant ovarian cancer in women <20 yr old. Both environmental and genetic factors may contribute to their development.

ASSESSMENT
Benign ovarian tumors: Depending on the type of tumor, common symptoms include abdominal enlargement and complaints of abdominal fullness.
Solid ovarian tumors: Abdominal enlargement and pressure; vague gastrointestinal symptoms (e.g., dyspepsia, indigestion; pelvic pressure and discomfort).
Signs and symptoms for both classifications: Amenorrhea, postmenopausal vaginal bleeding and other menstrual irregularities; urinary frequency and urgency; GI complaints, such as nausea, anorexia, and constipation. Usually there are no early signs in ovarian cancer, or they may be mild, including digestive disturbances.
Physical assessment: Abdominal distention and ascites; palpable inguinal lymph nodes; an enlarged ovary, which is highly suspicious in prepubertal and

postmenopausal women. Benign masses are commonly smooth, mobile, unilateral, and <8 cm in size. Malignant masses are irregular, fixed, and commonly bilateral.

DIAGNOSTIC TESTS

Abdominal ultrasound: (Especially by vaginal probe) may reveal an ovarian mass.

Elevated serum markers: CA-125 is elevated in 80%-85% of ovarian cancers. If germ cell tumor is suspected, human chorionic gonadotropin (HCG) and α-fetoprotein (AFP) will be elevated.

Laparoscopy: Use of a laparoscope, an instrument with a telescope and light source, to visualize the pelvic organs and take biopsy specimens of suspicious areas through an incision made near the umbilicus. This procedure is done with the patient under general or regional anesthesia, usually on an outpatient basis.

Cytologic examination of the pelvic washings/ascites: May show presence of malignant cancerous cells.

Other diagnostic testing: May be done preoperatively when ovarian cancer is suspected; chest x-ray, CT scan of the abdomen, intravenous pyelogram (IVP), barium enema, upper GI series, and endoscopic bowel examination may be done, depending on symptoms.

Staging of ovarian tumors (dependent on surgical exploration):   The following guidelines are used, based on clinical classification by the International Federation of Gynecology and Obstetrics (FIGO):

- *Stage I:* tumor limited to the ovaries.
  - —*Stage IA:* growth limited to one ovary; no ascites; capsule intact.
  - —*Stage IB:* tumors limited to both ovaries; no ascites; capsule intact.
  - —*Stage IC:* tumor IA or IB but with tumor on the surface, ruptured capsule; with ascites containing malignant cells; or with positive peritoneal washings.
- *Stage II:* tumors involving one or both ovaries with pelvic extension.
  - —*Stage IIA:* involvement of uterus or fallopian tubes.
  - —*Stage IIB:* extension to other pelvic tissues.
  - —*Stage IIC:* tumor IIA or IIB with ascites or positive peritoneal washings; tumor on surface of the ovary or ovary with ruptured capsule.
- *Stage III:* tumors involving one or both ovaries with metastasis outside the pelvis or positive retroperitoneal nodes. Tumor limited to retroperitoneal lymph nodes. Malignant cells found in small bowel omentum or superficial liver metastasis.
  - —*Stage IIIA:* tumor grossly limited to the true pelvis with negative nodes but with microscopic seeding of abdominal peritoneal surfaces.
  - —*Stage IIIB:* tumor of one or both ovaries with abdominal or peritoneal implants ≤2 cm; negative nodes.
  - —*Stage IIIC:* abdominal implants >2 cm and/or positive retroperitoneal or inguinal nodes.
- *Stage IV:* tumors involving one or both ovaries with metastasis to distant organs (e.g., pleural effusion with positive cytology; parenchymal live metastasis).

COLLABORATIVE MANAGEMENT

For benign tumors

Wedge resection: Surgical procedure in which a benign tumor is removed, leaving normal ovarian tissue. It is done with the patient under general anesthesia, using an abdominal approach; depending on size, laparoscopic surgery may be used.

Salpingo-oophorectomy: Removal of the ovary and fallopian tube on the affected side. It is performed with the patient under general anesthesia, using an abdominal approach.

For malignant tumors

Cytoreductive surgery: Involves resection of as much abdominal and pelvic disease as possible to increase the effectiveness of radiation and chemotherapy, which are more successful when the residual tumor is minimized.

Paraaortic and pelvic lymphadenectomy: For staging of the disease when it is grossly confined to the ovary.

Total hysterectomy and bilateral salpingo-oophorectomy: Along with omental removal. Partial colectomy or small bowel resection may be necessary to debulk the tumor.

Chemotherapy and radiation: Used depending on the stage of the disease. Chemotherapy is indicated for stages III and IV and for some high-risk stage I and II patients. Chemotherapeutic medications usually are used in combination and may include (among others) cisplatin (the most active), doxorubicin, melphalan, paclitaxel (Taxol), and cyclophosphamide. Intraperitoneal administration may be used in women with minimal or microscopic residual disease (<2 cm). This form of chemotherapy applies treatment directly to the tumor and decreases general toxicity. The role of radiation therapy has not been clearly established; when used, it involves the whole abdomen.

NURSING DIAGNOSES AND INTERVENTIONS

See "Cancer of the Cervix" for **Pain,** p. 636; **Risk for fluid volume deficit** (bleeding), p. 636; **Altered pattern of urinary elimination,** p. 637; **Grieving,** p. 637; Appendix One, "Caring for Preoperative and Postoperative Patients," p. 717; "Caring for Patients With Cancer and Other Life-disrupting Illnesses," p. 747, for nursing diagnoses and interventions.

PATIENT-FAMILY TEACHING AND DISCHARGE PLANNING

When providing patient-family teaching, focus on sensory information; avoid giving excessive information; and initiate a visiting nurse referral for necessary follow-up teaching. Consider including verbal and written information about the following:

- Medications, including drug name, dosage, schedule, purpose, precautions, drug/drug and food/drug interactions, and potential side effects.
- Importance of reporting indicators of infection (depending on the surgery) to the health care provider: fever; vaginal bleeding, odor, or discharge; abdominal pain and distention; and incisional redness, tenderness, purulent drainage, local warmth, and swelling.
- Activity restrictions related to heavy lifting (>10 lb), exercise, sexual intercourse, or housework, as directed by health care provider (usually 6 wk).
- Necessity of follow-up appointments; confirm date and time of next appointments for health care provider, radiation therapy, and chemotherapy.
- Phone numbers to call if questions or concerns arise about therapy or disease after discharge. Additional general information can be obtained by contacting the following organizations:

The American Cancer Society
1599 Clifton Road NE
Atlanta, GA 30329   (800) ACS-2345
WWW address: *http://www.cancer.org*

National Cancer Institute Information Service (CIS)
Bldg. 31, Room 10A16
9000 Rockville Pike
Bethesda, MD 20892   (800) 422-6237
WWW address: *http://wwwicic.nic.nih.gov/*

- Phone numbers to call if questions or concerns arise following oopherectomy. Additional general information can be obtained by contacting the following organization:

  Hysterectomy Educational Resources and Services (HERS) Foundation
  422 Bryn Mawr Ave.
  Bala Cynwyd, PA 19004   (610) 667-7757
  e-mail: *74053.2441@compuserve.com*

Endometrial cancer

Endometrial (uterine) cancer is the most common type of female genital cancer in the United States and is one of the six leading causes of cancer deaths in women. Typically it occurs in postmenopausal women age 50-70 yr. Risk factors for developing uterine cancer include a diet high in fat, obesity, nulliparity, late menopause (after age 52 yr), hypertension, diabetes mellitus, unopposed menopausal estrogen therapy (i.e., giving estrogen without progestin), infertility as a result of failure to ovulate, and dysfunctional uterine bleeding during menopause. The tumor can be found in any location within the uterus, as either a focal lesion or a diffuse condition. The invasive stages of uterine cancer can involve spread to the vagina, pelvic lymph nodes, ovaries, and, less often, through the vascular system to the lungs, bones, and liver. Recurrence most frequently is seen in the vagina. When an early diagnosis is made, the prognosis is very good because the tumor tends to be localized and well differentiated. *Adenocarcinoma* is the most common endometrial cancer.

ASSESSMENT

Signs and symptoms: Uterine bleeding in the postmenopausal woman (occurs in 90%); irregular, heavy, and prolonged menses and intermenstrual spotting in the premenopausal woman; watery, purulent, or blood-tinged vaginal drainage; suprapubic discomfort; lower abdominal or lumbosacral pain.
Physical assessment: Presence of a palpable uterine mass, softened uterus, uterine polyps; obvious increase in uterine size in advanced disease.

DIAGNOSTIC TESTS

Endometrial biopsy: An office procedure used to obtain specimens from the endometrium.
Hysteroscopy: Examination via an endoscope, which enters the uterus through the vagina, allowing visualization, biopsy, and photography with a camera. The patient is anesthetized with a paracervical block. This procedure can be used for diagnosis and staging.
Dilation and curettage (D&C):   Surgical procedure done with the patient under general anesthesia in which the cervical opening is widened by a dilator and the uterine lining is scraped with a curette to obtain an endometrial specimen for examination. Fractional D&C involves individual curettage of each quadrant of the uterus with each specimen separated from the others to identify the area of abnormal tissue within the uterus.
Other diagnostic testing: Chest x-ray, intravenous pyelogram, sigmoidoscopy, ultrasound, CT scan, or MRI may be done to evaluate adnexal involvement, uterine size, lymphadenopathy, local invasion, and degree of myometrial invasion.
Serum markers: CA-125 is drawn to determine elevation.
Staging of the disease: The following guidelines are used, based on clinical classification by FIGO:
- *Stage IA:* tumor limited to endometrium.
- *Stage IB:* less than half the myometrium involved.
- *Stage IC:* more than half the myometrium involved.

- *Stage IIA:* involvement of endocervical gland only.
- *Stage IIB:* invasion of cervical stroma.
- *Stage IIIA:* invasion of serosa and/or adnexae and/or positive peritoneal cytologic findings.
- *Stage IIIB:* metastasis to vagina.
- *Stage IIIC:* metastasis to paraaortic and/or pelvic lymph nodes.
- *Stage IVA:* invasion to bladder and/or bowel mucosa.
- *Stage IVB:* distant metastasis.

COLLABORATIVE MANAGEMENT

Surgery is the standard therapy for endometrial cancers confined to the uterus. More aggressive tumors with extension require more complex treatment. Treatment is individualized and can vary from progestin therapy to surgery. **Hysterectomy with bilateral salpingo-oophorectomy (with or without radiation):** With cytologic examination of peritoneal washings; possible pelvic and aortic lymphadenectomy.
Radiation therapy (either internal or external): Usually reserved for high-virulence tumors. If an implant is used, the applicator is positioned in the uterus through the vagina while the patient is anesthetized. After the patient returns to her room, the radioisotope is placed in the applicator by a radiologist. External radiation of the uterus and pelvic nodes is performed on an outpatient basis for a period of time that is determined by the radiologist.
Chemotherapy: Used for advanced or recurrent disease for poorly differentiated tumors that are not hormone dependent. Chemotherapeutic drugs include doxorubicin, cisplatin, and cyclophosphamide. Combinations of drugs and the dosage and length of treatment are determined by the patient's response to treatment and the severity of recurrence.
Hormone therapy: Used for recurrent and advanced endometrial cancers. A progestin is usually used. This therapy is more effective when the tumor has a large number of progesterone receptors.

NURSING DIAGNOSES AND INTERVENTIONS

See "Cancer of the Cervix," p. 636.

PATIENT-FAMILY TEACHING AND DISCHARGE PLANNING

See "Cancer of the Cervix," p. 638.

Vulvar cancer

Vulvar cancers represent 5% of the cancers of the female reproductive tract. Nearly 50% of newly diagnosed patients with carcinoma in situ (intraepithelial neoplasia) are 20-40 yr old. Older women (>60 yr) are more likely to develop invasive cancer. Squamous cell carcinoma accounts for 90%-95% of primary vulvar tumors; the 5-yr survival rate is approximately 50% because of late diagnosis and involvement of the inguinal lymph nodes. The following have been associated with vulvar cancer: chronic granulomatous venereal disease, herpes simplex virus type 2, human papillomavirus, and history of cervical cancer. Vulvar cancer is more commonly found in obese, hypertensive, or diabetic women.

ASSESSMENT

Signs and symptoms: Pruritus (in about two thirds of cases); lesions in the labia majora, clitoris, and/or periurethral areas; dysuria; ulceration of lesions in advanced disease; vulvar pain or burning; and discharge or bleeding. About 20% of cases are asymptomatic. Early cutaneous lesions appear white, lichenified, or hyperpigmented; mucous membrane lesions are gray or erythematous.

DIAGNOSTIC TESTS

Vulvar biopsy: A Keyes cutaneous punch often is used to perform the biopsy on any suspicious lesions, confluent masses, or warts. Colposcopy of the cervix and upper vagina may be used to identify lesions for biopsy.

Staging: The following clinical stages of invasive vulvar carcinoma are adapted from the FIGO and the American Joint Committee on Cancer (AJCC) classification systems:

* *Stage 0:* carcinoma in situ; intraepithelial carcinoma.
* *Stage 1:* maximum diameter of lesions ≤2 cm; confined to the vulva or perineum.
* *Stage II:* diameter of lesions >2 cm; confined to the vulva or perineum.
* *Stage III:* extension of lesions to the lower urethra, anus, perineum, or vagina, without grossly positive groin lymph nodes; *or* lesions of any size confined to the vulva with unilateral regional lymph node involvement.
* *Stage IV:* presence of lesions with fixed or ulcerative lymph nodes in both groins. Lesions involving rectal, bladder, or the upper urethral mucosa or fixed to bone. All cases with pelvic or distant metastases.

COLLABORATIVE MANAGEMENT

Carcinoma in situ: Depending on the size, multiplicity of foci, lesion location, and age of the patient, lesions may be treated by topical application of chemotherapeutic cream, wide local excision, cryosurgery, laser therapy, or vulvectomy. Wide local excision can use either primary-closure skin flaps or skin grafts. Skinning vulvectomy may involve incision of the vulvar skin and preservation of fat, muscle, and glands with a split-thickness skin graft.

Invasive carcinoma: May involve multimodal therapy with surgery and irradiation to avoid extremely radical treatments. Tumor size, location, remaining vulvar tissue, and lymph node involvement determine the management.

* *Stages I and II:* radical vulvectomy and bilateral lymphadenectomy. For single lesions in an otherwise healthy vulva, wide local excision is used. Ipsilateral groin lymphadenectomy is needed for >1-mm stromal invasion.
* *Stage III:* involves the previous treatment plus femoral and groin lymphadenectomy. More extensive surgery to allow for tumor-free margins may necessitate removal of urethra, vagina, or anus.
* *Stage IV:* pelvic exenteration (removal of the entire female reproductive tract along with both urinary and fecal diversions) may be necessary in addition to radical vulvectomy. If the disease is very advanced, therapy may consist of conservative surgery and irradiation. Chemotherapy, in conjunction with radiation, preoperatively may permit a more conservative approach rather than exenteration.

NURSING DIAGNOSES AND INTERVENTIONS

Sexual dysfunction related to fear after surgical procedure, grafting, excision of all or part of the reproductive tract, and/or pain

Desired outcome: Within the 24-hr period before hospital discharge, patient communicates concerns with partner and verbalizes a plan for satisfying sexual activity.

* Determine patient's need to communicate fears and concerns regarding sexual functioning following treatment of vulvar cancer.
* As indicated, teach patient that vulvectomy does not diminish sexual responsiveness; however, sexual functioning may be changed, depending on the procedure used and the patient's individual psychosocial adjustment. Introital stenosis may follow simple vulvectomy, and radical vulvectomy includes removal of the clitoris.
* Advise patient to use analgesics or relaxation techniques (e.g., hot shower) before sexual activity to help prevent discomfort.

- If vaginal lubrication is decreased, suggest that patient use a water-soluble lubricant with intercourse, such as Astroglide.
- Suggest the female superior position during coitus to control depth of penetration.
- Suggest alternative sexual practices, depending on the couple's values. Options include vibrators, touching, massage, and anal stimulation.
- As indicated, advise patient that sexual intercourse usually can be resumed after healing has occurred.

NIC: Anticipatory Guidance; Coping Enhancement; Counseling; Sexual Counseling; Teaching: Sexuality

---

See Also: "Cancer of the Cervix," p. 636, for other nursing diagnoses and interventions.

PATIENT-FAMILY TEACHING AND DISCHARGE PLANNING
See "Cancer of the Cervix," p. 638.

Section Three: Disorders of the Female Pelvis

Endometriosis is often seen in younger women, whereas cystocele, rectocele, and uterine prolapse more often are associated with women who are postmenopausal. These conditions occur when there is misplacement of structures or tissue within the female pelvis.

Endometriosis

Endometriosis is a benign condition in which endometrial tissue is present outside the uterus. This process occurs primarily in women of higher socioeconomic status and is uncommon in African-American women. Endometriosis has an estimated prevalence of 15% in the general population and 25%-50% in the infertile population. The mean age of diagnosis is 25-30 yr. Typically endometriosis is found on the ovaries or in the peritoneal cul-de-sac. It also can be found on any surface of structures in the pelvic peritoneum (e.g., fallopian tubes, serosal surface of the uterus, uterosacral ligaments, rectovaginal septum, bladder, large or small bowel). In extreme cases ectopic endometrium has been found in the lungs, umbilicus, breasts, and other areas of the body. The histologic origin of endometriosis is speculated to involve a combination of factors (e.g., a genetic defect, an immunologic reaction, and retrograde menstruation with implantation via the fallopian tubes).

ASSESSMENT
Signs and symptoms: Dysmenorrhea 5-7 days before and 2-3 days after menses, hypermenorrhea (prolonged, excessive, and/or frequent menses), infertility, painful defecation during menses, lower abdominal pain, sacral backache, and dyspareunia. Patient may be asymptomatic.
Physical assessment: Presence of a tender, fixed, retroverted uterus. Bimanual palpation of the peritoneal cul-de-sac and ovaries may reveal presence of tender nodules, masses, or fixation. The pelvic examination is performed several days before the menstrual cycle.

DIAGNOSTIC TESTS
Laparoscopy: Confirms presence of endometriomas on pelvic organs by passing a lighted instrument through an incision made near the umbilicus and

visualizing (e.g., bluish brown implants, "powder-burn" lesions on the peritoneal surface, and/or unexplained adhesions).

Pharmacology: Pain relief within 1 mo of initiating therapy with a gonadotropin-releasing hormone (GnRH) agonist, in the absence of other causes of pelvic pain, such as PID, ovarian cysts, pelvic varicosities, myomas, cervical stenosis, and malignancy.

COLLABORATIVE MANAGEMENT

Pharmacotherapy: *Danazol* (400 mg bid), an androgen, is a hormone inhibitor that acts by suppressing ovulation and hence hormone stimulation of endometrial tissue, allowing endometriomas to atrophy. *Progestin* (norethynodrel, norethindrone, hydroxyprogesterone caproate, medroxyprogesterone) treatment results in atrophy of endometrial tissues, improving symptoms but not curing the disease. Estrogen is commonly added to reduce break-through bleeding. This production of a pseudopregnancy state may be maintained for 6-12 mo and is successful in approximately 80% of patients. *GnRH agonists* also suppress ovulation (anovulation) and induce amenorrhea. *Gestrinone,* an orally administered, antiprogestational steroid, may reduce symptoms and decrease pain.

Surgical procedures: Determined by the patient's age and desire to have children and by extent and symptoms of the disease. They are performed if medical treatment is unsuccessful.

For women without extensive disease who wish to have children: One of the following is performed: laser vaporization or cauterization of endometrial implants, uterine suspension, lysis of adhesions, or removal of endometrial implants. These procedures are usually performed through a laparoscope. Open laparotomy may be required for more extensive involvement.

For women who are not menopausal but do not wish to have children: A hysterectomy may be performed, leaving the ovaries intact so that normal hormonal balance is maintained.

For women with extensive disease: A total hysterectomy with bilateral salpingo-oophorectomy is performed. The ovaries are removed because they are hormone-producing organs that influence the development and progression of the disease.

NURSING DIAGNOSES AND INTERVENTIONS

Anticipatory grieving related to potential for reproductive infertility

Desired outcome: Within the 24-hr period before hospital discharge, patient and significant other express grief, participate in decisions about the future, and communicate their concerns to the health care team and to each other.

- Assess for and accept patient's stage in the grieving process and behavioral response. Expect reactions such as disbelief, denial, grief, ambivalence, and depression. Recognize that the patient and significant other may move from one stage to another, depending on the circumstance (i.e., desire for a child, type of treatment recommended, or stage of endometriosis and subsequent likelihood of infertility).

- Assess religious and sociocultural expectations related to the loss (e.g., Is childbearing of primary importance in the relationship? What are the desires of the family for offspring? Has there been a lifelong desire to have children?).

- Encourage patient and significant other to explore and communicate feelings about the anticipated loss of fertility. Recognize that the woman often feels a greater sense of loss than the man feels. Infertility can place a strain on the relationship; treatment options may be expensive and time consuming and may raise ethical issues.

- Assess the couple's coping strategies. Suggest other ways of handling grief if their strategies are ineffective. Common strategies include increasing the space between themselves and reminders of their infertility (i.e., keeping busy), regaining control (seeking information, keeping a positive attitude), giving in to feelings (crying, indulging), and sharing their burden with each other and others.

- Demonstrate empathy. Provide an open and supportive atmosphere. The patient often is exposed to persons who have children and do not value the experience. Recognize that the patient may feel hostility toward persons who are fertile.
- Assess support systems, and describe and provide addresses of groups that share a common interest (e.g., RESOLVE). It also may be helpful to arrange referrals to specialists with knowledge of infertility (e.g., psychiatric nurse clinician, psychologist).
- For additional interventions, see Appendix One, "Caring for Patients With Cancer and Other Life-disrupting Illnesses" for **Anticipatory grieving,** p. 796.

NIC: Active Listening; Counseling; Family Integrity Promotion; Grief Work Facilitation; Support System Enhancement

---

See Also: "Cancer of the Cervix" for **Pain,** p. 636; **Risk for fluid volume deficit** (bleeding), p. 636; Appendix One, "Caring for Preoperative and Postoperative Patients," p. 717, for nursing diagnoses and interventions.

PATIENT-FAMILY TEACHING AND DISCHARGE PLANNING
See "Ovarian Tumors," p. 641.

Cystocele

A cystocele is the bulging of the posterior bladder wall into the vagina. It is caused by stretching and tearing of the pelvic connective tissue during childbirth, especially of a very large baby, or after several deliveries. Symptoms usually do not appear until menopausal or postmenopausal age. A rectocele (see p. 648) also may be present.

ASSESSMENT
Signs and symptoms: Sensation of vaginal fullness or of bearing down, inability to empty bladder with voiding, urinary frequency, dysuria, stress incontinence, incontinence resulting from urgency, and recurrent cystitis.
Physical assessment: Manual pelvic examination reveals a soft mass that bulges into the anterior vagina. The mass increases in size with coughing or straining.

DIAGNOSTIC TESTS
Urine culture and sensitivity: May reveal bladder infection.
Urodynamic evaluation: Involves study of the flow of urine from the bladder through the urethra to differentiate stress incontinence from urgency incontinence. A combination of tests is used, including voiding flow rate, urethral pressure profile, urethroscopy, and cystometrogram.

COLLABORATIVE MANAGEMENT
Urinary catheterization: To empty a distended bladder. This is an emergency measure rather than a permanent correction.
Antibiotics: Given if urinary retention results in an infection.
Estrogen therapy: A regimen of conjugated estrogen (Premarin) and a progesterone sometimes is given in small daily doses to postmenopausal women to maintain hormonal levels. Administration may be topical (creams or

suppositories) or systemic (oral forms or intramuscular injections of long-acting estrogen). A lack of hormones may result in weakness of the anterior vaginal wall, which allows the development of a cystocele.

Kegel isometric exercises: To help with bladder control (see p. 183).

Anterior colporrhaphy: Surgical procedure via vaginal approach to suspend the bladder. It involves separating the anterior vaginal wall from the bladder and urethra, excising the redundant thinned vaginal wall, urethropexy (urethral suspension), plication of the bladder neck, and suturing the remaining vagina to provide support for the bladder. Vaginal hysterectomy may also be done at this time. If both a cystocele and rectocele (see below) are present, an anterior and posterior colporrhaphy (A&P repair) is performed.

Laparoscopic Burch colposuspension: Elevates and attaches the proximal urethra to Cooper's ligament to relieve stress incontinence. Requires four laparoscopic portals and has the advantages of decreased voiding dysfunction, reduced blood loss, shortened hospitalization, and reduced postoperative recovery.

Pessary: Provides intravaginal support of descending pelvic structures and relief of symptoms; especially useful in patients with high surgical risk (see discussion in "Uterine Prolapse," p. 650). A Smith-Hodge device often is used if a cystocele exists.

NURSING DIAGNOSES AND INTERVENTIONS

See "Urinary Incontinence," p. 180, for related nursing diagnoses; "Cancer of the Cervix" for **Risk for fluid volume deficit** (bleeding), p. 636; Appendix One, "Caring for Preoperative and Postoperative Patients," p. 717, for nursing diagnoses and interventions.

PATIENT-FAMILY TEACHING AND DISCHARGE PLANNING

When providing patient-family teaching, focus on sensory information; avoid giving excessive information; and initiate a visiting nurse referral for necessary follow-up teaching. Consider including verbal and written information about the following:

- Medications, including drug name, purpose, dosage, schedule, precautions, drug/drug and food/drug interactions, and potential side effects.
- Activity limitations during the first 6 wk or as directed, including no heavy lifting (>10 lb) or strenuous exercises.
- Abstinence from sexual intercourse for 6 wk or as prescribed if vaginal surgery was performed. Discuss alternate methods of sexual expression.
- If discharged with a suprapubic catheter, teach the need to monitor postvoiding residual and how to attach the tubing to a drainage bag overnight.
- Notifying health care provider of the following indicators of infection: fever; persistent pain; local warmth; purulent, foul-smelling drainage; urinary retention.
- Kegel exercises (see p. 183) to improve sphincter control.
- Importance of follow-up appointments; confirm date and time of next appointment if known.

Rectocele

A rectocele is a rectovaginal hernia that develops when the connective tissue between the rectum and vagina (i.e., rectovaginal septum) is weak. Congenital weakness; pregnancy and subsequent trauma; menopause; straining with defecation; obesity; heavy lifting; and surgical trauma can contribute to this condition. The symptoms of this condition often do not become apparent until the woman is 35-40 yr old.

ASSESSMENT

Signs and symptoms: Continuous urge to have a bowel movement, sensation of rectal and vaginal fullness, constipation, difficulty generating pressure to pass stool (intravaginal digital pressure may be needed to facilitate defecation), incontinence of flatus or feces, and the presence of hemorrhoids or fecal impaction.

Physical assessment: A nontender fullness can be felt by depressing the perineum as the patient strains; manual rectal examination reveals a rectocele.

DIAGNOSTIC TESTS

Barium enema: Reveals a rectocele. As the hernia increases in size, the wall of the anterior rectum tends to be pushed into the vagina.

Defecography: Dynamic rectal examination using radiographic dye and fluoroscopy to identify rectoanal function during defecation.

COLLABORATIVE MANAGEMENT

Promotion of bowel elimination: With a high-fiber diet, fluids, stool softeners, and laxatives. If not contraindicated, walking is encouraged as a means of exercise to promote elimination.

Kegel isometric exercises: To help strengthen pelvic floor musculature (see p. 183).

Posterior colporrhaphy: To separate the posterior vaginal wall from the rectum, excise redundant vaginal tissue, and rejoin the rectovaginal septum with sutures to reduce the rectal herniation. If both a cystocele and a rectocele are present, an A&P repair is performed (see "Cystocele," p. 647).

NURSING DIAGNOSES AND INTERVENTIONS

Constipation related to restriction against straining, low-residue diet, or pain with defecation secondary to surgical procedure

Desired outcomes: After the early postoperative period, patient relates the presence of bowel movements within her normal pattern and with minimal discomfort. Patient verbalizes knowledge of the rationale for alerting staff before and after bowel movements and for not straining during defecation.

- Administer stool softeners or mild laxatives as prescribed. Ensure the patient drinks a full 8-10 oz of water with each dose.
- Unless otherwise contraindicated, push fluids to >2500 ml/day.
- The patient will be on a low-residue diet during the early postoperative period to minimize the potential for disruption of the surgical site. As indicated after the early postoperative period, consult health care provider about introducing high-residue foods to promote bowel movements.
- Instruct patient to avoid straining when having a bowel movement, because this can disrupt the surgical repair.
- Advise patient that defecation may be painful and to alert staff as soon as the urge to defecate is felt so that she can be medicated before the bowel movement.
- Avoid the use of enemas or rectal tubes, which can disrupt the surgical repair.
- Provide sitz baths as a comfort measure after bowel movements.
- Request that the patient notify staff after each bowel movement; document accordingly.

NIC: Bowel Management; Constipation/Impaction Management; Diet Staging; Fluid Management; Rectal Prolapse Management

---

See Also: "Cancer of the Cervix" for **Risk for fluid volume deficit** (bleeding), p. 636; Appendix One, "Caring for Preoperative and Postoperative Patients," p. 717, for nursing diagnoses and interventions.

PATIENT-FAMILY TEACHING AND DISCHARGE PLANNING

When providing patient-family teaching, focus on sensory information; avoid giving excessive information; and initiate a visiting nurse referral for necessary follow-up teaching. Consider including verbal and written information about the following:

- Medications, including drug name, purpose, dosage, schedule, precautions, drug/drug and food/drug interactions, and potential side effects.
- Limitation of activities during the first 6 wk as directed by health care provider, including heavy lifting (>10 lb) and exercising. Abstinence from sexual intercourse is usually recommended for 6 wk. Discuss alternate forms of sexual expression with patient. Advise patient that initially coitus may be painful.
- Indicators of infection: abdominal or rectal pain, foul-smelling vaginal discharge, and fever.
- Kegel exercises (see p. 183) to aid in defecation.
- Importance of a regular bowel elimination pattern to prevent constipation and straining.
- Importance of a high-fiber diet and a fluid intake of at least 2-3 L/day (unless this is contraindicated by a renal, hepatic, or cardiac disorder). High-fiber foods include bran, whole grains, nuts, and raw and coarse vegetables and fruits with skins.
- Importance of follow-up care; confirm date and time of next medical appointment if known.

Uterine prolapse

A uterine prolapse is a bulging of the uterus through the pelvic floor into the vagina. It results from an injury to the cardinal and uterosacral ligaments, which can occur with childbirth, surgical trauma, or atrophy of the supportive tissue during menopause. A prolapse can develop also as a result of uterine tumor, diabetic neuropathy, neurologic injury to the sacral nerves, obesity, or ascites. A prolapse will progress unless surgically repaired.

A prolapse is graded in the following way:

- *Grade I:* cervix remains within the vagina; the uterus partially descends into the vagina (first-degree prolapse).
- *Grade II:* cervix protrudes through the entrance to the vagina (second-degree prolapse).
- *Grade III:* entire uterus protrudes through the entrance of the vagina, and the vagina is inverted (third-degree prolapse, or procidentia). Occurs most frequently in postmenopausal, multiparous women and often along with a rectocele, cystocele, and enterocele (a hernia containing a loop of small intestine or the sigmoid colon, which bulges into the upper posterior vagina).

ASSESSMENT

Signs and symptoms: Complaints of heaviness in the pelvis, low backache (more severe by the end of the day), dragging sensation in the inguinal region, dyspareunia or lack of sensation with intercourse, and bulging at the introitus.

Physical assessment: Pelvic examination performed with patient either standing or supine. As patient bears down, a firm mass can be palpated in the lower vagina. This examination also can confirm diagnosis of a rectocele and cystocele if present. Diagnosis may be aided with the insertion of a Smith-Hodge pessary (i.e., reduced symptoms after insertion increase the likelihood that symptoms are related to uterine prolapse).

COLLABORATIVE MANAGEMENT

Placement of a vaginal pessary: A rubber, plastic, or silicone device that is inserted into the vagina to support the pelvic structures. It may be used if there is first- or second-degree prolapse or if surgery is contraindicated or unwanted by patient.

Topical estrogen (suppositories or creams): To maintain tone of the pelvic floor.

Antibiotics: If patient has a urinary tract infection.

High-fiber diet: To aid in bowel elimination.

Kegel exercises: Daily sets at frequent intervals to increase pelvic floor musculature (see p. 183).

Hysterectomy: To correct uterine prolapse; may be total abdominal or vaginal hysterectomy. Laparoscopic-assisted vaginal hysterectomy is used in some centers. For severe prolapse with rectocele and cystocele, a hysterectomy with an anterior and posterior colporrhaphy is performed.

NURSING DIAGNOSES AND INTERVENTIONS

See "Cancer of the Cervix" for **Risk for fluid volume deficit** (bleeding), p. 636; **Grieving** (if a hysterectomy is performed), p. 637; "Vulvar Cancer" for **Sexual dysfunction**, p. 644; "Rectocele" for **Constipation,** p. 649; Appendix One, "Caring for Preoperative and Postoperative Patients," p. 717, for nursing diagnoses and interventions.

PATIENT-FAMILY TEACHING AND DISCHARGE PLANNING

See "Rectocele," p. 650.

Section Four: Interruption of Pregnancy

The following conditions or surgical procedures involve women of childbearing age and can result in continued problems with childbearing or sterilization.

Spontaneous abortion

A spontaneous abortion, or miscarriage, occurs in approximately 15% of pregnancies. The primary causes of spontaneous abortion are *fetal,* including defective development and faulty implantation of the fertilized ovum and accounting for the majority of spontaneous abortions; and *maternal,* including infection, malnutrition, endocrine abnormalities, and incompetent cervix. Spontaneous abortion is defined as the expulsion of the products of conception (POC) before the twentieth week of gestation, and it is classified in the following ways.

Threatened abortion: Vaginal bleeding or cramping during the first half of the pregnancy. There is no tissue loss, and the cervix is closed. Either the symptoms disappear or an abortion occurs.

Inevitable abortion: Vaginal bleeding, cramping, rupture of membranes, and dilation and effacement of the cervix; cannot be halted.

Incomplete abortion: Partial expulsion of POC, with continued vaginal bleeding.

Complete abortion: Expulsion of all POC, with decrease in or cessation of vaginal bleeding and pain following expulsion.

Missed abortion: Presence of a nonviable fetus in the uterus for ≥2 mo.

Recurrent (habitual) abortion: Three or more pregnancies that are spontaneously aborted during the first trimester.

ASSESSMENT

Signs and symptoms: Vaginal bleeding, cramping, low back pain, signs of pregnancy, no progressive increase in size of uterus.

Physical assessment: A pelvic examination reveals the size of the uterus, location of pain, dilation of the cervix, presence of the POC at the os, and the amount of bleeding.

DIAGNOSTIC TESTS

CBC: Reveals a decrease in Hgb and Hct. There is a potential for elevation in leukocyte count, which would signal an infection.

Blood type and screen: To determine if the woman is Rh negative and thus a candidate for Rh_o (D) immune globulin (RhoGAM).

Laboratory examination of POC: To confirm presence of POC.

Ultrasound: Will confirm the presence of a nonviable fetus, as evidenced by absence of fetal heart motion. This test may be performed abdominally or transvaginally. Allows determination of the need for follow-up D&C; that is, endometrial thickness of ≤10 mm is consistent with complete abortion.

Endocrine studies: Human chorionic gonadotropin (HCG) will be minimal or absent with pregnancy loss; a 66% rise is expected within 48 hr in viable pregnancy. Progesterone level <5 ng/ml may suggest ectopic pregnancy, whereas >25 ng/ml indicates an intrauterine pregnancy.

COLLABORATIVE MANAGEMENT

Management depends on the type of abortion. The following are examples of treatment options.

Administration of blood or blood products: For excessive blood loss.

Parenteral fluid administration: For excessive fluid loss.

Analgesics: For pain management.

Antibiotics: When indicated, to prevent development of infection.

D&C: Procedure done in the first trimester to remove POC. With the patient under general or local anesthesia, the canal of the cervix is dilated to allow a catheter to pass through the cervix into the uterus and suction any POC that remain.

IV oxytocin: Used as an alternative to D&C to aid in the passage of POC. Oxytocin contracts the uterus by stimulating the smooth muscles.

Cervical cerclage: Performed early in the second trimester to manage an incompetent cervix when patient has a history of repeated painless, second-trimester abortions. With this technique, the cervix is reinforced with a suture (using McDonald, Shirodkar, or transabdominal cervicoisthmic cerclage procedure). The suture is released at term (or immediately if labor begins) to allow a vaginal delivery. This procedure is best performed before 18 wk or as early as 12 wk in the presence of cervical changes.

RhoGAM: An Rh_o (D) immune globulin that is given to prevent Rh sensitization in Rh-negative women.

Other: When the pregnancy is viable, observation by ultrasound and quantitative HCG levels may assist in monitoring progress of pregnancy. Although not empirically demonstrated to alter outcomes, bedrest often is recommended. Other treatments may depend on the probable cause. If POC are passed, instruct the patient to save them and bring them to the health care provider.

NURSING DIAGNOSES AND INTERVENTIONS

Risk for fluid volume deficit with risks related to abortive or postsurgical bleeding

Desired outcome: Patient is normovolemic as evidenced by BP ≥90/60 mm Hg; HR 60-100 bpm; urinary output ≥30 ml/hr; RR ≤20 breaths/min with normal pattern and depth (eupnea); warm and dry skin; and orientation to person, place, and time.

- Assess and document BP, HR, and RR at frequent intervals (typically q15min × 4; q30min × 2; q1-2hr until stable; and then q4hr). Notify health

care provider of significant changes. Be alert to hypotension; changes in mental status or LOC; cool and clammy skin; and increasing HR and RR.
- Monitor I&O at least q4hr. Be alert to decreasing urinary output, which can signal the onset of shock.
- Administer parenteral fluids, blood, and blood products as prescribed.
- If prescribed, administer oxytocin to assist with the contraction of the uterus and expulsion of the fetus.
- Inspect perineal pads, and note and document the amount and quality of bleeding. If vaginal bleeding increases or POC are expelled, notify health care provider at once. Save any tissue or clots that are expelled. **Note:** Bleeding is considered excessive if one or more perineal pads is saturated in 1 hr and there are symptoms of orthostasis (i.e., fainting or dizziness upon standing, diaphoresis, pallor).
- After POC are expelled, palpate the uterine fundus to assess its tone. If it feels soft and boggy, provide light massage using a circular motion. **Caution:** Avoid massaging a well-contracted uterus because this can result in muscle fatigue and uterine relaxation.

NIC: Bleeding Reduction: Antepartum Uterus; Blood Products Administration; Fluid Management; High-Risk Pregnancy Care; Intravenous (IV) Therapy

Pain related to uterine contractions
Desired outcomes: Within 30 min of intervention, patient's subjective perception of pain decreases, as documented by a pain scale. Subjective indicators, such as grimacing, are absent or diminished.
- Monitor and document frequency and duration of contractions. Assess and document patient's level of pain and response to management, using a scale of 0 (no pain) to 10 (worst pain).
- Administer analgesics as prescribed. Provide back rubs, which are especially relaxing.
- Instruct patient to request analgesic before pain becomes severe.
- Instruct patient in alternative methods of pain relief, including deep breathing, relaxation techniques, and guided imagery.
- For additional interventions, see Appendix One, "Caring for Preoperative and Postoperative Patients" for **Pain,** p. 719.

NIC: Analgesic Administration; Distraction; Pain Management; Simple Massage; Simple Relaxation Therapy

Risk for infection with risks related to retention of some or all of the POC
Desired outcome: Patient is free of infection, as evidenced by normothermia and absence of foul-smelling vaginal discharge and abdominal tenderness.
- Assess temperature q4hr; notify health care provider if an elevation occurs.
- Be alert to the presence of foul-smelling vaginal discharge, a signal of infection.
- Administer antibiotics as prescribed.
- Ensure that perineal care is performed after every voiding and bowel movement.

NIC: Infection Control; Infection Protection; Postpartal Care; Vital Signs Monitoring

Altered role performance related to fetal loss
Desired outcome: Patient verbalizes change in her role as wife or childbearer or verbalizes plans for adaptation.
- Provide emotional support for patient and significant other. Provide time and a supportive atmosphere for patient to feel comfortable with expressing feelings and concerns. Do not minimize patient's feelings of loss. Conversely, if the pregnancy was not desired, she may experience feelings of relief or guilt regarding the loss.

- Assist patient in identifying concerns, if present, with role performance as a wife or childbearer. Assist patient in developing plans for adaptation. Provide referral for genetic counseling if genetics was a factor in the pregnancy loss.
- Involve social services if needed.

NIC: Coping Enhancement; Emotional Support; Normalization Promotion; Role Enhancement

Grieving related to anticipated or actual fetal loss
Desired outcome: Before hospital discharge, the patient expresses her feelings about the loss (actual or potential) and shares her grief with significant other.

- Assess the stage of grieving that patient is experiencing. Be aware that feelings may be complicated by emotions that preceded the actual or impending fetal loss (e.g., if the woman experienced joy about her pregnancy, her grief may be more than anticipated; conversely, if the pregnancy was viewed negatively, she may experience feelings of guilt and self-blame).
- Do not minimize patient's feelings of loss. Recognize that an early pregnancy loss may take longer to resolve because the grieving process is complicated by the absence of a recognizable body.
- Assist patient and significant other with acknowledging the loss by taking the time to sit and talk with them.
- Offer emotional support, and encourage patient and significant other to discuss the loss among themselves as well.
- Ensure privacy for patient and significant other.
- Refer patient to community-based parent support group.
- Provide for pastoral or other supportive care if indicated.
- See psychosocial nursing diagnoses for patients and families in Appendix One, "Caring for Patients With Cancer and Other Life-disrupting Illnesses," p. 791.

NIC: Active Listening; Counseling; Emotional Support; Grief Work Facilitation; Grief Work Facilitation: Perinatal Death; Support System Enhancement

PATIENT-FAMILY TEACHING AND DISCHARGE PLANNING

When providing patient-family teaching, focus on sensory information; avoid giving excessive information; and initiate a visiting nurse referral for necessary follow-up teaching. Consider including verbal and written information about the following:

- Medications, including drug name, purpose, dosage, schedule, precautions, drug/drug and food/drug interactions, and potential side effects.
- Vaginal bleeding, which should change in color (red to brown) and taper gradually during the first 10 days. Advise patient that consistently red drainage or increasing bleeding is abnormal and necessitates medical attention.
- Indicators of infection that necessitate medical attention: temperature ≥37.7° C (100° F), foul-smelling vaginal discharge, and/or abdominal tenderness or pain.
- Activity limitations as directed by health care provider, including strenuous exercise and sexual relations.
- Importance of follow-up care; confirm date and time of next medical appointment.
- Names and addresses of community resources.

Ectopic pregnancy

An ectopic pregnancy is a fertilized ovum implanted outside the uterus. The most common site is the fallopian tube; it occurs less commonly in the peritoneum, ovary, or cervix. In the fallopian tube, the implanted ovum causes a weakening of the tubal wall, resulting in a rupture that can cause bleeding into the peritoneum, a medical emergency. Factors that predispose a woman to ectopic pregnancy include pelvic inflammatory disease, intrauterine device (IUD) usage, prior surgical procedure of the fallopian tube, history of infertility, previous ectopic pregnancy, and smoking. These pathologic conditions may interfere with the structure and function of the fallopian tube and cause a delay in the passage of the ovum into the uterus, which can result in ectopic pregnancy. Ectopic pregnancies occur in approximately 1 of every 72 pregnancies—a nearly threefold increase from 1970 statistics.

ASSESSMENT

Signs and symptoms: Indications of pregnancy (i.e., amenorrhea, nausea, fatigue, breast enlargement, urinary frequency), uterine bleeding or spotting, and abdominal pain. Most symptoms appear 6-8 wk after the last menstrual period. The following acute symptoms may develop before or may accompany rupture: mild to moderate vaginal bleeding with unilateral lower abdominal cramping that becomes increasingly sharp and constant, referred shoulder pain caused by irritation of the diaphragm from the pooling of blood in the peritoneum, and a falling Hct and Hgb. **Caution:** Immediate intervention is necessary to prevent loss of blood, which can lead to shock and death.

Physical assessment: Abdominal palpation may reveal a unilateral lower quadrant tenderness as well as size and date discrepancy. **Caution:** If ectopic pregnancy is suspected, pelvic examination is deferred to minimize the risk of tubal rupture.

DIAGNOSTIC TESTS

CBC: May reveal a decreased Hgb and Hct and an increased leukocyte count.

Serum human chorionic gonadotropin (HCG): Serial levels will plateau and then diminish. There will be lower than normal levels of serum progesterone and urinary metabolites of serum progesterone.

Ultrasound: May identify the location of pregnancy via transvaginal probe. Doppler ultrasound using color identifies the direction of blood flow in relationship to the transducer; abnormal flow patterns in the adnexa may allow identification of ectopic pregnancy.

Culdocentesis: May reveal the presence of blood in the peritoneum. In this test, fluid is aspirated from the vaginal cul-de-sac.

Laparoscopy: Will confirm the presence of ectopic pregnancy and allow immediate treatment.

COLLABORATIVE MANAGEMENT

Administration of whole blood or packed cells: To replace loss if necessary.

Broad-spectrum IV antibiotics: May be administered prophylactically.

Analgesics/narcotics: For pain management.

Laparoscopy: Performed using an endoscope inserted through a small opening (portal) in the abdomen with additional portals for instruments to accomplish tissue retraction and cautery. Often it is used in conjunction with tubal sparing procedures.

Laparotomy with unilateral salpingectomy (removal of the fallopian tube) or salpingo-oophorectomy (removal of the fallopian tube and ovary): May be necessary if the ectopic pregnancy ruptures. A ruptured ectopic pregnancy is considered a surgical emergency because of the inevitable loss of blood into the peritoneum. The type of surgical procedure used depends on the extent of structural involvement.

Methotrexate: Drug that is often used in chemotherapy. Can be given to select patients with unruptured tubes early in diagnosis in whom surgery is contraindicated or future fertility is desired. Methotrexate, a folinic acid antagonist, induces abrupt tubal abortion.

Rh$_o$ (D) immune globulin (RhoGAM): If indicated, is given to Rh-negative mothers after ectopic pregnancy.

NURSING DIAGNOSES AND INTERVENTIONS

Risk for fluid volume deficit with risks related to bleeding or hemorrhage with ectopic rupture

Desired outcome: Patient is normovolemic, as evidenced by urinary output ≥30 ml/hr, BP ≥90/60 mm Hg, RR ≤20 breaths/min with normal depth and pattern (eupnea), HR ≤100 bpm, warm and dry skin, and absent or scant vaginal bleeding.

- Assess VS at frequent intervals, noting changes in BP, HR, and RR. Be alert to hypotension, increases in HR and RR, and cool and clammy skin as indicators of impending shock.
- Assess the amount and quality of vaginal bleeding. Bright red, frank bleeding, along with abnormal VS, should be reported to the health care provider at once.
- Review results of CBC, noting values of Hgb and Hct that are decreased with blood loss. Optimal values are Hct ≥37% and Hgb ≥12 g/dl.
- Infuse parenteral and blood products as prescribed.

NIC: Bleeding Reduction: Antepartum Uterus; Blood Products Administration; Hypovolemia Management; Intravenous (IV) Therapy; Shock Management: Volume

---

See Also: "Spontaneous Abortion" for **Grieving,** p. 653; **Altered role performance,** p. 653; "Endometriosis" for **Anticipatory grieving,** p. 646; Appendix One, "Caring for Preoperative and Postoperative Patients," p. 717, for nursing diagnoses and interventions; "Caring for Patients With Cancer and Other Life-disrupting Illnesses," p. 791, for psychosocial nursing diagnoses and interventions for patient and significant other.

PATIENT-FAMILY TEACHING AND DISCHARGE PLANNING

When providing patient-family teaching, focus on sensory information; avoid giving excessive information; and initiate a visiting nurse referral for necessary follow-up teaching. Consider including verbal and written information about the following, depending on the type of surgical procedure:

- Medications, including drug name, purpose, dosage, schedule, precautions, drug/drug and food/drug interactions, and potential side effects.
- Importance of monitoring vaginal drainage, including the amount, color, consistency, and odor and reporting significant findings to the health care provider.
- Activity limitations as directed by the health care provider, including strenuous exercise, housework, and sexual relations.
- Indicators of incisional infection, including persistent redness, swelling, local warmth, fever, purulent discharge, and incisional/abdominal pain.
- Importance of follow-up care and purpose for serial HCG levels (with the more conservative treatment) or methotrexate management; confirm time and date of next medical visit if known.

Section Five: Disorders and Surgeries of the Male Pelvis

Benign prostatic hypertrophy

The prostate is an encapsulated gland that surrounds the male urethra below the bladder neck and produces a thin, milky fluid during ejaculation. As a man ages, the prostate gland grows larger. Although the exact cause of the enlargement is unknown, one theory is that hormonal changes affect the estrogen/androgen balance. This noncancerous enlargement is common in men older than 50 yr, and as many as 80% of men older than 65 yr are believed to have symptoms of prostatic enlargement. Treatment is given when symptoms of bladder outlet obstruction appear.

ASSESSMENT

Chronic indicators: Urinary frequency, hesitancy, urgency, and dribbling or postvoid dribbling; decreased force and caliber of stream; nocturia (several times each night); hematuria.

Acute indicators/bladder outlet obstruction: Anuria, nausea, vomiting, severe suprapubic pain, severe and constant urgency, flank pain during micturition.

Physical assessment: Bladder distention, kettledrum sound with percussion over the distended bladder. Rectal examination reveals a smooth, firm, symmetric, and elastic enlargement of the prostate.

DIAGNOSTIC TESTS

Urinalysis: Checks for the presence of WBCs, leukocyte esterase, WBC casts, bacteria, and microscopic hematuria.

Urine culture and sensitivity: Verifies presence of an infecting organism, identifies the type of organism, and determines the organism's antibiotic sensitivities.

> **Note:** All urine specimens should be sent to the laboratory immediately after they are obtained, or they should be refrigerated if this is not possible (specimens for urine culture should *not* be refrigerated). Urine left at room temperature has a greater potential for bacterial growth, turbidity, and alkaline pH, any of which can distort the test results.

Hct and Hgb: Decreased values may signal mild anemia from local bleeding.

Blood urea nitrogen (BUN) and creatinine: To evaluate renal and urinary function. **Note:** BUN can be affected by the patient's hydration status, and the results must be evaluated accordingly: fluid volume excess reduces BUN levels, whereas fluid volume deficit will increase them. Serum creatinine may not be a reliable indicator of renal function in the older adult because of decreased muscle mass and decreased glomerular filtration rate; results of this test must be evaluated along with those of urine creatinine clearance, other renal function studies, and the patient's age.

Prostate-specific antigen (PSA): Elevated above normal (0-4.0 ng/ml; normal range may increase with age) correlates well with positive digital examination findings. This glycoprotein is produced only by the prostate and reflects prostate size.

Cystoscopy: To visualize the prostate gland, estimate its size, and ascertain the presence of any damage to the bladder wall secondary to an enlarged prostate. **Note:** Because patients undergoing cystoscopy are susceptible to septic shock, this procedure is contraindicated in patients with acute urinary tract infection (UTI) because of the possible danger of hematogenic spread of gram-negative bacteria.

Transrectal ultrasound (TRUS): Assesses the size and shape of the prostate via a probe inserted into the rectum.

Pelvic ultrasound: Demonstrates residual urine in the bladder.

COLLABORATIVE MANAGEMENT

Catheterization: To relieve urinary retention. Because of the high incidence of bacteriuria from indwelling catheterization (50% after the first 24 hr), intermittent catheterization is preferred.

Antibiotics and antimicrobial agents: To treat infection if one is present.
α_1-**Adrenergic receptor blockers (doxazosin, prazosin, terazosin):**   Relieve
symptoms of outflow obstruction by acting to relax the bladder neck and
prostatic smooth muscle. **Note:** When beginning therapy, warn patient that
these agents may result in orthostatic changes leading to postural dizziness or
syncope; advise patient to change positions slowly to avoid dizziness.
Androgen hormone inhibitor (finasteride):   To inhibit the conversion of
testosterone to the potent androgen dihydrotachysterol (DHT), which is responsible for development of the prostate; can eventually reduce the size of the
prostate and thus reduce symptoms. **Note:** When necessary, inform the patient
that pregnant women should not handle this medication or semen from a male
taking this medication; finasteride may adversely affect the developing fetus.
Restriction of rapid intake of fluids: Particularly alcohol, which can result
in episodes of acute urinary retention from loss of bladder tone secondary to
rapid distention.
Balloon dilation: Insertion of a balloon catheter into the prostatic urethra,
using fluoroscopy, cystoscopy, ultrasound, or MRI. The balloon is inflated with
sterile water or contrast material, using topical pressure to compress the prostate
gland allowing enlargement of the urethral lumen. This procedure is indicated
for individuals who are poor surgical risks.
Stents: Placement of a small metal coil, via cystoscopy, into the prostatic
urethra to maintain a patent urethra for improved urination. This procedure is
usually restricted to patients who are a high surgical risk.
Thermotherapy: Use of heat to reduce prostatic overgrowth. Transurethral
microwave thermotherapy (TUMT) uses a special urethral catheter introduced
into the prostatic urethra. Transrectal hyperthermia (THT) is applied to the
prostate through the rectum via a specially designed rectal probe.
Transurethral incision of the prostate (TUIP):   Incisions made into the
prostatic urethra via cystoscopy to release bladder neck stricture and improve
bladder emptying. This procedure is used in symptomatic men with small
prostate (<30 g).
Transurethral needle ablation (TUNA) of the prostate: Introduction of a
special probe into the prostatic urethra through which heat and low radio frequency waves are directed to selected prostatic areas. These waves do not injure
the prostatic urethra while destroying underlying prostatic tissue. This is done
to relieve outlet obstructive symptoms and is usually an outpatient procedure.
Prostatectomy: Removal of enlarged prostatic tissue.
Transurethral resection of the prostate (TURP):   Resection of prostatic tissue
via cystoscopy. This is the most common approach, especially in patients who
are poor surgical risks. It is done with the patient under general or spinal
anesthesia.
Suprapubic transvesical prostatectomy/retropubic extravesical prostatectomy/
perineal resection: Removal of prostatic tissue via an incision high in the
bladder (abdominal approach), a low abdominal incision without entry into the
bladder, or an incision between the scrotum and rectum. These procedures are
indicated for a large prostate (≥40 g) that cannot be removed transurethrally.
These approaches may be used if large bladder diverticula or calculi exist that
can be corrected at the time of surgery, in the presence of a severe urethral
stricture, and with orthopedic conditions that contraindicate positioning for
other approaches.
Laser prostatectomy: Use of a laser probe, via cystoscopy, to excise
overgrown prostatic tissue to widen the urethra and reduce symptoms.
Coagulation necrosis of affected tissue sloughs off and is voided with urine over
the following weeks.

NURSING DIAGNOSES AND INTERVENTIONS

Risk for fluid volume deficit with risks associated with postsurgical
bleeding/hemorrhage

Desired outcomes: Patient is normovolemic as evidenced by balanced I&O, HR ≤100 bpm (or within patient's normal range), BP ≥90/60 mm Hg (or within patient's normal range), RR ≤20 breaths/min, and skin that is warm, dry, and of normal color. Following instruction, patient relates actions that may result in hemorrhage of the prostatic capsule and participates in interventions to prevent them.

- On patient's return from the recovery room, monitor VS as the patient's condition warrants or per agency protocol. Be alert to increasing pulse, decreasing BP, diaphoresis, pallor, and increasing respirations, which can occur with hemorrhage and impending shock.
- Monitor and document I&O q8hr. Subtract the amount of fluid used with continuous bladder irrigation (CBI) from the total output.
- Monitor catheter drainage closely for the first 24 hr. Watch for dark red drainage that does not lighten to reddish pink or drainage that remains thick in consistency after irrigation, which can signal bleeding within the operative site. Drainage should lighten to pink or blood tinged within 24 hr after surgery.
- Be alert to bright red, thick drainage at any time, which can occur with arterial bleeding within the operative site.
- Do not measure temperature rectally or insert tubes or enemas into the rectum. Instruct patient not to strain with bowel movements or sit for long periods. Any of these actions can result in pressure on the prostatic capsule and may lead to hemorrhage. Obtain prescription for and provide stool softeners or cathartics as necessary. Encourage a diet high in fiber, and increase fluid intake to aid in producing soft stool.
- The surgeon may establish traction on the indwelling urethral catheter in the operating room to help prevent bleeding. Maintain the traction for 4-8 hr after surgery or as directed. **Note:** Urethral catheters used after prostatic surgery commonly have a large retention balloon (30 ml).
- Also monitor patient for signs of disseminated intravascular coagulation, which can result from the release of large amounts of tissue thromboplastins during a TURP. Watch for active bleeding (dark red) without clots and unusual oozing from all puncture sites. Report significant findings promptly if they occur. For more information, see "Disseminated Intravascular Coagulation," p. 535.

◎ **NIC:** Bleeding Precautions; Fluid Monitoring; Hemorrhage Control; Postanesthesia Care; Shock Prevention

Risk for infection (septic shock) with risks related to invasive procedure (cystoscopy or TURP) resulting in risk of introducting gram-negative bacteria, leading to septic shock

Desired outcome: Patient is free of gram-negative infection as evidenced by normothermia; urinary output ≥30 ml/hr; RR 12-20 breaths/min; HR and BP within patient's normal range; no mental status changes; and orientation to person, place, and time (within patient's normal range).

> **Note:** Accurate assessment of the patient in the early (warm) stage of septic shock greatly improves the prognosis.

- Monitor patient's VS and mentation status at frequent intervals for indicators of the early (warm) stage of septic shock. During the first 24 hr after surgery, be alert to temperatures of 38.3°-40.0° C (101°-104° F), which occur in the presence of infection caused by increased metabolic activity and release of pyrogens. Also assess for moderately increased RR and HR and decreased BP. Classic circulatory signs of collapse occur in the late (cold) stage of septic shock, including profoundly decreased BP (because of decreased stroke volume), greatly increased and weakened HR (compensatory mechanism to maintain cardiac output), and decreased RR (because of respiratory center depression). Mental status changes of inappropriate behavior, personality changes, restlessness, increasing lethargy, and disorientation may signal hypoxia caused by decreased cerebral perfusion.

- Monitor patient's skin for flushing and warmth, which are early signs of septic shock caused by vasodilation. In the cold stage of septic shock, skin becomes clammy, cool, and pale because of sustained vasoconstriction.
- Monitor patient's urinary output for decrease and for increased concentration (normal specific gravity is 1.010-1.030).
- Notify health care provider promptly if septic shock is suspected. Prepare for the following if septic shock is confirmed: IV infusion (e.g., lactated Ringer's or normal saline); oxygen administration; specimens for WBC, ABG, and electrolyte values; and administration of antibiotics.
- Teach the indicators of infection and early septic shock to patient, and stress the importance of notifying staff promptly if they occur after cystoscopy or TURP.

NIC: Infection Protection; Medication Management; Surveillance; Teaching: Disease Process; Vital Signs Monitoring

Fluid volume excess (or risk for same) related to absorption of irrigating fluid during surgery (TURP syndrome)

> **Note:** Large amounts of fluid, commonly plain sterile water, are used to irrigate the bladder during operative cystoscopy to remove blood and tissue to allow visualization of the surgical field. Over time, this fluid may be absorbed through the bladder wall into the systemic circulation.

Desired outcomes: Following surgery, patient is normovolemic as evidenced by balanced I&O (after subtraction of irrigant from total output); orientation to person, place, and time with no significant changes in mental status; BP and HR within patient's normal range; absence of dysrhythmias; and electrolyte values within normal range. Urinary output is ≥30 ml/hr.

- Monitor and record VS. Watch for sudden increases in BP with corresponding decrease in HR. Monitor pulse for dysrhythmias, including irregular rate and skipped beats.
- Monitor and record I&O. To determine the true amount of urinary output, subtract the amount of irrigant (CBI) from the total output. Report discrepancies, which can signal fluid retention or loss.
- Monitor the patient's mental and motor status. Assess for the presence of muscle twitching, seizures, and changes in mentation. These are signs of water intoxication and electrolyte imbalance, which can occur within 24 hr after surgery because of the high volumes of fluid used as irrigation.
- Monitor electrolyte values, in particular those of Na^+, for evidence of hyponatremia. Normal range for Na^+ is 137-147 mEq/L.
- Promptly report indications of fluid overload and electrolyte imbalance to the health care provider.

NIC: Cardiac Care; Electrolyte Management: Hyponatremia; Fluid/Electrolyte Management; Neurologic Monitoring; Urinary Elimination Management

Pain related to bladder spasms
Desired outcomes: Within 1 hr of intervention, patient's subjective perception of pain decreases, as documented by a pain scale. Objective indicators, such as grimacing, are absent or diminished.

- Assess and document the quality, location, and duration of pain. Devise a pain scale with patient, rating pain from 0 (no pain) to 10 (worst pain).
- Medicate patient with prescribed analgesics, narcotics, and antispasmodics as appropriate; evaluate and document the patient's response, using the pain

scale. For individuals in whom the retropubic approach has been used, suppositories (e.g., belladonna and opium [B&O] suppositories) are *contra-indicated.* Oral anticholinergics, such as oxybutynin, are used instead.

- Instruct patient to request analgesic before pain becomes severe.
- Provide warm blankets or heating pad to affected area to increase regional circulation and relax tense muscles.
- Monitor for leakage around the catheter, which can signal the presence of bladder spasms.
- If patient has spasms, assure him that they are normal and can occur from irritation of the bladder mucosa by the catheter balloon or from a clot that results in backup of urine into the bladder with concomitant irritation of the mucosa. Encourage fluid intake to help prevent spasms. If the health care provider has prescribed catheter irrigation for the removal of clots, follow instructions carefully to prevent discomfort and injury to patient.
- Monitor for the presence of clots in the tubing. If clots are present for the patient with CBI, adjust the rate of bladder irrigation to maintain light red urine (with clots). Total output should be greater than the amount of irrigant instilled. If output equals the amount of irrigant or the patient complains that his bladder is full, the catheter may be clogged with clots. If clots inhibit the flow of urine, irrigate the catheter by hand according to agency or health care provider's directive.

NIC: Analgesic Administration; Bladder Irrigation; Distraction; Pain Management; Progressive Muscle Relaxation; Tube Care: Urinary

Risk for impaired skin integrity with risks related to wound drainage from suprapubic or retropubic prostatectomy
Desired outcome: Patient's skin remains nonerythemic and intact.

- Monitor incisional dressings frequently during the first 24 hr, and change or reinforce as needed. If the incision has been made into the bladder, irritation can result from prolonged contact of urine with the skin.
- Use Montgomery straps or gauze net (Surginet) rather than tape to secure the dressing.
- If the drainage is copious after drain removal, apply a wound drainage or ostomy pouch with a skin barrier over the incision. Use a pouch with an antireflux valve to prevent contamination from reflux.

NIC: Incision Site Care; Ostomy Care; Skin Care: Topical Treatments; Skin Surveillance; Wound Care

Sexual dysfunction related to fear of impotence caused by lack of knowledge about postsurgical sexual function
Desired outcome: Following intervention/patient teaching, patient discusses concerns about sexuality and relates accurate information about sexual function.

- Assess patient's level of readiness to discuss sexual function; provide opportunities for patient to discuss fears and anxieties.
- Assure patient who has had a simple prostatectomy that ability to attain and maintain an erection is unaltered. Retrograde ejaculation (backward flow of seminal fluid into the bladder, which is eliminated with the next urination) or "dry" ejaculation will occur in most patients, but this probably will end after a few months. However, it will not affect ability to achieve orgasm.
- Encourage communication between patient and his significant other.
- Be aware of your own feelings about sexuality. If you are uncomfortable discussing sexuality, request that another staff member take responsibility for discussing feelings and concerns with the patient.
- As indicated, encourage continuation of counseling after hospital discharge. Confer with health care provider and social services to identify appropriate referral.

NIC: Active Listening; Anxiety Reduction; Sexual Counseling; Teaching: Preoperative; Teaching: Sexuality

Constipation related to postsurgical discomfort or fear of exerting excess pressure on the prostatic capsule
Desired outcome: By the third to fourth postoperative day, patient relates the presence of a bowel pattern that is normal for him with minimal pain or straining.

> Note: A patient who states that he needs to have a bowel movement during the first 24 hr after surgery may have clots in the bladder that are creating pressure on the rectum. Assess for the presence of clots (see **Pain,** earlier), and irrigate the catheter as indicated.

- Document the presence or absence and quality of bowel sounds in all four abdominal quadrants.
- Gather baseline information on patient's normal bowel pattern, and document findings.
- Unless contraindicated, encourage patient to drink 2-3 L of fluid/day on the day after surgery.
- Consult health care provider and dietitian about need for increased fiber in patient's diet.
- Teach patient to avoid straining when defecating to prevent excess pressure on the prostatic capsule.
- Encourage patient to ambulate and be as active as possible.
- Consult health care provider about use of stool softeners for patient during the postoperative period.
- See Appendix One, "Caring for Patients on Prolonged Bedrest" for **Constipation,** p. 743, for more information.

NIC: Activity Therapy; Bowel Management; Fluid Management; Teaching: Prescribed Diet

Urge incontinence related to urethral irritation after removal of urethral catheter
Desired outcome: Patient reports increasing periods of time between voidings by the second postoperative day and regains normal pattern of micturition within 4-6 wk after surgery.
- Before removing the urethral catheter, explain to patient that he may void in small amounts for the first 12 hr after catheter removal because of irritation from the catheter.
- Instruct patient to save urine in a urinal for the first 24 hr after surgery. Inspect each voiding for color and consistency. First urine specimens can be dark red from the passage of old blood. Each successive specimen should be lighter in color.
- Note and document the time and amount of each voiding. Initially the patient may void q15-30min, but the time interval between voidings should increase toward a more normal pattern.
- Encourage the patient to drink 2.5-3.0 L/day.
- Before hospital discharge, inform patient that dribbling may occur for the first 4-6 wk after surgery because of disturbance of the bladder neck and urethra during prostate removal. As muscles strengthen and healing occurs (the urethra reaches normal size and function), the dribbling stops.
- Teach patient Kegel exercises (see p. 183) to improve sphincter control.

NIC: Fluid Management; Mutual Goal Setting; Pelvic Floor Exercise; Teaching: Prescribed Activity/Exercise; Urinary Habit Training

Acute confusion (or risk for same) related to fluid volume deficit secondary to postsurgical bleeding/hemorrhage; fluid volume excess secondary to absorption of irrigating fluid during surgery; or cerebral hypoxia secondary to infectious process or sepsis

Desired outcomes: Patient's mental status returns to normal for patient within 3 days of treatment. Patient exhibits no evidence of injury as a result of his altered mental status.

- Assess patient's baseline LOC and mental status on admission. Ask patient to perform a three-step task (i.e., "Raise your right hand, place it on your left shoulder, and then place the right hand by your side."). Test short-term memory by showing patient how to use the call light, having patient return the demonstration, and then waiting 5 min before having patient demonstrate use of the call light again. Inability to remember beyond 5 min indicates poor short-term memory. Document patient's response.
- Document patient's actions in behavioral terms. Describe the "confused" behavior.
- Obtain description of prehospital functional and mental status from sources familiar with patient (e.g., patient's family, friends, personnel at nursing home or residential care facility).
- Identify cause of acute confusion. Assess oximetry or request ABG values to determine oxygenation levels; check serum or fingerstick glucose to determine glucose levels; and request current serum electrolytes and CBC to ascertain imbalances and/or presence of elevated WBC count as a determinant of infection. Assess hydration status by reviewing I&O records after surgery. Note any imbalances either way; output should match intake. Assess legs for presence of dependent edema, which can signal overhydration with poor venous return. Assess cardiac and lung status for presence of abnormal heart sounds or rhythms and presence of crackles (rales) in lung bases, which can indicate fluid excess. Assess mouth for furrowed tongue and dry mucous membranes, which are signals of fluid deficit.
- For oximetry readings $\leq 92\%$, anticipate initiation of oxygen therapy to increase oxygenation.
- As appropriate, anticipate initiation of antibiotics in the presence of sepsis; diuretics to increase diuresis; increased fluid intake by mouth or IV to rehydrate patient.
- As appropriate, have patient wear glasses and hearing aid, or keep them close to the bedside and within patient's easy reach.
- Keep patient's urinal and other frequently used items within easy reach. If patient has a short-term memory problem, do not expect him to use the call light.
- As indicated by the patient's mental status, check on patient frequently or every time you pass by the room.
- If indicated, place patient close to nurse's station if possible. Provide an environment that is nonstimulating and safe. Provide music, but avoid use of TV (individuals who are acutely confused regarding place and time often think the action on the TV is happening in the room).
- Attempt to reorient patient to surroundings as needed. Keep a clock and calendar at the bedside, and remind patient verbally of the date and place.
- Encourage patient or significant other to bring items familiar to patient to provide a foundation for orientation. These items can be simple and include blankets, bedspreads, and pictures of family or pets.
- If the patient becomes belligerent, angry, or argumentative while you are attempting to reorient him, *stop this approach.* Do not argue with patient or patient's interpretation of the environment. State "I can understand why you may (hear, think, see) that."
- If the patient displays hostile behavior or misperceives your role (e.g., nurse becomes thief, jailer), leave the room. Return in 15 min. Introduce yourself to the patient as though you have never met. Begin dialogue anew. Patients who are acutely confused have poor short-term memory and may not remember the previous encounter or that you were involved in that encounter.

- If the patient attempts to leave the hospital, walk with him and attempt distraction. Ask patient to tell you about the destination (e.g., "That sounds like a wonderful place! Tell me about it."). Keep tone pleasant and conversational. Continue walking with patient away from exits and doors around the unit. After a few minutes, attempt to guide patient back to his room.
- If the patient has permanent or severe cognitive impairment, check on him frequently and reorient to baseline mental status as indicated; however, do not argue with patient about his perception of reality. This can cause a cognitively impaired person to become aggressive and combative. **Note:** Patients with severe cognitive impairments (e.g., Alzheimer's disease, dementia) also can experience acute confusional states (i.e., delirium) and can be returned to their baseline mental state.

NIC: Calming Technique; Delirium Management; Elopement Precautions; Environmental Management: Safety; Hallucination Management; Physical Restraint; Reality Orientation; Security Enhancement; Surveillance: Safety

---

See Also: "Cancer of the Bladder" for **Altered urinary elimination** related to obstruction of suprapubic catheter, p. 176; "Prostatic Neoplasm" for **Stress incontinence,** p. 668; Appendix One, "Caring for Preoperative and Postoperative Patients," p. 717, for nursing diagnoses and interventions.

PATIENT-FAMILY TEACHING AND DISCHARGE PLANNING

When providing patient-family teaching, focus on sensory information; avoid giving excessive information; and initiate a visiting nurse referral for necessary follow-up teaching. Consider including verbal and written information about the following:

- Medications, including drug name, purpose, dosage, schedule, precautions, drug/drug and food/drug interactions, and potential side effects.
- Necessity of reporting the following indicators of UTI to health care provider: chills; fever; hematuria; flank, CVA, suprapubic, low back, buttock, or scrotal pain; cloudy and foul-smelling urine; frequency; urgency; dysuria; and increasing or recurring incontinence.
- Care of incision, if appropriate, including cleansing, dressing changes, and bathing. Advise patient to be aware of indicators of infection: persistent redness, increasing pain, edema, increased warmth along incision, or purulent or increased drainage.
- Care of catheters or drains if patient is discharged with them.
- Daily fluid requirement of at least 2-3 L/day in nonrestricted patients.
- Importance of increasing dietary fiber or taking stool softeners to soften stools. This will minimize risk of damage to the prostatic capsule by preventing straining with bowel movements. Caution patient to avoid using suppositories or enemas for treatment of constipation.
- Use of a sofa, reclining chair, or footstool to promote venous drainage from the legs and to distribute weight on the perineum, not the rectum.
- Avoiding the following activities for the period of time prescribed by health care provider: sitting for long periods, heavy lifting (>10 lb), and sexual intercourse.
- Kegel exercises to help regain urinary sphincter control for postoperative dribbling. See discussion on p. 183.
- As appropriate, refer patients to the U.S. Agency for Health Care Policy and Research (AHCPR) publication, "Treating your Enlarged Prostate," available by calling the AHCPR Publications Clearinghouse at (800) 358-9295.

- For patients experiencing impotence, provide the following information, as appropriate:

  Impotents Anonymous (IA)
  119 South Ruth Street
  Maryville, TN 37803-5746   (615) 983-6092

Prostatic neoplasm

Cancer of the prostate is the most common reproductive cancer in men older than 50 yr. Most prostatic neoplasms develop in the posterior portion of the gland and can be detected by digital rectal examination (DRE) in the early stages of development. Although age is a critical risk factor, familial incidence also increases a man's risk of developing this form of cancer. Thus, for men with a positive family history, the American Cancer Society (ACS) recommends a DRE and prostate-specific antigen (PSA) screening as part of the annual health checkup in men older than 40 yr. For men with a negative family history, the ACS recommends annual DRE after the age of 40 yr and annual PSA after the age of 50 yr. Elevations of PSA indicate the presence of cancer before symptoms develop or a tumor can be palpated. When detected early, prostatic cancer usually can be treated successfully. Unfortunately, medical treatment often is not sought until the tumor has affected the urinary pattern or caused hip or back pain, recurring cystitis, or urinary obstruction. These symptoms indicate that metastasis has occurred, which dramatically decreases the survival rate.

ASSESSMENT

Signs and symptoms (in the later stages of development):   Dribbling, incontinence, decreased caliber and strength of stream, hesitancy, complaints of incomplete bladder emptying, anuria, hematuria, nocturia, burning with urination (dysuria), urgency, chills, fever, cloudy and foul-smelling urine, decreased urinary output, and lower back pain.

Physical assessment: Bladder distention; kettledrum sound with percussion over distended bladder. Rectal examination may reveal a large, hard, fixed prostate with irregular nodules.

DIAGNOSTIC TESTS

Urinalysis and urine culture: To verify or rule out the presence of WBCs, leukocyte esterase, WBC casts, RBCs (usually as microscopic hematuria), bacteria, and pH >8.0, which would signal infection.

> **Note:**   All urine specimens should be sent to the laboratory immediately after they are obtained, or they should be refrigerated if this is not possible (specimens for culture are *not* refrigerated). Urine left at room temperature has a greater potential for bacterial growth, turbidity, and alkalinity, any of which can distort the test results.

CBC: May reveal marked anemia in the presence of metastatic disease.
BUN and creatinine: May be elevated if renal function is compromised.
Note: BUN values are affected by the patient's hydration status and should be evaluated accordingly. Fluid volume excess decreases the value, whereas fluid volume deficit increases it. In the older adult, decreased muscle mass and a decreased glomerular filtration rate may affect the values of serum creatinine. Therefore these values must be evaluated along with those of urine creatinine clearance, other renal function studies, and the patient's age.

Serum acid phosphatase (also known as prostatic acid phosphatase [PAP]): To monitor disease progress. Values will be elevated if metastasis has occurred (normal adult/elderly level: 0.11-0.60 U/L). Because prostate tissue is rich in this enzyme, the spread of the disease results in an increase in the amount of acid phosphatase in the blood.

Serum alkaline phosphatase: Will be elevated if metastasis has spread to the bones. **Note:** This enzyme is predominately produced by liver and bone tissues and thus is not specific to prostatic metastasis.

Prostate-specific antigen (PSA): Elevation above normal (0.0-4.0 ng/ml; normal range may increase with age) correlates well with positive digital examination findings. This glycoprotein is produced only by the prostate and reflects prostate size. Elevated PSA levels in the presence of a normal DRE may indicate cancer. PSA is assessed for routine screening and staging and to observe progress of the disease.

> **Note:** Serum acid phosphatase and PSA must be drawn before a rectal examination or initiation of urinary catheterization. Both procedures stimulate the prostate to secrete more of these substances and thus raise blood levels.

Intravenous pyelogram (IVP)/excretory urogram: Evaluates the structure and function of the kidneys, ureters, and bladder. Other findings may include ureteral obstruction caused by metastasis to the pelvic lymph nodes or direct invasion by the tumor. (See discussion of the complications of IVP in the testicular cancer section, p. 670.)

Biopsy of the prostate

Transperineal/transrectal needle core biopsy: Performed with the patient under general or spinal anesthesia. The biopsy needle is inserted through the perineal skin or via the rectum directly into the area that contains the tumor. The sample is aspirated and sent to the laboratory for analysis.

Transrectal fine-needle aspiration: Performed with the patient under local anesthesia; biopsy needle is passed into the tumor through the rectum. The sample is aspirated, transferred to slides, and sent to the laboratory for analysis.

Transrectal ultrasonography (TRUS): To assess the size and shape of the prostate, including tumor growth. This test is especially useful in recognizing and localizing intracapsular prostatic tumors and in monitoring response of the tumor to therapy.

COLLABORATIVE MANAGEMENT

Staging of the disease: Based on the TNM system of the American Joint Committee on Cancer (AJCC), an international standard for staging many forms of cancer. The T represents tumor size; N refers to the identified number of involved lymph nodes; and M stands for metastasis (i.e., the presence or absence of known metastasis beyond the prostate and associated lymph nodes).

Grading of the cancer: Based on the number of abnormal cells seen under microscope. The higher the number, the more invasive and aggressive the cancer. Usually the Gleason grading system is used; grades range between 2 and 10.

External radiation therapy: Performed for both curative and palliative therapy, depending on the stage of the neoplasm. Treatment occurs over a 6-wk period, and patients can expect to remain sexually potent after treatment. This therapy also is used to shrink the tumor, thereby relieving obstruction in the urinary tract.

Interstitial irradiation of the prostate: Uses radioactive gold, chromium, or iodine needles or seeds implanted in the prostate to destroy the prostate tumor at its origin. This therapy will not, however, affect other areas if metastasis has occurred.

Cryosurgical ablation: Freezing of the prostate via cryoprobes inserted into the prostate and surrounding tissues using fluoroscopy. Liquid nitrogen is used to cool the probes and freeze adjacent prostatic tissues. An indwelling urinary catheter irrigated with warm (44° C [111.2° F]) irrigant is used to maintain body temperature.

Hormonal therapy: To block the production of testosterone, which is thought to play a role in the development of prostatic cancer. The following therapies may be used alone or in combination with each other.

Luteinizing hormone–releasing hormone (LHRH) agonists (i.e., leuprolide acetate): To block the release of testosterone. Leuprolide acetate must be given either IM monthly or SC daily and is expensive.

Estrogens (e.g., diethylstilbestrol [DES]): Block the release of LHRH. Approximately 25% of patients using estrogen develop side effects, of which the more serious are heart failure, thrombophlebitis, and myocardial infarction.

Antiandrogens (i.e., flutamide, bicalutamide): To block male hormones from reaching the prostate.

Chemotherapy: Might be used as either a curative or palliative measure.

Surgical procedures

Prostatectomy (transurethral resection of the prostate [TURP]): Resection of prostatic tissue via cystoscopy; used when the tumor is in a beginning stage and is well differentiated. For additional information, see "Benign Prostatic Hypertrophy," p. 658.

Radical prostatectomy: With or without pelvic node dissection. Either the perineal or retropubic approach is used to remove the entire prostate gland along with the seminal vesicles and a portion of the bladder neck, part of the vas deferens, and adjacent lymph nodes. This procedure is done for tumors that are large or not well differentiated. Erectile dysfunction occurs in 85%-90% of males having this procedure. However, this side effect can be avoided if periprostatic autonomic nerves are spared. Urinary incontinence also occurs in the majority of patients after removal of the indwelling catheter. In a radical prostatectomy, all of the prostate and its capsule are removed (as opposed to the TURP, in which the apex of the prostate and its capsule remain). As a result, the following can occur to cause incontinence: (1) the external sphincter can be damaged because of surgical trauma to the bladder neck and prostate capsule, or (2) portions of the bladder neck are removed as are portions of the urethra in an effort to remove all of the cancer. This damage may take up to 6 mo to heal, and the incontinence subsides 6 mo after surgery in 85%-90% of this patient population.

Nerve-sparing radical prostatectomy: Used in patients with negative lymph nodes, no elevated serum acid phosphatase, and no evidence of extracapsular extension. This procedure involves the use of a longitudinal, rather than a transverse, incision through the periprostatic fascia and a careful dissection along a longitudinal plane from the prostate to the urethra, thus avoiding damage to the neurovascular bundles that affect potency.

Bilateral orchiectomy: May be used with estrogen therapy to depress testosterone production.

NURSING DIAGNOSES AND INTERVENTIONS

Sexual dysfunction related to erectile dysfunction (risk is 85%-90%) after radical prostatectomy

Desired outcome: Patient verbalizes feelings about sexuality within 3 days after surgery.

- Assess patient's readiness to discuss sexual concerns. Encourage verbalization, and, as indicated, use facilitative communication techniques, such as open-ended questions, reflective statements, and rephrasing of patient's statements for clarification.

- Be alert to signs of grief, such as hostility, depression, and demanding behavior, and to signs of denial, such as inappropriate affect or accepting the diagnosis too well.
- As appropriate, arrange for caregivers who have established rapport with the patient to spend time with him and encourage verbalization of his concerns.
- Be alert to the needs of the patient and significant other for more information about sexual functioning.
- As indicated, inform health care provider about patient's need for more information so that counseling can be reinforced.
- Confer with health care provider and social services to identify appropriate referrals for counseling after hospital discharge.

NIC: Active Listening; Anxiety Reduction; Grief Work Facilitation; Sexual Counseling; Teaching: Sexuality

Knowledge deficit: Side effects of antiandrogen therapy or bilateral orchiectomy
Desired outcome: Within the 24-hr period before hospital discharge, patient verbalizes knowledge about the extent and duration of body changes.
- Inform patient of side effects of estrogen therapy and orchiectomy (e.g., breast enlargement, breast tenderness, loss of sexual desire, impotence). As indicated, teach him about the side effects of hormone therapy (e.g., LHRH agonists, antiandrogens), including hot flashes, impotence, or diarrhea.
- For patients taking estrogen therapy, provide instruction about symptoms related to complications of heart failure, thrombophlebitis, and myocardial infarction, which should be reported to the health care provider (e.g., SOB; orthopnea; dyspnea; pedal edema; unilateral leg swelling or pain; left arm, left jaw, or left-sided chest pain). Provide reassurance that most side effects will disappear after therapy has been discontinued.
- If appropriate, explain to patient that before initiating estrogen therapy, health care provider may prescribe radiation therapy to the areolae of the breasts to minimize painful gynecomastia. However, this procedure will not decrease other side effects.
- Assure patient undergoing orchiectomy that the procedure will not affect his ability to have an erection and orgasm but that he will not ejaculate.

NIC: Discharge Planning; Teaching: Disease Process; Teaching: Individual; Teaching: Prescribed Medication

Stress incontinence related to temporary loss of muscle tone in the urethral sphincter after radical prostatectomy
Desired outcome: Within the 24-hr period before hospital discharge, patient relates understanding of the cause of the temporary incontinence and the regimen that must be observed to promote bladder control.
- Explain to patient that there is a potential for urinary incontinence after prostatectomy but that it should resolve within 6 mo. Describe the reason for the incontinence, using aids such as anatomic illustrations.
- Encourage patient to maintain an adequate fluid intake of at least 2-3 L/day (unless contraindicated by an underlying cardiac dysfunction or other disorder). Explain that dilute urine is less irritating to the prostatic fossa.
- Instruct patient to avoid fluids that irritate the bladder, such as caffeine-containing drinks. Explain that caffeine has a mild diuretic effect, which would make bladder control even more difficult.
- Establish a bladder routine with patient before hospital discharge (see "Urinary Incontinence," p. 180).
- Teach patient Kegel exercises to enhance sphincter control (see "Urinary Incontinence," p. 183).

- Remind patient to discuss any incontinence problems with health care provider during follow-up examinations.
- NIC: Fluid Management; Pelvic Floor Exercise; Teaching: Prescribed Activity/Exercise; Urinary Bladder Training; Urinary Habit Training

> **See Also:**   "Benign Prostatic Hypertrophy" for **Risk for fluid volume deficit** (bleeding/hemorrhage), p. 658; **Pain,** p. 658; **Risk for infection,** p. 659; **Risk for impaired skin integrity,** p. 661; **Constipation,** p. 662; **Acute confusion,** p. 662; Appendix One, "Caring for Preoperative and Postoperative Patients," p. 717; "Caring for Patients With Cancer and Other Life-disrupting Illnesses," p. 747, for nursing diagnoses and interventions.

PATIENT-FAMILY TEACHING AND DISCHARGE PLANNING

When providing patient-family teaching, focus on sensory information; avoid giving excessive information; and initiate a visiting nurse referral for necessary follow-up teaching. Consider including verbal and written information about the following:

- For patients with radical prostatectomy, referral to a counselor or counseling agency as necessary, and discussion about incontinence following removal of indwelling catheter.
- Medications, including drug name, purpose, dosage, schedule, precautions, drug/drug and food/drug interactions, and potential side effects.
- Phone numbers to call if questions or concerns arise about therapy or disease after discharge. Additional general information can be obtained by contacting the following organizations:

The American Cancer Society
1599 Clifton Road NE
Atlanta, GA 30329   (800) ACS-2345
WWW address: *http://www.cancer.org*

National Cancer Institute Information Service (CIS)
Bldg. 31, Room 10A16
9000 Rockville Pike
Bethesda, MD 20892   (800) 422-6237
WWW address: *http://wwwicic.nic.nih.gov/*

- See this section in "Benign Prostatic Hypertrophy," p. 664, for more information.

Testicular neoplasm

Cancer of the testes is most often found in men in their 20s and 30s. Usually it is discovered by accident, often after a traumatic injury to the groin for which professional examination is warranted. Self-examination is the best method of early detection for this disorder. It is believed that men with an undescended testicle are at higher risk than the general male population. Individuals who have had surgery at an early age (before 2 yr) to correct an undescended testicle virtually eliminate the potential of developing the cancer. However, these men are better able to check for lumps and thickening in the testis after it has been surgically descended.

   The most common testicular tumors are seminomas, which spread slowly through the lymphatic system to the iliac and periaortic nodes. Embryonal tumors or nonseminoma types, on the other hand, metastasize quickly. Nonseminoma types include teratocarcinoma, adult teratoma, choriocarcinoma, and Leydig cell. Most testicular cancers are combinations of two forms of cancer, which can make treatment difficult. However, with treatment, prognosis for all forms of this cancer is good.

ASSESSMENT

Signs and symptoms: Lump the size of a pea or thickening of the testis. There may be an aching or heaviness in the testis caused by swelling of the scrotum as a result of an accumulation of fluid or blood. Pain usually is not a symptom. In the later stages of the disease, the patient may experience abdominal pain caused by bowel or ureteral obstruction, coughing caused by metastasis to the lungs, weight loss, or anorexia. Breast enlargement may occur because of reduction in testosterone.

Physical assessment: Palpation of symmetric, firm scrotal mass; presence of supraclavicular or abdominal mass caused by enlargement of lymph nodes in those areas.

DIAGNOSTIC TESTS

Hct and Hgb: Drawn preoperatively to assess for anemia, which can occur because of metastasis.

Serum liver function tests (alanine aminotransferase [ALT], aspartate aminotransferase [AST], lactic dehydrogenase [LDH], K-glutamyl transpeptidase [GGTP]):   To assess adequacy of liver function for patients needing chemotherapy and for presence of abnormalities, which may indicate metastasis. ALT and AST detect hepatocellular obstruction or liver damage. LDH becomes elevated with liver disease or malignant tumors. Serum GGTP also rises in the presence of liver damage or disease.

Serum renal function tests (creatinine and electrolytes, e.g., Na^+ and K^+):   To help determine adequacy of renal function for the patient needing chemotherapy; abnormalities may signal metastatic ureteral obstruction.

Serum α-fetoprotein (AFP):   Used as a tumor marker and to identify the type of carcinoma. AFP is rarely elevated in a seminoma, but it will be elevated with nonseminomas. Response to treatment and assessment for recurrence can be evaluated based on comparison with the baseline value of this test.

Human chorionic gonadotropin (HCG) levels: Used as a tumor marker and for identification of the type of carcinoma. Normally, HCG is found in the maternal circulation during pregnancy, and it is an abnormal finding in the male. However, it is found with most testicular cancers. As with AFP, response to treatment and assessment for recurrence can be evaluated based on comparison with the baseline value of this test.

Chest x-ray: May show presence of metastasis to the lungs.

Intravenous pyelogram (IVP)/excretory urogram: May show displacement of the kidney or ureters by masses of carcinomatous lumbar lymph nodes, which may also cause ureteral obstruction.

Lymphangiograms: May reveal enlarged iliac and periaortic lymph nodes if disease has spread. In this procedure, contrast medium is injected into the dorsal aspects of the feet to outline the lymphatic vessels. The contrast medium will discolor the patient's urine and stool for 24-48 hr after the procedure. The injection of this substance might be uncomfortable, and the injection site will be tender for a few days.

> **Note:**   Two complications of IVP and lymphangiogram are allergic reactions to the dye and contrast medium–induced acute renal failure. Exposure to contrast medium may worsen existing renal or cardiac insufficiency, especially in older, dehydrated, or diabetic patients. Before the study, query the patient about allergies to shellfish and iodine and reactions to previous dye studies. After the test, monitor patient for indicators of renal failure.

COLLABORATIVE MANAGEMENT

Classification and staging of the disease: Following orchiectomy, the primary tumor is classified using the TNM classification system of the American Joint Committee on Cancer (AJCC). In the TNM classification system, the T represents tumor size; N refers to the identified number of involved lymph nodes; and M stands for metastasis (i.e., the presence or absence of known metastasis beyond the testicle and associated lymph nodes).

Biopsy: To confirm the presence of malignancy. In the absence of malignancy, the abnormal benign lump is removed but the testicle is left. If the lump proves to be malignant, an orchiectomy is performed to remove the diseased testicle. Incisional biopsy of the testicle is rarely used.

Orchiectomy: A small incision is made at the inguinal area on the affected side rather than in the scrotum itself. This permits high ligation of the cord at the inguinal ring to allow for removal of the whole testis, which other approaches do not allow. The patient may return from surgery with an indwelling catheter and incisional drain for removal of excess exudate.

Retroperitoneal lymph node dissection or lymphadenectomy: Patients with seminomas undergo a lymphadenectomy *only* if the disease has spread beyond the scrotal sac and does not respond to irradiation. Patients with nonseminomatous tumors receive lymphadenectomy as part of a treatment regimen that includes orchiectomy, radiation therapy, and chemotherapy. It is performed at the time of the orchiectomy or a few days later. Lymph nodes are removed from the kidney to the inguinal area on the affected side.

Chemotherapy: Used if cancer has spread outside the testicle or retroperitoneal lymph nodes. It is used for radio-resistant tumors (choriocarcinoma), with or without surgery. Most types of testicular carcinomas appear to be sensitive to chemotherapy, particularly to cisplatin, vinblastine sulfate, and bleomycin. Doxorubicin may be used before irradiation to treat metastases to retroperitoneal nodes.

Radiation therapy: Most commonly used for patients with seminomas. Use of this therapy varies with the type and stage of the cancer. In the absence of metastasis, lymph nodes often are irradiated to prevent microscopic spread of the seminoma. Low-dose radiation is used to minimize complications.

Serial AFP and HCG levels: Drawn routinely over a a 2-yr period. Levels drop toward normal if the neoplasm has been eradicated and rise if it has not.

NURSING DIAGNOSES AND INTERVENTIONS

Sexual dysfunction related to body changes that occur with orchiectomy

Desired outcome: Before hospital discharge, patient verbalizes feelings and frustrations about the orchiectomy and relates realistic knowledge about changes that will occur.

- Provide a calm, unhurried atmosphere for patient and significant other. Use facilitative communication techniques, such as open-ended questions, reflective statements, and rephrasing of patient's statements for clarification.
- Encourage communication between patient and significant other.
- Encourage patient to verbalize feelings, fears, and frustrations about sexual attractiveness, feared impotence, and infertility. Explain that the *surgery* will not impair fertility or potency; however, fertility may be compromised by radiation therapy or chemotherapy and can last for 2 yr.
- For patient undergoing lymphadenectomy, explain that ejaculatory failure may occur if the sympathetic nerve is damaged but that erection and orgasm will be possible. Explain that if ejaculatory failure does occur, artificial insemination is possible because the semen flows back into the urine, from which it can be extracted, enabling the ovum to become impregnated artificially.
- If appropriate, explain that a silicone prosthesis may be placed in the scrotum to achieve a normal appearance. Consult health care provider about the potential for this procedure.

- For patient undergoing radiation or chemotherapy, explain that he can store sperm in a sperm bank. The rate of pregnancy is only 50% by this method, however, because some sperm do not survive the freezing process.

NIC: Active Listening; Anxiety Reduction; Grief Work Facilitation; Sexual Counseling; Teaching: Sexuality

Pain related to scrotal swelling secondary to orchiectomy or lymphadenectomy
Desired outcomes: Within 1-2 hr of intervention, patient's subjective perception of pain decreases, as documented by a pain scale. Objective indicators, such as grimacing, are absent or diminished.
- Assess and document the quality, duration, and location of the pain. Ask patient to rate the pain on a scale of 0 (no pain) to 10 (worst pain).
- Administer prescribed analgesics as indicated. Note and document patient's response, using the pain scale to evaluate the improvement.
- Instruct patient to request analgesic before pain becomes severe.
- Adjust scrotal support as needed to enhance patient comfort. The scrotal support elevates and supports the scrotum to minimize edema.
- Apply ice gloves or packs to the scrotum to reduce swelling.
- Encourage patient to ambulate as soon as possible. Explain that exercise reduces swelling and pain by improving circulation.

NIC: Activity Therapy; Analgesic Administration; Distraction; Heat/Cold Application; Pain Management; Progressive Muscle Relaxation

Risk for fluid volume deficit with risks related to postsurgical bleeding or hemorrhage
Desired outcome: Patient remains normovolemic as evidenced by BP ≥90/60 mm Hg (or within patient's normal range), HR ≤100 bpm (or within patient's normal range), balanced I&O, urinary output ≥30 ml/hr, RR ≤20 breaths/min, and warm, dry skin.
- Monitor patient's VS q15min for 30 min after return from the recovery room. Once stable, assess VS as indicated by patient's condition or hospital protocol.
- Be alert to increasing HR, decreasing BP, diaphoresis, cool and clammy skin, pallor, decreasing urinary output, and increasing RR, which signal hemorrhage and impending shock.
- Monitor I&O. Immediately after surgery, administer IV fluids and then advance to oral fluids.
- Measure and document urine, gastric tube, and drainage system output; record output amounts separately. Optimally, drainage amounts will decrease gradually and then cease.
- Check dressing at frequent intervals after surgery, changing it when it becomes damp. Document color and amount of drainage. Notify health care provider if drainage is heavy (saturates dressings within 1 hr after changing), becomes bright red, or forms clots on the dressings, any of which can occur with arterial or venous bleeding.
- Notify health care provider if output from drainage systems appears suspicious (i.e., bright red drainage) or exceeds 50 ml/hr for 2 hr.

NIC: Bleeding Precautions; Fluid Monitoring; Hemorrhage Control; Postanesthesia Care; Shock Prevention; Tube Care

See Also: Appendix One, "Caring for Preoperative and Postoperative Patients," p. 717; "Caring for Patients With Cancer and Other Life-disrupting Illnesses," p. 747, for nursing diagnoses and interventions.

PATIENT-FAMILY TEACHING AND DISCHARGE PLANNING

When providing patient-family teaching, focus on sensory information; avoid giving excessive information; and initiate a visiting nurse referral for necessary

follow-up teaching. Consider including verbal and written information about the following:

- Medications, including drug name, purpose, dosage, schedule, precautions, drug/drug and food/drug interactions, and potential side effects.
- Care of incision, including cleansing and dressing changes. Advise patient to be alert to signs of infection, such as fever, persistent redness, swelling, pain, warmth or puffiness along incision, and purulent or persistent drainage.
- Care of drains or catheters if patient is discharged with them.
- Review of postoperative activity restrictions as directed by health care provider, such as no heavy lifting (>10 lb), driving, or sexual intercourse for 4-6 wk.
- Necessity of continued care (e.g., radiation therapy, chemotherapy, serial laboratory work); confirm date and time of next appointment if known.
- Importance of self-examination of remaining testicle, since it is possible to get unrelated cancer in the remaining testis.
- Phone numbers to call if questions or concerns arise about therapy or disease after discharge. Additional general information can be obtained by contacting the following organizations:

The American Cancer Society
1599 Clifton Road NE
Atlanta, GA 30329   (800) ACS-2345
WWW address: *http://www.cancer.org*

National Cancer Institute Information Service (CIS)
Bldg. 31, Room 10A16
9000 Rockville Pike
Bethesda, MD 20892   (800) 422-6237
WWW address: *http://wwwicic.nic.nih.gov/*

Selected Bibliography

Averette HE, Nguyen H: Gynecologic cancer. In Murphy GP, Lawrence W, Lenhard RE, editors: *American cancer society textbook of clinical oncology,* ed 2, Atlanta, 1995, American Cancer Society.

Beck RP: Abnormalities of support in the female genital tract: genital prolapse. In Copeland L, editor: *Textbook of gynecology*, Philadelphia, 1993, Saunders.

Boone T: Physical medicine and management of impotence in physically disabled men, *Phys Med Rehabil* 9(2):523-537, 1995.

Bostwick D et al: *Prostate cancer: what every man and his family needs to know,* New York, 1996, American Cancer Society.

Brakey M: Myths & facts ... about testicular cancer, *Nursing* 24(9):24, 1994.

Brenner Z, Krenzer M: Update on cryosurgical ablation for prostate cancer, *Am J Nurs* 95(4):44-49, 1995.

Butler R, Whitehead D: Love and sex after 60: how to evaluate and treat the impotent man, *Geriatrics* 49(10):27-32, 1994.

Dale PS, Williams JT, IV: Axillary staging utilizing selective sentinel lymphadenectomy for patients with invasive breast carcinoma, *Am Surg* 64(1):28-31, 1998.

De Stefano MS, Bertin-Matson K: Gynecologic cancers. In McCorkle R et al, editors: *Cancer nursing: a comprehensive textbook*, ed 2, Philadelphia, 1996, Saunders.

Donovan JF, Williams RD: Urology. In Way LW, editor: *Current surgical diagnosis and treatment*, ed 10, Norwalk, Conn, 1994, Appleton & Lange.

Gerber G, Rukstalis D: Laparoscopic approach to retroperitoneal lymph node dissection, *Semin Surg Oncol* 12(2):121-125, 1996.

Gross J, Johnson B: *Handbook of oncology nursing,* ed 3, Boston, 1998, Jones & Bartlett.

Harris JR et al, editors: *Diseases of the breast*, ed 3, Philadelphia, 1996, Lippincott-Raven.

Henderson IC: Breast cancer. In Murphy GP et al, editors: *American Cancer Society textbook on clinical oncology,* ed 2, Philadelphia, 1996, Saunders.

Horne MM, Heitz UE, Swearingen PL: *Pocket guide to fluid, electrolyte, and acid-base balance,* ed 3, St Louis, 1997, Mosby.

Interqual: *The ISD-A review system with adult ISD criteria,* Northhampton, NH, and Marlboro, Mass, August 1992, Interqual.

Jacobs SL: Using GnRH agonists to diagnose endometriosis in chronic pelvic pain patients, *Contemp Obstet Gynecol* 41(2):78-87, 1996.

Kim MJ et al: *Pocket guide to nursing diagnoses,* ed 7, St Louis, 1997, Mosby.

Knobf MT: Breast cancers. In McCorkle R et al, editors: *Cancer nursing: a comprehensive textbook,* ed 2, Philadelphia, 1996, Saunders.

Kohl N, Miklos JR: Laparoscopic Burch colposuspension: a modern approach, *Contemp Obstet Gynecol* 42(1):36-56, 1997.

Lemcke DP et al, editors: *Primary care of women,* Norwalk, Conn, 1995, Appleton & Lange.

McCloskey JC, Bulechek GM, editors: *Nursing interventions classification (NIC),* ed 2, St Louis, 1996, Mosby.

Nichol J et al: Efficacy and safety of finasteride therapy for benign prostatic hyperplasia: results of a 2-year randomized controlled trial (the PROSPECT study), *Can Med Assoc J* 155(9):1251-1259, 1996.

Parker SL et al: Cancer statistics, 1997, *CA Cancer Clin* 47:5-27, 1997.

Perk AJ et al: Silicone gel–filled breast implants and connective tissue diseases, *Plast Reconstr Surg* 101(2):261-268, 1998.

Roumen RM, Valkenburg JG, Geuskens LM: Lymphoscintigraphy and feasibility of sentinel node biopsy in 83 patients with primary breast cancer, *Eur J Surg Oncol* 23(6):495-502, 1997.

Speights V et al: Evaluation of age-specific normal ranges for prostate-specific antigen, *Urology* 45(3):454-458, 1995.

Stewart KC, Lyster DM: Interstitial lymphoscintigraphy for lymphatic mapping in surgical practice and research, *J Invest Surg* 10(5):249-262, 1997.

Tierney L et al, editors: *Current medical diagnosis and treatment,* ed 36, Stamford, Conn, 1997, Appleton & Lange.

Wiersma TG et al: Dynamic rectal examination (defecography), *Baillieres Clin Gastroenterol* 8(4):729-741, 1994.

◎ 10 PROVIDING CARE FOR PATIENTS WITH SPECIAL NEEDS

Section One: Caring for Individuals With Human Immunodeficiency Virus Disease

Acquired immunodeficiency syndrome (AIDS) is a life-threatening illness caused by the human immunodeficiency virus (HIV). AIDS is characterized by the disruption of cell-mediated immunity. This breakdown of the immune system is manifested by opportunistic infections such as *Pneumocystis carinii* pneumonia (PCP) or tumors such as Kaposi's sarcoma (KS).

The three confirmed routes of HIV transmission are the following:

- Sexual contact that involves an exchange of body fluids.
- Parenterally via receipt of contaminated blood or blood products or injecting drug use.
- From an infected mother to a child during the perinatal period.

It is estimated that the average time span between infection with HIV and seroconversion (development of a positive HIV antibody test) is 6-8 wk, although antibody response may be absent for 1 yr or more. Therefore a negative test does not guarantee the absence of infection. Individuals with a recent history of high-risk behavior and a negative HIV antibody test should be retested at 6-mo intervals for 1 yr and follow the guidelines for safer sex practices (Table 10-1). Anyone with a positive HIV antibody test must be considered infectious and capable of transmitting the virus.

Although the Centers for Disease Control and Prevention (CDC) continues, for epidemiologic reasons, to identify "exposure categories" (Table 10-2), the epidemiologic focus no longer is on groups but on high-risk behaviors. HIV infection has transcended all racial, social, sexual, and economic barriers, and it is primarily high-risk behaviors that are responsible for its transmission. Table 10-3 details the behaviors that place an individual at the greatest risk for HIV infection.

To a minimal extent, health care workers who come into contact with the body substances of patients also are at some risk. Understanding and practicing Standard Precautions or variations, such as Body Substance Isolation, are essential for all health care workers. Review Table A-19, p. 818, for a discussion of the handling of blood and body fluids for all patients.

AIDS is the terminal phase of HIV infection. It is a chronic viral disease that covers a wide spectrum of illnesses and symptoms for a variable course of

675

TABLE 10-1　Safer Sex Guidelines

Safer sexual practices
   Social (dry) kissing
   French (wet) kissing
   Hugging
   Massage
   Mutual masturbation
   Body-to-body contact (except mucous membrane areas)
   Activities not involving direct body contact

Sexual practices of questionable safety
   Anal-oral contact (rimming) using a latex barrier
   Anal or vaginal intercourse using latex condoms*
   Fellatio (mouth to penis) without ejaculation
   Cunnilingus (mouth to vaginal area)
   Water sports (enemas, urination)

Unsafe sex practices
   Anal or vaginal intercourse without latex condom
   Oral contact with body fluids (semen, urine, feces, vaginal secretions)
   Contact with blood
   Oral-anal contact (rimming)
   Manual anal/vaginal penetration (fisting)
   Sharing of sexual aids or needles

*Petroleum-based lubricants have been shown to increase the risk of condom rupture. Water-based products, such as K-Y Jelly and similar products, are preferred.
Use of viricidal spermicides, such as nonoxynol-9, is strongly urged as added protection.

TABLE 10-2　Exposure Categories and Their Percentages for Contracting HIV Disease

Group	Percent
Men who have sex with men	45
Injecting drug users	27
Men who have sex with men and inject drugs	5
People with hemophilia/coagulation disorders	1
People with heterosexual contact	10
Recipients of blood transfusions, blood components, or tissue	2
People with multiple modes of exposure	6
Undetermined	4

time. There is no classic disease progression (e.g., some individuals proceed from an asymptomatic, seropositive state to AIDS, whereas others may experience the symptoms for many years). Therefore HIV disease should be considered a continuum of infection. The stages of illness are described under "Assessment," p. 677.

The mortality rate for those diagnosed with HIV disease is grim but slowly improving. Early recognition and treatment of the complications of HIV infections, as well as promising experimental drug therapies, have given patients not only increased survival times but also a better quality of life.

TABLE 10-3 High-Risk Sexual Behaviors

Unprotected anonymous sex
Unprotected oral sex with transfer of body fluids
Unprotected receptive anal/vaginal sex
Unprotected oral-anal contact (rimming)
Manual anal/vaginal penetration (fisting)
Sharing sexual aids or needles
Unprotected sex with multiple partners

Maintenance of a positive attitude by the patient and caregivers is an essential element in the therapeutic plan, but an honest approach to the realities of any life-threatening illness also must prevail.

ASSESSMENT

The four stages of HIV infection can be categorized as acute infection, asymptomatic stage, AIDS-related complex (ARC—a now obsolete term that still is used to define symptoms for this stage), and AIDS.

Acute infection: A mononucleosis-like syndrome.

Signs and symptoms: Fever, malaise, muscle aches, night sweats, headache, nausea.

Laboratory results: HIV antibody test may not yet be positive.

Asymptomatic stage: May range from 5 yr to much longer.

Signs and symptoms: Generally none but may have persistent, generalized lymphadenopathy.

Laboratory results: Positive HIV antibody test; CD4 T lymphocyte count usually >400/mm^3.

ARC

Signs and symptoms: Persistent fever, involuntary weight loss, chronic diarrhea, fatigue, night sweats, thrush, hairy leukoplakia.

Laboratory results: Positive HIV antibody test, CD4 T lymphocyte or helper lymphocyte count usually <400/mm^3, anemia, thrombocytopenia, leukopenia, or lymphopenia.

AIDS: Diagnosed by the presence of one or more of these "indicator" diseases as defined by CDC: cryptosporidiosis with diarrhea lasting >1 mo; cytomegalovirus of an organ other than the liver, spleen, or lymph nodes; isosporiasis; KS; lymphoma of the brain (primary); lymphoid interstitial pneumonia or pulmonary lymphoid hyperplasia; *Pneumocystitis carinii* pneumonia; progressive multifocal leukoencephalopathy; toxoplasmosis of the brain; candidiasis of the esophagus, trachea, bronchi, or lungs; coccidioidomycosis; extrapulmonary cryptococcosis; herpes simplex virus infection causing an ulcer that persists >1 mo; histoplasmosis; pulmonary tuberculosis; other mycobacterioses; salmonellosis; other bacterial infection; HIV encephalopathy; Burkitt's lymphoma; immunoblastic sarcoma; *Mycobacterium avium* complex; recurrent pneumonia; HIV wasting syndrome; and invasive cervical cancer.

Signs and symptoms: Depend on the presenting opportunistic infection.

Laboratory results: Positive HIV antibody test, CD4 T lymphocyte count usually <200/mm^3, or total lymphocytes <14%, hematologic disorders (see "ARC," above), multiple chemistry abnormalities.

History: If the patient is suspected of having HIV infection, the history would be incomplete without detailed social and sexual interviews, with special focus on determining high-risk behaviors. A complete review of body systems with careful attention to the common symptoms of HIV infection should be performed.

Physical assessment: The following indicators are seen frequently with HIV infection.

General: Fever, cachexia, weight loss.

Cutaneous: Herpes zoster or simplex infection(s); seborrheic or other dermatitis; fungal infections of the skin (moniliasis, candidiasis) or nail beds (onychomycosis); KS lesions; petechiae.

Head/neck: "Cotton-wool" spots visualized on funduscopic examination; oral KS; candidiasis (thrush); hairy leukoplakia; aphthous ulcers; enlarged, hard, and occasionally tender lymph nodes.

Respiratory: Tachypnea, dyspnea, diminished or adventitious breath sounds (crackles [rales], rhonchi, wheezing).

Cardiac: Tachycardia, friction rub, gallops, murmurs.

Gastrointestinal: Enlargement of liver or spleen, diarrhea, constipation, hyperactive bowel sounds, abdominal distention.

Genital/rectal: KS lesions, herpes, candidiasis, fistulas.

Neuromuscular: Flattened affect, apathy, withdrawal, memory deficits, headache, muscle atrophy, speech deficits, gait disorders, generalized weakness, incontinence, neuropathy.

DIAGNOSTIC TESTS

Individuals with HIV disease may experience many signs and symptoms, as previously stated. The health care provider may prescribe other evaluations than the commonly performed diagnostic tests listed below.

HIV antibody: The initial test for HIV is the enzyme-linked immunosorbent assay (ELISA), which tests for presence of antibody to the virus that causes HIV disease. A positive result signals the individual's infection with HIV and ability to transmit HIV to others, not the presence of AIDS. An initially reactive ELISA should be repeated twice on the same specimen. If one or both repeats are reactive, the ELISA is considered repeatedly reactive and should be confirmed by another test, usually the Western blot (WB).

Western blot: A confirmatory test used to detect immune response to the specific viral proteins of HIV. A reactive WB is defined by a specific pattern of protein bands separated by electrophoresis on a strip of nitrocellulose paper; three of the following bands must be present for reactivity: p24 (see below), gp41, and gp210 or gp160.

p24 Antigen test: Detects HIV p24 antigen in serum, plasma, and cerebrospinal fluid (CSF) of infected individuals. Its advantage is that it detects viral antigen (HIV p24) early in the course of infection before seroconversion.

Viral load tests: Provide a more direct measure of disease progression via the amount of HIV RNA (genetic material) in the blood. These include RT-PCR (quantitative polymerase chain reaction), bDNA (branched chain deoxyribonucleic acid), and NASBA (nucleic acid sequence-based amplification). These tests are reported in copies per milliliter. Fewer than 10,000 copies/ml is associated with a low risk for disease progression; 10,000-100,000 copies/ml is associated with moderate risk; >100,000 copies/ml is associated with a high risk for disease progression.

Immunofluorescence assay: Tests for HIV antibody; has three distinct advantages over the WB test: more sensitive, less expensive, and less technically demanding.

Urinalysis: Tests for beta$_2$, a microglobulin that has been used as a marker for proximal tubule dysfunction; also detects cytomegalovirus (CMV).

Biopsy: Used for both esophageal and KS lesions; helps distinguish invasive pathogens from secondary colonizers.

COLLABORATIVE MANAGEMENT

Medical management is limited primarily to chemotherapeutic intervention in an attempt to arrest the progression of the disease. Currently, no single drug or

T A B L E   1 0 - 4   Retroviral Drugs

Drug name	Dosage	Instructions
Nucleoside analogs (NRTIs)		
Zidovudine (Retrovir, AZT, ZDV)	300 mg bid	Take all these on an empty stomach
Didanosine (Videx, ddI)	200 mg bid	
Zalcitabine (HIVID, ddC)	0.75 mg tid	
Stavudine (Zerit, d4T)	40 mg bid	
Lamivudine (Epivir, 3TC)	150 mg bid	
Protease inhibitors (PIs)		
Siquinavir (Invirase)	600 mg tid	Take with a high-fat meal
Ritonavir (Norvir)	600 mg bid	Refrigerate
Indinavir (Crixivan)	800 mg q8h/L	Take on an empty stomach
Nonnucleoside reverse transcriptase inhibitor (NNRTI)		
Nevirapine (Viramune)	200 mg bid	Do not take concomitantly with PIs (above)

combination of drugs has restored immunocompetence to afflicted patients. Medical treatment is palliative.

Retroviral drugs: Commonly used in combination, three classes of retroviral agents are available (Table 10-4). Although not a cure for HIV, some combinations have demonstrated ability to reduce viral load of HIV in plasma. Reduced viral load has been associated with improved clinical outcomes, including longer life and reduced incidence of opportunistic infections. Specific patient education is needed about administration and side effects of these agents.

Surgical interventions: May include resection of tumors; placement of venous access devices for total parenteral nutrition (TPN), chemotherapy, or frequent blood withdrawals; or, in selected instances, splenectomy for idiopathic thrombocytopenic purpura (ITP). **Note:** IV gammaglobulin or prednisone therapy is also used for ITP.

NURSING DIAGNOSES AND INTERVENTIONS

Risk for infection with risks related to inadequate secondary defenses of the immune system, malnutrition, or side effects of chemotherapy

Desired outcome: Patient is free of additional infections during hospitalization, as evidenced by appropriate cultures or biopsies.

- Assess for indicators of opportunistic infections (e.g., persistent fevers, night sweats, fatigue, involuntary weight loss, persistent and dry cough, persistent diarrhea, headache). See Table 10-5 for the common opportunistic infections and organisms that infect individuals with HIV disease.
- Monitor laboratory data, especially CBC, differential, erythrocyte sedimentation rate (ESR), and cultures, to evaluate the course of infection. Be alert to abnormal results, and notify health care provider of significant findings.
- Maintain strict sterile technique for all invasive procedures to prevent introduction of new pathogens.
- Assist patient in maintaining meticulous body hygiene to prevent spread of organisms from body secretions into skin breaks, especially if patient has diarrhea.

TABLE 10-5	Opportunistic Infections and Organisms Infecting Individuals With HIV Disease		
Viral	**Fungal**	**Protozoal**	**Bacterial**
Herpes (1 and 2)	*Candida*	*Pneumocystis carinii*	*Treponema pallidum* (syphilis)
Cytomegalovirus	*Histoplasma capsulatum*	*Toxoplasma gondii*	*Neisseria gonorrhoeae*
Varicella	*Cryptococcus*	*Entamoeba histolytica*	*Shigella*
Epstein-Barr	*Coccidioides*	*Giardia lamblia*	*Salmonella*
Hepatitis A, B		*Cryptosporidium enteritisdis*	*Mycobacterium avium-intracellulare* (MAI) *Mycobacterium tuberculosis*
Hepatitis non-A/ non-B			

- Monitor temperature and VS at frequent intervals for evidence of fever or sepsis. In addition to increased temperature, be alert to diaphoresis, confusion or mental status changes, decrease in LOC, increased HR, and decreased BP secondary to the vasodilator effect of the increased body temperature. Perform a complete physical assessment at least q8hr to identify changes from baseline assessment. Assess for changes in breath sounds, which may indicate an increasing level of infiltrates.
- Promote pulmonary toilet by encouraging patient to engage in frequent breathing or incentive spirometry exercises. Use caution when performing postural drainage and chest physiotherapy, if prescribed, because patients may be too ill to tolerate these activities.
- Monitor sites of invasive procedures for signs of infection, including erythema, swelling, local warmth, tenderness, and purulent exudate.
- Enforce good hand-washing techniques before contact with patient to minimize risk of transmitting infectious organisms from staff and other patients.
- Teach patient home care considerations for infection prevention after hospital discharge (see "Patient-Family Teaching and Discharge Planning," p. 686).

◎ You may also wish to refer to the following interventions from the Nursing Interventions Classification (NIC):

NIC: Infection Protection; Respiratory Monitoring; Surveillance; Vital Signs Monitoring

Impaired gas exchange related to altered oxygen supply secondary to presence of pulmonary infiltrates, hyperventilation, and sepsis
Desired outcomes: After treatment/intervention, patient has adequate gas exchange as evidenced by RR 12-20 breaths/min with normal depth and pattern (eupnea) and absence of adventitious sounds, nasal flaring, and other clinical indicators of respiratory dysfunction. By hospital discharge, patient's oximetry demonstrates an O_2 saturation >92% or ABG results as follows: Pao_2 ≥80 mm Hg; $Paco_2$ 35-45 mm Hg; pH 7.35-7.45.

- Assess patient's respiratory status q2hr during patient's awake period, noting rate, rhythm, depth, and regularity of respirations. Observe for use of accessory muscles, flaring of nares, presence of adventitious sounds, cough, changes in the color or character of sputum, or cyanosis, which occur with respiratory dysfunction.
- As indicated, assess O_2 saturation via oximetry. Report O_2 saturation <92% to the health care provider.
- Monitor ABG results closely for decreased $Paco_2$ (<35 mm Hg) and increased pH (>7.40), which can occur with hyperventilation.
- Adjust oxygen therapy to attain optimal oxygenation, as determined by ABG values.
- Instruct patient to report changes in cough, as well as dyspnea that increases with exertion.
- To maintain adequate tidal volume, provide chest physiotherapy as prescribed; encourage use of incentive spirometry at frequent intervals.
- Reposition patient q2hr to help prevent stasis of lung fluids.
- Monitor for changes in the color or character of sputum; obtain sputum for culture and sensitivity as indicated.
- Group nursing activities to provide patient with uninterrupted periods of rest, optimally 90-120 min at a time.
- When administering sulfa for PCP, monitor closely for side effects, such as rash or bone marrow suppression (leukopenia, neutropenia). If administering pentamidine, be alert to side effects such as hypotension or hypoglycemia, which necessitate frequent BP checks and fingersticks for blood sugar levels.
- To relieve mucous membrane irritation, which can predispose patient to coughing spells, deliver humidified oxygen to patient.
- Administer sedatives and analgesics judiciously to help prevent or minimize respiratory depression.

Caution: Wear a high-efficiency mask and protect mucous membranes when caring for patients diagnosed as having active tuberculosis. See p. 26 for more information.

NIC: Bedside Laboratory Testing; Chest Physiotherapy; Infection Control; Medication Management; Oxygen Therapy; Respiratory Monitoring

Altered nutrition: Less than body requirements related to diarrhea and nausea associated with side effects of medications, malabsorption, anorexia, dysphagia, and fatigue

Desired outcome: By hospital discharge, patient has adequate nutrition as evidenced by stable weight, serum albumin 3.5-5.5 g/dl, transferrin 180-260 mg/dl, thyroxine-binding prealbumin 20-30 mg/dl, retinol-binding protein 4-5 mg/dl, and a state of nitrogen (N) balance or a positive N state.

- Assess nutritional status daily, noting weight, caloric intake, and protein and albumin values. Be alert to progressive weight loss, wasting of muscle tissue, loss of skin tone, and decreases in both total protein and albumin, which can adversely affect wound healing and impair the patient's ability to withstand infection.
- Provide small, frequent, high-caloric, high-protein meals, allowing sufficient time for patient to eat. Offer supplements between feedings. As a rule, these patients are kept in a slightly positive N state (after resolution of the critical phases of this illness) by ensuring daily caloric intake equal to 50 kcal/kg of ideal body weight with an additional 1.5 g of protein per kilogram (e.g., a man weighing 70 kg should receive 3500 kcal plus 105 g of protein per day).
- Provide supplemental vitamins and minerals as prescribed to replace deficiencies.
- To minimize anorexia and help treat stomatitis, which can occur as a side effect of chemotherapy, provide oral hygiene before and after meals.

- If patient feels isolated socially, encourage significant other to visit at mealtimes and bring patient's favorite high-caloric, high-protein foods from home.
- If patient is nauseated, provide instructions for deep breathing and voluntary swallowing, which help decrease stimulation of vomiting center. Administer antiemetics as prescribed. Encourage patients to request medication before discomfort becomes severe.
- If patient is dysphagic, encourage intake of fluids that are high in calories and protein; provide different flavors and textures for variation.
- As prescribed, deliver isotonic tube feeding for patients unable to eat. Isotonic fluids will help prevent diarrhea associated with hypertonic or hypotonic fluids. Check placement of gastric tube before each feeding; assess absorption by evaluating amount of residual feeding q4hr. Do not deliver feeding if residual is >50-100 ml. Keep HOB elevated 30 degrees while feeding, and position patient in a right side-lying position to facilitate gastric emptying.
- If patient's caloric intake is insufficient, discuss the potential need for TPN with health care provider.

NIC: Diet Staging; Enteral Tube Feeding; Nutrition Management; Nutritional Counseling; Tube Care: Gastrointestinal

Diarrhea related to gastrointestinal (GI) infection, chemotherapy, or tube feeding intolerance
Desired outcome: By the time of hospital discharge, patient has formed stools and a bowel elimination pattern that is normal for him or her.

- Ensure minimal use of antidiarrheal medications, which promote intestinal concentration of infectious organisms.
- Teach patient to avoid large amounts (>300 mg/day) of caffeine, which increases peristalsis and can promote diarrhea.
- Maintain accurate I&O records to monitor changes in fluid volume status. Be alert to signs of hypovolemia, such as cool and clammy skin, increased HR (>100 bpm), increased RR (>20 breaths/min), and decreased urinary output (<30 ml/hr).
- Assess stool for the presence of blood, fat, and undigested materials.
- Monitor stool cultures for evidence of new infectious organisms.
- Monitor patient for indicators of electrolyte imbalance, such as anxiety, confusion, muscle weakness, cramps, dysrhythmias, weak pulse, and decreased BP.
- If patient is being given tube feedings, dilute strength or decrease rate of infusion to prevent "solute drag" (concentrated solutions that pull water into the lumen of the bowel), which may be the cause of the diarrhea.
- Encourage foods high in potassium (K^+) (see Table 3-4, p. 146) and sodium (Na^+) (see Table 3-2, p. 133) to replace any decrements of these ions.
- Protect anorectal area by keeping it cleansed and using compounds such as zinc oxide to prevent or retard skin excoriation.

NIC: Diarrhea Management; Fluid/Electrolyte Management; Perineal Care; Self-Care Assistance: Toileting

Impaired tissue integrity (or risk for same) related to cachexia and malnourishment, diarrhea, side effects of chemotherapy, KS lesions, negative N state, and decreased mobility caused by arthralgia and fatigue
Desired outcome: At hospital discharge patient's tissue is intact.

- Assess and document skin integrity, noting temperature, moisture, color, vascularity, texture, lesions, and areas of excoriation or poor wound healing. Evaluate KS lesions for location, dissemination, weeping, or significant changes. Note and record the presence of herpes lesions, especially those that are perirectal.

- Avoid prolonged pressure on dependent body parts by turning and positioning patient q2hr; encourage patient to change position frequently.
- Provide patient with a pressure relief mattress, as indicated.
- Teach patient to use mild, hypoallergenic, nondrying soaps or lanolin-based products for bathing and to pat rather than rub the skin to dry it. When appropriate, use lotions and emollients to soften and relieve itching of dry, flaky skin.
- Use soft sheets on the bed, avoiding wrinkles. If patient is incontinent, use some type of rectal device (e.g., fecal incontinence bags, rectal tube) to protect the skin and prevent perirectal excoriation and skin breakdown.
- To enhance skin and tissue healing, assist patient toward a state of N balance by promoting adequate amounts of protein and carbohydrates (see discussion under **Altered nutrition,** p. 681).
- Ensure that patient receives minimum daily requirements of vitamins and minerals; supplement them as necessary.
- Encourage ROM and weight-bearing mobility, when possible, to increase circulation to skin and tissue.

NIC: Nutritional Counseling; Perineal Care; Pressure Ulcer Prevention; Skin Care: Topical Treatments; Skin Surveillance

Pain related to physical and chemical factors associated with prolonged immobility, side effects of chemotherapy, infections, peripheral neuropathy, and frequent venipunctures
Desired outcomes: Within 1 hr of intervention, patient's subjective perception of pain decreases, as documented by a pain scale. Nonverbal indicators of discomfort, such as grimacing, are absent or diminished.
- Assess and record the following: location, onset, duration, and factors that precipitate and alleviate patient's pain. With patient, establish a pain scale, rating pain from 0 (no pain) to 10 (worst pain). Use the scale to evaluate degree of pain and to document the degree of relief achieved.
- Administer analgesic as prescribed. Encourage patient to request medication before the pain becomes severe.
- Provide heat or cold applications to affected areas (e.g., apply heat to painful joints and cold packs to reduce swelling associated with infections or multiple venipunctures).
- Encourage patient to engage in diversional activities as a means of increasing pain tolerance and decreasing its intensity (e.g., soothing music; quiet conversation; reading; slow, rhythmic breathing).
- To reduce pain intensity, teach patient techniques that decrease skeletal muscle tension, such as deep breathing, biofeedback, and relaxation exercises (see **Health-seeking behaviors:** Relaxation technique effective for stress reduction, p. 59).
- If frequent venipunctures cause the patient discomfort, discuss with health care provider the desirability of a capped venous catheter for long-term blood withdrawal.
- Administer anticonvulsant agents as prescribed for relief of peripheral neuropathy.
- Promote relaxation and comfort with back rubs and massage.
- For other interventions, see Appendix One, "Caring for Preoperative and Postoperative Patients" for **Pain**, p. 719.

NIC: Analgesic Administration; Anxiety Reduction; Distraction; Heat/Cold Application; Pain Management; Simple Guided Imagery; Simple Relaxation Therapy

Activity intolerance related to generalized weakness secondary to fluid and electrolyte imbalance, arthralgia, myalgia, dyspnea, fever, pain, hypoxia, and effects of chemotherapy

Desired outcome: Before hospital discharge, patient rates perceived exertion at ≤3 on a 0-10 scale and exhibits tolerance to activity as evidenced by HR ≤20 bpm over resting HR, RR ≤20 breaths/min, and systolic BP ≤20 mm Hg over or under resting systolic BP.

- Assess patient's tolerance to activity by assessing HR, RR, and BP before and immediately after activity, and ask patient to rate his or her perceived exertion. See Appendix One, "Caring for Patients on Prolonged Bedrest" for **Activity intolerance,** p. 738, for details about perceived exertion.
- Plan adequate (90- to 120-min) rest periods between patient's scheduled activities. Adjust activities as appropriate to reduce energy expenditures.
- As much as possible, encourage regular periods of exercise to help prevent cardiac intolerance to activities, which can occur quickly after periods of prolonged inactivity.
- Monitor electrolyte levels to ensure that patient's muscle weakness is not caused by hypokalemia.
- Monitor oximetry or ABG values to ensure that patient is oxygenated adequately; adjust oxygen delivery accordingly.
- Advise patient to keep anecdotal notes (perhaps in journal format) on exacerbation and remission of signs and symptoms.
- For more information, see Appendix One, "Caring for Patients on Prolonged Bedrest" for **Activity intolerance,** p. 738.

NIC: Energy Management; Environmental Management; Exercise Promotion; Teaching: Prescribed Activity/Exercise

Anxiety related to threat of death and social isolation
Desired outcome: Following intervention, patient expresses feelings and is free of harmful anxiety as evidenced by HR ≤100 bpm, RR ≤20 breaths/min with normal depth and pattern (eupnea), and BP within patient's normal range.

- Monitor patient for verbal or nonverbal expressions of the following: inability to cope, apprehension, guilt for past actions, uncertainty, concerns about rejection and isolation, and suicidal ideation.
- Spend time with patient, and encourage expression of feelings and concerns.
- Support effective coping patterns (e.g., by allowing patient to cry or talk rather than denying his or her legitimate fears and concerns).
- Provide accurate information about HIV disease and related diagnostic procedures.
- If patient hyperventilates, teach him or her to mimic your normal respiratory pattern (eupnea).

NIC: Anticipatory Guidance; Anxiety Reduction; Coping Enhancement; Crisis Intervention; Emotional Support; Suicide Prevention

Body image disturbance related to biophysical changes secondary to KS lesions, chemotherapy, and emaciation
Desired outcome: Before hospital discharge, patient expresses positive feelings about self to family, significant other, and primary nurse.

- Encourage patient to express feelings, especially the way he or she views or feels about self.
- Provide patient with positive feedback; help patient focus on facts rather than myths or exaggerations about self.
- Provide patient with access to clergy, psychiatric nurse, social worker, psychologist, or HIV counselor as appropriate.
- Encourage patient to join and share feelings with HIV support group.
- For additional information, see Appendix One, "Caring for Patients With Cancer and Other Life-disrupting Illnesses" for **Body image disturbance,** p. 799.

NIC: Body Image Enhancement; Counseling; Emotional Support; Self-Esteem Enhancement

Knowledge deficit: Disease process, prognosis, life-style changes, and treatment plan
Desired outcome: Before hospital discharge, patient verbalizes accurate information about the disease process, prognosis, behaviors that increase the risk of transmitting the virus to others, and treatment plan.

- Assess patient's knowledge about HIV disease, including pathophysiologic changes that will occur, ways the disease is transmitted, necessary behavioral changes, and side effects of treatment. Correct misinformation and misconceptions as necessary.
- Inform patient of private and community agencies that are available to help with tasks such as handling legal affairs, cooking, house cleaning, and nursing care. Provide telephone numbers and addresses for HIV support groups and self-help groups.
- Provide literature that explores the myths and realities of the HIV disease process.
- Teach patient the importance of informing sexual partners of HIV condition and modifying high-risk behaviors known to transmit the virus (see Table 10-3).
- Involve significant other in the teaching and learning process.
- Provide patient and significant other with the names and addresses or phone numbers of HIV resources (see "Patient-Family Teaching and Discharge Planning," p. 686).

NIC: Learning Facilitation; Learning Readiness Enhancement; Teaching: Disease Process; Teaching: Individual; Teaching: Prescribed Medication; Teaching: Procedure/Treatment

Social isolation related to altered state of wellness, societal rejection, loss of support system, feelings of guilt and punishment, fatigue, and changed patterns of sexual expression
Desired outcome: Before hospital discharge, patient communicates and interacts with others.

- Keep patient and significant other well informed about patient's status and treatment plan.
- Provide private periods of time for patient to communicate and interact with significant other.
- Encourage significant other to share in care of the patient.
- Encourage physical closeness between patient and significant other. Provide privacy as much as possible.
- Involve patient in unit or group activities as appropriate.
- Explain significance of isolation precautions to patient.

NIC: Active Listening; Emotional Support; Socialization Enhancement; Support System Enhancement

Impaired environmental interpretation syndrome related to physiologic changes and impaired judgment secondary to infection, space-occupying lesion in the central nervous system (CNS), or HIV dementia
Desired outcomes: Following intervention, patient verbalizes orientation to person, place, and time. Optimally, by hospital discharge patient correctly completes exercises in logical reasoning, memory, perception, concentration, attention, and sequencing of activities.

- Assess patient for minor alterations in personality traits that cannot be attributed to other causes, such as stress or medication.
- Assess patient for signs of dementia, which would include a slowing of all cognitive functioning, with problems in attention, concentration, memory, perception, logical reasoning, and sequencing of activities.
- Encourage patient to report persistent headaches, dizziness, or seizures, which may signal CNS involvement.

- Note any cranial nerve involvement that differs from patient's past medical history. Most commonly the fifth (trigeminal), seventh (facial), and eighth (acoustic) nerves are involved in infectious processes of the CNS.
- Assess patient for signs of mental aberration, blindness, aphasia, hemiparesis, or ataxia, which may signal the presence of a demyelinating disease.
- Divide activities into small, easily accomplished tasks.
- Maintain a stable environment so patient is able to familiarize self with the immediate surroundings (i.e., do not change the location of furniture in room).
- Write notes as reminders; maintain a calendar of appointments.
- Provide some mechanism (e.g., pill box) to ensure that patient takes medications as prescribed.
- Teach patient the importance of reporting changes in neurologic status (e.g., increasing severity of headaches, blurred vision, gait disturbances, or blackouts). Notify health care provider of all significant findings.

NIC: Cognitive Stimulation; Delirium Management; Environmental Management; Neurologic Monitoring; Reality Orientation; Surveillance: Safety

---

See Also: "Section Two: Providing Nutritional Support," p. 687; "Section Three: Managing Wound Care," p. 704; Appendix One, "Caring for Patients on Prolonged Bedrest," p. 738; "Caring for Patients With Cancer and Other Life-disrupting Illnesses," p. 747, for other nursing diagnoses and interventions.

PATIENT-FAMILY TEACHING AND DISCHARGE PLANNING

When providing patient-family teaching, focus on sensory information; avoid giving excessive information; and initiate a visiting nurse referral for necessary follow-up teaching. Consider including verbal and written information about the following:

- Importance of avoiding use of recreational drugs, which are believed to potentiate the immunosuppressive process and lower resistance to infection.
- Significance and importance of refraining from donating blood.
- Necessity of modifying high-risk sexual behaviors. See Table 10-3 for specific information.
- Principles and importance of maintaining a balanced diet; ways to supplement diet with multivitamins and other food sources, such as high-caloric substances (e.g., Isocal, Ensure). Because of increased susceptibility to food-borne opportunistic organisms, fruits and vegetables should be washed thoroughly; meats should be cooked thoroughly at appropriate temperatures; and raw eggs, raw fish (sushi), and unpasteurized milk should be avoided.
- Because of decreased resistance to infection, the importance of limiting contact with individuals known to have active infections. In addition, pets may harbor various fungal, protozoal, and bacterial organisms in their excrement. Therefore contact with bird cages, cat litter, and tropical fish tanks should be avoided.
- Necessity for meticulous hygiene to prevent spread of any extant or new infectious organisms. To avoid exposure to fungi, damp areas in bathrooms (e.g., shower) should be cleaned with solutions of bleach; refrigerators should be cleaned thoroughly with soap and water; and leftover foodstuffs should be disposed of within 2-3 days.
- Techniques for self-assessment of early signs of infection (e.g., erythema, tenderness, local warmth, swelling, purulent exudate) in all cuts, abrasions, lesions, or open wounds.
- Care of venous access device, including technique for self-administration of TPN or medications (see "Providing Nutritional Support," p. 700); care of gastric tube and administration of enteral tube feedings if appropriate.

- Importance of avoiding fatigue by limiting participation in social activities, getting maximum amounts of rest, and minimizing physical exertion.
- Prescribed medications, including drug name, food/drug and drug/drug interactions, dosage, purpose, and potential side effects. Instruct the patient and significant other in the necessity of taking antiretroviral medications as prescribed to avoid viral resistance (especially in the case of protease inhibitors).
- Importance of maintaining medical follow-up appointments.
- Advisability of keeping anecdotal notes (perhaps in journal format) on exacerbation and remission of signs and symptoms.
- Importance of reporting changes in neurologic status (e.g., increasing severity of headaches, blurred vision, gait disturbances, blackouts).
- Advisability of sharing feelings with significant other or within a support group.
- Referral to hospice or agency that provides home help. This should occur before discharge planning begins to ensure continuity of care between the hospital and home or hospice.
- Phone numbers to call if questions or concerns arise about hospice after discharge. Information for these patients can be obtained by contacting the following organization:

  National Hospice Association
  1901 North Moore St., Suite 901
  Arlington, VA 22209   (703) 243-5900; (703) 525-5762 FAX
  WWW address: *http://www.nho.org*

- In addition, provide the following information regarding HIV resources:

  Public Health Service AIDS Hotline: (800) 342-AIDS or
  (800) 342-2437

  AZT Information Hotline: (800) 843-9388

  National Gay Task Force AIDS Information Hotline: (800) 221-7044

  National Sexually Transmitted Diseases Hotline/American Social
  Health Association: (800) 227-8922

  Local Red Cross *or*
  American Red Cross AIDS Education Office
  1730 D Street, N.W.
  Washington, DC 20006   (202) 737-8300

  CDC National AIDS Clearinghouse
  P.O. Box 6003
  Rockville, MD 20849-6003   (800) 243-7012
  WWW address: *http://www/cdcnac.aspensys.com:86/*

  National AIDS Network
  729 Eighth Street, S.E., Suite 300
  Washington, DC 20003   (202) 546-2424

  Association of Nurses in AIDS Care (ANAC)
  11250 Roger Bacon Drive, Suite 8
  Reston, VA 20190-5202   (703) 437-4377

Section Two: Providing Nutritional Support

Hospitalized patients are at high risk for developing protein-energy malnutrition. Studies have shown that 40%-50% of hospitalized surgical patients have insufficient nutrient intake. This situation may be seen in surgical patients who are given IV dextrose/electrolyte solutions alone for extended periods and in patients kept fasting for diagnostic procedures. If this state lasts longer than 5-7 days or if the duration of illness is expected to last longer than 10-14 days, nutritional support should be given.

Nutritional assessment

Because no single sensitive and comprehensive nutritional assessment factor exists, multiple sources of information are used, including any of the following: historical data, nutritional history, anthropometric data, biochemical analysis of blood and urine, and the duration of the disease process.

DIETARY HISTORY

A dietary history is compiled to reveal the adequacy of usual and recent food intake. Be alert to excesses or deficiencies of nutrients and any special eating patterns (e.g., various types of vegetarian or prescribed diets), use of fad diets, and excessive supplementation. Note anything that impairs adequate selection, preparation, ingestion, digestion, absorption, and excretion of nutrients. Include the following:

- Three-day review (including a weekend day) of the patient's usual dietary intake. Identify any food allergies, food aversions, and use of nutritional supplements.
- Recent unplanned weight loss or gain.
- Chewing or swallowing difficulties.
- Nausea, vomiting, or pain with eating.
- Altered pattern of elimination (e.g., constipation, diarrhea).
- Chronic disease affecting utilization of nutrients (e.g., malabsorption, pancreatitis, diabetes mellitus).
- Surgical resection; disease of the gut or accessory organs of digestion (i.e., pancreas, liver, gallbladder).
- Use of medications (e.g., laxatives, antacids, antibiotics, antineoplastic drugs) or alcohol. Long-term use of drugs may affect appetite, digestion, or utilization or excretion of nutrients.

PHYSICAL ASSESSMENT

Most physical findings are not specific to a particular nutritional deficiency. Compare current assessment findings with past assessments, especially related to the following:

- Loss of muscle and adipose tissue.
- Work and muscle endurance.
- Changes in hair, skin, or neuromuscular function.

ANTHROPOMETRIC DATA

Anthropometric science entails measuring the body or its parts. It is helpful to remember that 1 L of fluid equals approximately 2 lb. To convert pounds (lb) and inches (in) to metric measurements, use the following formulas:

Divide *lb* by 2.2 to convert to kilograms (kg).

Divide *in* by 39.37 to convert to meters (m).

Height: Used to determine ideal weight and body mass index (BMI). If patient's height is unavailable or it is not possible to measure, obtain estimate from family or significant other or compare patient's recumbent length with known length of the mattress.

Weight: A readily available and practical indicator of nutritional status that can be compared with previous weight and ideal weight or used to calculate BMI. Changes may reflect fluid retention (edema, diuresis, third spacing), diuresis, dehydration, surgical resections, traumatic amputations, or weight of dressings or equipment (Table 10-6).

T A B L E 1 0 - 6 Height and Weight Guidelines for Men and Women

Height	Men			Women		
	Small frame (lb)	Medium frame (lb)	Large frame (lb)	Small frame (lb)	Medium frame (lb)	Large frame (lb)
4 ft 10 in	—	—	—	102-111	109-121	118-131
4 ft 11 in	—	—	—	103-113	111-123	120-134
5 ft	—	—	—	104-115	113-126	122-137
5 ft 1 in	—	—	—	106-118	115-129	125-140
5 ft 2 in	128-134	131-141	138-150	108-121	118-132	128-143
5 ft 3 in	130-136	133-143	140-153	111-124	121-135	131-147
5 ft 4 in	132-138	135-145	142-156	114-127	124-138	134-151
5 ft 5 in	134-140	137-148	144-160	117-130	127-141	137-155
5 ft 6 in	136-142	139-151	146-164	120-133	130-144	140-159
5 ft 7 in	138-146	142-154	148-168	123-136	133-147	143-163
5 ft 8 in	140-148	145-157	152-172	126-139	136-150	146-167
5 ft 9 in	142-151	148-160	156-176	129-142	139-153	149-170
5 ft 10 in	144-154	151-163	158-180	132-145	142-156	152-173
5 ft 11 in	146-157	154-166	161-184	135-148	145-159	155-176
6 ft	149-160	157-170	164-188	138-151	148-162	158-179
6 ft 1 in	152-164	160-174	168-192	—	—	—
6 ft 2 in	155-168	164-178	172-197	—	—	—
6 ft 3 in	158-172	167-182	176-202	—	—	—
6 ft 4 in	162-176	171-187	181-207	—	—	—

Data courtesy Metropolitan Life Insurance Company, 1983. Ages 25 through 59 yr include 5 lb indoor clothing for men and 3 lb indoor clothing for women and 1-inch heels for both.

Body mass index: Used to evaluate the weight of adults. One calculation and one set of standards are applicable to both men and women:

$$\text{BMI (kg/m}^2) = \frac{\text{Weight}}{\text{Height (m}^2)}$$

BMI values of 20-25 are optimum; values >25 indicate obesity; and values <20 indicate underweight status.

Fat-fold or skinfold measurement: Measurement of subcutaneous fat provides an accurate estimate of total body fat. Triceps skinfold (TSF) thickness is easily accessible and is measured by trained health care providers using a standard protocol and reliable instrumentation (calipers).

BIOCHEMICAL DATA

Protein status: Evaluated via the following tests, with normal values in parentheses: serum albumin (3.5 g/dl), transferrin (180-260 mg/dl), thyroxine-binding prealbumin (20-30 mg/dl), and retinol-binding protein (4-5 mg/dl). Normal values may vary somewhat with different laboratory procedures and standards. Albumin and transferrin have relatively long half-lives of 19 days and 9 days, respectively, whereas thyroxine-binding prealbumin and retinol-binding protein have very short half-lives of 24-48 hr and 10 hr, respectively. If hydration status is normal and anemia is absent, albumin and transferrin levels can be used as baseline indicators of adequacy of protein intake and synthesis. For evidence of response to nutritional therapy, values for the short turnover proteins—thyroxine-binding prealbumin (although very expensive) and retinol-binding protein—are the most useful.

Iron status: Measurement of RBC size, that is, mean corpuscular volume (MCV) (normal: 80-95 μm^3), aids in determining the type of nutrient anemia. In iron-deficiency anemia, RBCs are smaller than normal, whereas in folate or vitamin B_{12} deficiencies, RBCs are larger than normal.

Total lymphocyte count (TLC):   Protein depletion depresses immune function and thus decreases lymphocyte production. TLC (mm^3) = WBC (mm^3) × % lymphocytes

Creatinine/height index: Compares the patient's 24-hr urinary creatinine excretion with a predicted urinary creatinine excretion for individuals of the same height as an evaluation of body muscle mass. The amount of creatinine produced is directly related to the amount of skeletal muscle wasting. Accuracy can be affected by inadequate urine collection and the lack of age-referenced norms.

ESTIMATING NUTRITIONAL REQUIREMENTS

The primary goal of nutritional support is to meet the needs for body temperature, metabolic processes, and tissue repair. Having collected all the data, energy needs now can be estimated using the following options.

Indirect calorimetry: Performed using a bedside metabolic cart. Specialized personnel are required to provide accurate results. Carts are an expense most patient care units cannot justify.

Harris and Benedict equations: To determine basal energy expenditure (BEE). BEE can be calculated using the following equations developed by Harris and Benedict:

$$\text{BEE (male)} = 66.5 + (13.8 \times W) + (5 \times H) - (6.8 \times A)$$

$$\text{BEE (female)} = 655.1 + (9.6 \times W) + (1.9 \times H) - (4.7 \times A)$$

where W = weight in kilograms; H = height in centimeters; and A = age in years. BEE is then multiplied by the appropriate correction factors to allow for the patient's activity level and condition:

Activity factor =
1.20 for bedridden patient
1.30 for ambulatory patient

Injury factor =
1.20 for minor surgery
1.35 for trauma (blunt or skeletal)
1.60 for sepsis

BEE × Activity factor × Injury factor = Total energy expenditure (TEE)

Distribution of calories: A relatively normal distribution of calories is adequate. Percentages of total calories from carbohydrates, protein, and fat should equal approximately 60%, 10%, and 30%, respectively.

Protein requirements: Usually 0.8-1.5 g/kg/day.

Carbohydrate requirements: Daily glucose administration of 9-15 g/kg is a suitable amount in critical care. Carbohydrates provided in excess of this amount are not well utilized and may lead to hyperglycemia, excessive CO_2 production, hypophosphatemia, and fluid overload.

Fat requirements: If protein and glucose are supplied as outlined, the remainder of needed calories can be supplied as fat. Fat can be administered in minimal quantities to satisfy needs for essential fatty acids, or it can be provided in larger quantities, as tolerated, to meet energy needs. Abnormal liver function often occurs in patients given total parenteral nutrition (TPN) longer than 3 wk. Usually the enzymes return to normal upon cessation of TPN. Giving cyclic TPN, in which the patient receives TPN for 12-16 hr out of 24 hr, sometimes helps.

Special diets for organ-specific pathologic conditions: Costly, and the metabolic advantages of some products remain unproven.

Hepatic failure: Branched-chain amino acids in combination with reduced aromatic amino acid concentrations are used to alleviate encephalopathy secondary to hepatic failure.

Renal disease: High percentages of essential amino acids are used to improve nitrogen use and decrease urea formation.

Respiratory disease: A low-protein, low-carbohydrate diet decreases CO_2 production and consequently the work of breathing (WOB).

Vitamin and essential trace mineral requirements: In general, follow the recommended daily allowances (RDAs) to provide minimum quantities of vitamins, minerals, and essential fatty acids. For specific patients, supplement specific vitamins or minerals needed in increased amounts for existing disease states (e.g., zinc and vitamins A and C for burns; thiamine, folate, and vitamin B_{12} for chronic alcohol ingestion).

Fluid requirements: Many factors affect fluid balance. Under usual circumstances an estimate of fluid needs can be made by providing 1 ml of free water for each calorie provided, or 30-50 ml/kg body weight. The daily loss of water includes approximately 1400 ml in urine (60 ml/hr), 350 ml via respiration, 350 ml as evaporative losses through skin, 100 ml in sweat, and about 200 ml in feces. If loss by any of these routes is increased, fluid needs will increase; if loss by any of these routes is impaired, fluid restriction may be necessary. All sources of intake (oral, enteral, intravenous, and medications) as well as output (urine, stool, drainage, emesis, fluid shifts, and respiratory and evaporative losses) must be considered. **Note:** Urine output may be as high as 2-3 L under normal conditions. This represents a range of 80-125 ml/hr.

Nutritional support modalities

Specialized nutritional support refers to the provision of a special formula via the enteral or parenteral route for the treatment or prevention of malnutrition. Enteral nutrition is preferred over parenteral nutrition because it resembles normal functioning more closely, has fewer side effects, and is less costly.

ENTERAL PRODUCTS

Enteral products are composed of standard and modular formulas and can be used for oral and/or tube feeding (Table 10-7).

Formula types

Standard: *Blended whole food diets,* which are less costly but have problems that include possible bacterial growth, solids that settle out, variation in nutrient composition, and the necessity of a large-bore tube for the viscous formula; and *commercial formulas,* which are sterile, homogeneous, and suitable for small-bore feeding tubes and have a fixed nutrient composition.

Modular: Consist of a single nutrient that may be combined with other modules (nutrients) to form a package tailor-made for an individual's specific deficits (e.g., carbohydrate, fat, protein, and vitamin modules).

Nutritional composition

Carbohydrates: The most easily digested and absorbed component in enteral formulas; 80% of all carbohydrates is broken down and absorbed as simple glucose in the normal intestine.

LACTASE DEFICIENCY: Lack of this enzyme, which aids in digestion of lactose, is most commonly found in African Americans, Asians, Native Americans, and people of Jewish descent. A secondary form also may be found in individuals who receive large amounts of lactose in a milk-based diet. Symptoms include watery diarrhea, abdominal cramps, flatulence, fullness, nausea, stool with a pH of <6, and stool that tests positive for glucose.

Fiber: Recently included in many commercial preparations because it is helpful in the control of bowel disorders such as diverticulosis, decreases hyperlipidemia, and controls blood glucose. These preparations are highly viscous, and use of a large-bore feeding tube (10 Fr) or an infusion pump is helpful. Begin the infusion slowly to reduce transient symptoms of gas and abdominal distention.

Protein: Three forms commonly are used.

POLYMERIC: Protein found in complete and original form (e.g., blenderized whole food diets that require normal levels of pancreatic enzymes).

HYDROLYZED: Protein that is broken down into smaller forms to assist absorption. It is helpful in short bowel syndrome or pancreatic insufficiency.

ELEMENTAL: Protein that requires no further digestion and is ready for absorption. It is most helpful in hepatic and renal disorders.

Fat: Two forms are the primary sources.

LONG-CHAIN TRIGLYCERIDES (LCTs):   A major source of essential fatty acids, fat-soluble vitamins, and calories.

MEDIUM-CHAIN TRIGLYCERIDES (MCTs):   Foster the absorption of both types of fat but have fewer side effects of nausea and vomiting, abdominal distention, and diarrhea.

Types of feeding tubes and sites: See also Tables 10-8 and 10-9.

Soft, small-bore feeding tube: Polyurethane or silicone with or without a tungsten tip (for weight to aid in placement); size 6-12 Fr; length 36-45 inches. Trade names are Keofeed, Dobhoff.

Rigid tube or tube with rigid guide: Inner silicone tube may be contained within a stiff outer tube that is removed, leaving inner soft tube in place. An advantage is the ease of placement.

Large-bore stiff tube: Rubber or polyvinyl chloride; size 10-18 Fr; used for gastric decompression. It can be used for short-term feeding of highly viscous fluids. Trade names are Levine, Salem. The Salem sump is a double-lumen tube, with one lumen providing an airway that facilitates gastric decompression by limiting excessively compressive suction on the stomach.

Gastric feeding tube: Tube that is placed through the naris (nasogastric [NG]) or mouth (orogastric) into the stomach for feeding purposes.

Nasointestinal feeding tube: Tube that is placed through the naris into the intestine for decompression (with small bowel obstruction) or to provide tube feedings. Trade names are Miller-Abbott, Cantor.

TABLE 10-7 Types of Enteral Formulations

Enteral formula	Description
Blenderized diet Compleat, Compleat Modified, Vitaneed	Nutritionally complete, requiring complete digestive capabilities; composed of natural foods, including meat, vegetables, milk, and fruit
Milk-based formula Meritene, Sustagen, Carnation Instant (if mixed with milk)	Nutritionally adequate diet for general nutritional support
Lactose-free formula Ensure, Entrition 1, Isocal, Osmolite	Nutritionally adequate, liquid preparation; used for general nutritional support; isoosmolar or hypoosmolar; all except Osmolite are low residue
Elemental or chemically defined	Nutrients tailored for specific needs
Criticare HN	Low-Na$^+$, lactose-free, high-N diet; 40% protein supplied as small peptides; nutritionally adequate; used for general nutritional support
Travasorb HN	Nutritionally adequate; used for general nutritional support; contains additional hydrolyzed protein that is readily digested and absorbed
Specialty formulas *Hepatic failure* Hepatic Travasorb	Nutritionally complete; has a greater ratio of branched chain to aromatic amino acids while restricting total amino acid concentrations and adding nonprotein calories
Hepatic-Aid II	Nutritionally incomplete powder diet with essential nutrients in easily digestible form; high in branched chain amino acids; low in aromatic amino acids and methionines
Renal failure Renal Travasorb	Electrolyte, lactose, fat-soluble, vitamin-free; high in calories; contains mostly essential amino acids; restricted total protein content may reduce or postpone need for dialysis
Amin-Aid	Nutritionally incomplete supplement with essential nutrients in readily digestible form with minimal electrolytes
Respiratory insufficiency Pulmocare	Nutritionally complete; contains a higher proportion of fat to carbohydrates; reduces CO_2 production
Hypermetabolic and trauma states Trauma-Aid HB	High in branched chain amino acids; readily digestible essential nutrients
Trauma Cal	Nutritionally adequate with high proportions of protein and calories in a limited volume
Modular formulas	Offer highly flexible tailoring of nutrients (e.g., fat [Lipomul], protein [Pro Mod], and carbohydrates [Moducal]) for specific patient needs

Modified from Webber KS. In Swearingen PL, Keen JH, editors: *Manual of critical care: applying nursing diagnoses to adult critical illness*, ed 3, St Louis, 1995, Mosby.

T A B L E 1 0 - 8   Methods and Typical Rates of Administration for Enteral Products

Type	Typical rate of administration	Comments
Bolus	250-400 ml 4-6 times/day	May cause cramping, bloating, nausea, diarrhea, aspiration; not recommended
Intermittent	120 ml isotonic formula with 30-50 ml H$_2$O; flush over 30-60 min	Starting regimen
	Advancement: increase formula q8-12hr by 60 ml if residual less than one-half volume of previous feeding	Should not exceed 30 ml/min; may cause cramping, nausea, bloating, diarrhea, aspiration
Continuous	Full-strength isotonic formula, 40-50 ml/hr	Starting regimen
	Advancement: if serum albumin levels <2.5 g/dl, or initial loose stools, dilute formula to 150 mOsm	Allows more time for absorption of nutrients

Modified from Webber KS. In Swearingen PL, Keen JH, editors: *Manual of critical care: applying nursing diagonses to adult critical illness,* ed 3, St Louis, 1995, Mosby.

T A B L E 1 0 - 9   Nursing Implications for Use of Gastric Tubes

Size	Nursing implications
Small bore	Ensure that x-ray confirms placement. Auscultation not a reliable method of determining placement; aspiration of stomach contents through tube often causes tube walls to collapse (use slow gentle pressure)
	Tubes are easily dislocated proximally in GI tract, but there may be no external signs, and tube still may be taped in position
	Use elemental formula for lower viscosity
	Flush after each feeding/medication administration with 50-150 ml water
	Use manufacturer's recommended suggestions regarding syringe size when irrigating tube
Large bore	Use smallest-bore tube possible to minimize chance of ulceration, pharyngitis, and fistula formation
	Aspirate stomach contents, and check pH of returns to ensure correct stomach placement. Stomach contents have a pH <5 (acidic)
	When taping tube, ensure that no traction is applied to patient's skin
	Flush after each feeding/medication with 50-150 ml water

Modified from Webber KS. In Swearingen PL, Keen JH, editors: *Manual of critical care: applying nursing diagonses to adult critical illness,* ed 3, St Louis, 1995, Mosby.

Gastrostomy tube: A soft, latex or silicone tube inserted through the abdominal wall into the stomach either temporarily or permanently for feeding purposes. A *gastrostomy button* is any of several forms of "low profile" gastrostomy tubes shown to decrease many of the disadvantages of gastrostomy tubes, such as site problems, leakage, mobility, and catheter occlusion and displacement.

Jejunostomy tube: A silicone or latex tube inserted through the abdominal wall into the jejunum that is not easily dislodged, requires continuous feeding (thus is not convenient for the home care patient), and can be worn under clothes. Needle catheter (Witzel) jejunostomy is an alternative method of nutrient delivery.

Percutaneous endoscopic gastrostomy (PEG) tube: Soft tube inserted into the stomach via the esophagus and then drawn through the abdominal wall using a small incision.

Accessory materials: Y-ports, either built in as part of the system or added as a small adapter, allow concurrent administration of fluids or medications without interrupting the tube feeding. Some feeding pumps permit routine, automatic administration of flush solutions as programmed into the machine by the nurse (e.g., flush with 100 ml q2hr).

Selection of feeding sites

Stomach: Easiest for tube placement, simulates normal GI function, may be used for intermittent or continuous feedings, and best reserved for patients who are alert with intact gag and cough reflexes. Tubes may be placed through the nose (nasogastric), mouth (orogastric), or directly into the stomach through the abdominal wall (gastrostomy).

Small bowel (duodenum or jejunum): Used for patients with diminished protective pharyngeal reflexes. Small bowel tube placement is more difficult, and feeding requires elemental formula for easier absorption. Continuous feedings are necessary because bolus feedings are not well tolerated and continuous feedings simulate normal function. The Moss tube is a dual-lumen tube that allows decompression of the stomach while providing tube feedings into the distal duodenum or jejunum.

Infusion rates: See Table 10-8.

Collaborative management of complications: See Tables 10-10 and 10-12.

PARENTERAL NUTRITION

Parenteral nutrition (PN) provides some or all nutrients by peripheral venous catheter (PVC), peripherally inserted central catheter (PICC), or central venous catheter (CVC). PN is used to provide complete nutrition for patients who cannot receive enteral feedings or to supplement the nutritional needs of patients who are unable to absorb sufficient calories via the GI tract. Although PN usually is considered more effective than enteral nutrition, it also is more expensive and has more complications.

Parenteral solutions: Solutions of combinations of dextrose (carbohydrate), protein (amino acids), fat (lipids), electrolytes, vitamins, and trace elements. Because of the concentrations of solutions and the wide variety of ingredients used, PN should be administered through a filter to prevent a precipitant from entering the bloodstream and becoming an embolus.

Carbohydrates: Dextrose solutions 5%-50% used to meet the patient's energy needs. When hypertonic solutions are infused, insulin demand and O_2 consumption are increased. In addition, CO_2 production is increased, which may lead to respiratory distress and hypermetabolism, especially in patients with low pulmonary reserve. Because of the administration of concentrated carbohydrate solutions, patients receiving PN should be carefully monitored for fluctuations in their serum glucose via glucometry q6hr.

Protein: Synthetic crystalline essential and nonessential amino acid formulations available in concentrations of 3%-10%. Special amino acid formulations

TABLE 10-10 Management of Complications in the Tube-Fed Patient

Complication/possible causes	Suggested management strategy
Nausea and vomiting	
Fast rate	Decrease rate
Fat intolerance	Fat should compose no more than 30%-40% of total intake
Lactose intolerance	As prescribed, change to lactose-free product
Delayed gastric emptying	See "Risk for Aspiration," p. 700
Product odor	Mask with flavoring
Blocked tube	
Viscous formula/medications; inadequate flushing	Flush tube with 50-150 ml water after each feeding/medication administration. Flush q4hr with 30 ml water
Instillation of crushed medications	Do not instill crushed medications into small-bore tubes. Substitute liquid preparations after consulting pharmacist and health care provider, or crush into a fine powder and dissolve in 30 ml water. Incompatibility between drugs and with feeding formula is possible

Modified from Webber KS. In Swearingen PL, Keen JH, editors: *Manual of critical care: applying nursing diagonses to adult critical illness,* ed 3, St Louis, 1995, Mosby.

for specific disorders (e.g., liver, renal disease) are also available (see "Estimating Nutritional Requirements," p. 690).

Fat: Lipid 10%-20% is an isotonic solution providing essential fatty acids and a source of concentrated calories. For best use and tolerance, lipids should be infused with carbohydrates and protein over no fewer than 8 hr. This is especially useful for patients at home. The most common symptoms of an adverse reaction include febrile response, chills and shivering, and pain in the chest and back. A second type of adverse reaction occurs with prolonged use of IV fat emulsions and may result in transient increase in liver enzymes, kernicterus, eosinophilia, and thrombophlebitis. To prevent sepsis, infuse fat emulsions for no longer than 12 hr. Keep the infusion rate at 1 ml/min for the first 15-30 min and then increase it to 80-100 ml/hr for the remainder of the first infusion.

Total nutrient admixtures (TNAs): Provide dextrose, fat, and amino acids combined in one container. Because these mixtures would trap lipid molecules, an in-line filter cannot be used. **Note:** If separation of the lipids and other ingredients occurs, called "cracking," the solution should not be used.

Selection of administration site

CVC or PICC: Used for infusion of larger amounts of nutrients or electrolytes with smaller fluid volumes (hypertonic solutions) vs. the amount of nutrients and volume (isotonic) provided via peripheral parenteral nutrition. Solution is delivered through a large-diameter vein, usually the superior vena cava via the subclavian or jugular vein. The volume of blood flow rapidly dilutes the hypertonic solutions and decreases the irritation of vein walls. However, there are more complications with CVC or PICC than with the peripheral route.

PVC: The need for low-osmolality solution (<800 mOsm/L) limits the types of infusions that can be used. However, combined solutions of dextrose, amino

TABLE 10-11 **Catheters Used in Parenteral Nutrition**

Catheter	Description
Subclavian/jugular	Inserted at bedside. Multiple uses for specimen retrieval, feeding, and medication administration increase the risk of infection, especially in compromised patients
Multilumen	Inserted at bedside. Dedication of one lumen in this catheter is common practice, enabling other lumen(s) to be used for medication administration and laboratory monitoring
Right atrial (e.g., Hickman, Broviac)	Composed of silicone rubber with plastic external segment, which is implanted in OR. Its safety enables use by home care patients
Implantable (e.g., Infuse-a-Port, Port-a-Cath)	Implanted in OR. Designed for repeated access, making the need for repeated venipuncture unnecessary

TABLE 10-12 **Management of Complications in Patients Receiving Parenteral Nutrition**

Potential complications	Management strategy
Pneumothorax	Ensure that x-ray is done immediately after insertion. Determine placement of catheter before initiating feeding by monitoring for diminished or unequal breath sounds, tachypnea, dyspnea, and labored breathing
Subclavian artery injury	If pulsatile bright red blood returns into the syringe, assist health care provider with immediate removal of the needle and apply pressure for 10 min anteriorly and posteriorly at point of penetration
Catheter occlusion	If solution is infusing sluggishly, flush line with heparinized saline. Check to see if line or tubing is kinked. If line is occluded, try to aspirate clot and contact health care provider, who may prescribe a thrombolytic agent

Modified from Webber KS. In Swearingen PL, Keen JH: *Manual of critical care: applying nursing diagonses to adult critical illness,* ed 3, St Louis, 1995, Mosby.

acids, and lipids (TNAs) lower osmolality, providing a concentrated energy source that can be safely delivered via a peripheral vein, usually of the hand or forearm. They are reserved for individuals with a need for nutritional support for short time periods, with small nutritional requirements, and for whom CVC access is unavailable.

Types of catheters: See Table 10-11.

Monitoring infusion rates: Using an infusion pump, PN is given at a consistent rate, with gradual acceleration of the infusion rate over a 3-day period to avoid wide fluctuations in blood glucose. A typical rate is 50-100 ml/hr, with increases of 25-50 ml/hr each day, depending on patient status.

Managing complications: See Tables 10-12 and 10-13.

T A B L E 1 0 - 1 3   Possible Electrolyte Imbalances in Enteral and Parenteral Nutrition

Sodium: Daily requirement is 60-150 mEq. Sodium is the primary extracellular cation in maintaining concentration and volume of extracellular fluid.

Complication	Pathophysiology/strategy
Hypernatremia	In PCM, patients have increased sodium because of extravascular volume expansion and intravascular volume depletion. Monitor sodium levels as depletion resolves, edema decreases, and diuresis occurs. Hypernatremia also occurs in patients receiving hypertonic tube feedings without adequate water supplements.
	Sources: Amino acid solutions contain varying amounts of sodium (up to 70 mEq/L); some antibiotics (e.g., sodium penicillin) also have a high sodium content (31-2000 mEq/dl). Corticosteroids may cause sodium retention, and blood products can contain increased levels (130-160 mEq/L).
Hyponatremia	Can be a problem in patients with gastric suctioning and in those receiving diuretic agents or those with SIADH.
	Replacement: TPN solutions can replace sodium by using acetate, phosphate, or chloride salt form, depending on underlying disease state. Phosphate form should not be used in patients with renal failure. In acidemia, the acetate form is preferred to correct the imbalance.

Potassium: Daily requirement is 50-100 mEq. Potassium is the major intracellular cation required for neurotransmission, protein synthesis, cardiac and renal function, and carbohydrate metabolism.

Complication	Pathophysiology/strategy
Hyperkalemia	May be caused by excessive parenteral or enteral potassium supplementation or increased tissue catabolism, especially in renal insufficiency.
	Sources: Amino acid solutions contain potassium. Elevated potssium levels occur in patients receiving ACE inhibitors, heparin, cyclosporin, and potassium-sparing diuretics.
Hypokalemia	May occur during anabolism (tissue synthesis) in patients being refed. Potassium shifts into intracellular space, and patients require supplementation. It also may occur in patients with high GI losses or increased loss from diuretics. Potassium levels in patients with acid-base disorders may be misleading; potassium decreases by 0.4-1.5 mEq/L for every 0.1 increase in pH.
	Replacement: In daily TPN solutions, 80-120 mEq may be given to patients without renal problems. Potassium can be replaced using acetate, phosphate, and chloride forms, depending on underlying disease state, but it should be titrated separately to avoid wasting TPN solutions. Infusion rates >0.5 mEq/kg/hr are associated with cardiac irregularities.

Phosphorus: Daily requirement is 2.5-4.5 mg/dl. Phosphorus is required for release of oxygen from hemoglobin in the form of 2,3-diphosphoglycerate and for bone deposition, calcium regulation, and synthesis of carbohydrates, fats, and protein.

Complication

Pathophysiology/strategy

Hyperphosphatemia

Occurs in catabolic stress, renal failure, and hypocalcemia. Treatment involves ingestion of aluminum antacids, which bind phosphate in the intestine.

Sources: Phosphorus-rich solutions, antacids, antacids, diuretic agents, and steroids.

Hypophosphatemia

A complication with a high mortality, often found in malnourished patients on refeeding. As patient receives fluids containing dextrose, phosphorus shifts rapidly into intracellular space, causing hypophosphatemia.

Replacement: Phosphate-rich TPN solutions.

Magnesium: Daily requirement is 18-30 mEq. Magnesium is required for carbohydrate and protein metabolism and enzymatic reactions.

Complication

Pathophysiology/strategy

Hypermagnesemia

Transient elevations can occur with use of diuretics or extracellular volume depletion.

Source: Magnesium-containing antacids.

Hypomagnesemia

Low levels commonly occur in patients with severe malnutrition or lower GI losses and in those given insulin for hyperglycemia. For anabolism to occur, the body requires 2 mEq of magnesium per gram of nitrogen.

Replacement: Parenteral magnesium.

Calcium: Daily requirement is 1000-1500 mg. Calcium is a necessary ingredient of the cells that play a major role in neurotransmission and bone formation.

Complication

Pathophysiology/strategy

Hypercalcemia

Occurs in thiazide diuretic use, prolonged immobilization, and decreased excretion.

Source: Side effect of diuretic use.

Hypocalcemia

May occur from reduced total body calcium or reduced ionized calcium. It also occurs with hyperphosphatemia. A deficit can be misleading, inasmuch as serum calcium is bound to protein and varies with changing albumin levels. Also, in acidosis, a lower pH results in release of more calcium from protein, which elevates serum calcium levels. The opposite is true as pH rises.

Replacement: Calcium-rich parenteral solutions.

PCM, Protein-calorie malnutrition; *SIADH,* syndrome of inappropriate antidiuretic hormone; *TPN,* total parenteral nutrition; *ACE,* angiotensin-converting enzyme; *GI,* gastrointestinal.

TRANSITIONAL FEEDING

A period of adjustment is needed before discontinuing nutritional support. Taper nutritional supplements for patients receiving enteral nutrition as oral intake increases. Similarly, patients receiving PN may have some mucosal atrophy of the bowel and will need a period of adjustment before the bowel can fully resume its usual functions of digestion and absorption.

NURSING DIAGNOSES AND INTERVENTIONS

Altered nutrition: Less than body requirements related to inability to ingest, digest, or absorb nutrients

Desired outcome: Patient has adequate nutrition as evidenced by stabilization of weight at desired level or steady weight gain of ½ to 1 lb/wk; improved or normal measures of protein stores (serum albumin 3.5-5.5 g/dl, transferrin 180-260 mg/dl, thyroxine-binding prealbumin 20-30 mg/dl, retinol-binding protein 4-5 mg/dl); presence of wound granulation (i.e., pinkish white tissue around wound edges that grows to fill in wound); and absence of infection (see **Risk for infection,** p. 703).

For oral nutrition

- Ensure nutritional screening and assessment of patient within 72 hr of admission; document and reassess weekly. See guidelines, p. 688.
- Position patient in high Fowler's position for eating; assist with preparation of food for eating as needed. Involve significant other in meal rituals for companionship.
- Provide small, frequent feedings of diet compatible with disease state and patient's ability to ingest foods.
- Respect food aversions, and try to maximize food preferences.
- Provide liquid nutritional supplements as prescribed. Serve them cold or over ice to enhance palatability.
- Document intake via calorie counts.
- Weigh weekly.
- Provide psychologic support.

For enteral or parenteral nutrition

- Ensure nutritional screening and assessment of patient within 72 hr of admission; document and reassess weekly. For guidelines, see p. 688.
- Administer formula within 10%-20% of prescribed rate. Check infused volume and rate hourly.
- Monitor laboratory data daily: blood glucose, BUN, and electrolytes. Ensure that trace elements, as well as serum albumin, transferrin, or prealbumin, are monitored weekly. Document findings.
- Record I&O carefully, tracking fluid balance trends.
- Weigh patient twice weekly, and consistently document findings.
- Ensure that patient receives prescribed caloric intake.
- Assess for fluid imbalance, especially fluid excess, via monitoring for peripheral edema and for adventitious breath sounds, especially crackles (rales).

NIC: Enteral Tube Feeding; Fluid/Electrolyte Management; Nutrition Management; Teaching: Prescribed Diet; Total Parenteral Nutrition (TPN) Administration; Tube Care: Gastrointestinal; Weight Gain Assistance

Aspiration (or risk for same) related to GI feeding (via nasogastric, nasoenteric, gastrostomy, or enterostomy tube), site of the feeding tube, or delayed gastric emptying

Desired outcome: Patient is free of aspiration problems as evidenced by auscultation of clear lung sounds, VS within patient's normal limits, and absence of signs of respiratory distress.

- Determine placement of feeding tube before each tube feeding. After initial insertion, check x-ray for position of feeding tube. Insufflation with air and aspiration of stomach contents do not always confirm placement of small-bore feeding tubes. Mark to determine tube migration, and secure tubing in place; reassess q4hr and before each feeding.
- Assess respiratory status q4hr for unexplained pulmonary infiltrates, noting respiratory rate and effort, and for adventitious breath sounds.
- Monitor VS q4hr; promptly report fever of unexplained origin.
- Auscultate bowel sounds, percuss abdomen, and assess abdominal contour and girth q8hr. Consult health care provider if bowel sounds are absent or high pitched, the abdomen becomes distended, the patient complains of nausea, or vomiting occurs.
- Elevate HOB ≥30 degrees during and 1 hr after feeding. If this is not possible or comfortable for patient, turn patient to a slightly elevated right side-lying position to enhance gravity flow from the greater stomach curvature to the pylorus.
- Consult health care provider if the residual feeding is >50% of the hourly infusion rate or >100 ml for intermittent/bolus feeding. Hold feeding for 1 hr, and recheck residual.
- Stop tube feeding ½-1 hr before chest physical therapy, suctioning, or placing patient supine.
- Discuss with health care provider the possibility of advancing the feeding tube well beyond the pylorus to reduce the risk of aspiration.
- As prescribed, administer metoclopramide HCl to promote gastric motility and emptying.

NIC: Aspiration Precautions; Enteral Tube Feeding; Gastrointestinal Intubation; Respiratory Monitoring; Vital Signs Monitoring

Constipation related to inadequate fluid and fiber in diet
Desired outcome: Patient states relief from constipation by having a soft bowel movement within 3-4 days of this diagnosis (or within patient's usual pattern).
- Recommend change of formula to one that has fiber added. .
- Assess intake of free water. Optimally water intake should be 1 ml/calorie of intake or 30-50 ml/kg body weight.
- Give free water q2hr or as prescribed. Request feeding pumps that allow automatic cycling of free water through the system at pre-programmed intervals.
- For other interventions, see Appendix One, "Caring for Patients on Prolonged Bedrest" for **Constipation,** p. 743.

NIC: Bowel Management; Constipation/Impaction Management; Fluid Management; Nutrition Management

Diarrhea (or risk for same) related to bolus feedings, lactose intolerance, bacterial contamination, osmolality intolerance, medications, and low-fiber content
Desired outcome: Patient has formed stools within 2-3 days of intervention.
- Assess abdomen and GI status: bowel sounds, distention, consistency and frequency of bowel movements, cramping, skin turgor, urine specific gravity, and other indicators of hydration.
- Monitor I&O status carefully.
- Bolus feeding: switch to intermittent or continuous feeding methods.
- Lactose intolerance: as prescribed, switch to lactose-free products.
- Bacterial contamination:
  —Obtain a stool specimen for culture and sensitivity.
  —Use aseptic technique when handling feeding tube, enteral products, and feeding sets.
  —Change all equipment q24hr.
  —Refrigerate all opened products, but discard after 24 hr.

- Osmolality intolerance: determine osmolality of feeding formula. Most are isotonic (plasma osmolality 300 mOsm). If hypertonic, reduce infusion rate. If problem continues, dilute to ½ formula and ½ water, but maintain rate.
- Medications:
  —Monitor use of antibiotics, antacids, antidysrhythmics, aminophylline, cimetidine, and potassium chloride and use of sorbitol in liquid medications.
  —As prescribed, administer *Lactobacillus acidophilus* to restore GI flora or use antidiarrheal agents to reduce GI motility.
- Low-fiber content: add bulk-forming agents (psyllium or fiber agents) to the formula. Jevity tube feeding incorporates psyllium in the formula.

NIC: Bowel Management; Diarrhea Management; Fluid/Electrolyte Management; Perineal Care

Risk for impaired swallowing related to decreased or absent gag reflex, facial paralysis, mechanical obstruction, fatigue, and decreased strength or excursion of muscles involved in mastication

Desired outcome: Before foods or fluids are initiated, patient demonstrates adequate cough and gag reflexes and the ability to ingest foods via the phases of swallowing as instructed.

- Assess oral motor function within 72 hr of patient's admission or upon progression to oral diet.
- Assess cough and gag reflexes before the first feeding. Initially liquids and solids may be difficult for the patient to manage. Offer semisolid foods, and progress to thicker texture as tolerated. Assist patient through the phases of ingesting food: opening the mouth, inserting food, closing lips, chewing, transferring food from side to side in the mouth and then to the back of the oral cavity, elevating the tongue to the roof of the mouth (hard palate), and swallowing between breaths.
- Order extra sauces, gravies, or liquids if dryness of the oral cavity impairs patient's swallowing ability. Suggest that patient moisten each bite of food with these substances.
- If tolerated, keep patient in high Fowler's position for ½ hr to minimize the risk of aspiration.
- Provide mouth care before and after meals and dietary supplements.
- Provide small, frequent meals; six feedings per day may be more tolerable than three feedings.
- Provide foods at temperatures acceptable to patient.
- Respect food aversions; honor food preferences whenever possible.
- Provide oral supplements or tube feeding supplements as prescribed. Advise patient of transition status, and praise his or her progress.
- In conjunction with speech, physical, or occupational therapist, assist in retraining or facilitating patient's swallowing.
- Monitor and record patient's intake (via calorie count, daily weight) and output.

NIC: Airway Suctioning; Aspiration Precautions; Diet Staging; Feeding; Surveillance; Swallowing Therapy

Impaired tissue integrity (or risk for same) related to mechanical irritant (presence of enteral tube)
Desired outcome: At time of hospital discharge, patient's tissue is intact, with absence of erosion around orifices, excoriation, skin rash, mucous membrane breakdown, or decubitus ulcers.

For gastric/enteral tube
- Assess skin for irritation or tenderness q8hr.
- Use tube with smallest bore possible.

- If long-term support is needed, discuss potential for using gastrostomy or jejunostomy tube with health care provider.
- Give ice chips, chewing gum, or hard candies prn if permitted.
- Apply petrolatum ointment to lips q2hr.
- Have patient brush teeth and tongue q4hr.
- Apply water-soluble lubricant to naris prn.
- Alter position of tube prn to avoid pressure on underlying tissue. Use hypoallergenic tape to anchor tube.

For gastrostomy/jejunostomy tube
- Assess site for erythema, drainage, tenderness, and odor q4hr.
- Secure tube so there is no tension on patient's tissue and skin.
- For new sites, cleanse skin with sterile normal saline. Dress with split 4 × 4s, and tape with paper or hypoallergenic tape.
- For healed sites, cleanse skin with soap and water daily; pat dry.
- If necessary, dress site with split 4 × 4s and tape with paper or hypoallergenic tape.

NIC: Gastrointestinal Intubation; Skin Care: Topical Treatments; Skin Surveillance; Wound Care

Risk for infection with risks related to invasive procedures, malnutrition, or suppressed immune system
Desired outcome: Patient is free of infection as evidenced by VS within normal range, total lymphocytes 25%-40% (1500-4500/mm^3), WBC count ≤11,000/mm^3, and absence of clinical signs of sepsis: erythema and swelling at catheter insertion site, chills, fever, and glucose intolerance.
- Ensure adequate nutritional support, based on the individual's needs; reassess weekly. For guidelines see p. 688.
- Twice weekly and prn, monitor total lymphocyte count, WBC count, and differential for values outside normal range.
- Check blood glucose via fingerstick glucometry for values outside normal range.
- Examine catheter insertion sites q8hr for erythema, swelling, or purulent discharge.
- Use meticulous sterile technique when changing central line dressing, containers, or lines. Cleanse insertion sites with tincture of iodine (1%-2%) followed with 70% alcohol or povidone-iodine solution.
- Do not use central line that is being used for nutritional support to draw blood, monitor pressure, or administer medications or other fluids.
- Change all administration sets within the time frame established by the agency.
- Infuse fat emulsion for time frame established by the agency.

NIC: Infection Control; Infection Protection; Intravenous (IV) Therapy; Total Parenteral Nutrition (TPN) Administration

Altered cardiopulmonary tissue perfusion (or high risk for same) related to interruption of arterial flow (air embolus)
Desired outcome: Patient has adequate cardiopulmonary tissue perfusion as evidenced by VS, ABG values, and oximetry readings within patient's normal limits, and absence of dyspnea, tachypnea, cyanosis, chest pain, tachycardia, and hypertension.
- Administer D$_5$W solution until chest x-ray verifies proper catheter position.
- Place patient in Trendelenburg position when changing tubing or when neck vein catheters are inserted or removed.
- If possible, teach patient Valsalva's maneuver for use during tubing changes, or apply abdominal pressure.
- Use Luer-Lok connectors on all connections.

- Tape all tubing connections longitudinally to prevent disconnection.
- Monitor patient for chest pain, tachycardia, tachypnea, cyanosis, and hypotension. If air embolus is suspected, listen for characteristic "mill-wheel" murmur.
- If air embolus is suspected, clamp the catheter and turn patient to left side-lying Trendelenburg position to trap air in the right ventricle. Give oxygen, and monitor VS. Notify health care provider immediately.
- Use occlusive dressing over insertion site for 24 hr after catheter is removed to prevent air entry via catheter-sinus tract.

NIC: Positioning; Surveillance; Teaching: Individual; Vital Signs Monitoring

Fluid volume deficit (or risk for same) related to failure of regulatory mechanisms, hyperglycemia, and hyperosmolar hyperglycemic nonketotic (HHNK) syndrome

Desired outcome: Patient's hydration status is adequate, as evidenced by baseline VS, serum glucose <300 mg/dl, balanced I&O, urine specific gravity 1.010-1.025, and serum electrolytes within normal limits.

- Assess rate and volume of nutritional support hourly. Reset to prescribed rate as indicated. To minimize the risk of HHNK, increase rate by no more than 10%-20%.
- Weigh patient daily; monitor I&O hourly.
- Consult health care provider for urine output <1 ml/kg/hr.
- Check urine specific gravity; consult physician for value >1.035.
- Monitor serum osmolality and electrolytes daily and prn; consult health care provider for abnormalities. See Table 10-13 for assessment of associated electrolyte imbalances.
- Monitor for circulatory overload during fluid replacement, for example, peripheral edema, jugular distention, adventitious lung sounds (especially crackles [rales]).
- Monitor for assessments of hyperglycemia. Perform fingerstick glucometry q6hr or prn until stable. Administer insulin (commonly sliding scale) as prescribed to keep blood glucose levels <220 mg/dl.
- Provide 1 ml of free water for each calorie of enteral formula provided (or 30-50 ml/kg of body weight).

NIC: Bedside Laboratory Testing; Fluid/Electrolyte Management; Fluid Monitoring; Medication Management; Surveillance

Section Three: Managing Wound Care

A wound is a disruption of tissue integrity caused by trauma, surgery, or an underlying medical disorder. Wound management is directed at preventing infection and deterioration in wound status and promoting healing.

Wounds closed by primary intention

Clean, surgical, or traumatic wounds whose edges are closed with sutures, clips, or sterile tape strips are referred to as wounds closed by *primary intention.* Impairment of healing most frequently manifests as dehiscence, evisceration, or infection. Individuals at high risk for disruption of wound healing include those who are obese, diabetic, elderly, malnourished, receiving steroids, or undergoing chemotherapy or radiation therapy.

ASSESSMENT

Optimal healing: Warm, reddened, indurated, tender incision line immediately after injury. After 1 or 2 days, wound fluid on the incision line dries,

TABLE 10-14   Assessment of Healing by Primary Intention

Normal findings	Abnormal findings
Edges well approximated	Edges not well approximated
Good initial inflammatory response: redness, warmth, induration, pain	Diminished or no inflammatory response, or response persists or occurs after day 5
No drainage 48 hr after closure	Drainage continues >48 hr after closure
Healing ridge present by postoperative day 7-9	No healing ridge by postoperative day 9; hypertrophic scar or keloid developing

forming a scab that subsequently falls off and leaves a pink scar. After 7-9 days, a healing ridge—a palpable accumulation of scar tissue—forms. See Table 10-14. In patients who undergo cosmetic surgery, the healing ridge is purposely avoided to minimize scar formation.

Impaired healing: Lack of an adequate inflammatory response manifested by absence of initial redness, warmth, and induration or inflammation that persists or occurs after the fifth post-injury day; continued drainage from the incision line 2 days after injury (when no drain is present); absence of a healing ridge by the ninth day after injury; presence of purulent exudate. See Table 10-14.

DIAGNOSTIC TESTS

WBC with differential: To assess for infection.

Gram stain of drainage: If infection is suspected, to identify the offending organism and aid in the selection of preliminary antibiotics.

Culture and sensitivity of tissue by biopsy or swab: To determine optimal antibiotic. Infection is said to be present when there are 10^5 organisms/g of tissue or when there is fever and drainage.

COLLABORATIVE MANAGEMENT

Application of a sterile dressing in surgery: To protect wound from external contamination and trauma or provide pressure. Usually, surgeon changes the initial dressing.

Regular (house) diet: To promote positive nitrogen (N) state for optimal wound healing.

Multivitamins, especially vitamin C: To promote tissue healing.

Minerals, especially zinc and iron: May be prescribed, depending on patient's serum levels.

Supplemental O_2:   Empirically, 2-4 L/min in high-risk patients. After injury, wound Po_2 is low, and administration of O_2 may promote healing.

Insulin: As needed to control glucose levels in persons with diabetes.

Local or systemic antibiotics: Given when infection is present and sometimes used prophylactically as well.

Incision and drainage: To drain pus when infection is present and localized. This allows healing by secondary intention. The wound may be irrigated with antiinfective agents, such as dilute Dakin's solution.

NURSING DIAGNOSES AND INTERVENTIONS

Impaired tissue integrity of wound related to altered circulation, metabolic disorders (e.g., diabetes mellitus [DM]), alterations in fluid volume and nutrition, and medical therapy (chemotherapy, radiation therapy, steroid administration)

Desired outcome: Patient exhibits the following signs of wound healing: well-approximated wound edges; good initial postinjury inflammatory response (erythema, warmth, induration, pain); no inflammatory response past the fifth day after injury; no drainage (without drain present) 48 hr after closure; healing ridge present by postoperative day 7-9.

- Assess wound for indications of impaired healing, including absence of a healing ridge, presence of drainage or purulent exudate, and delayed or prolonged inflammatory response. Monitor VS for signs of infection, including elevated temperature and HR. Document findings.
- Follow Standard Precautions (see p. 817) and sterile technique when changing dressings. If a drain is present, keep it sterile, maintain patency (e.g., empty drainage reservoir and recharge suction on closed drainage systems as needed), and handle it gently to prevent it from becoming dislodged. If wound care will be necessary after hospital discharge, teach the dressing change procedure to patient and significant other.
- Maintain blood glucose within normal range for persons with DM by performing serial monitoring of capillary glucose and administering insulin to keep glucose level <200 mg/dl.
- Explain to patient that deep breathing promotes oxygenation, which enhances wound healing. Encourage deep breathing and coughing q2hr while awake. Splint incision as needed. If indicated, provide incentive spirometry at least 4 times/day. Stress the importance of position changes and activity as tolerated to promote ventilation. As indicated, monitor oximetry, report O_2 saturation <92%, and consult health care provider about administration of O_2.
- Monitor perfusion status by checking BP, HR, capillary refill time in the tissue adjacent to incision, peripheral pulses as appropriate, moisture of mucous membranes, skin turgor, volume and specific gravity of urine, and I&O.
- For nonrestricted patients, ensure a fluid intake of at least 2-3 L/day.
- Encourage ambulation or ROM exercises as allowed to enhance circulation to the wound.
- To promote wound healing, provide a diet with adequate protein, vitamin C, and calories. If patient complains of feeling full with three meals per day, give more frequent small feedings. Encourage between-meal high-protein supplements (e.g., yogurt, milk shakes). Monitor serum albumin (<3.5 g/dl) and total lymphocyte counts (<1800/mm^3), and report decreases; consult health care provider about high-protein nutrition supplements.

NIC: Incision Site Care; Nutrition Management; Respiratory Monitoring; Wound Care; Wound Care: Closed Drainage; Wound Irrigation

PATIENT-FAMILY TEACHING AND DISCHARGE PLANNING

When providing patient-family teaching, focus on sensory information; avoid giving excessive information; and initiate a visiting nurse referral for necessary follow-up teaching. Consider including verbal and written information about the following:

- Local wound care, including type of equipment necessary, wound care procedure, and therapeutic and negative side effects of topical agents used. Have patient or significant other demonstrate dressing change procedure before hospital discharge.
- Signs and symptoms of improvement in wound status (see Table 10-14).
- Signs and symptoms of deterioration in wound status, including those that necessitate notification of health care provider or clinic (see Table 10-14).
- Diet that promotes wound healing. Discuss the importance of adequate protein and calorie intake. See "Section Two: Providing Nutritional Support," p. 687. Involve dietitian, patient, and significant other as necessary.
- Activities that maximize ventilatory status: a planned regimen for ambulatory patients, and deep breathing and turning (at least q2hr) for those on bedrest.

- Importance of taking multivitamins, antibiotics, and supplements of iron and zinc as prescribed. For all medications to be taken at home, provide the following: drug name, purpose, dosage, schedule, precautions, drug/drug and food/drug interactions, and potential side effects.
- Importance of follow-up care with health care provider; confirm time and date of next appointment if known.
- If needed, arrange for a visit by a home health nurse before hospital discharge.

Surgical or traumatic wounds healing by secondary intention

Wounds healing by secondary intention are those with tissue loss or heavy contamination that form granulation tissue and contract in order to heal. Most often, impairment of healing is caused by contamination and inadequate perfusion, oxygenation, and nutrition. Individuals at risk for impaired healing include those who are obese, diabetic, malnourished, elderly, taking steroids, or undergoing radiation therapy or chemotherapy.

ASSESSMENT

Optimal healing: Initially the wound edges are inflamed, indurated, and tender. At first, granulation tissue on the floor and walls is pink, progressing to a deeper pink and then to a beefy red; wound tissues should be moist. Epithelial cells from the tissue surrounding the wound gradually migrate across the granulation tissue. As healing occurs, the wound edges become pink, the angle between surrounding tissue and the wound becomes less acute, and wound contraction occurs. Occasionally a wound has a tract or sinus that gradually decreases in size as healing occurs. The time frame for healing depends on the size and location of the wound and on the patient's physical and psychologic status. See Table 10-15.

Impaired healing: Exudate appears on the floor and walls of the wound and does not abate as healing progresses. It is important to note the distribution, color, odor, volume, and adherence of the exudate. The skin surrounding the wound should be assessed for signs of tissue damage, including disruption, discoloration, swelling, local increased warmth, and increasing pain. When a drain is in place, the volume, color, and odor of the drainage should be evaluated. See Table 10-15.

TABLE 10-15   Assessment of Healing by Secondary Intention

Normal findings	Abnormal findings
Initially after injury, wound edges inflamed, indurated, and tender; with epithelialization, edges become pink	Initially after injury, decreased inflammatory response or inflammation around wound that continues past day 5 after injury; epithelialization slowed or mechanically disrupted and not continuous around wound
Granulation tissue initially avascular and moist and then turns pink; becomes beefy red over time	Granulation tissue remains pale or is excessively dry or moist
No odor	Odor
No exudate or necrotic tissue	Exudate or necrotic tissue

DIAGNOSTIC TESTS

CBC with WBC differential: To assess hematocrit (Hct) level and for presence of infection. Increased WBC count signals infection, whereas a decrease occurs with immunosuppression. Watch the differential for a shift to the left, which indicates infection. Monitor the lymphocyte count and serum albumin: $\leq 1800/mm^3$ and <3.5 g/dl, respectively, are signs of malnutrition. For optimal healing, the Hct should be >20%.

Gram stain of drainage: To determine the characteristics of the offending organism, if present, and aid in selection of the preliminary antibiotic.

Tissue biopsy or culture and sensitivity of drainage: To determine presence of infection and the optimal antibiotic, if appropriate.

Ultrasound, sonogram, or sinogram: To determine wound size, especially when abscesses or tracts are suspected. (A sinogram involves instillation of a radiopaque dye into a sinus tract to determine its direction and length.)

COLLABORATIVE MANAGEMENT

Debriding enzymes: To soften and remove necrotic tissue (e.g., fibrinolysin plus deoxyribonuclease [Elase]).

Dressings: To provide débridement, keep healthy wound tissue moist, or provide antiseptic agent to decrease wound surface bacterial counts. See Table 10-16.

Hydrophilic agents: To remove contaminants and excess exudate (e.g., dextran beads or paste [Envisan], polymer flakes [Bard Absorption Dressing]).

Hydrotherapy: To soften and remove debris mechanically.

Wound irrigation with or without antiinfective agents: To dislodge and remove bacteria and loosen necrotic tissue, foreign bodies, and exudate. Antiinfective agents work locally to kill organisms.

IV fluids: To ensure adequate perfusion for patients unable to take adequate oral fluids.

Topical or systemic vitamin A: As needed to reverse adverse effects of steroids on healing. Use is limited to 7-10 days.

Drain(s): To remove excess tissue fluid or purulent drainage.

Surgical débridement: To remove dead tissue and reduce debris and fibrotic tissue.

Skin graft: To provide coverage of wound if necessary.

Tissue flaps: To fill tissue defect and provide wound closure with its own blood supply.

Regular diet, supplemental O_2, multivitamins and minerals, insulin, and incision and drainage: See discussion in "Wounds Closed by Primary Intention," p. 705.

NURSING DIAGNOSES AND INTERVENTIONS

Impaired tissue integrity of wound related to presence of contaminants, metabolic disorders (e.g., DM), medical therapy (e.g., chemotherapy, radiation therapy), altered perfusion, or malnutrition

Desired outcomes: Patient's wound exhibits the following signs of healing: initially after injury, wound edges are inflamed, indurated, and tender; with epithelialization, edges become pink within 1 wk of injury; granulation tissue develops (identified by pink tissue that becomes beefy red) within 1 wk of injury; and there is no odor, exudate, or necrotic tissue. Patient or significant other successfully demonstrates wound care procedure before hospital discharge, if appropriate.

- Monitor for the following signs of impaired healing: initially after injury, decreased inflammatory response or inflammatory response that lasts >5 days; epithelialization slowed or mechanically disrupted and noncontinuous around the wound; granulation tissue remaining pale or excessively dry or moist; presence of odor, exudate, and/or necrotic tissue.

TABLE 10-16   Dressings Used for Wound Care

Dressing	Advantages	Limitations
Moist to moist* (insert and remove moist)	Provides topical antiinfective agent; no wound desiccation; good débridement; removal painless; inexpensive	If too wet, can cause tissue maceration; if dries out, must be moistened before removal
Xeroform gauze	Provides antiseptic; keeps tissue hydrated; minimal pain with removal	If too moist, can cause tissue maceration
Porcine skin dressing	Can provide topical antibiotic; keeps tissue hydrated; removal painless; often used before closure of wound with tissue grafts	Expensive; usually stored in refrigerator until use
Transparent dressing (e.g., Op-Site, Tegaderm, Biocclusive)	Prevents loss of wound fluid; protects wound from external contamination; protects from friction and fluid loss; minimal pain with removal	Cannot be used with heavily draining wounds
Hydrocolloid dressing (e.g., Duoderm, Restore, Intact)	Maintains moist wound surface while minimizing pooling; easy to apply; minimal pain with removal	Wound cannot be directly assessed without removing dressing; "melts" when used under radiant heat; limited absorption
Hydrogel (e.g., Vigilon, Intrasite Gel)	Maintains moist wound surface; nonadherent; absorbs some exudate; compatible with topical medications; easy to apply; minimal pain with removal	Maceration with direct contact with normal tissue; may require frequent changing; minimal absorption of exudate
Alginates (e.g., Sorbsan)	Physiologic; maintains moisture; removal painless	Not good for dry wounds
Foams (e.g., Lyofoam, Allevin)	Maintains moist wound surface; insulates wound; nonadherent	Poor barrier; not good for wounds with copious drainage

*Dressings are sterile, coarse mesh gauze without cotton fiber fill and are covered with a dry, sterile outer layer to prevent ingress of organisms. When moisture is prescribed, it is provided with an antiinfective agent or physiologic solution.

- Apply prescribed dressings (see Table 10-16) following Standard Precautions (see p. 818). Insert dressing into all tracts to promote gradual closure of those areas. Ensure good handwashing before and after dressing changes, and dispose of contaminated dressings appropriately.
- When a drain is used, maintain its patency, prevent kinking of the tubing, and secure the tubing to prevent the drain from becoming dislodged. Use sterile technique when caring for drains. With closed drainage systems, empty drainage reservoir and recharge suction as needed.

- To help prevent contamination, cleanse drainage or secretions from the skin surrounding the wound with a mild disinfectant (e.g., soap and water). Do not use friction with cleansing if tissue is friable.
- If irrigation is prescribed for reducing contaminants, employ high-pressure irrigation using a 35-ml syringe with an 18-gauge Angiocath, and follow Standard Precautions. If the tissue is friable or the wound is over a major organ or blood vessel, use extreme caution with the irrigation pressure. To remove contaminants effectively, use a large volume of irrigant (e.g., 100-150 ml). Generally, irrigation is done until returns are as clear as possible.
- Topically applied antiinfective agents, such as neomycin and iodophors, are absorbed by the wound and can produce systemic side effects. When these agents are used, be alert to side effects, such as toxicity to cells in the wound, nephrotoxicity, and acidosis.
- When a hydrophilic agent such as dextranomer (Debrisan) is prescribed, remove it with high-pressure irrigation. If removed with a 4 × 4 or surgical sponge, the friction would disrupt capillary budding and delay healing.
- When topical enzymes are prescribed, use them on necrotic tissue only and follow package directions carefully. Be aware that some agents, such as povidone-iodine, deactivate the enzymes. Protect surrounding undamaged skin with zinc oxide or aluminum hydroxide paste.
- Teach patient or significant other the prescribed wound care procedure, if indicated.

NIC: Incision Site Care; Nutrition Management; Pressure Ulcer Care; Respiratory Monitoring; Wound Care; Wound Care: Closed Drainage; Wound Irrigation

PATIENT-FAMILY TEACHING AND DISCHARGE PLANNING
See teaching and discharge planning interventions in "Wounds Closed by Primary Intention," p. 707.

Pressure ulcers

Pressure ulcers result from a disruption in tissue integrity and are caused most often by excessive tissue pressure, friction, or shear or altered circulation. High-risk patients include older persons and those who have decreased mobility, decreased LOC, impaired sensation, debilitation, incontinence, sepsis/elevated temperature, or malnutrition.

ASSESSMENT
High-risk individuals should be identified upon admission assessment, with daily assessments during hospitalization using a standard assessment schema. When pressure ulcers are present, their severity can be staged on a scale of I to IV (Table 10-17). See also "Surgical or Traumatic Wounds Healing by Secondary Intention," p. 707, for other assessment data.

DIAGNOSTIC TESTS
See "Diagnostic Tests," p. 708, in "Surgical or Traumatic Wounds Healing by Secondary Intention."

COLLABORATIVE MANAGEMENT
Debriding enzymes: To soften and remove necrotic tissue.
Dressings: To provide débridement, keep healthy tissue moist, or apply an antiinfective agent. See Table 10-16.
Hydrophilic agents: To remove contaminants and excess moisture.

TABLE 10-17   Staging of Pressure Ulcers

Stage	Description
I	Nonblanchable erythema of intact skin; in people with dark skin, heat may be only indication of a grade I pressure ulcer
II	Partial-thickness skin loss that involves epidermis or dermis or both; seen as an abrasion, blister, or shallow crater
III	Full-thickness skin loss that involves subcutaneous tissue but does not extend through fascia
IV	Full-thickness injury that involves muscle, bone, or supporting structures

Wound irrigation with antiinfective agents: To reduce contamination.

Hydrotherapy: To soften and remove debris mechanically.

Diet: Adequate protein and calories to promote positive nitrogen (N) state for rapid wound healing.

Supplemental vitamins and minerals: As needed.

Supplemental O_2:   Usually 2-4 L/min to promote wound healing for high-risk patients or those with delayed wound healing.

Surgical débridement: Removal of devitalized tissue with a scalpel to reduce the amount of debris and fibrotic tissue.

Tissue flaps: To provide wound closure with its own blood supply.

Cultured keratinocytes: To provide cover for the wound in the form of a sheet of skin cells grown from a biopsy of the patient's own skin.

Growth factors: Naturally occurring proteins that stimulate new cell formation (e.g., platelet-derived growth factor, insulin).

Hyperbaric O_2:   Used with difficult wounds to support oxidative processes in healing.

NURSING DIAGNOSES AND INTERVENTIONS

Impaired tissue integrity (or risk for same) related to excessive tissue pressure, friction, shear, or altered circulation

Desired outcomes: Patient's tissue remains intact. Patient participates in preventive measures and verbalizes understanding of the rationale for these interventions.

- Identify individuals at risk, and systematically assess skin over bony prominences daily; document.
- Establish and post a position-changing schedule.
- Assist patient with position changes. There is an inverse relationship between pressure and time in ulcer formation; therefore heavier patients need to change position more frequently. Position changes include turning the bed-bound patient q1-2hr and having the wheelchair-bound patient (who is able) perform pushups in the chair q15min to ensure periodic relief from pressure on the buttocks. Use pillows, foam wedges, or gel pads to protect bony prominences from direct pressure. In addition, patients with history of previous tissue injury will require pressure-relief measures more frequently. Because high Fowler's position results in increased shearing, use low Fowler's position and alternate supine position with prone and 30-degree elevated side-lying positions.
- For immobile patients, totally relieve pressure on heels by raising them off the bed surface via pillows inserted under the length of the lower leg.

- Minimize friction and shear on tissue during activity. Lift rather than drag patient during position changes and transferring; use a draw sheet to facilitate patient movement. Do not massage over bony prominences, because this can result in tissue damage.
- Minimize skin exposure to moisture. Cleanse at the time of soiling and at routine intervals. Use moisture barriers and disposable briefs as needed.
- Use a mattress that reduces pressure, such as foam, low air loss, alternating air, gel, or water.
- To enhance circulation, encourage patient to maintain current level of activity.

NIC: Activity Therapy; Bathing; Perineal Care; Positioning; Positioning: Wheelchair; Pressure Ulcer Prevention

Impaired tissue integrity: Presence of pressure ulcer, with increased risk for further breakdown related to altered circulation and presence of contaminants or irritants (chemical, thermal, or mechanical)
Desired outcomes: Stages I and II are healed within 7-10 days; stages III and IV may require months to heal. Following intervention and instruction, patient verbalizes causes and preventive measures for pressure ulcers and successfully participates in the plan of care to promote healing and prevent further breakdown.

- Evaluate stage of pressure ulcer (see Table 10-17) and wound status (see Table 10-15).
- Maintain a moist physiologic environment to promote tissue repair and minimize contaminants. Change dressings as prescribed, using Standard Precautions (see p. 818).
- Be sure patient's skin is kept clean with regular bathing, and be especially conscientious about washing urine and feces from the skin. Soap should be used and then thoroughly rinsed from the skin.
- If the patient has excessive perspiration, ensure frequent bathing and change bedding as needed.
- To absorb moisture and prevent shearing when the patient is moved, apply heel and elbow protection as needed.
- Use lamb's wool to keep the areas between the toes dry. Change wool periodically, depending on the amount of moisture present.
- Do not use a heat lamp, because it dries tissues and increases the metabolic rate of the tissues, resulting in increased demand for blood flow in an area with impaired perfusion. As a result, ulcer diameter and depth can be increased.
- Teach patient and significant other the importance of and measures for preventing excess pressure as a means of preventing pressure ulcers.
- Provide wound care as needed (described under "Surgical or Traumatic Wounds Healing by Secondary Intention" earlier).

NIC: Activity Therapy; Bathing; Perineal Care; Positioning; Pressure Ulcer Prevention

---

See Also: "Surgical or Traumatic Wounds Healing by Secondary Intention" for **Impaired tissue integrity,** p. 708.

PATIENT-FAMILY TEACHING AND DISCHARGE PLANNING

When providing patient-family teaching, focus on sensory information; avoid giving excessive information; and initiate a visiting nurse referral for necessary

follow-up teaching. Consider including verbal and written information about the following:

* Location of local medical supply stores that have pressure-reducing mattresses and wound care supplies.
* Planning a schedule for changing patient positions.

See Also: "Wounds Closed by Primary Intention," p. 707, for other teaching and discharge planning interventions.

Selected Bibliography

A.S.P.E.N. Board of Directors: Guidelines for the use of parenteral and enteral nutrition in adult and pediatric patients, *J Parenteral Enteral Nutr* 17(4): 1SA-25SA, 1993.

Bankhead RR: Commonly asked questions about nutrition care, *Am J Nurs* 95(10):70-74, 1995.

Carpenter CJ et al: Antiretroviral therapy for HIV infection in 1996: recommendations of the International Panel, *JAMA* 276:146-154, 1996.

Gianino S, St John R: Nutritional assessment of the patient in the intensive care unit, *Crit Care Nurs Clin North Am* 5(1):1-16, 1993.

Gianino S et al: The ABCs of TPN, *RN,* pp 42-48, February 1996.

HIV infection, *Am J Nurs* 97(1):45-52, 1996.

Hoppe B: Central venous catheter-related infections: pathogenesis, predictors, and prevention, *Heart Lung* 24(4):333- 339, 1995.

Interqual: *The ISD-A review system with adult ISD criteria,* Northhampton, NH, and Marlboro, Mass, August 1992, Interqual.

Kim MJ et al: *Pocket guide to nursing diagnoses,* ed 7, St Louis, 1997, Mosby.

Konstantinides NN, Lehmann S: The impact of nutrition on wound healing, *Crit Care Nurs* 13(5):25-33, 1993.

McCloskey JC, Bulechek GM, editors: *Nursing interventions classification (NIC),* ed 2, St Louis, 1996, Mosby.

Mellors JW et al: *Prognostic value of plasma HIV-RNA quantification in seropositive adult men.* Presented at AI International Conference on AIDS, July 10, 1996.

Metheny N: Minimizing respiratory complications of nasoenteric tube feedings: state of the science, *Heart Lung* 22(3):213-223, 1993.

Panel on the treatment of pressure ulcers: *Treatment of pressure ulcers: clinical practice guideline,* no. 15. Pub no. 95-0652, Rockville, Md, 1994, U.S. Department of Health and Human Services, Agency for Health Care Policy Research.

Stotts NA: Impaired wound healing. In Keene JH, Swearingen PL, editors: *Mosby's critical care consultant,* St Louis, 1997, Mosby.

Viall C: Taking the mystery out of TPN, *Nurs 95* 15(4):34-41, 1995.

Webber KS: Providing nutritional support. In Horne MM, Heitz UE, Swearingen PL, editors: *Pocket guide to fluid, electrolyte, and acid-base balance,* ed 3, St Louis, 1997, Mosby.

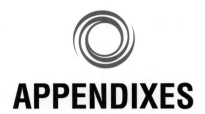

APPENDIXES

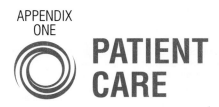

PATIENT
CARE

Section One: Caring for Preoperative and Postoperative Patients

Knowledge deficit: Surgical procedure, preoperative routine, and postoperative care

Desired outcome: Patient verbalizes knowledge about the surgical procedure, including preoperative preparations and sensations and postoperative care and sensations, and demonstrates postoperative exercises and use of devices before surgical procedure or during the immediate postoperative period for emergency surgery.

- Assess patient's understanding about the diagnosis, surgical procedure, preoperative routine, and postoperative regimen. Evaluate patient's desire for knowledge about the diagnosis and procedure (some individuals find detailed information helpful; others prefer very brief and simple explanations). Assess for factors that would affect the patient's ability to learn. Determine past surgical experiences and their positive or negative effect on patient. Assess nature of any concerns or fears related to surgery. Document and communicate these assessment data to others involved in the patient's care.
- Based on your assessment, clarify and explain diagnosis and surgical procedure accordingly. When possible, emphasize associated sensations (i.e., dry mouth, thirst, muscle weakness). This information often is helpful in reducing stress and anxiety. Provide ample time for instruction and clarification, and reinforce health care provider's explanation of the procedure. Use anatomic models, diagrams, and other audiovisual aids when possible. Provide simply written information to reinforce learning. Provide written and verbal information in the patient's native language for non-English-speaking patients. **Note:** Evaluate patient's reading comprehension before providing written materials.
- Explain the perioperative course of events. Review the following with the patient and significant other:
  - —Where the patient will be before, during, and immediately after surgery (i.e., postanesthesia care unit [PACU], ICU, other specialty unit). Clarify sounds and other sensations (e.g., sore throat, cool temperature, hard stretcher) the patient may experience during the immediate postoperative period. If possible, take the patient to the new unit and introduce him or her to the nursing staff.
  - —Preoperative medications and timing of surgery (scheduled time, expected duration).
  - —If indicated, preoperative bowel preparation.
  - —Pain management, including sensations to expect and methods of relief. If patient-controlled analgesia (PCA) will be prescribed, have patient return demonstration of the use of delivery device.
  - —Placement of tubes, catheters, drains, cooling systems (Cryocuff), continuous passive motion (CPM) units, oxygen delivery devices, and similar

devices routinely used for the patient's surgery. Enable patient to see these devices when possible.

—Use of antiembolism stockings, sequential compression devices (SCDs), pneumatic foot pumps, or similar devices.

—Dietary alterations and progression, including NPO status followed by clear liquids until return of full gastrointestinal (GI) function.

—Restrictions of activity and positions, as indicated by specific surgical procedure (e.g., total hip arthroplasty positional limitations).

—Need to refrain from smoking during the perioperative period.

—Visiting hours and location of waiting room.

- Explain the postoperative activities, exercises, and precautions. Have patient return demonstration of the following devices and exercises, as appropriate:

—Deep-breathing and coughing exercises (see **Ineffective airway clearance,** p. 725). **Caution:** Individuals for whom increased intracranial, intrathoracic, or intraabdominal pressure is contraindicated should not cough.

—Use of incentive spirometry and other respiratory devices.

—Calf-pumping, ankle-circling, and footboard-pressing exercises to enhance circulation and prevent thrombophlebitis in the lower extremities (see "Venous Thrombosis/Thrombophlebitis," p. 125, for more information).

—Use of PCA device.

—Movement in and out of bed.

- Before patient is discharged, teach the prescribed activity precautions, such as getting maximum amounts of rest, increasing activities gradually to tolerance, avoiding heavy lifting (>10 lb), avoiding driving a car (often for as long as 4-6 wk). Include restrictions on sexual activity as indicated by the surgical procedure.

- Provide time for patient to ask questions and express feelings of anxiety; be reassuring and supportive. Be certain to address the individual's main concerns.

You may also wish to refer to the following interventions from the Nursing Interventions Classification (NIC):

NIC: Learning Facilitation; Learning Readiness Enhancement; Preparatory Sensory Information; Surgical Preparation; Teaching: Preoperative

Risk for injury with risks related to exposure to pharmaceutical agents and other external factors during the perioperative period

Desired outcome: Patient does not experience injury or untoward effects of pharmacotherapy.

- Assess the need for holding, administering, or adjusting the patient's maintenance medications before or immediately after surgery. Some medications, such as anticonvulsants and cardiac medications, should be continued throughout the perioperative period. Sometimes the patient needs to be weaned from medications for the perioperative period, such as baclofen (Lioresal). Other medications may require increased dosages during surgery or alternative routes (i.e., hydrocortisone [Solu-Cortef] in place of prednisone and with an increased dosage for steroid-dependent patients). The health care provider and pharmacist should be consulted as necessary.

- Verify completion of preoperative activities and procedures, and document on the preoperative checklist or nursing documentation.

- Ensure that the consent has been signed and witnessed and that the patient appears to understand what the procedure involves. Answer questions, or call the health care provider to answer the patient's questions. Ensure the patient's ID bracelet, blood transfusion bracelet, and allergy alert bracelets are in place. Review the medical record to ensure all appropriate documentation is present; report untoward findings (e.g., abnormal ECG, suspicious chest radiograph, abnormal laboratory findings) to the health care provider.

- Prepare the surgical site as prescribed (e.g., shower with surgical soap, shave, or depilatory preparation, and/or surgical scrub). Accomplish additional presurgical procedures as indicated (e.g., douche, enemas, eye drops).
- Administer preoperative analgesia, sedation, or other medications as prescribed. Ensure that medications, especially antibiotics, are given promptly to ensure adequate serum levels. Make provisions for patient safety following administration (e.g., bed in lowest position, side rails up, and reminding the patient not to get out of bed without assistance).

NIC: Preoperative Coordination; Surgical Preparations; Teaching: Preoperative

Pain or chronic pain related to disease process, injury, or surgical procedure
Desired outcomes: Patient's subjective perception of discomfort decreases within 1 hr of intervention, as documented by a pain scale. Patient does not exhibit nonverbal indicators of pain (Table A-1). Autonomic indicators (Table A-2) are diminished or absent. Verbal responses, such as crying or moaning, are absent.

- Develop a systematic approach to pain management for each patient. The primary nurse should collaborate with the surgeon, anesthesiologist, and patient for optimal management of pain. See Figures A-1 and A-2 for pain treatment flow charts.
- Monitor patient at frequent intervals for the presence of discomfort. Use a formal method of assessing pain. One method is to have the patient rate discomfort on a scale of 0 (no discomfort) to 10 (worst pain). Other methods may be used, but the method selected should be used consistently.

TABLE A-1   Nonverbal Indicators of Pain

Masklike, grimacing, tense facial expression
Guarding or protective behavior
Restlessness or increase in motor activity
Withdrawal or decrease in motor activity
Skeletal muscle tension
Short attention span
Irritability
Anxiety
Sleep disturbances

TABLE A-2   Autonomic Indicators of Pain

Diaphoresis
Vasoconstriction
Increased systolic and diastolic BP
Increased pulse rate (>100 bpm)
Pupillary dilation
Change in respiratory rate (usually increased, >20 breaths/min)
Muscle tension or spasm
Decreased intestinal motility, evidenced by nausea, vomiting, abdominal distention, and possibly ileus
Endocrine imbalance, evidenced by sodium and water retention and mild hyperglycemia

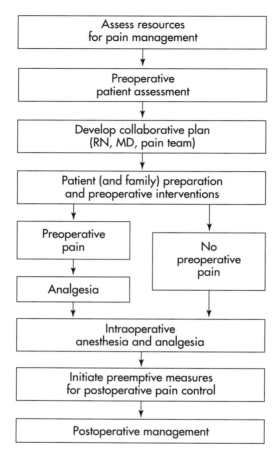

Figure A-1: Pain treatment flow chart: preoperative and intraoperative phases. (From U.S. Department of Health and Human Services: *Acute pain management: operative or medical procedures and trauma.* AHCPR pub. no. 92-0032, Rockville, Md, 1992, U.S. Department of Health and Human Services.)

- Evaluate patients with acute and chronic pain for nonverbal indicators of discomfort (see Table A-1).
- Evaluate patients with acute pain for autonomic indicators of discomfort (see Table A-2). Be aware that patients with chronic pain (>6 mo) may not exhibit an autonomic response.
- Evaluate patient's health history for evidence of alcohol and drug (prescribed and nonprescribed) use. A positive history of addiction to alcohol or drugs affects effective doses of analgesics (i.e., patient may require more or less). Ensure that the surgeon, anesthesiologist, and other health care providers are aware of any significant findings. Consult a pain management team if available. All care providers must be consistent in setting limits while

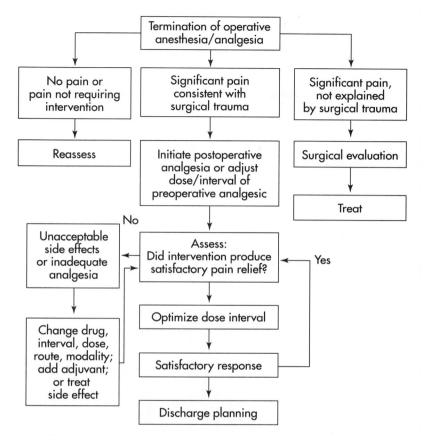

Figure A-2: Pain treatment flow chart: postoperative phase. (From U.S. Department of Health and Human Services: *Acute pain management: operative or medical procedures and trauma.* AHCPR pub. no. 92-0032, Rockville, Md, 1992, U.S. Department of Health and Human Services.)

providing effective pain control through pharmacologic and nonpharmacologic methods. Psychiatric consultation may be necessary.

• Administer opioid (e.g., morphine) and related mixed agonist-antagonist (e.g., butorphanol) analgesics as prescribed (Table A-3). When possible, morphine or related "mu" (µ) receptor agonists are preferred to meperidine (Demerol) because bioaccumulation of the active metabolites of meperidine may result in toxicity, especially in older patients or patients with renal impairment. Monitor for side effects, such as respiratory depression, excessive sedation, nausea, vomiting, and constipation. Be aware that meperidine may produce excitation, muscle twitching, and seizures, especially in conjunction with phenothiazines. **Note:** Do not administer mixed agonist-antagonist analgesics concurrently with morphine or other pure agonists, because reversal of analgesic effects may occur.

TABLE A-3   Use of Opioid and Agonist-Antagonist Analgesia

Route	Commonly prescribed medications	Advantages	Disadvantages
Continuous infusion	Morphine, fentanyl (Sublimaze)	Useful for severe, predictable pain or as a basal dose with bolus supplements for fluctuating pain Relieves pain with lower doses than IV bolus Avoids peaks and valleys of pain found with IV bolus and IM injections	Requires frequent observation to monitor flow rate VS must be monitored often
IV bolus	Morphine, meperidine (Demerol), fentanyl	Useful for severe, intermittent pain (i.e., for procedures, treatments) Rapid onset of action; may be controlled by patients using specialized pump; very effective when used with basal (continuous) dosing plus PCA mode	Relatively short duration of pain relief Fluctuating levels Possibility of excessive sedation as drug levels peak
Epidural	Morphine, fentanyl, hydromorphone, meperidine	Very effective relief of moderate to severe pain Delivery close to opiate receptors provides pain control with small doses May be delivered with local anesthetic (e.g., bupivacaine) for increased effectiveness	Catheter must be inserted by anesthetist or anesthesiologist Specialized delivery system must be used Side effects include urinary incontinence, hypotension, respiratory depression, pruritus, nausea, and vomiting

Route	Medications	Advantages	Disadvantages
Patient-controlled analgesia	Morphine, meperidine, fentanyl, buprenorphine (Buprenex)	Useful for moderate to severe pain; Enables titration by patient for effective analgesia without excessive sedation; Relief of pain with lower dosages of medication; Immediate delivery of medication; Patient's sense of self-control lowers anxiety; Less nursing time spent preparing medications	Pumps necessary to deliver drug are expensive; Patient must have clear mental status; Health care provider resistance to self-administration by patient
IM injection	Meperidine, morphine, pentazocine (Talwin), nalbuphine (Nubain), butorphanol (Stadol), buprenorphine	Useful for moderate to severe pain; Longer duration of action than with IV route; Used for postoperative pain	Variable absorption and fluctuating levels, especially in hypotensive and critically ill patients; Possibility of excessive sedation as drug levels peak; Potential delay in administration
Oral	Codeine, oxycodone (Percodan), meperidine, pentazocine, propoxyphene (Darvon), hydromorphone (Dilaudid), morphine (MS Contin)	Useful for mild to moderate acute pain or chronic severe pain (large doses necessary)	Variable absorption; Cannot be used until GI function returns; lengthy interval before onset of action
Transdermal	Fentanyl (Duragesic)	Long duration of action (3 days); Useful when pain is moderate to severe and constant for prolonged periods	Delayed onset of action (up to 36 hr); Prolonged effects after removal; Must be used with rapid-action supplement for variable pain; Not usually appropriate for postoperative pain control unless patient using system preoperatively

VS, Vital signs; *IV*, intravenous; *IM*, intramuscular; *PCA*, patient-controlled analgesia; *GI*, gastrointestinal.

TABLE A-4 Common Nonnarcotic and Nonsteroidal Antiinflammatory Analgesics	
Nonsteroidal antiinflammatory drugs	Nonnarcotic drugs
Acetylsalicylic acid (aspirin)	Acetaminophen (Tylenol, Tempra)
Ibuprofen (Motrin, Advil, Nuprin)	
Indomethacin (Indocin)	
Ketorolac (Toradol)	
Naproxen (Naprosyn, Anaprox)	

- Assess patients receiving opioid analgesics at frequent intervals for evidence of excessive sedation when awake or respiratory depression (i.e., RR <10 breaths/min or Sao_2 <85%). In the presence of respiratory depression, reduce the amount or frequency of the dose as prescribed. Have naloxone (Narcan) readily available to reverse severe respiratory depression. **Caution:** Use reduced doses and titrate carefully in patients with limited pulmonary reserve (i.e., COPD, asthma) or hepatic or renal insufficiency and in older adults.
- Administer nonnarcotic drugs (acetaminophen [Tylenol, Tempra]) and nonsteroidal antiinflammatory drugs (NSAIDs) (acetylsalicylic acid [aspirin], ibuprofen [Motrin, Advil, Nuprin], indomethacin [Indocin], naproxen [Naprosyn, Anaprox], ketorolac [Toradol]) as prescribed for relief of mild to moderate pain during postoperative recovery (Table A-4). NSAIDs are especially effective when pain is associated with inflammation and soft tissue injury. Be certain that GI function has returned before administering oral agents. Ketolorac may be given IM or IV for patients unable to tolerate oral agents. Monitor for side effects, such as epigastric pain, nausea, dyspepsia, and gastric bleeding. Be aware that NSAIDs affect platelet adhesiveness and may contribute to bleeding. **Note:** Because NSAIDs have peripheral effects and a different mechanism of action, they are very effective when combined or used with centrally acting opioid analgesics.
- Check the patient's analgesic record for the last dose and amount of medication given during surgery and in the postanesthesia recovery room. Be careful to coordinate timing and dose of postoperative analgesics with previously administered medication. **Note:** Combined fentanyl and droperidol (Innovar) anesthesia potentiates the effects of opiates for up to 10 hr after administration, and the patient should be monitored carefully when opioid analgesia is used.
- Administer prn analgesics before pain becomes severe. Consider conversion to scheduled dosing with supplemental prn analgesics. Prolonged stimulation of pain receptors results in increased sensitivity to painful stimuli and will increase the amount of drug required to relieve pain. Be aware that addiction to opioids occurs infrequently in hospitalized patients.
- Plan to administer intermittently scheduled analgesics before painful procedures, before ambulation, and at bedtime. Schedule them so that their peak effect is achieved at the inception of the activity or procedure.
- Augment analgesic therapy with sedatives and tranquilizers to prolong and enhance analgesia. Avoid substituting sedatives and tranquilizers for analgesics.
- Wean patient from opioid analgesics by decreasing dose or frequency of the drug. Convert to oral therapy as soon as possible. When changing route of

administration or medication, be certain to use equianalgesic doses (Table A-5) of the new drug.
- Augment action of the medication by using nonpharmacologic methods of pain control (Table A-6). Many of these techniques may be taught to and implemented by the patient and significant other.
- Maintain a quiet environment to promote rest. Plan nursing activities to enable long periods of uninterrupted rest at night.
- Evaluate for and correct nonoperative sources of discomfort (i.e, position, full bladder, infiltrated IV site).
- Position patient comfortably, and reposition at frequent intervals to relieve discomfort caused by pressure and improve circulation.
- Sudden or unexpected changes in pain intensity can signal complications, such as internal bleeding or leakage of visceral contents. Carefully evaluate the patient, and notify the health care provider immediately.
- Document efficacy of analgesics and other pain control interventions, using the pain scale or other formalized method.

NIC: Analgesic Administration; Anxiety Reduction; Environmental Management: Comfort; Meditation; Pain Management; Progressive Muscle Relaxation; Simple Massage; Simple Relaxation Therapy

Ineffective airway clearance related to increased tracheobronchial secretions secondary to effects of anesthesia; ineffective coughing secondary to central nervous system (CNS) depression or pain and muscle splinting; and possible laryngospasm secondary to endotracheal tube or allergic reaction to anesthetics
Desired outcome: Patient's airway is clear as evidenced by normal breath sounds to auscultation, RR 12-20 breaths/min with normal depth and pattern (eupnea), normothermia, normal skin color, and O_2 saturation $\geq 92\%$.
- Assess respiratory status, including breath sounds, q1-2hr during the immediate postoperative period and q8hr during recovery. Note and report the presence of rhonchi that do not clear with coughing, labored breathing, tachypnea (RR >20 breaths/min), mental status changes, restlessness, cyanosis, and the presence of fever ($\geq 38.3° C$ [$101° F$]).
- Use oximetry to assess oxygen saturation as indicated, and report saturation <92% to health care provider. Especially consider use of oximetry in patients with COPD, respiratory or cardiovascular disease, cardiothoracic surgery, major surgery, prolonged general anesthesia, and surgery for a fractured pelvis or long bone, as well as debilitated patients and older patients.
- Encourage deep breathing and coughing q2hr or more often for the first 72 hr postoperatively. In the presence of fine crackles (rales) and if not contraindicated, have patient cough to expectorate secretions. Facilitate deep breathing and coughing by demonstrating how to split the abdominal and thoracic incisions with the hands or a pillow. If indicated, medicate patient ½ hr before deep breathing, coughing, or ambulation to enhance compliance. **Caution:** Vigorous coughing may be contraindicated for some individuals (e.g., those undergoing intracranial surgery, spinal fusion, eye and ear surgery, and similar procedures). Coughing after a herniorrhaphy and some thoracic surgeries should be done in a controlled manner, with the incision supported carefully.
- Be certain that emergency airway equipment (i.e., intubation tray, endotracheal tubes, suctioning equipment, tracheostomy tray) is readily available in the event of sudden airway obstruction or ventilatory failure.
- Administer humidified oxygen as prescribed to prevent further drying of respiratory passageways and secretions.

NIC: Airway Management; Chest Physiotherapy; Cough Enhancement; Oxygen Therapy; Respiratory Monitoring

Risk for aspiration with risks related to entry of secretions, food, or fluids into the tracheobronchial passages secondary to CNS depression, depressed cough

TABLE A-5 Dosing Data for Opioid Analgesics*†

Drug	Approximate equianalgesic oral dose	Approximate equianalgesic parenteral dose	Recommended starting dose (adults >50-kg body weight)		Recommended starting dose (children and adults <50-kg body weight)‡	
			Oral	Parenteral	Oral	Parenteral
Opioid agonist						
Morphine§	30 mg q3-4hr (around-the-clock dosing) 60 mg q3-4hr (single dose or intermittent dosing)	10 mg q3-4hr	30 mg q3-4hr	10 mg q3-4hr	0.3 mg/kg q3-4hr	0.1 mg/kg q3-4hr
Codeine‖	130 mg q3-4hr	75 mg q3-4hr	60 mg q3-4hr	60 mg q2hr (intramuscular/subcutaneous)	1 mg/kg q3-4hr‖	Not recommended
Hydromorphone§ (Dilaudid)	7.5 mg q3-4hr	1.5 mg q3-4hr	6 mg q3-4hr	1.5 mg q3-4hr	0.06 mg/kg q3-4hr	0.015 mg/kg q3-4hr
Hydrocodone (in Lorcet, Lortab, Vicodin, others)	30 mg q3-4hr	Not available	10 mg q3-4hr	Not available	0.2 mg/kg q3-4hr‖	Not available
Levorphanol (Levo-Dromoran)	4 mg q6-8hr	2 mg q6-8hr	4 mg q6-8hr	2 mg q6-8hr	0.04 mg/kg q6-8hr	0.02 mg/kg q6-8hr
Meperidine (Demerol)	300 mg q2-3hr	100 mg q3hr	Not recommended	100 mg q3hr	Not recommended	0.75 mg/kg q2-3hr
Methadone (Dolophine, others)	20 mg q6-8hr	10 mg q6-8hr	20 mg q6-8hr	10 mg q6-8hr	0.2 mg/kg q6-8hr	0.1 mg/kg q6-8hr

| Oxycodone (Roxi-codone, also in Percocet, Percodan, Tylox, others) | 30 mg q3-4hr | Not available | 10 mg q3-4hr | Not available | 0.2 mg/kg q3-4hr‖ | Not available |
| Oxymorphone§ (Numorphan) | Not available | 1 mg q3-4hr | Not available | 1 mg q3-4hr | Not recommended | Not recommended |

Opioid agonist-antagonist and partial agonist

Buprenorphine (Buprenex)	Not available	0.3-0.4 mg q6-8hr	Not available	0.4 mg q6-8hr	Not available	0.004 mg/kg q6-8hr
Butorphanol (Stadol)	Not available	2 mg q3-4hr	Not available	2 mg q3-4hr	Not available	Not recommended
Nalbuphine (Nubain)	Not available	10 mg q3-4hr	Not available	10 mg q3-4hr	Not available	0.1 mg/kg q3-4hr
Pentazocine (Talwin, others)	150 mg q3-4hr	60 mg q3-4hr	50 mg q4-6hr	Not recommended	Not recommended	Not recommended

From Acute Pain Management Guideline Panel: *Acute pain management: operative or medical procedures and trauma. Clinical practices guideline.* AHCPR pub. no. 92-0032, Rockville, Md, 1992, Agency for Health Care Policy and Research, Public Health Service, U.S. Department of Health and Human Services.

*Note: Published tables vary in the suggested doses that are equianalgesic to morphine. Clinical response is the criterion that must be applied for each patient; titration to clinical response is necessary. Because there is not complete cross tolerance among these drugs, it is usually necessary to use a lower than equianalgesic dose when changing drugs and to retitrate to response.

†Caution: Recommended doses do not apply to patients with renal or hepatic insufficiency or other conditions affecting drug metabolism and kinetics.

‡Caution: Doses listed for patients with body weight <50 kg cannot be used as initial starting doses in babies younger than 6 mo. Consult the *Clinical Practice Guideline for Acute Pain Management: Operative or Medical Procedures and Trauma* section on management of pain in neonates for recommendation.

§For morphine, hydromorphone, and oxymorphone, rectal administration is an alternate route for patients unable to take oral medications, but equianalgesic doses may differ from oral and parenteral doses because of pharmacokinetic differences.

‖Caution: Codeine doses >65 mg often are not appropriate because of diminishing incremental analgesia with increasing doses but continually increasing constipation and other side effects.

¶Caution: Doses of aspirin and acetaminophen in combination opioid nonsteroidal antiinflammatory drug (NSAID) preparations must also be adjusted to the patient's body weight.

TABLE A-6   Common Nonpharmacologic Methods of Pain Control*

Sensory interventions

Massage: to relax muscular tension and increase local circulation; back and foot massages are especially relaxing

Range-of-motion (ROM) exercises (passive, assisted, or active): to relax muscles, improve circulation, and prevent pain related to stiffness and immobility

Applications of heat or cold: cold used initially to diminish tissue injury response and alter pain threshold; heat used to facilitate clearance of tissue toxins and mobilize fluids

Transcutaneous electrical nerve stimulation (TENS): battery-operated device used to send weak electrical impulses via electrodes placed on the body; reduces sensation of pain during and sometimes after treatment

Emotional interventions

Prevention and control of anxiety: limiting anxiety reduces muscle tension and increases patient's pain tolerance; anxiety and fear contribute to autonomic stimulation and pain responses; progressive relaxation exercises and slow, controlled breathing may be helpful

Promoting self-control: feelings of helplessness and lack of control contribute to anxiety and pain; techniques such as patient-controlled analgesia (PCA) and promoting self-helping behavior contribute to feelings of self-control

Cognitive interventions

Cognitive preparations: preparing patient by explaining what can be expected, thereby reducing stress and anxiety (e.g., preoperative teaching)

Patient education: teaching methods for preventing or reducing pain (e.g., suggesting comfortable postoperative positions, methods of ambulation, and splinting of incisions when coughing)

Distraction: encouraging patient to focus on something unrelated to pain (e.g., conversing, reading, watching TV or videos, listening to music, employing relaxation techniques [see **Health-seeking behaviors:** Relaxation technique effective for stress reduction, p. 59])

Humor: can be an excellent distraction and may help patient cope with stress

Guided imagery: patient uses a mental process that uses images to alter a physical or emotional state; a technique that promotes relaxation and reduces pain sensations

*Many of these techniques can be taught to and implemented by the patient and significant other.

and gag reflexes, decreased GI motility, abdominal distention, recumbent position, presence of gastric tube, and possible impaired swallowing in individuals with oral, facial, or neck surgery

Desired outcome: Patient's upper airway remains unobstructed as evidenced by clear breath sounds, RR 12-20 breaths/min with normal depth and pattern (eupnea), normal skin color, and O_2 saturation $\geq 92\%$.

- See first four interventions under **Ineffective airway clearance,** p. 725.
- If the sedated patient experiences nausea or vomiting, turn him or her immediately into a side-lying position. Fully alert patients may remain in an upright position. As necessary, suction the oropharynx with a Yankauer or similar suction device to remove vomitus.
- Check placement and patency of gastric tubes q8hr and before instillation of feedings and medications. **Note:** Use caution when irrigating and otherwise manipulating the GI tubes of patients with recent esophageal, gastric, or

duodenal surgery because the tube may be displaced or the surgical incision disrupted by such activity. Consult health care provider before irrigating tubes for these individuals.

- Assess patient's abdomen q4-8hr by inspection, auscultation, palpation, and percussion for evidence of distention (increasing size, firmness, increased tympany, decreased bowel sounds). Notify health care provider if distention is of rapid onset or if it is associated with pain.
- Encourage early and frequent ambulation to improve GI motility and reduce abdominal distention caused by accumulated gases.
- Introduce oral fluids cautiously, especially in patients with oral, facial, and neck surgery.
- Administer antiemetics, histamine H_2-receptor blocking agents, omeprazole (Prilosec), metoclopramide (Reglan), and similar agents as prescribed.
- For additional information see "Providing Nutritional Support" for **Risk for aspiration,** p. 700.

NIC: Airway Management; Airway Suctioning; Medication Management; Oxygen Therapy; Postanesthesia Care

Ineffective breathing pattern (or risk of same) related to decreased lung expansion secondary to CNS depression, pain, muscle splinting, recumbent position, and effects of anesthesia
Desired outcome: Patient exhibits effective ventilation as evidenced by relaxed breathing, RR 12-20 breaths/min with normal depth and pattern (eupnea), clear breath sounds, normal color, O_2 saturation ≥92%, Pao_2 ≥80 mm Hg, pH 7.35-7.45, $Paco_2$ 35-45 mm Hg, and HCO_3^- 22-26 mEq/L.
- See interventions under **Ineffective airway clearance,** p. 725.
- Perform a preoperative baseline assessment of patient's respiratory system, noting rate, rhythm, degree of chest expansion, quality of breath sounds, cough, and sputum production. Note preoperative O_2 saturation and ABG values if available.
- If appropriate, encourage patient to refrain from smoking for at least 1 wk after surgery. Explain the effects of smoking on the body.
- Monitor O_2 saturation continuously via oximetry in high-risk patients (e.g., patients who are heavily sedated, patients with preexisting lung disease, older adults) and at periodic intervals in other patients as indicated. Notify health care provider of O_2 saturation <92%.
- Evaluate ABG values, and notify health care provider of low or decreasing Pao_2 and high or increasing $Paco_2$.
- Assist patient with turning and deep-breathing exercises q2hr for the first 72 hr postoperatively to promote lung expansion. Be aware that opioid analgesics depress the respiratory system.
- If patient has an incentive spirometer, provide instructions and ensure compliance with its use q2hr or as prescribed.
- Unless contraindicated, assist patient with ambulation by the second postoperative day to enhance ventilation.
- For other interventions, see "Atelectasis" for **Ineffective breathing pattern,** p. 2.

NIC: Airway Management; Chest Physiotherapy; Cough Enhancement; Oxygen Therapy; Postanesthesia Care; Respiratory Monitoring

Risk for fluid volume deficit with risks related to postoperative bleeding/hemorrhage
Desired outcomes: Patient is normovolemic as evidenced by BP ≥90/60 mm Hg (or within patient's preoperative baseline), HR 60-100 bpm, RR 12-20 breaths/min with normal depth and pattern (eupnea), brisk capillary refill (<2 sec), warm extremities, distal pulses >2+ on a 0-4+ scale, urinary output ≥30 ml/hr, and urine specific gravity <1.030. Patient does not demonstrate

significant mental status changes and verbalizes orientation to person, place, and time.

- Monitor VS at frequent intervals during the first 24 hr of the postoperative period. Be alert to indicators of internal hemorrhage and impending shock, including decreasing pulse pressure (difference between systolic and diastolic BP), decreasing BP, increasing HR, and increasing RR.
- Assess patient at frequent intervals during the first 24 hr of the postoperative period for indicators of internal hemorrhage and impending shock, including pallor, diaphoresis, cool extremities, delayed capillary refill, diminished intensity of distal pulses, restlessness, agitation, mental status changes, and disorientation. Also note subjective complaints of thirst, anxiety, or a sense of impending doom.
- Monitor and measure urinary output q4-8hr during the initial postoperative period. Report average hourly output <30 ml/hr. Assess urinary specific gravity, and report specific gravity ≥1.030 to the health care provider.
- Inspect surgical dressing for evidence of frank bleeding (i.e., rapid saturation of dressing with bright red blood). Record saturated dressings, and report significant findings to the health care provider. If the initial postoperative dressing becomes saturated, reinforce and notify the health care provider because he or she may wish to perform the initial dressing change.
- Monitor wound drains and drainage systems for excessive drainage (>50 ml/hr for 2-3 hr), and report findings to the health care provider.
- Note the amount and character of drainage from gastric and other tubes at least q8hr. If drainage appears to contain blood (e.g., bright red, burgundy, or dark coffee ground appearance), perform an occult blood test. If the test is newly or unexpectedly positive, report results to the health care provider. **Note:** After gastric and some other GI surgeries, the patient will have small amounts of bloody or blood-tinged drainage for the first 12-24 hr. Be alert to large or increasing amounts of bloody drainage.
- Review CBC values for evidence of bleeding: decreases in hemoglobin (Hgb) from normal (male 14-18 g/dl; female 12-16 g/dl); and decreases in hematocrit (Hct) from normal (male 40%-54%; female 37%-47%).
- Maintain a patent 18-gauge or larger IV catheter for use if hemorrhagic shock develops. See "Cardiac and Noncardiac Shock," p. 92, for management.

NIC: Bedside Laboratory Testing; Fluid Management; Incision Site Care; Intravenous (IV) Therapy; Wound Care; Wound Care: Closed Drainage

Risk for fluid volume deficit with risks related to *active loss* secondary to presence of indwelling drainage tubes, wound drainage, or vomiting; *inadequate intake of fluids* secondary to nausea, NPO status, CNS depression, or lack of access to fluids; or *failure of regulatory mechanisms* with third spacing of body fluids secondary to the effects of anesthesia, endogenous catecholamines, blood loss during surgery, and prolonged recumbency

Desired outcomes: Patient is normovolemic as evidenced by BP ≥90/60 mm Hg (or within patient's preoperative baseline), HR 60-100 bpm, distal pulses >2+ on a 0-4+ scale, urinary output ≥30 ml/hr, urine specific gravity ≤1.030, stable or increasing weight, good skin turgor, warm skin, moist mucous membranes, and normothermia. Patient does not evidence significant mental status changes and verbalizes orientation to person, place, and time.

- Monitor VS q4-8hr during the recovery phase. Be alert to indicators of dehydration, including decreasing BP, increasing HR, and slightly increased body temperature.
- Assess patient's physical status q4-8hr. Be alert to indicators of dehydration, including dry skin, dry mucous membranes, excessive thirst, diminished intensity of peripheral pulses, and alteration in mental status. Assess skin turgor by lifting a section of skin along the forearm, abdomen, or calf. Release the skin, and watch its return to the original position. With good hydration, it will return quickly; with dehydration, the skin will remain in the

lifted position (tenting) or return slowly. **Note:** This test may be less reliable in the older adult because of decrease in skin elasticity and subcutaneous fat.

- Monitor urinary output q4-8hr. Be alert to a concentrated urine (specific gravity >1.030) and low or decreasing output (average normal output is 60 ml/hr, or 1400-1500 ml/day).
- Measure, describe, and document any emesis. Be alert to and document excessive perspiration. Include your assessment of both with the documentation of urinary, fecal, and other drainage for a total estimation of the patient's fluid balance.
- Measure and record output from drains, ostomies, wounds, and other sources. Ensure patency of gastric and other drainage tubes. Record quality and quantity of output. Report and replace excessive losses.
- Monitor patient's weight daily, using the results as an indicator of the patient's hydration and nutritional status. Always weigh the patient at the same time every day, using the same scale and same type and amount of bed clothing. Be aware that this method is not useful in detecting intravascular fluid loss due to third spacing.
- If nausea and vomiting are present, assess the potential causes, including administration of opioid analgesics, loss of patency of the gastric tube, and environmental factors (e.g., unpleasant odors or sights). Administer antiemetics (e.g., hydroxyzine, ondansetron, prochlorperazine, promethazine), metoclopramide (Reglan), or similar agents as prescribed to combat nausea and vomiting. Instruct patient to request medication *before* the nausea becomes severe.
- Monitor serum electrolytes. Be alert to low potassium levels (K^+ <3.5 mEq/L) and the following signs and symptoms of hypokalemia: lethargy, irritability, anorexia, vomiting, muscle weakness and cramping, paresthesias, weak and irregular pulse, and respiratory dysfunction. Also assess for low calcium levels (Ca^{++} <8.5 mg/dl) and the following signs and symptoms of hypocalcemia: tetany, muscle cramps, fatigue, irritability, personality changes, and Trousseau's or Chvostek's sign. Trousseau's sign is elicited by applying a BP cuff to the arm, inflating it to slightly higher than the systolic BP, and leaving it inflated for 1-4 min. Carpopedal spasms are indicative of hypocalcemia. Chvostek's sign is assessed by tapping the face just below the temple (where the facial nerve emerges). The sign is positive if twitching occurs along the side of the nose, lip, or face.
- Administer and regulate IV fluids and electrolytes as prescribed until patient is able to resume oral intake. When IV fluids are discontinued, encourage intake of oral fluids, at least 2-3 L/day in the nonrestricted patient. As possible, respect patient's preference in oral fluids, and keep them readily available in patient's room.

NIC: Bedside Laboratory Testing; Fluid/Electrolyte Management; Medication Management; Surveillance; Vital Signs Monitoring

Fluid volume excess related to compromised regulatory mechanisms after major surgery
Desired outcome: Following intervention/treatment, patient becomes normovolemic as evidenced by BP within normal range of patient's preoperative baseline, distal pulses <4+ on a 0-4+ scale, presence of eupnea, clear breath sounds, absence of or barely detectable edema (≤1+ on a 0-4+ scale), urine specific gravity >1.010, and body weight near or at preoperative baseline.

- Assess for and report any indicators of fluid overload, including elevated BP, bounding pulses, dyspnea, crackles (rales), and pretibial or sacral edema.
- Maintain record of 8-hr and 24-hr I&0. Note and report significant imbalance. Monitor urinary specific gravity, and report consistently low (<1.010) findings. Remember that normal 24-hr output is 1400-1500 ml and normal 1-hr output is 60 ml/hr.

- Weigh patient daily, using the same scale and same type and amount of bed clothing. Note significant weight gain. Remember that 1 L of fluid equals approximately 2.2 lb.
- Anticipate postoperative diuresis approximately 48-72 hr after surgery because of mobilization of third-space (interstitial) fluid.
- Administer furosemide (Lasix) as prescribed to mobilize interstitial fluid. **Note:** Diuretic therapy may cause dangerous K^+ depletion. See **Risk for fluid volume deficit** on p. 730 for signs and symptoms of hypokalemia.
- Be aware that older adults and individuals with cardiovascular disease are at risk for developing postoperative fluid volume excess.

NIC: Bedside Laboratory Testing; Fluid/Electrolyte Management; Medication Management; Surveillance; Vital Signs Monitoring

Risk for infection with risks related to inadequate primary defenses (broken skin, traumatized tissue, decrease in ciliary action, stasis of body fluids), invasive procedures, or chronic disease

Desired outcome: Patient is free of infection as evidenced by normothermia; HR ≤100 bpm; RR ≤20 breaths/min with normal depth and pattern (eupnea); negative cultures; clear and normal-smelling urine; clear and thin sputum; no significant mental status changes; orientation to person, place, and time; and absence of unusual tenderness, erythema, swelling, warmth, or drainage at the surgical incision.

- Monitor VS for evidence of infection, such as elevated HR and RR and increased body temperature. Notify health care provider if these are new findings.
- Evaluate mental status, orientation, and LOC q8hr. Consider infection if altered mental status or LOC is unexplained by other factors, such as age, medication, or disease process.
- Encourage and assist patient with coughing, deep breathing, incentive spirometry, and turning q2-4hr, and note quality of breath sounds, cough, and sputum.
- Evaluate IV sites for evidence of infection (erythema, warmth, swelling, tenderness, unusual drainage). Change IV line and site if evidence of infection is present and according to agency protocol (q48-72hr).
- Evaluate patency of all surgically placed tubes or drains. Monitor insertion sites for indications of infection (erythema, warmth, swelling, tenderness, unusual drainage). Irrigate or attach to low-pressure suction as prescribed. Promptly report unrelieved loss of patency.
- Note color, character, and odor of all drainage. Report the presence of foul-smelling, creamy, or abnormal drainage.
- Evaluate incisions and wound sites for evidence of infection: unusual erythema, warmth, tenderness, swelling, delayed healing, and purulent or excessive drainage.
- Change dressings as prescribed, using sterile technique. Prevent cross-contamination of wounds in the same patient by changing one dressing at a time and washing hands between dressing changes.
- Suspect evisceration if the patient complains of a feeling of "letting go" or there is a sudden profusion of serous drainage on the dressing or a bulge in the dressing. If patient develops evisceration, do not reinsert tissue or organs. Place a sterile, saline-soaked gauze over eviscerated tissues and cover with a sterile towel until the wound can be evaluated by the health care provider. Maintain the patient on bedrest, usually in semi-Fowler's position with the knees slightly bent for comfort, to prevent further evisceration. Begin to prepare the patient for surgical repair: especially keep the patient NPO, and anticipate the need for IV therapy.
- When appropriate, encourage use of intermittent catheterization q4-6hr instead of an indwelling catheter.

- Prevent reflux of urine into the bladder by keeping drainage collection container below the level of patient's bladder. Help prevent urinary stasis by avoiding kinks or obstructions in the drainage tubing.
- Do not open closed urinary drainage system unless absolutely necessary; irrigate catheter only with health care provider's prescription and when obstruction is the known cause.
- Assess for indicators of urinary tract infection (UTI), including chills; fever (>37.7° C [100° F]); dysuria; urgency; frequency; flank, low back, suprapubic, buttock, inner thigh, scrotal, or labial pain; and cloudy or foul-smelling urine.
- Encourage intake of 2-3 L/day in nonrestricted patients to minimize the potential for UTI by diluting the urine and maximizing urinary flow.
- Ensure that the patient's perineum and meatus are cleansed during the daily bath and that the perianal area is cleansed after bowel movements. Do not hesitate to remind patient of these hygiene measures. Be alert to indicators of meatal infection, including swelling, purulent drainage, and persistent meatal redness. Intervene if the patient is unable to perform self-care.
- Change the catheter according to established protocol or sooner if sandy particles can be felt in the distal end of the catheter or patient develops UTI. Change the drainage collection container according to established protocol or sooner if it becomes foul smelling or leaks.
- Obtain cultures of suspicious drainage or secretions (e.g., sputum, urine, wound) as prescribed. For urine specimens, be certain to use the sampling port, which is at the proximal end of the drainage tube. Cleanse the area with an antimicrobial wipe, and use a sterile syringe with a 25-gauge needle to aspirate the urine.
- Prevent transmission of infectious agents by washing hands well before and after caring for patient and by wearing gloves when contact with blood, drainage, or other body substance is likely.
- Use contact precautions (see Appendix Two, p. 818) for patients colonized with MRSA, VRE, or other epidemiologically important organisms.

NIC: Bathing; Cough Enhancement; Infection Control; Infection Protection; Perineal Care; Wound Care: Closed Drainage

Constipation related to immobility, opioid analgesics and other medications, effects of anesthesia, lack of privacy, disruption of abdominal musculature, or manipulation of abdominal viscera during surgery
Desired outcome: Patient returns to his or her normal bowel elimination pattern as evidenced by return of active bowel sounds within 48-72 hr after most surgeries, absence of abdominal distention or sensation of fullness, and the elimination of soft, formed stools.

- Monitor for and document the elimination of flatus or stool, which signals returning intestinal motility.
- Assess for evidence of decreased GI motility, including abdominal distention, tenderness, absent or hypoactive bowel sounds, and sensation of fullness. Report gross distention, extreme tenderness, and prolonged absence of bowel sounds.
- To stimulate peristalsis, encourage in-bed position changes, exercises, and ambulation to patient's tolerance unless contraindicated.
- If a nasogastric (NG) tube is in place, perform the following:
  —Check placement of the tube after insertion, before any instillation, and q8hr. For a larger-bore tube, aspirate gastric contents and assess for pH <5 for gastric tube placement. If the tube is in the trachea, the patient will exhibit signs of respiratory distress and the tube should be repositioned immediately. Once assured of placement, mark the tube to easily assess tube migration, and secure tubing in place. For smaller-bore

tubes, check a recent x-ray to confirm position before instilling anything into the tube.

—Prevent migration of the tube by keeping it securely taped to the patient's nose and reinforcing placement by attaching the tube to the patient's gown with a safety pin or tape.

—Measure and record the quantity and quality of output. Typically the color will be green. For patients who have undergone gastric surgery, the output may be brownish initially because of small amounts of bloody drainage but should change to green after about 12 hr. Test reddish, brown, or black output for the presence of blood, which can signal gastrointestinal bleeding. Reposition the tube as necessary. **Note:** For patient with gastric, esophageal, or duodenal surgery, notify health care provider before manipulating the tube.

—Maintain patency of the NG tube with gentle instillation of normal saline as prescribed. Ensure low, intermittent suction of gastric sump tubes by maintaining patency of sump port (usually blue). If sump port becomes occluded by gastric contents, flush sump port with air until a *whoosh* sound is heard over the epigastric area. **Caution:** Never clamp or otherwise occlude sump port, because excessive pressure may accumulate and damage gastric mucosa. For patient with gastric, esophageal, or duodenal surgery, notify health care provider before irrigating tube.

—When the tube is removed, monitor patient for abdominal distention, nausea, and vomiting.

• Monitor and document patient's response to diet advancement from clear liquids to a regular or other prescribed diet.

• Encourage oral fluid intake (>2500 ml/day), especially of prune juice.

• Administer stool softeners, mild laxatives, and enemas as prescribed. As appropriate, encourage a high-bulk diet (fresh vegetables and fruits). Monitor and record results.

• Arrange periods of privacy during patient's attempts at bowel elimination.

NIC: Bowel Management; Constipation/Impaction Management; Diet Staging; Fluid Management; Nutrition Management; Tube Care: Gastrointestinal

Sleep pattern disturbance related to preoperative anxiety, stress, postoperative pain, noise, and altered environment

Desired outcome: Following intervention/treatment, patient relates minimal or no difficulty with falling asleep and describes a feeling of being well rested.

• Administer sedative/hypnotic (Table A-7) as prescribed. Be aware that these agents may cause CNS depression and contribute to the respiratory depressant effects of opioid analgesics. Also be aware that active metabolites of many of the benzodiazepines may accumulate and result in greater physiologic effects or toxicity. **Note:** Use special caution when administering sedative/hypnotic to patients with COPD because of its respiratory depres-

TABLE A-7 Sedatives and Hypnotics Used Perioperatively	
Antihistamine sedatives	Benzodiazepines
Diphenhydramine (Benadryl)	Alprazolam (Xanax)
Hydroxyzine (Vistaril)	Chlordiazepoxide (Librium)
	Diazepam (Valium)
	Lorazepam (Ativan)
	Oxazepam (Serax)
	Temazepam (Restoril)

sant effects. Monitor respiratory function, including oximetry, at frequent intervals in these individuals.

- After administering sedative/hypnotic, be certain to raise side rails, lower the bed to its lowest position, and caution patient not to smoke in bed.
- Administer analgesics at bedtime to reduce pain and augment effects of hypnotic.
- Be certain that consent for surgery is signed before administering sedative/hypnotic.
- Use nonpharmacologic measures to promote sleep (Table A-8).

◎ NIC: Environmental Management: Comfort; Medication Management; Simple Relaxation Therapy; Sleep Enhancement

Impaired physical mobility related to postoperative pain, decreased strength and endurance secondary to CNS effects of anesthesia or blood loss, musculoskeletal or neuromuscular impairment secondary to disease process or surgical procedure, perceptual impairment secondary to disease process or surgical procedure (e.g., ocular surgery, neurosurgery), or cognitive deficit secondary to disease process or effects of opioid analgesics and anesthetics
Desired outcome: Optimally, by hospital discharge (depending on type of surgery), patient returns to preoperative baseline physical mobility as evidenced by the ability to move in bed, transfer, and ambulate independently or with minimal assistance.

- Assess patient's preoperative physical mobility by evaluating coordination and muscle strength, control, and mass. Be aware of medically imposed restrictions against movement, especially with conditions or surgeries that are orthopedic, neurosurgical, or ocular.

TABLE A-8	Nonpharmacologic Measures to Promote Sleep
Activity	Examples
Mask or eliminate environmental stimuli	Use eye shields or ear plugs; play soothing music; dim lights at bedtime; mask odors from dressings/drainage; change dressing or drainage container as indicated
Promote muscle relaxation	Encourage ambulation as tolerated throughout the day; teach and encourage in-bed exercises and position changes; perform back massage at bedtime; if not contraindicated, use heating pad
Reduce anxiety	Ensure adequate pain control; keep patient informed of progress and treatment measures; avoid overstimulation by visitors or other activities immediately before bedtime; avoid stimulant drugs (e.g., caffeine)
Promote comfort	Encourage patient to use own pillows and bedclothes if not contraindicated; adjust bed; rearrange linens; regulate room temperature
Promote usual presleep routine	Offer oral hygiene at bedtime; provide warm beverage at bedtime; encourage reading or other quiet activity
Minimize sleep disruption	Maintain quiet environment throughout the night; plan nursing activities to allow long periods (at least 90 min) of undisturbed sleep; use dim lights when checking on patient during the night

- Evaluate and correct factors limiting physical mobility, including oversedation with opioid analgesics, failure to achieve adequate pain control, and poorly arranged physical environment.
- Initiate movement from bed to chair and ambulation as soon as possible after surgery, depending on postoperative prescriptions, type of surgery, and patient's recovery from anesthetics (usually 12-24 hr after surgery). Assist patient with moving slowly to a sitting position in bed and then standing at bedside before attempting ambulation. For more information, see **Altered cerebral tissue perfusion,** p. 743. **Note:** Many anesthetic agents depress normal vasoconstrictor mechanisms and can result in sudden hypotension with quick changes in position.
- Encourage frequent movement and ambulation by postoperative patients. Provide assistance as indicated.
- Explain the importance of movement in bed and ambulation in reducing postoperative complications, including atelectasis, pneumonia, thrombophlebitis, and depressed GI motility.
- Instruct the patient in performance of in-bed exercises (e.g., gluteal and quadriceps muscle sets [isometrics], ankle circling, calf pumping).
- For additional information, see "Caring for Patients on Prolonged Bedrest" for **Risk for activity intolerance,** p. 738, and **Risk for disuse syndrome,** p. 740.

NIC: Activity Therapy; Exercise Therapy: Ambulation; Exercise Therapy: Joint Mobility; Surveillance: Safety; Teaching: Prescribed Activity/Exercise

Risk for trauma with risks related to weakness, balancing difficulties, and reduced muscle coordination secondary to anesthetics and postoperative opioid analgesics
Desired outcome: Patient does not fall and remains free of trauma as evidenced by absence of bruises, wounds, or fractures.

- Orient and reorient patient to person, place, and time during the initial postoperative period. Inform patient that surgery is over. Repeat information until patient is fully awake and oriented (usually several hours but may be days in heavily sedated or otherwise obtunded individuals).
- Maintain side rails on stretchers and beds in upright and locked positions. Be aware that some individuals experience agitation and thrash about as they emerge from anesthesia.
- Secure all IV lines, drains, and tubing to prevent dislodgment.
- Maintain bed in its lowest position when leaving patient's room.
- Be certain that the call mechanism is within patient's reach; instruct patient about its use.
- Identify patients at risk for falling by assessing the following. Correct or compensate for risk factors.
  —*Time of day:* night shift, peak activity periods such as meals, bedtime.
  —*Medications:* opioid analgesics, sedatives, hypnotics, and anesthetics.
  —*Impaired mobility:* individuals requiring assistance with transfer and ambulation.
  —*Sensory deficits:* diminished visual acuity caused by disease process or environmental factors; changes in kinesthetic sense because of disease or trauma.
- Use restraints and protective devices if necessary and prescribed.

NIC: Environmental Management: Safety; Fall Prevention; Physical Restraint; Surveillance: Safety; Teaching: Individual

Risk for impaired skin integrity with risks related to presence of secretions/excretions around percutaneous drains and tubes
Desired outcome: Patient's skin around percutaneous drains and tubes remains intact and nonerythematous.

- Change dressings as soon as they become wet. The health care provider may prefer to perform the first dressing change at the surgical incision. Use sterile technique for all dressing changes.
- Keep the area around drains as clean as possible (e.g., intestinal secretions, bile, and similar drainage can lead quickly to skin excoriation). Sterile normal saline or a solution of saline and hydrogen peroxide or other prescribed solution may be used to clean around the drain site.
- If some external drainage is present, position a pectin-wafer skin barrier around the drain or tube. Ointments, such as zinc oxide, petrolatum, and aluminum paste, also may be used. Consult enterostomal therapy (ET) nurse if drainage is excessive or skin excoriation develops. For additional information, see "Managing Wound Care," p. 704.

NIC: Incision Site Care; Infection Protection; Skin Surveillance; Wound Care

Altered oral mucous membrane related to NPO status and/or presence of NG or endotracheal tube
Desired outcome: At the time of hospital discharge, patient's oral mucosa is intact, without pain or evidence of bleeding.
- Provide oral care and oral hygiene q4hr and prn. Arrange for patient to gargle, brush teeth, and cleanse the mouth with sponge-tipped applicators as necessary to prevent excoriation and excessive dryness.
- Use a moistened cotton-tipped applicator to remove encrustations. Carefully lubricate the lips and nares with an antimicrobial ointment, petroleum jelly, or emollient cream.
- If the patient's throat is irritated from the presence of an NG tube, obtain a prescription for a lidocaine gargling solution.
- For additional information, see "Stomatitis" for **Altered oral mucous membrane,** p. 780.

NIC: Oral Health Maintenance; Oral Health Restoration

See Also: "Atelectasis," p. 1; "Pneumonia," p. 3; "Venous Thrombosis/Thrombophlebitis," p. 124; "Urinary Retention," p. 185; "Providing Nutritional Support," p. 687; "Managing Wound Care," p. 704; "Caring for Patients on Prolonged Bedrest," p. 738, for additional information about the prevention of surgical complications; "Caring for Patients With Cancer and Other Life-disrupting Illnesses," p. 791, for psychosocial nursing diagnoses and interventions.

Selected Bibliography

Acute Pain Management Guideline Panel: *Acute pain management: operative or medical procedures and trauma. Clinical practices guideline.* AHCPR pub. no. 92-0032, Rockville, Md, 1992, Agency for Health Care Policy and Research, Public Health Service, U.S. Department of Health and Human Services.

Interqual: *The ISD-A review system with adult ISD criteria,* Northhampton, NH, and Marlboro, Mass, August 1992, Interqual.

Keen JH: Pain. In Keen JH, Swearingen PL, editors: *Mosby's critical care consultant,* ed 3, St Louis, 1997, Mosby.

Kim MJ et al: *Pocket guide to nursing diagnoses,* ed 7, St Louis, 1997, Mosby.

McCloskey JC, Bulechek GM, editors: *Nursing interventions classification (NIC),* ed 2, St Louis, 1996, Mosby.

Pasero C, McCaffery M: Managing postoperative pain in the elderly, *Am J Nurs* 96(10):38-45, 1996.

Stannard D et al: Clinical judgement and management of postoperative pain in critical care patients, *Am J Crit Care* 5(6):433-441, 1996.

Section Two: Caring for Patients on Prolonged Bedrest

Risk for activity intolerance with risks related to deconditioned status (Table A-9)

Desired outcomes: Patient exhibits cardiac tolerance to activity or exercise as evidenced by HR ≤20 bpm over resting HR, systolic BP ≤20 mm Hg over or under resting systolic BP, RR ≤20 breaths/min with normal depth and pattern (eupnea), normal sinus rhythm, warm and dry skin, and absence of crackles (rales), new murmurs, new dysrhythmias, gallop, or chest pain. Patient rates perceived exertion (RPE) at ≤3 on a scale of 0 (none) to 10 (maximal).

- Perform ROM exercises 2-4 times per day on each extremity. Individualize the exercise plan based on the following guidelines:
  —*Mode or type of exercise:* begin with passive exercises, moving the joints through the motions of abduction, adduction, flexion, and extension. Progress to active-assisted exercises in which you support the joints while the patient initiates muscle contraction. When the patient is able, supervise him or her in active isotonic exercises, during which the patient contracts a selected muscle group, moves the extremity at a slow pace, and then relaxes the muscle group. Have the patient repeat each exercise 3-10 times.

> **Caution:** Stop any exercise that results in muscular or skeletal pain. Consult a physical therapist (PT) about necessary modifications. Avoid isometric exercises in cardiac patients.

  —*Intensity:* begin with 3-5 repetitions as tolerated by the patient. Assess exercise tolerance by measuring HR and BP at rest, peak exercise, and 5 min after exercise. If HR or systolic BP increases >20 bpm or >20 mm Hg over the resting level, decrease the number of repetitions. If HR or systolic BP decreases >10 bpm or >10 mm Hg at peak exercise, this could be a sign of left ventricular failure, denoting that the heart cannot meet this work load. For other adverse signs and symptoms, see *Assessment of exercise tolerance,* p. 739.
  —*Duration:* begin with 5 min or less of exercise. Gradually increase the exercise to 15 min as tolerated.
  —*Frequency:* begin with exercises 2-4 times per day. As the duration increases, the frequency can be reduced.

T A B L E   A - 9   Physiologic Effects of Prolonged Bedrest (Deconditioning)

Increased HR and BP for submaximal work load
Decrease in functional capacity
Decrease in circulating volume
Orthostatic hypotension
Reflex tachycardia
Modest decrease in pulmonary function
Increase in thromboemboli
Loss of muscle mass
Loss of muscle contractile strength
Decreased periarticular tissue elasticity
Negative protein state
Negative nitrogen (N) state

—*Assessment of exercise tolerance:* be alert to signs and symptoms that the cardiovascular and respiratory systems are unable to meet the demands of the low-level ROM exercises. Excessive SOB may occur if (1) transient pulmonary congestion occurs secondary to ischemia or left ventricular dysfunction; (2) lung volumes are decreased; (3) oxygen-carrying capacity of the blood is reduced; or (4) there is shunting of blood from the right to the left side of the heart without adequate oxygenation. If cardiac output does not increase to meet the body's needs during modest levels of exercise, systolic BP may fall; the skin may become cool, cyanotic, and diaphoretic; dysrhythmias may be noted; crackles (rales) may be auscultated; or a systolic murmur of mitral regurgitation may occur. If the patient tolerates the exercise, increase the intensity or number of repetitions each day.

- Ask the patient to rate perceived exertion experienced during exercise, basing it on the following scale developed by Borg (1982):

  0—nothing at all
  1—very weak effort
  2—weak (light) effort
  3—moderate
  4—somewhat stronger effort
  5—strong effort
  7—very strong effort
  9—very, very strong effort
  10—maximal effort

The patient should not experience an RPE >3 while performing ROM exercises. Reduce the intensity of the exercise and increase the frequency until an RPE of ≤3 is attained.

- As the patient's condition improves, increase activity as soon as possible to include sitting in a chair. Assess for orthostatic hypotension, which can occur as a result of decreased plasma volume and difficulty in adjusting immediately to postural change. Prepare the patient for this change by increasing the amount of time spent in high Fowler's position and moving the patient slowly and in stages. The following describes activity progression in hospitalized patients:

Level I: Bedrest	Flexion and extension of extremities 4 times/day, 15 times each extremity; deep breathing 4 times/day, 15 breaths; position change from side to side q2hr
Level II: Out of bed to chair	As tolerated, 3 times/day for 20-30 min; may perform ROM exercises 2 times/day while sitting in chair
Level III: Ambulate in room	As tolerated, 3 times/day for 3-5 min
Level IV: Ambulate in hall	Initially, 50-200 ft 2 times/day; progressing to 600 ft 4 times/day; may incorporate slow stair climbing in preparation for hospital discharge
Signs of activity intolerance:	Decrease in BP >20 mm Hg; increase in heart rate to >120 bpm (or >20 bpm above resting HR in patients receiving beta-blocker therapy)

- Increase activity level by having patient perform self-care activities such as eating, mouth care, and bathing as tolerated.
- Teach significant other the purpose and interventions for preventing deconditioning. Involve him or her in patient's plan of care.
- To help allay fears of failure, pain, or medical setbacks, provide emotional support to patient and significant other as patient's activity level is increased.

NIC: Cardiac Care: Rehabilitative; Energy Management; Exercise Promotion: Stretching; Exercise Therapy: Joint Mobility; Exercise Therapy: Muscle Control; Mutual Goal Setting; Teaching: Prescribed Activity/Exercise

Risk for disuse syndrome with risks related to paralysis, mechanical immobilization, prescribed immobilization, severe pain, or altered LOC
Desired outcome: Patient exhibits complete ROM of all joints without pain, and limb girth measurements are congruent with or increased over baseline measurements.

Note: ROM exercises should be performed at least twice per day for all immobilized patients with *normal* joints. Modification may be required for patient with flaccidity (i.e., immediately after cerebrovascular accident [CVA] or spinal cord injury [SCI]) to prevent subluxation; or for patient with spasticity (i.e., during the recovery period for patient with CVA or SCI) to prevent an increase in spasticity. Consult physical therapist (PT) or occupational therapist (OT) for assistance in modifying the exercise plan for these patients. Also, be aware that ROM exercises are restricted or contraindicated for patients with rheumatologic disease during the inflammatory phase and for joints that are dislocated or fractured.

- Be alert to the following areas that are especially susceptible to joint contracture: *shoulder,* which can become "frozen" to limit abduction and extension; *wrist,* which can "drop," prohibiting extension; *fingers,* which can develop flexion contractures that limit extension; *hips,* which can develop flexion contractures that affect the gait by shortening the limb or develop external rotation or adduction deformities that affect the gait; *knees,* in which flexion contractures can develop to limit extension and alter the gait; and *feet,* which can "drop" as a result of plantar flexion, which limits dorsiflexion and alters the gait.
- Ensure that patient changes position at least q2hr. Post a turning schedule at patient's bedside. Position changes will not only maintain correct body alignment, thereby reducing strain on the joints, but also prevent contractures, minimize pressure on bony prominences, decrease venostasis, and promote maximal chest expansion.
  —Try to place patient in a position that achieves proper standing alignment: head neutral or slightly flexed on the neck, hips extended, knees extended or minimally flexed, and feet at right angles to the legs. Maintain this position with pillows, towels, or other positioning aids.
  —To prevent hip flexion contractures, ensure that patient is prone or side-lying, with the hips extended, for the same amount of time patient spends in the supine position or, at a minimum, three times per day for 1 hr.
  —When the HOB must be elevated 30 degrees, extend patient's shoulders and arms, using pillows to support the position, and allow the fingertips to extend over the edge of the pillows to maintain normal arching of the hands. **Caution:** Because elevating the HOB promotes hip flexion, ensure that patient spends time with the hips in extension (see preceding intervention).
  —When patient is in the side-lying position, extend the lower leg from the hip to help prevent hip flexion contracture.
  —When able to place patient in the prone position, move patient to the end of the bed and allow the feet to rest between the mattress and footboard. This will prevent not only plantar flexion and hip rotation, but also injury to the heels and toes. Place thin pads under the angles of the axillae and lateral aspects of the clavicles to prevent internal rotation of the shoulders and maintain anatomic position of the shoulder girdle.
- To maintain the joints in neutral position, use the following as indicated: pillows, rolled towels, blankets, sandbags, antirotation boots, splints, and

orthotics. When using adjunctive devices, monitor the involved skin at frequent intervals for alterations in integrity, and implement measures to prevent skin breakdown.
- Assess for footdrop by inspecting the feet for plantar flexion and evaluating patient's ability to pull the toes upward toward the head. Because the feet lie naturally in plantar flexion, be particularly alert to the patient's inability to pull the toes up. Document this assessment daily.
- Teach patient and significant other the rationale and procedure for ROM exercises, and have patient return the demonstrations. Review **Risk for activity intolerance,** earlier, to ensure that patient does not exceed his or her tolerance. Provide passive exercises for patients unable to perform active or active-assisted exercises. In addition, incorporate movement patterns into care activities, such as position changes, bed baths, getting the patient on and off the bedpan, or changing the patient's gown. Ensure that joints especially prone to contracture are exercised more stringently. Provide patient with a handout that reviews the exercises and lists the repetitions for each. Instruct significant other to encourage patient to perform exercises as required.
- Perform and document limb girth measurements, dynamography, and ROM, and establish exercise-baseline limits to assess patient's existing muscle mass and strength and joint motion.
- Explain to patient that muscle atrophy occurs because of disuse or failure to use the joint that is often caused by immediate or anticipated pain. Eventually disuse may result in a decrease in muscle mass and blood supply and a loss of periarticular tissue elasticity, which in turn can lead to increased muscle fatigue and joint pain with use.
- Emphasize the importance of maintaining or increasing muscle strength and periarticular tissue elasticity through exercise. If unsure about patient's complicating pathologic condition, consult health care provider about the appropriate form of exercise for patient.
- Explain the need to participate maximally in self-care as tolerated to help maintain muscle strength and enhance a sense of participation and control.
- For noncardiac patients needing greater help with muscle strength, assist with resistive exercises (e.g., moderate weight lifting to increase the size, endurance, and strength of the muscles). For patients in beds with Balkan frames, provide the means for resistive exercise by implementing a system of weights and pulleys. First determine patient's baseline level of performance on a given set of exercises, and then set realistic goals with the patient for repetitions (e.g., if the patient can do 5 repetitions of lifting a 5-lb weight with the biceps muscle, the goal may be to increase the repetitions to 10 within 1 wk, to an ultimate goal of 20 within 3 wk, and then advance to 7.5-lb weights).
- If the joints require rest, isometric exercises can be used. With these exercises, teach patient to contract a muscle group and hold the contraction for a count of 5 or 10. The sequence is repeated for increasing counts or repetitions until an adequate level of endurance has been achieved. Thereafter, maintenance levels are performed.
- Provide a chart to show patient's progress, and combine this with large amounts of positive reinforcement. Post the exercise regimen at the bedside to ensure consistency by all health care personnel. Instruct significant other in the exercise regimen, and elicit his or her support and encouragement of patient's performance of the exercises.
- As appropriate, teach transfer or crutch-walking techniques and use of a walker, wheelchair, or cane so that patient can maintain the highest possible level of mobility. Include significant other in the demonstrations, and stress the importance of good body mechanics.

- Provide periods of uninterrupted rest between exercises/activities to enable patient to replenish energy stores.
- Seek a referral to a PT or OT as appropriate.

○ **NIC:** Exercise Promotion: Stretching; Exercise Therapy: Ambulation; Exercise Therapy: Joint Mobility; Medication Management; Mutual Goal Setting; Teaching: Prescribed Activity/Exercise

Altered peripheral tissue perfusion related to interrupted venous flow secondary to prolonged immobility
Desired outcomes: At least 24 hr before hospital discharge, patient has adequate peripheral perfusion as evidenced by normal skin color and temperature and adequate distal pulses (>2+ on a 0-4+ scale) in peripheral extremities. Patient performs exercises independently, adheres to the prophylactic regimen, and maintains an intake of 2-3 L/day of fluid unless contraindicated.

- Teach patient that pain, redness, swelling, and warmth in the involved area and coolness, edema, unnatural color or pallor, and superficial venous dilation distal to the involved area are all indicators of deep vein thrombosis (DVT) and should be reported to staff member promptly if they occur.
- Monitor for the indicators just listed, along with routine VS checks. If patient is asymptomatic for DVT, assess for positive Homans' sign: flex the knee 30 degrees and dorsiflex the foot. Pain elicited with the dorsiflexion may be a sign of DVT, and patient should be referred to health care provider for further evaluation. Additional signs of DVT may include fever, tachycardia, and elevated erythrocyte sedimentation rate (ESR). Normal ESR (Westergren method) in males younger than 50 yr is 0-15 mm/hr and older than 50 yr is 0-20 mm/hr; in females younger than 50 yr it is 0-20 mm/hr and older than 50 yr it is 0-30 mm/hr.
- Teach patient calf-pumping (ankle dorsiflexion–plantar flexion) and ankle-circling exercises. Instruct patient to repeat each movement 10 times, performing each exercise hourly during extended periods of immobility, provided that patient is free of symptoms of DVT. Help promote circulation by performing passive ROM or encouraging active ROM exercises.
- Encourage deep breathing, which increases negative pressure in the lungs and thorax to promote emptying of large veins.
- When not contraindicated by peripheral vascular disease (PVD), ensure that patient wears antiembolism hose, pneumatic foot pump devices, or pneumatic sequential compression stockings. Remove them for 10-20 min q8hr, and inspect underlying skin for evidence of irritation or breakdown. Reapply hose after elevating patient's legs at least 10 degrees for 10 min.
- Instruct patient not to cross the feet at the ankles or knees while in bed, because doing so may cause venous stasis. If patient is at risk for DVT, elevate the foot of the bed 10 degrees to increase venous return.
- In nonrestricted patient, increase fluid intake to at least 2-3 L/day to reduce hemoconcentration, which can contribute to the development of DVT. Educate patient about the need to drink large amounts of fluid (9-14 eight-ounce glasses). Monitor I&O to ensure compliance.
- Patients at risk for DVT, including those with chronic infection and a history of PVD and smoking, as well as older, obese, and anemic patients, may require pharmacologic interventions such as aspirin, sodium warfarin, phenindione derivatives, heparin, or low-molecular-weight heparin (e.g., enoxaparin sodium). Administer medication as prescribed, and monitor appropriate laboratory values (e.g., prothrombin time [PT], partial thromboplastin time [PTT]). Educate patient to self-monitor for and report bleeding (epistaxis, bleeding gums, hematemesis, hemoptysis, melena, hematuria, hematochezia, menometrorrhagia, ecchymoses).
- In patients prone to DVT, acquire bilateral baseline measurements of the mid-calf, knee, and mid-thigh, and record them on patient's Kardex. Monitor

these measurements daily, and compare them with the baseline measurements to rule out extremity enlargement caused by DVT.

◎ NIC: Bed Rest Care; Circulatory Care; Embolus Precautions; Exercise Therapy: Joint Mobility; Laboratory Data Interpretation; Surveillance

Altered cerebral tissue perfusion (orthostatic hypotension) related to interrupted arterial flow to the brain secondary to prolonged bedrest

Desired outcome: When getting out of bed, patient has adequate cerebral perfusion as evidenced by HR <120 bpm and BP ≥90/60 mm Hg (or within 20 mm Hg of patient's normal range) immediately after position change, dry skin, normal skin color, and absence of vertigo and syncope, with return of HR and BP to resting levels within 3 min of position change.

- Assess patient for factors that increase the risk of orthostatic hypotension because of fluid volume changes (recent diuresis, diaphoresis, or change in vasodilator therapy), altered autonomic control (diabetic cardiac neuropathy, denervation after heart transplant, or advanced age), or severe left ventricular dysfunction.
- Explain the cause of orthostatic hypotension and measures for preventing it.
- Application of antiembolism hose, which are used to prevent DVT, may be useful in preventing orthostatic hypotension once the patient is mobilized. For patients who continue to have difficulty with orthostatic hypotension, it may be necessary to supplement the hose with elastic wraps to the groin when the patient is out of bed. Ensure that these wraps encompass the entire surface of the legs.
- When patient is in bed, provide instructions for leg exercises as described under **Risk for activity intolerance,** p. 738. Encourage patient to perform leg exercises immediately before mobilization to facilitate venous return.
- Prepare patient for getting out of bed by encouraging position changes within necessary confines. It is sometimes possible and advisable to use a tilt table to reacclimate patient to upright positions.
- Follow these guidelines for mobilization:
  —Check the BP in any high-risk patient for whom this will be the first time out of bed. Instruct the patient to immediately report symptoms of lightheadedness or dizziness.
  —Have the patient dangle legs at the bedside. Be alert to indicators of orthostatic hypotension, including diaphoresis, pallor, tachycardia, hypotension, and syncope. Question patient about the presence of lightheadedness or dizziness. Again, encourage performance of leg exercises.
  —If indicators of orthostatic hypotension occur, check the VS. A drop in systolic BP of 20 mm Hg and an increased pulse rate, combined with symptoms of vertigo and impending syncope, signal the need for return to a supine position.
  —If leg dangling is tolerated, have patient stand at the bedside with two staff members in attendance. If no adverse signs or symptoms occur, have patient progress to ambulation as tolerated.

◎ NIC: Cardiac Care; Cerebral Perfusion Promotion; Circulatory Precautions; Fluid/Electrolyte Management; Vital Signs Monitoring

Constipation related to less than adequate fluid or dietary intake and bulk, immobility, lack of privacy, positional restrictions, and use of narcotic analgesics

Desired outcomes: Within 24 hr of this diagnosis, patient verbalizes knowledge of measures that promote bowel elimination. Patient relates the return of normal pattern and character of bowel elimination within 3-5 days of this diagnosis.

- Assess patient's bowel history to determine normal bowel habits and interventions that are used successfully at home.

- Monitor and document patient's bowel movements, diet, and I&O. Be alert to the following indications of constipation: fewer than patient's usual number of bowel movements, abdominal discomfort or distention, straining at stool, and patient complaints of rectal pressure or fullness. Fecal impaction may be manifested by oozing of liquid stool and confirmed via digital examination.
- Auscultate each abdominal quadrant for at least 1 min to determine the presence of bowel sounds. Normal sounds are gurgles occurring at a rate of 5-34/min. **Note:** Bowel sounds are decreased or absent with paralytic ileus. High-pitched rushing sounds or "tinkles" may be heard during abdominal cramping, indicating an intestinal obstruction.
- If a rectal impaction is suspected, use a gloved, lubricated finger to remove stool from the rectum. This stimulation may be adequate to stimulate bowel movement. Oil retention enemas may soften impacted stool.
- Teach patient the importance of a high-fiber diet and a fluid intake of at least 2-3 L/day (unless this is contraindicated by a renal, hepatic, or cardiac disorder). High-fiber foods include bran, whole grains, nuts, and raw and coarse vegetables and fruits with skins.
- Maintain patient's normal bowel habits whenever possible by offering the bedpan, ensuring privacy, and timing medications, enemas, or suppositories so that they take effect at the time of day patient normally has a bowel movement. Provide warm fluids before breakfast, and encourage toileting to take advantage of gastrocolic or duodenocolic reflexes.
- To promote peristalsis, maximize patient's activity level within the limitations of endurance, therapy, and pain.
- Request pharmacologic interventions from health care provider when necessary. To help prevent rebound constipation, make a priority list of interventions to ensure minimal disruption of patient's normal bowel habits. The following is a suggested hierarchy of interventions:
  - Bulk-building additives (psyllium), bran
  - Mild laxatives (apple or prune juice, Milk of Magnesia)
  - Stool softeners (docusate sodium, docusate calcium)
  - Potent laxatives and cathartics (bisacodyl, cascara sagrada)
  - Medicated suppositories
  - Enemas
- Discuss the role that narcotic agents and other medications have in constipation. Teach alternative methods of pain control (see Table A-6).

NIC: Bowel Management; Constipation/Impaction Management; Diet Staging; Flatulence Reduction; Fluid Management; Medication Management; Nutrition Management

Diversional activity deficit related to prolonged illness and hospitalization
Desired outcome: Within 24 hr of intervention, patient engages in diversional activities and relates the absence of boredom.
- Be alert to patient indicators of boredom, including wishing for something to read or do, daytime napping, and expressed inability to perform usual hobbies because of hospitalization.
- Assess patient's activity tolerance as described on p. 739.
- Collect a database by assessing patient's normal support systems and relationship patterns with significant other. Question patient and significant other about patient interests, and explore diversional activities that may be suitable for the hospital setting and patient's level of activity tolerance.
- Personalize the patient's environment with favorite objects and photographs of significant others.
- Provide low-level activities commensurate with patient's tolerance (e.g., books or magazines pertaining to patient's recreational or other interests, computer games, television, writing for short intervals).

- Initiate activities that require little concentration, and proceed to more complicated tasks as patient's condition allows (e.g., if reading requires more energy or concentration than patient is capable of, suggest that significant other read to patient or bring audiotapes of books).
- Encourage discussion of past activities or reminiscence as a substitute for performing favorite activities during convalescence.
- As patient's endurance improves, obtain appropriate diversional activities, such as puzzles, model kits, handicrafts, and computerized games and activities; encourage patient to use them.
- Encourage significant other to visit within limits of patient's endurance and to involve patient in activities that are of interest to him or her, such as playing cards or backgammon. Encourage significant other to stagger visits throughout the day.
- Spend extra time with patient.
- Suggest that significant other bring a radio, or, if appropriate, rent a television or radio from the hospital, if not part of the standard room charge.
- If appropriate for patient, arrange for hospital volunteers to visit, play cards, read books, or play board games.
- As appropriate for patient who desires social interaction, consider relocation to a room in an area of high traffic.
- As patient's condition improves, assist him or her with sitting in a chair near a window so that outside activities can be viewed. When patients are able, provide opportunities to sit in a solarium so that they can visit with other patients. If the physical condition and weather permit, take patient outside for brief periods.
- Request consultation from social services, OT, pastoral services, and psychiatric nurse for interventions as appropriate.
- Increase patient's involvement in self-care to provide a sense of purpose, accomplishment, and control. Performing in-bed exercises (e.g., deep breathing, ankle circling, calf pumping), keeping track of I&O, and similar activities can and should be accomplished routinely by these patients.

NIC: Art Therapy; Environmental Management; Music Therapy; Pass Facilitation; Patient Contracting; Play Therapy; Recreation Therapy; Self-Esteem Enhancement; Visitation Facilitation

Altered sexuality patterns related to actual or perceived physiologic limitations on sexual performance secondary to disease, therapy, or prolonged hospitalization

Desired outcome: Within 72 hr of this diagnosis, patient relates satisfaction with sexuality and/or understanding of the ability to resume sexual activity.

- Assess patient's normal sexual function, including the importance placed on sex in the relationship, frequency of interaction, normal positions used, and the couple's ability to adapt or change to meet requirements of patient's limitations.
- Identify patient's problem diplomatically, and clarify it with patient. Indicators of sexual dysfunction can include regression, acting-out with inappropriate behavior such as grabbing or pinching, sexual overtures toward the hospital staff, self-enforced isolation, and similar behaviors.
- Encourage patient and significant other to verbalize feelings and anxieties about sexual abstinence, having sexual relations in the hospital, hurting the patient, or having to use new or alternative methods for sexual gratification. Develop strategies in collaboration with the patient and significant other.
- Encourage acceptable expressions of sexuality by the patient (e.g., in a woman this could involve wearing makeup and jewelry).
- Inform patient and significant other that it is possible to have time alone together for intimacy. Provide that time accordingly by putting a "Do Not Disturb" sign on the door, enforcing privacy by restricting staff and visitors to the room, or arranging for temporary private quarters.

- Encourage patient and significant other to seek alternate methods of sexual expression when necessary. This may include mutual masturbation, altered positions, vibrators, and identification of other erotic areas for the partner.
- Refer patient and significant other to professional sexual counseling as necessary.

NIC: Behavior Management: Sexual; Body Image Enhancement; Self-Esteem Enhancement; Sexual Counseling; Teaching: Sexuality

Altered role performance: Dependence vs. independence
Desired outcome: Within 48 hr of this diagnosis, patient collaborates with caregivers in planning realistic goals for independence, participates in own care, and takes responsibility for self-care.

- Encourage patient to be as independent as possible within limitations of endurance, therapy, and pain. Be aware, however, that temporary periods of dependence are appropriate because they enable the individual to restore energy reserves needed for recovery.
- Ensure that all health care providers are consistent in conveying their expectations of eventual independence.
- Alert patient to areas of excessive dependence, and involve him or her in collaborative goal setting to achieve independence.
- Do not minimize patient's expressed feelings of depression. Allow patient to express emotions, but provide support, understanding, and realistic hope for a positive role change.
- If indicated, provide self-help devices to increase patient's independence with self-care.
- Provide positive reinforcement when patient meets or advances toward goals.

NIC: Caregiver Support; Coping Enhancement; Mutual Goal Setting; Normalization Promotion; Role Enhancement; Self-Esteem Enhancement

---

See Also: "Respiratory Disorders" for interventions related to prevention of atelectasis (p. 2) and pneumonia (p. 4); "Stomatitis," p. 403, for interventions for patients with altered oral mucous membrane; "Pressure Ulcers" for **Impaired tissue integrity** (for patients without pressure ulcers who are at risk because of immobility), p. 711; "Caring for Patients With Cancer and Other Life-disrupting Disorders," p. 791, for psychosocial nursing diagnoses and interventions.

Selected Bibliography

American Association of Cardiovascular and Pulmonary Rehabilitation: *Guidelines for cardiac rehabilitation programs,* ed 2, Champaign, Ill, 1996, Human Kinetic Books.

Interqual: *The ISD-A review system with adult ISD criteria,* Northhampton, NH, and Marlboro, Mass, August 1992, Interqual.

Borg GV: Psychophysical basis of perceived exertion, *Med Sci Sports Exerc* 14:377-381, 1982,

Kim MJ et al: *Pocket guide to nursing diagnoses,* ed 7, St Louis, 1997, Mosby.

McCloskey JC, Bulechek GM, editors: *Nursing interventions classification (NIC),* ed 2, St Louis, 1996, Mosby.

Noble BS, Roberston RJ: *Perceived exertion,* Champaign, Ill, 1996, Human Kinetics.

Swearingen PL, Howard CA: *Addison-Wesley photo-atlas of nursing procedures,* ed 3, Redwood City, Calif, 1996, Addison-Wesley.

Wenger NK et al: *Cardiac rehabilitation.* Clinical Practice Guideline no. 17. ACPHR pub. no. 96-0672, Rockville, Md, 1995, U.S. Department of Health and Human Services, Agency for Health Care Policy and Research, and the National Heart, Lung and Blood Institute.

Section Three: Caring for Patients With Cancer and Other Life-disrupting Illnesses

Chemotherapy and immunotherapy

Risk for injury (to staff, patients, and environment) with risks related to preparation, handling, administration, and disposal of chemotherapeutic agents
Desired outcome: Chemotherapy exposure to staff and environment is minimized by proper preparation, handling, administration, and disposal by individuals familiar with these agents.

- Make sure that chemotherapy is prepared by pharmacists or specially trained and supervised personnel and administered by nurses familiar with the agents. Keep institutional guidelines readily available for safe preparation, handling, and potential complications, such as spills or individual contact with these drugs. **Note:** A chemotherapy approval course and guided clinical experience are highly recommended for nurses who will be administering these drugs.
- Ensure that pregnant nurses exercise extreme caution when handling these agents. Check with individual agencies for policies about administration of these drugs by women who are pregnant and/or breast-feeding or by employees, male or female, considering a pregnancy.
- Implement measures to minimize aerosolization and direct contact with these drugs during preparation. These measures include using a biologic safety cabinet (laminar flow hood); an absorbent, plastic-backed, pad placed on the work area; latex gloves (powder free and a minimum of 0.007 inch thick); full-length impervious (nonabsorbent) gown with cuffed sleeves and back closure; and goggles. Gloves and gowns should be worn during all handling and disposing of these agents.
- Prime IV tubing with diluent, not with fluid containing the chemotherapy agent.
- Use syringes and IV administration sets with Luer-Lok fittings.
- When removing the IV administration set, wear latex gloves and wrap sterile gauze around the needle to prevent direct or aerosol contact with the drug. Place all needles (noncrushed, clipped, or recapped), drugs, drug containers, and related material in a puncture-proof container that is clearly marked *Biohazardous Waste.* **Note:** Follow this procedure for disposal of immunotherapy waste as well.
- Wear latex gloves (and impermeable gown and goggles if splashing is possible) when handling all body excretions for 48 hr after chemotherapy because the drug is excreted through urine and feces.
- Specially trained personnel will clean up a chemotherapy spill. Double-gloves, eye protection, and an appropriate, full-length gown will be worn. Absorbent pads are used to absorb liquid; solid waste is picked up with moist absorbent gauze; glass fragments are collected with a small scoop—never with hands. These areas are cleansed three times with a detergent solution. All waste is put in a biohazardous waste container.
- To prevent oral contamination with the drug, avoid any activity in which the hand goes to the mouth (e.g., eating, drinking, smoking) in any area in which the chemical is given or prepared.
- In the event of skin contact with the drug, wash the affected area with soap and water. Notify health care provider for follow-up care.
- If eye contact occurs, irrigate the eye with water for 15 min and notify health care provider for follow-up care.

◎ NIC: Chemotherapy Management; Environmental Management: Worker Safety; Medication Administration; Medication Administration: Parenteral; Risk Identification

Impaired tissue integrity (or risk for same) related to extravasation of vesicant or irritating chemotherapy agents
Desired outcome: Patient's tissue remains intact without evidence of inflammation or pain along the injection site.

Note: The following vesicant agents have the potential to produce tissue damage: dactinomycin, daunomycin, doxorubicin, mitomycin C, epirubicin, estramustine, idarubicin, mechlorethamine, mitoxantrone, paclitaxel, vinblastine, vincristine, vindesine, and vinorelbine. The following irritants have the potential to produce pain along the injection site with or without inflammation: amsacrine, bleomycin, carmustine, dacarbazine, doxorubicin liposome, etoposide, ifosfamide, plicamycin, streptozocin, docetaxel, and teniposide. See Table A-10 for more information.

- Make sure that vesicant chemotherapy is administered by a nurse who is experienced in venipuncture and knowledgeable about chemotherapy.
- Select the IV site carefully, using a new site if possible. Avoid sites such as the antecubital fossa, wrist, or dorsal side of the hand, in which there is an increased risk of damage to underlying tendons or nerves.
- Check patency of the IV line before and during administration of the drug. Instruct patient to report burning or pain immediately.
- When possible, give infusions of vesicant drugs through a central venous catheter to minimize risk of extravasation. Assess the entry site at frequent intervals. Pain, burning, and stinging are common with extravasation, as are erythema and swelling around the needle site. Do not use blood return as an indicator that extravasation has not occurred, because blood return is possible in the presence of extravasation. Instruct patient to report discomfort at the site promptly.
- Keep an extravasation kit readily available, along with institutional guidelines for extravasation management.
- In the event of extravasation, follow these general guidelines:
  —Stop the infusion immediately, and aspirate any remaining drug from the needle. To do this, first apply latex gloves, and then attach the syringe to the tubing and aspirate the drug.
  —Consult the health care provider.
  —Leave the needle in place if an antidote is to be used with the extravasated drug.
  —Attach a syringe containing the recommended antidote, and instill the antidote. Remove the IV needle from the site.
  —If recommended, inject the extravasated site with the antidote, using a tuberculin (TB) syringe and a 25- to 27-gauge needle.
  —Do not apply pressure to the site. Apply a sterile occlusive dressing, elevate the site, and apply heat or cold as recommended.
  —Document the incident, noting the date, time, insertion site of the needle, venous access device type and size, drug, concentration of the drug, approximate amount of drug that extravasated, patient symptoms, management of the extravasation, and appearance of the site. Check institutional guidelines regarding necessity of photo documentation. Monitor the site at frequent intervals.
  —Provide patient with information about site care and follow-up appointments for evaluation of the extravasation. If appropriate, collaborate with health care provider regarding a plastic surgery consultation.

NIC: Heat/Cold Application; Intravenous (IV) Insertion; Intravenous (IV) Therapy; Medication Administration: Parenteral; Venous Access Devices (VAD) Maintenance

Knowledge deficit: Chemotherapy and the purpose, expected side effects, and potential toxicities related to chemotherapy drugs; appropriate self-care measures for minimizing side effects; and available community and educational resources

Desired outcome: Before specific chemotherapeutic drugs are administered, patient and significant other verbalize knowledge about their potential side effects and toxicities, appropriate self-care measures for minimizing the side effects, and available community and educational resources.

- Establish patient's and significant other's current level of knowledge about patient's health status and prescribed therapies.
- Assess patient's and significant other's cognitive and emotional readiness to learn.
- Recognize barriers to learning, such as ineffective communication, inability to read, neurologic deficit, sensory alterations, fear, anxiety, or lack of motivation. In particular, clarify misunderstandings about the side effects and toxicities of chemotherapy. Define all terminology as needed. Correct any misconceptions.
- Assess patient's and significant other's learning needs and establish short-term and long-term goals with these individuals. Identify their preferred methods of learning and the amount of information they would like to receive. Develop a teaching plan based on this information.
- Use individualized verbal and audiovisual strategies to promote learning and enhance understanding. Give simple, direct instructions; reinforce this information frequently.
- Provide an environment that is free from distractions and conducive to teaching and learning.
- Discuss the treatment plan and goals of treatment with patient and significant other.
- Discuss the drugs the patient will receive, including route of administration, duration of treatment, schedule, frequency of laboratory tests, most common side effects and toxicities, follow-up care, and appropriate self-care (see Table A-10). Provide both written and verbal information.
- Provide emergency phone numbers for use if the patient has any questions or develops a fever or other side effects.
- Provide materials from educational resources such as the American Cancer Society, National Cancer Institute, and drug companies. Make sure that materials are at a reading level appropriate for the patient. Explain that the National Cancer Institute has a booklet entitled "Chemotherapy and You" that gives a general overview of chemotherapy, side effect management, and ways for patients to help themselves during chemotherapy.
- Identify appropriate community resources that assist with transportation, costs of care, and skilled care as appropriate.

NIC: Chemotherapy Management; Learning Facilitation; Learning Readiness Enhancement; Teaching: Individual; Teaching: Prescribed Medication

Knowledge deficit: Immunotherapy and its purpose, potential side effects and toxicities, appropriate self-care measures to minimize side effects, and available community and education resources

Desired outcome: Before immunotherapy is administered, patient and significant other verbalize understanding of its purpose, potential side effects and toxicities, appropriate self-care measures to minimize side effects, and available community and education resources.

- See first six interventions under preceding **Knowledge deficit.**
- Discuss treatment plan and goals of treatment with patient and significant other.
- Discuss the drugs the patient will receive, including information about the route of administration, the expected action, duration of treatment, schedule, frequency of laboratory tests, appropriate self-care, follow-up care, and

Text continued on p. 768

TABLE A-10 Common Chemotherapy and Immunotherapy Agents and Colony-Stimulating Factors

Classification (generic/trade name)	Route of administration	Dosage	Acute toxicity	Delayed toxicity	Special precautions
Chemotherapy *Alkylating agents* Carboplatin/ Paraplatin	IV	360-400 mg/m²/day; repeat q28days 100 mg/m²/day × 3; repeat q28days	Nausea and vomiting Anorexia Allergic reaction	Hair loss (rare) Taste alterations Mild, reversible increase in liver enzymes Electrolyte abnormalities (Ca^{++}, Mg^{++}, Na^+, K^+) Myelosuppression Thrombocytopenia Neutropenia	Contraindicated in patients with cisplatin allergy Have epinephrine, corticosteroids, and antihistamine available Check liver function tests before treatment Check electrolyte, BUN, and creatinine levels before each cycle; maintain oral intake Creatinine clearance done initially; reduced dosage indicated if creatinine clearance <60 ml/min Myelosuppression is a dose-limiting side effect Avoid aluminum needle since it reacts with the drug to form a precipitate Drug stable at room temperature for 24 hr

| Carmustine/ BCNU | IV | 40 mg/m^2 for 5 days; 150–200 mg/m^2 in single dose | Nausea and vomiting; Flushing of skin if infused too rapidly; Pain at injection site | Hepatic toxicity; Delayed bone marrow depression; Skin hyperpigmentation; Pulmonary fibrosis; Renal damage; *Rare:* dizziness, stomatitis, alopecia | Premedicate with antiemetics; Report symptoms of pulmonary fibrosis (see p. 43) promptly; Do not exceed cumulative dose of 1400 mg/m^2; Monitor liver function tests, BUN, creatinine, CBC, and platelets before each treatment; Monitor creatinine clearance, BUN, serum creatinine, Mg^{++}, Ca^{++}, and K$^+$ before each treatment |

Continued

Note: This table is not meant to be comprehensive but rather to provide a quick reference for the most common drugs in clinical practice, including the route of administration, dose, side effects, and precautions. Because the drug dose and schedule of administration vary with each protocol, check individual protocols for additional information and guidelines.

IV, Intravenous; *Ca^{++},* calcium; *Mg^{++},* magnesium; *Na$^+$,* sodium; *K$^+$,* potassium; *BUN,* blood urea nitrogen; *CBC,* complete blood count; *PO,* by mouth; *I&O,* intake and output; *SIADH,* syndrome of inappropriate antidiuretic hormone; *IM,* intramuscular; *SQ,* subcutaneous; *CNS,* central nervous system; *NaCl,* sodium chloride; *BP,* blood pressure; *PVC,* polyvinyl chloride; *VS,* vital signs; *ASA,* acetylsalicylic acid; *NSAIDs,* nonsteroidal antiinflammatory drugs; *LDH,* lactic dehydrogenase; *SGOT,* serum glutamicoxaloacetic transaminase; *SGPT,* serum glutamic-pyruvic transaminase; *ANC,* absolute neutrophil count.

*Irritant drug: an agent that produces pain along the injection site with or without an inflammatory reaction.

†Given along with certain chemotherapy agents to minimize toxicity.

‡Vesicant drug: an agent capable of producing tissue damage.

TABLE A-10 Common Chemotherapy and Immunotherapy Agents and Colony-Stimulating Factors—cont'd

Classification (generic/trade name)	Route of administration	Dosage	Acute toxicity	Delayed toxicity	Special precautions
Chemotherapy—cont'd					
Alkylating agents—cont'd					
Cisplatin/Platinol	IV; intraarterial; intraperitoneal	20 mg/m² for 5 days; 120 mg/m² in single dose	Severe nausea and vomiting Anaphylaxis (uncommon)	Nephrotoxicity, neurotoxicity, ototoxicity Bone marrow depression Electrolyte imbalances	Maintain adequate hydration before, during, and after treatments Maintain urine output at 100 ml/hr before administration and for at least 4 hr after; keep fluid intake > output Premedicate with antiemetics before treatment Keep the following emergency drugs readily available: epinephrine, hydrocortisone, antihistamines This drug precipitates; do not use aluminum needles
Dacarbazine/ DTIC*	IV	50-250 mg/m² for 5 days; 375 mg/m² in single dose	Severe nausea and vomiting Pain at injection site Possible tissue damage with extravasation	Bone marrow depression Flu-like symptoms Elevated liver enzymes Facial flushing, facial paresthesia *Rare:* alopecia, anaphylaxis	Stable for 8 hr at room temperature Premedicate with antiemetics Check CBC, platelets, and liver function enzymes before treatment Keep emergency drugs readily available In the event of extravasation, apply ice for 24 hr

Drug	Route	Dose		Toxicity	Nursing considerations
Cyclophosphamide/ Cytoxan	PO; IV; intraarterial	50-200 mg/m² PO daily; 500-1500 mg/m² IV q3-4wk	Nausea and vomiting Nasal congestion, headache with high doses that are infused rapidly	Bone marrow depression Alopecia Hemorrhagic cystitis Amenorrhea and sterility Stomatitis Potentiation of doxorubicin Cardiotoxicity Interstitial pulmonary fibrosis Liver dysfunction SIADH with high doses Development of secondary cancer	Fluid intake should be at least 2-3 L/day after treatment Voiding should be frequent to avoid bladder irritation Administer early in day to minimize risk of bladder irritation from not voiding at night High doses (>1.5 g) may require IV hydration Maintain I&O for 48 hr after treatment Test urine for blood Initiate oral care/saline rinses qid Monitor CBC, liver function tests, BUN, and creatinine before and after treatment
Ifosfamide/Ifex	IV	1.2 g/m²/day for 5 consecutive days	Nausea and vomiting	Bone marrow depression Alopecia Hematuria/hemorrhagic cystitis Confusion, lethargy *Rare:* renal impairment, liver dysfunction	Hydrate with at least 2-3 L/day Administer mesna before treatment and 4 and 8 hr after (or as continuous infusion) to minimize hemorrhagic cystitis Test urine for blood

Continued

TABLE A-10 Common Chemotherapy and Immunotherapy Agents and Colony-Stimulating Factors—cont'd

Classification (generic/trade name)	Route of administration	Dosage	Acute toxicity	Delayed toxicity	Special precautions
Chemotherapy—cont'd					
Alkylating agents—cont'd					
Mesna/Mesnex†	IV PO	20% of ifosfamide dose given just before and 4 and 8 hr after ifosfamide (total mesna dose = 60% of ifosfamide dose)	Bad taste in mouth Nausea and vomiting	Diarrhea Rash Long-term administration: possible pulmonary dysfunction	Give 15 min before ifosfamide, then again after 4 and 8 hr May cause false-positive test for urinary ketones Lifetime dose: 1400 mg/m^2
Lomustine/CCNU	PO	100-130 mg/m^2 q6wk	Nausea and vomiting Anorexia	Anorexia Bone marrow depression *Rare:* hepatic toxicity, stomatitis, alopecia	Give before bed and on an empty stomach to minimize nausea and vomiting Monitor CBC, platelets, and liver function tests
Mechlorethamine/ nitrogen mustard‡	IV Intracavitary Topical	1.6 mg/m^2 q3-4wk 0.8 mg/m^2 10 mg dissolved in 50 ml sterile water	Severe nausea and vomiting Burning sensation around injection site; tissue damage with extravasation Chills, fever, and diarrhea may occur immediately after drug administration	Bone marrow depression Amenorrhea Skin rash Secondary cancers	Premedicate with antiemetics before administration Never give IM or SQ because severe tissue necrosis would occur Extravasation management (antidote for vesicant): Mix 4 ml 10% sodium thiosulfate with 6 ml sterile water for injection

Drug	Route	Dose	Side effects	Nursing considerations
Antibiotics				
Bleomycin/ Blenoxane	IV; IM; SQ Intraarterial, bladder instillation, intracavitary, intrapleural	10-20 mg/m²/wk or q2wk 60 U/m²	Mild nausea and vomiting Anaphylaxis Fever and chills Skin reactions, including rash, dermatitis, hyperpigmentation Stomatitis Alopecia Pulmonary fibrosis	Inject 5-6 ml IV through existing IV line and then SQ with multiple injections Repeat dosing over next several hr Apply cold compresses Mix immediately before use; use within 1 hr Administer test dose of 1-2 U before treatment Premedicate with acetaminophen and diphenhydramine Pulmonary toxicity is dose related; suggested total cumulative dose is 400 U Monitor pulmonary function tests before treatment and after every 100 U Initiate oral care/saline rinses qid
Doxorubicin/ Adriamycin‡	IV	15 mg/m²/wk; 20-30 mg/m² for 3 days; 50-75 mg/m² q3wk	Moderate nausea and vomiting Tissue damage if extravasation occurs Local erythematous streaking with rapid infusion ("adria flare") Red urine Alopecia Bone marrow depression Stomatitis Cardiomyopathy Potentiates radiation-induced skin damage	Cardiac toxicity is dose related; suggested total cumulative dose is 550 mg/m² Modify dose during radiation to minimize skin reaction Initiate oral care/saline rinses qid Extravasation management: apply ice

Continued

TABLE A-10 Common Chemotherapy and Immunotherapy Agents and Colony-Stimulating Factors—cont'd

Chemotherapy—cont'd
Antibiotics—cont'd

Classification (generic/trade name)	Route of administration	Dosage	Acute toxicity	Delayed toxicity	Special precautions
Mitomycin C‡	IV	10-20 mg/m^2; repeated once in 6-8 wk	Moderate nausea and vomiting Extravasation causes tissue damage	Bone marrow depression Mouth ulcers Hemolytic-uremic syndrome Pulmonary fibrosis	Extravasation management; apply ice Initiate oral care/saline rinses qid Report symptoms of pulmonary fibrosis (see p. 43)
Dexrazoxane/ Zinecard† (protective agent for doxorubicin-induced cardiotoxicity)	IV	Dosage ratio of Zinecard/ doxorubicin is 10:1	Nausea and vomiting Anorexia	Alopecia Stomatitis Fever	May add to myelosuppression caused by other chemotherapy drugs Doxorubicin should be given at the completion of the Zinecard infusion and within 30 min of the beginning of Zinecard infusion
Antimetabolites					
5-Fluorouracil/ 5-FU	IV	1000 mg/m^2 over 24 hr for 4-5 days 300 mg/m^2/day indefinitely 300-450 mg/m^2 for 5 days; 300-750 mg/m^2 qwk	Mild nausea and vomiting	Bone marrow depression Stomatitis Diarrhea Photosensitivity Hyperpigmentation Excessive lacrimation Nail changes	Initiate oral care/saline rinses qid Instruct patient in use of sunscreen to protect skin Instruct patient on interventions if stomatitis or diarrhea occurs

	Intraarterial	20-30 mg/kg/day for 4 days, followed by 15 mg/kg for 17 days	Hand-foot syndrome (paresthesia, erythema, and swelling of palms and soles of feet)	
Methotrexate/ Amethopterin	PO, IV, IM	50 mg/m² qwk; 20-40 mg/m² qwk or q2wk (solid tumors); 200-500 mg/m² q2-4wk (leukemias and lymphomas)	Nausea and vomiting; Bone marrow depression; Stomatitis; Diarrhea; Photosensitivity; Infertility; CNS reaction with intrathecal administration; *Rare:* hepatic, renal toxicity	Do not administer to patients with BUN >25; Use with caution in patients with third-spacing of fluids because elimination will be decreased, thereby enhancing toxicity; Administer high-dosage (>80 mg/m²) with leucovorin to minimize toxicity; Ensure adequate hydration before, during, and after high-dose administration; Ensure alkaline urine (pH >7) to promote excretion; Teach use of sunscreen during sun exposure; Check serum BUN, creatinine, CBC, platelets, and liver function tests before and after administration
	Intrathecal	6-15 mg as a single dose or repeated weekly or 2 times/wk		

Continued

TABLE A-10 Common Chemotherapy and Immunotherapy Agents and Colony-Stimulating Factors—cont'd

Chemotherapy—cont'd
Antimetabolites—cont'd

Classification (generic/trade name)	Route of administration	Dosage	Acute toxicity	Delayed toxicity	Special precautions
Fludarabine/ Fludara	IV	25 mg/m²/day × 5; repeat q4wk	Mild nausea and vomiting	Bone marrow depression Constipation, abdominal cramping Skin rashes Edema Fever CNS toxicities	Mild, transient elevated ALT (SGOT) May cause tumor lysis syndrome in patients with large tumor burden Pulmonary reactions (e.g., cough, dyspnea, interstitial pulmonary infiltrates)
Leucovorin/ Wellcovorin (given with high-dose methotrexate)†	PO, IM, IV	Dose calculated based on methotrexate dose, methotrexate serum levels, and serum creatinine			Dose usually begins 24 hr after infusion of methotrexate Stress importance of taking all doses as prescribed; give written instructions about dose and schedule Provide emergency number in case patient is unable to take doses
Cytarabine/cytosine arabinoside/ara-C	IV Intrathecal SQ	100-200 mg/m²; high dose = 1.5-4.5 g/m² 1 mg/kg q12h for 5-7 days 10-30 mg/m² up to 3 times wk	Mild to moderate nausea and vomiting	Bone marrow depression Stomatitis, esophagitis Diarrhea Hepatotoxicity Rash Ocular toxicity	Initiate oral care/saline rinses qid SQ injection may cause pain at injection site; apply warm compresses Administer high doses over 1 hr to minimize neurologic toxicity

	Route	Dosage	Side effects/Toxicity	Nursing implications
		100 mg/m² IV or SQ twice daily for 5 days q28days; 10 mg/m² SQ q12hr for 15-21 days	Neurotoxicity with high doses Flu-like symptoms Metallic taste Bone pain Gastrointestinal ulceration	Perform neurologic examination before high-dose administration and report signs of cerebellar dysfunction Steroid eye drops usually given with high doses to minimize ocular toxicity
Plant alkaloids Vinblastine/Velban‡	IV	5-10 mg/m²/wk or q2wk	Nausea and vomiting Tissue damage with extravasation Bone marrow depression Alopecia Neurotoxicity (peripheral neuropathy) Constipation Infertility Stomatitis	Assess for neurotoxicity before administration Initiate prophylactic bowel regimen to minimize constipation Extravasation management: Mix 1 ml NaCl with 150 U hyaluronidase Inject 1-6 ml (150-900 U) SQ into extravasated site with multiple injections Repeat dose SQ over next several hr
Vincristine/Oncovin‡	IV	0.5-2.0 mg/m²/wk or q2wk	Neurotoxicity (peripheral neuropathy) Tissue damage with extravasation Constipation	Do not exceed 2.5 mg/dose Assess for neurotoxicity before administration

Continued

TABLE A-10 Common Chemotherapy and Immunotherapy Agents and Colony-Stimulating Factors—cont'd

Classification (generic/trade name)	Route of administration	Dosage	Acute toxicity	Delayed toxicity	Special precautions
Chemotherapy—cont'd					
Plant alkaloids—cont'd					
Vinorelbine/ Navelbine‡	IV PO	30 mg/m²/wk 50-80 mg/m²/wk	Nausea and vomiting	Bone marrow depression Peripheral neuropathy Mild alopecia Constipation Dyspnea Cystitis Elevated liver enzymes SIADH Chest pain	Evaluate neurologic status routinely Monitor liver enzymes Initiate prophylactic bowel regimen Administer properly diluted dose in 6-10 min to decrease irritation to vein; then adequately flush vein after administration
Etoposide (VP-16)*	IV PO	50-150 mg/m² for 3-5 days, repeated q3-4wk Twice the IV dose rounded to the nearest 50 mg	Hypotension with rapid infusion Mild nausea and vomiting	Jaw pain Alopecia Bone marrow depression Stomatitis Hypotension Peripheral neuropathy *Rare:* anaphylaxis	Maximum concentration is 0.4 mg/ml to prevent precipitation Initiate prophylactic bowel regimen to minimize constipation Extravasation management: see vinblastine, p. 759 Administer over 1-hr period to minimize hypotension Monitor BP q15min during infusion Extravasation management: see vinblastine, p. 759

Topoisomerase I inhibitors			
Topotecan/ Hycamptin	IV	1.3-2 mg/m²/day × 5 days	Nausea and vomiting	Bone marrow suppression Diarrhea Alopecia Rash Headache Dizziness, lightheadedness Peripheral neuropathy Fever	Monitor alkaline phosphatase, ALT (SGOT), and bilirubin levels
CPTII/irinotecan, Camptosar	IV	Several regimens have been evaluated 125 mg/m²/wk × 4 followed by 2-wk rest	Nausea and vomiting Diarrhea Flushing	Bone marrow suppression Mucositis Alopecia Diaphoresis Abdominal pain Diarrhea	Collaborate with physician on use of atropine for early-onset diaphoresis, abdominal cramping, diarrhea Educate patient on extreme importance of diarrhea management Instruct on specific management schedule Educate patient on importance of adequate hydration

Continued

TABLE A-10 Common Chemotherapy and Immunotherapy Agents and Colony-Stimulating Factors—cont'd

Classification (generic/trade name)	Route of administration	Dosage	Acute toxicity	Delayed toxicity	Special precautions
Chemotherapy—cont'd					
Antimicrotubule agents/taxanes					
Paclitaxel/Taxol	IV	Various doses 135-250 mg/m² over 3 hr q3wk	Acute hypersensitivity reaction	Bone marrow depression	Have emergency medications on hand (e.g., antihistamines, epinephrine, corticosteroids, bronchodilators)
			Nausea and vomiting	Alopecia	Premedicate with dexamethasone, diphenhydramine (Benadryl), and famotidine (Pepcid), cimetidine, or ranitidine
	Intraperitoneal	Maximum 175 mg/m²	Vesicant potential	Mucositis	Do not use PVC bags and infusion sets because of leaching of toxic plasticizer DEHP (diethylhexyl phthalate)
				Abdominal pain	
				Extremity pain	
				Peripheral neuropathy	
				Myalgias and arthralgias	Glass bottles and plastic bags (polypropylene, polyolefin) and nitroglycerin infusion sets/ polyethylene-lined administration sets must be used
				Rash	
				Hypotension	
				Bradycardia	Dilute to concentration of 0.3-1.2 mg/ml
				Cardiac dysrhythmias	
				Elevated renal and hepatic function test values	Monitor VS including BP closely during infusion, especially in first hr

Taxotere/Docetaxel	IV	60-100 mg/m² over at least 1 hr q3wk	Hypersensitivity reaction Nausea and vomiting Irritant potential Bone marrow depression Alopecia Mucositis Diarrhea Rash Potential severe edema Paresthesia Asthenia Nail changes Myalgias Localized erythema with edema followed by desquamation has been observed (most often in extremities)	Administer oral corticosteroids as prescribed for 5 days starting day 1 before taxotere to reduce severity of fluid retention and hypersensitivity reaction Have emergency medications on hand Glass bottles and plastic bags (polypropylene, polyolefin) and nitroglycerin infusion sets/polyethylene-lined administration sets must be used
Miscellaneous agents Hydroxyurea/ Hydrea	PO	60-75 mg/m²/day	Nausea and vomiting Bone marrow depression Renal insufficiency	Ensure adequate hydration (at least 2 L/day)

Continued

TABLE A-10 Common Chemotherapy and Immunotherapy Agents and Colony-Stimulating Factors—cont'd

Classification (generic/trade name)	Route of administration	Dosage	Acute toxicity	Delayed toxicity	Special precautions
Chemotherapy—cont'd *Miscellaneous agents—cont'd*					
L-Asparaginase/ Elspar	IV, IM, SQ	200-1000 IU/kg/day or 2 times/wk	Anaphylaxis Nausea and vomiting	Hepatotoxicity Fever, malaise CNS toxicity Renal dysfunction	Have emergency drugs readily available before administration Skin test recommended before initial dose and when there are 7 days or more between treatments Physician should be available in case of anaphylaxis; drug should be administered during the day in hospital setting Record baseline VS; record VS 15 min into infusion and following infusion
Procarbazine/ Matulane	PO	100-200 mg/m²/ day × 14 days q14wk	Nausea and vomiting	Bone marrow depression CNS depression Peripheral neuropathy Amenorrhea Dermatologic reactions Hypotension, tachycardia Syncope	Avoid foods with high tyramine content (bananas, fava beans, aged cheeses, yogurt, beer, Chianti wine, chocolate, coffee, cola, yeast)

Gemcitabine hydrochloride/ Gemzar	IV	1000 mg/m²/wk up to 7 wk followed by 1-wk rest; subsequent dosage q3wk followed by 1 wk respite	Nausea and vomiting Flu-like symptoms (e.g., fever, headache, chills, myalgia, asthenia) Bone marrow depression Diarrhea Stomatitis Transient elevations of serum transaminases Mild proteinuria/ hematuria Rash Pruritus Dyspnea Edema Mild alopecia	Do not administer over more than 60 min Determine results of CBC with differential before each dose
Immunotherapy *Biologic response modifiers* Interferon/Intron	IM IV SQ, intra-lesional	2-3 × 10⁶ U 3 times/wk 30 × 10⁶ U/day	Flu-like symptoms (fever, chills, fatigue, malaise, lessen with continued treatment) Anorexia Bone marrow depression CNS toxicity Skin rash/injection site reactions *Rare:* nausea and vomiting, hypotension	Avoid ASA and NSAIDs Premedicate with acetaminophen; administer q4hr Anorexia may be dose related: arrange for nutritional consultation Refrigerate

Continued

TABLE A-10 Common Chemotherapy and Immunotherapy Agents and Colony-Stimulating Factors—cont'd

Classification (generic/trade name)	Route of administration	Dosage	Acute toxicity	Delayed toxicity	Special precautions
Colony-stimulating factors					
Granulocyte colony-stimulating factor					
G-CSF/filgrastim	SQ, IV	5 μg/kg/day	Bone pain (sternum or lower back) Erythema, burning at injection site	Exacerbations of preexisting inflammatory conditions Transient increase in uric acid, LDH, alkaline phosphatase Mild headache	Initiate 24 hr after completion of chemotherapy; stop 24 hr before administration of chemotherapy Bone pain usually controlled with acetaminophen or ibuprofen; if lasts >24 hr, further investigation needed for cause of pain Solution must be refrigerated, but use at room temperature to minimize erythema and burning at site Patient should take drug at about same time every day Monitor CBC 2-3 times/wk; stop if ANC >10,000/mm^3 after the expected chemotherapy-induced nadir

Granulocyte-macrophage colony-stimulating factor

GM-CSF/ sargramostim	IV infusion × 2-4 hrs SQ	250 mg/m^2	Hypersensitivity reactions Mild flu-like symptoms: fever, myalgia, fatigue, anorexia, chills, rigors Erythema or phlebitis at injection site Bone pain	Generalized rash Headache Abnormal taste Increased LDH, alkaline phosphatase, ALT (SGOT), AST (SGPT)	Monitor CBC 2-3 times/wk; stop if ANC >20,000/mm^3 Initiate 24 hr after completion of chemotherapy
Erythropoietin/ epogen/Procrit	SQ	50-300 U/kg 3 times/wk	Rare nausea and vomiting	Flu-like symptoms Arthralgias/myalgias Headache Hypertension Rash Edema	Monitor CBC for response

potential side effects. Because these patients often give their own injections of interferon, instruct them in the proper technique and site rotation schedule. Teach patient to record the site of injection, time of administration, side effects, self-management of side effects, and any medications taken. Teach proper disposal of needles.

- Instruct on proper handling and storage of medication (e.g., refrigeration). If necessary, arrange for pharmacy delivery of medication because of the need for refrigeration. As appropriate, arrange for community nursing follow-up for additional supervision and instruction.
- Teach patient and significant other to be alert to the following side effects of interferon: fever, chills, and flu-like symptoms. Suggest that patient take acetaminophen, with health care provider's approval, to manage these symptoms, but avoid aspirin and NSAIDs because they may interrupt the action of interferon.
- Teach patient to monitor and record temperature 2 times/day and drink extra fluids. Anorexia and weight loss, which are dose related, are other common side effects of interferon. Provide information about nutritional supplementation.
- Provide both verbal and written information and educational materials.

NIC: Chemotherapy Management; Learning Facilitation; Learning Readiness Enhancement; Teaching: Individual; Teaching: Prescribed Medication; Teaching: Psychomotor Skill

Venous access devices

Knowledge deficit: Purpose, type, and management of venous access device (VAD)

Desired outcome: Within the 24-hr period before hospital discharge, patient and significant other verbalize understanding about the VAD, including its purpose, appropriate management measures, and potential complications.

> Note: Three types of VADs are generally used: tunneled catheters, nontunneled catheters, and implanted ports.

- Determine patient's and significant other's level of understanding of the purpose of a VAD. As appropriate, explain that the device can be used for administration of drugs, fluids, and blood products and drawing of blood samples and that it eliminates the need for frequent venipunctures.
- Show patient a model of the device, and explain the insertion procedure. Nontunneled catheters can be inserted at the bedside or in the clinic with the patient under local anesthesia. Tunneled central venous catheters and implanted ports are inserted in the operating room with the patient under local anesthesia. There may be mild discomfort, similar to a toothache, for 48 hr after the procedure. Reassure patient that the discomfort responds readily to mild pain medication.
- If possible, introduce patient and significant other to another individual who has the device so that they can see firsthand what the VAD looks like and discuss their concerns.
- Teach patient about VAD maintenance care. Provide both verbal and written instructions, including educational materials provided by the VAD manufacturer. Have patient or significant other demonstrate dressing care, flushing technique, and cap-changing routine before hospital discharge. Make sure patient has 24-hr emergency number to call in case of problems.
    —*Nontunneled catheters:* inserted by venipuncture into the vessel of choice, usually the basilic, cephalic, or medial cubital vein near or at the

antecubital area or the jugular or subclavian vein in the upper thorax. A peripherally inserted central catheter (PICC) is an example of a nontunneled catheter. Maintenance involves flushing daily and after use with normal saline and heparinized solution and sterile dressing and cap changes. Refer to institutional policies for specific instructions.

—*Tunneled central venous catheters:* inserted into a central vein with a portion of the catheter tunneled through subcutaneous tissue and exiting the body at a convenient area, usually the chest. A Dacron cuff encircles the catheter about 2 inches from the exiting end of the catheter. Tissue grows into this cuff, helping to prevent catheter dislodgment and decreasing the risk that microorganisms can migrate along the surface of the catheter and enter the bloodstream. Single-lumen or multi-lumen catheters can be used. Examples of tunneled central venous catheters include Broviac, Hickman, and Groshong. Maintenance involves daily flushing or after each use with saline or heparinized saline solution (Groshong catheters are flushed weekly or after use with plain saline; no heparinized solution is used); sterile dressing changes until the insertion site is healed; and sterile cap changes. Refer to institutional policies for specific instructions.

—*Implanted venous access ports:* consist of a catheter inserted into a central or peripheral vein attached to a plastic or metal port sutured in place in a surgically created subcutaneous pocket, most commonly on the chest. Venous access ports are completely embedded under the skin. They may have single or multiple access ports. Access to the port may be from the top or side, depending on the type. Noncoring needles **must** be used to access the port to allow the system to reseal when the needle is removed. There are many types of implanted venous access ports, such as Port-a-cath and P.A.S. Port. Maintenance involves preparation of the site for access with an antibacterial preparation solution (e.g., povidone-iodine solution) and flushing at least monthly or after each use with normal saline and heparinized solution. Refer to institutional policies for specific instructions.

- Discuss potential complications associated with VADs, along with appropriate self-management measures.
    - —*Infection:* teach patient to assess exit site for erythema, swelling, local increased temperature, discomfort, purulent drainage, and fever >38° C (>100.4° F).
    - —*Bleeding:* teach patient to apply pressure to the site. Instruct patient to notify health team member if bleeding does not stop in 5 min.
    - —*Clot in the catheter:* teach patient to flush the catheter without using excessive pressure, which could damage or dislodge the catheter (particularly an implanted port). If flushing does not dislodge the clot, instruct patient to notify health team member. **Note:** It is not unusual for small blood clots or fibrin sheaths to develop on the end of the catheter. The most common manifestation of a fibrin sheath is the ability to infuse fluids with the inability to aspirate blood. Both fibrin sheaths and small blood clots respond readily to urokinase therapy. The usual dose of urokinase is 5,000-10,000 U. The suggested dwell time in the catheter is ≥30-60 min.
    - —*Disconnected cap:* instruct patients to tape all connections and to carry hemostats or alligator clamps with them at all times. Instruct patient and significant other on measures to take if the cap becomes disconnected (i.e., clamp the tubing and go to a local health care institution for cleansing of the catheter).
    - —*Extravasation:* although this is a relatively rare complication, it can cause severe damage if a sclerosing agent such as adriamycin is involved. Therefore it is important to instruct patients to report pain, burning, and

stinging in the chest, clavicle, or port pocket or along the subcutaneous tunnel during drug administration.

NIC: Learning Readiness Enhancement; Peripherally Inserted Central (PIC) Catheter Care; Teaching: Prescribed Procedure/Treatment; Teaching: Psychomotor Skill; Venous Access Devices (VAD) Maintenance

Radiation therapy

Risk for injury (to staff, other patients, and visitors) related to risk of exposure to sealed sources of radiation, such as cesium-137 (^{137}Cs), gold-198 (^{198}Au), iridium-192 (^{192}Ir), iodine-125 (^{125}I), radium-226 (^{226}Ra), or strontium-90 (^{90}Sr); or unsealed sources of radiation, such as iodine-131 (^{131}I), phosphorus-32 (^{32}P), or strontium-90 (^{90}Sr)

Desired outcome: Staff and visitors verbalize understanding about the potential dangers of radiation therapy and the measures that must be taken to ensure safety.

> **Note:** Most institutions have a radiation safety committee that assists in providing and enforcing guidelines that minimize radiation risks to employees and the environment (committee guidelines should be kept readily available). The committee approves certain rooms that can be used for patients undergoing radioactive treatment to minimize exposure to employees and other patients.

- Assign the patient a private room (with private bathroom), and place an appropriate radiation precaution sign on patient's chart, door, and ID bracelet.
- Follow radiologist or agency protocol for visitor restrictions. Visitors usually are restricted to 1 hr/day and should stand 6 ft from the bed.
- Ensure that pregnant women and children younger than 18 yr do not enter the room.
- To ensure optimal care planning, recognize the type and amount of the radiation source. The two major principles are time and distance:
  —*Time:* plan care to minimize the amount of time spent in the patient's room. Staff members should not spend more than 30 min/shift with patient and should not care for more than two patients with implants at the same time. Staff should perform nondirect care activities in the hall (e.g., opening food containers, preparing food tray, opening medications). Linen should be changed only when it is soiled, rather than routinely, and complete bed baths should be avoided.
  —*Distance:* maximize distance from the implant (e.g., if the implant is in the patient's prostate, stand at the head of bed [HOB]).
- Wear gloves when in contact with secretions and excretions of all patients treated with unsealed radiation sources, which are radioactive. Flush toilet several times after depositing urine or feces from commode.

> **Note:** Urine from individuals with sealed radiation is *not* radioactive and can be discarded in the usual manner. However, patients with implanted ^{125}I seeds should save all urine so that it can be assessed for the presence of seeds.

- Save all linen, dressings, and trash from patients with sealed sources of radiation. They will be analyzed by the safety committee representative before discarding to ensure that seeds have not been misplaced.
- Keep long, disposable forceps and a sealed box in the room at all times in case displaced seeds are found. Caution all staff members to use forceps but never the hands to pick up the seeds.

- Use disposable products for all patients with unsealed radiation. These patients will be radioactive for several days. Cover all articles in the room with paper to prevent their contamination.
- Attach a radiation badge (dosimeter) to your clothing before entering the room to monitor the amount of radiation exposure. According to federal regulations, radiation should not exceed 400 mrem/month. Nurses who care for patients with radiation implants rarely receive this much exposure.

NIC: Environmental Management: Worker Safety; Radiation Therapy Management; Risk Identification; Surveillance: Safety

Knowledge deficit: Type of, procedure for, and purpose of radiation implant (internal radiation) and the measures for preventing and managing complications
Desired outcome: Before radiation implant is inserted, patient and significant other verbalize understanding of its type and of the implant procedure and identify measures for preventing and managing complications.
- Determine patient's and significant other's level of understanding of the radiation implant. Explain the following, as indicated:
  —*Afterloading:* the implant carrier is inserted in the operating room, and the radioactive source is inserted later.
  —*Preloading:* radioactive source is implanted with the carrier.
- Explain that the implant is used to provide high doses of radiation therapy to one area, thereby sparing normal tissue.
- Explain that radiation precautions (see **Risk for injury** earlier) are required to protect health care team, other patients, and visitors.
- Explain the following assessment guidelines and management interventions for specific types of implants.

Gynecologic implants
- Explain that the following can occur: vaginal drainage, bleeding, or tenderness; impaired bowel or urinary elimination; and phlebitis. Instruct patient to report any of these, or associated signs and symptoms.
- Explain that complete bedrest is required to prevent displacement of the implants. The HOB may be elevated to 30-45 degrees, and the patient can log roll from side to side. A urinary catheter is placed to facilitate urinary elimination. Generally a bowel clean-out (oral cathartics and/or enemas until clear) is prescribed. A low-residue diet and medications to prevent bowel elimination may be prescribed to prevent bowel movements during the implant period.
- Teach patient to perform isometric exercises while on bedrest to minimize the risk of contractures or muscle atrophy.
- Encourage patient to take analgesics routinely for pain or to request analgesic before pain becomes severe.
- Explain the importance and rationale for wearing antiembolism hose and performing calf-pumping and ankle-circling exercises while on bedrest. If prescribed, describe the rationale for and use of sequential compression devices or pneumatic foot pumps to prevent lower extremity venostasis.
- Explain that ambulation will be increased gradually when bedrest no longer is required (see "Caring for Patients on Prolonged Bedrest," p. 738, for guidelines after prolonged immobility).
- Explain that after the radiation source has been removed, patient should dilate the vagina via either sexual intercourse or a vaginal dilator to prevent fibrosis or stenosis.

Head and neck implants
- After a complete nutritional assessment and assessment of the oropharyngeal area, discuss measures for nutritional support during the implantation,

such as a soft or liquid diet, a high-protein diet, and optimal hydration (>2500 ml/day).
- Teach the signs and symptoms of infection: fever, pain, swelling, local increased warmth, erythema, and purulent drainage at the site of implantation.
- When appropriate, instruct the patient on the need for careful and thorough oral hygiene while the implant is in place. **Note:** When implants are placed within the tongue, palate, or other structures of the buccal cavity, the patient should not perform oral hygiene; oral hygiene will be specifically prescribed by the health care provider and generally accomplished by the nurse.
- Encourage patient to take analgesics routinely for pain or to request analgesic before pain becomes severe.
- Use a humidifier to aid in maintaining moist mucous membranes.
- Identify alternative means for communication if patient's speech deteriorates (e.g., cards, Magic Slate, pencil and paper, picture boards). Consult speech therapist as appropriate.

Breast implants
- Teach the signs of infection that may appear in the breast: pain, fever, swelling, erythema, warmth, and drainage at the insertion site.
- Teach the importance of avoiding trauma at the implant site and keeping the skin clean and dry to help maintain skin integrity.
- Encourage patient to take analgesics routinely for pain or to request analgesic before pain becomes severe.

Prostate implants
- Explain the need for the patient to use a urinal for voiding so that urinary output can be measured every shift and to allow a staff member to inspect urine for the presence of radiation seeds.
- Instruct the patient or significant other to report dysuria, decreasing caliber of stream, difficulty urinating, voiding small amounts, feelings of bladder fullness, or hematuria.
- Caution that patient's linen, dressings, and trash will be saved and examined for the presence of seeds.
- Encourage patient to take analgesics routinely for pain or to request analgesic before pain becomes severe.
- Explain that caregivers will limit the amount of time spent close to the implant site.

NIC: Environmental Management: Worker Safety; Learning Facilitation; Learning Readiness Enhancement; Radiation Therapy Management; Teaching: Procedure/Treatment implant site.

Knowledge deficit: Purpose and procedure for external beam radiation therapy, appropriate self-care measures after treatment, and available educational and community resources
Desired outcome: Before external radiation beam therapy is initiated, patient and significant other identify its purpose and describe the procedure, appropriate self-care measures, and available educational and community resources.
- See first six interventions under **Knowledge deficit:** Chemotherapy, p. 749.
- Provide information about treatment schedule, duration of each treatment, and number of treatments planned.
  —Radiation therapy usually is given 5 days/wk, Monday through Friday.
  —The treatment itself lasts only a few minutes; the majority of the time is spent preparing patient for treatment. Immobilization devices and shields are positioned before treatment to ensure proper delivery of radiation and minimize radiation to surrounding normal tissue.

- Explain that the skin will be marked to facilitate delivery of radiation to the desired area. Usually small skin tatoos (small pinpoint marks) are used. These tatoos are permanent and are used to ensure precise delivery of the radiation. However, if gentian violet is used, explain the importance of not washing the marks (see **Impaired skin/tissue integrity,** p. 787, for more information). Caution patient that it is important not to use skin lotions or soaps unless approved by the radiation therapy provider.
- Discuss side effects that may occur with radiation treatment and the appropriate self-care measures. Systemic side effects include fatigue and anorexia; however, the most commonly occurring side effects appear locally (e.g., side effects associated with head and neck radiation include mucositis, xerostomia, altered taste sensation, dental caries, sore throat, hoarseness, dysphagia, headache, and nausea and vomiting). See subsequent nursing diagnoses and interventions for more detail about local side effects.
- Provide patient with a written copy of the side effects for his or her site of radiation therapy. Explain that the National Cancer Institute has a booklet entitled "Radiation and You" that lists side effects and side effect management.
- Provide information about community resources for transportation to and from the radiation center and for skilled nursing care, as needed.

NIC: Learning Facilitation; Learning Readiness Enhancement; Teaching: Disease Process; Teaching: Individual; Teaching: Procedure/Treatment

General care of patients with cancer

Activity intolerance related to decreased oxygen-carrying capacity of the blood secondary to anemia occurring with some chemotherapeutic drugs, radiation therapy, or chronic disease

> Note: For desired outcome and interventions, see this nursing diagnosis in "Lymphoma," p. 543. Review the anemia disorders (p. 514) discussed in "Hematologic Disorders." Advise patient that fatigue and activity intolerance are temporary side effects of chemotherapy or radiation therapy and will abate when therapy has been completed. Stress the importance of good nutrition, vitamin and iron supplements, and intake of foods high in iron such as liver and other organ meats, seafood, green vegetables, cereals, nuts, and legumes. As prescribed, administer erythropoietin (see Table A-10) for chemotherapy-related anemia.

Body image disturbance related to alopecia secondary to radiation therapy to the head and neck or administration of some chemotherapeutic agents
Desired outcome: Patient discusses the effects that alopecia may have on self-concept, body image, and social interaction and identifies measures that prevent, minimize, or enable adaptation to alopecia.

> Note: Common chemotherapeutic agents that cause alopecia include actinomycin D, amsacrine, bleomycin, cyclophosphamide, daunomycin, docetaxel, doxorubicin, epirubicin, etoposide (VP-16), topotecan (Hycamtin), idarubicin, ifosfamide, irinotecan (CPT-11), paclitaxel, teniposide, vinblastine, and vincristine.

- Discuss the potential for hair loss with the patient before treatment:
  —Radiation therapy of 1500-3000 cGy to the head and neck will produce either partial or complete hair loss. Explain that this hair loss is temporary and that onset usually occurs within 5-7 days, with regrowth beginning 2-3 mo after the final treatment.
  —Radiation therapy >4500 cGy usually results in permanent hair loss.

—Hair loss associated with chemotherapy is temporary and related to the specific agent, dose, and duration of administration. Hair loss is commonly delayed until about 2 wk after administration of chemotherapy. Regrowth usually begins 1-2 mo after the last treatment. However, the hair often grows back a different color or texture.

- Explore the impact hair loss has on the patient's self-concept, body image, and social interaction. Recognize that alopecia is an extremely stressful side effect for most patients.
- Encourage the following measures that will minimize the impact or severity of alopecia: using a mild shampoo, hair conditioner, soft-bristle hair brush, or wide-tooth comb; sleeping on a silk pillowcase to minimize hair tangles; decreasing frequency of hair washing; and avoiding irritants, such as dyes, permanent wave solutions, hair dryers, curling irons, clips, and hair sprays.
- Explain that scalp hypothermia and tourniquet applications during IV infusion may decrease the severity of hair loss. In particular, a significant decrease in alopecia has been found in individuals who use a hypothermia cap. These techniques are contraindicated in hematologic malignancy and in solid tumors with scalp metastasis because they may prevent adequate absorption of the drug where it is needed.
- Suggest measures that may help minimize the psychologic impact of hair loss: cut the hair short before treatment; select a wig before hair loss occurs, which will enable patients to match color and style of their own hair; wear a hair net or turban during hair loss to collect hair that falls out; use scarves, hats, caps, and turbans to cover the head; use makeup and accessories to enhance self-concept. **Note:** Wigs are tax deductible and often are reimbursed by insurance with the appropriate prescription.
- Inform patient that hair loss may occur on body parts other than the head, including the axillae, groin, legs, face, and eyes (eyelashes and eyebrows).
- Instruct patient to keep head covered during the summer to minimize sunburn and during the winter to prevent heat loss.
- Provide information about alopecia available through community resources, such as the American Cancer Society's "Look Good, Feel Better" national program.

NIC: Body Image Enhancement; Chemotherapy Management; Coping Enhancement; Heat/Cold Application; Self-Care Assistance: Bathing/Hygiene; Self-Esteem Enhancement

Ineffective breathing pattern related to decreased lung expansion secondary to fluid accumulation in the lungs (pleural effusion)

Note: For desired outcome and interventions, see this nursing diagnosis in "Pleural Effusion," p. 13. Patients at increased risk for pleural effusion are those with corresponding cancers, including lymphoma, leukemia, mesothelioma, lung and breast cancers, and metastasis to the lung from other primary cancers.

NIC: Airway Management; Cough Enhancement; Pain Management; Positioning; Respiratory Monitoring; Tube Care: Chest

Ineffective breathing pattern related to decreased lung expansion secondary to pulmonary fibrosis

Note: For desired outcome and interventions, see this nursing diagnosis in "Pulmonary Fibrosis," p. 44. Some chemotherapeutic agents (e.g., bleomycin sulfate, busulfan, carmustine, chlorozotocin, cytarabine, 1-asparaginase, semustine) can cause pulmonary toxicity, an inflammatory reaction that results in fibrotic lung changes, cellular damage, and decreased lung capacity. Pulmonary toxicity also can occur, although much more rarely, with use of cyclophosphamide, chlorambucil, melphalan, mitomycin, methotrexate, mercaptopurine, procarbazine hydrochloride, and zinostatin.

NIC: Emotional Support; Energy Management; Exercise Promotion; Oxygen Therapy; Respiratory Monitoring; Teaching: Procedure/Treatment

Chronic pain related to direct tumor involvement; infiltration of tumor into nerves, bones, or hollow viscus; or postchemotherapy or postradiotherapy syndrome

Desired outcome: Patient participates in a prescribed pain regimen and reports that pain associated with direct involvement or infiltration of the tumor and side effects associated with the prescribed therapy are reduced or at an acceptable level within 1-2 hr of intervention, based on a pain assessment tool (e.g., descriptive, numeric [on a scale of 0-10], or visual scale).

* After patient has undergone a complete medical evaluation of the cause of the pain (Tables A-11 and A-12) and the most effective strategies for pain relief, review the evaluation and pain-relief strategies with patient and significant other to determine their level of understanding.
* Ongoing assessment of pain is essential. Assessment should occur at regularly scheduled intervals. Any change in pain pattern or new complaints of pain should be promptly reported to the health care provider. Pain assessment should include the following:
  —*Characteristics* (e.g., "burning" or "shooting" often describes nerve pain).
  —*Location and sites of radiation.*
  —*Onset and duration.*
  —*Severity:* use a pain scale that is comfortable for the patient (e.g., descriptive, numeric, or visual scale). For example, use of a numeric scale would require the patient to rate pain from 0 (none) to 10 (worst).
  —*Aggravating and relieving factors.*
  —*Previous use of strategies that have worked to relieve pain.*
* Assess patient's and significant other's attitudes and knowledge about the pain medication regimen. Many patients and their families have fears related to patient's ultimate addiction to narcotics. Dispel any misperceptions about narcotic-induced addiction when chronic pain therapy is necessary.
* Pharmacologic management of pain is often the mainstay of treatment of chronic cancer pain. Incorporate the following principles:
  —*Administer nonnarcotic and narcotic analgesics in the correct dose, at the correct frequency, and via the correct route.* Chronic cancer analgesia often is administered orally, and if pain is present most of the day, it should be given around the clock (at scheduled intervals) rather than as needed.

TABLE A-11   Physiologic Causes of Acute Pain in Cancer Patients

Tumor compression or infiltration of nerves

Tumor obstruction of hollow viscera or ductal system

Infiltration/obstruction of blood vessels

Exacerbation of altered body functions unrelated to cancer (e.g., preexisting conditions such as chronic headaches, arthritis)

Pain associated with treatments

Postsurgical pain, stomatitis, or peripheral neuropathies

TABLE A-12 Physiologic Causes of Chronic Pain in Cancer Patients

Tumor unresponsive to therapy
Postsurgical pain
Postchemotherapy pain
Postradiation pain
Postherpetic neuralgia
Altered body functions (e.g., chronic arthritis, back pain, or any musculoskeletal disorder)

—*Recognize and treat side effects of narcotic analgesia early.* Side effects include nausea and vomiting, constipation, sedation, itching, and respiratory depression. The presence of these side effects does not necessarily preclude continued use of the drug.

—*Use prescribed adjuvant medications to help increase efficacy of narcotics.* These include tricyclic antidepressants, antihistamines, dextroamphetamines, steroids, phenothiazines, and anticonvulsants.

—*Monitor for signs and symptoms of tolerance, and when it occurs discuss treatment with health care provider.* Patients with chronic pain often require increasing doses of narcotics. Respiratory depression occurs rarely in these patients.

—*Be aware of the potential for physical dependence in patients taking narcotics for a prolonged period.* Narcotics should not be stopped abruptly in these patients, because withdrawal may occur.

—*Evaluate the effectiveness of analgesics at regular and frequent intervals after administration, particularly after the initial dose.*

—*Use nonpharmacologic approaches (see Table A-6) when appropriate.* See discussion in **Pain,** p. 719.

NIC: Analgesic Administration; Environmental Management: Comfort; Pain Management; Patient-Controlled Analgesia (PCA) Assistance; Simple Guided Imagery; Simple Relaxation Therapy

Constipation related to treatment with certain chemotherapy agents, narcotic analgesics, tranquilizers, and antidepressants; less than adequate intake because of anorexia; hypercalcemia; spinal cord compression; mental status changes; decreased mobility; or colonic disorders

> **Note:** For desired outcomes and interventions, see "General Care of Patients With Neurologic Disorders" for **Constipation,** p. 339; "Caring for Preoperative and Postoperative Patients" for **Constipation,** p. 733; "Caring for Patients on Prolonged Bedrest" for **Constipation,** p. 743.

> **Note:** Patients with cancer should not go more than 2 days without having a bowel movement. Patients receiving *Vinca* alkaloids are at risk for ileus in addition to constipation. Preventive measures, such as use of senna products (Senokot) or docusate calcium with casanthranol, especially for patients taking narcotics, are highly recommended. In addition, all individuals taking narcotics should receive a prophylactic bowel regimen.

NIC: Bowel Management; Constipation/Impaction Management; Diet Staging; Fluid Management; Teaching: Disease Process

Diarrhea related to chemotherapeutic drugs, especially antimetabolite agents; antacids containing magnesium; radiation therapy to the abdomen or pelvis;

tube feedings; food intolerance; and bowel dysfunction, such as tumors, Crohn's disease, ulcerative colitis, and fecal impaction

> **Note:** For desired outcomes and interventions, see **Diarrhea,** p. 418; **Risk for fluid volume deficit** related to diarrhea, p. 419, in "Malabsorption/Maldigestion." See "Ulcerative Colitis" for **Risk for impaired perineal/perianal skin integrity** related to prolonged diarrhea, p. 448. For patients receiving chemotherapy with potential for causing diarrhea (e.g., 5-fluorouracil, CPT-11), instruct the patient about the need for having an appropriate antidiarrheal medication (loperamide) available and other methods used to combat the effects of diarrhea (fluid replacement, addition of psyllium to the diet to provide bulk to stool, careful perineal hygiene). Instruct patient to notify health care provider if experiencing more than three loose stools per day.

NIC: Diarrhea Management; Fluid/Electrolyte Management; Perineal Care; Surveillance; Teaching: Prescribed Diet

Risk for infection with risks related to inadequate secondary defenses (neutropenia) secondary to malignancy, chemotherapy, radiation therapy, or immunotherapy

Desired outcomes: Patient is free of infection as evidenced by normothermia, BP $\geq$90/60 mm Hg, and HR $\leq$100 bpm. Patient identifies risk factors for infection, verbalizes early signs and symptoms of infection and reports them promptly to health care professional if they occur, and demonstrates appropriate self-care measures to minimize the risk of infection.

- Identify patients at risk for infection by obtaining the absolute neutrophil count (ANC). Calculate ANC by using the following formula:

  ANC = (% of segmented neutrophils + % of bands) $\times$ Total WBC count

—ANC of 1500-2000/mm^3 = No significant risk.
—ANC of 1000-1500/mm^3 = Minimal risk.
—ANC of 500-1000/mm^3 = Moderate risk. Initiate neutropenic precautions.
—ANC of <500/mm^3 = Severe risk. Initiate neutropenic precautions.

- Assess each body system thoroughly to determine potential and actual sources of infection.
- Monitor VS and temperature q4hr. Be alert to temperature $\geq$38° C (100.4° F) $\times$ 2, temperature <35.5° C (<96° F) $\times$ 1, temperature >38.3° C (>101° F) $\times$ 1, increased HR, decreased BP, and the following clinical signs of infection: tenderness, erythema, warmth, swelling, and drainage at invasive sites; chills; and malaise. **Note:** Signs of infection may be absent in the presence of neutropenia; a fever of $\geq$ 38° C ($\geq$100.4° F) may be the *only* sign of infection in the neutropenic patient.
- Place sign on patient's door indicating that neutropenic precautions are in effect for patients with ANC $\leq$1000/mm^3.
- Instruct all persons entering patient's room to wash hands thoroughly.
- Restrict individuals from entering who have transmissible illnesses, such as colds, influenza, chickenpox, or herpes zoster.
- Instruct patient to wear a mask when out of the hospital room.
- Encourage patient to practice good personal hygiene.
- Notify health care provider immediately if patient's temperature is >38° C (>100.4° F) $\times$ 2, temperature >38.3° C (>101° F) $\times$ 1, or temperature <35.5° C (<96° F) $\times$ 1. Initiate antibiotic therapy as prescribed within 1 hr when ANC is $\leq$500/mm^3.
- Implement oral care routine to minimize the risk of infection caused by nonintact mucosa or tongue. Teach patient to use a soft-bristle toothbrush after meals and before bed (bristles may be softened even more by running

them under hot water). Inspect oral cavity daily, noting presence of white patches on the tongue or mucous membrane. Nystatin (Mycostatin) swish and swallow or swish and spit may be prescribed to prevent the development of oral candidiasis. Individuals with prolonged neutropenia are at risk for candidiasis and other bacterial and viral infections. Monitor for vesicles, crusted lesions that may signal herpes simplex. Acyclovir may be prescribed to prevent or minimize herpetic infections in patients with prolonged neutropenia who are at risk for herpes.

- Avoid use of rectal suppositories, rectal temperature, or enemas to minimize the risk of traumatizing the rectal mucosa, thereby increasing the risk of infection. Be aware that patients with prolonged neutropenia are at increased risk for perirectal infection; monitor for it accordingly. Caution patient to avoid straining at stool. Suggest use of stool softener.
- Implement measures that maintain skin integrity, and instruct patient accordingly: use electric shaver rather than razor blade; avoid vaginal douche and tampons; use emery board rather than clipper for nail care; check with health care provider before dental care; avoid all invasive procedures; use antimicrobial skin preparations before injections; change IV sites q48hr; use steel-tipped rather than plastic catheters (minimizes the risk of infection).
- Instruct patient to use water-soluble lubricant before sexual intercourse and avoid oral and anal manipulation during sexual activities. Patients should abstain from sexual intercourse during periods of severe neutropenia.
- Teach patient to avoid potential sources of infection during periods of neutropenia (e.g., avoid foods with high bacterial count [raw eggs, raw fruits and vegetables, foods prepared in a blender that cannot adequately be cleaned]; bird, cat, and dog excreta; plants, flowers, and sources of stagnant water).
- Be alert to signs of impending sepsis, including subtle changes in mental status: restlessness or irritability; warm and flushed skin; chills, fever, or hypothermia; increased urine output; bounding pulse; tachypnea; and glycosuria. These symptoms often precede the classic signs of septic shock: cold, clammy skin; thready pulse; decreased BP; and oliguria.
- As prescribed, administer colony-stimulating factors (see Table A-10) to minimize the risk of myelosuppression with chemotherapy, especially for patients with a history of neutropenia with severe infections in the past.

NIC: Environmental Management; Infection Protection; Oral Health Maintenance; Risk Identification; Self-Care Assistance: Bathing/Hygiene; Vital Signs Monitoring

Altered nutrition: Less than body requirements related to nausea and vomiting or anorexia occurring with chemotherapy, radiation therapy, or disease
Desired outcome: At least 24 hr before hospital discharge, patient has adequate nutrition as evidenced by stable weight and a positive or balanced nitrogen (N) state.

For anorexia
- Monitor for clinical signs of malnutrition. See "Providing Nutritional Support" for **Altered nutrition,** p. 700. Weigh patient daily.
- Assess patient's food likes and dislikes, as well as cultural and religious preferences related to food choices.
- Explain that anorexia can be caused by pathophysiology of cancer, surgery, and side effects of chemotherapy and radiation therapy.
- Teach the importance of increasing caloric intake to increase energy and minimize weight loss.
- Teach the importance of increasing protein intake to facilitate repair and regeneration of cells.
- Suggest that patient eat several small meals at frequent intervals throughout the day.

TABLE A-13   Antineoplastic Agents With Emetic Action

Mild emetic action	Moderate emetic action	Severe emetic action
L-Asparginase	Hexamethylmelamine	Nitrosourea
Bleomycin	Azacytidine	Dactinomycin
Chlorambucil	Daunorubicin	Cisplatin
Hydroxyurea	Doxorubicin	Cyclophosphamide
Melphalan	Etoposide (VP-15)	Dacarbazine
Mercaptopurine	5-Fluorouracil (5-FU)	Mitomycin C
Tamoxifen	Procarbazine	Methotrexate
Thioguanine	Streptozocin	Plicamycin (Mithramycin)
Thiotepa	Carboplatin	Mechlorethamine
Vinblastine	Mitoxantrone	
Vincristine	Ifosfamide	
Steroids		
Cytarabine		
L-Phenylalanine		
Lomustine		
Paclitaxel		

- Encourage use of nutritional supplements.
- Consider use of megestrol acetate or hydrazine sulfate medications. These agents have proven to have a positive influence on appetite stimulation and weight gain in individuals with cancer. Consult patient's health care provider accordingly.

For nausea and vomiting

- Assess patient's pattern of nausea and vomiting: onset, frequency, duration, intensity, and amount and character of emesis.
- Explain to patient that nausea and vomiting can be side effects of chemotherapy and radiation therapy. (Nausea and vomiting also can occur with advanced cancer, bowel obstruction, some medications, or metabolic abnormalities.) See Table A-13 for a list of antineoplastic agents with known emetic action.
- Administer antiemetics (Table A-14) as prescribed. Teach patient to take antiemetic 1-12 hr before chemotherapy as prescribed. Continue to take the drug as prescribed to cover the expected emetogenic period of the chemotherapy agent given; also consider the duration of previous nausea and vomiting episodes following chemotherapy.
- Teach patient to eat cold foods or food served at room temperature because the odor of hot food may aggravate nausea.
- Suggest intake of clear liquids and bland foods.
- Teach patient to avoid sweet, fatty, highly salted, and spicy foods, as well as foods with strong odors, any of which may increase nausea.
- Minimize stimuli such as smells, sounds, or sights, all of which may promote nausea.
- Encourage patient to eat sour or mint candy during chemotherapy to decrease the unpleasant, metallic taste.
- Encourage patient to experiment with various dietary patterns:
  —Avoid eating or drinking for 1-2 hr before and after chemotherapy.
  —Follow a clear liquid diet for 1-2 hr before and 1-24 hr after chemotherapy.
  —Avoid contact with food while it is being cooked; avoid being around people who are eating.
  —Eat small, light meals at frequent intervals (5-6 times/day).

TABLE A-14 Common Antiemetic Agents

Agent	Generic name	Trade name
Phenothiazine	Prochlorperazine	Compazine
Steroids	Dexamethasone	Decadron
Antihistamine	Diphenhydramine	Benadryl
Butyrophenone derivatives	Haloperidol	Haldol
Benzodiazepines	Lorazepam	Ativan
Benzamide	Metoclopramide*	Reglan
Cannabinoids	Dronabinol	Marinol
	Granisetron	Kytril
Serotonin antagonist	Ondansetron	Zofran

*Metoclopramide blocks the neurotransmitter sites to reduce stimulation of an area in the medulla known as the chemoreceptor trigger zone.

- Suggest that patient sit near an open window to breathe fresh air when feeling nauseated.
- Help patient find an appropriate distraction technique (e.g., music, television, reading).
- Teach patient to use relaxation techniques. See **Health-seeking behaviors:** Relaxation technique effective for stress reduction, p. 59. This technique also may help prevent anticipatory nausea and vomiting.
- Teach patient to maintain NPO status for 4-8 hr if frequent episodes of vomiting occur.
- Instruct patient to sip clear liquids, such as broth, ginger ale, cola, tea, or gelatin, slowly; suck on ice chips; and avoid large volumes of water.

○ **NIC:** Diet Staging; Distraction; Nutritional Counseling; Simple Guided Imagery; Simple Relaxation Therapy; Teaching: Prescribed Diet

Altered oral mucous membrane related to treatment with chemotherapy agents (especially antitumor antibiotics), antimetabolites, and *Vinca* alkaloids; radiation therapy to head and neck; ineffective oral hygiene; gingival diseases; and poor nutritional status
Desired outcomes: Patient complies with therapeutic regimen within 12-24 hr of instruction. Patient's oral mucosal condition improves as evidenced by intact mucous membrane; moist, intact tongue and lips; and absence of pain and lesions.

- With myelosuppression, caution the patient not to floss teeth.
- For moderate to severe stomatitis, patient may require parenteral analgesics, such as morphine.
- Patients with xerostomia (dryness of the mouth from a lack of normal salivary secretion) caused by radiation may benefit from chewing sugarless gum, sucking sugarless candy, or taking frequent sips of water. Saliva substitutes are another option, although they are expensive and do not last long.
- Close dental follow-up is essential because the lack of or decrease in salivary fluid predisposes the patient to dental caries. Fluoride treatment is recommended for these patients.

○ **NIC:** Oral Health Maintenance; Oral Health Promotion; Oral Health Restoration; Teaching: Disease Process; Teaching: Procedure/Treatment

Pain related to the presence of cancer or its treatments

Note: For desired outcome and interventions, see this nursing diagnosis in "Caring for Preoperative and Postoperative Patients," p. 719. Explain that acute pain is of short duration and that relief will occur when the underlying cause is treated.

NIC: Analgesic Administration; Coping Enhancement; Environmental Management: Comfort; Pain Management; Simple Guided Imagery; Simple Relaxation Therapy

Impaired physical mobility related to musculoskeletal or neuromuscular impairment secondary to bone metastasis or spinal cord compression; pain and discomfort; intolerance to activity; or perceptual or cognitive impairment

Note: For desired outcome and interventions, see this nursing diagnosis in "Osteoarthritis," p. 556, and "Osteomyelitis," p. 583. See discussions of care of patients at risk for pressure ulcers, p. 710, and "Caring for Patients on Prolonged Bedrest," p. 738.

NIC: Energy Management; Exercise Promotion: Stretching; Exercise Therapy: Joint Mobility; Exercise Therapy: Muscle Control; Mutual Goal Setting; Teaching: Prescribed Activity/Exercise

Altered protection related to risk of bleeding/hemorrhage secondary to thrombocytopenia (for all patients receiving chemotherapy and radiation therapy, as well as those with cancer, particularly involving the bone marrow)
Desired outcome: Patient is free of signs and symptoms of bleeding as evidenced by negative occult blood tests, HR $\leq$100 bpm, and systolic BP $\geq$90 mm Hg.
- Identify platelet counts that place individuals at increased risk for bleeding:
   —Platelets 150,000-300,000/mm^3 = normal risk for bleeding.
   —Platelets <50,000/mm^3 = moderate risk for bleeding. Initiate thrombocytopenic precautions.
   —Platelets <20,000/mm^3 = severe risk of bleeding. Patient may develop spontaneous bleeding; initiate thrombocytopenic precautions.
   —Platelets <10,000/mm^3 = **critical** risk of bleeding.
- Perform a baseline physical assessment, monitoring for evidence of bleeding, including petechiae, ecchymosis, hematuria, coffee ground emesis, tarry or bloody stools, hemoptysis, heavy menses, headaches, somnolence, mental status changes, confusion, and blurred vision. Also monitor VS every shift, being alert to hypotension and tachycardia. Avoid use of rectal thermometer, which can cause rectal bleeding (use a tympanic thermometer when available).
- Test all secretions and excretions for occult blood.
- Perform a psychosocial assessment, including patient's past experience with thrombocytopenia; the effect of thrombocytopenia on patient's life-style; and changes in patient's work pattern, family relationships, and social activities. Identify learning needs and necessity of skilled care after hospital discharge.
- Place a sign on patient's door, indicating that thrombocytopenia precautions are in effect for patients with platelet count <50,000/mm^3.
- In the presence of bleeding, begin pad count for heavy menses (discourage use of tampons, which may cause trauma during placement); measure quantity of vomiting and stool; elevate (when possible) and apply direct pressure and ice to site of bleeding (VAD, venipuncture); and deliver platelet transfusion as prescribed.
- Initiate oral care at frequent intervals to promote integrity of gingiva and mucosa. Advise patient to brush with soft-bristle toothbrush after meals and

before bed (hot water run over bristles may soften them further). In the presence of gum bleeding, teach patient to use sponge-tipped applicator rather than toothbrush, avoid dental floss, and avoid mouthwash with more than 6% alcohol content. Suggest use of normal saline solution mouthwashes 4 times/day and water-based ointment for lubricating the lips.

- Implement bowel program, and check with patient daily for bowel movement. Assess need for stool softeners or psyllium to prevent constipation; encourage adequate hydration (at least 2500 ml/day) and high-fiber foods to promote bowel function; and avoid use of rectal suppositories, enemas, or harsh laxatives to minimize the risk of bleeding.
- Implement measures that prevent bleeding. Teach patient to use electric shaver; apply direct pressure and elevation for 3-5 min after injections and venipuncture; and avoid vaginal douche and tampons, constrictive clothing, aspirin or aspirin-containing products because of aspirin's antiplatelet action, alcohol ingestion, anticoagulants, and indomethacin (Indocin), which is a GI irritant. Caution patient to perform gentle nose blowing, use emery board rather than clippers for nail care, check with health care provider before seeking dental care, and avoid bladder catheterization if possible.
- When appropriate, instruct patient to abstain from sexual intercourse when the platelet count is <50,000/mm^3. Instruct patient to use water-soluble lubrication during sexual intercourse.
- Caution patient to avoid activities that predispose to trauma or injury; remove hazardous objects or furniture from patient's environment. Assist with ambulating if patient's physical mobility is impaired. When the patient's platelet count is <20,000/mm^3, teach patient to avoid activities involving Valsalva's maneuver, which increases intracranial pressure. These activities include moving up in bed, straining at stool, bending at the waist, and lifting heavy objects (>10 lb). Suggest bedrest if patient's platelet count is <10,000/mm^3.
- See "Thrombocytopenia," p. 529, for more information.

- **NIC:** Bleeding Precautions; Bleeding Reduction; Blood Products Administration; Environmental Management: Safety; Hemorrhage Control; Shock Management: Volume; Shock Prevention

Sensory/perceptual alterations: Auditory and kinesthetic impairment related to use of cisplatin, cytarabine, 5-fluorouracil, high-dose methotrexate, nitrosoureas, paclitaxel, or *Vinca* alkaloids
Desired outcome: Patient reports early signs and symptoms of ototoxicity and peripheral neuropathy; measures are implemented promptly to minimize these side effects.

- Explain that tinnitus or decreased hearing can occur with use of cisplatin. It is usually dose related and a result of cumulative side effects. Most commonly, high-frequency hearing loss occurs, although with cumulative doses, speech-frequency hearing range also may be affected. Affected individuals may have difficulty hearing speech in the presence of background noise. Suggest that the patient face the speaker and watch the speaker's lips during conversation. A hearing aid also may be helpful, or it may amplify background noise and worsen speech comprehension; suggest patients use hearing aids for a trial before purchase. In instances of hearing loss from cisplatin, which is usually irreversible, refer patient to community resources for hearing-impaired persons.
- Monitor patient for the development of peripheral neuropathy, which can occur with cisplatin, paclitaxel, and vincristine use. The first symptom usually is numbness and tingling of the fingers and toes, which can progress to difficulty with fine motor skills, such as buttoning shirt or picking up objects. The most severely affected individuals may lose sensation at hip level and have difficulty with balance and ambulation. Instruct patient to

report early signs and symptoms. Suggest consultation with PT or OT to assist with maintaining function.

- Monitor bowel elimination daily in individuals at risk for paralytic ileus associated with the neuropathy (i.e., those taking vincristine, vinblastine). Administer stool softeners, psyllium, or laxatives daily if patient has not had a bowel movement within a 48-hr period or as prescribed. Instruct patient in the need to increase fluid intake to >2400 ml/day.

NIC: Bowel Management; Communication Enhancement: Hearing Deficit; Fluid Management; Peripheral Sensation Management; Teaching: Individual

Sexual dysfunction (impaired sexual self-concept and infertility) related to the disease process; psychosocial issues; radiation therapy to the lower abdomen, pelvis, and gonads; or chemotherapeutic agents, especially actinomycin D, alkylating agents, amsacrine, bleomycin, cytarabine, daunorubicin, epirubicin, methotrexate, mitomycin, procarbazine, and vinblastine
Desired outcome: Following instruction, patient identifies potential treatment side effects on sexual and reproductive function and acceptable methods of contraception during treatment.

- Initiate discussion about the effects of treatment on sexuality and reproduction. The PLISSIT model provides an excellent framework for discussion. This 4-step model includes the following: (1) **P**ermission—give the patient permission to discuss issues of concern; (2) **L**imited **I**nformation—provide patient with information about expected treatment effects on sexual and reproductive function, without going into complete detail; (3) **S**pecific **S**uggestions—provide suggestions for managing common problems that occur during treatment; and (4) **I**ntensive **T**herapy—although most individuals can be managed by nurses using the first 3 steps in this model, some patients may require referral to an expert counselor.
- Assess the impact of the diagnosis and treatment on the patient's sexual functioning and self-concept.
- Determine the possibility of pregnancy before treatment is initiated. Pregnancy will cause a delay in treatment. If treatment cannot be delayed, a therapeutic abortion may be recommended.
- Discuss the possibility of decreased sexual response or desire, which may result from side effects of chemotherapy. Encourage patients to maintain open communication with their partner about needs and concerns. Explore alternate methods of sexual fulfillment, such as hugging, kissing, talking quietly together, or massage. In the presence of symptoms related to therapy, such interventions as taking a nap before sexual activity or use of pain or antiemetic medication may help decrease symptoms. Other suggestions include using a water-based lubricant if dyspareunia or fatigue is a problem, changing the usual time of day for intimacy, or using supine or side-lying positions, which require the least expenditure of energy.
- Discuss the possibility of temporary or permanent sterility resulting from treatment. Explore the possibility of sperm banking for men before chemotherapy treatment or oophoropexy (surgical displacement of the ovaries outside the radiation field) for women undergoing abdominal radiation therapy.
- Teach patients the importance of contraception during treatment. Discuss, with patients and significant others, issues related to the timing of pregnancy after treatment.
- Inform patients that healthy offspring have been born from parents who have received radiation therapy or chemotherapy, but long-term effects have not been clearly identified. Suggest that patients have genetic counseling before becoming parents, as indicated.

NIC: Preconception Counseling; Pregnancy Termination Care; Risk Identification: Childbearing Family; Sexual Counseling; Teaching: Individual

Impaired skin integrity related to pigmentation changes (malignant skin lesions)

Desired outcome: Following instruction, patient verbalizes measures that promote comfort and skin integrity.

- Identify populations at risk for malignant lesions: individuals with primary tumors of the breast, lung, colon/rectum, ovary, or oral cavity; and individuals with malignant melanoma, lymphoma, or leukemia.
- Identify common sites of cutaneous metastases: anterior chest, abdomen, head (scalp), and neck.
- Inspect skin lesions, and note and document the following: general characteristics, location and distribution, configuration, size, morphologic structure (e.g., nodule, erosion, fissure), drainage (color, amount, character), and odor.
- Monitor for indicators of infection: local warmth, swelling, erythema, tenderness, purulent drainage.
- Perform the following skin care for nonulcerating lesions, and teach these interventions to the patient and significant other, as indicated:
  - —Wash affected area with tepid water, and pat dry.
  - —Avoid pressure on the area.
  - —Apply dry dressing to protect the area from exposure to irritants and mechanical trauma (e.g., scratching, abrasion).
  - —To enhance penetration of topical medications, apply occlusive dressings, such as Telfa, using paper tape.
  - —Teach patient to avoid wearing irritating fabrics, such as wool and corduroy.
- Perform the following skin care for ulcerating lesions, and teach these interventions to the patient and significant other, as indicated.

For cleansing and debriding
- Use ½-strength hydrogen peroxide and normal saline solution for irrigation, followed by a normal saline rinse.
- Use cotton swabs or sponges to apply gentle pressure, thereby debriding the ulcerated area.
- As necessary, if the ulcerated area is susceptible to bleeding, gently irrigate only, using a syringe.
- Use soaks (wet dressings) of saline, water, Burow's solution (aluminum acetate), or hydrogen peroxide for débridement. **Note:** Failure to rinse hydrogen peroxide or aluminum acetate off the skin may cause further skin breakdown.
- As necessary, use wet-to-dry dressings for gentle débridement.

For prevention and management of local infection
- Irrigate and scrub with antibacterial agents, such as acetic acid solution or povidone-iodine.
- Collect wound cultures as prescribed.
- Apply topical antibacterial agents (e.g., sulfadiazine cream, bacitracin ointment) to open areas susceptible to infection as prescribed.
- Administer systemic antibiotics as prescribed.

To maintain hemostasis
- For capillary oozing, use silver nitrate sticks for cautery.
- For larger surface area bleeding, use oxidized cellulose or pack the wound with Gelfoam or similar product.

To control odor
- Cleanse wound and change dressings as frequently as necessary.
- Collect specimens for culture and sensitivity of the wound drainage, as prescribed.

- Use antiodor agents (e.g., open a bottle of oil of peppermint or place a tray of activated charcoal) in patient's room.
- Collaborate with an enterostomal nurse as needed on wound-healing techniques.
- Also see "Providing Nutritional Support," p. 687, and "Managing Wound Care," p. 704.

NIC: Bleeding Precautions; Health Screening; Infection Control; Skin Care: Topical Treatments; Skin Surveillance; Specimen Management

Impaired skin integrity or **impaired tissue integrity** (or risk for same) related to treatment with chemical irritants (chemotherapy)
Desired outcome: Before the chemotherapy, patient identifies the potential side effects of chemotherapy on the skin and tissue and measures that will maintain skin integrity and promote comfort.

> **Note:** Alterations of the skin or nails that occur in conjunction with chemotherapy are a result of the destruction of the basal cells of the epidermis (general) or of cellular alterations at the site of chemotherapy administration (local). The reactions are specific to the agent used and vary in onset, severity, and duration. The skin reactions include the following: transient erythema/urticaria, hyperpigmentation, telangiectasis, photosensitivity, hyperkeratosis, acnelike reaction, ulceration, and radiation recall.

Transient erythema/urticaria
Transient erythema/urticaria may be generalized or localized at the site of chemotherapy administration. Usually it occurs within several hours after chemotherapy and disappears in several hours. It is caused by the following agents: doxorubicin hydrochloride (Adriamycin), bleomycin, l-asparaginase, mithramycin, and mechlorethamine.
- Perform and document a pretreatment assessment of the patient's skin for posttreatment comparison.
- Assess the onset, pattern, severity, and duration of the reaction after treatment.
- Compare posttreatment findings with those from the pretreatment assessment to determine if the cause of the erythema/urticaria is related to the chemotherapy or to herpes zoster, bacterial or fungal embolic lesions, skin metastasis, allergic reaction, or parasitic infestation.

Hyperpigmentation
Hyperpigmentation is believed to be caused by increased levels of epidermal melanin-stimulating hormone. It can occur on the nail beds, on the oral mucosa, or along the veins used for chemotherapy administration, or it can be generalized. It is caused by the following chemotherapeutic agents: doxorubicin hydrochloride (Adriamycin), carmustine, bleomycin, cyclophosphamide, daunorubicin, fluorouracil, and melphalan. In addition, it can occur with tumors of the pituitary gland.
- Inform the patient before treatment that this reaction is to be expected and that it will disappear gradually when the course of treatment is finished.

Telangiectasis (spider veins)
Telangiectasis is believed to be caused by destruction of the capillary bed and occurs as a result of applications of topical carmustine and mechlorethamine.
- Inform patient that this reaction is permanent but that the configuration of the veins will become less severe over time.

Photosensitivity

Photosensitivity is enhanced when the skin is exposed to ultraviolet light. Acute sunburn and residual tanning can occur with short exposure to the sun. Photosensitivity can occur during the time the agent is administered, or it can reactivate a skin reaction caused by sun exposure when the agent is administered in close proximity to the sun exposure. It is caused by bleomycin, dacarbazine, dactinomycin, daunorubicin, doxorubicin hydrochloride, fluorouracil, methotrexate, and vinblastine.

- Assess onset, pattern, severity, and duration of the reaction.
- Teach patient to avoid exposing skin to the sun. Advise patient to wear protective clothing and use an effective sun-screening agent (SPF of 15 or greater).
- In the event that burning takes place, advise patient to treat it like a sunburn (e.g., tepid bath, moisturizing cream, consultation with health care provider).

Hyperkeratosis

Hyperkeratosis presents as a thickening of the skin, especially over the hands, feet, face, and areas of trauma. It is disfiguring and causes loss of fine motor function of the hands. It occurs with bleomycin administration and should be considered an indicator of more severe fibrotic changes in the lungs. This condition is reversible when treatment with bleomycin is discontinued.

- For patients taking bleomycin, assess for the presence of skin thickening and loss of fine motor function of the hands.
- In the presence of skin thickening, be aware that fibrotic changes may be present in the lungs. Assess for this condition accordingly (see "Pulmonary Fibrosis," p. 42).
- Reassure patient that this condition is reversible when bleomycin has been discontinued.

Acnelike reaction

An acnelike reaction presents as erythema, especially of the face, and progresses to papules and pustules, which are characteristic of acne. It occurs with administration of dactinomycin and will disappear when the drug is discontinued.

- Reassure patient that this reaction disappears when treatment with dactinomycin is discontinued.
- Suggest that patient use a commercial preparation, such as benzoyl peroxide lotion, gel, or cream, to conceal these blemishes.
- Teach patient about proper skin care:
  —Avoid hard scrubbing.
  —Avoid use of antibacterial soap because the removal of nonpathogenic bacteria on the skin results in replacement by pathogens, which are implicated in the genesis of acne. Use a plain soap, such as Ivory or Camay.
  —Avoid oil-based cosmetics.

Ulceration

Ulceration presents as a generalized, shallow lesion of the epidermal layer. It is caused by bleomycin, methotrexate, and mitomycin C.

- Assess for ulceration.
- If present, cleanse the ulcers with a solution of ¼-strength hydrogen peroxide and ¾-strength normal saline q4-6hr; rinse with normal saline solution.
- Expose the ulcer to the air, if possible.
- Be alert to the presence of infection at the ulcerated site, as evidenced by local warmth, swelling, tenderness, erythema, and purulent drainage.
- Teach patient assessment and treatment interventions.

Radiation recall reaction
Radiation recall reaction occurs when chemotherapy is given at the same time or after treatment with radiation therapy. It presents as erythema, followed by dry desquamation. More severe reactions can progress to vesicle formation and wet desquamation. After the skin heals, it is permanently hyperpigmented. This reaction is caused by bleomycin, cyclophosphamide, dactinomycin, doxorubicin, fluorouracil, hydroxyurea, and methotrexate.

- Teach patient the following skin care routine:
  —Cleanse the skin gently at the site of recall reaction, using mild soap, tepid water, and a soft cloth; pat dry.
  —Use A&D ointment on areas with dry desquamation.
  —Apply topical steroid creams or ointments as prescribed.
  —If edema and wet desquamation are present, cleanse the area with $\frac{1}{2}$-strength hydrogen peroxide and normal saline, and rinse with normal saline solution.
  —To promote healing, use moisture-permeable and vapor-permeable dressings, such as hydrocolloids and hydrogels, on noninfected areas.
- Teach patient to protect the skin at the site of recall reaction in the following ways:
  —Avoid wearing tight-fitting clothes.
  —Avoid trauma to the area.
  —Avoid harsh fabrics, such as wool or corduroy.
  —Use mild detergents, such as Ivory Snow.
  —Avoid exposing the site of recall reaction to heat and cold.
  —Avoid swimming in salt water or chlorinated pools.
  —Avoid use of all medications (except A&D ointment and topical steroids), deodorants, perfumes, powders, or cosmetics on the skin at the recall site.
  —For pruritus, use corticosteroid cream (triamcinolone acetonide 0.1%). Diphenhydramine (25 mg q6hr) may be prescribed for severe pruritus.
  —Avoid shaving the site of recall reaction; if shaving is absolutely necessary, use an electric razor.

NIC: Skin Care: Topical Treatments; Skin Surveillance; Teaching: Procedure/ Treatment; Wound Care; Wound Irrigation

Impaired skin integrity and impaired tissue integrity related to radiation therapy
Desired outcome: Within 24 hr of instruction, patient identifies potential skin reactions and the management interventions that will promote comfort and skin integrity.

- Assess the degree and extensiveness of the skin reaction as follows:
  Stage I: inflammation, mild erythema, slight edema.
  Stage II: inflammation; dry desquamation; dry, scaly, itchy skin.
  Stage III: inflammation, edema, wet desquamation, blisters, peeling.
  Stage IV: skin ulceration and necrosis, permanent loss of hair in the treatment field, suppression of sebaceous glands. *Late effects:* fibrosis and atrophy of the skin, fibrosis of the lymph glands.
- Teach patient the following skin care for the treatment field:
  —Cleanse skin gently and in a patting motion, using a mild soap, tepid water, and a soft cloth. Rinse the area, and pat it dry.
  —Apply cornstarch; A&D ointment; ointments containing aloe or lanolin; or mild topical steroids as prescribed to skin with stage II reaction.
- For patients with stage III skin reaction, teach the following regimen:
  —Cleanse the area with $\frac{1}{2}$-strength hydrogen peroxide and normal saline, using an irrigation syringe. Rinse with saline or water, and pat dry gently.
  —Use nonadhesive absorbent dressings, such as Telfa or Adaptic and an ABD pad for draining areas. Be alert to indicators of infection.
  —To promote healing, use moisture-permeable and vapor-permeable dressings, such as hydrocolloids and hydrogels, on noninfected areas.

- Teach the following interventions for protecting the patient's skin:
  —Avoid tight-fitting clothing.
  —Avoid wearing harsh fabrics, such as wool or corduroy.
  —Avoid sun exposure.
  —Use gentle detergents (e.g., Ivory Snow).
  —Avoid exposure to heat and cold.
  —Avoid swimming in chlorinated pools or salt water.
  —Avoid using medications, deodorants, perfumes, powders, or cosmetics on the skin in the treatment field.
  —Avoid shaving the hair on the skin in the treatment field; if shaving is absolutely necessary, use an electric razor.
  —Moist desquamation is more likely to occur in areas of skin prone to apposition and moisture, such as skin folds. Encourage patient cleansing 3-4 times daily and exposure to air for 10-15 min at least 3 times daily.
  —For pruritus, use corticosteroid cream (triamcinolone acetonide 0.1%). Diphenhydramine (25 mg q6hr) may be prescribed for severe pruritus.
- For stage IV reaction, teach the following interventions:
  —Topical antibiotics (e.g., sulfadiazine cream, bacitracin ointment) may be applied to open areas prone to infection.
  —Debride the wound of eschar (necessary before healing can occur).
  —After removing eschar (results in yellow-colored wound), keep the wound clean to prevent infection. Wet-to-moist dressings often are used to keep the wound clean.
  —Collaborate with an enterostomal nurse as needed on wound-healing techniques.
  —See interventions for alopecia under **Body image disturbance,** p. 773.

NIC: Skin Care: Topical Treatments; Skin Surveillance; Teaching: Procedure/Treatment; Wound Care; Wound Irrigation

Impaired swallowing related to esophagitis secondary to radiation therapy to the neck, chest, and upper back or use of chemotherapy agents, especially the antimetabolites; or obstruction (tumors of the esophagus)
Desired outcomes: Before food or fluids are given, patient exhibits the gag reflex and is free of symptoms of aspiration as evidenced by RR 12-20 breaths/min with normal depth and pattern (eupnea), normal skin color, and the ability to speak. Following instruction, patient verbalizes the early signs and symptoms of esophagitis, alerts health care team as soon as they occur, and identifies measures for maintaining nutrition and comfort.
- Monitor patient for evidence of impaired swallowing with concomitant respiratory difficulties.
- Teach patient the early signs and symptoms of esophagitis and the importance of reporting them promptly to the staff if they occur: sensation of lump in the throat with swallowing, difficulty with swallowing solid foods, discomfort or pain with swallowing.
- Monitor patient's dietary intake, and provide the following guidelines: maintain a high-protein diet; eat foods that are soft and bland; add milk or milk products to the diet to coat the esophageal lining (for individuals without excessive mucus production); and add sauces and creams to foods, which may facilitate swallowing.
- Ensure an adequate fluid intake of at least 2 L/day.
- Implement the following measures that promote comfort, and discuss them with the patient accordingly:
  —Use a local anesthetic, as prescribed, to minimize pain with meals. Lidocaine 2% and diphenhydramine may be taken via swish and swallow before eating. **Caution:** These anesthetics may decrease the patient's gag reflex.
  —Suggest that patient sit in an upright position during meals and for 15-30 min after eating.

—Mild analgesics, such as liquid ASA or acetaminophen, can be very helpful. Administer them as prescribed.

—For severe discomfort, narcotic analgesics may be required. Administer as prescribed. **Note:** If pain is severe or persistent, a barium swallow may be performed to evaluate for the presence of an infection. Common causative agents are *Candida* and herpes. Appropriate medical treatment, such as low-dose amphotericin, ketoconazole, or acyclovir, may be initiated.

—Encourage frequent oral care with normal saline or sodium bicarbonate solution.

—Teach patient to avoid irritants, such as alcohol, tobacco, and alcohol-based commercial mouthwashes.

• Keep suction equipment readily available in case patient experiences aspiration. Educate patient about ways to manage oral secretions.

—Suction mouth as needed, using low, continuous suction equipment.

—Expectorate saliva into tissues, and dispose of tissues in nearby waste cans.

NIC: Aspiration Precautions; Medication Management; Nutrition Management; Nutrition Therapy; Oral Health Maintenance; Swallowing Therapy

Altered cardiopulmonary tissue perfusion related to interrupted blood flow secondary to pericardial tamponade
Desired outcome: During activity, patient rates perceived exertion at ≤3 on a 0-10 scale and exhibits cardiac tolerance to activity, as evidenced by systolic BP within 20 mm Hg of resting BP, RR ≤20 breaths/min, HR ≤20 bpm above resting HR, and absence of chest pain or new dysrhythmia.

> **Note:** Pericardial tamponade may be caused by an accumulation of fluid in the pericardial space, tumor, invasion of the mediastinum, pericardial fibrosis, or effusion from radiotherapy. Patients at increased risk for pericardial tamponade include those with corresponding cancers, such as mesothelioma, sarcoma, leukemia, lymphoma, melanoma, primary GI cancer, and metastatic lung and breast tumors.

• Monitor patient for evidence of activity intolerance, and ask patient to rate perceived exertion. For further information see "Caring for Patients on Prolonged Bedrest" for **Activity intolerance,** p. 739.

• Make sure patient maintains bedrest during febrile period and understands the rationale for doing so.

• Anticipate patient's needs by placing personal articles within easy reach.

• Advise patient about the importance of frequent rest periods during convalescence.

• Monitor vital signs for changes indicating cardiac or pulmonary decompensation: decreasing BP, increasing HR and RR.

NIC: Energy Management; Surveillance; Teaching: Prescribed Medication; Vital Signs Monitoring

Altered peripheral tissue perfusion related to interrupted blood flow secondary to lymphedema
Desired outcome: Following intervention/treatment, patient exhibits adequate peripheral perfusion as evidenced by edema <2+ on a 0-4+ scale, peripheral pulses >2+ on a 0-4+ scale, normal skin color, decreasing or stable circumference of edematous site, bilaterally equal sensation, and ability to perform complete ROM in the involved extremity.

> **Note:** Patient populations at risk include those who have had a radical mastectomy, lymph node dissection (upper and lower extremities), blockage of the lymphatic system from tumor burden, radiation therapy to the lymphatic system, or any combination of these.

- Assess the involved extremity for the degree of edema, quality of the peripheral pulses, color, circumference, sensation, and ROM.
- Assess for signs of infection: tenderness, erythema, and warmth at the edematous site.
- Elevate and position the involved extremity on a pillow in slight abduction.
- Encourage wearing loose-fitting clothing.
- Consult PT and health care provider about development of exercise plan for ensuring mobility. Suggest use of elastic bandages to promote a decrease in mild, chronic lymphedema or use of compressive bandages or sequential compression devices for more severe cases of swelling.

NIC: Circulatory Precautions; Peripheral Sensation Management; Positioning; Teaching: Disease Process

Altered urinary elimination related to hemorrhagic cystitis secondary to cyclophosphamide/ifosfamide treatment; oliguria or renal toxicity secondary to cisplatin or high-dose methotrexate administration; renal calculi secondary to hyperuricemia; or dysuria secondary to cystitis

Desired outcomes: Patients receiving cyclophosphamide/ifosfamide test negative for blood in their urine, and patients receiving cisplatin exhibit urine output of ≥100 ml/hr 1 hr before treatment and 4-12 hr after treatment. Patients with leukemia and lymphomas and those taking methotrexate exhibit urine pH ≥7.5.

- Ensure adequate hydration during treatment and for at least 24 hr after treatment for patients taking cyclophosphamide (Cytoxan), ifosfamide, methotrexate, and cisplatin. Teach patient the importance of drinking at least 2-3 L/day. IV hydration also may be required, especially with high-dose chemotherapy.
- Administer cyclophosphamide early in the day to minimize the retention of antimetabolites in the bladder during the night. Encourage patients to void q2hr during the day and before going to bed. Test urine for the presence of blood, and report positive results to health care provider. Monitor I&O q8hr during high-dose treatment for 48 hr after treatment. Be alert to decreasing urinary output.
- Mesna is administered before ifosfamide and then 4 hr and 8 hr after the infusion (or via a continuous infusion) to minimize the risk of hemorrhagic cystitis. Test all urine for the presence of blood. Promote fluid intake to maintain urine output approximately 100 ml/hr. Monitor I&O during infusion and for 24 hr after therapy to ensure that this level of urinary output is attained.
- For patients receiving cisplatin, prehydrate with IV fluid (150-200 ml/hr). Cisplatin can be administered as soon as the patient's urine output is ≥100-150 ml/hr. Monitor I&O hourly for 4-12 hr after therapy to ensure that urine output is maintained at ≥100-150 ml/hr. Patients may require diuretics to maintain this output. Promote fluid intake to ensure a positive fluid state for at least 24 hr after treatment, especially for patients taking diuretics. Notify health care provider promptly if urine output drops to <100 ml/hr. Urine output should be kept at a relatively high level because nephrotoxicity can occur as a side effect of this treatment.
- An alkaline urine will enhance excretion of methotrexate and of the uric acid that results from tumor lysis, which is associated with leukemia and lymphoma. Monitor I&O q8hr, being alert to a decreasing output, and test urine pH with each voiding to ensure that it is ≥7.5. Sodium bicarbonate or acetazolamide (Diamox) is used to alkalinize the urine. Allopurinol prevents uric acid formation and is often administered before chemotherapy for patients with leukemia or lymphoma.
- Urinary calculi can occur as a result of hyperuricemia caused by chemotherapy treatment for leukemia and lymphoma, which causes rapid cell lysis and increased excretion of uric acid. For more information, see "Ureteral Calculi," p. 164.

- Teach patient the signs of cystitis, which can occur as a result of cyclophosphamide and ifosfamide treatment: fever, pain with urination, malodorous or cloudy urine, and urinary frequency and urgency. Instruct patient to notify health care professional if these signs and symptoms occur.

NIC: Bedside Laboratory Testing; Fluid Management; Intravenous (IV) Therapy; Medication Management; Teaching: Disease Process

See Also: "Atelectasis," p. 2 (for patients with myelosuppression); Nursing diagnoses and interventions in "Pneumonia," p. 9; "Pulmonary Fibrosis," p. 42 (for patients receiving bleomycin therapy); "Heart Failure," p. 68 (for patients experiencing cardiotoxicity and who are taking chemotherapeutic agents, such as doxorubicin or daunorubicin); "Hepatic and Biliary Disorders," p. 476 (for patients taking hepatotoxic medications, such as cyclophosphamide and methotrexate).

Psychosocial care for the patient

Knowledge deficit: Current health status and therapies
Desired outcome: Before invasive procedure, surgical procedure, or hospital discharge (as appropriate), patient verbalizes understanding about his or her current health status and therapies.

- Assess patient's current level of knowledge about his or her health status.
- Assess cognitive and emotional readiness to learn.
- Recognize barriers to learning, such as ineffective communication, neurologic deficit, sensory alterations, fear, anxiety, or lack of motivation.
- Assess learning needs, and establish short-term and long-term goals.
- Use individualized verbal or written information to promote learning and enhance understanding. Give simple, direct instructions. As indicated, use audiovisual tools as supplemental information.
- Encourage significant other to reinforce correct information about diagnosis and therapies to the patient.
- As appropriate, facilitate referral of neurologically impaired patient to neurologic clinical nurse specialist or neuropsychologist.
- Encourage patient's interest in health care information by planning care collaboratively. Explain rationale for care and therapies.
- Talk frequently with patient to evaluate comprehension of information given. Ask patient to repeat what he or she has been told. Individuals in crisis often need repeated explanations before information can be understood. Also be aware that many individuals may not understand seemingly simple medical terms (e.g., *terminal, malignant, constipation*). Provide written information to reinforce teaching.
- As appropriate, assess understanding of informed consent. Assist patient to use information he or she receives to make informed health care decisions (e.g., about invasive procedures, surgery, resuscitation).

NIC: Anxiety Reduction; Learning Readiness Enhancement; Teaching: Disease Process; Teaching: Individual; Teaching: Preoperative; Teaching: Prescribed Activity

Anxiety related to actual or perceived threat of death, change in health status, threat to self-concept or role, unfamiliar people and environment, or the unknown
Desired outcome: Within 1-2 hr of intervention, patient's anxiety has resolved or decreased as evidenced by patient's verbalization of same, HR ≤100 bpm, RR ≤20 breaths/min, and absence of or decreased irritability and restlessness.

- Engage in honest communication with the patient; provide empathetic understanding. Listen closely, and establish an atmosphere that allows free expression.
- Assess the patient's level of anxiety. Be alert to verbal and nonverbal cues.
  —*Mild:* restlessness, irritability, increase in questions, focusing on the environment.
  —*Moderate:* inattentiveness, expressions of concern, narrowed perceptions, insomnia, increased HR.
  —*Severe:* expressions of feelings of doom, rapid speech, tremors, poor eye contact. Patient may be preoccupied with the past; may be unable to understand the present; and may have tachycardia, nausea, and hyperventilation.
  —*Panic:* inability to concentrate or communicate, distortion of reality, increased motor activity, vomiting, tachypnea.
- For patients with severe anxiety or panic state, refer to psychiatric clinical nurse specialist, case manager, or other health team members as appropriate.
- If patient is hyperventilating, encourage slow, deep breaths by having patient mimic your own breathing pattern and have patient concentrate on a focal point.
- Validate the nursing assessment of anxiety with the patient (e.g., "You seem distressed; are you feeling uncomfortable now?").
- After an episode of anxiety, review and discuss with patient the thoughts and feelings that led to the episode.
- Identify the patient's current coping behaviors (e.g., denial, anger, repression, withdrawal, daydreaming, or dependence on narcotics, sedatives, or tranquilizers). Review coping behaviors patient has used in the past. Assist patient with using adaptive coping to manage anxiety (e.g., "I understand that your wife reads to you to help you relax. Would you like to spend a part of each day alone with her?").
- Encourage patient to express fears, concerns, and questions (e.g., "I know this room looks like a maze of wires and tubes; please let me know when you have any questions.").
- Reduce sensory overload by providing an organized, quiet environment (see **Sensory/perceptual alterations,** p. 793).
- Introduce self and other health care team members; explain each individual's role as it relates to the patient's care.
- Teach patient relaxation and imagery techniques. See **Health-seeking behaviors:** Relaxation technique effective for stress reduction, p. 59.
- Enable support persons to be in attendance whenever possible.
- Engage in and promote awareness of touch to significant other when appropriate. Kinds of touch are described in Table A-15.

NIC: Active Listening; Anxiety Reduction; Calming Technique; Coping Enhancement; Crisis Intervention; Presence; Touch

Impaired verbal communication related to neurologic or anatomic deficit, psychologic or physical barriers (e.g., tracheostomy, intubation), or cultural or developmental differences

Desired outcome: At the time of intervention, patient communicates needs and feelings and reports decreased or absent feelings of frustration over communication barriers.

- Assess cause of the impaired communication (e.g., tracheostomy, cerebrovascular accident, cerebral tumor, Guillain-Barré syndrome).
- Involve patient and significant other in assessing patient's ability to read, write, and understand English. If patient speaks a language other than English, collaborate with English-speaking family member or an interpreter to establish effective communication.
- When communicating with patient, face the patient, make direct eye contact, and speak in a clear, normal tone of voice.

TABLE A-15   Kinds of Touch

Instrumental touch
>   Task or procedure related
>   May be negatively perceived but accepted as impersonal

Affective touch
>   Expressive, personal
>   Caring
>   Comforting
>   May be positively or negatively perceived
>   Influenced by cultural patterns

Therapeutic touch
>   A deliberate intervention to accomplish a purpose (e.g., massage, acupressure)

- If patient cannot speak because of a physical barrier (e.g., tracheostomy, wired mandibles), provide reassurance and acknowledge his or her frustration (e.g., "I know this is frustrating for you, but please do not give up. I want to understand you.").
- Provide slate, word cards, pencil and paper, alphabet board, pictures, or other device to assist patient with communication. Adapt the call system to meet the patient's needs. Document the meaning of the signals used by the patient to communicate.
- Explain the source of the patient's communication impairment to significant other; teach significant other effective communication alternatives (see above).
- Be alert to nonverbal messages, such as facial expressions, hand movements, and nodding of the head. Validate their meaning with patient.
- Recognize that the inability to speak may foster maladaptive behaviors. Encourage patient to communicate needs; reinforce independent behaviors.
- Be honest with patient; do not pretend to understand if you are unable to interpret patient's communication.

NIC: Active Listening; Communication Enhancement: Hearing Deficit; Communication Enhancement: Speech Deficit; Communication Enhancement: Visual Deficit; Referral

Sensory/perceptual alterations related to therapeutically or socially restricted environment; psychologic stress; altered sensory reception, transmission, or integration; or chemical alteration
Desired outcome: At the time of intervention, patient verbalizes orientation to person, place, and time; reports the ability to concentrate; and expresses satisfaction with the degree and type of sensory stimulation being received.
- Assess factors contributing to patient's sensory-perceptual alteration:
    —*Environmental:* excessive noise in the environment; constant, monotonous noise; restricted environment (immobility, traction, isolation); social isolation (restricted visitors, impaired communication); therapies.
    —*Physiologic:* altered organ function, sleep or rest pattern disturbance, medication, previous history of altered sensory perception.
- Determine sensory stimulation appropriate for the patient, and plan care accordingly.
- Manage factors that contribute to environmental overload (e.g., avoid constant lighting [maintain day/night patterns]; reduce noise whenever possible [decrease alarm volumes, avoid loud talking, keep room door closed, provide earplugs]).

- Provide meaningful sensory stimulation:
  - —Display clocks, large calendars, and meaningful photographs and objects from home.
  - —Depending on patient preference, provide a radio, music, reading materials, and tape recordings of family and significant other. Earphones help to block out external stimuli.
  - —Position patient to look toward window when possible.
  - —Discuss current events, time of day, holidays, and topics of interest during patient care activities (e.g., "Good morning, Mr. Smith. I'm Ms. Stone, your nurse for the afternoon and evening, 3 PM to 11 PM. It's sunny outside. Today is the first day of summer.").
  - —As needed, orient patient to surroundings. Direct patient to reality as necessary.
  - —Establish personal contact by touch to help promote and maintain patient's contact with the real environment.
  - —Encourage significant other to communicate with patient frequently, using a normal tone of voice.
  - —Convey concern and respect for the patient. Introduce yourself, and call patient by name.
  - —Stimulate patient's vision with mirrors, colored decorations, and pictures.
  - —Stimulate patient's sense of taste with sweet, salty, and sour substances as allowed.
  - —Encourage use of eyeglasses and hearing aids.
- Inform patient before initiating therapies and using equipment.
- Encourage patient to participate in health care planning and decision making whenever possible. Allow for choice when possible.
- Assess patient's sleep/rest pattern to evaluate its contribution to the sensory/perceptual disorder. Make sure that patient attains at least 90 min of uninterrupted sleep as often as possible. For more information, see next nursing diagnosis.

NIC: Communication Enhancement: Visual Deficit; Energy Management; Environmental Management; Medication Administration; Medication Management; Simple Relaxation Therapy

Sleep pattern disturbance related to environmental changes, illness, therapeutic regimen, pain, immobility, or psychologic stress
Desired outcomes: After discussion, patient identifies factors that promote sleep. Within 8 hr of intervention, patient attains 90-min periods of uninterrupted sleep and verbalizes satisfaction with his or her ability to rest.

- Assess patient's usual sleeping patterns (e.g., bedtime routine, hours of sleep per night, sleeping position, use of pillows and blankets, napping during the day, nocturia).
- Explore relaxation techniques that promote patient's rest/sleep (e.g., imagining relaxing scenes, listening to soothing music or taped stories, using muscle relaxation exercises).
- Identify causative factors and activities that contribute to patient's insomnia, awaken patient, or adversely affect sleep patterns (e.g., pain, anxiety, therapies, depression, hallucinations, medications, underlying illness, sleep apnea, respiratory disorder, caffeine, fear).
- Organize procedures and activities to allow for 90-min periods of uninterrupted rest/sleep. Limit visiting during these periods.
- Whenever possible, maintain a quiet environment by providing earplugs or reducing alarm volume. White noise (i.e., low-pitched, monotonous sounds: electric fan, soft music) may facilitate sleep. Dim the lights for a period of time each day by drawing the drapes or providing blindfolds.
- If appropriate, put limitations on patient's daytime sleeping. Attempt to establish regularly scheduled daytime activity (e.g., ambulation, sitting in chair, active ROM), which may promote nighttime sleep.

- Investigate and provide nonpharmacologic comfort measures that are known to promote patient's sleep (see Table A-8).

NIC: Energy Management; Environmental Management: Comfort; Medication Administration; Medication Management; Simple Relaxation Therapy; Sleep Enhancement

Fear related to separation from support systems, unfamiliarity with environment or therapeutic regimen, or loss of sense of control
Desired outcome: Following intervention, patient expresses fears and concerns and reports feeling greater psychologic and physical comfort.
- Assess patient's perceptions of the environment and health status and determine factors contributing to patient's feelings of fear. Evaluate patient's verbal and nonverbal responses.
- Acknowledge patient's fears (e.g., "I understand that this equipment frightens you, but it is necessary to help you breathe.").
- Provide opportunities for patient to express fears and concerns (e.g., "You seem very concerned about receiving more blood today."). Listen closely to the patient. Recognize that anger, denial, occasional withdrawal, and demanding behaviors may be coping responses.
- Encourage patient to ask questions and gather information about the unknown. Provide information about equipment, therapies, and routines according to patient's ability to understand.
- To promote an increased sense of control, encourage patient to participate in and plan care whenever possible. Provide continuity of care by establishing a routine and arranging for consistent caregivers whenever possible. Appoint a case manager or primary nurse and associate nurses.
- Discuss with health care team members the appropriateness of medication therapy for patients with disabling fear or anxiety.
- Explore patient's desire for spiritual or psychologic counseling.
- When there is a question of the patient surviving the illness or surgery, consult health care provider about a visit by another individual with the same disorder or situation who has survived the surgery or disorder.

NIC: Anxiety Reduction; Coping Enhancement; Support Group; Support System Enhancement; Teaching: Disease Process

Ineffective individual coping related to health crisis, sense of vulnerability, or inadequate support systems
Desired outcome: Within 24 hr of this diagnosis, patient verbalizes feelings, identifies strengths and coping behaviors, and does not demonstrate ineffective coping behaviors.
- Assess patient's perceptions and ability to understand current health status.
- Establish honest communication with the patient (e.g., "Please tell me what I can do to help you."). Help patient to identify strengths, stressors, inappropriate behaviors, and personal needs.
- Support positive coping behaviors (e.g., "I see that reading that book seems to help you relax.").
- Provide opportunities for the patient to express concerns; gather information from nurses and other support persons or systems. Provide patient with explanations about prescribed routine, therapies, and equipment. Acknowledge patient's feelings and assessment of current health status and environment.
- Identify factors that inhibit patient's ability to cope (e.g., unsatisfactory support system, knowledge deficit, grief, fear).
- Recognize maladaptive coping behaviors (e.g., severe depression; dependence on narcotics, sedatives, or tranquilizers; hostility; violence; suicidal ideation). Confront patient about these behaviors (e.g., "You seem to be requiring more pain medication. Are you having more physical pain, or does

it help you cope with your situation?''). Refer patient to psychiatric liaison, clinical nurse specialist, case manager, or clergy as appropriate.
- As patient's condition allows, assist with reducing anxiety. See **Anxiety,** p. 791.
- Help reduce patient's sensory overload by maintaining an organized, quiet environment. See **Sensory/perceptual alterations,** p. 793.
- Encourage regular visits by significant other. Encourage him or her to talk with patient to help minimize patient's emotional and social isolation.
- Assess significant other's interactions with patient. Attempt to mobilize support persons or systems by involving them in patient care whenever possible.
- As appropriate, explain to significant other that increased dependency, anger, and denial may be adaptive coping behaviors used by patient in early stages of crisis until effective coping behaviors are learned.

NIC: Anxiety Reduction; Coping Enhancement; Decision-Making Support; Presence; Support Group; Support System Enhancement

Anticipatory grieving related to perceived potential loss of physiologic well-being (e.g., expected loss of body function or body part, changes in self-concept or body image, illness, death)
Desired outcome: Following intervention, patient and significant other express grief, participate in decisions about the future, and discuss concerns with health care team members and each other.
- Assess factors contributing to anticipated loss.
- Assess and accept patient's behavioral response. Expect reactions such as disbelief, denial, guilt, anger, and depression. Determine patient's stage of grieving as described in Table A-16.
- Assess spiritual, religious, and sociocultural expectations related to loss (e.g., "Is religion an important part of your life? How do you and your family deal with serious health problems?"). Refer to the clergy or community support groups as appropriate.

T A B L E   A - 1 6   Stages of Grieving

Protest stage	Denial: "No, not me"
	Disbelief: "But I just saw her this morning"
	Anger
	Hostility
	Resentment
	Bargaining to postpone loss
	Appeal for help to recover loss
	Loud complaints
	Altered sleep and appetite
Disorganization	Depression
	Withdrawal
	Social isolation
	Psychomotor retardation
	Silence
Reorganization	Acceptance of loss
	Development of new interests and attachments
	Restructuring of life-style
	Return to preloss level of functioning

- Encourage patient and significant other to share their concerns (e.g., "Is there anything you'd like to talk about today?"). Also respect their desire not to speak.
- Demonstrate empathy (e.g., "This must be a very difficult time for you and your family."). Touch when appropriate (see Table A-15).
- In selected circumstances, explain the grieving process. This approach may help the patient and family better understand and acknowledge their feelings.
- Assess grief reactions of patient and significant other, and identify those individuals with potential for dysfunctional grieving reactions (e.g., absence of emotion, hostility, avoidance). If the potential for dysfunctional grieving is present, refer the individual to psychiatric clinical nurse specialist, case manager, clergy, or other source of counseling as appropriate.
- When appropriate, assess patient's wishes about tissue donation.

NIC: Active Listening; Counseling; Family Support; Grief Work Facilitation; Presence; Spiritual Support

Dysfunctional grieving related to loss of physiologic well-being or chronic fatal illness
Desired outcomes: Within 24 hr of this diagnosis, patient and significant other express grief, explain the meaning of the loss, and communicate concerns with each other. The patient completes necessary self-care activities.

- Assess grief stage (see Table A-16) and previous coping abilities. Discuss with patient and significant other their feelings, the meaning of the loss, and their goals (e.g., "How do you feel about your condition/illness? What do you hope to accomplish in these next few days/weeks?").
- Acknowledge and permit anger; set limits on the expression of anger to discourage destructive behavior (e.g., "I understand that you must feel very angry, but for the safety of others, you may not throw equipment.").
- Identify suicidal behavior (e.g., severe depression, statements of intent, suicide plan, previous history of suicide attempt). Ensure patient safety, and refer patient to psychiatric clinical nurse specialist, psychiatrist, clergy, or other support persons or system.
- Encourage patient and significant other to participate in ADL and diversional activities. Identify physiologic problems related to loss (e.g., eating or sleeping disorders), and intervene accordingly.
- If there is a question of the patient's surviving the illness, consult health care provider about a visit by another individual with the same disorder who has survived the surgery or illness.

NIC: Activity Therapy; Emotional Support; Grief Work Facilitation; Spiritual Support; Suicide Prevention; Surveillance: Safety

Powerlessness related to health care environment or illness-related regimen
Desired outcome: Within 24 hr of this diagnosis, patient makes decisions about care and therapies and reports an attitude of realistic hope and a sense of self-control.

- Assess with patient personal preferences, needs, values, and attitudes.
- Before providing information, assess patient's knowledge and understanding of his or her condition and care.
- Recognize patient's expressions of fear, lack of response to events, and lack of interest in information, any of which may signal patient's sense of powerlessness.
- Evaluate caregiver practices, and adjust them to support patient's sense of control (e.g., if the patient always bathes in the evening to promote relaxation before bedtime, modify the care plan to include an evening bath rather than follow the hospital routine of giving a morning bath).
- Ask patient to identify activities he or she can perform independently.

- Whenever possible, offer alternatives related to routine hygiene, diet, diversional activities, visiting hours, and treatment times.
- Ensure patient's privacy and preserve his or her territorial rights whenever possible (e.g., when distant relatives and casual acquaintances request information about the patient's status, check with patient and family members before sharing that information).
- Discourage patient's dependency on staff. Avoid overprotection and parenting behaviors toward patient. Instead, act as an advocate for the patient and significant other.
- Assess support systems; involve significant other in patient care whenever possible.
- Offer realistic hope for the future. On occasion, encourage patient to direct his or her thoughts beyond the present.
- Determine the patient's wishes about end-of-life decisions, and document advanced directives as appropriate.
- Refer to clergy and other support persons or systems as appropriate.

NIC: Activity Therapy; Emotional Support; Mutual Goal Setting; Self-Esteem Enhancement; Self-Responsibility Facilitation

Spiritual distress related to separation from religious ties or cultures or challenged belief and value system
Desired outcome: Within 24 hr of this diagnosis, patient verbalizes his or her religious beliefs and expresses hope for the future, the attainment of spiritual well-being, and resolution of conflicts.

- Assess patient's spiritual or religious beliefs, values, and practices (e.g., "Do you have a religious preference? How important is it to you? Are there any religious or spiritual practices you wish to participate in while in the hospital?"). If the patient expresses a desire, volunteer to read scripture or other religious literature.
- Inform patient and significant other of the availability of spiritual resources, such as a chapel or volunteer chaplain.
- Display a nonjudgmental attitude toward patient's religious or spiritual beliefs and values. Attempt to create an environment that is conducive to free expression.
- Identify available support persons or systems that may assist in meeting the patient's religious or spiritual needs (e.g., clergy, fellow church members, support groups).
- Be alert to comments related to spiritual concerns or conflicts (e.g., "I don't know why God is doing this to me." "I'm being punished for my sins.").
- Listen closely and ask questions to help patient resolve conflicts related to spiritual issues (e.g., "I understand that you want to be baptized. We can arrange to do that here.").
- Provide privacy and opportunities for religious practices, such as prayer and meditation.
- If spiritual beliefs and therapeutic regimens are in conflict, provide patient with honest, concrete information to encourage informed decision making (e.g., "I understand that your religion discourages receiving blood transfusions. Do you understand that by refusing blood you make your condition more difficult to treat?").
- Refer patient or significant other to an ethics committee to assist in resolving care dilemmas, if appropriate.

NIC: Active Listening; Decision-Making Support; Emotional Support; Family Support; Referral; Spiritual Support; Values Clarification

Social isolation related to altered health status, inability to engage in satisfying personal relationships, altered mental status, body image change, or altered physical appearance

TABLE A-17   Indicators Suggesting Body Image Disturbance

Nonverbal indicators

Missing body part—internal or external (e.g., splenectomy, amputated extremity)

Change in structure (e.g., open, draining wound)

Change in function (e.g., colostomy)

Avoidance of looking at or touching body part

Hiding or exposing body part

Verbal indicators

Expression of negative feelings about body

Expression of feelings of helplessness, hopelessness, or powerlessness

Personalization or depersonalization of missing or mutilated part

Refusal to acknowledge change in structure or function of body part

---

Desired outcome: Within 24 hr of this diagnosis, patient demonstrates interaction and communication with others.

- Assess factors contributing to patient's social isolation:
  - —Restricted visiting hours.
  - —Absence of or inadequate support system.
  - —Inability to communicate (e.g., presence of intubation/tracheostomy).
  - —Physical changes that affect self-concept.
  - —Denial or withdrawal.
  - —Hospital environment.
- Recognize patients at risk for social isolation: older adults; disabled, chronically ill, or economically disadvantaged persons.
- Assist patient to identify feelings associated with loneliness and isolation (e.g., "You seem very sad when your family leaves the room. Can you tell me more about your feelings?").
- Determine patient's need for socialization, and identify available and potential support person or systems. Explore methods for increasing social contact (e.g., TV, radio, tapes of loved ones, intercom system, more frequent visitations, scheduled interaction with nurse or support staff).
- Provide positive reinforcement for socialization that lessens the patient's feelings of isolation and loneliness (e.g., "Please continue to call me when you need to talk to someone. Talking will help both of us to better understand your feelings.").
- Facilitate patient's ability to communicate with others (see **Impaired verbal communication,** p. 792).

NIC: Activity Therapy; Counseling; Emotional Support; Environmental Management; Normalization Promotion; Socialization Enhancement

Body image disturbance related to loss or change in body parts or function or physical trauma

Desired outcomes: Within the 24-hr period before hospital discharge, patient acknowledges body changes and demonstrates movement toward incorporating changes into self-concept. Patient does not demonstrate maladaptive response, such as severe depression.

- Establish open, honest communication with the patient. Promote an environment conducive to free expression (e.g., "Please feel free to talk to me whenever you have any questions."). Assess patient for indicators suggesting body image disturbance (Table A-17).
- When planning patient's care, be aware of therapies that may influence patient's body image (e.g., medications or invasive procedures and monitoring).

- Assess patient's knowledge of the pathophysiologic process that has occurred and his or her present health status. Clarify any misconceptions.
- Discuss the loss or change with the patient. Recognize that what may seem to be a small change may be of great significance to the patient (e.g., arm immobilizer, catheter, hair loss, ecchymoses, facial abrasions).
- Explore with patient concerns, fears, and feelings of guilt (e.g., "I understand that you are frightened. Your face looks very different now, but you will see changes and it will improve. Gradually you will begin to look more like yourself.").
- Encourage patient and significant other to interact with one another. Help family to avoid reinforcement of their loved one's unhappiness over a changed body part or function (e.g., "I know your son looks very different to you now, but it would help if you speak to him and touch him as you would normally.").
- Encourage patient to participate gradually in self-care activities as he or she becomes physically and emotionally able. Allow for some initial withdrawal and denial behaviors (e.g., when changing dressings over traumatized part, explain what you are doing but do not expect the patient to watch or participate initially).
- Discuss opportunities for reconstruction of the loss or change (e.g., surgery, prosthesis, grafting, PT, cosmetic therapies, organ transplant).
- Recognize manifestations of severe depression (e.g., sleep disturbances, change in affect, change in communication pattern). As appropriate, refer to psychiatric clinical nurse specialist, case manager, clergy, or support group.
- Help patient attain a sense of autonomy and control by offering choices and alternatives whenever possible. Emphasize patient's strengths, and encourage activities that interest patient.
- Offer realistic hope for the future.

NIC: Body Image Enhancement; Coping Enhancement; Counseling; Emotional Support; Self-Esteem Enhancement

Risk for violence with risks related to sensory overload, suicidal behavior, rage reactions, temporal lobe epilepsy, perceived threats, or toxic reaction to medications
Desired outcome: Patient does not harm self or others.
- Assess factors that may contribute to or precipitate violent behavior (e.g., medication reactions, inability to cope, suicidal behavior, confusion, hypoxia, postictal states).
- Attempt to eliminate or treat causative factors (e.g., provide patient teaching, reorient patient, ensure delivery of prescribed oxygen therapy, reduce or prevent sensory overload; see **Sensory/perceptual alterations,** p. 793).
- Assess for history of physical aggression or family violence as maladaptive coping behaviors.
- Monitor for early signs of increasing anxiety and agitation (e.g., restlessness, verbal aggressiveness, inability to concentrate). Assess for body language that is indicative of violent behavior: clenched fists, rigid posture, increased motor activity.
- Approach patient in a positive manner, and encourage verbalization of feelings and concerns (e.g., "I understand that you are frightened. I will be here from 3 PM to 11 PM to care for you.").
- Offer patient as much personal and environmental control as the situation allows (e.g., "Let's discuss the care you will need today. What fluids would you like to drink? Would you prefer a bath in the morning or evening?").
- Help patient distinguish reality from altered perceptions. Orient patient to person, place, and time. Alter the environment to promote reality-based thought processes (e.g., provide clocks, calendars, pictures of loved ones, familiar objects).

- For patients with acute confusion who become aggressive, do not attempt to reorient them and avoid arguing with them. Instead, state, "I can understand why you may [hear, think, see] that." Use nonthreatening mannerisms, facial expressions, and tone of voice.
- Initiate measures that prevent or reduce excessive agitation:
  —Reduce environmental stimuli (e.g., alarms, loud or unnecessary talking).
  —Before touching patient, explain procedures and care, using short, concise statements.
  —Speak quietly (but firmly, as necessary), and project a caring attitude toward the patient (e.g., "We are very concerned for your comfort and safety. Can we do anything to help you feel more relaxed?").
  —Avoid crowding (e.g., of equipment, visitors, health care personnel) in patient's personal environment.
  —Avoid direct confrontation.
- Explain and discuss patient's behavior with significant other. Acknowledge frustration, concerns, fears, and questions. Review safety precautions with significant other (see next intervention).
- In the event of violent behavior, institute safety precautions as discussed in Table A-18.

NIC: Anger Control Assistance; Behavior Management; Calming Technique; Environmental Management: Violence Prevention; Support System Enhancement; Surveillance: Safety

Hopelessness related to prolonged isolation or activity restriction, failing or deteriorating physiologic condition, long-term stress, or loss of faith in God or belief system
Desired outcome: Within the 24-hr period before hospital discharge, patient verbalizes hopeful aspects of health status and reports that feelings of despair are absent or lessened.

- Develop open, honest communication with the patient. Listen closely, provide empathetic understanding of fears and doubts, and promote an environment that is conducive to free expression.

TABLE A-18	Safety Precautions in the Event of Violent Behavior
Patient safety	Remove harmful objects from the environment, such as heavy objects, scissors
	Apply padding to side rails according to agency protocol
	Use restraints as necessary and prescribed; monitor patient's neurovascular status at frequent intervals
	Set limits on patient's behavior, using clear and simple commands
	As prescribed, consider chemical sedation when unable to control patient's behavior by other means
	Explain safety precautions to patient and family
Caregiver safety	Alert hospital security department when risk of violence is present
	Do not approach violent patient without adequate assistance from others
	Never turn your back on a violent patient
	Maintain a calm, matter-of-fact tone of voice
	Monitor security measures often
	Remain alert

- Assess patient's and significant other's understanding of patient's health status and prognosis; clarify any misperceptions.
- Assess for indicators of hopelessness: unwillingness to accept help, pessimism, withdrawal, lack of interest, silence, loss of gratification in roles, previous history of hopeless behavior, hypoactivity, inability to accomplish tasks, expressions of incompetence, closing eyes, and turning away.
- Provide opportunities for the patient to feel cared for, needed, and valued by others (e.g., emphasize importance of relationships by saying "Tell me about your grandchildren." "It seems that your family loves you very much.").
- Support significant other who seems to spark or maintain patient's feelings of hope (e.g., "Your husband's mood seemed to improve after your visit.").
- Recognize discussions and factors that promote patient's sense of hope (e.g., discussions about family members, reminiscing about better times).
- Explore patient's coping mechanisms; assist patient in expanding positive coping behavior (see **Ineffective individual coping,** p. 795).
- Assess patient's spiritual state and needs (see **Spiritual distress,** p. 798).
- Promote anticipation of positive events (e.g., mealtime, grandchildren's visits, bath time, extubation, discontinuation of traction).
- Help patient recognize that although there may be no hope for returning to original life-style, there *is* hope for a new, but different life.
- Avoid insisting that the patient assume a positive attitude. Encourage hope for the future, even if it is the hope for a peaceful death.
- Set realistic, attainable goals, and reward achievement.

NIC: Emotional Support; Hope Instillation; Mood Management; Presence; Socialization Enhancement

Psychosocial care for the patient's family and significant other

Altered family processes related to situational crisis (patient's illness)

Desired outcome: Following intervention, significant other demonstrates effective adaptation to change/traumatic situation as evidenced by seeking external support when necessary and sharing concerns within the family unit.

- Assess the family's character: social, environmental, ethnic, and cultural factors; relationships; and role patterns. Identify family developmental stage (e.g., the family may be dealing with other situational or maturational crises, such as an elderly parent or a teenager with a learning disability).
- Assess previous adaptive behaviors (e.g., "How does your family react in stressful situations?"). Discuss observed conflicts and communication breakdown (e.g., "I noticed that your brother would not visit your mother today. Has there been a problem we should be aware of? Knowing about it may help us better care for your mother.").
- Acknowledge the family's involvement in patient care, and promote strengths (e.g., "You were able to encourage your wife to turn and cough. That is very important to her recovery."). Encourage family to participate in patient care conferences. Promote frequent, regular patient visits by family members.
- Provide the family with information and guidance related to the critically ill patient. Discuss the stresses of hospitalization, and encourage the family to discuss feelings of anger, guilt, hostility, depression, fear, or sorrow (e.g., "You seem to be upset since being told that your husband is not leaving the hospital today."). Refer to clergy, clinical nurse specialist, or social services as appropriate.
- Evaluate patient and family responses to one another. Encourage family to reorganize roles and establish priorities as appropriate (e.g., "I know your husband is concerned about his insurance policy and seems to expect you to investigate it. I'll ask the financial counselor to talk with you.").

- Encourage the family to schedule periods of rest and activity outside the hospital and to seek support when necessary (e.g., "Your neighbor volunteered to stay in the waiting room this afternoon. Would you like to rest at home? I'll call you if *anything* changes.").

◎ NIC: Family Integrity Promotion; Family Process Maintenance; Family Therapy; Normalization Promotion; Support System Enhancement

Family coping: Potential for growth related to use of support persons or systems, referrals, and choosing experiences that optimize wellness
Desired outcomes: At the time of the patient's diagnosis, significant other expresses intent to use support persons or systems and resources and identifies alternative behaviors that promote family communication and strengths. Significant other expresses realistic expectations and does not demonstrate ineffective coping behaviors.

- Assess family relationships, interactions, support persons or systems, and individual coping behaviors. Permit movement through stages of adaptation. Encourage further positive coping.
- Acknowledge family expressions of hope, future plans, and growth among family members.
- Encourage development of open, honest communication within the family. Provide opportunities in a private setting for family interactions, discussions, and questions (e.g., "I know the waiting room is very crowded. Would your family like some private time together?").
- Refer the family to community or support groups (e.g., ostomy support group, head injury rehabilitation group).
- Encourage the family to explore outlets that foster positive feelings (e.g., periods of time outside the hospital area, meaningful communication with the patient or support individuals, and relaxing activities such as showering, eating, exercising).

◎ NIC: Family Integrity Promotion; Family Involvement; Family Mobilization; Family Support; Spiritual Support

Ineffective family coping: Compromised related to inadequate or incorrect information or misunderstanding, temporary family disorganization and role change, exhausted support persons or systems, unrealistic expectations, fear, or anxiety
Desired outcome: Following intervention, significant other verbalizes feelings, identifies ineffective coping patterns, identifies strengths and positive coping behaviors, and seeks information and support from the nurse or other support persons or systems outside the family.

- Establish open, honest communication within the family. Assist the family in identifying strengths, stressors, inappropriate behaviors, and personal needs (e.g., "I understand your mother was very ill last year. How did you manage the situation?" "I know your loved one is very ill. How can I help you?").
- Assess family members for ineffective coping (e.g., depression, chemical dependency, violence, withdrawal), and identify factors that inhibit effective coping (e.g., inadequate support system, grief, fear of disapproval by others, knowledge deficit). For example, "You seem to be unable to talk about your husband's illness. Is there anyone with whom you can talk about it?"
- Assess the family's knowledge about the patient's current health status and treatment. Provide information frequently, and allow sufficient time for questions. Reassess the family's understanding at frequent intervals.
- Provide opportunities in a private setting for family to talk and share concerns with nurses. If appropriate, refer family to psychiatric clinical nurse specialist for therapy.
- Offer realistic hope. Help the family to develop realistic expectations for the future and to identify support persons or systems that will assist them with planning for the future.

- Assist family with reducing anxiety by encouraging diversional activities (e.g., period of time outside the hospital) and interaction with support persons or systems outside the family (e.g., "I know you want to be near your son, but if you would like to go home to rest, I will call you if *any* changes occur.").

NIC: Family Involvement; Family Support; Presence; Spiritual Support

Ineffective family coping: Disabling related to unexpressed feelings, ambivalent family relationships, or disharmonious coping styles among family members
Desired outcome: Within the 24-hr period before hospital discharge, significant other verbalizes feelings, identifies sources of support as well as ineffective coping behaviors that create ambivalence and disharmony, and does not demonstrate destructive behaviors.

- Establish open, honest communication and rapport with family members (e.g., "I am here to care for your mother and to help your family as well.").
- Identify ineffective coping behaviors (e.g., violence, depression, substance misuse, withdrawal). For example, "You seem to be angry. Would you like to talk to me about your feelings?" Refer to psychiatric clinical nurse specialist, case manager, clergy, or support group as appropriate.
- Identify perceived or actual conflicts (e.g., "Are you able to talk freely with your family members?" "Are your brothers and sisters able to help and support you during this time?").
- Assist family in search for healthy functioning within the family unit (e.g., facilitate open communication among family members and encourage behaviors that support family cohesiveness). For example, "Your mother enjoyed your last visit. Would you like to see her now?"
- Assess the family's knowledge about patient's current health status. Provide opportunities for questions; reassess family's understanding at frequent intervals.
- Assist family members in developing realistic goals, plans, and actions. Refer them to clergy, psychiatric nurse, social services, financial counseling, and family therapy as appropriate.
- Encourage family members to spend time outside the hospital and to interact with support individuals. Respect the family's need for occasional withdrawal.
- Include family members in the patient's plan of care. Offer them opportunities to become involved in patient care (e.g., ROM exercises, patient hygiene, comfort measures such as back rub).

NIC: Family Involvement; Family Process Maintenance; Family Support; Family Therapy; Spiritual Support

Fear related to patient's life-threatening condition and knowledge deficit
Desired outcome: Following intervention, significant other reports that fear has lessened.

- Assess the family's fears and their understanding of the patient's clinical situation. Evaluate verbal and nonverbal responses.
- Acknowledge the family's fear (e.g., "I understand these tubes must frighten you, but they are necessary to help nourish your son.").
- Assess the family's history of coping behavior (e.g., "How does your family react to difficult situations?"). Determine resources and significant others available for support (e.g., "Who usually helps your family during stressful times?").
- Provide opportunities for family members to express fears and concerns. Recognize that anger, denial, withdrawal, and demanding behavior may be adaptive coping responses during initial period of crisis.
- Provide information at frequent intervals about patient's status, treatments, and equipment used. Demonstrate a caring attitude.

- Encourage the family to use positive coping behaviors by identifying fears, developing goals, identifying supportive resources, facilitating realistic perceptions, and promoting problem solving.
- Recognize anxiety, and encourage family members to describe their feelings (e.g., "You seem very uncomfortable tonight. Can you describe your feelings?").
- Be alert to maladaptive responses to fear: potential for violence, withdrawal, severe depression, hostility, and unrealistic expectations for staff or of patient's recovery. Provide referrals to psychiatric clinical nurse specialist or other staff member as appropriate.
- Offer *realistic* hope, even if it is hope for the patient's peaceful death.
- Explore the family's desire for spiritual or other counseling.
- Assess your own feelings about the patient's life-threatening illness. Acknowledge that your attitude and fear may be reflected to the family.
- For other interventions, see **Altered family processes** and **Ineffective family coping**, listed earlier.

NIC: Anxiety Reduction; Coping Enhancement; Presence; Security Enhancement; Teaching: Group

Knowledge deficit: Patient's current health status or therapies
Desired outcome: Following intervention, significant other verbalizes knowledge and understanding about the patient's current health status or treatment.
- At frequent intervals, inform the family about the patient's current health status, therapies, and prognosis. Use individualized verbal, written, and audiovisual strategies to promote family's understanding.
- Evaluate the family at frequent intervals for understanding of information that has been provided. Assess factors for misunderstanding, and adjust teaching as appropriate. Some individuals in crisis need repeated explanations before comprehension can be assured (e.g., "I have explained many things to you today. Would you mind summarizing what I've told you so that I can be sure you understand your husband's status and what we are doing to care for him?").
- Encourage family to relay correct information to the patient. This also will reinforce comprehension for family and patient.
- Ask family members if their needs for information are being met (e.g., "Do you have any questions about the care your mother is receiving or about her condition?").
- Help family members use the information they receive to make health care decisions about the patient (e.g., surgery, resuscitation, organ donation).
- Promote family's active participation in patient care when appropriate. Encourage family to seek information and express feelings, concerns, and questions.

NIC: Family Support; Health System Guidance; Support Group; Teaching: Group; Truth Telling

Selected Bibliography

Armstrong T et al: Neurological, pulmonary, and cutaneous toxicities of high dose chemotherapy, *Oncol Nurs Forum Suppl* 24(1):22-33, 1997.

Berg D: New chemotherapy treatment options and implications for nursing care, *Oncol Nurs Forum Suppl* 24(1):5-12, 1997.

Boyle D, Engelking C: Vesicant extravasation: myths and realities, *Oncol Nurs Forum* 22:57-67, 1995.

Brogden J, Nevidjon B: Vinorelbine tartrate (navelbine): drug profile and nursing implications of a new vinca alkaloid, *Oncol Nurs Forum* 22(4):635-646, 1995.

Bucholtz J, editor: *Guidelines for radiation safety,* Pittsburgh, 1995, Oncology Nursing Society.

Hall P: Critical care nursing: psychosocial aspects of care. In Burrell L et al, editors: *Adult nursing: acute hospital and community care,* ed 2, Norwalk, Conn, 1997, Appleton & Lange.

Interqual: *The ISD-A review system with adult ISD criteria,* Northhampton, NH, and Marlboro, Mass, August 1992, Interqual.

Kim MJ et al: *Pocket guide to nursing diagnoses,* ed 7, St Louis, 1997, Mosby.

Korinko A, Yurick A: Maintaining skin integrity during radiation therapy, *Am J Nurs* 97(2):40-44, 1997.

Management of Cancer Pain Guideline Panel: *Clinical practice guideline: management of cancer pain,* AHCPR pub. no. 94-0592, Rockville, Md, 1994, Agency for Health Care Policy and Research, Public Health Service, U.S. Department of Health and Human Services.

McCloskey JC, Bulechek GM, editors: *Nursing interventions classification (NIC),* ed 2, St Louis, 1996, Mosby.

Oncology Nursing Society: *Cancer chemotherapy guidelines and recommendations for practice,* Pittsburgh, 1996, Oncology Nursing Press.

Rieger RT, Haeuber D: A new approach to managing chemotherapy-related anemia: nursing implications of epoetinal, *Oncol Nurs Forum* 22(1):71-81, 1995.

Rogers B: Taxol: a promising new drug of the '90s, *Oncol Nurs Forum* 20(10):1483-1489, 1993.

Sandstrom SK: Nursing management of patients receiving biological therapy, *Semin Oncol Nurs* 12(2):152-162, 1996.

Skalla K: The interferons, *Semin Oncol Nurs* 12(2):97-105, 1996.

Section Four: Caring for Older Adults

Risk for aspiration with risks related to decreased masticatory muscle function secondary to age-related changes

Desired outcomes: Patient swallows independently without choking. Patient's airway is patent and lungs are clear to auscultation both before and after meals.

- Assess patient's LOC on admission and then routinely during hospital stay.
- Assess patient's ability to swallow by asking if he or she has any difficulty swallowing or if any foods or fluids are difficult to swallow or cause gagging. If patient is unable to answer, consult patient's caregiver or significant other. Document findings.
- Assess for the gag reflex by *gently* touching one side and then the other of the posterior pharynx. Document both findings.
- Place patient in an upright position while eating or drinking, and support this position with pillows on patient's sides.
- Monitor patient when he or she is swallowing. Watch for limited lip, tongue, or jaw movement as indicated by drooling of saliva or food or an inability to close lips around a straw. Check for retention of food in sides of mouth, which is an indication of poor tongue movement.
- Monitor patient for coughing or choking before, during, or after swallowing. This may occur up to several minutes following placement of food or fluid in the mouth. This signals aspiration of material into the airway.
- Monitor patient for a wet or gurgling sound when talking after a swallow. This indicates aspiration into the airway and signals a delayed or absent swallow reflex and a delayed or absent gag reflex.
- For patients with poor swallowing reflex, tilt their head forward 45 degrees during swallowing. This will help prevent inadvertent aspiration by closing

off the airway. **Note:** For patients who have hemiplegia, tilt head toward the unaffected side.
- As indicated, request evaluation by speech therapist for further assessment of gag and swallow reflex.
- Anticipate swallowing video fluoroscopy in evaluation of the patient's gag and swallow reflex. Using four consistencies of barium, the radiologist and speech therapist watch for the presence of reduced or ineffective tongue function, reduced peristalsis in the pharynx, delayed or absent swallow reflex, and poor or limited ability to close the epiglottis that protects the airway. This procedure is used to determine whether the patient is aspirating, the consistency of the materials most likely to be aspirated, and the cause of the aspiration.
- Based on results of the swallowing video fluoroscopy, thickened fluids may be prescribed. Agents are added to the fluid to make it more viscous and easier for the patient to swallow. Similarly, mechanical soft, pureed, or liquid diets may be prescribed to allow the patient to ingest food with less potential for aspiration.
- Provide adequate rest periods before meals. Fatigue increases the risk of aspiration.
- Monitor intake of food. Document consistencies and amounts of food patient eats, where patient places food in the mouth, how patient manipulates or chews before swallowing, and the length of time before patient swallows the bolus of food.
- Remind patients with dementia to chew and swallow with each bite.
- Ensure that patient has dentures in place, if appropriate, and that they fit correctly.
- Ensure that someone stays with patient during meals or fluid intake.
- Provide patient with adequate time to eat and drink. Generally, patients with swallowing deficits require twice as much time for eating and drinking as those whose swallowing is adequate.
- Monitor patient for signs of aspiration, including changes in lung auscultation (e.g., crackles [rales], wheezes, rhonchi), SOB, dyspnea, decreasing LOC, increasing temperature, and cyanosis.
- Be aware of location of suction equipment to be used in the event of aspiration. If the patient is at increased risk for aspiration, suction equipment should be available at the bedside.
- If patient aspirates, implement the following:
  —Follow American Heart Association (AHA) standards if patient displays characteristics of complete airway obstruction (i.e., choking).
  —For partial airway obstruction, encourage patient to cough as needed.
  —For partial airway obstruction in the unconscious or nonresponsive individual who is not coughing, suction the airway with a large-bore catheter such as the Yankauer or tonsil suction tip.
  —For either a complete or partial aspiration, inform health care provider and obtain prescription for chest x-ray.
  —Protect patient by implementing NPO status until diagnosis is confirmed.
  —Monitor breathing pattern and RR q1-2hr after a suspected aspiration for alterations (i.e., increased RR) that signal a change in the patient's condition.
  —Anticipate use of antibiotics to prevent infection.
  —Encourage patient to cough and deep breathe q2hr while awake and q4hr during the night to promote expansion of available lung tissue.
- **NIC:** Airway Management; Aspiration Precautions; Chest Physiotherapy; Cough Enhancement; Neurologic Monitoring; Respiratory Monitoring

Constipation related to changes in diet, activity, and psychosocial factors secondary to hospitalization

Desired outcomes: Patient states that bowel habit has returned to the patient's stated normal pattern within 3-4 days of this diagnosis. Stool appears soft, and patient does not strain in passing stools.

- On admission, assess and document patient's normal bowel elimination pattern. Include frequency, time of day, associated habits, and successful methods used to correct constipation in the past. Consult patient's caregiver or significant other if patient is unable to provide this information.
- Inform patient that changes that occur with hospitalization may increase the potential for constipation. Urge patient to institute successful nonpharmacologic methods used at home as soon as this problem is noticed or prophylactically as needed.
- Teach patient the relationship between fluid intake and constipation. Unless otherwise contraindicated, encourage fluid intake that exceeds 2500 ml/day. Monitor and record bowel movements (date, time, consistency, amount).
- Teach patient the relationship between types of foods consumed and constipation. When possible, encourage patient to include roughage as a part of each meal (e.g., raw fruits and vegetables, whole grains, nuts, fruits with skins). For the patient unable to tolerate raw foods, encourage intake of bran via cereals, muffins, and breads. Titrate the amount of roughage to the degree of constipation.
- Teach patient the relationship between constipation and activity level. Encourage optimum activity for all patients. Establish and post an activity program to enhance participation; include devices necessary to enable independence.
- Advise patient about the need to maintain normal bowel elimination pattern. Provide any materials or support environments the patient normally uses (e.g., cup of coffee on arising, privacy, short walk).
- Ask patient if the toilet seat height seems the same as that at home. If the toilet is higher, provide a footstool to raise patient's feet off the floor comfortably. A high-rise toilet seat may be used to increase the toilet's height.
- Schedule interventions to coincide with the patient's habit. If the patient's bowel movement occurs in the early morning, use the patient's gastrocolic or duodenocolic reflex to promote colonic emptying. If the patient's bowel movement occurs in the evening, ambulate the patient just before the appropriate time. Digital stimulation of the inner anal sphincter also may facilitate bowel movement.
- Attempt to use methods the patient has used successfully in the past. Follow the maxim "go low, go slow" (i.e., use the lowest amount of nonnatural intervention and advance to more powerful interventions slowly). Older persons tend to focus on the loss of habit as an indicator of constipation rather than on the number of stools. Do not intervene pharmacologically until the older adult has not had a stool for 3 days.
- When requesting a pharmacologic intervention, use the more benign, oral methods first. The following hierarchy is suggested:
  —Bulk-building additives such as psyllium or bran.
  —Mild laxatives (apple or prune juice, Milk of Magnesia).
  —Stool softeners (docusate sodium, docusate calcium).
  —Potent laxatives or cathartics (bisacodyl, cascara sagrada).
  —Medicated suppositories (glycerin, bisacodyl).
  —Enema (tap water, saline, sodium biphosphate/phosphate).
- After diagnostic imaging of the GI tract with barium, ensure that the patient receives postexamination laxative to facilitate removal of the barium. After any procedure involving a bowel clean-out, there may be rebound constipation from the severe disruption of bowel habit. Monitor hydration status for signs of dehydration, which can occur from osmotic agents used. Emphasize diet, fluid, activity, and resumption of routines. If no bowel movement occurs in 3 days, begin with mild laxatives to try to regain normal pattern.

- See also "Caring for Patients on Prolonged Bedrest," for **Constipation,** p. 743.

NIC: Bowel Management; Constipation/Impaction Management; Diet Staging; Fluid Management; Teaching: Disease Process

Risk for fluid volume deficit with risks related to inability to obtain fluids by self secondary to illness, placement of fluid, or presence of chronic illness; or related to use of osmotic agents during radiologic tests

Desired outcomes: Patient's mental status, VS, and urine specific gravity, color, consistency, and concentration remain within normal limits for patient. Patient's mucous membranes remain moist, and there is no "tenting" of skin. Patient's intake equals output.

- Monitor fluid intake. In nonrestricted individuals, encourage fluid intake of 2-3 L/day. Specify intake goals for day, evening, and night shifts.
- Assess and document skin turgor. Check hydration status by pinching skin over sternum or forehead. Skin that remains in the lifted position (tenting) and returns slowly to its original position indicates dehydration. A furrowed tongue is a signal of severe dehydration.
- Assess and document urine specific gravity and color q8hr.
- Assess and document color, amount, and frequency of any fluid output, including emesis, urine, diarrhea, or other drainage.
- Monitor patient's orientation, ability to follow commands, and behavior. Loss of ability to follow commands, decrease in orientation, and confused behavior can signal a dehydrated state.
- Weigh patient daily at the same time of day (preferably before breakfast) using the same scale and bedclothing. Be alert to wide variations in weight (e.g., ≥2.5 kg [5 lb]).
- In the patient who is dehydrated, anticipate elevation in serum Na^+, blood urea nitrogen (BUN), and serum creatinine levels.
- If the patient is receiving IV therapy, monitor cardiac and respiratory systems for signs of overload, which could precipitate heart failure or pulmonary edema. Assess the apical pulse and listen to lung fields during every VS assessment. A rising HR and crackles and bronchial wheezes in the lungs can be signals of heart failure or pulmonary edema.
- Carefully monitor I&O when the patient is receiving tube feedings or dyes for contrast. These agents act osmotically to pull fluid into the interstitial tissue. Watch for evidence of third spacing of fluids, including increasing peripheral edema, especially sacral; output significantly less than intake (1:2); and urine output <30 ml/hr.
- Offer patient fluid whenever in the room. Older persons have a decreased sense of thirst and need encouragement to drink. Offer a variety of drinks the patient likes, but limit caffeine, because caffeine tends to act as a diuretic.
- Assess patient's ability to obtain and drink fluids by self. Place fluids within easy reach. Use cups with tops to minimize concern over spilling.
- Ensure access to toilet, urinal, commode, or bedpan at least q2hr when patient is awake and q4hr at night. Answer the call light quickly. The time between recognition of the need to void and urination decreases with age.

NIC: Diarrhea Management; Fluid/Electrolyte Management; Perineal Care; Teaching: Prescribed Diet; Urinary Elimination Management

Impaired gas exchange (or risk for same) related to decreased functional lung tissue secondary to age-related changes

Desired outcomes: Patient's respiratory pattern and mental status remain normal for patient. Patient's ABG or pulse oximetry values are within patient's normal limits.

- Assess and document the following upon admission and routinely thereafter: respiratory rate, pattern, and depth; breath sounds; cough; sputum; and sensorium.

- Assess patient for subtle changes in mentation such as increased restlessness, anxiety, disorientation, and presence of hostility. If available, monitor oxygenation status via ABG findings (optimally Pao_2 ≥80%-95%) or pulse oximetry (optimally ≥92%).
- Assess lungs for the presence of adventitious sounds. **Note:** The aging lung has decreased elasticity. The lower part of the lungs is no longer adequately aerated. As a result, crackles commonly are heard in individuals 75 yr of age and older. This sign alone does not mean that a pathologic condition is present. Crackles (rales) that do not clear with coughing in an individual with no other clinical signs (e.g., fever, increasing anxiety, changes in mental status, increasing respiratory depth) are considered benign.
- Encourage patient to cough and breathe deeply to promote alveolar expansion and clear secretions from the bronchial tree. When appropriate, instruct patients in the use of incentive spirometry. Encourage fluid intake >2.5 L/day to ensure less viscous pulmonary secretions that are more easily mobilized.
- Reduce the potential for patient's increased oxygen consumption by treating fevers promptly, decreasing pain, minimizing pacing activity, and lessening anxiety.
- Instruct patient in the use of support equipment such as oxygen masks or cannulas.
- Schedule and pace patient's activities according to tolerance. Document patient's ability to accomplish ADL.

◎ NIC: Chest Physiotherapy; Cough Enhancement; Fluid Management; Oxygen Therapy; Respiratory Monitoring

Hopelessness related to slow recovery from illness or surgery secondary to decreased physiologic reserve
Desired outcome: Within 2-4 days of interventions, patient verbalizes knowledge of his or her strengths, feelings about health, and the understanding of a potentially long recovery.

- Monitor patient for signs of depression, such as refusal to participate in own care; refusal to answer questions; and statements such as "I don't care," "Leave me alone," and "Let me die."
- Encourage patient to verbalize feelings of despair, frustration, fear, and anger and concerns regarding hospitalization and health. Reassure patient and significant other that such feelings and concerns are normal.
- Discuss normal age changes with patient. Inform patient and significant other that recovery periods are longer for older adults because of decreased physiologic reserve. More energy is spent in maintaining normal status, and thus the body has less capacity to rebuild strength and endurance.
- Encourage short-term goals and praise small steps, such as participation in own care.
- Arrange a care conference to discuss discharge requirements specific to the patient. Involve patient and significant other in the conference. Set realistic goals with patient based on patient's condition and desires.

◎ NIC: Complex Relationship Building; Emotional Support; Hope Instillation; Presence; Reminiscence Therapy; Socialization Enhancement; Spiritual Support

Hypothermia related to age-related changes in thermoregulation and/or environmental exposure
Desired outcome: Patient's temperature and mental status remain within patient's normal limits or they return to patient's normal limits, at a rate of 1° F/hr, after interventions.

- Monitor patient's temperature, using a low-range thermometer if possible. Be aware that older adults can have a normal temperature of 35.5° C (96° F).

- Assess patient's temperature rectally since this will provide the most accurate assessment of the patient's core temperature. If necessary, assess temperature orally by placing the thermometer far back in the mouth. To ensure proper placement, slide the thermometer along the buccal membrane and position it under the back of the tongue. **Note:** Do not take axillary temperature in the older adult because older persons have decreased peripheral circulation and loss of subcutaneous fat in the axillary area, resulting in formation of a pocket of air that may make readings inaccurate. If unable to measure patient's temperature orally, measure temperature via ear but note that the reliability of the electronic tympanic thermometers may be inconsistent because of improper use.
- Assess and document patient's mental status. Increasing disorientation, mental status changes, or the presence of atypical behavior can signal hypothermia.
- Be alert to the following patients who are at risk for environmental hypothermia: those taking sedatives, hypnotics (including anesthetics), and muscle relaxants because these drugs decrease shivering. In addition, all older adults are at risk for environmental hypothermia at ambient temperatures of 22.22°-23.89° C (72°-75° F).
- Ensure that patients going for testing or x-rays are sent with enough blankets to keep warm.
- If patient is mildly hypothermic, initiate slow rewarming using external methods, such as raising room temperature to at least 23.89° C (75° F). Other methods of external warming include use of warm blankets, head covers, and warm circulating air blankets.
- If patient's temperature falls below 35° C (95° F), warm patient internally by administering warm oral or IV fluids. Also anticipate use of warmed saline gastric or rectal irrigations or introduction of warmed humidified air into the airway.
- Be alert to signs of too rapid rewarming: irregular HR, dysrhythmias, and very warm extremities caused by vasodilation in the periphery, which causes heat loss from the core.
- If patient's temperature fails to rise 1° F/hr using these techniques, suspect a cause other than environmental. In this event, anticipate laboratory tests, including WBC count for possible sepsis, thyroid test for hypothyroidism, and glucose level for hypoglycemia.
- As prescribed, administer antibiotics for sepsis, initiate thyroid therapy, or administer glucose for hypoglycemia. The patient's temperature will not return to normal unless the underlying condition has been treated.

NIC: Environmental Management; Hypothermia Treatment; Oxygen Therapy; Respiratory Monitoring; Skin Surveillance; Temperature Regulation

Risk for infection with risks related to age-related changes in immune and integumentary systems; related to suppressed inflammatory response secondary to long-term medication use (e.g., antiinflammatory agents, steroids, analgesics); related to slowed ciliary response; or related to poor nutrition
Desired outcome: Patient remains free of infection as evidenced by orientation to person, place, and time and behavior within patient's normal limits; respiratory rate and pattern within patient's normal limits; urine that is straw colored, clear, and of characteristic odor; core temperature and HR within patient's normal limits; sputum that is clear to whitish in color; and skin that is intact and of normal color and temperature for patient.

Note: WBC count ≥11,000/mm^3 can be a late sign of infection in older patients because the immune system is slow to respond to insult.

- Assess patient's baseline VS, including LOC and orientation. A change in mentation is a leading sign of infection in older patients. Also be alert to HR >100 bpm and RR >24 breaths/min. Auscultate lung fields for adventitious sounds. Be aware, however, that crackles (rales) may be a normal finding when heard in the lung bases.
- Monitor patient's temperature, using a low-range thermometer if possible. Be aware that a temperature of 35.5° C (96° F) may be normal for the patient. In that case, a patient with a temperature of 36.67°-37.22° C (98°-99° F) may be considered febrile.
- To ensure that the patient's core temperature is being accurately determined, obtain temperature readings rectally if the oral reading does not match the clinical picture (i.e., patient's skin is very warm, patient is restless, mentation is depressed), or if the temperature reads ≥36.11° C (97° F). If temperature measurement is done using a tympanic thermometer, note that the reliability of the electronic tympanic thermometer may be inconsistent because of improper use.
- Assess patient's skin for tears, breaks, redness, or ulcers. Document condition of the patient's skin on admission and as an ongoing assessment (refer to **Risk for impaired skin integrity,** p. 813).
- Assess the quality and color of the patient's urine. Urinary tract infections (UTIs), as manifested by cloudy, foul-smelling urine, without painful urination, are the most common infection in older adults. Document changes when noted, and report findings to the health care provider. Also be alert to urinary incontinence, which can signal UTI.
- Because of the increased risk of infection, avoid insertion of urinary catheters when possible.
- Obtain drug history in reference to use of antiinflammatory or immunosuppressive drugs or long-term use of analgesics or steroids, because these drugs mask fever.
- If infection is suspected, anticipate initiation of IV fluid therapy for maintenance of fluid balance; blood cultures, urinalysis, and urine culture to isolate bacteria type; and WBC count to determine immune response. Expect a chest x-ray to rule out pneumonia if patient's chest sounds are not clear. If infection is present, prepare for initiation of broad-spectrum antibiotic therapy, oxygen therapy to maintain adequate oxygenation to the brain, and use of acetaminophen to decrease temperature and cardiac output, which will decrease cardiac load.

NIC: Cough Enhancement; Infection Protection; Oxygen Therapy; Respiratory Monitoring; Surveillance; Wound Care

Powerlessness related to hospital environment
Desired outcome: Within 2-4 days after interventions, patient participates in care and verbalizes feelings of control over his or her environment.
- Encourage patient to verbalize feelings about hospitalization and illness.
- Assist patient in identifying factors that contribute to feelings of powerlessness.
- Encourage patient to participate in ADL as much as possible. Provide adequate time for patient to complete ADL.
- As often as possible, enable patient to participate in scheduling of activities.
- Discuss with patient and significant other realistic goals of care, and encourage patient's participation in care planning.
- Explain procedures and routines to patient. Inform patient when changes in the plan of care are necessary.
- Provide flexibility in patient's plan of care when possible (e.g., if patients want to wear their own clothes, enable them to do so).

NIC: Cognitive Restructuring; Crisis Intervention; Health System Guidance; Learning Facilitation; Patient Contracting; Self-Esteem Enhancement

Risk for impaired skin integrity with risks related to decreased subcutaneous fat and decreased peripheral capillary networks secondary to age-related changes in the integumentary system
Desired outcome: Patient's skin remains nonerythemic and intact.

- Assess patient's skin on admission and routinely thereafter. Note any areas of redness or any breaks in the skin surface.
- Ensure that patient turns frequently (at least q2hr). Lift or roll patient across sheets when repositioning. Pulling, dragging, or sliding patient across sheets can lead to shear (cutaneous or subcutaneous tissue) injury.
- Monitor skin over bony prominences (i.e., sacrum, scapulae, heels, spine, hips, pelvis, greater trochanter, knees, ankles, costal margins, occiput) for erythema. Use pillows or pads around bony prominences to protect the overlying skin, even when patient is up in a wheelchair or sits for long periods. The ischial tuberosities are prone to breakdown when patient is in the seated position. Gel pads for chair or wheelchair seats aid in distributing pressure.
- Use lotions on dry skin to promote moisture and suppleness. Lanolin-containing lotions are especially useful.
- Use alternating-pressure mattress, air-fluidized mattress, waterbed, air bed, or other pressure-sensitive mattress for older patients who are on bedrest or unable to get out of bed, to protect skin from injury caused by prolonged pressure.
- Avoid placing tubes under patient's limbs or head. Excess pressure from tubes can create a pressure ulcer. Place pillow or pad between patient and tube for cushioning.
- Optimize patient mobility; get patient out of bed as often as possible. Liberally use mechanical lifting devices to aid in safe patient transfers. If patient is unable to get out of bed, assist with position changes q2hr. Establish and post a turning schedule on the patient care plan and at the bedside.
- At a minimum, ensure that patient's face, axillae, and genital areas are cleansed daily. Complete baths dry out older adults' skin and should be given every other day instead. Use tepid water (90°-105° F [32.2°-40.5° C]) and super-fatted, nonperfumed soaps, which help decrease dry skin. Avoid hot water, which can burn older adults, who have decreased pain sensitivity and decreased sensation to temperature.
- Minimize use of plastic protective pads under patient. These pads trap moisture and heat and can lead to skin breakdown. When used, place at least one layer of cloth (drawsheet) between the patient and the plastic pad to absorb moisture.
- Document percentage of food intake with meals. Encourage significant other to provide patient's favorite foods. Suggest snacks high in protein and vitamin C if patient's diet is not restricted.
- Obtain nutritional consultation with dietitian as needed.
- Monitor serum albumin for evidence of protein status (normal value is 3.0 g/dl for older adults).
- For more information, see "Providing Nutritional Support," p. 687; "Managing Wound Care," p. 710.

NIC: Nutrition Management; Perineal Care; Pressure Ulcer Prevention; Skin Care: Topical Treatments; Skin Surveillance; Teaching: Prescribed Activity/Exercise

Sleep pattern disturbance related to unfamiliar surroundings and hospital routines
Desired outcomes: Within 24 hr of interventions, patient reports the attainment of adequate rest. Mental status remains normal for the patient.

- Assess and document patient's sleeping pattern, obtaining information from patient or patient's caregiver or significant other. Ask questions about naps and activity levels. Individuals who take naps and have a low level of activity frequently sleep only 4-5 hr/night.

- Determine patient's usual nighttime routine, and attempt to emulate it.
- Inform patient of necessary interruptions during hospitalization.
- Attempt to group together activities such as medications, VS, and toileting to reduce the number of interruptions.
- Provide comfort measures at bedtime, such as pain medications, back rub, and conversation.
- Provide patient with compatible roommate when possible.
- Monitor patient's activity level. If patient complains of being tired after activities or displays behaviors such as irritability, yelling, or shouting, encourage napping after lunch or early in the afternoon. Otherwise, discourage daytime napping by involving patient in care or activities.
- Avoid stimulants such as coffee, cola, and tea after 6 pm.
- Provide a quiet environment by avoiding loud noises and use of overhead lights and minimizing interruptions during sleep hours.

NIC: Calming Technique; Environmental Management: Comfort; Music Therapy; Progressive Muscle Relaxation; Simple Relaxation Therapy; Sleep Enhancement

Altered thought processes related to decreased cerebral perfusion secondary to age-related decreased physiologic reserve or cardiac dysfunction; electrolyte imbalance secondary to age-related decreased renal function; altered sensory/perceptual reception secondary to poor vision or hearing; or decreased brain oxygenation secondary to illness state and decreased functional lung tissue
Desired outcomes: Patient's mental status returns to normal for the patient within 3 days of treatment. Patient sustains no evidence of injury or harm as a result of mental status.

- Assess patient's baseline LOC and mental status on admission. Ask patient to perform a 3-step task (e.g., "Raise your right hand, place it on your left shoulder, and then place the right hand by your right side."). Test short-term memory by showing patient how to use the call light, having the patient return the demonstration, and then waiting at least 5 min before having patient demonstrate use of call light again. Inability to remember beyond 5 min indicates poor short-term memory. Document patient's response.
- Document patient's actions in behavioral terms. Describe the "confused" behavior.
- Obtain preconfusion functional and mental status abilities from significant other.
- Identify cause of acute confusion (e.g., consult health care provider regarding oximetry or ABG values to assess oxygenation levels; serum glucose or fingerstick glucose to determine glucose level; and electrolytes and CBC to ascertain imbalances and/or presence of elevated WBC count as a determinant of infection). Assess hydration status by pinching skin over the sternum or forehead for turgor and checking for dry mucous membranes and furrowed tongue.
- Review cardiac status. Assess apical pulse, and notify health care provider of an irregular pulse that is new to the patient. If patient is on a cardiac monitor or telemetry, watch for dysrhythmias; notify health care provider accordingly.
- Review current medications, including OTC drugs, with the pharmacist. Toxic levels of certain medications, such as digoxin or theophylline, cause acute confusion. Drugs that are anticholinergic also can cause confusion, as can drug interactions.
- Monitor I&O at least q8hr. Output should match intake. Anticipate/encourage a creatinine clearance test to assess renal function. **Note:** BUN and serum creatinine are affected by hydration status. Serum creatinine is affected by the aging process because lower muscle mass produces lower creatinine. Normal

serum creatinine levels in a well-hydrated older adult can therefore signal renal insufficiency.

- Have patient wear glasses and hearing aid, or keep them close to the bedside and within easy reach for patient use.
- Keep patient's urinal and other routinely used items within easy reach for the patient. If patient has short-term memory problems, do not expect him or her to use the call light. Toilet or offer patient urinal or bedpan q2hr while awake and q4hr during the night. Establish a toileting schedule, and post it on the patient care plan and, inconspicuously, at the bedside.
- Check on the patient at least q30min and every time you pass the room.
- Place patient close to the nurses' station if possible. Provide an environment that is nonstimulating and safe. Provide music but not TV (patients who are confused regarding place and time often think the action on TV is happening in the room).
- Attempt to reorient patient to surroundings as needed. Keep a clock with large numerals and large print calendar at the bedside, and verbally remind patient of the date and day as needed.
- Tell patient in simple terms what is occurring (e.g., "It's time to eat breakfast," "This medicine is for your heart," "I'm going to help you get out of bed.").
- Encourage patient's significant other to bring items familiar to patient, including blanket, bedspread, pictures of family and pets.
- If patient becomes belligerent, angry, or argumentative while you are attempting to reorient, **stop this approach.** Do not argue with patient or patient's interpretation of the environment. State, "I can understand why you may (hear, think, see) that."
- If patient displays hostile behavior or misperceives your role (nurse becomes, e.g., thief, jailer), leave the room. Return in 15 min. Introduce yourself to the patient as though you had never met. Begin dialogue anew. Patients who are acutely confused have poor short-term memory and may not remember the previous encounter or that you were involved in that encounter. When you return, enable patient to share feelings about the previous encounter as appropriate.
- If patient attempts to leave the hospital, walk with patient and attempt distraction. Ask patient to tell you about the destination (e.g., "That sounds like a wonderful place! Tell me about it."). Keep tone pleasant and conversational. Continue walking with patient away from exits and doors around the unit. After a few minutes, attempt to guide patient back to the room. Offer refreshments and a rest (e.g.,"We've been walking for a while and I'm a little tired. Why don't we sit and have some juice while we talk?").
- If the patient has a permanent or severe cognitive impairment, check on her or him at least q30min and reorient to baseline mental status as indicated; however, do not argue with patient about his or her perception of reality. This can cause a cognitively impaired person to become aggressive and combative. **Note:** Individuals with severe cognitive impairment (e.g., Alzheimer's disease or dementia) also can experience acute confusional states (i.e., delirium) and can be returned to their baseline mental state.
- If the patient tries to climb out of bed, he or she may need to use the toilet; offer the urinal or bedpan, or assist to the commode. Alternately, if patient is not on bedrest, place him or her in chair or wheelchair at nurses' station for added supervision.
- Bargain with patient. Try to establish an agreement to stay for a defined period of time, such as until the health care provider, breakfast or lunch, or significant other arrives.
- Have patient's significant other talk with patient by phone or come in and sit with patient if patient's behavior requires checking more often than q30min.
- If patient is attempting to pull out tubes, hide the tubes (e.g., under blankets). Put stockinette mesh dressing over IV lines. Tape feeding tubes to the side of

the face using paper tape, and drape the tube behind patient's ear. Remember: out of sight; out of mind.

- Evaluate continued need for therapy that may have become an irritating stimulus (e.g., if the patient is now drinking, discontinue IV line; if the patient is eating, discontinue feeding tube; if the patient has an indwelling urethral catheter, discontinue catheter and begin toileting routine).
- Use restraints with caution. Patients can become more agitated when wrist and arm restraints are used.
- Use medications cautiously for controlling behavior. Neuroleptics, such as haloperidol, can be used successfully in calming patients with dementia or psychiatric illness (contraindicated for individuals with parkinsonism). However, if the patient is experiencing acute confusion or delirium, short-acting benzodiazapines (e.g., lorazepam) are more effective in reducing anxiety and fear. Anxiety or fear usually triggers destructive or dangerous behaviors in the acutely confused older patient. A short-acting benzodiazapine, such as lorazepam, will decrease feelings of anxiety and calm the patient after 1 or 2 doses. **Note:** Neuroleptics can cause akathisia, an adverse drug reaction evidenced by increased restlessness.

NIC: Area Restriction; Behavior Management: Overactivity/Inattention; Cerebral Perfusion Promotion; Cognitive Restructuring; Cognitive Stimulation; Elopement Precautions; Environmental Management: Safety; Family Support; Hallucination Management; Patient Rights Protection; Physical Restraint; Reality Orientation; Security Enhancement; Surveillance: Safety

Selected Bibliography

Abrams W et al: *The Merck manual of geriatrics,* ed 2, Whitehouse Station, NJ, 1995, Merck.

American Pharmaceutical Association (Semia T et al, editors): *Geriatric dosage handbook,* Cleveland, 1993, LexiComp.

Brody G: Hyperthermia and hypothermia in the elderly, *Clin Geriatr Med* 10(1):213-227, 1994.

Forrest J: Assessment of acute and chronic pain in older adults, *J Gerontol Nurs* 21(10):15-20, 1995.

Hall G, Wakefield B: Confusion: what to do when the clouds roll in, *Nursing* 26(7):32-37, 1996.

Harvell J, Malbach H: Percutaneous absorption and inflammation in aged skin: a review, *J Acad Dermatol* 31:1015-1021, 1994.

Interqual: *The ISD-A review system with adult ISD criteria,* Northhampton, NH, and Marlboro, Mass, August 1992, Interqual.

Juaradeh S: Neurophysiology of swallowing in the aged, *Dysphagia* 98:218-220, 1994.

Kim MJ et al: *Pocket guide to nursing diagnoses,* ed 7, St Louis, 1997, Mosby.

Knox D, Martof M: Effects of drug therapy on renal function of healthy older adults, *J Gerontol Nurs* 21(4):35-40, 1995.

Matteson M et al: *Gerontological nursing: concepts and practice,* ed 2, Philadelphia, 1996, Saunders.

McCloskey JC, Bulechek GM, editors: *Nursing interventions classification (NIC),* ed 2, St Louis, 1996, Mosby.

Pals J et al: Clinical triggers for detection of fever and dehydration: implications for long term care, *J Gerontol Nurs* 21(4):13-19, 1995.

Resnick N: Geriatric medicine. In Tierney L et al, editors: *Current medical diagnosis and treatment,* ed 3, Stamford, Conn, 1997, Appleton & Lange.

Van Ort S, Phillips L: Nursing interventions to promote functional feeding, *J Gerontol Nurs* 21(10):6-14, 1995.

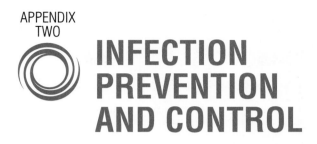

INFECTION
PREVENTION
AND CONTROL

For several decades, infection prevention and control have focused on the use of barriers (e.g., gloves, gowns, masks) to interrupt transmission of organisms among and between patients and health care workers. These barriers are a major component of various systems of isolation precautions.

Systems of isolation precautions

Five different systems of isolation precautions commonly have been used in hospitals. The Centers for Disease Control and Prevention (CDC) revised its guidelines for isolation precautions in 1996 to meet the following objectives: (1) to be epidemiologically sound, (2) to recognize the importance of all body fluids, secretions, and excretions in the transmission of nosocomial pathogens, (3) to ensure adequate precautions for infections transmitted by the airborne, droplet, and contact routes of transmission, (4) to be as simple and user friendly as possible, and (5) to use new terms to avoid confusion with existing infection control and isolation systems. The 1996 guideline contains two tiers of precautions (Table A-19): **Standard Precautions,** which are designed for the care of all patients in hospitals regardless of their diagnosis or presumed infection status, and **Transmission-Based Precautions,** which are used for patients known to be or suspected of being infected or colonized with epidemiologically important pathogens that can be transmitted by airborne or droplet transmission or by contact with dry skin or contaminated surfaces.

The 1996 guideline replaces the 1983 guideline for isolation precautions in hospitals, which offered three options: a Category-Specific system, a Disease-Specific system, and a Hospital-Designed system. Body Substance Isolation (BSI) is a Hospital-Designed system that has been adopted by many hospitals in the United States and elsewhere. In 1987-1988, the CDC introduced Universal Precautions to reduce health care workers' risk of being exposed to bloodborne pathogens. The 1996 Standard Precautions system synthesizes the major features of Universal Precautions and Body Substance Isolation and applies to (1) blood, (2) all body fluids, secretions, and excretions, except sweat, regardless of whether they contain visible blood, (3) nonintact skin, and (4) mucous membranes. Standard Precautions are designed to reduce the risk of transmission of microorganisms from both recognized and unrecognized sources of infection in hospitals.

The 1996 Transmission-Based Precautions are designed for patients documented to be or suspected of being infected or colonized with organisms transmitted by the airborne route, by droplet, and by organisms that are epidemiologically important. Transmission-Based Precautions replace the 1983 Category-Specific and Disease-Specific systems.

Thus, beginning in 1996, all hospitals were encouraged to review and consider adoption of Standard Precautions and Transmission-Based Precautions

Text continued on p. 824

817

TABLE A-19 Recommendations for Isolation Precautions in Hospitals

	Standard Precautions	Transmission-Based Precautions: airborne	Transmission-Based Precautions: droplet	Transmission-Based Precautions: contact
When to use	All patients	Use in addition to Standard Precautions for patients known to be or suspected of being infected with microorganisms transmitted by airborne droplet nuclei (≤5 μm) of evaporated droplets containing microorganisms that can remain suspended in the air and can be widely dispersed by air currents	Use in addition to Standard Precautions for patients known to be or suspected of being infected with microorganisms transmitted by droplets (>5 μm) that can be generated during coughing, sneezing, talking, or performance of procedures	Use in addition to Standard Precautions for specified patients known to be or suspected of being infected or colonized with epidemiologically important microorganisms that can be transmitted by direct contact with patient, such as occurs during patient care activities, or by indirect contact, such as touching surfaces or equipment in patient's environment
Hand washing	Wash hands after touching blood, body fluids, secretions, excretions, and contaminated items, regardless of whether gloves are worn; wash hands immediately after gloves are removed, between patient contacts, and to prevent transfer of microorganisms to other patients or environment; use plain			Wash hands with an antimicrobial agent or a waterless antiseptic agent

	Standard Precautions	Airborne Precautions	Droplet Precautions	Contact Precautions
Gloves	(nonantimicrobial) soap for routine hand washing. Wear nonsterile gloves when touching blood, body fluids, secretions, excretions, and contaminated items; put on clean gloves just before touching mucous membranes and nonintact skin; remove gloves promptly after use, before touching noncontaminated items or environmental surfaces, and before going to another patient; wash hands immediately to avoid transfer of microorganisms to other patients or environment			In addition to glove use as described in Standard Precautions, wear gloves when entering the room and during patient care; change gloves after contact with infective material (e.g., fecal material or wound drainage). After glove removal and hand washing, do not touch items in room
Mask, eye protection, face shield	Wear mask and eye protection or face shield to protect mucous membranes of eyes, nose, and mouth during procedures and patient care activities likely to generate splashes or sprays	Wear respiratory protection when entering room of patient known to have or suspected of having tuberculosis (a type of particulate respirator is recommended)	Wear a mask when working within 3 ft of patient	

Continued

TABLE A-19 Recommendations for Isolation Precautions in Hospitals—cont'd

	Standard Precautions	Transmission-Based Precautions: airborne	Transmission-Based Precautions: droplet	Transmission-Based Precautions: contact
Mask, eye protection, face shield—cont'd		Do not enter room of patient known to have or suspected of having measles (rubeola) or varicella (chickenpox) if susceptible to these infections		
Gown	Wear clean, nonsterile gown to protect skin and prevent soiling of clothing during procedures and patient care activities likely to generate splashes or sprays of blood, body fluids, secretions, or excretions, or to cause soiling of clothing; remove gown promptly when tasks are completed; wash hands			Wear clean, nonsterile gown when entering room if substantial contact is anticipated with patient, surfaces, or items in environment; wear gown when entering room if patient is incontinent or has diarrhea, an ileostomy, colostomy, or uncontained wound drainage; remove gown carefully when tasks are completed; wash hands
Patient care equipment	Handle used patient care equipment in manner that prevents skin and mucous membrane exposures, contamination of clothing, and environmental soiling			When possible, dedicate use of noncritical patient care equipment to a single patient to avoid sharing among patients; if common equipment or items must be shared, adequately clean and disinfect them between uses

Linen	Handle, transport, and process used linen in manner that prevents skin and mucous membrane exposure, contamination of clothing, and environmental soiling
Patient placement	Place patient who contaminates environment or who does not (or cannot) assist in maintaining appropriate hygiene or environmental control in private room, if possible; consult infection control professionals for other alternatives	Place patient in private room that has (1) monitored negative air pressure in relation to surrounding areas, (2) 6-12 air exchanges per hour, and (3) appropriate discharge of air outdoors or monitored high-efficiency filtration of room air before air is circulated to other areas of the hospital; keep room door closed when patient is in room When a private room is not available, patient may be placed in room with another patient who has an active infection with the same microorganism; consult infection control professionals for alternatives	Place patient in private room; when a private room is not available, cohort* infected patients or maintain spatial separation of at least 3 ft between infected patient and other patients and visitors; consult infection control professional for other alternatives	Place patient in private room; when a private room is not available, cohort* infected patients; consult infection control professionals for selection of suitable roommates or other alternatives

---

Cohorting is a term used when patients share a room if infected by the same microorganism, provided they are not infected with other potentially transmissible microorganisms and the likelihood of reinfection with the same organism is minimal. Cohorting is used when there is a shortage of private rooms and may be useful during outbreaks.

Continued

TABLE A-19   Recommendations for Isolation Precautions in Hospitals—cont'd

	Standard Precautions	Transmission-Based Precautions: airborne	Transmission-Based Precautions: droplet	Transmission-Based Precautions: contact
Patient transport		Limit movement and transport of patient from room to essential purposes only; if transport or movement is necessary, minimize patient dispersal of droplet nuclei by placing surgical mask on patient if possible	Limit movement and transport of patient from room to essential purposes only; if transport or movement is necessary, minimize patient dispersal of droplets by placing surgical mask on patient if possible	Limit movement and transport of patient from room to essential purposes only; if transport is necessary, ensure that precautions are maintained to minimize contamination of environmental surfaces or equipment
Environmental control	Ensure that hospital has adequate procedures for routine care, cleaning, and disinfection of environment and patient care items			Ensure that patient care items, bedside equipment, and frequently touched surfaces receive daily cleaning
Occupational Safety and Health Administration (OSHA) Bloodborne Pathogens Standard (1991)	Take care to prevent injuries when using needles, scalpels, and other sharp instruments or devices; when handling sharp instruments after procedures; when cleaning used instruments; and when disposing of used needles			

Never recap used needles or otherwise manipulate them using both hands or use any other technique that involves directing the point of a needle toward any part of the body

Use either one-handed "scoop" technique or mechanical device designed for holding needle sheath if recapping is required by procedure

Do not remove used needles from disposable syringes by hand; do not bend, break, or manipulate used needles by hand

Place used sharps in appropriate puncture-resistant containers located as close as practical to location of use

Use mouthpieces, resuscitation bags, or other ventilation devices as an alternative to mouth-to-mouth resuscitation methods in areas where need is predictable and discontinue use of the older forms of isolation precautions. As always, the CDC offers hospitals the option of modifying the recommendations according to their needs and circumstances and as directed by federal, state, or local regulations. For example, the Occupational Safety and Health Administration's Bloodborne Pathogens Standard (1991) is still operable, and all facilities are required to comply with its provisions. The CDC's 1996 Standard Precautions incorporate all requirements of the OSHA Bloodborne Pathogens Standard.

Isolation precautions for patients with pulmonary or laryngeal TB

In response to the increasing incidence of pulmonary tuberculosis (TB) in the United States, the CDC in 1990 published guidelines for preventing the transmission of TB in the health care setting. These guidelines were revised in 1994. A component of these guidelines is Airborne Precautions for persons diagnosed with or suspected of having pulmonary or laryngeal tuberculosis that can be transmitted to others via the airborne route. These guidelines focus on early identification and treatment of persons with a diagnosis or suspected diagnosis of active tuberculosis. In addition, the CDC defined requirements for special ventilation and use of masks that provide better filtration and a tighter fit than standard surgical masks. Masks of this type are called *particulate respirators (PRs)* and were originally developed for industrial use to protect workers from dust, fumes, and other hazardous substances that could affect the respiratory tract. The efficacy of PRs in protecting susceptible persons from infection with TB has not been demonstrated; however, research is in progress. Meanwhile, OSHA is in the process of developing a Tuberculosis Control Standard for health care settings that will include requirements for risk assessment, respiratory protection, environmental controls, special ventilation, PRs, skin testing programs, exposure management, training programs, and other elements similar to those of OSHA's Bloodborne Pathogens Standard of 1991. The proposed OSHA TB Control Standards are being evaluated with the expectation that a final Standard will be forthcoming by 1999.

Management of devices and procedures to reduce risk of nosocomial infection

Use of barriers is but one of many strategies that can reduce the risk of nosocomial infection among patients and personnel. In fact, studies from the CDC show that significant gains can be made in reducing infection risks by focusing on the management of devices and procedures frequently used in patient care. For example, many patients need intravascular devices that deliver therapeutic medications, but they are put at risk for site infections and bacteremias when these devices are used. It is well known that rotating the access site at appropriate intervals reduces these risks to the patient, and catheter materials that are more "vein friendly" also reduce trauma to the vascular system. In addition, use of needles to deliver medications and fluids to patients through these intravascular devices can put the health care worker at risk for puncture injury. Needleless or needle-free IV access devices now are used to access line ports so that it is not necessary to use needles once the intravascular catheter has entered the vascular system. Thus the use of newer and safer intravascular devices and procedures can benefit both the patient and health care worker by reducing their risk of nosocomial infection. Research studies of interventions to reduce nosocomial infection risks are published in general and specialty journals and presented at professional meetings each year. Infection control practitioners and hospital epidemiologists use these studies to make recommendations about changes in nursing and medical practice. The Joint Commission on Accreditation of Healthcare Organizations (JCAHO) requires that all accredited facilities have a person qualified to provide infection surveillance, prevention, and control services. The national associations for these professionals are the Association for Professionals in Infection Control and Epidemiology, Inc. (APIC), which publishes the *American Journal of Infection Control,* and the Society for Healthcare Epidemiology of America (SHEA), which publishes the journal *Infection Control and Hospital Epidemiology.*

Selected Bibliography

Association for Professionals in Infection Control and Epidemiology: *APIC infection control and applied epidemiology: principles and practice,* St Louis, 1996, Mosby.

Bennett JV, Brachman PS, editors: *Hospital infections,* ed 4, Boston, 1998, Lippincott-Raven.

Centers for Disease Control: Guideline for isolation precautions in hospitals, *Infect Control* 4:245-325, 1983.

Centers for Disease Control: Recommendations for prevention of HIV transmission in health-care settings, *MMWR Morb Mortal Wkly Rep* 36 (suppl 2):1-18, 1987.

Centers for Disease Control: Update: Universal Precautions for prevention of transmission of human immunodeficiency virus and other bloodborne pathogens in health-care settings, *MMWR Morb Mortal Wkly Rep* 37:377-388, 1988.

Centers for Disease Control: Guidelines for preventing the transmission of tuberculosis in health-care settings, with special focus on HIV-related issues, *MMWR Morb Mortal Wkly Rep* 39(no. RR 1-17), 1990.

Centers for Disease Control and Prevention: Guidelines for preventing the transmission of *Mycobacterium tuberculosis* in health-care facilities, *MMWR Morb Mortal Wkly Rep* 43(no. RR-13):1-133, 1994.

Centers for Disease Control and Prevention: Guideline for isolation precautions in hospitals, *Infect Control Hosp Epidemiol* 17:53-80, 1996.

Department of Labor, Occupational Safety and Health Administration: Occupational exposure to bloodborne pathogens: final rule, 29 CFR part 1910:1030, *Federal Register* 56:64003-64182, December 6, 1991.

Jackson MM: Infection prevention and control, *Crit Care Nurs Clin North Am* 4(3):401-409, 1992.

Jackson MM, Lynch P: Infection control: too much or too little? *Am J Nurs* 84:208-210, 1984.

Jackson MM, Lynch P: In search of a rational approach, *Am J Nurs* 90(10):65-73, 1990.

Jackson MM, Lynch P: An attempt to make an issue less murky: a comparison of four systems for infection precautions, *Infect Control Hosp Epidemiol* 12:448-450, 1991.

Jackson MM, Lynch P: Developing a numeric scale to assess health-care worker risk for bloodborne pathogen exposure, *Am J Infect Control* 23:13-21, 1995.

Jackson MM et al: Why not treat all body substances as infectious? *Am J Nurs* 87:1137-1139, 1987.

Lynch P et al: Implementing and evaluating a system of generic infection precautions: body substance isolation, *Am J Infect Control* 18:1-12, 1990.

Lynch P et al: Rethinking the role of isolation practices in the prevention of nosocomial infections, *Ann Intern Med* 107:243-246, 1987.

Martone WJ, Garner JS, editors: Proceedings of the Third Decennial International Conference on Nosocomial Infections, *Am J Med* 91(3B): 1-333, 1991.

Mayhall CG, editor: *Hospital epidemiology and infection control,* Baltimore, 1996, Williams & Wilkins.

Pugliese G et al, editors: *Univerisal Precautions: policies, procedures, and resources,* Chicago, 1990, American Hospital Publishing.

Wenzel RP: *Prevention and control of nosocomial infections,* ed 2, Baltimore, 1993, Williams & Wilkins.

HEART AND BREATH SOUNDS

TABLE A-20 Assessing heart sounds

Sound	Auscultation site	Timing	Pitch	Clinical occurrence	End-piece/patient position
S_1 (M_1 T_1)	Apex	Beginning of systole	High	Closing of mitral and tricuspid valves; normal sound	Diaphragm/patient supine
S_1 split	Apex	Beginning of systole	High	Ventricles contracting at different times because of electrical or mechanical problems (e.g., a longer time span between M_1 and T_1 caused by right bundle-branch heart block, or reversal [T_1 M_1] caused by mitral stenosis)	Same as S_1
S_2 (A_2 P_2)	A_2 at second ICS, RSB; P_2 at second ICS, LSB	End of systole	High	Closing of aortic and pulmonic valves; normal sound	Diaphragm/patient supine
S_2 physiologic split	Second ICS, LSB	End of systole	High	Accentuated by inspiration; disappears on expiration. Sound that corresponds with the respiratory cycle caused by normal delay in closure of pulmonic valve during inspiration. It is accentuated during exercise or in individuals with thin chest walls; heard most often in children and young adults	Same as S_2
S_2 persistent (wide) split	Second ICS, LSB	End of systole	High	Heard throughout the respiratory cycle; caused by late closure of pulmonic valve or early closure of aortic valve. Occurs in atrial septal defect, right ventricular failure, pulmonic stenosis, hypertension, or right bundle-branch heart block	Same as S_2

Sound	Location	Timing	Pitch	Description	
S_2 paradoxic (reversed) split ($P_2 A_2$)	Second ICS, LSB	End of systole	High	Because of delayed left ventricular systole, the aortic valve closes after the pulmonic valve rather than before it. (Normally during expiration the two sounds merge.) Causes may include left bundle-branch heart block, aortic stenosis, severe left ventricular failure, MI, and severe hypertension	Same as S_2
S_2 fixed split	Second ICS, LSB	End of systole	High	Heard with equal intensity during inspiration and expiration because of split of pulmonic and aortic components, which are unaffected by blood volume or respiratory changes. May be heard in pulmonary stenosis or atrial septal defect	Same as S_2
S_3 (ventricular gallop)	Apex	Early diastole just after S_2	Dull, low	Early and rapid filling of ventricle, as in early ventricular failure, heart failure. Common in children, during last trimester of pregnancy, and possibly in healthy adults >50 yr of age	Bell/patient in left lateral or supine position
S_4 (atrial gallop)	Apex	Late in diastole just before S_1	Low	Atrium filling against increased resistance of stiff ventricle, as in heart failure, coronary artery disease, cardiomyopathy, pulmonary artery hypertension, ventricular failure. May be normal in infants, children, and athletes	Same as S_3

ICS, Intercostal space; *LSB*, left sternal border; *RSB*, right sternal border; *MI*, myocardial infarction.

TABLE A-21 Commonly Occurring Heart Murmurs

Type	Timing	Pitch	Quality	Auscultation site	Radiation
Pulmonic stenosis	Systolic ejection	Medium-high	Harsh	Second ICS, LSB	Toward left shoulder, back
Aortic stenosis	Midsystolic	Medium-high	Harsh	Second ICS, RSB	Toward carotid arteries
Ventricular septal defect	Late systolic	High	Blowing	Fourth ICS, LSB	Toward RSB
Mitral insufficiency	Holosystolic	High	Blowing	Fifth or sixth ICS, left MCL	Toward left axilla
Tricuspid insufficiency	Holosystolic	High	Blowing	Fourth ICS, LSB	Toward apex
Aortic insufficiency	Early diastolic	High	Blowing	Second ICS, RSB	Toward sternum
Pulmonary insufficiency	Early diastolic	High	Blowing	Second ICS, LSB	Toward sternum
Mitral stenosis	Mid-late diastolic	Low	Rumbling	Fifth ICS, left MCL	Usually none
Tricuspid stenosis	Mid-late diastolic	Low	Rumbling	Fourth ICS, LSB	Usually none

ICS, Intercostal space; *LSB*, left sternal border; *RSB*, right sternal border; *MCL*, midclavicular line.

TABLE A-22　Assessing Normal Breath Sounds

Type	Normal site	Duration	Characteristics
Vesicular	Peripheral lung	I > E	Soft and swishing sounds. Abnormal if heard over the large airways
Bronchial	Trachea and bronchi	E > I	Louder, coarser, and of longer duration than vesicular. Abnormal if heard over peripheral lung
Bronchovesicular	Sternal border of major bronchi	E = I	Moderate in pitch and intensity. Abnormal if heard over peripheral lung

I, Inspiration; *E*, expiration.

TABLE A-23 Assessing Adventitious Breath Sounds

Type	Waveform	Characteristics	Possible clinical condition
Coarse crackle		Discontinuous, explosive, interrupted. Loud; low in pitch	Pulmonary edema; pneumonia in resolution stage
Fine crackle		Discontinuous, explosive, interrupted. Less loud than coarse crackles, lower in pitch, and of shorter duration	Interstitial lung disease; heart failure; atelectasis
Wheeze		Continuous, of long duration, high pitched, musical, hissing	Narrowing of airway; bronchial asthma; COPD
Rhonchus		Continuous, of long duration, low pitched, snoring	Production of sputum (usually cleared or lessened by coughing or suctioning)
Pleural friction rub		Grating, rasping noise	Rubbing together of inflamed parietal linings; loss of normal pleural lubrication

COPD, Chronic obstructive pulmonary disease.

TABLE A-24   Assessing Respiratory Patterns

Type	Waveform	Characteristics	Possible clinical condition
Eupnea		Normal rate and rhythm for adults and teenagers (12-20 breaths/min)	Normal pattern while awake
Bradypnea		Decreased rate (<12 breaths/min); regular rhythm	Normal sleep pattern; opiate or alcohol use; tumor; metabolic disorder
Tachypnea		Rapid rate (>20 breaths/min); hypoventilation or hyperventilation	Fever; restrictive respiratory disorders; pulmonary emboli
Hyperpnea		Depth of respirations greater than normal	Meeting increased metabolic demand (e.g., sepsis, MODS, SIRS, and exercise)
Apnea		Cessation of breathing; may be intermittent	Intermittent with CNS disturbances or drug intoxication; obstructed airway; respiratory arrest if it persists
Kussmaul's		Deep, rapid (>20 breaths/min), sighing, labored	Renal failure, DKA, sepsis, shock
Cheyne-Stokes		Alternating patterns of apnea (10-20 sec) with periods of deep and rapid breathing. Lesions located bilaterally and deep within cerebral hemispheres	Heart failure; opiate or hypnotic overdose, thyrotoxicosis, dissecting aneurysm, subarachnoid hemorrhage, IICP, aortic valve disorders; may be normal in older adults during sleep

MODS, Multiple organ dysfunction syndrome; *SIRS,* systemic inflammatory response syndrome; *CNS,* central nervous system; *DKA,* diabetic ketoacidosis; *IICP,* increased intracranial pressure.

Continued

TABLE A-24 Assessing Respiratory Patterns—cont'd

Type	Waveform	Characteristics	Possible clinical condition
Central neurogenic hyperventilation		Rapid (>20 breaths/min), deep, regular. Lesions of midbrain or upper pons thought to be source of pattern	Primary injury (ischemia, infarction, space-occupying lesion); secondary injury (IICP, metabolic disorders, drug overdose)
Apneustic		Deep, prolonged inspiration, followed by 20- to 30-sec pause and short expiration. Lesion located in lower pons	Anoxia, meningitis, basilar artery occlusion
Cluster		Irregular breaths occurring in clusters with periods of apnea. Overall pattern irregular. Lesion located in lower pons or upper medulla	Primary and secondary injury as above may produce this respiratory pattern
Ataxic (Biot's)		Irregular deep or shallow breaths. No discernible pattern. Lesion located in medulla	Primary and secondary injury as above may produce this respiratory pattern

APPENDIX
FOUR

LABORATORY TESTS DISCUSSED IN THIS MANUAL: NORMAL VALUES*

TABLE A-25

Complete blood count (CBC)	Adult normal values
Hemoglobin (Hgb)	Male: 14-18 g/dl
	Female: 12-16 g/dl
Hematocrit (Hct)	Male: 40%-54%
	Female: 37%-47%
Red blood cell (RBC) count	Male: 4.5-6.0 million/mm^3
	Female: 4.0-5.5 million/mm^3
RBC indices	
Mean corpuscular volume	80-95 μm^3
Mean corpuscular hemoglobin	27-31 pg/cell
Mean corpuscular hemoglobin concentration	32-36 g/dl
WBC count	4,500-11,000/mm^3
Neutrophils	54%-75%
Band neutrophils	3%-8%
Lymphocytes	20%-40%
Monocytes	2%-8%
Eosinophils	1%-4%
Basophils	0.5%-1.0%
Platelet count	150,000-400,000/mm^3

TABLE A-26

Serum, plasma, and whole blood chemistry	Adult normal values
Adrenocorticotropic hormone (ACTH)	8-10 AM <100 pg/ml
Antidiuretic hormone (ADH; vasopressin)	1-5 pg/ml
Albumin	3.5-5.5 g/dl

Continued

---

*Normal values may vary significantly with different laboratory methods of testing.

835

TABLE A-26—cont'd

Serum, plasma, and whole blood chemistry	Adult normal values
Aldosterone	Male: 6-22 ng/dl Female: 4-31 ng/dl
Alanine aminotransferase (ALT; formerly called serum glutamic-pyruvic transaminase [SGPT])	5-35 IU/L
Ammonia	15-110 µg/dl
Amylase	60-180 Somogyi U/dl
Aspartate aminotransferase (AST; formerly called serum glutamic-pyruvic transaminase [SGOT])	8-20 U/L; 5-40 IU/L (values slightly higher in older adults and slightly lower in females than in males)
Base, total	145-160 mEq/L
Bicarbonate	22-26 mEq/L
Bilirubin	Total: 0.3-1.4 mg/dl
Blood gases, arterial	
pH	7.35-7.45
Pa_{CO_2}	35-45 mm Hg
Pa_{O_2}	80-95 mm Hg
O_2 saturation (Sa_{O_2})	95%-99%
Blood urea nitrogen (BUN)	6-20 mg/dl
CA-125 cancer marker	0-35 U/ml
Calcitonin	<100 pg/ml
Calcium	8.5-10.5 mg/dl; 4.3-5.3 mEq/L
Carcinoembryonic antigen (CEA)	<5 ng/ml
Chloride (Cl^-)	95-108 mEq/L
Cortisol	8-10 AM: 5-25 µg/dl 4 PM–Midnight: 2-18 µg/dl
CO_2 content (total CO_2^-)	22-28 mEq/L
Creatinine	0.6-1.5 mg/dl
Creatinine clearance	Male: 107-141 ml/min Female: 87-132 ml/min
Creatinine phosphokinase (CPK)	Male: 55-170 U/L Female: 30-135 U/L
CPK isoenzyme (MB)	<5% of total CPK activity
Erythrocyte sedimentation rate (ESR) (Westergren method)	Male: up to 15 mm/hr Female: up to 20 mm/hr
Fibrin split products (FSPs, FDPs)	<10 µg/ml
Folic acid (folate)	5-20 µg/ml
Follicle-stimulating hormone (FSH, follitropin)	
Adult female	Premenopausal 4-30 mIU/ml Postmenopausal 40-250 mIU/ml
Adult male	4-25 mIU/ml 4-25 IU/L
Free thyroxine index (FTI)	0.9-2.4 ng/dl

TABLE A-26—cont'd

Serum, plasma, and whole blood chemistry	Adult normal values
Globulins, total	1.5-3.5 g/dl
Glucose, fasting	True glucose: 60-120 mg/dl
	All sugars: 80-120 mg/dl
Glucose, 2-hr postprandial	<145 mg/dl
Glucose tolerance	
Intravenous	Fasting: 60-120 mg/dl
	5 min: maximum 250 mg/dl
	60 min: decrease
	2 hr: <120 mg/dl
	3 hr: 65-110 mg/dl
Oral	Fasting: 60-120 mg/dl
	30 min: <155 mg/dl
	1 hr: <165 mg/dl
	2 hr: <120 mg/dl
	3 hr: ≤60-120 mg/dl
Growth hormone (GH)	<10 ng/ml
Insulin	11-240 μIU/ml
	4-24 μU/ml
Iron	Total: 60-200 μg/dl
	Male, average: 125 μg/dl
	Female, average: 100 μg/dl
	Older adult: 60-80 μg/dl
Total iron-binding capacity	25-420 μg/dl
Ketone bodies	2-4 μg/dl
Lactic acid	Arterial: 0.5-1.6 mEq/L
	Venous: 1.5-2.2 mEq/L
Lactic dehydrogenase	45-90 U/L; 115-225 IU/L
Lipase	0-110 U/L
Magnesium	1.8-3.0 mg/dl
	0.65-1.05 mmol
Osmolality	280-300 mOsm/kg H_2O
Parathyroid hormone	<2000 pg/ml
Partial thromboplastin time	Normal: 60-70 sec
	On anticoagulant therapy: 1.5-2.5 × control value
Phosphatase, acid	0-1.1 U/ml (Bodansky)
	1-4 U/ml (King-Armstrong)
	0.13-0.63 U/ml (Bessey-Lowery)
Phosphatase, alkaline	1.5-4.5 U/dl (Bodansky)
	4-13 U/dl (King-Armstrong)
	0.8-2.3 U/ml (Bessey-Lowery)
Phosphorus	2.5-4.5 mg/dl; 1.7-2.6 mEq/L
Potassium (K^+)	3.5-5.0 mEq/L
Prolactin	2-15 ng/ml
Prothrombin time (PT)	11-12.5 sec

Continued

TABLE A-26—cont'd

Serum, plasma, and whole blood chemistry	Adult normal values
Renin	Normal sodium intake:
	Supine (4-6 hr): 0.5-1.6 ng/ml/hr
	Sitting (4 hr): 1.8-3.6 ng/ml/hr
	Low sodium intake:
	Supine (4-6 hr): 2.2-4.4 ng/ml/hr
	Sitting (4 hr): 4.0-8.1 ng/ml/hr
Reticulocyte count	0.5%-2% of total erythrocytes
Reticulocyte index	1.0
Retinol-binding protein	4-5 mg/dl
Sodium (Na^+)	137-147 mEq/L
Thyroid-stimulating hormone	2-10 mU/L
Thyroxine-binding prealbumin	20-30 mg/dl
Transferrin	200-400 mg/dl
Triiodothyronine (T_3)	110-230 ng/dl
Urea clearance	Serum/24-hr urine:
	64-99 ml/min (maximum)
	41-65 ml/min (standard)
Uric acid	Male: 2.0-7.5 mg/dl
	Female: 2.0-6.5 mg/dl

TABLE A-27

Urine chemistry	Adult normal values
Albumin	Random: negative
	24-hr: 10-100 mg
Amylase	Mayo clinic method 10-80 U/hr
	Somogyi method 26-950 U/24 hr
Bilirubin	Random: negative
Calcium (Ca^{++})	Random: 1+; <40 mg/dl
	24-hr: 50-300 mg
Creatinine	24-hr: Male: 20-26 mg/kg
	Female: 14-22 mg/kg
Creatinine clearance	Male: 107-141 ml/min/1.73 m^2
	Female: 87-132 ml/min/1.73 m^2
Glucose	Random: negative
	24-hr: 130 mg
Ketone	24-hr: negative: 0.3-2.0 mg/dl
Osmolality	Random: 350-700 mOsm/kg H_2O
	24-hr: 300-900 mOsm/kg H_2O
	Physiologic range: 50-1400 mOsm/kg H_2O
pH	Random: 4.6-8.0
Phosphorus	24-hr: 0.9-1.3 g; 0.2-0.6 mEq/L

TABLE A-27—cont'd

Urine chemistry	Adult normal values
Protein	Random: negative: 2-8 mg/dl
	24-hr: 40-150 mg
Sodium (Na^+)	Random: 50-130 mEq/L
	24-hr: 40-220 mEq
Specific gravity	Random: 1.010-1.020
	After fluid restriction: 1.025-1.035
Sugar	Random: negative
Urea clearance	24-hr: 64-99 ml/min (maximum)
	41-65 ml/min (standard)
Urea nitrogen	24-hr: 6-17 g

Index

Page numbers followed by *t* indicate tables.

ABBREVIATIONS USED IN THIS MANUAL

ABD: abdominal
ABG: arterial blood gas
ABI: ankle-brachial index
ac: before meals
AC: acromioclavicular
ACBaE: air contrast barium enema
ACE: angiotensin-converting enzyme
ACL: anterior cruciate ligament
ACS: American Cancer Society
ACTH: adrenocorticotropic hormone
AD: autonomic dysreflexia
ADA: American Diabetes Association
ADH: antidiuretic hormone
ADL: activities of daily living
AEH: antiembolism hose
AFB: acid-fast bacillus
AFP: α (alpha)-fetoprotein
AHA: American Heart Association; American Hospital Association
AHCPR: Agency for Health Care Policy and Research
AICD: automatic implantable cardioverter-defibrillator
AIDS: acquired immunodeficiency syndrome
AIPC: Association for Professionals in Infection Control and Epidemiology, Inc.
AJCC: American Joint Committee on Cancer
AKA: above-knee amputation
ALG: antilymphocyte globulin
ALL: acute lymphoblastic leukemia
ALS: amyotrophic lateral sclerosis
ALT: alanine aminotransferase
AML: acute myelocytic leukemia
ANC: absolute neutrophil count
ANS: autonomic nervous system
AP: anteroposterior
APECED: autoimmune polyendocrinopathy-candidiasis-ectodermal dystrophy
APR: abdominoperineal resection
APSAC: anisoylated plasminogen streptokinase activator complex
ARC: AIDS-related complex
ARDS: adult respiratory distress syndrome
ARF: acute renal failure; acute respiratory failure
ASA: acetylsalicylic acid (aspirin)
5-ASA: 5-aminosalicylic acid
AST: aspartate aminotransferase
ATCS: anterior tibial compartment syndrome
ATGAM: antilymphocyte sera
atm: atmosphere (measure of pressure)
ATN: acute tubular necrosis
A-V: atrioventricular
AVM: arteriovenous malformation
AZT: azidothymidine

BAER: brainstem auditory evoked responses
B&O: belladonna and opium
BCG: bacillus Calmette-Guérin
BCNU: carmustine
bDNA: branched-chain DNA
BEE: basal energy expenditure
bid: twice a day
BKA: below-knee amputation
BMI: body mass index
BMT: bone marrow transplant

BP: blood pressure
BPH: benign prostatic hypertrophy
bpm: beats per minute
BRM: biologic response modifiers
BSA: body surface area
BSE: breast self-examination
BUN: blood urea nitrogen

C: cervical
Ca/Ca²⁺/Ca⁺⁺: calcium
CABG: coronary artery bypass grafting
CAD: coronary artery disease
CAPD: continuous ambulatory peritoneal dialysis
CAVH: continuous arteriovenous hemofiltration
CBC: complete blood count
CBF: cerebral blood flow
CBI: continuous bladder irrigation
CCNU: lomustine
CCPD: continuous cycling peritoneal dialysis
CCU: coronary care unit
2-cdA: cladribine
CDC: Centers for Disease Control and Prevention
CDCA: chenodeoxycholic acid
CDE: common duct exploration
CEA: carcinoembryonic antigen
CIE: counterimmunoelectrophoresis
CIN: cervical intraepithelial neoplasia
CK: creatinine phosphokinase
Cl/Cl⁻: chloride
CLL: chronic lymphocytic leukemia
cm: centimeter
CMC: carpometacarpal
CML: chronic myelocytic leukemia
CMV: cytomegalovirus
CNS: central nervous system
CO₂: carbon dioxide
COMT: catechol-O-methyl-transferase
COPD: chronic obstructive pulmonary disease
CPK: creatinine phosphokinase
CPK-MB: creatinine phosphokinase with MB isoenzymes
CPM: continuous passive movement
CPP: cerebral perfusion pressure; coronary perfusion pressure
CPR: cardiopulmonary resuscitation
CPZ: chlorpromazine
CRF: chronic renal failure
CROS: contralateral routing of signal
CSF: cerebrospinal fluid
CSII: continuous subcutaneous insulin infusion
CT: computerized axial tomography
CV: costovertebral
CVA: cerebrovascular accident; costovertebral angle
CVC: central venous catheter
CVP: central venous pressure

D: dorsal
D₅₀: 50% dextrose
D&C: dilation and curettage
DAI: diffuse axonal injury
DCA: directional coronary atherectomy
DDAVP: desmopressin

2D-ECHO: two-dimensional echocardiogram
DES: diethylstilbestrol
DHT: dihydrochysterol
DI: diabetes insipidus
DIC: disseminated intravascular coagulation
DIP: distal interphalangeal
DJD: degenerative joint disease
DKA: diabetic ketoacidosis
dl: deciliter
DM: diabetes mellitus
DMARD: disease-modifying antirheumatic drug
DNA: deoxyribonucleic acid
DOE: dyspnea on exertion
DPL: diagnostic peritoneal lavage
DPT: diphtheria, pertussis, and tetanus (vaccine)
DRE: digital rectal examination
DSA: digital subtraction angiography
DT: diphtheria and pertussis toxoids, pediatric type
DTR: deep tendon reflex
DTs: delirium tremens
DVT: deep vein thrombosis
D₅NS: 5% dextrose in normal saline
D₅W: 5% dextrose in water

E: expiration
EBV: Epstein-Barr virus
ECA: external carotid artery
ECC: endocervical curettage
ECF: extracellular fluid
ECG: electrocardiogram
EEG: electroencephalogram
EF: ejection fraction
e.g.: for example
EHDP: etidronate disodium
ELISA: enzyme-linked immunosorbent assay
EMB: ethambutol (antituberculin agent)
EMG: electromyography
EP: evoked potential
EPA: eicosapentaenoic acid
EPO: erythropoietin
EPS: electrophysiologic study
ERCP: endoscopic retrograde cholangiopancreatogram (cholangiopancreatogram)
ERT: estrogen replacement therapy
ESR: erythrocyte sedimentation rate
ESRD: end-stage renal disease
ESWL: extracorporeal shock wave lithotripsy
ET: endotracheal; enterostomal therapy
EV: evoked potentials

F: Fahrenheit
FAP: familial adenomatous polyposis
FBS: fasting blood sugar
FDA: U.S. Food and Drug Administration
FDP: fibrin degradation product
FEF: forced mid-expiratory flow
FES: functional electrical stimulation
FEV: forced expiratory volume
FEV₁: forced expiratory volume for 1 sec

Continued

ABBREVIATIONS USED IN THIS MANUAL—cont'd

FFA: free fatty acid
FFP: fresh frozen plasma
FIGO: International Federation of Gynecology and Obstetrics
Fio₂: fraction of inspired oxygen
FNA: fine needle aspiration
Fr: French
FSH: follicle-stimulating hormone
FSP: fibrin split product
ft: foot or feet
FTI: free thyroxine index
FU: fluorouracil
FVC: forced vital capacity

g: gram
μg: microgram
GBS: Guillain-Barré syndrome
GDNF: glial-cell-line derived neurotrophic factor
GFR: glomerular filtration rate
GGTP: γ-glutamyl transpeptidase
GH: growth hormone
GI: gastrointestinal
γ-Globulin: gamma-globulin
GN: glomerulonephritis
GnRH: gonadotropin-releasing hormone
GOT: glutamic oxaloacetic transaminase
GPEF: gated pool ejection fraction
GU: genitourinary

hr: hour
HA: hepatitis A
HAV: hepatitis A virus
HB: hepatitis B
HbAIC: glycohemoglobin
HBeAG: hepatitis B e antigen
HBIG: hepatitis B immune globulin
HBP: high blood pressure/hypertension
HBsAg: hepatitis B specific antigen
HBV: hepatitis B virus
HCG: human chorionic gonadotropin
HCl: hydrochloric acid
HCO₃/HCO₃: bicarbonate
Hct: hematocrit
HCV: hepatitis C virus
HD: Hodgkin's disease
HDV: hepatitis D virus
HEV: hepatitis E virus
Hgb: hemoglobin
Hgb AS: sickle cell trait
Hgb SS: sickle cell disease
HHHT: hypervolemic, hypertensive, hemodilution therapy
HHNK: hyperosmolar hyperglycemic nonketotic (syndrome)
HI: head injury
HIDA: radioisotopic scan
HIV: human immunodeficiency virus
HKA: hip-knee-ankle orthosis
HLA: human leukocyte antigen
H₂O: water
HOB: head of bed
HR: heart rate
hs: hour of sleep
HTLV-I: human T-cell leukemia virus I
HVWP: hepatic vein wedge pressure

I: inspiration
ICAM-1: intercellular adhesion molecule 1
ICD: implantable cardioverter-defibrillator
ICF: intracellular fluid
ICP: intracranial pressure
ICS: intercostal space
ICSH: interstitial cell–stimulating hormone
ICU: intensive care unit
ID: identification
IDDM: insulin-dependent diabetes mellitus
i.e.: that is
IG: immune globulin
IgA: immunoglobulin A
IgG: immunoglobulin G
IgM: immunoglobulin M
IGT: impaired glucose tolerance
IICP: increased intracranial pressure
IL-1: interleukin-1
IL-6: interleukin-6
IL-10: interleukin-10
IM: intramuscular
in: inch or inches
INH: isoniazid
INR: International Normalized Ratio (used to monitor oral anticoagulant therapy)
I&O: intake and output
IPD: intermittent peritoneal dialysis
IPOP: immediate postoperative prosthesis
IPPB: intermittent positive-pressure breathing
IRMA: immunoradiometric assay
ISI: International Sensitivity Index
ITP: idiopathic thrombocytopenic purpura
IU: international unit
IUD: intrauterine device
IV: intravenous
IVIgG: intravenous immunoglobulin G
IVP: intravenous pyelogram
IVUS: intravascular ultrasound

JCAHO: Joint Commission on Accreditation of Healthcare Organizations

K/K⁺: potassium
KCl: potassium chloride
kg: kilogram
KS: Kaposi's sarcoma
KUB: kidney, ureter, bladder

L: liter; lumbar
LAD: left arterial descending
LATS: long-acting thyroid stimulator
lb: pound
LCT: long-chain triglyceride
LDH: lactic dehydrogenase
LEEP: loop electrosurgical excision procedure
LES: lower esophageal sphincter
LH: luteinizing hormone
LHRH: luteinizing hormone–releasing hormone; leuprolide
LLQ: left lower quadrant
LMN: lower motor neuron
LOC: level of consciousness
LP: lumbar puncture

LPA: latex particle agglutination
LSB: left sternal border
LTH: luteotropic hormone
LUQ: left upper quadrant
LVH: left ventricular hypertrophy

m: meter (s)
μm: micrometer
m²: square meter
μm³: cubic micrometer
MAI: *Mycobacterium avium-intracellulare*
MAO: monoamine oxidase
MAP: mean arterial pressure
MCHC: mean corpuscular hemoglobin concentration
MCL: midclavicular line
MCP: metacarpophalangeal
MCT: medium-chain triglyceride
MCV: mean corpuscular volume
MDI: metered dose inhaler; multiple daily injections
mEq: milliequivalent
mg: milligram
Mg/Mg²⁺/Mg⁺⁺: magnesium
mi: mile (s)
MI: myocardial infarction
min: minute
ml: milliliter
mm: millimeter
mm Hg: millimeters of mercury
mmol: millimole
MODS: multiple organ dysfunction syndrome
mOsm: milliosmol
6-MP: mercaptopurine
MR: mitral regurgitation
MRC: Medical Research Council
MRI: magnetic resonance imaging
MRSA: methicillin-resistant *Staphylococcus aureus*
MS: multiple sclerosis
MSG: monosodium glutamate
MSH: melanocyte-stimulating hormone
MSU: monosodium urate
MTP: metatarsophalangeal
MTX: methotrexate
MUGA scan: multiple-gated acquisition scan

N: nitrogen
Na/Na⁺: sodium
NaCl: sodium chloride
NaHCO₃: sodium bicarbonate
NASBA: nucleic acid sequence-based amplification
NCV: nerve conduction velocity
ng: nanogram
NG: nasogastric
NHL: non-Hodgkin's lymphoma
NIC: Nursing Intervention Classification
NIDDM: non-insulin-dependent diabetes mellitus
NNRTI: nonnucleoside reverse transcriptase inhibitor
NPH: neutral protamine Hagedorn; isophane insulin suspension
NPO: nothing by mouth
NRTI: nucleoside reverse transcriptase inhibitor
NS: nephrotic syndrome
NSAID: nonsteroidal antiinflammatory drug
NSCLC: non-small-cell lung cancer